Perinatology

AF829840

Renato Augusto Moreira de Sá •
Eduardo Borges da Fonseca
Editors

Perinatology

Evidence-Based Best Practices in Perinatal Medicine

Volume I

Springer

Editors
Renato Augusto Moreira de Sá
Maternal and Child Department
Fluminense Federal University
Niterói, Rio de Janeiro
Brazil

Eduardo Borges da Fonseca
Federal University of Paraíba
João Pessoa, Paraíba
Brazil

ISBN 978-3-030-83436-4 ISBN 978-3-030-83434-0 (eBook)
https://doi.org/10.1007/978-3-030-83434-0

© Springer Nature Switzerland AG 2022
This work is subject to copyright. All rights are reserved by the Publisher, whether the whole or part of the material is concerned, specifically the rights of translation, reprinting, reuse of illustrations, recitation, broadcasting, reproduction on microfilms or in any other physical way, and transmission or information storage and retrieval, electronic adaptation, computer software, or by similar or dissimilar methodology now known or hereafter developed.
The use of general descriptive names, registered names, trademarks, service marks, etc. in this publication does not imply, even in the absence of a specific statement, that such names are exempt from the relevant protective laws and regulations and therefore free for general use.
The publisher, the authors, and the editors are safe to assume that the advice and information in this book are believed to be true and accurate at the date of publication. Neither the publisher nor the authors or the editors give a warranty, expressed or implied, with respect to the material contained herein or for any errors or omissions that may have been made. The publisher remains neutral with regard to jurisdictional claims in published maps and institutional affiliations.

This Springer imprint is published by the registered company Springer Nature Switzerland AG
The registered company address is: Gewerbestrasse 11, 6330 Cham, Switzerland

Rodrigo, Alice, and Isadora, our children
and our hope for a better world.

Foreword

As one of the founders of perinatal medicine, it is my particular pleasure to write this foreword and to support the current activities in this fascinating new field of human medicine.

A particular highlight is to do it together with Ana Bianchi, the scientific daughter of my old friend and supporting pioneer in fetal medicine Roberto Caldeyro-Barcia from Uruguay. He in heaven and I still on earth are grateful to the younger, currently so active, and successful generation for continuing what we started and founded decades ago.

Perinatal medicine is very versatile because its main part, the prenatal block – this means everything that happens before birth – was to a high degree, up to the beginning of the 1960s, a medically unexplored space. In the meantime, the evolution has been explosive.

Perinatal medicine is subject to its special characteristics, namely to be interdisciplinary. This means that the cooperation with other important disciplines should be essential. The closest connection exists between obstetrics and neonatology in advanced centres even more than between obstetrics and gynecology.

I wish good success.

Erich Saling
"Professor Emeritus" of Perinatal Medicine at the Charité,
Humboldt-University Berlin - Germany
The Father of Perinatal Medicine

Ana Bianchi
President of Caldeyro-Barcia Foundation - Uruguay

Preface

Perinatal period is defined as *"the period of time between 22 weeks after fertilization and 7 days after parturition."*[1]

Usually, authors specializing in obstetrics and maternal-fetal medicine are invited to write chapters of perinatology books and to express themselves about problems related to perinatology. Consequently, the set of written productions includes strictly obstetric texts, most often intended for prenatal care, or works written by pediatricians and intended for neonatal care.

At the development stage of this book, our desire was to follow the idea of Erich Saling from the book ***The Child in the Field of Obstetrics*** (Das Kind im Bereich der Geburtshilfe) [2]. In the 1950s, "The Father of Perinatal Medicine," exhorts the antenatal care importance, reinforcing the innovative achievement of another pioneer on perinatal care, Roberto Caldeyro-Barcia.

The progressive specialization in the field of medicine has led us to bring two specialties, materno-fetal medicine and neonatology. The improvement in the assessment of fetal well-being and *in-utero* treatment and the advancements in neonatal intensive care have greatly improved the chances of babies' long-term survival. Therefore, to avoid unnecessary confusion for the purposes of this book, the perinatal period will be extended from 20 completed weeks (140 days) of gestation to 28 completed days after birth. This extended definition is accepted by many authors and medical specialty societies.

Keeping in mind the original proposal of the pioneers of perinatology, which correspond with our convictions, we accepted the invitation of Springer to bring together in this book renowned authors of the two great specialties involved in the field of perinatology: obstetrics and neonatology.

---

[1] 1. World Health Organization. ICD-11 for mortality and morbidity statistics. Version: 2020 September. Available from: https://icd.who.int/browse11/l-m/en#/http://id.who.int/icd/entity/914150644. Assessed in February 2021.

[2] Dudenhausen JW. Erich Saling - The Father of Prenatal and Perinatal Medicine-Dedication to his 90th birthday. J Perinat Med. 2015 Jul;43(4):379.

This work was not without its difficulties. The main one comes from the fact that this type of book organization gathers varied chapters in form and content, and is at risk of becoming a "patchwork" that leaves the reader disoriented.

Such inconvenience was overcome by the editors, who were careful to put the texts in consistent thematic blocks, managing to make the book reflect the themes related to pediatrics and obstetrics in an integrated way to allow a better understanding of perinatology. So, our aim was to avoid transmitting an overly integrated and closed view of one of the specialties, leaving to our reader space for their own reflection on the themes and for the development of self-interpretations.

We are grateful to chapter authors and the support by the notable Professors Erich Saling, Asim Kurjak, and Ana Bianchi.

We dedicate this book to our children Rodrigo, Alice, and Isadora, who are the biggest motivation of our lives.

Rio de Janeiro, RJ, Brazil — Renato Augusto Moreira de Sá
Niteroi, RJ, Brazil
João Pessoa, Paraíba, Brazil — Eduardo Borges da Fonseca

Acknowledgement

Prof Asim Kurjak, for supporting the Perinatal Medicine activities all around the world.

Contents

Contributors

Daniela Aires Moreira University of Medical Sciences, João Pessoa, Paraíba, Brazil

Maternal Fetal Medicine Group, Nova Diagnóstico por Imagem, João Pessoa, Brazil

Melania M. Amorim Post-Graduate Program in Instituto de Medicina Integral Professor Fernando Figueira, Recife, Brazil

Obstetrics & Gynecology, Federal University of Campina Grande, Campina Grande, Brazil

Ana Espinosa Institution Matersur, Teaching and Research, Bahía Blanca, Buenos Aires, Argentina

Carla Betina Andreucci Department of Medicine, Center of Biological and Health Sciences, Federal University of São Carlos, São Carlos, Brazil

L. Atzori Clinical Metabolomics Unit, Department of Biomedical Sciences, University of Cagliari, Cagliari, Italy

Diogo Ayres-De-Campos Departamento de Obstetrícia, Ginecologia e Medicina da Reprodução, Faculdade de Medicina da Universidade de Lisboa, Centro Hospitalar Universitário Lisboa Norte – Hospital de Santa Maria, Lisbon, Portugal

Arnaldo Prata Barbosa Instituto D'Or de Pesquisa e Ensino – IDOR, Rio de Janeiro, Brazil

Lara Spalldi Barišić Fetal and Maternal Medicine, Private Clinic Veritas, Zagreb, Croatia

Renato José Bauer Department of Obstetrics, Faculty of Medicine of Pontifical University of Sao Paulo, City of Sorocaba, SP, Brazil

Michael W. Bebbington Washington University School of Medicine in St. Louis, Louis, US

Matheus Cabral L. Beleza Maternal-Fetal Medicine Department, NEXUS Institute, Brasília, Federal District, Brazil

Augusto César Garcia Saab Benedeti FATESA – Faculdade de Tecnologia em Saúde, Ribeirão Preto, SP, Brazil

Leticia Benítez BCNatal - Barcelona Center for Maternal-Fetal and Neonatal Medicine (Hospital Clínic and Hospital Sant Joan de Deu), University of Barcelona, Barcelona, Spain

Lisandra Stein Bernardes Department of Obstetrics and Gynecology, University of São Paulo, São Paulo, Brazil

Sepaco Hospital, São Paulo, Brazil

School of Medicine, Faculdade Israelita de Ciências da Saúde Albert Einstein, São Paulo, Brazil

Carlos A. Bhering Departamento de Neonatologia do Instituto Fernandes Figueira/ FIOCRUZ, Rio de Janeiro, Brazil

Pediatria da Universidade de Vassouras, Vassouras, Brazil

Ana B. Bianchi Perinatal Department, Pereira Rossell Hospital, Montevideo, Montevideo, Uruguay

M. F. Blasina Department of Neonatology, Hospital de Clínicas, Facultad de Medicina, Universidad de la República, Montevideo, Uruguay

Fernando Javier Rojas Bravo Clínica Universidad de los Andes, Las Condes, Chile

Ingrid Schwach Werneck Britto Department of Obstetrics and Gynecology, Faculty of Medical Sciences of Santa Casa of São Paulo, São Paulo, São Paulo, Brazil

Isabela Bussade Pontifícia Universidade Católica (PUC), Rio de Janeiro, RJ, Brazil

Gabriel Martins Cruz Campos Fetal Medicine Residence – Hospital das Clínicas da UFMG, Belo Horizonte, Brazil

José Carlos Carraro-Eduardo Department of Internal Medicine, School of Medicine, Universidade Federal Fluminense (UFF), Niterói, Rio de Janeiro, Brazil

Ricardo Carvalho Cavalli Department of Obstetrics and Gynecology, Ribeirão Preto Medical School, University of São Paulo, São Paulo, SP, Brazil

Department of Obstetrics and Gynecology, Hospital das Clínicas, Faculty of Medicine, University of São Paulo, FMUSP, São Paulo, SP, Brazil

Frank A. Chervenak Department of Obstetrics and Gynecology, Zucker School of Medicine of Hofstra/Northwell, Lenox Hill Hospital, New York, NY, USA

Luciana C. Cima Perinatal/Rede D'or, Rio de Janeiro, RJ, Brazil

V. Corda Department of Prenatal and Preimplantation Genetic Diagnosis and Fetal Therapy, Ospedale Pediatrico Microcitemico "A. Cao", Cagliari, Italy

Egle Couto Department of Obstetrics and Gynecology, University of Campinas (UNICAMP), Campinas, SP, Brazil

Pontifical Catholic University of Campinas, Campinas, Brazil

Antonio José Cunha Faculdade de Medicina da Universidade Federal do Rio de Janeiro, Rio de Janeiro, Brazil

Bartolomeu Expedito da Câmara França Materno-Infantil, Federal Fluminense University, Niteroi, RJ, Brazil

Gisele Passos da Costa Gribel Department of Anesthesiology, Hospital Maternidade Escola, Universidade Federal do Rio de Janeiro (UFRJ), Rio de Janeiro, RJ, Brazil

Eduardo Borges da Fonseca Maternal Fetal Medicine Group - Nova Diagnóstico por Imagem, João Pessoa, PB, Brazil

Ob/Gyn Department, Federal University of Paraiba, João Pessoa, PB, Brazil

Antonio Claudio Lucas da Nóbrega Laboratório de Ciências do Exercício, Instituto Biomédico, Universidade Federal Fluminense, Niterói, RJ, Brazil

Jair Roberto da Silva Braga Maternidade Escola da UFRJ, Universidade Federal do Rio de Janeiro, Rio de Janeiro, RJ, Brazil

Fabrício da Silva Costa Department of Obstetrics and Gynecology, Ribeirão Preto Medical School – University of São Paulo, Ribeirão Preto, São Paulo, Brazil

Fernanda Campos da Silva Department of Obstetrics, Universidade Federal do Estado do Rio de Janeiro (UNIRIO), Rio de Janeiro, RJ, Brazil

Marcos José Burle de Aguiar Medicine School, Federal University of Minas Gerais, Belo Horizonte, Brazil

Regina Amélia Lopes Pessoa de Aguiar Medicine School, Federal University of Minas Gerais, Belo Horizonte, Brazil

João Henrique Carvalho Leme de Almeida Neonatology Department, Instituto Nacional da Saúde da Mulher, da Criança e do Adolescente Fernandes Figueira, Fundação Oswaldo Cruz, Rio de Janeiro, RJ, Brazil

José Maria de Andrade Lopes Perinatal Maternity Hospital, Rio de Janeiro, Brazil

Eduardo Carvalho de Arruda Veiga Department of Obstetrics and Gynecology, Ribeirão Preto Medical School, University of São Paulo, São Paulo, SP, Brazil

Márcia Cristina de Azevedo Gomes Clínica Perinatal, Neonatal Intensive Care, Rio de Janeiro, RJ, Brazil

Mario Henrique Burlacchini de Carvalho Department of Obstetrics and Gynecology, Faculty of Medical Sciences of Santa Casa of São Paulo, São Paulo, São Paulo, Brazil

Paulo Roberto Nassar de Carvalho Instituto Fernandes Figueira, Rio de Janeiro, Fundação Oswaldo Cruz –FIOCRUZ, Rio de Janeiro, Brazil

IETECS – Instituto de Estudos de Tecnologia em Saúde, Rio de Janeiro, Brazil

Grupo Perinatal, Rio de Janeiro, Brazil

Victor Rocha de Castro Alves FATESA – Faculdade de Tecnologia em Saúde, Ribeirão Preto, SP, Brazil

Renata Rodrigues Teixeira de Castro Department of Cardiology, Hospital Naval Marcílio Dias & School of Medicine, Iguaçu University, Rio de Janeiro, RJ, Brazil

Fernando de Freitas Martins Neonatology Department, Fernandes Figueira Institute, Oswaldo Cruz Foundation, Neonatal Intensive Care Unit, Perinatal Clinic, Rio de Janeiro, RJ, Brazil

Guilherme Ramires de Jesús Department of Obstetrics, Universidade do Estado do Rio de Janeiro, Rio de Janeiro, Brazil

Nilson Ramires de Jesús Department of Obstetrics, Universidade do Estado do Rio de Janeiro, Rio de Janeiro, Brazil

José Roberto de Moraes Ramos Departamento de Neonatologia do Instituto Fernandes Figueira/FIOCRUZ, Rio de Janeiro, Brazil

Programa de Reanimação Neonatal da Sociedade Brasileira de Pediatria, Rio de Janeiro, Brazil

Roberto Magliano de Morais Filho Faculdade de Medicina Nova Esperança, Joao Pessoa, Paraiba, Brazil

Roberto Magliano de Morais Universidade Federal da Paraiba, Joao Pessoa, Paraiba, Brazil

Cristiane Alves de Oliveira Federal Fluminense University and Rio de Janeiro Federal University, Niteroi and Rio de Janeiro, Brazil

Elaine de Paula Fiod Costa Medicine Department, Federal University of Maranhão, Maranhão, Brazil

Helenilce de Paula Fiod Costa Neonatology Department, Institution Santa Joana/ Promatre Hospital Group, São Paulo, Brazil

Jorge de Rezende-Filho Maternidade Escola da UFRJ, Universidade Federal do Rio de Janeiro, Rio de Janeiro, RJ, Brazil

Renato Augusto Moreira de Sá Fernandes Figueira Institut - FIOCRUZ, Rio de Janeiro, RJ, Brazil

Danielle Negri de Souza Lopes Neonatology Department, Perinatal Maternity Hospital, Rio de Janeiro, RJ, Brazil

Evaldo Trajano de Souza Silva Filho Maternal-Fetal Medicine Department, NEXUS Institute, Brasília, Federal District, Brazil

J. L. Diaz-Rossello Department of Neonatology, Hospital de Clínicas, Facultad de Medicina, Universidad de la República, Montevideo, Uruguay

Flavia Cunha dos Santos Department of Obstetrics, Universidade do Estado do Rio de Janeiro, Rio de Janeiro, Brazil

Karina dos Santos Research Group on Maternal and Child Health (Grupo de Pesquisa em Saúde Materna e Infantil – GPSMI), Nutrition Institute, Federal University of Rio de Janeiro, Rio de Janeiro, RJ, Brazil

Joachim Dudenhausen Department of Obstetrics and Gynecology, Zucker School of Medicine at Hofstra/Northwell, New York, NY, USA

Siw Helen Westby Eger Department of Pediatrics and Adolescence Medicine, Oslo University Hospital, Oslo, Norway

D. P. Esteves Department of Cardiology, Pregnancy Heart Disease Sector, Hospital Federal dos Servidores do Estado, Rio de Janeiro, RJ, Brazil

Juliana Silva Esteves Hospital Federal dos Servidores do Estado - Ministry of Health, Rio de Janeiro, RJ, Brazil

Carlos Augusto Faria Department of Maternal and Child Health, School of Medicine, Universidade Federal Fluminense (UFF), Niterói, RJ, Brazil

Francesc Figueras BCNatal - Barcelona Center for Maternal-Fetal and Neonatal Medicine (Hospital Clínic and Hospital Sant Joan de Deu), University of Barcelona, Barcelona, Spain

Francisco Mauad Filho FATESA – Faculdade de Tecnologia em Saúde, Ribeirão Preto, SP, Brazil

Mario Julio Franco Florianópolis, SC, Brazil

Amos Grunebaum Department of Obstetrics and Gynecology, Zucker School of Medicine at Hofstra/Northwell, New York, NY, USA

Fernanda Hermeto Neonatology Department, Perinatal Maternity Hospital, Rio de Janeiro, RJ, Brazil

A. Iuculano Department of Prenatal and Preimplantation Genetic Diagnosis and Fetal Therapy, Ospedale Pediatrico Microcitemico "A. Cao", Cagliari, Italy

Edward Araujo Júnior Discipline of Fetal Medicine, Department of Obstetrics, Paulista School of Medicine –Federal University of São Paulo (EPM-UNIFESP), São Paulo, SP, Brazil

Joffre Amim Junior Maternidade Escola da Universidade Federal do Rio de Janeiro, Rio de Janeiro, Brazil

José Eleutério Junior Department of Women's, Child and Teenager Health, Federal University of Ceará, Fortaleza, Brazil

Mário Dias Corrêa Júnior Obstetrics and Gynecology Department – Faculdade de Medicina da UFMG, Belo Horizonte, Brazil

Renato Passini Junior Department of Obstetrics and Gynecology, University of Campinas (UNICAMP), Campinas, SP, Brazil

Leila Katz Catholic University of Pernambuco (UNICAP), Recife, Brazil

Post-Graduate Program in Instituto de Medicina Integral Professor Fernando Figueira, Recife, Brazil

Roxana Knobel Faculty of Medical Sciences, State University of Campinas – UNICAMP, Campinas, Brazil

Department of Obstetrics & Gynecology, Federal University of Santa Catarina (UFSC), Florianópolis, Brazil

Henri Augusto Korkes Department of Obstetrics, Faculty of Medicine of Pontifical University of Sao Paulo, City of Sorocaba, SP, Brazil

Regis Kreitchmann Department of Gynecology and Obstetrics, Federal University of Health Sciences of Porto Alegre, Porto Alegre, Brazil

Asim Kurjak Sarajevo School of Science and Technology, Sarajevo, Bosnia and Herzegovina

Department of Obstetrics and Gynecology, School of Medicine, University of Zagreb, Zagreb, Croatia

Marcela Ignacchiti Lacerda Department of Obstetrics, Universidade do Estado do Rio de Janeiro, Rio de Janeiro, Brazil

Roger Abramino Levy Immunology and Inflammation, GlaxoSmithKline (GSK), Upper Providence, PA, USA

Renata Bastos Lopes Neonatology Department, Perinatal Maternity Hospital, Rio de Janeiro, RJ, Brazil

Jürgen Lüthje Institute of Perinatal Medicine, Berlin-Neukölln, Germany

André Luiz Malavasi Pérola Byington Hospital, São Paulo, Brazil

Hospital do Servidor Público Municipal de São Paulo, São Paulo, Brazil

International Society on Thrombosis and Haemostasis, São Paulo, Brazil

Penélope Saldanha Marinho Maternidade Escola da Universidade Federal do Rio de Janeiro, Rio de Janeiro, Brazil

Judith Martínez BCNatal - Barcelona Center for Maternal-Fetal and Neonatal Medicine (Hospital Clínic and Hospital Sant Joan de Deu), University of Barcelona, Barcelona, Spain

Alexandra Matias Department of Obstetrics, Gynecology and Pediatrics, Faculty of Medicine University of Porto, Centro Hospitalar Universitário Hospital of S. João, Porto, Portugal

Laurence B. McCullough Department of Obstetrics and Gynecology, Zucker School of Medicine of Hofstra/Northwell, Lenox Hill Hospital, New York, NY, USA

Maria Dalva Barbosa Baker Méio Instituto Fernandes Figueira- Fiocruz, Rio de Janeiro, Brazil

Eva Meler BCNatal - Barcelona Center for Maternal-Fetal and Neonatal Medicine (Hospital Clínic and Hospital Sant Joan de Deu), University of Barcelona, Barcelona, Spain

Angelica Espinosa Miranda Department of Social Medicine, Federal Universty of Espírito Santo, Vitória, Brazil

Carolina Carvalho Mocarzel Department of Obstetrics, Hospital Federal dos Servidores do Estado, Rio de Janeiro, Rio de Janeiro, Brazil

G. Monni Department of Prenatal and Preimplantation Genetic Diagnosis and Fetal Therapy, Ospedale Pediatrico Microcitemico "A. Cao", Cagliari, Italy

Viviane P. Monteiro Instituto Fernandes Figueira/Fiocruz, Rio de Janeiro, RJ, Brazil

Maria Elisabeth Lopes Moreira Instituto Fernandes Figueira - Fiocruz, Clinica Perinatal Laranjeiras, Rio de Janeiro, RJ, Brazil

F. Murgia Clinical Metabolomics Unit, Department of Biomedical Sciences, University of Cagliari, Cagliari, Italy

Janaína Luz Narciso-Schiavon Florianópolis, SC, Brazil

Carlos Antonio Negrato Medical school from Faculdade de Odontologia de Bauru (FOB), Universidade de São Paulo, Bauru, São Paulo, Brazil

Antônio Rodrigues Braga Neto Materno-Infantil, Federal Fluminense University, Niteroi, RJ, Brazil

Luiza M. Neves Instituto NAcional de Saude da Mulher, da Criança e do Adolescente, FIOCRUZ, Rio de Janeiro, Brazil

Departamento de Oftalmologia, Universidade do Estado do Rio de Janeiro, Rio de Janeiro, Brazil

Ana Carla Zanchietta Nicolielo Maternidade Perinatal, Department of Obstetrícia, Rio de Janeiro, Rio de Janeiro, Brazil

Rone Peterson Cerqueira Oliveira Department of Gynecology, Obstetrics and Human Reproduction, Federal University of Bahia, Salvador, Bahia, Brazil

Mario S. F. Palermo Diagnomed Affiliated Institution Faculty of Medicine of Buenos Aires, Teaching and Research, Buenos Aires, Argentina

Viral Mahesh Pandya GHU Paris-Centre, Hôpital Necker-Enfants Malades, Paris, France

Mauro Romero Leal Passos Department of Microbiology and Parasitology, Fluminense Federal University, Niterói, Brazil

Alberto Borges Peixoto Department of Gynecology and Obstetrics, University of Uberaba (UNIUBE), Uberaba, Brazil

Department of Gynecology and Obstetrics, Federal University of Triângulo Mineiro (UFTM), Uberaba, Brazil

Fernando Barbosa Peixoto Department of Obstetrics and Gynecology, Ribeirão Preto Medical School, University of São Paulo, São Paulo, SP, Brazil

Fernando Maia Peixoto-Filho Instituto Fernandes Figueira, Rio de Janeiro, Fundação Oswaldo Cruz –FIOCRUZ, Rio de Janeiro, Brazil

IETECS – Instituto de Estudos de Tecnologia em Saúde, Rio de Janeiro, Brazil

Grupo Perinatal, Rio de Janeiro, Brazil

Miguel Pereira-Macedo Centro Hospitalar Universitário Lisboa Central, Lisbon, Portugal

Rafaela Cardoso Gil Pimentel FATESA – Faculdade de Tecnologia em Saúde, Ribeirão Preto, SP, Brazil

Priscila Chaves Pita Ultrasonography Residence – Hospital das Clínicas da UFMG, Belo Horizonte, Brazil

Cristos Pritsivelis Maternidade Escola da UFRJ, Universidade Federal do Rio de Janeiro, Rio de Janeiro, RJ, Brazil

Camila Luiza Meira Pucci Department of Obstetrics and Gynecology, University of São Paulo, São Paulo, Brazil

Sepaco Hospital, São Paulo, Brazil

Conrado Sávio Ragazini Department of Obstetrics and Gynecology, Ribeirão Preto Medical School – University of São Paulo, Ribeirão Preto, São Paulo, Brazil

Gustavo Mourão Rodrigues Department of Obstetrics, Universidade Federal do Estado do Rio de Janeiro (UNIRIO), Rio de Janeiro, Rio de Janeiro, Brazil

Miguel Ruoti University Asuncion, Asunción, Paraguay

Erich Saling Institute of Perinatal Medicine, Berlin-Neukölln, Germany

Susana Santo Departamento de Obstetrícia, Ginecologia e Medicina da Reprodução, Faculdade de Medicina da Universidade de Lisboa, Centro Hospitalar Universitário Lisboa Norte – Hospital de Santa Maria, Lisbon, Portugal

Nelson Sass Department of Obstetrics, Universidade Federal de São Paulo (Federal University of São Paulo) – UNIFESP, City of Sao Paulo, SP, Brazil

Ola Didrik Saugstad Ann & Robert H. Lurie Children's Hospital of Chicago and Prentice Women's Hospital, Division of Neonatology, Feinberg School of Medicine, Northwestern University, Chicago, IL, USA

Department of Pediatric Research, Oslo University Hospital and University of Oslo, Oslo, Norway

Cláudia Saunders Research Group on Maternal and Child Health (Grupo de Pesquisa em Saúde Materna e Infantil – GPSMI), Nutrition Institute, Federal University of Rio de Janeiro, Rio de Janeiro, RJ, Brazil

Matthew A. Shanahan Washington University School of Medicine in St. Louis, Louis, US

Jussara de Lima e Souza Neonatology and Palliative Medicine, University of Campinas – UNICAMP, Clinic of Neonatology, Women's Hospital – CAISM, University of Campinas (UNICAMP), Campinas, Brazil

Milan Stanojevic Clinical Hospital Sveti Duh, Department of Obstetrics and Gynecology Medical School University of Zagreb, Neonatal Unit, Zagreb, Croatia

Mariane T. Tauile Perinatal/Rede D'or, Rio de Janeiro, RJ, Brazil

Julio Cesar Teixeira Department of Gynecology and Obstetrics, Faculty of Medical Sciences, University of Campinas (UNICAMP), Campinas, SP, Brazil

Mónica Trasmonte Hospital Nacional Prof. Dr. A. Posadas, MATERNAL CHILD, Buenos Aires, Argentina

Lucas Trigo Maternal-Fetal Medicine Department, Fetal Medicine Research Center (BCNatal), Hospital Clinic and Hospital Sant Joan de Déu, University of Barcelona, Barcelona, Catalunya, Spain

Shamik Trivedi Ann & Robert H. Lurie Children's Hospital of Chicago and Prentice Women's Hospital, Division of Neonatology, Feinberg School of Medicine, Northwestern University, Chicago, IL, USA

Yves Ville GHU Paris-Centre, Hôpital Necker-Enfants Malades, Paris, France

Liliana Susana Voto Maternal and Childbirth Department, Hospital General de Agudos Dr. Juan A. Fernandez, School of Medicine, University of Buenos Aires, Buenos Aires, Argentina

Masami Yamamoto GHU Paris-Centre, Hôpital Necker-Enfants Malades, Paris, France

Lenita Zajdenverg Internal Medicine Department, Diabetes Division, Hospital Universitário Clementino Fraga Filho, Universidade Federal do Rio de Janeiro, Rio de Janeiro, Brazil

Moises Gabriel Zeitune Maternal and Childbirth Department, Hospital General de Agudos Dr. Juan A. Fernández, School of Medicine, University of Buenos Aires, Buenos Aires, Argentina

Andrea Zin Instituto NAcional de Saude da Mulher, da Criança e do Adolescente, FIOCRUZ, Rio de Janeiro, Brazil

Part I
Periconceptional Care

Chapter 1
Historical Preface: Early Stages of Perinatal Medicine

Erich Saling and Jürgen Lüthje

Obstetrical medicine and obstetrical science have a long history. Far in the past, the Greek gynecologist Soranos of Ephesos (98–138) wrote a textbook which was essential for centuries: "De arte obstetrica morbisque mulierum" [1]. However, since its beginning, obstetrics had been predominantly mother-oriented for a very long time until the middle of the twentieth century.

Although first attempts have been made in earlier decades to assess some signs of existence of the fetus (e.g., with auscultation of its heart rate, see below), very little was known about clinically useful parameters of the fetal condition.

The Fetus as a New Patient in Obstetrics

The most impressive evolutionary event in obstetrics was the great change from predominantly mother-oriented obstetrics with its considerable operative character, to a combined also embryo- and fetus-oriented widespread concept. This began in the 1960s, when for the first time also the unborn became accessible to applied routine medicine. In 1966, the two British pediatricians Dobbs and Gairdner wrote: "With the advent of the techniques of amnioscopy and foetal blood sampling developed by Saling, and of amniocentesis and foetal transfusion due to Bevis and to Liley, we witness the end of the long period of foetal inaccessibility and, we hopefully believe, the start of the science of foetal medicine" [2].

The development—particularly of the prenatal part of Perinatal Medicine—was explosive. In the meantime, it has achieved an enormous extent and has become widespread. It was started by obstetricians, and in the following years,

E. Saling (✉) · J. Lüthje
Institute of Perinatal Medicine, Berlin-Neukölln, Germany
e-mail: prof@saling-institut.de; http://www.saling-institut.de

© Springer Nature Switzerland AG 2022
R. A. Moreira de Sá, E. B. d. Fonseca (eds.), *Perinatology*,
https://doi.org/10.1007/978-3-030-83434-0_1

they came close together with open-minded pediatricians and colleagues from other interested disciplines. They created powerful interdisciplinary cooperation. In this context, in 1967, we coined the term "Perinatal Medicine" [3]. In this young medical subdiscipline, new methods for routine diagnosis and therapy were introduced, and its rapid development would not have been possible without new structures in clinical care as well as in scientific organization, research, and education.

Development of New Methods

Up to the end of the 1960s, in applied routine medicine the following main subfields had developed:

- Assessment of fetal heart activity
- Fetal blood analysis
- Examination of amniotic fluid
- Application of ultrasonography
- Neonatological assessment

Assessment of Fetal Heart Activity

Already in 1818, during a lecture, Mayor remarked on the existence of fetal heart sounds for the first time [4], and in 1821 Kergaradec reported in more detail on simple auscultation of fetal heart sounds [5]. In 1833, Kennedy from Dublin published a monumental monograph on the observations of obstetric auscultation of the fetal heart [6]. According to Goodlin, many of Kennedy's clinical impressions concerning various fetal heart rate patterns are compatible with current concepts. Kennedy included, for example, Bodson's statement that the most ominous fetal heart rate pattern was "slowness of its return when a contraction is passing on" [7]. The first measurement of intrauterine pressure during labor was done in Germany in 1872 by Schatz, using a transcervically inserted balloon [8].

Fetal cardiography, this means recording the fetal heartbeats, started in 1890 when Pestalozza recorded heartbeats by a sphygmograph for the first time [9]. Cremer was successful in recording the first fetal electrocardiogram in 1906 [10], in which the small fetal signals could be differentiated from the bigger ones of the mother. In 1908, Hofbauer and Weiss recorded the first phono-cardiogram [11]. Beruti from Buenos Aires developed a phonocardiograph that could be applied in clinical practice. He combined the microphone with a telephone and predicted already in 1927, that in the future, obstetricians would be able to monitor the pregnant patient from the distance [12].

The two outstanding pioneers of modern electronically based fetal heart rate surveillance are Edward Hon and Roberto Caldeyro-Barcia. In 1957, Hon succeeded in separating the fetal signals out of the abdominally recorded maternal and fetal complexes and thus laid the basis for modern cardiography [13, 14]. Roberto Caldeyro-Barcia was not only a main pioneer of cardiotocography but also of uterine physiology and pathophysiology. In 1958, Caldeyro-Barcia and his coworkers were the first who recorded the fetal heart rate in combination with uterine contractions [15, 16]. This was the initial step for modern heart rate monitoring. All these registrations required the usage of complicated huge equipment and could therefore only serve experimental purposes. They were hardly suitable for widespread routine clinical use.

The breakthrough leading to later practical clinical usage came in the 1960s when Hammacher in cooperation with Hewlett Packard was successful in developing suitable transportable equipment, called cardiotocograph (Fig. 1.1), which was based on the phonocardiographic principle [17]. Equipment for widespread use was not available until 1968. But from then on cardiotocography developed rapidly into a surveillance method used all over the world.

Other pioneers in cardiotocography, particularly in the use of Doppler CTG, were Kazuo Maeda from Japan [18] and Mosler from Germany [19].

When we met Caldeyro-Barcia in October 1964 in Montevideo, we performed the first combined examinations of three fetuses. That is, when pathological heart rate patterns were present, we examined the fetal acid–base situation with our fetal blood analysis, which had been developed 4 years earlier.

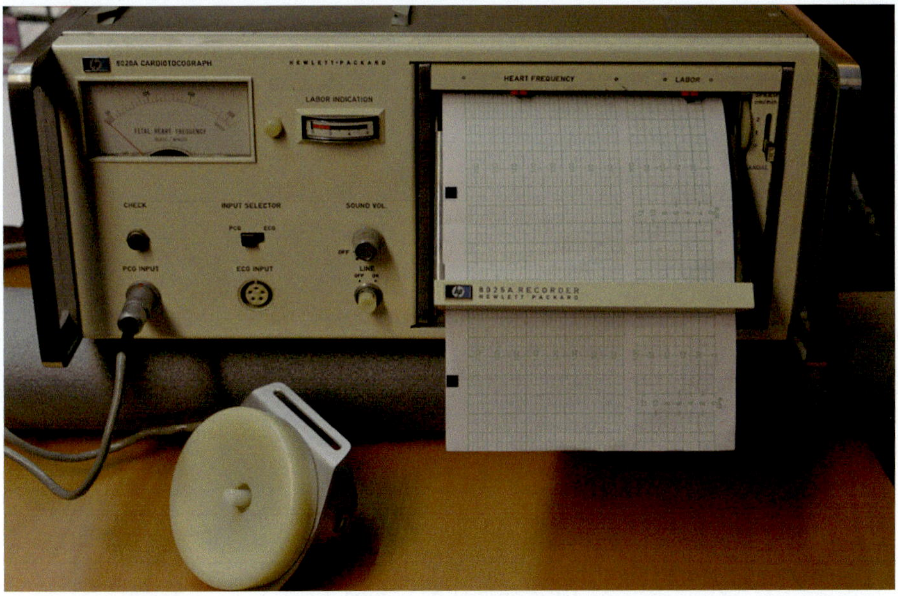

Fig. 1.1 Early model (8020A) of a transportable cardiotocograph developed by Hammacher in cooperation with Hewlett Packard, suitable for clinical use. (© Erich Saling)

Later, in 1968, when cardiotocography became available for routine use, in our department the very first real study of combined assessment of the fetus by cardiotocography and fetal blood analysis was conducted in 146 cases. In 1970, we presented the results from 489 cases at the second European Congress of Perinatal Medicine in London. We were surprised that in a number of cases, even with bradycardia, there were normal pH values. In 52 cases with bradycardia with less than 120 bpm, there were acidotic pH values only in 33% [20]. Many later studies have confirmed this weakness of cardiotocography, i.e., often yielding false-positive results.

Later considerable progress has been achieved particularly by the introduction of computer assessment of cardiotocograms. Pioneers in this field have been Geoffrey Dawes and his coworkers Visser and Redman, who already in 1978 started to evaluate different patterns of cardiotocograms by the use of computers, published in 1981 [21].

Fetal Blood Analysis

Eight years before, cardiotocography became available for widespread routine application, the first direct approach to the human fetus that could be used for routine clinical practice had been achieved. This can be considered as the moment of the birth of intrauterine medicine. It was in Berlin on June 21, 1960 (first published in 1961 [22, 23]) when we started sampling and examining the fetal blood from its presenting part (Fig. 1.2). First, there were serological and hematological examinations, followed by blood gas and acid–base analysis. Consequently, the fetus for the first time became a real patient apart from the mother, and obstetrics underwent an essentially new character.

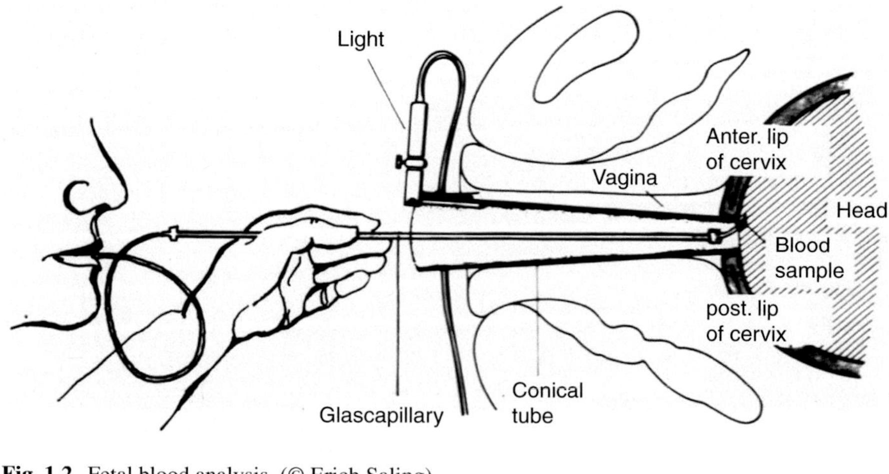

Fig. 1.2 Fetal blood analysis. (© Erich Saling)

Through the course of the years, fetal blood analysis became a gold standard of biochemical assessment of the fetus during labor. As fetal blood analysis only allows random tests, there have been attempts to also introduce continuous methods. But up to now, none of them has been successful for widespread use.

Examination of Amniotic Fluid

According to Goodlin [7], in 1833, Kennedy in his monography on obstetric auscultation already made accurate reflections about the significance of meconium-stained fluid [6].

Amniocentesis was regarded as a sacrilegious breach of the inner sanctum of the uterus. There were only occasional case reports of decompressing a polyhydramnios, for example, Lambl in 1881 [24] and Schatz in 1882 [25]. In 1930, Menees performed the first amniography [26]. In 1948, the first amniocentesis for measurement of intrauterine pressure has been published by H. Alvarez and R. Caldeyro-Barcia [27, 28]. In 1952, Bevis used amniocentesis for diagnosing Rh-erythroblastosis [29]. This was a prerequisite for two important methods developed by Liley in Australia:

- Spectrophotometric analysis of amniotic fluid in 1961 [30]
- Intrauterine treatment of severe Rh-disease afflicted fetuses in 1963 [31]

This treatment made Liley the pioneer of fetal therapy. From the 1960s onward with the help of amniocentesis, diagnosis of more diseases became possible.

Amnioscopy is a quite different amniotic fluid examination which we introduced in 1961 (published in 1962 [32]) and which enabled the obstetrician for the first time to assess amniotic fluid through the intact membranes at the forewaters during the last weeks of pregnancy (Fig. 1.3). Amnioscopy was the first method that made it possible to differentiate between the following:

- Fetuses at not increased risk concerning their respiratory supply from the mother (in cases with clear amniotic fluid)
- Fetuses with increased risk (e.g., when meconium-stained amniotic fluid or lack of amniotic fluid has been diagnosed)

Application of Ultrasonography

Another breakthrough that very much influenced modern obstetrics and perinatal medicine was the introduction of ultrasonic diagnostics into the obstetrical routine. The basic idea of making morphological structures visible by sound was born after the Titanic disaster in 1912. The technology was further developed during World War I to locate German submarines [33]. The attempt of the very first medical diagnostic application of ultrasound was done in 1942 by Dussik, but without success [34].

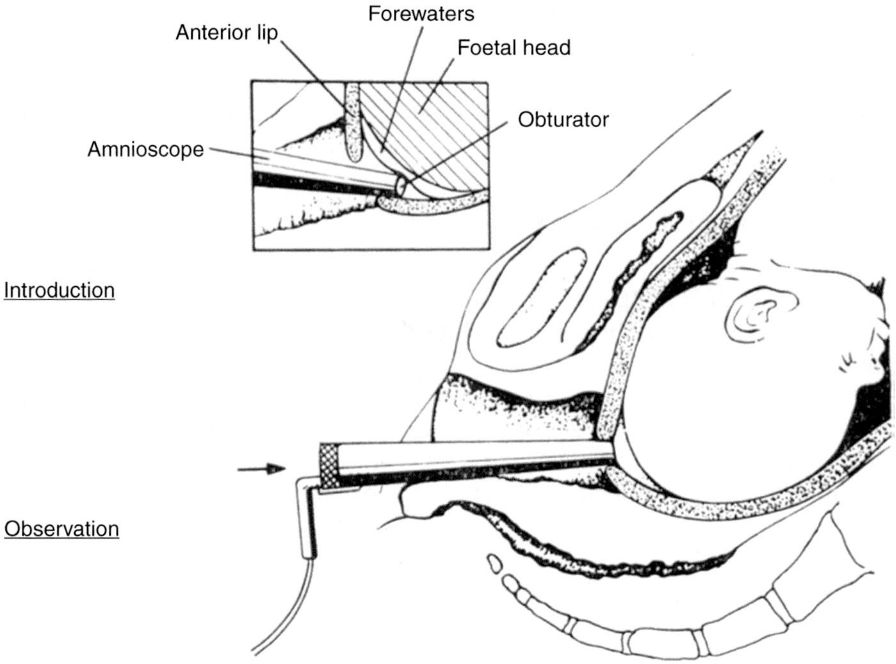

Fig. 1.3 Amnioscopy: Introduction of the tube (above) and observation of the forewaters (below). (© Erich Saling)

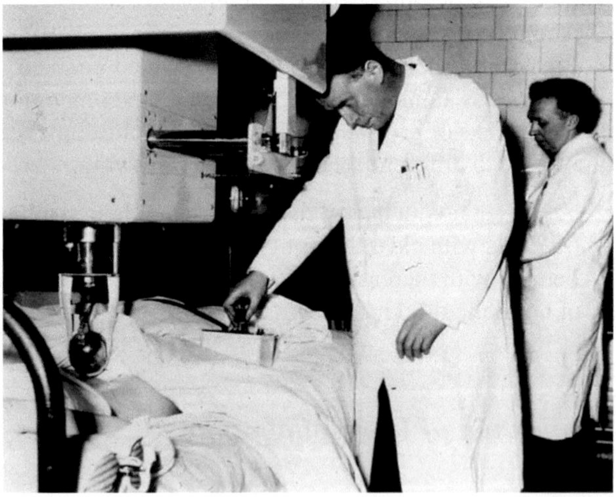

Fig. 1.4 Ian Donald examining a patient by a gigantic ultrasound scanner. (Photo taken in the Glasgow Western Infirmary in 1960. Reproduced with the kind permission of the British Medical Ultrasound Society)

In 1958, the British gynecologist Ian Donald published the first ultrasonographic scans of a fetus [35] (Fig. 1.4). The introduction of this new diagnostic tool enabled the obstetrician to receive a spectacular visual insight into the intrauterine milieu which was highly unknown before. The broad application of ultrasound diagnostics started in the late 1960s when suitable equipment for widespread routine use became available. The history of ultrasonography and its influence on the evolution of applied perinatal medicine would need a whole publication of its own. Here we can only mention some of the later pioneers:

- Doppler ultrasound in obstetrics was first used in 1964 by Callagan [36].
- Kratochwil described the usefulness of detecting fetal cardiac motion by M-mode [37].
- Hansmann described intrauterine transfusion under ultrasonic guidance [38].
- Campbell started diagnosis of fetal malformations. In 1972, he reported on an anencephalic fetus [39] and in 1975 on spina bifida [40].

The further development of ultrasonography led to unbelievable progress.

Neonatological Assessment

The introduction of a vitality score by the anesthesiologist Virginia Apgar in 1953 [41] was an important step for diagnosing the state of the newborn. However, a weakness of the Apgar score is its subjective influence. Improvements were achieved by her cooperation with Stanley James [42] and also by combination with pH measurements in umbilical blood, which we introduced in 1965 [43].

Development of Clinical Structures

The time for reforms of clinical structures was also overdue. John Ballantyne from Edinburgh had already proposed in 1901 a "pro-maternity hospital" for women with complicated pregnancies, and he was the first to have hospital beds for antenatal patients [44]. Ballantyne was apparently way ahead of his time.

In 1967, we recommended establishing a new subdiscipline within women's departments in Germany, concentrating on mother and fetus [3]. However, this initiative was not accepted and was blocked by the conservative older generation of colleagues.

In 1970, a center for perinatology with emphasis on scientific activities was founded in Montevideo, Uruguay [45]. It was the first Latin American Center of Perinatology (CLAP). In 1972, the first "Maternal-Fetal-Units" were established in the USA, and many other countries followed [46].

In contrast to former times, when many births took place at home, nowadays for instance in Germany fortunately about 98.5% of all births take place in a hospital [47]. This is highly recommendable for safety reasons.

Development of Scientific Publications

The above-mentioned changes in obstetrical medicine are reflected by the development of obstetrical publications. At the beginning of the 1960s, there were only single pages that concerned the state of the fetus.

In 1966, we published the first real book about this new field, with the literally translated title: "The Infant Within the Field of Obstetrics" [48]. In 1968, it was translated into English (unfortunately with an incorrect title) [49]. How immensely this field has grown since then is shown for instance by the huge "Textbook of Perinatal Medicine" whose first edition was edited by Asim Kurjak in 1998. It contained about 2000 pages, and more than 160 authors from many countries contributed to it [50].

In 1973, we founded the very first *Journal of Perinatal Medicine* in Berlin. Roberto Caldeyro-Barcia, Edward Hon, and Stanley James joined us as editors [51]. In the meantime, there are several other additional scientific journals in this field.

Development of Societies and Congresses

In 1963, we started international introductory 1-week courses in modern obstetrics and perinatal medicine in our hospital. In the first year, we had participants from eight European countries.

When Dr. Joseph Bieniarz, a German speaking coworker of Prof. Caldeyro-Barcia read our first publications, the team of Montevideo contacted us, and the subsequent result was the first international meeting on a high scientific level, which took place in Uruguay, in Montevideo in October 1964 (with a small group of participants including Caldeyro-Barcia, Hon, James, and Saling) (Fig. 1.5).

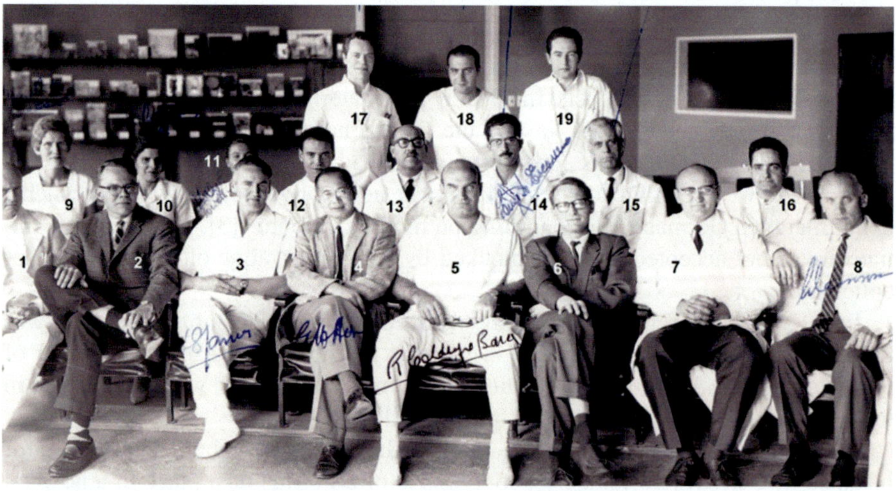

Fig. 1.5 Meeting in Montevideo in October 1964. First row, from left to right: (1) Juan Poseiro (Uruguay), (2) Edward Quilligan (USA), (3) L. Stanley James (USA), (4) Edward H. Hon (USA), (5) Roberto Caldeyro-Barcia (Uruguay), (6) F. Kubli (Germany), (7) Erich Z. Saling (Germany), (8) Karlis Adamsons (USA), Second row, from left to right: (9) Name unknown to us, (10) Name unknown to us, (11) Molly Towell (USA), (12) J. Esteban-Altirriba (Spain), (13) D. Fonseca (Uruguay),(14) L. Escarcena (Uruguay), (15) S. V. Pose (Uruguay), (16) C. Méndez-Bauer (Uruguay). Third row, from left to right: (17) O. Alvarez (Uruguay), (18) O. Althabe (Uruguay), (19) R. Schwarz (Argentina). (© of the original picture: Family of Prof. Caldeyro-Barcia, reproduced with the kind permission of Martin Caldeyro-Stajano, the son of Prof. Caldeyro-Barcia (numbers inserted by the authors)

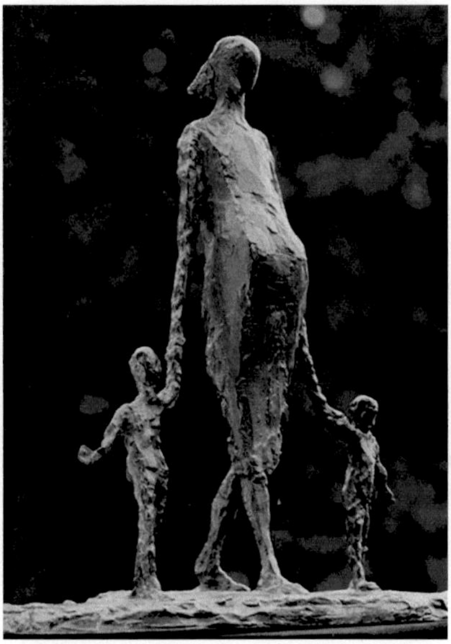

Europäischer Kongreß für Perinatale Medizin
28.–30. März 1968 Kongreßhalle, Berlin

European Congress of Perinatal Medicine
28th – 30th March, 1968 in the Congress Hall, Berlin

Congrès Européen de Médecine Périnatale
28 – 30 mars 1968, Palais des Congrès, Berlin

Wissenschaftliches Komitee - Scientific Committee - Comité scientifique

P. J. HUNTINGFORD, London, L. S. PROD'HOM, Lausanne, B. VEDRA, Praha, K. FISCHER, Hamburg, E. SALING, Berlin

Organisation - Organisation - Organisation

Arbeitsgruppe für perinatale Klinik und Forschung an der Städtischen Frauenklinik Berlin-Neukölln.
Assistenz: H. LISON und D. REICHWEIN

Fig. 1.6 Cover and title page of the program of the first European Congress of Perinatal Medicine. (© Erich Saling)

The very first national scientific society in cooperation with other closely related disciplines—mainly neonatology—was founded by us on February 6, 1967, in Berlin. It was the German Society of Perinatal Medicine. This point in time can be considered as the birth of the official public corporation of Perinatal Medicine. In November of the same year, we had the first national congress in Germany.

In 1968, the first international congress took place, the first European Congress of Perinatal Medicine in Berlin (Fig. 1.6). The first international interdisciplinary society was founded on March 30 during this congress, it was the European Association of Perinatal Medicine [52]. After 1968, a considerable number of national and international societies of this new field have been founded.

Twenty-three years later, in 1991, the first worldwide Congress of Perinatal Medicine was held in Tokyo, where the World Association of Perinatal Medicine was also founded [53].

Outlook

Now, in the year 2020, Perinatal Medicine is about 60 years old. It has grown from nearly nothing to a huge medical science which increasingly plays an important role not only before birth but also by means of epigenetics and perinatal programming for the whole life of the individual. We have the privilege of being witnesses of and contributors to this revolutionary period. Further vivid scientific and clinical progress can be expected.

References

1. Schubert C. Griechenland und die europäische Medizin. 500 v. Chr.–400 n. Chr. In: Schott H, editor. Die Chronik der Medizin. Gütersloh/München: Chronik-Verlag; 1997. p. 34–62.
2. Dobbs RH, Gairdner D. Foetal medicine - who is to practise it? Editorial. Arch Dis Child. 1966;41(219):453.
3. Saling E. Vorschläge zur Neuordnung der Geburtshilfe. Geburtsh Frauenheilk. 1967;27(6):572–85.
4. Gültekin-Zootzmann B. The history of monitoring the human fetus. J Perinat Med. 1975;3(3):135–44.
5. Kergaradec, Jean Alexandre Lejumeau de. Mémoire sur l'Auscultation appliquée à l'Etude de la Grossesse ou Recherches sur deux nouveaux signes propres á faire reconnaitre plusieurs circonstances de l'Etat de Gestation; lu à l'Académie royal de médecine, dans sa séance générale du 26 décembre 1821. Paris. 1822.
6. Kennedy E. Observations on obstetric auscultation. Dublin: Hodges and Smith; 1833.
7. Goodlin RC. History of fetal monitoring. Am J Obstet Gynecol. 1979;133(3):323–52.
8. Schatz F. Beiträge zur physiologischen Geburtskunde. Arch Gynakol. 1872;3:58–144, 174-182 (plus Tafel 1-5).
9. Pestalozza E. Graphische Darstellung des fötalen Herzimpulses. In: Dührssen, editor. Verhandlungen der gynäkologischen Section des X. internationalen medicin. Congresses in Berlin vom 4. bis 9. August 1890, 1891, p. 137.
10. Cremer M. Ueber die direkte Ableitung der Aktionsströme des menschlichen Herzens vom Oesophagus und über das Elektrokardiogramm des Fötus. Münch Med Wochenschr. 1906;53(17):811–3.
11. Hofbauer J, Weiss O. Photographische Registrierung der fötalen Herztöne. Zentralbl Gynakol. 1908;13:429–31.
12. Beruti JA. Fernauskultation und Registrierung der fetalen Herztöne. Gegenwärtiger Stand der Versuche. Arch Gynakol. 1927;132:52–7.
13. Hon EH, Hess OW. Instrumentation of fetal electrocardiography. Science. 1957;125(3247):553–4.
14. Hon EH. The electronic evaluation of the fetal heart rate. Preliminary report. Am J Obstet Gynecol. 1958;75(6):1215–30.
15. Caldeyro-Barcia R. Estudio de la anoxia fetal intrauterina mediante el ECG fetal y el registro continuo de la frecuencia cardiaca fetal. III Congr. Lat. Amer. Obst. Ginec., 1958, p. 388–90.
16. Poseiro JJ, Caldeyro-Barcia R. Estudio de la anoxia fetal intrauterina mediante el ECG fetal y el registro continuo de la frequencia cardiaca fetal. Archivos de Ginecologia y Obstetrica. 1958;XVI(4-6):105–11.
17. Hammacher K. Neue Methode zur selektiven Registrierung der fetalen Herzschlagfrequenz. Geburtsh Frauenheilk. 1962;22:1542–3.
18. Maeda K, Kimura S, Fukui Y, Shuichi O, Kosaka T, et al. Pathophysiology of the fetus. Fukuoka: Fukuoka printing; 1969.
19. Mosler KH. Dauerüberwachung der fetalen Herzaktion unter der Geburt mittels Ultraschall. Experientia. 1969;25(2):222–3.
20. Saling E. The measurement of fetal heart-rate and acid-base balance. In: Proc. 2nd Europ. Congr. Perinatal Medicine (London 1970). Basel: Karger; 1971. p. 13–22.
21. Dawes GS, Visser GH, Goodman JD, Redman CW. Numerical analysis of the human fetal heart rate: the quality of ultrasound records. Am J Obstet Gynecol. 1981;141(1):43–52.
22. Saling E. Neue Untersuchungsmöglichkeiten des Kindes unter der Geburt (Einführung und Grundlagen). Zentralbl Gynakol. 1961;83(47):1906–7.
23. Saling E. Neues Vorgehen zur Untersuchung des Kindes unter der Geburt. Einführung, Technik und Grundlagen. Vorgetragen am 10.3.61 vor der Berliner Gesellschaft für Geburtshilfe und Gynäkologie. Arch. Gynakol. 1962;197(1):108–22.
24. Lambl D. Ein seltener Fall von Hydramnios. Zentralbl Gynakol. 1881;5(14):329–34.

25. Schatz F. Eine besondere Art von einseitiger Polyhydramnie mit anderseitiger Oligohydramnie bei eineiigen Zwillingen. Arch Gynakol. 1882;19:329–69.
26. Menees TO, Miller JD, Holly LE. Amniography. Preliminary report. Am J Roentgenol. 1930;24(4):363–6.
27. Alvarez H, Caldeyro-Barcia R. Estudios sobre la fisiología de la actividad contráctil del utero humano. Primera comunicación. Nueva técnica para registrar la actividad contráctil del útero humano grávido Archivos de Ginecologia y Obstetrica. 1948;7(1–2):7–24.
28. Alvarez H, Caldeyro-Barcia R. Fisiologia de la Actividad contractil del utero humano gravido. Cuarta communicatión. Adaptacion del "Tono" Uterino, a las variaciones de volumen de su contenido. Archivos de Ginecologia y Obstetrica. 1948;VII(5–6):139–51.
29. Bevis DC. The antenatal prediction of haemolytic disease of the newborn. Lancet. 1952;259(6704):395–8.
30. Liley AW. Liquor amnii analysis in the management of the pregnancy complicated by resus sensitization. Am J Obstet Gynecol. 1961;82:1359–70.
31. Liley AW. Intrauterine transfusion of foetus in haemolytic disease. Br Med J. 1963;2(5365):1107–9.
32. Saling E. Die Amnioskopie, ein neues Verfahren zum Erkennen von Gefahrenzuständen des Feten bei noch stehender Fruchtblase. Geburtsh Frauenheilk. 1962;22(9):830–45.
33. Strunk H, Frentzel-Beyme B, Stuckmann G. Geschichte der diagnostischen Sonographie. Available: https://www.degum.de/degum/historie-museum/geschichte-der-diagnostischen-sonographie.html. Accessed 5 Mar 2020.
34. Woo J (2006) Karl Dussik. Available: http://www.ob-ultrasound.net/dussikbio.html. Accessed 19 March 2020.
35. Donald I, MacVicar J, Brown TG. Investigation of abdominal masses by pulsed ultrasound. Lancet. 1958;271(7032):1188–95.
36. Callagan DA, Rowland TC, Goldman DE. Ultrasonic Doppler observation of the fetal heart. Obstet Gynecol. 1964;23(4):637.
37. Kratochwil A. Ein neues Registrierverfahren des fetalen Ultraschall-Kardiogramms. Geburtsh Frauenheilk. 1968;28(10):949–53.
38. Hansmann M, Lang N. Intrauterine Transfusion unter Ultraschallkontrolle. Klin Wochenschr. 1972;50(19):930–2.
39. Campbell S, Johnstone FD, Holt EM, May P. Anencephaly: early ultrasonic diagnosis and active management. Lancet. 1972;300(7789):1226–7.
40. Campbell S, Pryse-Davies J, Coltart TM, Seller MJ, Singer JD. Ultrasound in the diagnosis of spina bifida. Lancet. 1975;305(7915):1065–8.
41. Apgar V. A proposal for a new method of evaluation of the newborn infant. Curr Res Anesth Analg. 1953;32(4):260–7.
42. James LS, Weisbrot IM, Prince CE, Holaday DA, Apgar V. The acid-base status of human infants in relation to birth asphyxia and the onset of respiration. J Pediatr. 1958;52(4):379–94.
43. Saling E. Zustandsdiagnose beim Neugeborenen unmittelbar nach der Geburt. Gynaecologia. 1965;160(3):133–56.
44. Ballantyne JW. A plea for a pro-maternity hospital. Br Med J. 1901;1(2101):813–4.
45. Stupin JH. History of clinical structures and development of the Perinatal Care System. In: Saling E, Dräger M, Stupin JH, editors. The beginnings of perinatal medicine. Berlin: Walter de Gruyter; 2014. p. 105–13.
46. Saling E. Birth and youth of prenatal and perinatal obstetrics. In: Kurjak A, Chervenak FA, editors. Textbook of perinatal medicine. London: Informa Healthcare; 2006. p. xxv–xxxiii.
47. Gesellschaft für Qualität in der außerklinischen Geburtshilfe e.V. Geburtenzahlen in Deutschland. 2019. Available: http://www.quag.de/quag/geburtenzahlen.htm. Accessed 18 Feb 2020.
48. Saling E. Das Kind im Bereich der Geburtshilfe. Eine Einführung in ausgewählte aktuelle Fragen. Stuttgart: Thieme; 1966.
49. Saling E. Foetal and neonatal hypoxia in relation to clinical obstetric practice. London: Edward Arnold (Publishers) Ltd; 1968.

50. Kurjak A, editor. Textbook of perinatal medicine. A comprehensive guide to modern clinical perinatology. London, New York: The Parthenon Publishing Group; 1998.
51. Hon EH, Caldeyro-Barcia R, Saling E. Editors' preface. J Perinat Med. 1973;1(1):3–6.
52. Saling E, Di Renzo GC. Perinatal care in Europe. A history of the European Association of Perinatal Medicine. New York: Parthenon Publishing Group; 1996.
53. Sakamoto S. Memories of the World Association of perinatal medicine. In: Kurjak A, Chervenak FA, editors. Textbook of perinatal medicine. London: Informa Healthcare; 2006. p. xxxiv–xxxvii.

Chapter 2
Professional Ethics in the Clinical Practice of Perinatal Medicine

Frank A. Chervenak and Laurence B. McCullough

Abbreviations

AAP	American Academy of Pediatrics
OPO	Organ Procurement Organization
ROSC	Restoration of Spontaneous Circulation

Introduction

Ethics is an essential component of perinatal clinical practice [1, 2]. The purposes of this chapter are to describe professional ethics in perinatal medicine and identify professionally responsible responses to ethical challenges in clinical practice.

Two Components of Professional Ethics in Perinatal Medicine

Perinatal medicine comprises obstetric management of the pregnant patient and fetal patient and pediatric management of the neonatal patient. Professional ethics in perinatal medicine, therefore, includes both professional ethics in obstetrics and professional ethics in pediatrics [1, 2]. Before describing these two components of professional ethics in perinatal medicine, we define key ethical terms and concepts.

F. A. Chervenak (✉) · L. B. McCullough
Department of Obstetrics and Gynecology, Zucker School of Medicine of Hofstra/Northwell, Lenox Hill Hospital, New York, NY, USA
e-mail: fchervenak@northwell.edu

© Springer Nature Switzerland AG 2022

R. A. Moreira de Sá, E. B. d. Fonseca (eds.), *Perinatology*,
https://doi.org/10.1007/978-3-030-83434-0_2

Key Ethical Terms and Concepts

Ethical Principles

Ethical principles provide practical guidance for deliberative (evidence-based, rigorous, transparent, and accountable [1, 2]) clinical judgment and clinical management based on such clinical judgment.

Two Kinds of Ethical Principles Some ethical principles are absolute, which means that they have no ethically justified exceptions. Some ethical principles are prima facie: they guide judgment and action unless another ethical principle can be shown in ethical reasoning to take priority. For example, a committed pacifist takes the view that the prohibition against killing another human being has no exceptions and is therefore absolute. Those who hold that the use of lethal means for self-defense is sometimes ethically justified take the view that the prohibition against killing another human being has ethically justified exceptions and is therefore prima facie. Professional ethics in perinatal medicine deploys two prima facie ethical principles [3].

The Ethical Principle of Beneficence The ethical principle of beneficence has a long pedigree in the global history of medical ethics. Perhaps the first occurrence of the word "beneficence" is in Medical Ethics by the English physician-ethicist, Thomas Percival (1740–1804) [1, 2]. This was the first book entitled "Medical Ethics" in the global history of medical ethics.

The ethical principle of beneficence creates the prima facie ethical obligation of a physician to identify and provide forms of clinical management that in deliberative clinical judgment are reliably predicted to result in net clinical benefit for the patient [1, 2]. By their very nature, beneficence-based clinical judgments are evidence based. This means that the strength of a beneficence-based ethical obligation varies directly with the strength of the evidence base for predicted net clinical benefit. Beneficence-based clinical judgment and management are designed to protect and promote the health-related interests of the patient. Forms of clinical management that are supported in evidence-based clinical judgment are known as medically reasonable forms of clinical management.

The Ethical Principle of Respect for Autonomy Perhaps the earliest expression of this ethical principle appeared in the professional ethics in medicine of the Scottish physician-ethicist, John Gregory (1724–1773) [1, 2]. Gregory held that every patient has "the right to speak" when his or her own life or health is concerned.

The ethical principle of respect for patient autonomy builds on the beneficence-based ethical obligation to identify the medically reasonable forms of clinical management for the patient's condition or diagnosis. Respect for autonomy in professional ethics in obstetrics creates the prima facie ethical obligation to empower the patient to make decisions on the basis of information about her condition or diagnosis, the medically reasonable forms of clinical management for her condition or diagnosis, and the clinical benefits and risks of each of these forms of clinical management [1, 2].

The Best Interests of the Child Standard The ethical principles of beneficence and respect for autonomy play a distinctive role in professional ethics in pediatrics. A core ethical concept of professional ethics in pediatrics is the best interests of the child standard [1]. The American Academy of Pediatrics (AAP) endorsed the best interests of the child standard in 1995 [4] and reaffirmed this endorsement in 2016 [5]. The standard is beneficence-based, the pediatric healthcare professional has the prima facie ethical obligation to identify and provide forms of clinical management that are supported in beneficence-based clinical judgment. In distinction from professional ethics in obstetrics, the clinical application of this beneficence-based standard does not require reference to the parents' beliefs and values. This standard has an important implication for parents: they have a parallel beneficence-based prima facie ethical obligation to authorize clinical management that is supported by the best interests standard. This ethical obligation places a constraint on parental autonomy. This is why the AAP calls for the use of "parental permission," rather than "parental consent." [4, 5] The ethical principle of respect for parental permission creates the prima facie obligation to empower the parents to make decisions about their child's clinical care by providing them with information about the medically reasonable alternatives for the clinical management of the child's condition and by supporting them in authorizing medically reasonable clinical management.

Two Components of Professional Ethics in Perinatal Medicine

Professional Ethics in Obstetrics

Professional ethics in obstetrics has three components in the perinatal clinical setting. The obstetrician has beneficence-based and autonomy-based prima facie ethical obligations to the pregnant patient and beneficence-based prima facie ethical obligations to the fetal patient [1, 2]. These three ethical obligations can become incompatible because of clinical circumstances or the expressed preference of the pregnant patient about the mode of delivery.

All three prima facie ethical obligations must be identified and taken into account in *all clinical circumstances*. Inasmuch as none of these obligations is absolute, incompatibility among them must be managed in deliberative, clinical ethical judgment that establishes an ethically justified priority among them. In particular, the views that autonomy-based ethical obligations to the pregnant patient are absolute or that beneficence-based ethical obligations to the fetal patient are absolute have no place in professional ethics in obstetrics [1, 2].

Professional Ethics in Pediatrics

Professional ethics in pediatrics is based on the best interest of the child standard and the principle of respect for parental permission, as explained above.

Professional Ethics in Obstetrics and Professional Ethics in Pediatrics Contrasted

Professional ethics in obstetrics has three components—prima facie beneficence-based and autonomy-based ethical obligations to the pregnant patient and prima facie beneficence-based ethical obligations to the fetal patient. In contrast, professional ethics in pediatrics has one component—prima facie beneficence-based to *one* patient—the child who is a patient.

Ethical Challenges in Clinical Practice

Counseling the Pregnant Patient About Intrapartum Management

In the past, it was common for an obstetrician to discuss cesarean delivery with a pregnant patient only when it becomes indicated during the intrapartum period. The patient may be experiencing pain and be distracted by the sudden rush of events as she is prepared for transfer to the operating room. These clinical factors can have an adverse effect on the adequacy of the informed consent process. For example, the patient's abilities to pay attention and to hear, process, and evaluate clinical information may be diminished. This clinical reality is much less likely to occur in the prepartum of antenatal care. It has, therefore, been proposed that obstetricians take a preventive ethics approach to counseling about intrapartum management [1, 2].

Every pregnant should be informed that before the intrapartum period that her pregnancy can, without warning, change from low- to high risk as a result of obstetric or fetal complications. The obstetrician should explain the concept that, when this becomes the case, decision-making about cesarean delivery may become urgent and constrained. The obstetrician should also explain that he or she will be recommending cesarean delivery when it is supported in evidence-based obstetric clinical judgment. Should the pregnant woman express concerns or reluctance about cesarean these should be addressed in advance and planning made on the shared value of having a good outcome for her pregnancy for her and her soon-to-be-born child. The patient should be asked to provide preliminary consent to cesarean delivery. This discussion and her consent should be documented. When this approach is taken, decision-making about the urgent need for cesarean delivery can begin with asking the pregnant women to recall the earlier discussion and her willingness to consent to cesarean delivery. The informed consent process should proceed and be appropriately documented.

Counseling the pregnant woman about intrapartum should be guided by professional ethics in obstetrics. When a neonatologist or other pediatric subspecialist participates in such counseling, he or she should think and speak like an obstetrician [1, 2]. The pregnant woman is the ultimate decision maker, a commonplace for the obstetrician but perhaps not for the pediatrician. For example, in pediatrics, it is commonly said that the "family" makes decisions, which is acceptable in pediatrics but not in obstetrics. In obstetrics, family members should be involved in decision-making only with the explicit authorization of the pregnant patient.

Counseling Prospective Parents About Neonatal Management

Counseling prospective parents about the clinical management of the neonatal patient should be guided by professional ethics in pediatrics and its best interests of the child standard. The decisions of parents are constrained by this standard, as explained above. Parents give permission, not consent. In obstetric management, the pregnant woman provides consent, not permission. The obstetrician, therefore, needs to think like a pediatrician, with counseling about neonatal management after live birth based on the best interests of the child standard [1, 2].

Counseling Parents About Setting Ethically Justified Limits on Neonatal Critical Care

Life-Sustaining Treatment as a Trial of Intervention The neonatologist should explain that the standard of care for the newborn patient is rapid evaluation followed by initiation of needed clinical management. Should the neonatal patient require resuscitation and admission to the neonatal critical care unit, the concept of a trial of management will guide decision-making. This means clinical interventions will be initiated and continued when they are supported by the best interests of the child standard. When the limits of clinical management to protect the health and life of the neonatal patient are approached, setting ethical justified limits on continued treatment becomes a medically reasonable alternative. In such clinical cases, discontinuation of life-sustaining treatment should be offered or recommended, depending on the probability of intact survival and iatrogenic risks of morbidity, disability, and mortality.

The General Concept of Futility The general clinical ethical concept of futility and its specifications can be used to guide clinical judgment about ethically justified limits on life-sustaining treatment and presenting this judgment to parents. The general concept of futility is that there is a very high predicted failure rate for a clinical intervention to produce the outcome for which that intervention was designed. The professionally responsible clinical application of this general concept of futility occurs in two steps [2].

The first step is to specify the failure rate. Insisting on a 100% failure rate would result in the general concept of futility having almost no clinical application. It would apply to attempted resuscitation of a totally decapitated patient because it is obvious that cardiopulmonary resuscitation will simply accelerate exsanguination and not restoration of spontaneous circulation (ROSC). Similarly, if a patient has been in asystole in the field for 1 hour, cardiopulmonary resuscitation will fail to produce ROSC. On the other hand, we should not set the failure rate too low because doing so could result in the death of some patients who would otherwise survive with acceptable functional status. Finally, setting the failure rate should take into account the clinical reality that when the incidence of survival is small in a gravely ill population, the disease-related and iatrogenic burdens may outweigh the benefit of survival with significantly impaired functional status.

In a landmark article Leslie Blackhall proposed that, to take account of these considerations, the failure rate should be set at 97–100% [6]. This can be understood as a cautiously prudent approach to decision-making about withholding or discontinuing life-sustaining treatment.

The second step is to specify the outcome. There are four beneficence-based specifications of the general concept of futility.

Anatomic Futility When in deliberative clinical judgment, a clinical intervention is predicted to have a failure rate of 97–100% of restoring normal anatomy, it is anatomically futile [2]. For example, there is no known surgical or medical correction of severely underdeveloped lungs caused by thanatophoric dysplasia.

Physiologic Futility When in deliberative clinical judgment a clinical intervention is predicted to have a failure rate of 97–100% of restoring normal physiology, it is physiologically futile [2]. This specification is invoked to discontinue cardiopulmonary resuscitation of newborn at 22 weeks.

Imminent-Demise Futility When in deliberative clinical judgment, a clinical intervention is predicted to have a failure rate of 97–100% of survival and no recovery of interactive capacity before death occurs, it is imminent-demise futile [2]. For example, a newborn with anencephaly may survive for a short time in the neonatal intensive care unit but never display any interactive capacity.

Interactive-Capacity Futility When in deliberative clinical judgment, a clinical intervention is predicted to result in survival, but with a failure rate of 97–100% of restoring interactive capacity, it is interactive-capacity futile [2]. For example, an infant with trisomy 13 can survive for quite some time with supportive care but never display interactive capacity during his or her lifetime.

Quality-of-Life Futility There is one autonomy-based specification of the general concept of futility: quality-of-life futility. The phrase "quality of life" entered the ethics of neonatology literature in the early 1970s but was never clearly articulated. As a consequence, the concept of quality of life has been applied with wide clinical variation, sometimes uncontrolled variation when the understanding of this concept varies from neonatologist to neonatologist. Patient safety and quality requires that the resulting risk of uncontrolled variation be managed in a professionally responsible, especially inasmuch as the life of the neonatal patient is at stake.

Getting clear about the concept of quality of life is the antidote to uncontrolled variation in its clinical application. Quality of life is a technical term of the social sciences that means engaging in life tasks and deriving satisfaction from doing so. A life task is a psychosocially complex undertaking. The specification of quality-of-life futility applies clinically when either a patient can no longer engage in valued life tasks or can but does not derive sufficient satisfaction from doing so. Quality-of-life futility judgments must be made by the patient himself or herself or a surrogate decision maker who is confident that he or she knows the patient well enough to make quality-of-life judgments for the patient.

In the professional ethics of perinatal medicine, the specification of quality-of-life futility does not apply to infants. This concept does apply to older children. For example, children entering school for the first time need to learn how to read, write, and do arithmetic. Younger children need to learn who to dress themselves and toilet unattended. These and other life tasks have goals and processes for achieving them. Infants do not yet have the neurologic capacity to have goals, much less undertake processes for achieving them. To be sure, infants have basic needs that must be met—but by others. Infants also lack the neurologic capacity to derive satisfaction from what they do, although infants can be happy, distressed, or in pain. These realities about the developmental capacity of infants mean that it is a clinical error to apply the concept of quality of life to an infant.

There are two further problems. The first is that studies of self-reported quality of life or persons with disabilities display no significant differences from self-reported quality of life of persons without disability. This means that a prediction that an infant with a future of disability will have a low quality of life lacks an evidence base and therefore should not be made. The second is that physicians are not reliable judges of the quality of life of their patients. A landmark study showed, indeed, that physicians underestimate the self-reported quality of life of patients. The specification of quality-of-life futility cannot reliably be invoked to justify withholding or discontinuing life-sustaining treatment from a neonatal patient.

A Clinical Variant of Interactive Capacity Futility We should note, however, that some neonatal conditions can be so severe that infants expend considerable energy in response to disease-related and iatrogenic morbidity. In a landmark paper, the Jesuit moral theologian, Richard McCormick (1922–2000), made the important clinical ethics observation that some neonatal conditions are so severe that an infant will expend *all* of his or her energy in the "struggle to survive." [7] The result is that whatever minimal interactive capacity the infant may have is overwhelmed by the combined clinical effects of disease-related and iatrogenic morbidity. This should be considered a clinical ethical variant of interactive-capacity futility. This clinically well-grounded specification of the general concept of futility should be used rather than quality-of-life futility. The observations and judgments of parents about their child's condition and its implications for interactive capacity should always be considered. If parents, the neonatologist, and the care team agree that a neonatal patient is only struggling to survive, it is ethically justified to withhold or discontinue life-sustaining treatment.

When Not Initiating or Discontinuing, Life-Sustaining Treatment Should Be Considered Medically Reasonable Not initiating neonatal life-sustaining treatment becomes medically reasonable when, in deliberative clinical judgment, it is predicted to be anatomically, physiologically, imminent-demise, or interactive-capacity futile. Discontinuing neonatal life-sustaining treatment becomes medically reasonable when, in deliberative clinical judgment, it has become anatomically, physiologically, imminent-demise, or interactive-capacity futile,

When either of these two deliberative clinical judgments applies, the perinatologist should explain this clinical judgment to the parents and explore with the parents their response to this clinical judgment. Questions should be encouraged and answered with the goal of meeting the parents' informational needs.

It will be important to be clear that parents can at the time love their child and acknowledge that it is time to set limits on life-sustaining treatment. The perinatologist should explain that, in such circumstances, the goal of treatment becomes palliative and hospice care. Psychosocial support for the parents should be marshalled including pastoral care for parents and family members who are religious or whose spiritual beliefs can be supported by pastoral care. The practices and rituals of faith communities during the dying process and after death should be supported. For neonatal patients who are potential sources of tissue or organs for transplantation, the organ procurement organization (OPO) that works with the hospital should be notified in a timely fashion, following organizational policy for doing so. OPO personnel should work closely with the neonatal care team to make clear and maintain the boundary between patient care, especially the distinction between determination that death has occurred by accepted cardiopulmonary or brain-function criteria and initiation of procurement procedures.

Conclusion

Professional ethics in perinatal medicine combines professional ethics in obstetrics and professional ethics in pediatrics. In perinatal clinical practice, it is important to distinguish these two forms of professional ethics in medicine. Professional ethics in obstetrics guides the counseling of the pregnant patient about intrapartum obstetric management. Professional ethics in pediatrics guides counseling prospective parents about neonatal clinical management. Professional ethics in pediatrics and its clinical ethical concept of futility guide counseling parents about setting ethically justified limits on life-sustaining treatment of the neonatal patient.

References

1. Chervenak FA, McCullough LB. The professional responsibility model of perinatal ethics. Berlin: Walter de Gruyter; 2014.
2. McCullough LB, Coverdale JH, Chervenak FA. Professional ethics in obstetrics and gynecology. Cambridge UK and New York: Cambridge University Press; 2020.
3. Beauchamp TL, Childress JF. Principles of biomedical ethics. 7th ed. New York: Oxford University Press; 2013.
4. American Academy of Pediatrics. Committee on Bioethics. Informed consent, parental permission, and assent in pediatric practice. Pediatrics. 1995;95:314–7.
5. American Academy of Pediatrics. Committee on Bioethics. Informed consent in decision-making in pediatric practice. Pediatrics. 2016;138:pii: e20161484. https://doi.org/10.1542/peds.2016-1484.
6. Blackhall LJ. Must we always use CPR? N Engl J Med. 1987;317:1281–5.
7. McCormick RA. To save or let die? The dilemma of modern medicine. JAMA. 1974;229:172–6.

Chapter 3
Guidance and Assessment of Preconception Risk

Amos Grunebaum, Joachim Dudenhausen, and Frank A. Chervenak

What Is Preconception Care?

Preconception care is a wide term which refers to the process of meeting with a woman and her partner, identifying risks to a woman's health, fertility, and pregnancy outcome as they relate to a woman becoming pregnant.

According to the Centers for Disease Control and Prevention (CDC) [1], preconception health refers to the health of women and men during their reproductive years, which are the years they can have a child. Part of preconception health is about people getting and staying healthy overall, throughout their lives. In addition, no one expects an unplanned pregnancy.

Preconception health care is the medical care a woman or man receives from the doctor or other health professionals that focuses on the parts of health that have been shown to increase the chance of having a healthy baby and the risks that may adversely affect a pregnancy.

The goals of preconception care are to: Identify potential risks to the mother, fetus, and pregnancy, educate the woman about these risks, options for intervention and management for risk reduction, and reproductive alternatives, and to initiate interventions to provide optimum maternal, fetal, and pregnancy outcomes.

The goal of preconception health care is to provide guidance, to identify and to address potential risks, reducing these risks, and providing an informed consent process to understand their risks prior to pregnancy [2]. In addition, preconception care allows for counseling about delaying pregnancy until risks have been reduced.

There is little knowledge in the medical profession about preconception care [4–6].

A. Grunebaum (✉) · J. Dudenhausen
Department of Obstetrics and Gynecology, Zucker School of Medicine at Hofstra/Northwell, New York, NY, USA

F. A. Chervenak
Department of Obstetrics and Gynecology, Zucker School of Medicine of Hofstra/Northwell, Lenox Hill Hospital, New York, NY, USA

© Springer Nature Switzerland AG 2022

R. A. Moreira de Sá, E. B. d. Fonseca (eds.), *Perinatology*,
https://doi.org/10.1007/978-3-030-83434-0_3

A preconception visit entails the initial gathering of information and providing feedback and should be an integral part of primary and preventive care for all women of childbearing age, especially those who present for a periodic health examination or for an ObGyn routine examination [1, 3].

Routinely addressing preconception issues in all women of childbearing potential is important for several reasons.

Preconception Risk Assessment

Preconception risk assessment is one of the major goals of preconception care. It includes the identification of risks to the mother and pregnancy, management to reduce risk, and initiate recommendations and interventions to provide optimum maternal, fetal, and pregnancy outcomes. In addition, preconception risk assessment allows for informed consent and for allowing the woman to wait with getting pregnant until her risks have improved. The key task in preconception risk assessment is to obtain a thorough history. One way to do this is with a structured checklist (Table 3.1: see below a sample which can be modified).

Table 3.1 Sample of preconception questionnaire

Family history
Has anyone in the mother's or father's family:
Been hospitalized for mental health reasons?
Had hearing loss/ear abnormalities?
Had blindness/severe vision problems?
Had mental retardation, learning disabilities, or fragile X syndrome?
Had miscarriages, stillbirths, or children who died soon after birth?
Had difficulty getting pregnant (trying for more than 1 year)
History of blood clots?
Are there genetic conditions in the patient and/or is there a family history of birth defects?
Cystic fibrosis?
Hemophilia?
Sickle cell diseases or trait?
Tay-Sachs disease
Canavan disease
Muscular dystrophy
Huntington chorea
Phenylketonuria
Diabetes
Alcohol abuse
Woman's/man's medical history
What is the mother's and the father's age?
Does the woman or her partner have a birth defect?

Table 3.1 (continued)

How much is their weight (underweight, normal, overweight, obese)
Are there chronic or acute medical problems?
Are there heart, lung, liver, kidney, thyroid diseases?
History of blood clots?
History of cancer?
Autoimmune diseases?
Is there diabetes or hypertension?
Which medications is she taking and are they needed and can they be potentially teratogenic?
Prior pregnancy outcomes
Is there smoking?
Is there substance abuse?
Depression/anxiety/bipolar screening; history of suicide?
Prior hospital admissions?
Any over-the-counter substances or dietary supplements?
Is there a history of infectious diseases?
Are vaccinations up to date?
Is the patient exercising regularly?
Nutritional status
Is the woman or her partner exposed to environmental hazards and toxins?
What kind of work do they do?
Are there social and mental health concerns
Dental issues?
Do you take folic acid and/or a multi-vitamin?
Immunizations/infections
Have you had or been immunized to:
Rubella (German measles)
Chicken pox
Hepatitis B
Mumps
Measles
Rubella
Tetanus
Diphtheria
Pertussis (whooping cough)
History of infections:
HIV/AIDS
Gonorrhea
Chlamydia
Urinary tract infections
Hepatitis A, B, C
Reproductive health
Do you know of any problems with your reproductive organs?

(continued)

Table 3.1 (continued)

Did you ever have epididymitis or an infection in your reproductive organs?
Have you ever had surgery on your penis or testicles?
Have you had any miscarriages?
Have any of your children been stillborn or died soon after birth?
Have you had any preterm births (before 37 completed weeks)?
Have any of your children weighed less than 5 1/2 pounds at birth?
Have any of your children weighed more than 9 pounds at birth?
Did any of your children need care in an intensive care nursery?
Did any of your children have to stay in the hospital after you or your partner went home from the delivery?
Do you have endometriosis?
Have you ever had surgery on your ovaries, uterus, cervix, fallopian
Tubes, or vagina?
Did you ever have pelvic inflammatory disease (PID) or an infection in your
Tubes or pelvis?
In any past pregnancies, did you have any problems (such as high blood pressure, diabetes, vaginal bleeding, premature labor, signs that the baby was in trouble, or difficult deliveries)?
Do you have a regular menstrual period?
Have you ever had abdominal surgery (for example, removal of the appendix)?
Have you had a child in the last year?
Have you been pregnant 5 or more times?
Have you had any abortions?
Have you delivered a baby early?
Nutrition
Are you happy with your weight?
Do you have or have you ever had an eating disorder (for example, anorexia or bulimia)?
Do you ever eat laundry starch, clay, dirt, or other things that are not foods?
Are you on a special diet (either to lose or gain weight, vegetarian, etc.)?
Do you skip meals?
Do you ever eat raw or very rare meats or fish?
Do you eat fish more than once a week?
Do you eat unpasteurized dairy products?
Do you eat soft cheeses such as feta, blue, brie, or Mexican style cheeses?
Are there foods that don't agree with you or that you are allergic to?
Do you eat a variety of foods (breads and cereals, fruits and vegetables, dairy products and meats)?
Work/home, or social issues
Do you work with metals or chemicals at work or at home (paint strippers, oven cleaners, ceramics or solder, pesticides, etc.)?
Are you exposed to high levels of heat at work or home or use hot tubs, whirlpool baths, or saunas?
Do you have a job that is physically hard work (heavy lifting, prolonged standing)?
Do you work with radiation or will you be exposed to x-rays?
Are you exposed to lead at home or work (through paint removal or remodeling, battery making, soldering, welding, radiator repair, or working at a firing range)?

Table 3.1 (continued)

Do you have contact with a cat litter box?
Has your drinking water been tested for lead, nitrates, or other contaminants?
If your drinking water was tested, were any contaminants found?
Are there family, friends, or work problems complicating things?
Do you smoke cigarettes? If yes, how many a day? #:__________ #: __________
Do you breathe second-hand smoke?
Do you drink beer, wine, or hard liquor?
How many drinks does it take to make you feel high? #:__________ #: __________
Have people annoyed you by criticizing your drinking?
Have you felt you ought to cut down on your drinking?
Have you ever had a drink first thing in the morning to steady your nerves or get rid of a hangover?
Do you use any recreational or street drugs (such as marijuana, cocaine, and crack)?

Modified from: http://publichealth.lacounty.gov/mch/ReproductiveHealth/PreconceptionHealth/PCHFiles/Becoming%20A%20Parent%20Preconception%20Checklist%20WAPC.pdf

Medical History

A thorough medical history is essential as medical problems can affect the pregnancy, and pregnancy can affect certain medical problems. Medical issues such as hypertension and diabetes can adversely affect the pregnancy and should optimally be controlled prior to pregnancy.

Diabetes or a history of diabetes or hypertension/preeclampsia in a prior pregnancy should be addressed and if necessarily treated. Diabetes should be optimally controlled prior to pregnancy [7–9]. Glycated hemoglobin (A1C) may be done in women with pregestational diabetes because good glucose control in early pregnancy reduces the risk of miscarriage and congenital anomalies. Women with a history of dyslipidemia and hypertension should undergo screening for occult type 2 diabetes as part of an overall cardiovascular risk assessment.

Hypertension should be controlled prior to conception. Women on antihypertensive drugs who have normal blood pressures or mild hypertension and no end-organ damage may be transitioned off of medication, with close monitoring of blood pressure response and reinstitution if blood pressure increases to potentially morbid levels. Patients who are on certain agents, such as angiotensin-converting enzyme (ACE) inhibitors and angiotensin receptor blockers (ARBs) in pregnancy, should be advised that these may be associated with adverse effects on the fetus and to switch to agents whose safety in pregnancy is established.

Asthma should be under good control prior to attempting conception. The use of steroids in pregnancy is generally safe, particularly when compared with the risk of maternal acid–base disturbance and fetal hypoxemia in the event of bronchospasm.

Thyroid disease can negatively affect the pregnancy and requires close monitoring of thyroid function as both hyper- and hypo-thyroidism can affect fertility and pregnancy outcome [10]. Women who receive radioiodine should defer pregnancy for at least 6 months.

Women with a history of seizures and women taking antiseizure drugs should receive thorough information about the risks of pregnancy for mother and fetus, adjustments in their drug regimen, and folic acid supplementation to reduce the risk of neural tube defects. Women with seizure disorder should take 4 mg folic acid daily [11]. Because of potentially adverse fetal teratogenic outcome, valproate should be discontinued prior to pregnancy if seizures can be adequately controlled with an alternative drug.

Pregnancy can pose additional risks to women with many cardiovascular diseases (congenital or acquired) that should be addressed before conception [12]. For women with some cardiac conditions, pregnancy can be life-threatening and should be avoided.

For women with systemic lupus erythematosus, the prognosis is best when the disease has been quiescent for at least 6 months prior to pregnancy and the patient's underlying renal function is stable and normal or near normal [13].

Women with inherited thrombophilias are at higher risk of thromboembolic complications during pregnancy because of pregnancy-associated changes in several coagulation factors; in some cases, they are at increased risk of adverse pregnancy outcome, as well. Indications for, and management of, anticoagulation should be addressed with a thrombosis specialist [14].

Nutrition, Diet, and Weight

Inadequate nutrition and extremes of body weight increase adverse outcomes [15]. Both nutrition and weight issues should be addressed when identified. Patients who are obese should lose weight to normal body mass index (BMI) levels (19.5–24.9) prior to pregnancy not only to improve fertility but also to prevent pregnancy complications associated with obesity.

All women planning pregnancy or capable of becoming pregnant should be counseled to take supplemental folic acid to reduce the risk of having an infant with a neural tube defect [16, 17], and possibly other congenital anomalies [18] and abruption [19]. The neural tube closes between 24 and 26 days after conception so folic acid supplementation after the diagnosis of pregnancy is usually too late to reduce the risk of neural tube defects. Folic acid supplementation and intake of folate fortified foods (400–800 mcg daily) and intake of fortified foods is recommended to reduce the risk of neural tube defects, and possibly other anomalies.

A healthy diet is generally similar to whether or not a woman is planning pregnancy, or not. High caffeine intake should be avoided and women who are attempting to conceive (or who are pregnant) should limit caffeine consumption to less than 200–300 mg per day (about 1–2 8 oz cups).

Megavitamins, nonessential dietary supplements, and herbal preparations should be discontinued. Megadoses of vitamin A taken during early pregnancy have been associated with birth defects [20, 21]. Multivitamin preparations containing more than 5000 international units of vitamin A should be avoided.

Obesity is associated with infertility, several adverse pregnancy outcomes, including birth defects, and an increased risk of maternal health consequences as well as long-term consequences on the offspring [22]. Weight reduction (for obese and overweight women) is recommended prior to pregnancy to achieve a normal body mass index (BMI) between 19.5 and 24.9.

Underweight women are at increased risk for infertility and pregnancy complications. In one large cohort study, women with a suboptimal body mass index had a 20% increase in risk for preterm birth and a 40% increase in risk of having a small gestational age infant [23].

Women and men trying to get pregnant should be informed that a safe level of alcohol intake during pregnancy has not been determined and therefore the only safe alcohol amount is zero.

Both nicotine and tetrahydrocannabinol (THC) have known negative impacts on pregnancy. Women who are planning pregnancy should stop smoking and/or vaping and to utilize smoking cessation resources.

Infertility Evaluation

The general consensus among infertility experts is that infertility evaluation should be undertaken for couples who have not been able to conceive after 12 months of unprotected and frequent intercourse, but earlier evaluation should be undertaken based on medical history and physical findings such as in women over 35 years of age, and those with certain issues such as irregular ovulation/menstrual cycles or other reproductive issues [24].

Prior Pregnancy Outcomes

One crucial part of risk assessment is to get information on prior pregnancy outcomes as adverse outcomes are more likely to recur.

Identifying and treating medical conditions prior to pregnancy and delaying pregnancy may be beneficial.

There are many adverse pregnancy outcomes that are more likely to recur in future pregnancies including:

- Miscarriages
- Preterm births
- Diabetes
- Hypertension and preeclampsia
- Macrosomia
- Intrauterine growth restriction

Maternal and Parental Age

As maternal age increases, the risk of infertility, fetal aneuploidy, miscarriage, gestational diabetes, preeclampsia, and stillbirth also increases [25]. Women should be aware of these risks and the consequences of delaying conception until they after 35 years of age should be known. Advanced paternal age also has some risks for offspring.

Environmental Exposures

Questions about the woman's work, travel, hobbies, pets, and home environment can identify potentially toxic exposures (including endocrine disruptors), such as mercury, lead, pesticides, air pollution, household cleaning products, unsafe sources of water, plastics used for food storage, and infection (e.g., Zika) [26]. In addition to occupational exposures, mercury may be found in fish and skin-lightening creams, and lead may be detected in paint (pre-1970), imported cosmetics/food additives/medicine, and clay [27].

Infections and Immunizations

The time prior to pregnancy is the optimal time to detect infections, discuss risks, and plan for immunizations.

Cytomegalovirus, zika, rubella, syphilis, toxoplasmosis, herpes simplex virus, and varicella are infections with teratogenic potential and should be treated optimally prior to pregnancy.

Preconception is an optimal time to test for sexually transmitted diseases such as chlamydia, gonorrhea, and human immunodeficiency virus (HIV).

Pregnant women with influenza and COVID-19 infections are more likely to develop severe illness and to die than the general population. Therefore, all women trying to get pregnant and those who are pregnant or might be pregnant during the influenza season should receive the inactivated influenza virus vaccine as soon as it becomes available. In addition, all all women trying to get pregnant and those who are pregnant should be vaccinated against COVID-19. Live vaccines (varicella, measles, mumps, rubella) should be administered more than month prior to pregnancy. The acellular pertussis vaccine is administered during pregnancy, rather than before conception to protect the infant from pertussis before it is eligible for vaccination [28]. Vaccination for pertussis is recommended between 27 and 36 weeks of gestation and at least 1 week before birth maximizes passive antibody transfer to the infant.

The CDC has issued a general overview of immunization in pregnancy [29].

Recommendations for Preconception Infection Testing

- Gonorrhea
- Chlamydia
- Syphilis
- Human immunodeficiency virus (HIV)
- Human papilloma virus (HPV)
- Hepatitis
- Other sexually transmitted infections according to standard guidelines

Immunity

- Document rubella immunity or lack of immunity
- Document varicella immunity or lack of immunity
- Confirm mumps, measles, rubella vaccination or immunity
- Parvovirus

A tuberculin skin test in high-risk populations to avoid exposing the fetus to treatment, if indicated, during pregnancy.

Intimate Partner Violence

The Centers for Disease Control and Prevention (CDC) define intimate partner violence (IPV) as actual or threatened physical or sexual violence, or psychological and emotional abuse, directed at a spouse, former spouse, current or former boyfriend or girlfriend, or dating partner [30].

Pregnant women who experience intimate partner violence during pregnancy may be about three times more likely to suffer fetal and neonatal death compared with women who do not experience intimate partner violence. It should be a priority to include intimate partner violence screenings or other detection strategies in pregnancy monitoring or family planning programs because these could help avoid preventable perinatal deaths [31].

Many women do not report IPV voluntarily. According to CDC data, 96% of all pregnant women seek prenatal care, making an average of 12 or 13 prenatal care visits during a pregnancy. These numbers demonstrate an ideal opportunity to screen for IVP.

Identifying intimate partner violence (IPV) in health care settings is becoming the standard of care.

There are several tools ranging from 5 to more questions that show the most sensitivity and specificity to screen for Intimate partner violence [32].

Here is a five-question tool to assess for intimate partner violence:

1. Have you been hit, kicked, punched, or otherwise hurt by someone in the past year and by whom?
2. Do you feel safe in your current relationship?
3. Is there a partner from a previous relationship who is making you feel unsafe now?
4. In general, how do you describe your relationship (with/without tension)?
5. Do you and your partner work out arguments with difficulties?

Genetics

Genetic carrier screening should be based individually on the woman's or partner's ethnicity, medical history or family history of heritable disease, or patient request [33].

For couples at increased risk of offspring with a heritable disease, referral to a specialist in genetics is usually warranted to discuss the results of screening tests, risk of the disease in the fetus, the natural course of the disease, options regarding preimplantation and prenatal diagnosis and intervention, and reproductive alternatives.

Africans should be tested for sickle cell, Jews for Tay-Sachs, and other genetic issues associated with their ethnicity.

Dental Issues

Dental and other oral and periodontal diseases are common and may be associated with pregnancy complications, such as preterm delivery; thus, referral to a dentist is appropriate [34]. Women should be advised to see a dentist prior to pregnancy and regularly during pregnancy.

Conclusions

Preconception interventions include health promotion education and counseling related to reproductive health risks, optimizing the control of medical disorders, and referral for specialized care, when appropriate. There is scant data on counseling for when to postpone pregnancy [35]. As part of preconception care, obstetricians should take a preventive ethics approach to the care of pregnant women with expectations for a perfect baby [36].

If pregnancy avoidance is desired, then contraceptive options should be discussed and a contraceptive chosen in line with the woman's planned timing of pregnancy.

References

1. https://www.cdc.gov/preconception/index.html.
2. Johnson K, Posner SF, Biermann J, et al. Recommendations to improve preconception health and health care--United States. A report of the CDC/ATSDR Preconception Care Work Group and the Select Panel on Preconception Care. MMWR Recomm Rep. 2006;55:1.
3. ACOG Committee Opinion No. 762: Prepregnancy Counseling. Obstet Gynecol. 2019;133:e78.
4. Moser R Jr, McCance KL, Smith KR. Results of a national survey of physicians' knowledge and application of prevention capabilities. Am J Prev Med. 1991;7:384.
5. Conway T, Mason E, Hu TC. Attitudes, knowledge, and skills of internal medicine residents regarding pre-conception care. Acad Med. 1994;69:389.
6. Conway T, Hu TC, Mason E, Mueller C. Are primary care residents adequately prepared to care for women of reproductive age? Fam Plan Perspect. 1995;27:66.
7. Hood KK. Preconception counseling for adolescent females with type 1 diabetes: the READY-Girls Program. Curr Diab Rep. 2010;10:393.
8. Temple RC, Aldridge VJ, Murphy HR. Prepregnancy care and pregnancy outcomes in women with type 1 diabetes. Diabetes Care. 2006;29:1744.
9. Tripathi A, Rankin J, Aarvold J, et al. Preconception counseling in women with diabetes: a population-based study in the north of England. Diabetes Care. 2010;33:586.
10. Stagnaro-Green A, Abalovich M, Alexander E, et al. Guidelines of the American Thyroid Association for the diagnosis and management of thyroid disease during pregnancy and postpartum. Thyroid. 2011;21:1081.
11. Neural tube defects. Practice Bulletin No. 187 ACOG. Obstet Gynecol. 2017;130:e279–290.
12. Adam K. Pregnancy in women with cardiovascular diseases. Methodist Debakey Cardiovasc J. 2017;13(4):209–15.
13. Fischer-Betz R, Specker C. Pregnancy in systemic lupus erythematosus and antiphospholipid syndrome. Best Pract Res Clin Rheumatol. 2017;31(3):397–414.
14. Silver RM, Warren JE. Preconception counseling for women with thrombophilia. Clin Obstet Gynecol. 2006;49(4):906–19.
15. Dudenhausen JW, Kunze M, Wittwer-Backofen U, Hagenah HP, Strauss A, Günther V, Alkatout İ, Grunebaum A, Voigt M. The relationship between maternal age, body mass index, and the rate of preterm birth. J Turk Ger Gynecol Assoc. 2018;19(4):182–6.
16. U.S. Preventive Services Task Force. Folic acid for the prevention of neural tube defects: U.S. Preventive Services Task Force recommendation statement. Ann Intern Med. 2009;150:626.
17. National Health Service. Vitamins and nutrition in pregnancy. http://www.nhs.uk/conditions/pregnancy-and-baby/pages/vitamins-minerals-supplements-pregnant.aspx. Accessed on 5 Nov 2012.
18. Goh YI, Bollano E, Einarson TR, Koren G. Prenatal multivitamin supplementation and rates of congenital anomalies: a meta-analysis. J Obstet Gynaecol Can. 2006;28:680.
19. Nilsen RM, Vollset SE, Rasmussen SA, et al. Folic acid and multivitamin supplement use and risk of placental abruption: a population-based registry study. Am J Epidemiol. 2008;167:867.
20. Oakley GP Jr, Erickson JD. Vitamin A and birth defects. Continuing caution is needed. N Engl J Med. 1995;333:1414.
21. Rothman KJ, Moore LL, Singer MR, et al. Teratogenicity of high vitamin A intake. N Engl J Med. 1995;333:1369.

22. Chandrasekaran S, Neal-Perry G. Long-term consequences of obesity on female fertility and the health of the offspring. Curr Opin Obstet Gynecol. 2017;29(3):180–7.
23. Tabet M, Flick LH, Tuuli MG, et al. Prepregnancy body mass index in a first uncomplicated pregnancy and outcomes of a second pregnancy. Am J Obstet Gynecol. 2015;213:548.e1.
24. https://www.acog.org/Patients/FAQs/Evaluating-Infertility?IsMobileSet=false.
25. Stubblefield PG, Coonrod DV, Reddy UM, et al. The clinical content of preconception care: reproductive history. Am J Obstet Gynecol. 2008;199:S373.
26. McDiarmid MA, Gardiner PM, Jack BW. The clinical content of preconception care: environmental exposures. Am J Obstet Gynecol. 2008;199:S357.
27. Sathyanarayana S, Focareta J, Dailey T, Buchanan S. Environmental exposures: how to counsel preconception and prenatal patients in the clinical setting. Am J Obstet Gynecol. 2012;207:463.
28. Waits JB, Smith L, Hurst DJ. Maternal pertussis vaccination during pregnancy. Am Fam Physician. 2019;99(7):454–5.
29. Prevention of measles, rubella, congenital rubella syndrome, and mumps, 2013: Summary recommendations of the Advisory Committee on Immunization Practices (ACIP). http://www.cdc.gov/mmwr/preview/mmwrhtml/rr6204a1.htm#Tab3
30. [https://www.cdc.gov/violenceprevention/intimatepartnerviolence/index.html].
31. Pastor-Moreno G, Ruiz-Pérez I, Henares-Montiel J, Petrova D. Intimate partner violence during pregnancy and risk of fetal and neonatal death: a meta-analysis with socioeconomic context indicators. Am J Obstet Gynecol. 2020;222(2):123–133.e5.
32. https://www.cdc.gov/violenceprevention/pdf/ipv/ipvandsvscreening.pdf.
33. American Society for Reproductive Medicine; American College of Obstetricians and Gynecologists' Committee on Gynecologic Practice. Prepregnancy counseling: Committee Opinion No. 762. Fertil Steril. 2019;111(1):32–42.
34. Boggess KA, Edelstein BL. Oral health in women during preconception and pregnancy: implications for birth outcomes and infant oral health. Matern Child Health J. 2006;10(5 Suppl):S169–74.
35. Dudenhausen JW, Grunebaum A, Staudinger UM. Optimization of women's health before conception when pregnancy has been postponed. J Perinat Med. 2013;41(1):23–5.
36. Chervenak FA, McCullough LB, Brent RL. The perils of the imperfect expectation of the perfect baby. Am J Obstet Gynecol. 2010;203(2):101.e1–5.

Chapter 4
Genetics for the Obstetrician: Bases of Genetic Counseling

Regina Amélia Lopes Pessoa de Aguiar and Marcos José Burle de Aguiar

Genetic counseling is one of the most important tools in medical genetics. It is characterized as a communication process that addresses problems related to the appearance or the risk of recurrence of a certain disease in a family [1]. The main objective of genetic counseling in obstetrics is to ensure that the woman or the couple has adequate information to exercise their autonomy in making reproductive decisions. In addition, during the counseling process, possible options should also be discussed, reducing anxiety and guilt and educating about a specific genetic disease, mainly when it is identified during pregnancy. This requires efficient communication about advantages, disadvantages, limitations, and risks for all prenatal screening and diagnosis options. Therefore, genetic counseling, in different situations, involves two distinct phases: pre- and post-test counseling [2].

Essential Features of Genetic Counseling

The essential feature of genetic counseling is not to be directive. This means that in genetic counseling we should not tell the woman or the couple or the family, in genetics called proband(s), what they should do, but rather provide the information in the clearest possible way for decision-making. In order to be successful, it is necessary to take into account the characteristics of the proband, such as age, education, religion, beliefs, among others, guaranteeing respect for their ethical concepts. Therefore, it is essential that the genetic counselor be limited to facts of the condition under analysis, avoiding, as much as possible, making value judgments, and ensuring that the decision be made by the proband [3–5].

R. A. L. P. de Aguiar (✉) · M. J. B. de Aguiar
Medicine School, Federal University of Minas Gerais, Belo Horizonte, Brazil

© Springer Nature Switzerland AG 2022

R. A. Moreira de Sá, E. B. d. Fonseca (eds.), *Perinatology*,
https://doi.org/10.1007/978-3-030-83434-0_4

Genetic Counseling Steps

For genetic counseling to be successful, some of these steps must be used and analyzed.

Problem Identification

The organization of the steps to be taken in genetic counseling depends on the correct identification of the problem that determined the need or indication for genetic counseling. Conducting a genetic counseling for a healthy 35-year-old woman who wants to know her reproductive risks is completely different from conducting a genetic counseling for an also healthy 35-year-old woman who has undergone a carrier screening test for gene disorders. The same if the woman had the result of a noninvasive prenatal test with a high risk for chromosome 21 trisomy in an ongoing pregnancy. It is also very different if what motivated the consultation was a history of previous stillborn with multiple malformations [6].

The Pedigree Construction

A detailed family history, with an emphasis on data suggestive of the occurrence of genetic diseases, remains a key piece in clinical genetics. The pedigree plays a key role in individualized planning and treatment, despite the increasing availability of sophisticated cytogenetic and molecular tests. A well-designed pedigree can clearly show an inheritance pattern, be it typical, as in Mendelian inheritance, or even in atypical patterns, such as in mitochondrial diseases, germ cell mosaicism, or multifactorial disease.

The identification of the pattern of inheritance is extremely important either for the diagnosis of a specific case or to search for other individuals of the same family at risk of the disease who may be benefited by specialized evaluation and genetic counseling [7].

It is important to understand that even in a simple situation as pretest counseling due to high maternal age, the construction of the pedigree is essential and, eventually, is possible to identify a risk situation for a specific genetic disease not previously noticed. The detection of several cases of intellectual disabilities in males in maternal family history "e.g." may suggest a risk for fragile X syndrome, or others X-linked diseases. In this case, the whole process and planning of genetic counseling will be very different.

Diagnostic Hypothesis

The degree of diagnostic certainty is an important factor to the quality of genetic counseling. Nevertheless, the possibility of an accurate diagnosis is not always common in clinical genetics, especially during pregnancy.

In some situations, an accurate diagnosis is not necessary. This is applicable either in the screening test for carrier status in Mendelian diseases, or in noninvasive screening tests for fetal diseases, or in invasive procedures to obtain fetal material for chromosomal study or molecular analysis. However, even in this context, it is essential to be able to inform the advantages, the limitations of each test, and the existing options in view of the possible results. So once again, it is essential that the professional be able to communicate the facts clearly and correctly, allowing the woman or couple to take informed choices [8].

On the other hand, in situations in which a pattern of fetal malformations has been identified, clinical reasoning for possible syndromic diagnosis is essential for planning diagnostic confirmation.

Genetic Counseling in Common Clinical Situations

It is increasingly common situations where the obstetrician is faced with issues related to genetic tests, both screening and diagnostic, in their clinical practice. The ethical principles of any medical–patient relationship take on even greater dimensions in this situation. Given the basic principles of genetic counseling, we report below some clinical situations in obstetrics where these principles are present. The objective here is not to exhaust the topic, but to show the applicability of genetic counseling in these conditions. The interested reader should refer to the specific chapters of each of these clinical entities.

Maternal Age Advanced

It is well established that maternal age correlates with the risk of aneuploidy in the fetus, especially trisomies. Although there is no age that determines no risk to genetic diseases, women aged 35 and over are considered to benefit from genetic counseling, ideally in the preconception period. For these women, information should be provided regarding the potential risks of fetal aneuploidies, the options for noninvasive screening (fetal aneuploidy screening in peripheral blood, ultrasound markers, biochemical screening) as well as invasive diagnostic techniques (chorionic villus biopsy and amniocentesis) [3, 4].

Repeated Pregnancy Losses

One of the etiological causes of repeated pregnancy losses is the existence of a structural chromosomal abnormality in one of the couple's members. Therefore, the history of two or more pregnancy losses, regardless of the gestational age at which they occurred, should alert to this possibility, generating not only the risk of new pregnancy losses but also the birth of children with congenital anomalies [3, 9].

Previous Child with Congenital Anomalies

Preconception genetic counseling is an effective measure for the reproductive planning of any woman or couple. When there is a history of previous pregnancy with fetal anomalies, the genetic counseling before a new gestation is imperative. If the couple has had a previous child with either developmental delay, or intellectual disabilities, or malformations, it is necessary that a previous genetic evaluation of the child affected, before the genetic counseling, due to the possibility of a syndromic diagnosis with a recurrence risk [4].

Couples with a history of stillbirth children or newborns who died after birth with multiple anomalies, without a well-established diagnosis will be benefited by the evaluation of a medical geneticist, in an attempt to define the etiological diagnosis and determine the risk of recurrence. In all situations, at least the couple's chromosomal study will be requested and, depending on the result, other specific tests may be indicated. In some cases, the pedigree, as well photos, X-ray studies, results of necropsies, and other complementary exams may lead to a possible etiological cause [9].

Isolated neural tube defects (anencephaly, meningomyelocele, meningocele, encephalocele) are relatively common and are usually multifactorial, with a risk of recurrence of around 4%. The most well-known risk factor for the occurrence of this anomaly is folic acid deficiency and the risk of recurrence can be reduced to less than 1%, with the woman's periconceptional use. However, it is necessary to remember that neural tube closure defects can be part of several syndromes and, in these cases, the risk of recurrence may be very different depending on the syndrome identified [4].

Isolated congenital heart diseases are also relatively common and may be determined by several mechanisms. However, most of the time, they have a multifactorial etiology. The risk of recurrence will depend on the type of heart disease and family history. It is important to note that heart diseases, as well as any congenital anomaly, can also be part of several syndromes. Therefore, the search for qualified information and the syndromic evaluation of each case is essential for the quality of reproductive counseling [4].

Monitoring the pregnancy of a couple with a previous child with congenital anomaly, counseling, and diagnostic options will depend on the type of anomaly presented and the gestational age of the current pregnancy. However, in all situations, the need for guidance on the benefits and limitations of ultrasonography, the possibilities of using invasive techniques for fetal chromosome studies or molecular biology exams is applied.

Mendelian Diseases in Relatives

There are numerous monogenic diseases and the type of counseling will be based on the data available on the pedigree and on the availability of complementary confirmatory tests. Currently, the use of platforms to identify carriers for recessive diseases (autosomal or X-linked) are quite useful tools in some situations [10, 11].

Exposure to Teratogens

Genetic counseling in an ongoing pregnancy with suspected exposure to a teratogen will depend on the type of teratogen, the stage of exposure, and the type of anomaly induced by the teratogen. For environmental factors that induce major anatomical malformations, guidance on the benefit of ultrasound for investigating fetal injury is relatively simple. However, it is essential that the woman or the couple understands that ultrasound is not a method capable of detecting all anatomical anomalies and is a very limited method for investigating functional anomalies [7].

Prescreening and Postscreening Counseling

The possibilities for noninvasive tests performed during pregnancy are increasing with the development of new techniques. Their aim is to identify the risk for genetic diseases or birth defects in ongoing pregnancies. In general, the pretest counseling may be done by the obstetrician. However, it is essential that the obstetrician know the indications and limitations of each test, including the rates of false positives and false negatives results, and carefully analyze the couple's reproductive risks [12, 13].

The screening tests identify, among all pregnancies, a group whose risk of fetal abnormalities is higher than expected in the general population. An abnormal screening test indicates a risky situation but does not establish a diagnosis. When it is altered, a specific diagnostic test is required. On the other hand, a normal screening test does not rule out the possibility of the disease searched.

In obstetrics, the most used prenatal screening tests are measurements of nuchal translucency and nasal bone, Doppler velocimetry of the venous duct, and the use of maternal blood to investigate fetal aneupolidias or to perform biochemical tests. These tests are directed to screen numerical chromosomal diseases, mainly chromosome 21 trisomy. However, tests for some microarrays chromosomal syndromes are already available through the analysis of free fetal DNA in maternal peripheral blood. In the specific chapters, the reader can consult details of each of these tests. The interested reader may found details of these tests in specific chapters.

As important as the prescreening counseling is the postscreening counseling. It is the opportunity to discuss with the woman or the couple the results of the tests and their meaning. It is also the moment to verify how the couple or woman receive the results and had understood them. Additionally, when the test is positive, it is time to discuss with the couple or the woman the possibilities of confirming the diagnosis and the best way forwarding, respecting the couple's or the woman's concerns [12, 13].

Abnormal Ultrasound Findings

Ultrasonography is an increasingly effective method for assessing fetal anatomy. Several studies have described the association of some detectable changes with ultrasound and some specific chromosomal syndromes, mainly Down's syndrome. These are called "chromosomal markers."

Ultrasonography is also able to identify major structural anomalies, such as hydrocephalus, hydranencephaly, neural tube closure defects, holoprosencephaly, microcephaly, macrocephaly, choroid plexus cysts, Dandy–Walker anomaly, cystic hygromas, various types of heart diseases, hernias diaphragmatic, omphalocele, gastroschisis, bladder and cloaca extrophies, digestive tract atresias, renal agenesis, hydronephrosis, polycystic kidneys, renal cysts, urethral obstructions with megabexiga, among others. It is possible to establish the diagnosis of some skeletal dysplasias or to call the attention for others ones. The same is possible to others osseous anomalies or dysostosis.

When a fetal anomaly is detected, a careful study of the fetal anatomy looking for other anomalies is indicated. In almost all situations, especially when there are multiple malformations, fetal chromosomal study is essential, since chromosomal diseases are associated with the most diverse congenital anomalies. Other genetic or genomic tests such as fluorescence in situ hybridization (FISH), quantitative polymerase chain reaction (qPCR), sequencing specific genes, new generation sequencing (NGS), array comparative genomic hybridization (aCGH), exome sequencing, and even genomic sequencing may be useful in specific situations [4].

Follow-Up of the Pregnancy

Sometimes, even using all the tools available, a certainty diagnosis is not possible. The follow-up of all cases after birth has the diagnosis established, or not, is part of genetic counseling. This monitoring has, as main objectives, to confirm the prenatal diagnosis or expanding the investigation for cases without diagnosis to provide the woman or couple the conclusion of counseling estimating reproductive risks for future pregnancies. Finally, and not least, contribute to the process of acceptance of the child by the parents.

When the birth of a child with a congenital defect or genetic disease occurs, a new stage begins, for the medical geneticist and the team, which is the approach of the family with a child with malformation and the planning of care and monitoring the sick child.

References

1. Human Genetics Society Australasia. Definition of genetic counselling. Disponível em https://www.hgsa.org.au/asgc/definition-of-genetic-counselling. Acessado em 11 de maio de 2020.
2. Resta R, Biesecker BB, Bennett RL, et al. A new definition of genetic counseling: National Society of Genetic Counselors' Task Force Report. J Genet Couns. 2006;2(15):77–83.
3. Gardner RJM, Amor DJ. Gardner and Sutherland's chromosome abnormalities and genetic counseling. 5th ed. New York: Oxford University Press; 2018. 1268p
4. Milunsky A, Milunsky JM. Genetic couseling: preconception, prenatal and perinatal. In: Milunsky A, Mylunsky JM, editors. Genetic disordes and the fetus. Diagnosis, prevention and treatment. 7th ed. New Jersey. USA: EUA; 2015.
5. Than NG, Papp Z. Ethical issues in genetic counseling. Best Pract Res Clin Obstet Gynaecol. 2017;43:32–49.
6. Walters L. Genetics and bioethics: how our thinking has changed since 1969. Theor Med Bioeth. 2012;33(1):83–95.
7. Nussbaum RL, McInnes RR, Willard HF. Thompson & Thompson genetics in medicine. 8th ed. Canada: Elsevier; 2016. 546p
8. O'Brien BM, Dugoff L. What education, background, and credentials are required to provide genetic counseling? Semin Perinatol. 2018;42(5):290–5.
9. Ioannides AS. Preconception and prenatal genetic counselling. Best Pract Res Clin Obstet Gynaecol. 2017;42:2–10.
10. Committee on Genetics. Committee Opinion No. 690: carrier screening in the age of genomic medicine. Obstet Gynecol. 2017;129(3):e35–40.
11. Committee on Genetics. Committee Opinion No. 691: carrier screening for genetic conditions. Obstet Gynecol. 2017;129(3):e41–55.
12. Rink BD, Kuller JA. What are the required components of pre- and post-test counseling? Semin Perinatol. 2018;42(5):287–9.
13. Nelson-Piercy C. Pre-pregnancy counselling. Curr Obstet Gynaecol. 2003;13:273–80.

Chapter 5
Screening for Chromosomal Anomalies

Fabrício da Silva Costa and Conrado Sávio Ragazini

Down syndrome is the most common aneuploidy in humans, occurring in 1 in 1000 to 1 in 1100 live births worldwide [1]. In the USA, the incidence is 1 in 700 born babies [2], which does not account for terminated pregnancies and miscarriages. Prenatal diagnosis of aneuploidies allows the pregnant woman/couple to decide either to terminate pregnancy (in locations where this practice is allowed) or to receive adequate antenatal care and newborn evaluation after birth.

Prenatal diagnosis, however, can only be truly determined by chorionic villus sampling (CVS) or amniocentesis, which are not risk free. Miscarriage rates are lower than previously thought but not absent [3]. This leads to the rationale that diagnostic procedures should only be offered for women who are at a high risk of having a newborn with a chromosomal anomaly. Prenatal screening helps counseling women and couples whether to have or not an invasive procedure, considering their risks and benefits, to allow a timely decision on termination of pregnancy (if allowed) or the correct assistance and follow-up of the child.

Screening for chromosomal anomalies started in 1971 and has evolved since then [4] to many different models: from maternal age alone to fetal cell-free DNA detection in maternal blood. This chapter will cover the most currently used models.

F. da Silva Costa (✉) · C. S. Ragazini
Department of Obstetrics and Gynecology, Ribeirão Preto Medical School – University of São Paulo, Ribeirão Preto, São Paulo, Brazil

© Springer Nature Switzerland AG 2022

R. A. Moreira de Sá, E. B. d. Fonseca (eds.), *Perinatology*,
https://doi.org/10.1007/978-3-030-83434-0_5

Isolated Markers

Maternal Age

As a woman ages, her chances of having an aneuploid fetus raises. Therefore, the first screenings for Down syndrome and other aneuploidies were first done considering maternal age and gestational age, since fetuses with chromosomal anomalies present higher in utero death rates. Considering the age of 35 as the cut-off for a high-risk pregnancy for aneuploidy, and setting a 5% false-positive rate, would yield a detection rate in modern days, when more women are getting pregnant after 35, of 50% of the affected fetuses [5]. It is important to notice that sex chromosome aneuploidies, such as Turner syndrome, do not have this relationship with maternal age.

Biochemical Markers

Many biochemical markers produced by the placenta and/or the fetus found in maternal serum differ in their concentrations between mothers of normal fetuses and aneuploid fetuses. Screening programs using these markers propose comparing such biomarkers levels in maternal serum to the expected levels of mothers with euploid fetuses. The most used are:

- Human Chorionic Gonadotrophin (β-hCG), especially the free β fraction
- Pregnancy-associated plasma protein-A (PAPP-A)
- Placental growth factor (PlGF)
- α-Fetoprotein (AFP)
- Inhibin A
- Unconjugated Estriol (uE3)

The behavior of β-hCG and PAPP-A levels in aneuploid pregnancies is presented in Table 5.1. Dosing the free β-subunit of hCG seems to yield better detection rates than total serum hCG [6], making it the preferred method of dosage.

Table 5.1 Biochemical and sonographic features of trisomies 21, 18, and 13

	Euploid	Trisomy 21	Trisomy 18	Trisomy 13
Median CRL-independent NT, mm	2.0	3.4	5.5	4.0
Median serum free β-hCG, MoM	1.0	2.0	0.2	0.5
Median serum PAPP-A, MoM	1.0	0.5	0.2	0.3
Absent nasal bone, %	2.5	60	53	45
Tricuspid regurgitation, %	1.0	55	33	30
Ductus venosus reversed a-wave, %	3.0	66	58	55

Adapted from Nicolaides [5]

NT nuchal translucency, *CRL* crown-rump length, *β-hCG* β-human chorionic gonadotrophin, *MoM* multiple of the median, *PAPP-A* Pregnancy-associated plasma protein-A

Individual screening performance of each of these biomarkers is low [7–9]. Hence, models using maternal serum biochemistry combine two or more markers to predict the risk of having an aneuploid fetus. They can be used in the first and/or second trimester, but biochemistry, alone, is currently only used in the second trimester in the so-called Quadruple test (see below).

Ultrasonographic Markers

There are many findings on fetal ultrasound evaluation in the first and second trimesters that raise the risks of aneuploidy (and other fetal malformations). The most reliable and used marker is the nuchal translucency (NT), defined as the fluid behind the fetal neck, which should be measured with a crown-rump length (CRL) of 45–84 mm, corresponding to 11–13 + 6 weeks. This timing is selected due to the ultrasound examination capacity at this age to detect early major fetal malformations that may not be associated with chromosomal abnormalities [10], and allow women and couples to choose for a safer termination of pregnancy if so desired.

The drawback of this marker is the need for trained and qualified personnel to perform the exam. Currently, the standards of how to measure are extensively promoted by The Fetal Medicine Foundation who also provides cost-free certification on correct measurement. Figure 5.1 shows a normal and Fig. 5.2 shows an abnormal nuchal translucency. It is important to guarantee the following requirements [11]:

- High magnification of the image, with only the upper thorax and head of the fetus in the picture
- Fetus in a neutral position (in order to avoid over and underestimation of the NT that happen due to flexion and extension of the neck)

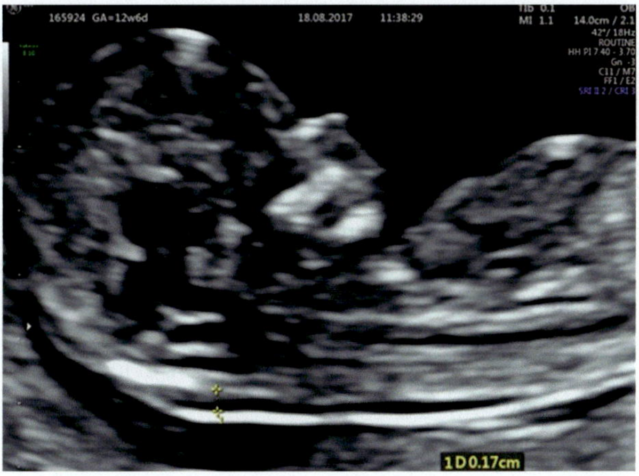

Fig. 5.1 Normal nuchal translucency. (Prof. Fabricio's personal archive)

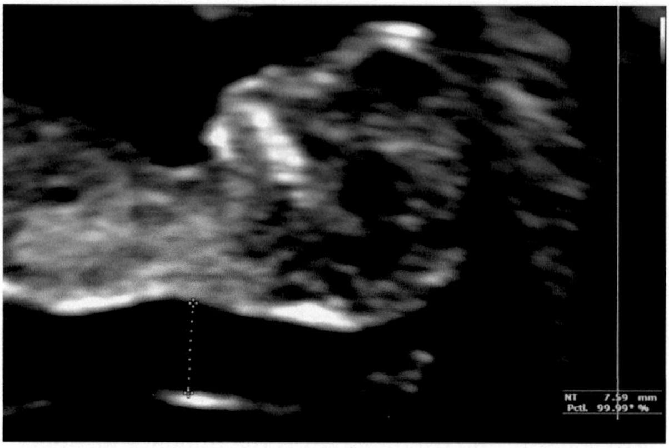

Fig. 5.2 Thickened nuchal translucency. (Prof. Renato de Sá's personal archive)

- The true mid-sagittal section of the fetus must include the echogenic tip of the nose, a rectangular shape of the palate anteriorly (must not contain the zygomatic process), the translucent diencephalon in the center, and the nuchal membrane posteriorly
- Measurement of the maximal thickness of nuchal translucency, with calipers placed *on* the two lines that represent the skin and soft tissue covering the cervical spine

A thickened NT may also be associated with cardiac malformations and genetic syndromes. Its performance as a marker for Down syndrome increases with gestational age (at a 5% false-positive rate, detection rates are 51% at 10 weeks and 62% at 12–13 weeks) [12]. The best performance of this marker is in association with biochemical markers (see below). However, fetuses with cystic hygroma (i.e., with septations in the NT) or very large NTs are already at a very high risk for aneuploidy, and these mothers should be directly offered a diagnostic procedure. The most used cut-off is 3.5 mm [13].

Other frequently cited first trimester markers that elevate the risk of aneuploidy are (Table 5.1):

- Absent nasal bone: nasal bone is considered present if it is seen as an echogenic line within the nasal bridge, brighter than the overlying skin (Fig. 5.3). If it is not visualized, or less echogenic than the skin, it is considered absent [14]. The efficiency of this marker is highly dependent of training [15], and therefore results of its performance vary among studies. Also, ethnicity plays a role, with absent nasal bone in the first trimester being more frequent in euploid fetuses of Afro-Caribbean origin when compared to Caucasians [16]
- Ductus venosus reversed a-wave: fetuses with this finding have a higher risk for aneuploidy [17, 18] and cardiac malformations [19]. As for other sonographic markers, proper training and certification are needed to ensure its usefulness in screening programs. However, there is evidence [18] supporting that adding it to the combined test (see below) increases the detection rates of aneuploidies. A normal image of a ductus venosus positive a-wave is depicted on Fig. 5.4

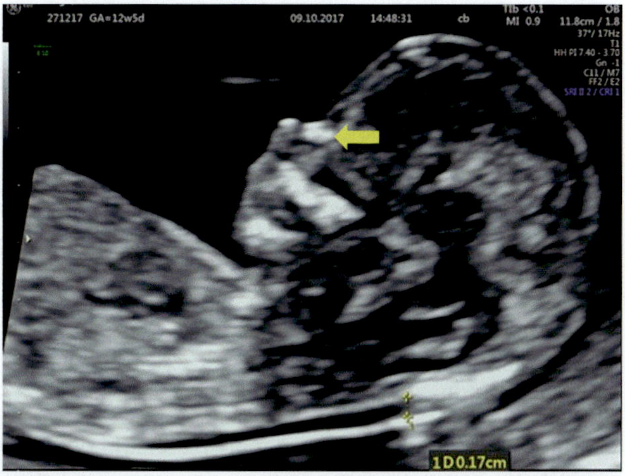

Fig. 5.3 Presence of nasal bone (arrow). (Prof. Fabricio's personal archive)

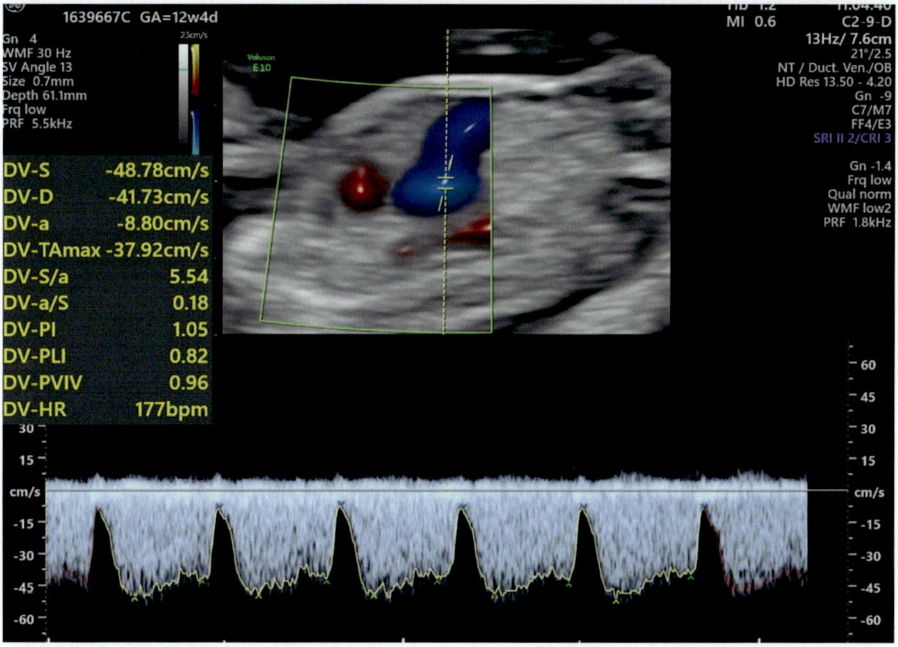

Fig. 5.4 Doppler velocimetry of the ductus venosus on a first-trimester scan. Notice the positive a-wave. Dr. Conrado's personal archive

- Tricuspid regurgitation: as for the ductus venosus, the presence of reflux through tricuspid valve during systole of at least 60 cm/s, is also a marker for aneuploidy [20], as well for cardiac defects [21]. It must, however, be used in addition to other markers in order to improve aneuploidies detection rates [20].

As for the second trimester, there are many findings that, despite having an association with aneuploidy, are also present in a significative amount of euploid fetuses [22]: the so-called soft markers. The most known soft markers are, among others:

- Absent or hypoplastic nasal bone
- Thickened nuchal fold
- Echogenic bowel
- Echogenic intracardiac focus/foci
- Pyelectasis
- Choroid plexus cysts
- Ventriculomegaly
- Short femur or humerus
- Single umbilical artery

One should notice that these markers should not be used in isolation to screen for aneuploidy; however, some of them are more predictive of chromosomal anomalies (e.g., thickened nuchal fold) than others (e.g., short femur) [23]. Finding one soft marker should prompt a thorough ultrasound examination. Managing the finding of a single soft marker depends on which marker has been found and the pregnancy's previous evaluation of aneuploidy risk, which can be recalculated after the scan, based on the findings [23]. Most cases will be reassured and will not need further evaluation. On the other hand, the finding of two or more soft markers should raise suspicion, and genetic counseling and/or diagnostic procedures should be considered [24].

Cell-Free DNA

Cell-free fetal DNA (cffDNA) can be successfully found in maternal plasma in the late first trimester (after 9–10 weeks), deriving mostly from the placenta, in small fragments. Next-generation sequencing technique allows the possibility of *screening* for aneuploidies. Although the test has very good sensitivity and specificity for trisomies 21 and other trisomies [25–27] (Table 5.2), it cannot be considered a diagnostic test because the tested conditions (aneuploidies) have very low prevalence and some biological factors (as confined placental mosaicism) may alter the results. In what concerns sex chromosome aneuploidies, in a recent meta-analysis [26], cffDNA had a detection rate (DR) of 95.8% for Monosomy X at a false-positive rate

Table 5.2 Detection rates and false-positive rates of cell-free DNA screening for common aneuploidies

Condition	Detection rate, %	False-positive rate, %
Trisomy 21	99.7	0.04
Trisomy 18	97.9	0.04
Trisomy 13	99.0	0.04
Monosomy X	95.8	0.14

Adapted from Gil et al. [26]

of 0.14%, whereas for other pooled sex chromosome aneuploidies, DR was 100% at 0.004% FPR.

It is important to consider that studies reporting these high performances have not included test failures. One important factor for test success is called fetal fraction, which is the proportion of cffDNA in the total amount of cell-free DNA in the mother's serum. Most laboratories require 4% of fetal fraction to run the test because a low fetal fraction can lead to a "no result" (i.e., test failure) or a false negative test.

Reasons for a low fetal fraction are maternal weight (with weight increase, plasma and maternal cfDNA also increase, whereas fetal cfDNA remains at a constant amount, leading to a low, diluted fetal fraction), early gestation (prior to 10 weeks, because fetal cfDNA amount is still very low), sample collection (that compromise methodology), and the fetal karyotype itself (trisomies 18, 13, trioploid fetuses have lower fetal fractions than euploid fetuses of the same age; trisomy 21 usually have a fetal fraction that is higher than that of an euploid fetus at the same gestational age).

Cell-free fetal DNA can be used as a single method for screening (i.e., primary screening) or in addition to other screening programs (i.e., secondary screening). Primary screening for all women with cffDNA carries a higher financial burden, and it is also not clear on how to proceed with women who have a test failure. The secondary screening, on the other hand, seems more rational and cost-effective: the so-called contingent model (see below).

Combined Tests

First Trimester Combined Test

This model combines both biochemical and ultrasound markers in the first trimester: free β-hCG, PAPP-A, and NT (associated with maternal age). It leads to a DR of 85% for Down syndrome with 5% of false positives [28, 29]. As discussed in previous sections, adding other sonographic markers can help improve the detection rates.

In places where NT is not available or reliable, combining four biochemical markers (free β-hCG, PAPP-A, PlGF, and AFP) in the first trimester could be an option for screening. This model leads to a DR of 74% (for Down syndrome) at 5% false-positive rate [30]. Another option for these women would be a serum integrated test, i.e., combining results from the first and the second trimesters (see below).

Second Trimester Quadruple Test

This model refers to combining AFP, uE3, β-hCG, and inhibin A in the second trimester. Before ultrasound popularization, this was a very useful tool for screening aneuploidies. Also, this is an available method for patients starting antenatal care on the second trimester. This method allows a 76% DR at 5% FPR for Down syndrome [31].

Integrated Tests

This model combines first and second trimesters markers to assess a fetus' risk for aneuploidy. PAPP-A and NT are measured in the first trimester while AFP, uE3, inhibin A, and β-hCG are measured in the second trimester ("fully integrated test"). This test can achieve 90% DR at 2% FPR [32]. Lowering the FPR is a beneficial result because less women may have a pregnancy loss of an euploid fetus related to a diagnostic procedure.

The drawback of this strategy is that results are obtained only in the second trimester, when it is harder to terminate a pregnancy. One way of (partially) solving this problem is to run the first-trimester measurements and offer a diagnostic procedure (CVS) for women considered at high-risk for aneuploidy. If the woman is not considered as so, she would not receive her results until completion of the second-trimester measurements.

Another approach of integrated tests is when NT is not available: to combine first and second trimesters biochemical markers. This is the second most-efficient method after the "fully integrated test."

Contingent Tests

In this setting, women are screened with usual tests (i.e., combined test) and those considered at high-risk are offered an invasive diagnostic test (they may have a cffDNA if they do not wish an invasive test upfront); low-risk women are reassured; and those considered to be at intermediate-risk for aneuploidies are offered the cffDNA test.

Cut-offs vary but the main idea is to not offer a costly screening procedure to every woman but also reduce the rates of invasive procedures.

References

1. United Nations: https://www.un.org/en/events/downsyndromeday/background.shtml
2. Mai CT, et al. National population-based estimates for major birth defects, 2010–2014. Birth Defects Res. 2019:1–16.
3. Akolekar R, et al. Procedure-related risk of miscarriage following amniocentesis and chorionic villus sampling: a systematic review and meta-analysis. Ultrasound Obstet Gynecol. 2015;45:16–26.
4. Renshaw R, et al. Antenatal screening for Down syndrome: a quantitative demonstration of the improvements over the past 20 years. J Health Serv Res Policy. 2013;18(4):195–201.
5. Nicolaides KH. Screening for aneuploidies at 11 to 13 weeks. Prenat Diagn. 2011;31:7–15.
6. Evans MI, et al. Meta-analysis of first trimester Down syndrome screening studies: free β-human chorionic gonadotropin significantly outperforms intact human chorionic gonadotropin in a multimarker protocol. Am J Obstet Gynecol. 2007;196(3):198–205.

7. Noble PL, et al. Maternal serum inhibin-A and free beta-hCG concentrations in trisomy 21 pregnancies at 10 to 14 weeks of gestation. Br J Obstet Gynaecol. 1997;104(3):367–71.
8. Brizot ML, et al. First trimester maternal serum alpha-fetoprotein in fetal trisomies. Br J Obstet Gynaecol. 1995;102(1):31–4.
9. Wright D, et al. First-trimester screening for trisomies 21, 18 and 13 by ultrasound and biochemical testing. Fetal Diagn Ther. 2014;35(2):118–26.
10. Souka AP, et al. Assessment of fetal anatomy at the 11-13-week ultrasound examination. Ultrasound Obstet Gynecol. 2004;24:730–4.
11. Nicolaides KH. The 11–13+6 weeks scan. London: Fetal Medicine Foundation; 2014.
12. Wald NJ, et al. SURUSS in perspective. BJOG. 2004;111:521.
13. Wright D, et al. A mixture model of nuchal translucency thickness in screening for chromosomal defects. Ultrasound Obstet Gynecol. 2008;31:376–83.
14. Sonek JD. Nasal bone evaluation with ultrasonography: a marker for fetal aneuploidy. Ultrasound Obstet Gynecol. 2003;22:11.
15. Cicero S, et al. Learning curve for sonographic examination of the fetal nasal bone at 11-14 weeks. Ultrasound Obstet Gynecol. 2003;22:135.
16. Cicero S, et al. Likelihood ratio for trisomy 21 in fetuses with absent nasal bone at the 11-14-week scan. Ultrasound Obstet Gynecol. 2004;23:218.
17. Mavrides E, et al. Screening for aneuploidy in the first trimester by assessment of blood flow in the ductus venosus. BJOG. 2002;109:1015.
18. Maiz N, et al. Ductus venosus Doppler in screening for trisomies 21, 18 and 13 and Turner syndrome at 11-13 weeks of gestation. Ultrasound Obstet Gynecol. 2009;33:512.
19. Maiz N, Plasencia W, Dagklis T, et al. Ductus venosus Doppler in fetuses with cardiac defects and increased nuchal translucency thickness. Ultrasound Obstet Gynecol. 2008;31:256.
20. Kagan KO, et al. Tricuspid regurgitation in screening for trisomies 21, 18 and 13 and Turner syndrome at 11 + 0 to 13 + 6 weeks of gestation. Ultrasound Obstet Gynecol. 2009;33:18–22.
21. Scala C, et al. Fetal tricuspid regurgitation in the first trimester as a screening marker for congenital heart defects: systematic review and meta-analysis. Fetal Diagn Ther. 2017;42:1–8.
22. Breathnach FM, et al. The second trimester genetic sonogram. Am J Med Genet Part C Semin Med Genet. 2006;145C:62–72.
23. Agathokleous M, et al. Meta-analysis of second-trimester markers for trisomy 21. Ultrasound Obstet Gynecol. 2013;41:247–61.
24. The American College of Obstetricians and Gynecologists. Practice Bulletin number 163 - screening for fetal aneuploidy. Obstet Gynecol. 2016;127:e123–37.
25. Mackie FL, et al. The accuracy of cell-free fetal DNA-based non-invasive prenatal testing in singleton pregnancies: a systematic review and bivariate meta-analysis. BJOG. 2017;124(1):32–46.
26. Gil MM, et al. Analysis of cell-free DNA in maternal blood in screening for aneuploidies: updated meta-analysis. Ultrasound Obstet Gynecol. 2017;50:302–14.
27. Taylor-Phillips S, et al. Accuracy of non-invasive prenatal testing using cell-free DNA for detection of Down, Edwards and Patau syndromes: a systematic review and meta-analysis. BMJ Open. 2016;6(1):e010002.
28. Nicolaides KH. Nuchal translucency and other first-trimester sonographic markers of chromosomal abnormalities. Am J Obstet Gynecol. 2004;191:45e67.
29. Veduta A, et al. The first trimester combined test for aneuploidies – a single center experience. J Matern Fetal Neonatal Med. 2017;31(16):2091–6.
30. Johnson J, et al. First-trimester Down syndrome screening using additional serum markers with and without nuchal translucency and cell-free DNA. Prenat Diagn. 2013;33:1044–9.
31. Wald NJ, et al. Antenatal screening for Down's syndrome. J Med Screen. 1997;4:181–246.
32. Wald NJ, et al. First and second trimester antenatal screening for Down's syndrome: the results of the Serum, Urine and Ultrasound Screening Study (SURUSS). Health Technol Assess. 2003;7(11):1.

Chapter 6
Protocol of Immunization of the Adult Woman

Julio Cesar Teixeira

Immunization is one of the low-cost measures with the greatest impact on preventing diseases and deaths [1]. Successes of immunization programs include the worldwide eradication of smallpox, polio control with a likelihood of eradication, and elimination of rubella in indigenous people in the United States [2, 3]. Immunization is the artificial process of inducing or promoting immunity, administering substances with immunobiological effects to protect the body from disease. Immunization can actively induce protection, that is, the body is stimulated to produce protective antibodies as occurs in vaccination. Or the immunization can be passive, where the body receives the effective antibodies, the immunoglobulins, as happens naturally in the antibody transference process from the mother to the fetus or newborn through transplacental or breastfeeding, or even artificially through immunoglobulin administration [4].

Vaccines are pharmaceutical products that contain one or more immunizing agents in various biological forms, such as live attenuated bacteria or viruses, inactivated viruses or dead bacteria, or purified and/or modified components of disease-causing substances, such as toxoids.

Access to vaccines is variable and, in general, the main ones are offered or subsidized by public care systems. You can take the opportunity to vaccinate and use more than one different vaccine at the same time. In this case, it is known that inactivated vaccines do not interfere with the immune system's response to other inactivated or live vaccines [5]. That is, an inactivated vaccine can be administered simultaneously or at any time before or after the application of another inactivated or live vaccine. In contrast, the administration of two different live

J. C. Teixeira (✉)
Department of Gynecology and Obstetrics, Faculty of Medical Sciences, University of Campinas (UNICAMP), Campinas, SP, Brazil
e-mail: juliotex@unicamp.br

© Springer Nature Switzerland AG 2022

R. A. Moreira de Sá, E. B. d. Fonseca (eds.), *Perinatology*,
https://doi.org/10.1007/978-3-030-83434-0_6

vaccines with a short interval between them can inhibit the immune response to the second vaccine [6]. Thus, it is recommended that different live vaccines be administered on the same day or after an interval of 4 weeks [5]. Examples are the oral vaccine against polio, measles, mumps, rubella, chickenpox, and yellow fever. The agent remains alive and multiplies in the host causing an infection like the disease which results in great protective capacity with just one dose and long-term immunity, possibly for life. The repetition of doses aims to cover any failures of the previous vaccination.

Routinely, the administration of two or more live vaccines at the same time is widely used and should preferably be carried out in different points, such as in different arms, or in the same arm, but with 3 cm between the injection sites [7]. Pregnant women and individuals with immunosuppression are contraindicated for a vaccination with live attenuated agents [8].

Passive artificial immunization through the administration of immunoglobulins provides faster protection. Heterologous immunoglobulins are antibodies obtained from the plasma of animals, in general horses, previously vaccinated, and the homologous immunoglobulins are antibodies obtained from the plasma of humans. Immunoglobulins against rabies, chickenpox, measles, tetanus, and hepatitis B are available for application. The protection obtained is maintained for about 3–6 months and should, in general, be administered in a hospital environment. Immunoglobulins do not affect the function of inactivated vaccines. However, vaccines with live and attenuated components must be postponed after the application of immunoglobulins, since immunoglobulins also inactivate these vaccine agents [9, 10].

A susceptible nonvaccinated individual exposed to an infectious agent the appropriate conduct needs to consider the incubation time of the agent. If the disease incubation time is short, immunoglobulins should be used because there will be not time enough for antibody formation. However, when the disease incubation time is longer than the time necessary for an adequate immune response to occur with antibody production, a postexposure vaccination can be employed, rather than the administration of immunoglobulins, a strategy used in cases of hepatitis A and B, chickenpox, and measles [9, 10].

Vaccination of Women at Reproductive Age

For the women health care assistance is essential that the health professional investigates the vaccination history, incomplete vaccination schedules, and the possibility of no seroconversion, even if a vaccination schedule compliance was achieved. The role of the health professional is to prescribe the necessary vaccine boosters and insert women for new vaccines in the programs. Thus, the woman's vaccination protocols will serve as a parameter for the health professional to define what vaccines are necessary according to the vaccination history and past infections, personalizing the prescription [4, 11].

Every effort should be made to ensure that the woman adheres to the vaccination schedule. However, when the vaccination schedule is incomplete, it is not necessary to restart it, even though the previous dose was a long time ago. The scheme should be continued with missing doses, that is, doses received will always be valid doses. When a woman does not present a valid document to prove previous vaccination, she must be considered as unvaccinated and advised to vaccinate with all the vaccines indicated for her age and situation [4, 12].

It is also recommended to ask about the intention to be pregnant, as the woman's immunization impacts on maternity planning, besides add individual protection.

The pregnant woman's own susceptibility to infectious conditions with worse evolution, as well as the maternal antibody's ability to offer neonatal protection, through its transplacental transfer, makes pregnancy a unique moment in which vaccination practice must be guaranteed [13]. Immunization of pregnant women plays a significant role in improving maternal and neonatal health protecting against various infectious diseases.

Maternal immunization is particularly important when considering diseases preventable by vaccination, for which there are no options for protecting babies in the first year of life [13, 14]. Primary immunization of infants is not complete before 6 months of life, in the vast majority of developed and developing countries, and after 14 months of life, in most underdeveloped countries [15].

In the context of vulnerability to infections of pregnant women and infants in the first months of life when the basic vaccination scheme cannot be completed yet, the maternal vaccination becomes a measure extremely important to promote child health. Maternal IgG antibodies cross the placenta and provide passive protection to the child up to approximately 15 months of life [16]. These antibodies are also transmitted through breastfeeding. A current example is the use of immunization of pregnant women against influenza and pertussis with significant impacts on the prevention of serious cases and death of newborns in the first months of life.

In this way, WHO in 2013 called for the development of a vaccine to be applied to pregnant women and prevent infant infection by the respiratory syncytial virus (RSV) and its complications in the first months of life. There are currently three vaccines in advanced stage of development, some starting phase 3 study, with the promise of possible licensing from 2021 [17, 18].

The adult woman's immunization protocols related to perinatal outcomes should consider two moments, a preconceptual orientation and during pregnancy or the puerperium. The basic protocol is shown in Table 6.1 and, below, there are some comments for each period.

Table 6.1 Vaccines recommended for adult women in the periconceptional period

Vaccine	Schedule	Previous doses	Actions	During pregnancy
Measles, Mumps and Rubella (MMR)	2 doses (interval > 30 days) Subcutaneous	0 or 1	To complete	Contraindicated
		2	Vaccinated	
Hepatitis A	2 doses (0–6 months) Intramuscular	0 or 1	To complete	Without theoretical risk Prefer to vaccinate out of pregnancy
		2	Vaccinated	
Hepatitis B	3 doses (0–1–6 months) Intramuscular	0, 1, or 2	To complete	Indicated
		3	Vaccinated	
	Immunity can be confirmed 30–60 days after the third dose with anti-HBs >10 mUnit/mL			
Hepatitis A and B	3 doses (0–1–6 months) Intramuscular	0, 1 or 2	To complete	See Hepatitis A
		3	Vaccinated	
Influenza	Annual dose (Protection after 2 weeks) Intramuscular		Annual dose	Recommended for each pregnancy
Diphtheria-tetanus-pertussis (dTpa)	3 doses (0–2–6 months) Booster each 10 years Intramuscular	Vaccinated (3 doses)	Booster with dTpa each 10 years	dTpa: 1 dose after gestational age 20 weeks to each pregnancy for immunization of the infant against pertussis
		Incomplete 0, 1, or 2	1 dose of dTpa and to complete with dT	To complete (30–60 days for doses interval; the last being up to 20 days before delivery) Attention: at least 1 dose should be dTpa, applied after 20 weeks to immunize the infant and, if necessary, complete with dT. For those not vaccinated: 1 dose of dTpa up to 45 days postpartum.
Varicella or chickenpox (if no previous history)	2 doses (interval 1–3 months) Subcutaneous	0 or 1	To complete	Contraindicated
		2	Vaccinated	
Meningococcal (C) *(in special situations)*	1 dose Intramuscular	0	1 dose	Indicated only in situations of epidemic risk
		Consider a booster every 5 years in immunocompromised and asplenic		

Table 6.1 (continued)

Vaccine	Schedule	Previous doses	Actions	During pregnancy
Meningococcal (ACWY) *(in special situations)*	1 dose 1 booster after 5 years Intramuscular	0	1 dose and 1 booster	Indicated only in situations of epidemic risk
		Consider 1 dose (booster) if more than 5 years of type C previous vaccination		
Yellow fever *(in special situations)*	1 dose (protection in 7–10 days) Intramuscular	0	1 dose	Contraindicated (Possible to use for unvaccinated in a high-risk and urgent situation. Do not breastfeed for 15 days)
		1	Vaccinated	

Preconceptional Counseling

Assessing the immunization of adult women during preconception counseling, it is important to check and update the vaccination, including boosters, particularly those vaccines that have a contraindication to be used during pregnancy. The goal is that the woman achieves a pregnancy status immunized. Vaccination of women is highly efficient in reducing the risk of congenital diseases due to infections, such as rubella, and in preventing the vertical transmission of infectious agents during labor and delivery, such as the hepatitis virus B. In addition, immunized women with circulating antibody levels can promote transplacental antibody transfer during pregnancy. This transference has a peak in the last 4–6 weeks of pregnancy and results in the protection of the newborn during the first year of life against diseases, such as influenza, whooping cough, hepatitis virus A, tetanus, yellow fever, among others.

In this situation, the vaccines considered essential are against rubella, hepatitis A and B, influenza, diphtheria, tetanus, and whooping cough. Attention: Regarding live attenuated virus vaccines (e.g., measles, mumps, and rubella(MMR) vaccine) for women planning to become pregnant, if the vaccination schedule is unknown or not performed, vaccination is recommended and the woman is advised to avoid pregnancy for 30 days.

Vaccination During Pregnancy and the Puerperium

After conception and during pregnancy, the goal of vaccination is to avoid diseases that reach greater severity when they occur in pregnant women, such as influenza, to prevent vertical transmission, such as Hepatitis B, and not least, to transfer antibodies to the newborn to gain protection in the first months of life, and until your own vaccination starts to work. Nowadays, the importance of vaccination against influenza, tetanus, and pertussis stands out. Thus, the basic vaccination protocol during pregnancy consists of the vaccines against influenza, hepatitis B, and the diphtheria-tetanus-pertussis vaccine (Table 6.1).

Other vaccines that can be used during pregnancy, but only in special situations, are the meningococcal vaccine and, in specific cases, the yellow fever vaccine.

In pregnancy, the risk of fetal abnormalities resulting from maternal vaccination is considered theoretical. Thus, there is no scientific evidence of risks to the pregnant woman or fetus after vaccination with inactivated viruses, bacterial vaccines, or toxoids [19]. On the other hand, live vaccines have a theoretical risk to the fetus and should be avoided during pregnancy.

Other Immunizations in Pregnant Women

Inactivated polio vaccine is indicated prior to travel to endemic areas and rabies vaccine is mandatory in case of exposure.

Use of Immunoglobulins

Chickenpox or varicella and pregnancy: unvaccinated pregnant women with no previous history of varicella are considered susceptible. In this case, after a chickenpox contact, the prevention should be achieved after the use of varicella-zoster immune globulin (VZIG). When performed within 10 days after the contact, it is possible to avoid or attenuate the clinical form of chickenpox in susceptible pregnant women [20]. VZIG is supplied in vials containing 125 units per vial and the recommended dose is 125 units per 10 kg body weight, up to a maximum dosage of 625 units [21]. For newborns, VZIG is indicated in the following situations [20, 21]:

- Term infant whose mother had chickenpox in the last 5 days prior to delivery or for up to 48 hours after delivery
- A preterm infant with gestational age 28 weeks or more whose mother did not have chickenpox
- A preterm infant with gestational age under 28 weeks or weighing less than 1000 grams at birth, regardless of maternal history of chickenpox

Hepatitis B and pregnant women: susceptible pregnant women who had contact with the hepatitis B virus (HBV) should receive Hepatitis B Immune Globulins (HBIG). In pregnant women with hepatitis B (HBsAg test positive), the prevention of vertical transmission to newborns must be done through vaccination and use of HBIG 0.5 mL, preferably in the first 12 hours after birth and, at most, within 7 days, applied to different muscle [22, 23]. Since 2018, there is a recommendation to add maternal antiviral therapy (lamivudine, telbivudine, and tenofovir) for a selected pregnant woman (HBV DNA is >200,000 IU/mL) and started at 28–32 weeks' gestation for the prevention of perinatal HBV transmission [24].

Puerperium

In the puerperal period, all vaccines except for the yellow fever vaccine can be administered to women, without restriction. The yellow fever vaccine can be administered to lactating women when the benefit is greater than the risk, but with the suspension of lactation for 10 days if the newborn age is less than 6 months [25, 26].

To conclude, it is recommended to take Table 6.1 for general guidance regarding the vaccines indicated for women in the periconceptional period.

References

1. Maciosek MV, Coffield AB, Edwards NM, et al. Priorities among effective clinical preventive services: results of a systematic review and analysis. Am J Prev Med. 2006;31:52–61.
2. Orenstein WA, Papania MJ, Wharton ME. Measles elimination in the United Estates. J Infect Dis. 2004;189(suppl 1):S1–3.
3. Centers for Disease Control and Prevention. Achievements in public health: elimination of rubella and congenital rubella syndrome— the United States, 1969–2004. MMWR. 2005;54:279–82.
4. Ballalai I. Conceitos básicos em imunizações. Manual Prático de Imunizações. Isabella Ballalai. - 1ª ed – Sao Paulo: AC Farmaceutica; 2013.
5. Centers for Disease Control and Prevention General Recommendations on Immunization: Recommendations of the Advisory Committee on Immunization Practice (ACIP). MMWR. 2006;55.
6. Petralli JK, Merigan TC, Wilbur JR. Action of endogenous interferon against vaccinia infection in children. Lancet. 1965;2:401–5.
7. Bergeson PS. Immunization in the deltoid region. Pediatrics. 1990;85:134–5.
8. American Academy of Pediatrics. Immunization in special clinical circumstances. In: Pickering LK, Baker CJ, Long SS, McMillan J, editors. Red book: 2006 report of the committee on infectious diseases. 27th ed. Elk Grove Village: American Academy of Pediatrics; 2006. p. 67–103.
9. American Academy of Pediatrics. Active and passive immunization. In: Pickering LK, et al., editors. Red book: report of the committee on infection diseases. 29th ed. Elk Grove Village: American Academy of Pediatrics; 2012. p. 1–110.
10. Plotkin SA, Orestein W, Offit PA, editors. Vaccines. 6th ed. Philadelphia: Elsevier; 2013.
11. FEBRASGO. Manual de Vacinação da Mulher. 1st ed. Neves NA; 2013.
12. Teixeira JC, Roteli-Martins CM, Ballalai I, Kfouri RA. Calendario de vacinação da mulher: recomendações FEBRASGO. In: Programa vacinal para mulheres. ed rev atual. Sao Paulo: Federação Brasileira das Associações de Ginecologia e Obstetricia; 2019. Cap. 3. p. 22–5.
13. Englund JAMI, Hammill H. Maternal immunization with influenza or tetanus toxoid vaccine for passive antibody protection in young infants. JID. 1993;168:647–56.
14. Edwards KM. Overview of pertussis: focus on epidemiology, sources of infection, and long term protection after infant vaccination. Pediatr Infect Dis J. 2005;24(6 Suppl):S104–8.
15. Omer SB. Maternal Immunization. N Engl J Med. 2017;376(13):1256–67.
16. Robinson DP, Klein SL. Pregnancy and pregnancy-associated hormones alter imune responses and disease pathogenesis. Horm Behav. 2012;62:263–71.
17. Higgins D, Trujillo C, Keech C. Advances in RSV vaccine research and development - a global agenda. Vaccine. 2016;34(26):2870–5.
18. Innis B, Khan S. Readying the world for maternal RSV vaccine. Gavi, The Vaccine Alliance. 18 January 2019. Available in: https://www.gavi.org/vaccineswork/readying-the-world-for-maternal-rsv-vaccine. Accessed: 20 Jan 2020.

19. Koren G, Pastuszak A, Ito S. Drugs in pregnancy. N Engl J Med. 1998;338:1128–37.
20. Brasil. Ministério da Saúde. Secretaria de Vigilância em Saúde. Departamento de Vigilância Epidemiológica. Manual dos centros de referência para imunobiológicos especiais (CRIEs) / Ministério da Saúde. 2006.
21. Marin M, Bialek SR, Seward JF. Updated recommendations for use of VariZIG - the United States, 2013. MMWR. 2013;62(28):574–6.
22. Sangkomkamhang US, Lumbiganon P, Laopaiboon M. Hepatitis B vaccination during pregnancy for preventing infant infection. Cochrane Database Syst Rev. In: The Cochrane Library. 2011;(4)
23. Komatsu H. Hepatitis B virus: where do we stand and what is the next step for eradication? World J Gastroenterol. 2014;20(27):8998–9016.
24. Schillie S, Vellozzi C, Reingold A, Harris A, Haber P, Ward JW, Nelson NP. Prevention of hepatitis B virus infection in the United States: recommendations of the advisory committee on immunization practices. MMWR. 2018;67(1):1–31.
25. Brasil. Programa Nacional de Imunizações. Available in: http://portalarquivos.saude.gov.br/images/pdf/2016/janeiro/14/Nota-Informativa-143-Febre-Amarela-Site-A-a-Z.pdf. Accessed: 20 Jan 2020.
26. WHO. Vaccines and vaccination against yellow fever WHO Position Paper – June 2013. Wkly Epidemiol Rec. 2013;88(27):269–84.

Chapter 7
Drugs in Pregnancy and Childbirth

Fernando Barbosa Peixoto, Eduardo Carvalho de Arruda Veiga, and Ricardo Carvalho Cavalli

Introduction

The drugs that are able to cross the placental barrier use different transport mechanisms which may depend or not depend on energy and on the physical and chemical properties of the agents themselves. In general, the common crossing mechanisms are based on endocytosis, active transport, facilitated diffusion, and simple diffusion. Extra-individual differences may occur in all cases, stimulated by genetic factors and by maternal health [1].

As pregnancy progresses, the placenta suffers a series of changes in structure and functionality, becoming increasingly finer. The ratio of cytotrophoblasts to syncythiotrophoblasts is reduced, with a consequent reduction of the thickness of the membrane, which becomes increasingly less continuous close to term, with greater chances of maternal-fetal exchanges, including drug exchanges. In general, the teratogenic risk increases starting from the second trimester of pregnancy [1].

Concern about the level of medicalization during pregnancy is basically due to the profile of metabolic exchanges in the mother-fetus binomium and to the often poorly understood potential teratogenic risk of certain drugs. However, there are countless situations in which pregnant women must use medications either owing to

F. B. Peixoto · E. C. de Arruda Veiga
Department of Obstetrics and Gynecology, Ribeirão Preto Medical School, University of São Paulo, São Paulo, SP, Brazil
e-mail: fernandopeixotonutricao@gmai.com; eduardo.veiga@fm.usp.br

R. C. Cavalli (✉)
Department of Obstetrics and Gynecology, Ribeirão Preto Medical School, University of São Paulo, São Paulo, SP, Brazil

Department of Obstetrics and Gynecology, Hospital das Clínicas, Faculty of Medicine, University of São Paulo, FMUSP, São Paulo, SP, Brazil
e-mail: rcavalli@fmrp.usp.br

© Springer Nature Switzerland AG 2022

R. A. Moreira de Sá, E. B. d. Fonseca (eds.), *Perinatology*,
https://doi.org/10.1007/978-3-030-83434-0_7

diseases preceding pregnancy or to complications occurring during the course of gestation. On this basis, it is necessary to study and control in depth the therapeutic alternatives in order to prevent or to minimize as much as possible any likely harmful effects on the fetus and consequently on the newborn.

The prevalence of women who use some type of medication during pregnancy may vary from 50% to 97% [2–4] between developed and developing countries, mainly occurring among pregnant women older than 29 years, with more than 11 years of schooling, who are married and who attend more than three prenatal visits, who have access to private health services and who have some health problem. About one-third of all pregnant women use at least one medication with unknown risks for the fetus, 6.5% used medications known to be teratogenic, and almost 30% use medication with suspected effects [2–4].

To facilitate the clinical and pharmacological conduct in this phase of life, in 1979 the Food and Drug Administration (FDA) [5] created a risk classification in the US based on categories A, B, C, D, and X for the prescription of medications to pregnant women. Category A represents the medications that did not show risks for the fetus at any time during gestation in controlled studies on pregnant women. Category B represents medications that were not studied in pregnant women but that did not pose risks to the fetus in animal studies, or that showed adverse effects on animal reproduction but not in studies on human beings. Category C represents medications that were not studied in animals or humans, or that showed a potential risk to the fetus when assayed in animals. Category D represents medications with positive evidence of risks to the fetus, although their benefits may be greater than the adverse effects on the fetus. Also category X includes medications with proven risks that exceed the benefits of the medication, thus being fully contraindicated [6].

However, this FDA classification of risk according to the category was discontinued after various criticisms regarding the difficulty in assessing the cost-benefit of each medication and the potential of creating doubts or misinterpretations. A new methodology was reformulated in 2014 with changes in the pregnancy and lactation sections and with the insertion of a new section on fertility. All medications will have to be brought up to date with the new description by June 2020 regarding the new information for indication in the leaflet [5].

Drug Teratogenesis During Pregnancy

Teratogenicity corresponds to the power of affecting any stage of embryo or fetal development through the maternal route, thus inducing irreversible changes. In general, a teratogen causes structural changes and may represent any chemical, physical, or biological agent that will act directly on the offspring by placental exchange, as is the case, for example, for medications [7].

In order to determine the teratogenicity of a drug, Shepard et al. [8] suggested a basic structure which is useful and which should still be considered today even though the entire proposal is not contemplated in some cases. According to Shepard et al. (1994), there are six fundamental points for determining when a drug is teratogenic:

1. A structural change, or anomaly, should be fully characterized so that its cause may be differentiated from genetic and environmental factors.
2. The substance responsible for teratogenicity should cross the placenta in a significant manner, i.e., its diffusion should be sufficient to cause any embryonic or fetal changes.
3. Exposure should occur within a critical phase of development, i.e., during the preímplantation period, during the embryonic period, or during the fetal phase.
4. There should be a plausible biological explanation supporting the hypothesis of teratogenicity.
5. Two consistent epidemiological reasons should exist, with two or more well-designed studies showing similar results, and a relative risk of at least 3.0 is proposed in order to strengthen the hypothesis.
6. The probable teratogen should cause anomalies in studies of animal reproduction.

It is fundamental to clearly consider these criteria when determining the possible teratogenic potential of drugs in order to avoid faulty conclusions about these medications, thus preventing unnecessary therapeutic gaps during pregnancy.

The Use of Drugs During Pregnancy

In view of the high prevalence of chronic pregestational conditions, the use of medication is often necessary during pregnancy. Furthermore, the physiology of pregnancy itself leads women to seek pharmacological alternatives for the relief of some conditions.

Gastrointestinal Symptoms

Various clinical complications affect the gastrointestinal system during pregnancy, such as nausea, vomiting, hyperemesis, gastroesophageal reflux, intestinal constipation, and diarrhea. These are all situations that cause discomfort for pregnant women, leading them to look for medicalization for symptom relief [9].

Antiemetics

Antiemetic drugs should be used with caution during pregnancy and only after 12–14 weeks of gestation. Among the best-known drugs are the phenothiazines, histamine receptor blockers, and dopamine antagonists. Among them, the phenothiazines have a greater fetotoxic potential since they are able to cross the placenta. Studies have suggested a higher incidence of congenital heart defects when dopamine antagonists are administered during the first trimester of gestation. However, metoclopramide is indicated for the treatment of vomiting and nausea in pregnant women since, even though it crosses the placenta, it has not been reported to have teratogenic effects in studies on animals and human beings [10, 11].

Thiamine, vitamins B1 and B6, and pyridoxin supplements are indicated for patients with nausea and vomiting and have proved to be effective against the symptoms and safe from a teratogenic viewpoint. Histamine receptor blockers, with no known adverse effects, are considered to be first-line drugs for the treatment of nausea and vomiting during pregnancy [10, 12].

Antacids

Antacids are the agents most extensively indicated for the treatment of gastroesophageal reflux (GR) since their action is considered to be nonsystemic and rapidly effective for symptom relief. Antacids consisting of calcium, magnesium, and aluminum are considered to be safe at traditional doses. In contrast, magnesium trisilicate compounds have been shown to cause cardiovascular involvement, hypotonia, and nephrolithiasis when administered at high doses for long periods of time [11, 13]. Sodium bicarbonate should be avoided since it may induce metabolic alkalosis in both pregnant women and their offspring [13].

Histamine receptor antagonists such as cimetidine and ranitidine have been long used as antacids for pregnant women and are considered to be effective and safe during gestation. And proton pump inhibitors are used as the most common pharmacological treatment of GR in pregnant women. Omeprazole, however, is still classified as a category C agent by the FDA due to its fetal mortality effects in rats and rabbits, even though it has not shown any teratogenic effect in assays on humans. Its use is limited to the treatment of GR with complications that do not respond to other therapies. Lansoprazole is the preferred drug for the treatment of GR [11, 13].

Laxative Agents

Another quite common condition during gestation is intestinal constipation, which is the second major gastrointestinal complaint of pregnant women. When behavioral changes are not effective for treatment, usually mass forming agents are preferred. Owing to their characteristics of local absorption, they are safe for pregnant women and can be used for long periods of time. However, their effects are not rapid, so that they may not be efficient for immediate symptom relief [14].

Osmotic drugs such as lactulose and glycols and stimulating drugs such as sennosides and bisacodyl, even though they do not show extensive systemic absorption, are classified as category C of the FDA and should be used with caution and for short periods because of the risk of diarrhea, abdominal pain, and electrolyte disorders [14, 15].

For this category of gastrointestinal complications, there are medications classified as category X by the FDA, i.e., drugs that are contraindicated for pregnant women. Among them are mineral oil, castor bean oil, and hyperosmotic saline agents. Mineral oil is associated with lower absorption of liposoluble vitamins and the consequen risk of hemorrhage. Castor bean oil induces premature uterine contractions and hyperosmotic agents promote fluid retention, thus also being contraindicated [15, 16].

Antidiarrheic Agents and Antibiotics

With a much lower prevalence among pregnant women compared to other gastrointestinal symptoms, diarrhea is usually caused by bacterial infections and by protozoa. When it is really necessary to stop diarrhea, loperamide is considered for treatment, although it was moved from Category B to Category C of the FDA after some studies reported a higher incidence of hypospadias, cesarean sections, and offspring of high gestational age [17].

Agents such as diphenoxylate with atropine and bismuth subsalicylates are contraindicated for pregnant women because of their teratogenic potential. Many antibiotics used for the treatment of infectious diarrheas are also contraindicated during the entire pregnancy or some parts of it, as is the case for quinolones, tetracyclins, sulfa preparations, and metronidazole. Under conditions of severe diarrhea with the necessity to use antibiotic therapy, erythromycin and ampicillin should be considered [18]. Cholestyramine, often used as an antidiarrheic agent for irritable bowel syndrome, is also contraindicated during pregnancy owing to its potential impairment of the absorption of liposoluble vitamins [19].

Hypoglycemic Agents

The teratogenicity of oral hypoglycemic agents has not been fully clarified, although some data have suggested that abnormal levels of circulating glucose are associated with a higher incidence of congenital abnormaities. In addition, the reduced glucose levels that characterize severe hypoglycemia have been detected in neonates born to mothers who had used hypoglycemic agents close to delivery [20].

Both regarding drugs of the biguanide class, such as metformin, and the sulfonylurea class, such as glyburide, there still is scarce evidence for a safe use of these medications during pregnancy, since these drugs cross the placenta, with fetal exposure remaining significant even with e-flux mechanisms. More recent studies of the offspring of women who had used metformin during pregnancy have suggested a possible effect of fetal programming for greater fat absorption and obesity among the offspring [20, 21].

Oral hypoglycemic drugs should be prescribed to pregnant women in cases in which their therapeutic effects would be more beneficial than the possible teratogenic complications they might cause. The preferential pharmacological treatment of diabetes during pregnancy, recommended by most professional classes, continues to be insulin therapy, for which no potential for placental diffusion has been demonstrated [20].

Antihypertensive Agents

Systemic arterial hypertension (SAH) is present in many pregnant women, possibly causing negative outcomes for mother and fetus, such as a high risk of eclampsia. For this reason and others, the control of SAH during pregnancy is essential. However, much care should be taken with pharmacological therapy since many hypotensive agents pose a teratogenic risk [22, 23].

A controlled randomized study published in *The Lancet* in 2019 evaluated the action of three oral antihypertensive agents for the control of severe SAH in pregnant women and their possible adverse effects on the fetus. The study concluded that the three drugs (nifedipine, labetalol, and methyldopa) were able to reduce SAH in the pregnant women, with nifedipine showing the greatest reducing power. The authors indicated that these three drugs may be an initial therapeutic alternative for the treatment of severe SAH in pregnant women when local resources are reduced [22].

A review of the phamacological characteristics of antihypertensive agents and their intrauterine impact concluded that severe SAH should be treated, whereas there is still no consensus in the literature about when to start treatment or which drugs should be used for mild conditions of the disease that do not generate injuries, mainly owing to the uncertainty of long-term results of intrauterine exposure to antihypertensive agents [23].

The antihypertensive agents indicated during pregnancy, which are not considered to be teratogenic, include betablockers α β, or adrenergic agents with a central action, calcium channel blockers, and methyldopa. However, there is no extensive evidence of the safety of any of them [23].

Other antihypertensive drugs are contraindicated during pregnancy by being associated with spontaneous abortion, fetal death, congenital heart defects, hydrocephalus, spina bifida, microcephaly, and craniofacial anomalies, among other maternal-fetal structural, and metabolic defects. Assigned to this group of contraindicated drugs are the inhibitors of the renin–angiotensin–aldosterone system, including angiotensin-converting enzyme (ACE) inhibitors, angiotensin receptor blockers, direct renin inhibitors, and fetotoxic agents, such as sacubitril/valsartan [23].

Hypolipidemic Agents

Drugs belonging to the statin group, traditionally used with efficacy for the reduction of cholesterol levels, have been reported to be teratogenic for pregnant women. Statins inhibit the synthesis of hepatic cholesterol by inhibiting the enzyme

HMG-CoA reductase, with the consequent reduction of plasma cholesterol levels. In addition, they increase the level of expression of low-density lipoproteins (LDL-cholesterol) at the hepatic level, also reducing circulating LDL [24].

HMG-CoA plays a fundamental role in placental development, especially during the first trimester of gestation, in addition to producing hormones that are essential for the maintenance of pregnancy. Thus, inhibition of this enzyme by lipid-lowering agents such as vastatins and statins may compromise embryonic and fetal development [24].

A review published by Maierean et al. has suggested that current evidence does not support the teratogenic role of statins, which, indeed, may have an important function in the prevention of pre-eclampsia since intrauterine exposure to cholesterol may significantly affect the offspring. Thus, the use of statins during pregnancy by women at risk for pre-eclampsia should be thoroughly discussed in terms of cost-benefit regarding the possible teratogenic and therapeutic potential of these agents [25].

So far, studies on humans have not detected a positive association between the use of statins during pregnancy and an increased incidence of births with congenital malformations. In studies on animals, sinvastatin has been found to be possibly responsible for an increased abortion rate. However, studies on both humans and animals are still quite scarce and inconclusive, a fact that has led the FDA to assign this group of drugs to category X, i.e., contraindicated [24, 26].

Anticoagulants

The use of anticoagulants of the warfarin class is also restricted during gestation since they may induce the known fetal warfarin syndrome or warfarin embryofetopathy, with the management of pregnant women under anticoagulation treatment representing a challenge [27].

Current guidelines suggest doses $\leq$5 mg/day when the use of the drug is necessary. However, although low warfarin doses suggest a lower risk of fetopathy, the risk of embryopathy seems not to be reduced [27]. Low molecular weight heparins are the most indicated drugs for pregnant women who require the prevention or treatment of venous thromboembolism since, in addition to being effective, they are safer than vitamin K antagonists in terms of teratogenic risk [28].

Anorexigenic Drugs and Anti-obesity Drugs

Anorexigenic drugs such as femproporex, amfepramone, and amphetamines are assigned to category X by the FDA and therefore are contraindicated for pregnant women. Studies on mouse pups and adolescents exposed to femproporex during pregnancy have concluded that the drug causes long-lasting toxicity regarding behavioral characteristics [29].

The use of amphetamine-derived drugs is believed to act directly on the transport of the neurotransmitters serotonin and dopamine, causing an excessive expression in the placenta and imbalance in amniotic fluid and in the fetal circulation. These changes may induce the development of preeclampsia, intrauterine growth restriction, placental detachment, premature birth, and low birth weight [30].

Antifungal Agents

The prescription of antifungal agents to pregnant women continues to be a challenge mainly owing to the lack of studies demonstrating the teratogenic potential of these drugs. Most antifungal drugs are assigned to categories B and C of the FDA. Amphotericin B by the pareneteral route continues to be the main choice even though its toxic effects have been clearly determined [31].

The literature has reported that the use of fluconazole during pregnancy is associated with a higher risk of stillbirth. However, cohort studies conducted on 1,485,316 Swedish and Norwegian pregnant women did not detect a higher risk of neonatal death or stillbirth with the use of fluconazole compared to a control group [32].

In general, antifungal agents of topical use are considered to be safer due to their limited absorption. Clotrimazole, miconazole, and nystatin are considered to be first-line drugs for the treatment of pregnant women. In contrast, butenafine, ciclopyrox, naftifine, oxiconazole, and terbinafine are indicated only after the first-line option. Economazole is indicated as a drug of restricted use during the first trimester of pregnancy and of cautious use during the second and third trimesters. Studies have suggested that ketoconazole and selenium sulfide are safe during pregnancy, although their use is indicated for small limited areas and for short periods of time [33].

Anticonvulsants

The drugs used for the treatment of convulsions, as in the case of epileptic patients, are known to be teratogenic. However, in view of the severity of the disease, their use often needs to be continued during pregnancy. Considering the risk of teratogenicity of the drugs used, strategies of dialogue with pregnant women are recommended. The drugs used for the treatment of epilepsy are assigned to categories C and D by the FDA [34].

Valproate is the best-known teratogen when used for the treatment of epilepsy since it is associated with negative neurological outcomes that are often incompatible with gestation. Phenytoin, carbamazepine, and lamotrigine show expected teratogenic effects when compared to valproate. Phenobarbital and topiramate induce negative cardiac outcomes at respective rates of 6% and 4%. Exposure to topiramate and zonisamide during pregnancy involves a well-known risk of low birth weight [34].

In the case of pregnant women under drug treatment for epilepsy or convulsive crises, the doctor will have to expose to the parents the risks related to treatment and the possible therapeutic options for each case. Studies have shown that monotherapy involves a lower prevalence of teratogencity than polytherapy [34, 35].

New generation drugs such as lamotrigine, levetiracetam, and oxcarbazepine suggest a possibly lower association with adverse teratogenic effects when taken during pregnancy. Studies have also suggested that the use of folic acid, even at higher doses than usual during pregnancy, as well as stimulation of breastfeeding should be encouraged since they show potentially positive postpartum effects [35, 36].

Conclusion

There is a clear and relevant concern about the need for careful prescription of medications during pregnancy in view of the substantially important topic of mother–child health. The scarcity of randomized, double-blind, and controlled studies on human beings eventually elicits more conservative conducts on the part of professional entities. Regarding mainly the theme of drug teratogenicity, it should be emphasized that it is of crucial importance for the prescribing professionals to be aware of the risks and benefits of given drugs and to have a clear and participative dialogue with pregnant women in order to assign proper responsibility to all the protagonists involved in this delicate scenario.

References

1. Al-Enazy S, et al. Placental control of drug delivery. Adv Drug Deliv Rev. 2017;116:63–72.
2. Costa DB, Coelho HLL, dos Santos DB. Medication use before and during pregnancy: prevalence and associated factors. Braz J Public Health. 2017;33:e00126215.
3. Gomes KRO, et al. Prevalence of medication use during pregnancy and relationships with maternal characteristics. Public Health J. 1999;2:246–54.
4. Waard M, et al. Medication use during pregnancy and lactation in a Dutch population. J Hum Lact. 2019;35(1):154–64.
5. FDA. Food and Drugs Administration. https://www.fda.gov/consumers/free-publications-women/medicine-and-pregnancy. Accessed Feb 2019.
6. Azevedo AA. The use of medications during pregnancy and the role of pharmacovigilance. 2019.
7. Raichand S, et al. Utilisation of teratogenic medicines before and during pregnancy in Australian women. Aust. N. Z. J. Obstet. Gynaecol. 2020;60(2):218–24.

8. Shepard TH. "Proof" of human teratogenicity. Teratology. 1994;50(2):97–8.
9. Body C, Christie JA. Gastrointestinal diseases in pregnancy: nausea, vomiting, hyperemesis gravidarum, gastroesophageal reflux disease, constipation, and diarrhea. Gastroenterol Clin. 2016;45(2):267–83.
10. Wegrzyniak LJ, Repke JT, Ural SH. Treatment of hyperemesis gravidarum. Rev Obstet Gynecol. 2012;5(2):78.
11. Richter JE. The management of heartburn in pregnancy. Aliment Pharmacol Ther. 2005;22(9):749–57.
12. Pope E, Maltepe C, Koren G. Comparing pyridoxine and doxylamine succinate-pyridoxine HCl for nausea and vomiting of pregnancy: a matched, controlled cohort study. J Clin Pharmacol. 2015;55(7):809–14.
13. Ali R, Raja A, Egan LJ. Gastroesophageal reflux disease in pregnancy. Best Pract Res Clin Gastroenterol. 2007;21(5):793–806.
14. Zielinski R, Searing K, Deibel M. Gastrointestinal distress in pregnancy. J Perinat Neonatal Nurs. 2015;29(1):23–31.
15. Christie J, Rose S. Constipation, diarrhea, hemorrhoids, and fecal incontinence. In: Pregnancy in gastrointestinal disorders. Bethesda: ACG Monograph American College of Physicians; 2007. p. 4–9. Available at: https://www.acg.gi.org.
16. Cullen G, O'Donoghue D. Constipation and pregnancy. Best Pract Res Clin Gastroenterol. 2007;21(5):807–18.
17. Källén B. Maternal use of drugs for intestinal problems, except intestinal inflammations, and infant congenital malformations. In: Maternal drug use and infant congenital malformations. Cham: Springer; 2019. p. 23–31.
18. Bonapace ES Jr, Fisher RS. Constipation and diarrhea in pregnancy. Gastroenterol Clin N Am. 1998;27(1):197–211.
19. Thukral C, Wolf JL. Therapy insight: drugs for gastrointestinal disorders in pregnant women. Nat Clin Pract Gastroenterol Hepatol. 2006;3(5):256–66.
20. Finneran MM, Landon MB. Oral agents for the treatment of gestational diabetes. Curr Diab Rep. 2018;18(11):119.
21. Feghali MN, Umans JG, Catalano PM. Drugs to control diabetes during pregnancy. Clin Perinatol. 2019;46(2):257–72.
22. Easterling T, et al. Oral antihypertensive regimens (nifedipine retard, labetalol, and methyldopa) for management of severe hypertension in pregnancy: an open-label, randomised controlled trial. Lancet. 2019;394(10203):1011–21.
23. Tamargo J, Caballero R, Delpón E. Pharmacotherapy for hypertension in pregnant patients: special considerations. Expert Opin Pharmacother. 2019;20(8):963–82.
24. Rounds M. Risks of statin use during pregnancy: a systematic review. J Obstet Gynaecol Can. 2007;29(11):906–8.
25. Maierean SM, et al. The potential role of statins in preeclampsia and dyslipidemia during gestation: a narrative review. Expert Opin Investig Drugs. 2018;27(5):427–35.
26. Ofori B, Rey E, Bérard A. Risk of congenital anomalies in pregnant users of statin drugs. Br J Clin Pharmacol. 2007;64(4):496–509.
27. Sousa AR, Barreira R, Santos E. Low-dose warfarin maternal anticoagulation and fetal warfarin syndrome. Case Rep. 2018;2018:bcr-2017.
28. Pieper PG. Use of medication for cardiovascular disease during pregnancy. Nat Rev Cardiol. 2015;12(12):718.
29. Moreira CQ, et al. Developmental exposure to fenproporex: reproductive and morphological evaluation. Hum Exp Toxicol. 2005;24(8):397–402.
30. Wright TE, et al. Methamphetamines and pregnancy outcomes. J Addict Med. 2015;9(2):111.
31. Pilmis B, et al. Antifungal drugs during pregnancy: an updated review. J Antimicrob Chemother. 2015;70(1):14–22.

32. Pasternak B, et al. Oral fluconazole in pregnancy and risk of stillbirth and neonatal death. JAMA. 2018;319(22):2333–5.
33. Patel VM, Schwartz RA, Lambert WC. Topical antiviral and antifungal medications in pregnancy: a review of safety profiles. J Eur Acad Dermatol Venereol. 2017;31(9):1440–6.
34. Harden C, Christine L. Epilepsy in pregnancy. Neurol Clin. 2019;37(1):53–62.
35. Viale L, et al. Epilepsy in pregnancy and reproductive outcomes: a systematic review and meta-analysis. Lancet. 2015;386(10006):1845–52.
36. Tomson T, Battino D, Perucca E. Teratogenicity of antiepileptic drugs. Curr Opin Neurol. 2019;32(2):246–52.

Part II
Prenatal Care

Chapter 8
Nutritional Aspects of Gestation and Puerperium

Cláudia Saunders and Karina dos Santos

Acronyms and Abbreviations

75 g OGTT	Oral glucose tolerance test – 75 g
AA	Arachidonic acid
ACOG	American College of Obstetricians and Gynecologists
ADA	American Diabetes Association
AGP	α-1 Acid glycoprotein
BMI	Body mass index
CI	Confidence interval
CRP	C-reactive protein
DASH diet	Dietary approaches to stop hypertension
DHA	Docosahexaenoic acid
DM	Diabetes mellitus
DM1	Type 1 diabetes
DM2	Type 2 diabetes
DNA	Deoxyribonucleic acid
EI	Energy intake
EPA	Eicosapentaenoic acid
FAO	Food and Agriculture Organization
GDM	Gestational diabetes mellitus
Hb	Hemoglobin
HDP	Hypertensive disorders of pregnancy

C. Saunders (✉) · K. dos Santos
Research Group on Maternal and Child Health (Grupo de Pesquisa em Saúde Materna e Infantil – GPSMI), Nutrition Institute, Federal University of Rio de Janeiro, Rio de Janeiro, RJ, Brazil
e-mail: claudiasaunders@nutricao.ufrj.br

© Springer Nature Switzerland AG 2022

R. A. Moreira de Sá, E. B. d. Fonseca (eds.), *Perinatology*,
https://doi.org/10.1007/978-3-030-83434-0_8

IADPSG	International Association of Diabetes and Pregnancy Study Groups
IDF	International Diabetes Federation
IOM	Institute of Medicine
IU	International Units
LGA	Large for gestational age
MCV	Mean corpuscular volume
NTD	Neural tube defects
OR	Odds ratio
PUFAs	Polyunsaturated fatty acids
RBP	Retinol-binding protein
DRI	Dietary Reference Intakes
RNA	Ribonucleic acid
SGA	Small for gestational age
TEV	Total energy value
WHO	World Health Organization

Highlights

- Preconception, gestation, and puerperium represent the window of opportunity for health professionals to implement nutritional interventions for women and their children.
- All women of reproductive age should receive nutritional counseling to promote the best obstetric and perinatal outcomes.
- Nutritional interventions leading to balanced diets and appropriate weight can improve maternal health and child development.
- Monitoring and counseling about gestational weight gain and postpartum weight retention should be an ongoing practice in prenatal and postnatal care as modifiable risk factors for obesity.

Introduction

Maternal nutrition during pregnancy and lactation is determinant for women's and child's health. Several physiological adaptations for fetal development depend on the adequate maternal response to intense metabolic changes, which deserve special needs of energy, water, macronutrients, and micronutrients. From conception to 6 months of age, it is assumed that the baby will be totally dependent on maternal nutrition Maternal nutrition: through placenta during pregnancy and through human milk during exclusive breastfeeding [169].

The "First 1100 days of life" is a crucial period for improving maternal and child health. It represents the 100 days of preconception, 270 days of pregnancy, and the first 730 days of extrauterine life (2 years). These days are considered a window of opportunity for health professionals to implement nutritional interventions that lead to intergenerational long-term benefits [72, 146].

At preconception, it is important to evaluate women's diet, weight, lifestyle (including physical activity, smoking, alcohol, and drug use), chronic diseases, vaccination status, obstetric history, job conditions, and potential harmful exposures (social and physical). Pregnancy planning enables nutritional counseling at opportune time to prescribe folic acid to prevent neural tube defects (NTD), at least a month before a woman gets pregnant [107].

During pregnancy, antenatal care is expected to offer a positive pregnancy experience, which includes the provision of effective clinical practices, relevant and timely information (including dietary and nutritional advice) and psychosocial and emotional support by health-care practitioners [297]. Pregnancy requires a healthy diet with an adequate intake of energy, protein, vitamins, and minerals to meet maternal and fetal needs. Monitoring gestational weight gain and nutritional status, carefully prescribing supplements, advice about common symptomatology and providing appropriate counseling in special situations are decisive for pregnancy outcomes [297].

After childbirth, nutritional counseling aims to advise about special needs of lactation (energy, nutrients, water, and supplements), promote healthy weight loss to avoid postpartum weight retention, and support breastfeeding. It may be a challenging time for health interventions because there is a lack of specific schedule of clinical appointments for women when the prenatal period ends [66]. Designing guidelines to widely offer adequate nutritional counseling to postpartum women is a critical demand to achieve better rates of breastfeeding (not only in duration but in quality of supply) and also to improve maternal and child health.

Nutritional Aspects of Gestation

Prenatal Care and Maternal Health

Prenatal care is an essential strategy for reducing maternal mortality among adult and adolescent pregnant women [283, 297]. The minimum schedule of prenatal consultations has been revised, and in 2016, the World Health Organization [297] started to recommend a minimum of eight consultations, to reduce perinatal deaths by up to 8 per thousand born compared with the minimum previously recommended, which for low-risk pregnant women was four consultations [297]. The committee also recommends that the first prenatal consultation takes place until the 12th week of gestation [283, 297]. Nicolaides [195] draws attention to the importance of consultations in the early stages of pregnancy (11–13 weeks), to identify high- and low-risk pregnant women.

The global estimates for the year 2017 indicate that there were 295,000 maternal deaths [292]. Maternal mortality can increase the chance of infant mortality, as newborns separated from their mothers will not receive maternal care and breastfeeding [226].

WHO [292] estimates that the majority (99%) of maternal death cases occur in low- and middle-income countries, with almost two-thirds (64%) occurring in the African region. The reduction of maternal mortality depends on the women's access to health and antenatal care before, during and after delivery [292, 297].

The main causes of maternal death in the world are hemorrhage, hypertensive disorders of pregnancy (HDP), sepsis, representing more than half of the causes of maternal death in the world [245, 292].

Nutritional Intervention During Pregnancy

In the context of prenatal care interventions, nutritional care deserves to be highlighted [297]. Studies show the positive effect of nutritional intervention on maternal health and conditions at birth. As an example, the risk of gestational diabetes mellitus (GDM) is reduced by a healthy diet and lifestyle advice, when these guidelines are provided by a nutritionist in the first or the beginning of the second gestational trimester [18, 137, 271]; calcium supplementation during pregnancy prevents preeclampsia [295–297], iron and folic acid supplementation during pregnancy prevents gestational anemia [297]; supplementation of folic acid preconception and in the first trimester of pregnancy reduces the chance of neural tube defects [297].

WHO [283] recognizes the importance of training nutritionists to face the main health and nutrition problems of the maternal and child group, such as anemia, malnutrition, overweight, obesity, and to encourage breastfeeding.

The organization of prenatal nutritional assistance provided by nutritionists, including four consultations with the nutritionist beginning concurrently with prenatal care and with monitoring throughout pregnancy, increases the chance of adequacy of total gestational weight gain, reduces the prevalence of gestational anemia and vitamin A deficiency – gestational night blindness [55, 194, 204, 238], and reduces the prevalence low birth weight [230]. Such scientific findings were obtained in studies carried out in a public maternity hospital in Rio de Janeiro, RJ, Brazil, with low-risk pregnant women.

In light of the above, nutritional guidance favors the adequacy of gestational weight gain and the importance of weight gain in the early stage of pregnancy (1st trimester) in the outcomes of birth weight and newborn weight index [46, 94, 203].

In a study in a basic health unit in Rio de Janeiro, RJ, Brazil, we tested three group prenatal care with a nutritionist, distributed throughout gestation with low-risk women. The group that received this intervention had a lower chance of gestational complications and inadequate gestational weight gain [155]. American College of Obstetricians and Gynecologists [11] and WHO [297] also describe that group prenatal consultations can be successfully adopted.

Another positive experience can be mentioned with the prenatal care of pregnant women with GDM. For this group, the calendar of five to six individual consultations with the nutritionist within the context of prenatal care specialized in a reference service, also had a positive effect, as it was associated with a low rate of macrosomia in the newborns of these pregnant women [253].

In quality prenatal nutritional care, a complete nutritional assessment must be carried out in all prenatal consultations, considering anthropometric, dietary, clinical, biochemical, sociodemographic, and obstetric assessments. This global assessment will provide the nutritional diagnosis for the individualized intervention, which must be reviewed at each visit [235].

Anthropometric Assessment

The determination of adequate weight gain for pregnant women associated with the best obstetric and perinatal outcome is a concern of researchers. Abrams et al. [2] reviewed the recommendations for gestational weight gain throughout the twentieth century and showed that the recommendations were controversial. The approaches adopted ranged from dietary restriction recommendations for weight gain restricted to more liberal weight gain for American women. The restriction of weight gain recommended by obstetricians was justified to avoid HDP, difficulty in labor, and maternal obesity [2].

In the 1960s, obstetricians recommended restricted maternal weight gain, ideally around 6.8 kg, requiring careful control and maternal dietary restriction. The restriction of gestational weight gain imposed at the time was associated with an increase in infant mortality rates, associated with low birth weight. With this, in the following decades, scientific evidence showed that the practice of restricting maternal weight gain should not be recommended and the weight gain range of 9–11.4 kg started to be recommended. As a consequence of this conduct, there was a real increase in the means of maternal weight gain, and consequently, in the means of birth weight and a reduction in infant mortality [2].

In view of the need to reassess the scientific evidence addressing the relationship between pregnancy, weight gain and the impact on maternal and fetal outcomes, the Institute of Medicine [129] of the National Academy of Sciences published in 1990 a report with gain ranges of gestational weight recommended specifically for each category of pregestational Body Mass Index (BMI; in kg/m^2), different from the recommendations published until then and adopted in practice, which was the same for all women. The cutoff points initially adopted by the committee [129] for the assessment of prepregnancy BMI were estimated specifically with anthropometric data from the American population, adopted by the Metropolitan Life Insurance Company's in the United States, dated 1959 [129].

The IOM [129] reports that this recommendation was designed for healthy American women living in the United States. This recommendation was very important and innovative, since it recommended different ranges of weight gain considering the presence of maternal weight deviation before pregnancy, aiming at a favorable gestational result, defined as term delivery (39–41 weeks of gestation), of newborns born weighing between 3 and 4 kg. These recommendations were widely adopted by several countries, but not universally accepted. In 2009, the IOM published a review, which recommends about a reduction in the weight gain range for the obesity category and started to recommend the cutoff points for pregestational BMI adopted by the World Health Organization [290].

The IOM's recommendation [129, 133] has been criticized over time and several researchers have evaluated its performance in identifying maternal and perinatal outcomes. Bodnar et al. [42] studied the association between the adequacy of gestational weight gain [133] in women with different degrees of obesity and perinatal outcomes. They found that weight loss or insufficient weight gain in all obesity categories (I, II, III) was associated with a greater chance of small for gestational age (SGA) and excessive weight gain in these women was associated with a greater chance of large for gestational age (LGA) also for all obesity classes.

Goldstein et al. [101] in a meta-analysis and metaregression to evaluate associations between gestational weight gain above or below the IOM guidelines [133] analyzed data from more than one million women (n = 1309 136). They found that 70% of the women had gestational weight gain below or above the recommended ranges. The gain of gestational weight below the recommendations was associated with a higher risk of SGA and premature but lower risk of LGA and macrosomia. In the same study, similar results were observed for pregnant women with obesity [101].

Feghali et al. [94] in a retrospective cohort study found that insufficient weight gain in the first and second trimesters of pregnancy [133] were associated with a greater chance of SGA and less chance of LGA. Excessive gestational weight gain at this early stage of pregnancy was associated with a greater chance of LGA and less chance of SGA. Excessive weight gain in the third trimester was associated with an increased risk of LGA, but the inadequacy of weight gain in this gestational period was not associated with SGA.

In 2013, the IOM [131, 132] revised the gestational weight gain ranges and defined the 1–3 kg range as adequate weight gain for the first trimester for pregnant women with low, adequate, and overweight pregestational BMI; for obese women, the defined weight gain range in that period was reduced to 0.2–2 kg. In 2013, the committee published a guideline to help disseminate the guidelines for weight gain and pregnancy, valuing the role of the health team in supporting women to achieve adequate gain in pregnancy, aiming to reduce obesity in reproductive age, and to improve the health of women and their children [131, 132].

Table 8.1 depicts the ranges recommended by the IOM [131] for adult women and adolescents of single fetus pregnancies. It is emphasized that the assessment of maternal anthropometric should occur in all consultations of prenatal care to guide nutritional care. The weekly and total gestational weight gain should be programmed according to the pregestational BMI and estimated for term delivery (40 weeks). The IOM (2009) [133] recommends for twin pregnancy (two fetuses), the intervals of total weight gain, according to the pre-pregnancy BMI values classified in Table 8.1, which are: for adults with normal BMI, the recommended weight gain is 17–25 kg (37–54 lbs); for overweight, the weight gain is 14–23 kg (31–50 lbs), and

Table 8.1 Recommendation for total and rate of weight gain (lbs/kg) for adult women and adolescents, during pregnancy, by prepregnancy BMI

Prepregnancy BMI (kg/m²)[a]	Total first trimester weight gain[b] *Range*	Rates of weight gain second and third trimesters, per gestational week (lbs/kg)[c,d] *Mean (range)*	Total weight gain (lbs/kg) *Range*
Underweight (<18.5)	2.2–6.6 lbs/1–3 kg	1 (1–1.3) lbs 0.51 (0.44–0.58) kg	28–40 lbs 12.5–18 kg
Normal weight (18.5–24.9)	2.2–6.6 lbs/1–3 kg	1 (0.8–1.1) lbs 0.42 (0.35–0.5) kg	25–35 lbs 11.5–16 kg
Overweight (25.0–29.9)	2.2–6.6 lbs/1–3 kg	0.6 (0.5–0.7) lbs/0.28 (0.23–0.33) kg	15–25 lbs 7–11.5 kg
Obese (≥30.0)	0.5–4.4 lbs 0.2–2 kg	0.5 (0.4–0.6) lbs/0.22 (0.17–0.27) kg	11–20 lbs 5–9 kg

Adaptation IOM [131, 133]
lbs – pounds; kg – kilograms
Comments:
[a]Ideally, the prepregnancy BMI is calculated with the informed prepregnancy weight, corresponding to a maximum of 2 months before conception, or with the weight measured before the 14th gestational week. If this is not possible, start the evaluation of the pregnant woman with the data from the first prenatal consultation, even if this occurs after the 14th gestational week, thus obtaining gestational BMI [32]. The IOM [131–133] recognizes the difficulty in adopting pediatric growth charts in clinical practice to assess adolescents, and that with the application of the same cutoff points indicated for adults, many adolescents will be classified as underweight. Consequently, adolescents will be oriented toward greater gestational weight gain. The IOM [133] declares that in this way, younger adolescents would benefit, as they need greater weight gain to improve conditions at birth. Alternatively, the cutoff points for prepregnancy BMI can be adopted [77, 285] and the specific classification for adolescents, considering the age in years and months of girls, thus minimizing the risk of improper classification of adolescents, especially older ones and with some degree of excess weight [234, 235]
[b]Total weight gain (kg) for the first trimester (up to the 14th week of gestation, [131]). In the 2009 guideline version [133], the recommended weight gain was 0.5–2 kg in the first trimester for all.
[c]Range weekly weight gain recommended from the 14th gestational week, and acceptable range in weight gain per week. This information is useful for assessing the adequacy of the weight gain obtained by the pregnant woman at each prenatal consultation
[d]The minimum value of the ranges for weekly weight gain can be adopted as the minimum expected weight gain for pregnant women with excessive weight gain or who have already achieved total weight gain in the second or third trimester of pregnancy [220]. Insufficient weight gain or weight loss during pregnancy should not be recommended even for obese women, due to the negative impact on birth conditions [42, 94, 101, 132]

for obese, it is 11–19 kg (25–42 lbs) at term. These proposed weight gain ranges aim at the birth of two newborns weighing ≥2.5 kg on average and with gestational age between 37 and 42 weeks.

Another recommendation for weight gain for twin pregnancies with two fetuses is the proposal by Luke et al. [165], which is a good alternative for application in clinical practice. In this proposal, weight gain is defined for the different gestational periods (Table 8.2).

Table 8.2 Weekly and total gain for twin pregnancies, according to prepregnancy BMI

Prepregnancy BMI (kg/m²)[a]	Ranges of weight gain (kg), per gestational week			Total weight gain (kg)
	0–20	20–28	28 until delivery	
Underweight (<18.5)	0.560–0.790	0.680–0.790	0.560	22.5–27.9
Normal weight (18.5–24.9)	0.450–0.680	0.560–0.790	0.450	18–24.3
Overweight (25.0–29.9)	0.450–0.560	0.450–0.680	0.450	17.1–21.2
Obese (≥30.0)	0.340–0.450	0.340–0.560	0.340	13–17.1

Adaptation: Luke et al. [165]; WHO [290]
[a]*BMI* Body mass index, *kg* kilograms

Dietary Assessment

The pregnant woman's dietary assessment must be detailed. In this assessment, the pattern of meals (number of meals, times and intervals between meals), eating habits, consumption of dietary products and sweeteners, food allergy and/or intolerance, dietary changes (inclusion/exclusion) due to pregnancy, and the presence of digestive symptoms should be investigated. As for foods with sweeteners, these should only be recommended for specific situations, when sucrose – sugar restriction is recommended (see section Diabetes Mellitus During Pregnancy).

Food consumption should be investigated according to the degree of processing (Table 8.3). The consumption of processed and ultra-processed foods should be discouraged and the consumption of fresh and minimally processed foods should be encouraged as a strategy to combat obesity and associated morbidities [181, 183].

The NOVA food classification system allows the identification of ultra-processed foods and beverages, which are low cost, hyperpalatable industrial formulations, with a long shelf life and their excessive consumption is driven by marketing [184].

Several studies have described the negative impact of excessive consumption of processed and ultra-processed foods on health, such as increased prevalence of obesity, chronic diseases, such as DM and hypertension, metabolic syndrome due to high levels of sugar, saturated and trans fats, cholesterol and sodium, in addition to high-caloric density, low content of fibers, proteins, micronutrients and bioactive compounds in food products/industrial formulations [161, 162, 183, 184, 206, 262].

Fardet [91] showed that the greater the degree of food processing, the greater the glycemic response and the lower its satiety potential. In a study developed with eutrophic and obese pregnant women, it was found that the increase of 1% of calories from the diet from ultra-processed foods was associated with an increase of 1.33 kg in gestational weight gain and with an increase in skin folds and the percentage of body adiposity of the newborn [225].

Table 8.3 Food groups defined according to the extent and purpose of food processing

Food groups	Examples
Unprocessed and minimally processed foods: natural foods (edible parts of plants or from animals) or altered by removal of inedible or unwanted parts, and also processes that include drying, crushing, powdering, fractioning, filtering, roasting, boiling, pasteurization, chilling, freezing, and packaging	Fruits: leafy and root vegetables; grains;legumes; starchy roots and tubers; fungi; meat, poultry, fish and seafood; eggs; milk; herbs and spices used in culinary preparations
Processed culinary ingredients: obtained from natural foods by industrial processes, such as pressing, centrifuging, refining, extracting or mining; used to prepare, season and cook	Vegetable oils, butter and lard, sugar, honey, salt
Processed foods: Products made by adding salt, oil or sugar to unprocessed or minimally processed foods, using preservation methods, such as canning and bottling, and, in the case of breads and cheeses, using nonalcoholic fermentation	Canned or bottled vegetables and legumes in brine; salted or sugared nuts and seeds; salted, dried, cured, or smoked meats and fish; canned fish; fruit in syrup; freshly made unpackaged breads and cheeses
Ultra-processed foods: Formulations of ingredients made by a series of industrial processes, many requiring sophisticated equipment and technology, using many types of additives, including those that imitate or enhance the sensory qualities of foods or culinary preparations made from foods. Sophisticated packaging, usually with plastic and other synthetic materials	Many ready-to-consume products, such as carbonated soft drinks; sweetened drinks; sweet or savoury packaged snacks; chocolate; cookies; pre-prepared ready-to-heat products (pies and pasta and pizza dishes); poultry and fish "nuggets" and "sticks," sausages

Source: MS [181]; Monteiro et al. [183]; PAHO [206]

In dietary assessment, eating disorders such as pica, bulimia, and anorexia should be investigated. Pica can be defined as the persistent intake of nonnutritive substances for a period of at least 1 month, or ingestion of nonnutritious substances that are unfit for health, or eating behavior that is not part of the culture practiced, or eating behavior that occurs exclusively during the course of a mental disorder [22, 71].

It is estimated that the worldwide prevalence of pica during pregnancy and/or the postpartum period is 27.8%, positively associated with the prevalence of anemia and negatively associated with women's education [93].

In clinical practice, these reports can be attributed to the wishes of the pregnant woman, and many report a feeling of satisfaction after practicing the pica [33]. Polypica can also occur during pregnancy (disorder that manifests itself through the persistent consumption of two or more nonnutritious substances, [160]). Considering the association of this practice with a negative impact on maternal and newborn health, pica should be considered as a proxy for high-risk pregnancies, given that it can be associated with anemia, pregnancy complications, intestinal obstruction, constipation, dental fractures, hyperkalaemia, heavy metal poisoning, iron deficiency, helminth infections, and digestive symptoms. In addition, pica may be associated with some degree of stress, anxiety, and depression during pregnancy [33, 71, 93, 160, 243].

Some reports of pica may be supported by cultural traditions. As an example, we can cite the geophagy (land consumption) associated with fertility and reproduction by women from Kenya and Nigeria. Geophagy is also practiced to relieve gastrointestinal discomfort (such as vomiting) in Nigeria, and geophagy is also believed to protect against infections and diseases during pregnancy [63, 93].

In adolescent pregnant women, the prevalence of pica may be higher than that described in adults. Lumish et al. [166] describe a 46% prevalence of pica among pregnant American teenagers and this disorder was associated with anemia and low concentrations of ferritin.

Chung et al. [63] reveals that pica is not limited to pregnancy and describes that 24% of Kenia women evaluated, reported pica during breastfeeding. In addition, they describe that geophagy, and the consumption of charcoal and/or ash was negatively associated with breastfeeding (OR = 0.38, 95% CI: 0.18–0.81) and amylophagy was associated with pregnancy (OR = 4.31, 95% CI: 1.24–14.96).

In view of the above, the investigation of pica should be part of the prenatal care routines and cases should be treated by a multidisciplinary team [71].

Biochemical and Clinical Evaluation

Biochemical assessment and routine exams of prenatal care can guide health professionals regarding the pregnant woman's health and nutrition status. The normality standards for the exams recommended during pregnancy consider the physiological adjustments of the period and assess whether the pregnancy has a normal course.

The useful parameters for assessing the pregnant woman's nutritional status are as follows: blood count (diagnosis of gestational anemia, [297]), fasting blood glucose (screening for DM, oral glucose tolerance (OGTT) – 75g), urine and culture (screening for urinary tract infection, proteinuria), proto parasitology (screening for parasitic infections and recommended tests especially in cases of anemia) [189]. In 2020, WHO [296] started recommending the evaluation of serum or plasma ferritin to identify the status of iron. In Table 8.4, some biochemical parameters are listed with values considered normal or altered during pregnancy.

The ultrasound examination, which is very useful during pregnancy, should be done between the 11th and 13th gestational week to certify gestational age, identification of the number of fetuses, identification of malformations, screening for aneuploidies and prediction of preeclampsia, and premature birth [185, 195]. During pregnancy, ultrasounds will allow the evaluation of fetal growth and development, evaluation of the placenta, umbilical cord and the amount of amniotic fluid. Breast examination aims to identify the type of nipple and possible problems that may interfere with breastfeeding, such as inverted or flat nipples [185].

Serial measurements of maternal weight (kg) allow the assessment of the speed of weekly and total weight gain per quarter; blood pressure assessment allows the detection of hypertension or hypotension. These measures should be evaluated in all prenatal consultations. The measurement of uterine height or waist circumference

Table 8.4 Laboratory test values considered normal or altered during pregnancy

Parameter	Cutoff points	References
Hemoglobin (Hb)		[289]
Absence of anemia	≥11 g/dl	
Mild anemia	10–10.9 g/dl	
Moderate anemia	7–9.9 g/dl	
Severe anemia	<7 g/l	
Hb: normal values per gestational trimester		[185]
1°. Trimester	≥11 g/dl	
2°. Trimester	≥10.5 g/dl	
3°. Trimester	≥11 g/dl	
Serum ferritin (iron deficiency)	<15 mg/L (first trimester)	[296]
Glycemia (screening for GDM). *One-step strategy*:* In women without a diagnosis of DM, perform the 75 g OGTT, measure the plasma glucose of the fasting pregnant woman and after 1 h and 2 h, between 24 and 28 weeks of gestation. The diagnosis of GDM is made when any of the following plasma glucose values are reached or exceeded:	Fasting plasma glucose: 5.1–6.9 mmol/L (92 mg/dL) 1 h plasma glucose: ≥10.0 mmol/L (180 mg/dL). 2 h plasma glucose: 8.5 mmol/L (153 mg/dL)	[18] *One-step strategy, based on the Hyperglycemia and Adverse Pregnancy Outcome [105]
Glycemia (screening for GDM) It should be diagnosed at any gestational age. It will be the case of GDM if one or more of the following criteria are met:	Fasting plasma glucose: 5.1–6.9 mmol/L (92–125 mg/dL) 1 h plasma glucose: ≥10.0 mmol/L (180 mg/dL) following a 75 g oral glucose load 2 h plasma glucose: 8.5–11.0 mmol/L (153–199 mg/dL) following a 75 g oral glucose load	[297]
Glycemia (screening for DM) It should be diagnosed at any gestational age. It will be the case of DM if one or more of the following criteria are met:	Fasting plasma glucose: ≥7.0 mmol/L (126 mg/dL) 2 h plasma glucose: ≥11,1 mmol/L (200 mg/dL) following a 75 g oral glucose load Random plasma glucose ≥11.1 mmol/L (200 mg/dL) in the presence of DM symptoms	[297]
Serum retinol (normal for the mother-infant group)	≥1.05μmol/L	[284]
Urine: Proteins (normal)	<300 mg/dia	[187]

Legend: *Hb* hemoglobin, *DM* diabetes mellitus, *GDM* gestational diabetes mellitus, *75 g OGTT* oral glucose tolerance test

allows the screening of restricted intrauterine growth [185]. The evaluation of edema during pregnancy is useful to identify possible cases of HDP. It is necessary to differentiate the type of edema, if physiological gravitational, limited to the ankles, which improves with the lateral decubitus, and generalized edema, characterized by sudden weight gain, associated with hypertension and proteinuria, suggestive of preeclampsia [186].

In the clinical evaluation, investigate the digestive symptoms that are due to the physiological adjustments of the pregnancy. The diagnosis of the cases and the intervention must be made as early as possible, because, depending on the severity of the condition, they can influence maternal food consumption, consequently, influence gestational weight gain and fetal development [13, 70].

Evaluate the presence of chronic diseases (chronic arterial hypertension, DM, heart disease, kidney diseases, endocrinopathies, among others) that can worsen during pregnancy.

Investigate the development of gestational complications, the most prevalent of which are GDM, HDP, urinary tract infection, nutritional deficiencies (anemias, vitamin A and D deficiency, among others).

Functional Assessment

The presence of vitamin A deficiency in pregnancy can be investigated with the application of a standardized and adapted interview [235, 288, 299] for the investigation of gestational night blindness, which is the first stage of xerophthalmia, eye symptom of vitamin A deficiency. This interview is a low-cost, low-invasive method that is easy to apply by any trained health professional. The interview is validated according to the biochemical indicator (serum retinol levels, [242], Table 8.5) and

Table 8.5 Standardized interview for diagnosis of gestational night blindness

1. Do you have difficulty seeing during the day?
2. Do you have difficulty seeing in low light or at night?
3. Do you have night blindness?
When the answer to question 1 is "no" and at least one answer to questions 2 or 3 is "yes," it is gestational night blindness, that is, those in which the pregnant woman reports difficulty in seeing in low light or at night and has no difficulty doing it during the day [235, 299]
This interview can also be applied to children and nursing mothers [299]
If the interviewee has an eye problem corrected by glasses or contact lenses, the ability to see with their use should be questioned
In question 3, the term night blindness can be replaced by a regional term that signifies such an eye symptom; or explain to the pregnant woman that the term night blindness refers to a change in the usual pattern of vision in low light or at night in the current pregnancy and the difficulty of adapting the vision in changing from a light to a dark environment, adopting it the night vision pattern in the pregestational period is used as a reference [235, 239]

must be applied in all prenatal consultations, allowing interventions to correct the deficiency still at a subclinical level.

In the case of gestational night blindness, the usual consumption of vitamin A source foods should be investigated to confirm the diagnosis of vitamin A deficiency [235]. If possible, measure the serum retinol concentration (Table 8.4).

Sociodemographic and Obstetric Assessment

WHO [297] recommends that all women and newborns receive quality care throughout pregnancy, childbirth, and the postnatal period, considering not only their physiological issues but also respecting sociocultural conditions and offering respectful and effective support, including its emotional and psychological aspects.

Maternal sociodemographic conditions can influence pregnancy outcomes, as they influence maternal health, access to and adherence to prenatal care, food consumption, and gestational weight gain [133].

In prenatal care, sociodemographic characteristics should be assessed: chronological age, skin color (by self-classification), education level, place of birth, professional occupation, marital status, number of family members living in the household, family income per capita, housing sanitation conditions, social habits (use of cigarettes, alcohol, and illegal drugs).

Regarding obstetric history, history of abortion and intergestion interval <24 months can increase the chance of gestational night blindness [237, 238] and failure to plan and/or accept pregnancy may influence adherence to prenatal care.

Nutritional Recommendations During Pregnancy

Energy and Macronutrients

The energy requirements of women during pregnancy are higher compared with the requirements of nonpregnant women [96, 123]. Ideally, women should conceive with adequate nutritional status, to obtain better obstetric results, and women with weight deviation (underweight or pregestational overweight/obesity) deserve greater attention [133, 297].

Dietary restriction and weight loss during pregnancy in women with pregestational overweight or obesity have not been proven to be beneficial strategies for improving the health of the mother–child binomial, nor for preventing pregnancy complications [42, 101, 123, 133, 190]. In cases of maternal excess weight, the estimate of the total energy value (TEV) must be adequate for the programmed weight gain according to the pregestational BMI (Table 8.1), thus guaranteeing the favorable obstetric and perinatal outcome [42, 101, 123, 133, 190].

The increased requirements in the gestational period are necessary for the synthesis of new tissues (fetus, placenta, and amniotic fluid) and growth of maternal tissues (uterus, breast, and maternal adipose), promotion of adequate gestational weight gain, meeting increased metabolic demands during pregnancy, providing additional energy to maintain maternal weight, body composition, and maternal physical activity. In addition, these increased requirements will allow the constitution of the energy reserve for the lactation period [96, 190].

The basal metabolic rate increases during pregnancy due to the metabolic contribution of the uterus and fetus and increased workload of the heart and lungs. The increase in basal metabolism is one of the main components of the increase in energy needs during pregnancy [120, 123].

Table 8.6 Daily recommendations for energy, macronutrients, fibers, and liquids for pregnant and lactating women

	Recommendation for pregnant women	Recommendation for lactating women	References
Additional energy (kcal/day)	1° trimester: 85 2° trimester: 285 3° trimester: 475	1° half: 500 a 670 2° half: 300 a 400	[96]
Carbohydrates (g)	50–75% of EI 175[a]	50–75% of EI 210[b]	[97] [123]
Proteins (g/kg[c]) Proteins (g)	1.1 71	1.1 71	[123]
	1° trimester: 0.8 g/kg + additional 1 g 2° trimester: 0.8 g/kg + additional 9 g 3° trimester: 0.8 g/kg + additional 31 g	1° half: 0.8 g/kg + additional 19 g 2° half: 0.8 g/kg + additional 12.5 g	[291]
Total lipids DHA (mg) EPA + DHA (mg) AA (mg) Trans fatty acids Linoleic acid (g) Alpha-linolenic acid (g)	20–35% of EI 200 (maximum 1 g) 300 (maximum 2.7 g) Maximum 800 Minimum feasible 13 1.4	20–35% of EI 200 (maximum 1 g) 300 (maximum 2.7 g) Maximum 800 Minimum feasible 13 1.3	[98] [123]
Fiber (g)	28	29	[123]
Liquids[d] (l)	3	3.8	[123]

AA arachidonic acid, *EPA* eicosapentaenoic acid, *DHA* docosahexaenoic acid, *EI* energy intake, *IOM* Institute of Medicine, *FAO* Food and Agriculture Organization, *WHO* World Health Organization

[a]Minimum amount needed to supply the central nervous system of the woman and the fetus during pregnancy

[b]Minimum amount needed to supply the woman's central nervous system and to produce breast milk during lactation

[c]Desirable weight, considering body mass index in the eutrophic range

[d]Including water content in food and drinks

The Food and Agriculture Organization committee [96] estimates that the gestational energy cost is 77,000 kcal, associated with an adequate total gestational weight gain, varying between 10 and 14 kg, with an average of 12 kg, for healthy and well-nourished women, with a greater chance of a newborn weighing 3.3 kg and lower rates of maternal–fetal complications. This energy surcharge represents a daily surcharge on the daily TEV during the 280 days of pregnancy ([96, 123]; Table 8.6).

The individualized calculation of the additional energy during pregnancy for a specific weight gain for a pregnant woman can be done considering the information: for the gestational weight gain of 12 kg, 77,000 kcal are needed, therefore for each 1 kg, 6.417 kcal [96, 240].

Good adherence to the nutritional guidelines of an individualized eating plan, with an estimate of the TEV, according to the recommendations of FAO/WHO/UNU [96], are associated with adequate weight gain during pregnancy [80].

For the calculation of individualized TEV, the international health committees [96, 123] present formulas that are easily applicable in prenatal care.

Energy intake has a close correlation with gestational weight gain, therefore, the TEV for the gestational period must be estimated individually in each prenatal consultation, considering the recommended weight gain until delivery, maternal age, gestational age (weeks), level of physical activity, pregestational BMI [96, 123, 240].

Macronutrients

The main recommendations for macronutrients, fibers, and liquids during pregnancy are summarized in Table 8.6. Protein needs during pregnancy aim to promote the constitution of maternal and fetal tissues, which show a significant increase in the second half of pregnancy [291]. Insufficient protein intake during pregnancy is associated with restricted intrauterine growth, impaired development of central fetal organs, such as heart and brain, and with a greater future predisposition to obesity, DM and cardiovascular diseases [142]. Consumption of 10–25% of total daily calories in the form of proteins is considered safe. Although the evidence is scarce, exceeding this limit may compromise fetal growth and weight gain, probably due to the saticty capacity of the high-protein diet, reducing the total energy consumption of the pregnant woman [190].

Lipids contribute up to 35% of the total daily energy and play a fundamental role in the formation of tissues, constituting cell membranes. The quality of dietary lipids gains special focus in pregnancy, as it determines what will be the composition of fatty acids available for the constitution of fetal tissues. In this sense, the importance of polyunsaturated fatty acid omega-3 is highlighted, especially docosahexaenoic acid (DHA) which has a direct effect on the development of the central nervous system and formation of the retina [98], as well as being associated with a lower risk of prematurity [177]. The main dietary source of DHA is the consumption of fish, avoiding those that present a higher risk of contamination by mercury, such as swordfish, tuna, shark, king mackerel, and tilefish. Vegetable oils may contain good amounts of alpha-linolenic acid, a precursor to DHA; however, bioconversion is quite restricted in humans, so direct sources should be prioritized during pregnancy [86].

However, the current dietary pattern in industrialized countries, characterized by high consumption of saturated and trans fatty acids, as well as much higher proportions of polyunsaturated fatty acid omega-6 in relation to omega-3, promotes excessive weight gain during pregnancy, maternal metabolic disorders and metabolic programming in offspring, with a greater predisposition to obesity and chronic diseases throughout life [142]. Therefore, the consumption of ultra-processed foods, rich in saturated and trans fatty acids, and fried foods or with excess of vegetable oils rich in polyunsaturated fatty acid omega-6 should be discouraged, associating with the increased consumption of polyunsaturated fatty acid omega-3, in order to favor the balance of the lipid composition for better maternal and child outcomes [86, 98].

In relation to carbohydrates, the main energy source in the diet, foods with a low glycemic index and with a higher fiber content seem to favor the adequacy of weight gain and glycemic control, especially in women at higher risk for GDM [307], and to reduce the occurrence of gestational hypertension [227]. Higher consumption of dietary fibers associated with polyunsaturated fatty acid omega-3 and polyphenols in pregnancy promotes variations in maternal intestinal microbiota and fetal microbial colonization with a systemic anti-inflammatory and protective effect against childhood obesity [99].

On the other hand, excessive dietary sugars can contribute to excessive weight gain, GDM, preeclampsia, and preterm birth, as well as representing a risk factor for obesity and metabolic disorders for the child throughout life [103]. Thus, the choice of carbohydrate source foods during pregnancy should be judicious, prioritizing cereals and whole grains, tubers, fruits and vegetables and limiting the consumption of refined cereals and sweetened foods and drinks that rapidly increase blood glucose [95].

Micronutrients

The main micronutrient recommendations for pregnant women are listed in Table 8.7. In general, daily needs are met through a healthy diet with a wide variety of foods from different groups: cereals and tubers, legumes, meat, dairy products, fruits, vegetables and fats [297]. Some micronutrients have a prominent role in pregnancy, such as folic acid, iron, calcium, and vitamins A and D.

Vitamin A

Vitamin A is a fat-soluble vitamin that participates in important biological processes. It plays an essential role in reproduction, fetal development, sperm formation, maintenance of the placenta, in the immune system, and maintenance of the

Table 8.7 Daily recommendations for micronutrients for pregnant and lactating women

Nutrients	Recommendation for pregnancy	Recommendation for lactating women	Food source
Thiamine/B1 (mg)[a]	1.4	1.4	Cereals, oilseeds, seeds, meat
Riboflavin/B2 (mg)[a]	1.4	1.6	Whole grains, milk, meat, eggs
Niacin/B3 (mg)[a]	18	17	Whole grains, meats
Pyridoxine/B6 (mg)[a]	1.9	2.0	Whole grains, meats, vegetables, legumes (beans, peas, soybeans, chickpeas, lentils)
Cyanocobalamin/ B12 (µg)[a]	2.6	2.8	Meat, eggs, milk and dairy products
Folate (µg)[a]	600	500	Dark green vegetables, legumes, citrus fruits
Vitamin C (mg)[b]	14–18 yr: 80 >19 yr: 85	14–18 yr: 115 >19 yr: 120	Citrus fruits, vegetables
Vitamin A (µg)[c]	14–18 yr:750 >19 yr: 770	14–18 yr: 1200 >19 yr: 1300	Provitamin A (dark green vegetables and yellow-orange fruits and vegetables; preformed vitamin A (animal foods: derived from whole milk, liver, fish oils and human milk)
Vitamin D (IU)[d]	600	600	Sun exposure, fish, egg yolk, mushrooms
Vitamin E (mg)[b]	15	19	Vegetable oils
Iron (mg)[c]	27	14–18 yr:10 > 19 yr: 9	Meat, legumes (beans, peas, soybeans, chickpeas, lentils), whole grains, cabbage
Zinc (mg)[c]	14–18 yr: 12 > 19 yr: 11	14–18 yr: 13 > 19 yr: 12	Meats, whole grains, legumes (beans, peas, soybeans, chickpeas, lentils), seeds, oilseeds.
Calcium (mg)[d]	14–18 yr: 1300 > 19 yr: 1000	14–18 yr: 1300 > 19 yr: 1000	Milk and dairy products, leafy green vegetables, nuts or fortified foods including flour and dairy alternatives (soya products)
Iodine (µg)[c]	220	290	Iodized salt, seafood
Selenium (µg)[b]	60	70	Meat, oilseeds

Source: IOM [124] [a], [126] [b], [125] [c], [122] [d]
IOM Institute of Medicine, *yr* years

integrity of mucous membranes and skin. It acts in the regulation of cell proliferation and differentiation and maintenance of skeletal tissue [284]. Vitamin A is necessary to maintain the integrity of the intestinal mucosa and regulate the expression of the mucin gene, and it improves several models of autoimmunity, including inflammatory bowel disease, rheumatoid arthritis, and others [74]. Vitamin A acts as one of the nuclear receptors and their activators that regulate the expression of several genes of the metabolism of several hormones (triiodothyronine (T3), estrogen, progesterone, cortisol, aldosterone, testosterone, and vitamin D), of the metabolism of cholesterol and fatty acids and of its antioxidant function [41, 190].

Evidence shows the role of vitamin A (retinoic acid) as an epigenetic modulator, capable of inducing epigenetic changes that produce various effects on the phenotype. It is suggested that retinoids act by promoting stem cell differentiation and thus altering the pattern of gene expression in tumor cells to make them more sensitive to therapies [74].

During pregnancy, placental transfer of vitamin A to the fetus is facilitated by the change in the proportion of circulating proteins of vitamin A holo and apo retinol-binding protein (RBP). In the case of low maternal body reserve in the preconception phase of vitamin A and persistent insufficient consumption of this vitamin during pregnancy, maternal liver reserve may be compromised, thus increasing the risk for the development of maternal vitamin A deficiency, as an example of gestational night blindness [125, 200, 246].

Maternal vitamin A deficiency, even at subclinical levels (serum retinol <1.05μmol/L), may be associated with lower hepatic reserve in the fetus and inadequate levels of serum retinol in the newborn [102], thereby increasing the risk of death in the first 6 months of life [61].

Deficient or excessive intake of vitamin A in humans can be associated with birth defects (including brain, eye, ear, genitourinary tract, heart and vascular system, depending on which system is in the differentiation phase at the time of exposure) due to changes in deoxyribonucleic acid (DNA) metabolism, which can cause embryo resorption and fetal death [200, 201]. In addition to changes in ribonucleic acid (RNA) metabolism, vitamin deficiency in pregnancy can be associated with a history of spontaneous abortions [102, 237, 238, 255].

Vitamin D

The cells of most organs of the human organism express receptors for vitamin D, which demonstrates its wide performance in biological processes with emphasis on calcium metabolism and maintenance of bone health [304], immune function [168], cognition [171], glucose metabolism [303], and blood pressure regulation [158].

In pregnancy, vitamin D acts in the transport of calcium to the fetus, as well as in maintaining adequate placental function. The inadequacy of the vitamin D nutritional status has been related to adverse outcomes such as preeclampsia, gestational diabetes, preterm birth, and low birth weight, in addition to impaired fetal bone formation. Effects on child health, such as the development of allergies and neurocognitive impairment have also been investigated, but the heterogeneity between the assessment methods used in the studies limits the conclusions [3, 277].

The main source of vitamin D is endogenous synthesis, dependent on sun exposure, in which the time required may vary according to geographic location, skin pigmentation, age and other individual characteristics. Foods such as fish, egg yolk, and some mushrooms contain vitamin D, but in small quantities; fortified foods also contain vitamin D [114]. Vitamin D supplementation during pregnancy has been recommended for maintaining serum 25-hydroxyvitamin D concentrations above 30 ng/ml [114, 222].

Complex B Vitamins

The B-complex vitamins are essential for the metabolism of macronutrients and energy production at the cellular level, as well as for the formation of blood cells, therefore, the daily recommendations are increased during pregnancy in relation to the nonpregnancy period. Due to the direct relationship with the folic acid cycle, the intake and consequent adequacy of the nutritional status of vitamin B12 is important for the formation of the neural tube [211]. Vitamin B12 deficiency is associated with a higher risk for preterm birth and low birth weight [224], and with depressive symptoms in pregnant women [209]. Vitamin B12 deficiency can also compromise children's cognitive performance when there is a shortage of other B complex vitamins simultaneously [52, 151].

Folate

Folate plays a central role in the synthesis of DNA and blood cells, in cell multiplication and in the regulation of gene expression through epigenetic mechanisms, being important in embryonic and fetal development [217]. The folate deficiency implies high concentrations of homocysteine, which may increase the risk for preeclampsia [256]. The adequacy of the nutritional status of folate in preconception and pregnancy is essential to prevent defects in the closure of the neural tube, a fact that supports the recommendation of generalized supplementation in this period, using its synthetic form of high bioavailability, the folic acid [15]. The importance of folate for adequate formation of the central nervous system supported the fortification of wheat and corn flours as a public health policy for the reduction of NTD in several countries [54].

Iron

Iron as an essential part of the hemoglobin molecule has its nutritional needs increased during pregnancy to meet the greater demand in the synthesis of erythrocytes and the consequent transport of oxygen to maternal and fetal tissues. Iron deficiency can be identified at an early stage by assessing serum ferritin. Serum concentrations below 15μg/dL in the first trimester of pregnancy (Table 8.4) indicate depletion of cellular iron stores, motivated by insufficient consumption, absorptive inefficiency and/or increased losses (parasitic infections, and hemorrhages) [296]. In advanced stages, the production of red blood cells is compromised, and anemia can be detected by hemoglobin concentrations $\leq$11 g/dL in the first and third trimesters and $\leq$10.5 g/dL in the second trimester [297].

The absorption of iron during pregnancy varies according to the gestational age. In the first trimester, there is a reduction in iron absorption, caused by the lower need for the nutrient in this period. With the expansion of blood volume caused by pregnancy, the rate of absorption in the second trimester is increased by 50% and in the third, the increase is even greater, that is fourfold. Despite this increase in the iron absorption rate, it is still not enough to meet the increased needs for the gestational period, even if the dietary consumption is adequate and with sources with high bioavailability [149, 215]. Thus, health committees recommend prophylactic iron supplementation in the case of anemia [149, 289].

Animal foods (beef, chicken, pork, and fish) contain heme iron, with an absorption rate of 15–35%, while those of plant origin offer nonheme iron, with less absorption efficiency (1–34%), but greater abundance in the diet, mainly through legumes and whole grains. The absorption of nonheme iron can be facilitated by the consumption of vitamin C and carotenoids in the same meal (for example, broccoli, tomatoes, pumpkin, and orange) [37].

Iodine

Iodine is an element that has an increased need by about 50% during pregnancy. Since it acts on the synthesis of thyroid hormones, it is essential for adequate fetal growth and development and for maternal endocrine-metabolic regulation. Severe deficiency can result in hypothyroidism, goiter, abortion, increased neonatal mortality, neurological damage, and intellectual impairment [308]. The WHO [291] presents a daily recommendation of 250µg of iodine during pregnancy, which in countries or regions where less than 90% of households have access to iodized salt must be obtained through supplementation.

Vitamins C and E, Selenium, and Zinc

Vitamins C and E, selenium, and zinc play an important systemic antioxidant action with a potential protective effect against negative outcomes related to inflammation and oxidative stress, such as preeclampsia and other placental disorders that compromise fetal nutrition and growth [24].

Calcium

Calcium is an essential nutrient involved in several biological processes, including signal transduction, muscle contraction, enzyme and hormone homeostasis, release of neurotransmitters, and cellular function. It is essential for bone mineralization and is an essential intracellular component for maintaining cell membranes [190]. In pregnancy, calcium is actively transported by the placenta and the changes in the metabolism of this nutrient aim to favor the transfer of this element to the fetus.

More efficient uptake and utilization of calcium occurs in pregnancy, including increased hormone-stimulated calcium absorption rate (vitamin D, estrogen, lactogen, and prolactin) and increased calcium retention by renal tubules [190]. The intestinal absorption rate is increased mainly from the second trimester, in the order of 54%, and 42% at term (40th gestational week).

Low maternal calcium intake can contribute to osteopenia, paraesthesia, muscle cramps, tetanus, and tremor in pregnant women, in addition to growth retardation, low birth weight and low fetal bone mineralization. But this last repercussion needs confirmation [190].

Evidence suggests that low calcium intake can cause high blood pressure by stimulating parathyroid hormone or releasing renin, thereby increasing intracellular calcium in vascular smooth muscle [38] and leading to vasoconstriction. Calcium supplementation reduces the stimulation of parathyroid hormone and intracellular calcium, thereby reducing smooth muscle contractility. The effect on reducing uterine smooth muscle contractility preventing premature delivery is also seen with calcium supplementation [280].

In a meta-analysis with randomized clinical trials published by Hofmeyr et al. [112, 113], they showed that high-dose calcium supplementation [42, 94, 101, 132] (≥1 g / day) can reduce the risk of preeclampsia and premature birth, especially in pregnant women with low consumption of calcium sources (<900 mg/day) and those with increased risk of preeclampsia. Women who receive calcium supplements are also less likely to die or have serious problems related to preeclampsia, high blood pressure, and premature birth.

The evidence further suggests that a relatively low dose of calcium may be effective in reducing preeclampsia, high blood pressure, and the admission of newborns to the intensive care unit. Thus, they concluded that in places where dietary calcium intake is low, supplementation is an important strategy for reducing the serious consequences of preeclampsia, including maternal death and premature birth [111, 113].

Use of Supplements During Pregnancy

Onc of the nutritional intervention strategies recommended by WHO [297] is healthy eating and physical activity during pregnancy, for women to stay healthy and prevent excessive weight gain. Multiple micronutrient supplementation is not recommended to improve maternal and perinatal outcomes [297]. The IOM [133] recommends supplementation during pregnancy only in case of nutritional deficiencies, especially iron, vitamin B12, folate, vitamin D, and calcium.

A discussion about the risks and benefits associated with the use of supplements for the health of women of reproductive age, pregnancy, and postpartum, is necessary, especially among the prenatal team, which provides nutrition counseling, such as nutritionists, doctors, and nurses. This individualized prescription is necessary, considering that many women do not consume adequate food in the preconception, pregnancy, and lactation phases, especially vegetables, meat, dairy products and fruits. As a result, the diet will be insufficient to meet the increased needs in the reproductive period, especially for women in low and middle-income countries, in which multiple nutritional deficiencies coexist, associated with unfavorable obstetric and perinatal results, which can be mitigated by interventions such as micronutrient supplementation [198, 246, 297].

Recognizing that prenatal care must prioritize health and well-being centered on women, not just on the prevention of morbidity and mortality [297], the prescription of nutritional supplementation should also be following this philosophy and be evaluated according to each case, considering the nutritional deficiencies of each woman. It is noteworthy that the excessive use of micronutrients that can occur with the concomitant use of more than one nutritional supplement can also have negative repercussions on the mother–child binomial, especially if used in the initial phase of pregnancy (embryonic period between the fourth and eighth gestational week, [148]).

In a meta-analysis published by Oh et al. [198], the effects of supplementation of some nutrients on pregnancy in healthy women were evaluated. The study analyzed 314 randomized controlled trials and quasi-experimental studies published and 451,723 women were studied. Among the results, there was little or no effect of multiple micronutrient supplementation on maternal, neonatal, perinatal, and infant mortality. They evidenced the association between multiple micronutrient supplementation and reduction in outcomes – premature birth, small-for-gestational age, and low birth weight compared with iron–folic supplementation. The reduction in maternal anemia and low birth weight was associated with iron–folic supplementation. The reduction of maternal anemia was also observed with iron supplementation alone. The positive effect of calcium supplementation in reducing the prevalence of preeclampsia/eclampsia was confirmed, and the reduction in premature births was associated with vitamin D supplementation. These findings highlight that micronutrient supplementation must be adapted to the specific needs of the groups.

The nutritional supplements recommended by the international health committees for the periconception and pregnancy periods are discussed in the following sections.

Vitamin A

Vitamin A supplementation during pregnancy is not recommended to prevent maternal and infant morbidity and mortality [200, 297]. Supplementation is recommended during pregnancy in specific settings to avoid night blindness, in places where vitamin A deficiency is a serious public health problem (≥5% of women in the population have a history of gestational night blindness in the most recent pregnancy, in the period of 3–5 years ending with a live birth, or if ≥20% of pregnant women have a serum retinol level <0.70μmol/L, [297]).

- Recommended dose: In areas where supplementation is indicated for vitamin A deficiency, it can be a dose of up to 10,000 IU of vitamin A per day or a weekly dose of up to 25,000 IU [297].

- A single dose of vitamin A supplement greater than 25,000 IU is not recommended, as it may have a teratogenic effect, especially if consumed between days 15 and 60 since conception [297].
- The benefit of using vitamin A supplements in populations with usual vitamin A intake greater than 8000 IU or 2400μg has not been demonstrated. The potential risk of adverse events increases with higher vitamin intake (above 10.000 IU) if supplements are routinely used by people in these populations [297].

The WHO [200] recommends the implementation of other nutritional interventions, such as food diversification and food fortification, which should be adopted together with vitamin A supplementation, in order to improve vitamin intake.

Calcium

Daily supplementation of 1.5–2.0 g of elemental calcium orally has been recommended for populations with low dietary calcium intake, aiming to reduce the risk of preeclampsia [295–297]. The WHO [295] recommends that calcium supplementation be prescribed at the first prenatal contact.

The WHO declares in 2020 that new evidence is needed to determine the effectiveness of supplementation before pregnancy and its continuity during pregnancy [112, 296]. Prepregnancy calcium supplementation to prevent preeclampsia is only recommended in the context of rigorous research [296].

Calcium supplementation scheme recommended by WHO [295, 296] for populations with low dietary calcium intake (<900 mg / day):

- Recommended dose: supplementation of 1.5–2.0 g/day, with the total dose divided into three doses, preferably taken with meals, in order to improve acceptability. Consider: 1 g of elemental calcium is equivalent to 2.5 g of calcium carbonate or 4 g of calcium citrate.
- Due to the possible negative interactions between iron and calcium supplements, the two supplements should be administered at different times, with several hours apart.
- Dietary advice for pregnant women should promote adequate calcium intake through the consumption of locally available calcium-rich foods.
- Calcium supplementation should be prescribed at the first prenatal visit.

When supplementation with high doses of calcium is not feasible or well tolerated by the pregnant woman, the option of supplement with a lower dose (500 milligrams –mg to 600 mg per day) may be an alternative for the prevention of preeclampsia [111, 113].

The WHO [296] recognizes that calcium requirements are increased during pregnancy and declares that the needs of this nutrient are easily achieved with the consumption of milk and dairy products. Dietary advice should be given to all women of childbearing age and consumption of source foods should be encouraged, considering the local availability of calcium-rich foods [296].

WHO [296] warns that a high salt diet lowers body calcium retention compared with a low salt diet. Another warning from WHO [297] is regarding the excessive consumption of caffeine present in soft drinks and energy drinks, as well as the protein-rich diet that can induce hypercalciuria, although to a lesser extent.

The committee [296] also recommends the fortification of staple foods with calcium as an important public health intervention in places where dietary calcium intake is low.

Iron

Insufficient consumption and the high prevalence of iron deficiency among women, support the recommendation for prophylactic supplementation during pregnancy to prevent anemia, puerperal sepsis, preterm birth, and low birth weight [178, 289].

The scheme for daily iron and folic acid supplementation in pregnant women is [289, 297]:

- Supplement composition Iron: 30–60 mg of elemental iron/one supplement daily (30 mg of elemental iron equals 90 mg of ferrous fumarate, 150 mg of ferrous sulfate heptahydrate or 250 mg of ferrous gluconate).
- Folic acid: 400μg (0.4 mg).
- Duration throughout pregnancy; supplementation with iron and folic acid should begin as early as possible.

In populations where anemia in pregnant women is a serious public health problem (prevalence greater than or equal to 40% of pregnant women with hemoglobin concentration <11.0 g/dL), the recommended daily dose is 60 mg of elemental iron ([289]).

In cases of anemia, the iron supplementation dose should be adjusted to 120 mg/day until maternal hemoglobin concentrations are normal, returning to the prophylactic dose [297].

If the daily iron supplementation scheme is not well tolerated because of side effects and in populations with anemia prevalence among pregnant women below 20%, alternatively, intermittent oral supplementation with 120 mg of elemental iron and 2800μg can be prescribed (2.8 mg) of folic acid, once a week [289].

As complementary strategies to iron supplementation, WHO [289] recommends dietary diversification with stimulating the consumption of foods that are sources of iron, vitamin A, vitamin B12, and folic acid, that is, with increased consumption of vegetables, fruits, and foods of animal origin such as meat, liver or other viscera, fish and chicken, turkey which are rich sources of bioavailable iron. Vegetable sources of iron are less bioavailable and the association with sources of organic citric, malic or ascorbic acids (vitamin C) in the same meal can improve the absorption of iron from these foods. And the use of nonheme iron inhibitors, such as polyphenols present in tea and coffee (can be consumed 1–2 hours after the big meal- lunch/dinner), calcium present in dairy products that should be consumed in small meals, should be avoided/snacks, and phytates present in oats, wheat germ, and lentils.

Folic Acid

The 400μg dose of folic acid supplementation in the preconception phase, started at least 1 month before fertilization and continued in the first trimester of pregnancy, is recommended to prevent NTD [15, 297]. The adequate folate levels at the time of pregnancy have been shown to decrease the incidence of NTD by 50–70% [36].

In women at higher risk (history of NTD in previous pregnancies, own or partner history), the dose is 4000μg, starting 3 months before conception. Women with obesity, DM or using antiepileptic drugs may be resistant to the protective effect of folic acid supplementation to NTD, even in higher doses [15].

Recommendations of folic acid supplementation apply to women and adolescent pregnant within the prenatal care:

- Folic acid: 400μg (0.4 mg)/daily oral and iron supplementation (30–60 mg of elemental iron) for pregnant women to prevent maternal anemia, puerperal sepsis, low birth weight, and preterm birth [289, 297].
- Duration throughout pregnancy: supplementation with iron and folic acid should begin as early as possible.

Continuing supplementation of folic acid associated with iron during pregnancy is recommended to prevent anemia, puerperal sepsis, preterm birth, and low birth weight [297].

In some countries, folic acid supplements contain up to 5 mg, and this has caused discussion about the potential impairment of overdoses in low-risk pregnancies for NTD [250]. In experimental models, high-dose folic acid supplementation has been linked to fetal metabolic disorders [272], while in humans, high concentrations of folate in early pregnancy appear to indicate a higher incidence of autism spectrum disorder [87], results that demonstrate the importance of more evidence to consolidate conclusions on the topic [250].

Vitamin D

The WHO [297] does not recommend vitamin D supplementation as a routine in prenatal care. However, this practice seems to reduce the risk for preeclampsia, GDM, maternal hemorrhage, and low birth weight [205], so it must be considered in an individualized and context-specific assessment to define necessary doses and period intervention during pregnancy [114, 222].

Considering the high prevalence of hypovitaminosis D among pregnant women [277], the recommendations of the Endocrine Society [114] recently corroborated by specialists from the Brazilian Association of Nutrology [222] include pregnant women in the risk group for hypovitaminosis D, considering serum 25-hydroxyvitamin D concentrations above 30 ng/ml as ideal during pregnancy. In order for these concentrations to be maintained, pregnant women need at least 600 IU daily of vitamin D, and even higher doses may be needed, such as 1500–2000 IU daily [114].

Nutritional supplements not recommended or recommended in specific contexts by WHO [297] are as follows:

Not Recommended

- In malnourished populations, supplements with high protein content are not recommended for pregnant women to improve maternal and perinatal outcomes [297].
- The supplementation of multiple micronutrients, vitamins B6 (pyridoxine), D, E and C are not recommended for pregnant women to improve maternal and perinatal outcomes [297].

Recommendations for Specific Contexts

- Zinc supplementation during pregnancy is only recommended in the context of rigorous research [297].
- For malnourished populations:
  - Promote nutritional education to increase daily energy and protein intake to reduce the risk of low birth weight [297].
  - Recommend a daily supplement with energy and proteins to reduce the risk of fetal death and of small newborns for gestational age [297].

Use of Probiotics in Pregnancy

Probiotics are living microorganisms that can promote health benefits to the host when administered in adequate amounts [109]. Pregnancy is a period of physiological adaptations that influence the composition of the intestinal microbiota. The use of probiotics in pregnancy appears to improve glycemic control, decreasing insulin resistance, with no significant effect on the incidence of gestational diabetes [170]. In women with GDM, the use of probiotics can improve insulin sensitivity, but the protection against adverse outcomes related to the condition is still controversial [207, 267, 306]. Protective effect of probiotic supplementation in pregnant women has been identified for eczema, atopic eczema, duration of pregnancy, necrotizing enterocolitis, and maternal mortality [147].

However, the effects of probiotics on human health are specific to each strain or its combinations and can interact with individual factors, making the definition of specific compositions, doses and intervention periods that can be extrapolated to clinical practice complex. *Lactobacillus* and *Bifidobacterium* strains are the most tested in studies with pregnant women, usually offered in capsules or added to dairy products [147, 170].

Nutritional Guidance in Common Situations During Pregnancy

Pregnant women should be advised that digestive signs and symptoms are frequent during pregnancy and that they can be resolved with simple dietary measures [185, 189].

Nausea and Vomiting

They are common in early pregnancy around 50–90% of pregnant women and may be related to increased levels of the hormone human chorionic gonadotropin and estrogen during pregnancy. Depending on the severity of the condition, it can cause anorexia [189].

Nausea and vomiting may be associated with an increase/decrease in food consumption, and replacement of healthy foods with ultra-processed foods, compromising the quality of the diet and causing weight loss or gain below the recommended [70].

Early treatment of nausea and vomiting should be employed to prevent the progression of the condition to hyperemesis gravidarum, which can be associated with severe weight loss during pregnancy, maternal nutritional deficiencies, restricted intrauterine growth, and even maternal death [13].

Management [185, 235, 297]

- Careful assessment of food consumption and dietary changes caused by the condition.
- Explain to the pregnant woman that there are frequent symptoms during pregnancy.
- Indicate fractional diet (6 meals per day) with less food volume per meal.
- Discourage the consumption of fatty foods, foods with a strong odor, and those that cause discomfort and/or intolerance.
- Suggest modification of the spices used in the preparations, avoiding the use of spicy condiments.
- Suggest consumption of more solid and high-carbohydrate foods (e.g., biscuits, toast, yogurt, and fruit jelly) in the first meal of the day.
- Encourage water and liquid intake between meals to avoid dehydration. Stimulate fruit consumption with broth.
- Avoid food monotony and encourage variation in food.
- Guide the pregnant woman to avoid lying down after large meals (lunch and dinner), to prevent reflux and worsening of the condition.

- As nonpharmacological therapies, ginger capsules (250 mg/oral, 4 times/day) and acupuncture have been recommended [4, 185, 297]. Eating ginger foods may be an option.

Heartburn

It is caused by the action of the hormone progesterone, which causes hypotonia of the favorite lower esophageal sphincter or gastrophageal reflux, and due to the pressure of the pregnant uterus on the stomach [185].

Management [185, 235, 287]

- Indicate fractional diet and small volumes.
- Discourage the consumption of coffee, tea, mate, sweets, fried foods, and alcohol and tobacco.
- Discourage the consumption of foods that cause discomfort/intolerance.
- Clarify that milk should be included in dietary planning, avoiding its use as a resource for gastric tamponade, since it is able to stimulate gastric secretion.
- Guide pregnant women to avoid lying in horizontal decubitus after meals and the position of the trunk curved forward when in the sitting position.

Ptyalism or Sialorrhea (Excessive Salivation)

Pregnant ptyalism is of unknown origin, usually occurs in the early stages of pregnancy and can be associated with nausea. Some researchers consider that the condition has a physiological and nonpsychological origin and that there is no effective medication. According to the reports of pregnant women affected by the condition, they describe difficulty in swallowing their saliva and prefer to spit it out. In clinical practice, it is observed that ptyalism can be increased with the ingestion of starch [185, 265].

Management [185, 235, 265]

- Indicate a fractional diet (five to six meals a day), with less volume.
- Stimulate the consumption of cold liquids.
- Stimulate fruit consumption with broth.
- Guide the swallowing of saliva.
- Orientation similar to that indicated for nausea and vomiting.

Intestinal Constipation and Flatulence

Constipation is a disorder resulting from decreased intestinal motility due to the action of the hormone progesterone and the pressure caused by the pregnant uterus causing displacement of the intestines.

Constipation symptoms started before pregnancy are usually due to dietary errors, low fluid intake and physical inactivity, and they can worsen during pregnancy. Flatulence can occur associated with constipation. And hemorrhoids can arise as a complication of intestinal constipation and by the compression of the large intestine by the enlarged uterus, so the prevention of constipation is the best way to prevent hemorrhoids [185, 235].

Management [185, 235, 297]

- Stimulate the consumption of water and liquids.
- Encourage increased fiber consumption: whole fruits and raw bagasse and vegetables, whole products (cereals, breads, biscuits, flour) and wheat or oat bran that should be eaten with liquids and should not be included in large meals (lunch and dinner), as they can interfere with the absorption of non-heme iron. To advise the pregnant woman that the effect of the fiber may not be immediate, as it is not a medication, but its prolonged use is effective. Wheat semolina or others can be used as an alternative, if there is no response to diet modification.
- Guide to observe tolerance to flatulent foods (garlic, sweet potato, broccoli, onion, cabbage, cauliflower, peas, beans, corn, egg, radish, cabbage, and among others).
- Avoid physical inactivity and adopt a healthy lifestyle by increasing physical activity, if there is no medical contraindication.
- Guide for the care of the rectal reflex. Create a daily sanitary habit, preferably in the morning, after breakfast.
- Guide for proper chewing of food, avoid talking during meals and eat slowly.

Pica

Pica is an eating disorder in which there is persistent ingestion of nonnutritive substances for a period of at least 1 month or ingestion of nonnutritious substances unsuitable for health or nonfood substances, unusual condiments, or atypical food combinations. This practice may be associated with stress, anxiety, anemia, pregnancy complications, intestinal obstruction, digestive symptoms among others [33, 71, 93, 160, 243].

The nonfood substances most often cited as consumed by adult pregnant women and adolescents are pagophagy (excessive intake of ice), geophagy (ingestion of earth/clay), amylophagy (ingestion of gum, mainly from laundry) and other substances such as hair, coal, ash, nail cuticle, enamel, antacid tablets, detergent, sponges, phosphorus, diaper, soot, gasoline, chalk, milk of magnesia, mothballs, burnt matchsticks, pieces of tube, stone and gravel, plastic, scented cleaning with pine, dog food, soap, dirt, paint, paper towel. And the most mentioned atypical combinations are green fruits with lemon and salt, sweet with bread [33, 71, 160, 243].

The cases must be investigated in all prenatal consultations and treated by a multidisciplinary team.

Management [33, 71, 235]

- Talk to the pregnant woman, investigating emotional or family problems that may be associated.
- Guide her to replace this practice by eating her favorite foods and avoid contact with the "desired" substance.
- Clarify that the practice can contribute to the occurrence or aggravation of anemia, impair the absorption of nutrients, leading to diseases such as parasites and pregnancy complications.

Vitamin A Deficiency

Vitamin A deficiency affects about 19 million (15.3%) of pregnant women worldwide [200]. Pregnancy deficiency can be associated with anemia [174, 192, 193, 212, 238, 269], premature birth, HDP, greater chance of maternal mortality from respiratory infection and other infections [59, 60]. The presence of gestational night blindness increases the chance of infant mortality in the first 6 months of life [61] in addition to a greater chance of low birth weight newborns and infant morbidities (diarrhea, dysentery and infection acute respiratory disease, [270]).

Despite these classic findings, randomized clinical trial studies have not shown the beneficial effect of prenatal vitamin A supplementation alone or combined with other micronutrients in reducing maternal or perinatal mortality [174, 200]. Evidence demonstrates the beneficial effect of prenatal vitamin A supplementation in preventing and treating gestational night blindness and in reducing maternal anemia in women living in areas where vitamin A deficiency is common [174, 200].

Among the factors associated with vitamin A deficiency, we have inadequate consumption of food sources of the vitamin, worse sociodemographic conditions [200], history of abortion, short intergestational interval (<24 months), low-number prenatal consultations (<6 consultations) and with the prenatal nutritionist, and use of cigarettes and alcohol during pregnancy [192, 200, 237, 238, 244] .

In prenatal care, the diagnosis of gestational night blindness can be made with the application of the standardized adapted interview, as given in Table 8.5 [200, 235, 242, 288], which must be applied in all prenatal consultations, to diagnose vitamin A deficiency in pregnant women, enabling interventions to correct the deficiency.

For the treatment of night blindness or inadequate serum retinol (<1.05μmol/L) in pregnant women or women of reproductive age, vitamin A supplementation is recommended orally, in liquid form based on retinyl palmitate oil or retinyl acetate, with daily oral dose of 10.000 IU or weekly dose of 25.000 IU weekly, doses considered safe for pregnant women at any gestational age. Treatment must be for at least 12 weeks during pregnancy and until delivery [200].

Supplementation with vitamin A in doses greater than 25.000 IU are not recommended for the gestational period, as they can have a teratogenic effect if consumed between days 15 and 60 after conception (day 0); 60 days after conception, the safety of a single dose of vitamin A above 25.000 IU is uncertain [200]. Women with high vitamin A intake through food, when exceeding 8.000 IU or 2.400 μgRE, should not use vitamin A supplements due to the potential risk of adverse events [297]. Therefore, in clinical practice, supplementation should be carefully prescribed and discussed by the team, considering all the vitamin supplements used by pregnant women and the consumption of source foods.

Bovine liver is an important dietary source of this vitamin, contains 14.574 μgRE [266] and can be indicated as an alternative for the use of supplementation, in the maximum amount of 100 g once a week, associated with regular nutritional monitoring during pregnancy, encouraging healthy eating for pregnancy ([55, 200, 266]).

The other intervention measures that should be employed in the prevention and treatment of gestational night blindness, according to WHO [297] are:

- Stimulate the consumption of source foods, reaching the dietary reference intake (DRI) for pregnancy (Table 8.7).
- Stimulate the preference for vitamin A fortified foods.
- Investigate gestational anemia and encourage adherence to the supplementation scheme prescribed for the prevention or treatment of anemia.
- Discourage the use of cigarettes and alcohol during pregnancy [244].
- Encourage pregnant women to follow the proposed antenatal consultation schedule.

Anemia

Anemia is considered a serious public health problem in 141 countries worldwide and the regions most affected are Africa and Southeast Asia [293]. Anemia is characterized by a low concentration of hemoglobin in the blood, which causes a decrease in the blood's ability to transport oxygen to the tissues, can cause fatigue, low productivity and shortness of breath among others [289].

Anemia affects more than 30% of pregnant women worldwide, with the majority of cases resulting from iron deficiency [294]. Maternal anemia can increase the risk of maternal infections and is associated with a higher risk of low birth weight, preterm birth, maternal, neonatal, and perinatal mortality [216]. The impairment of the nutritional status of iron in the newborn with impaired psychomotor development and cognitive function in childhood has also been associated with maternal anemia [100, 190, 289, 293].

Iron supplementation during pregnancy has been an effective strategy in the prevention and treatment of gestational anemia compared with placebo, but the effect on reducing low birth weight and premature birth remains to be confirmed [208].

The routine indication for iron supplementation to prevent anemia during pregnancy has been the subject of debate, as several countries adopt iron supplementation programs during pregnancy, even in cases of absence of anemia, which is associated with increased hemoglobin concentrations.

It is noteworthy that some studies show that high concentrations of hemoglobin in the second or third trimesters are associated with lower birth weight; fetal growth restriction and increased risk for admission to the prenatal intensive care unit [7, 65]. The authors suggest the beneficial effect of hemodilution and lower hemoglobin concentrations (without anemia diagnosis) in pregnancy for placental function, positively influencing birth weight. Other studies demonstrate an increase in oxidative stress, which can cause damage to the intestinal epithelium due to the increase in iron concentration associated with unnecessary iron supplementation during pregnancy [8, 51, 179].

The findings encourage reflection on the need for iron supplementation in pregnant women without anemia [261, 289, 297]. Oral prophylaxis with iron during pregnancy improves the stores of this nutrient and prevents iron deficiency anemia [179]. On the other hand, researchers have demonstrated the existence of a U-shaped curve for low and high concentrations of maternal hemoglobin and the risks of adverse outcomes to pregnancy and birth [44, 73].

The development of anemia is associated with three main mechanisms: ineffective erythropoiesis, hemolysis, and blood loss. Nutritional deficiencies, diseases and genetic disorders of hemoglobin are the most common mechanisms. Anemias are often classified according to the cause – nutritional anemias or hemolytic anemias, and can also be classified by the characteristics of red blood cells (erythrocytes) – size, shape and color.

The interpretation of mean corpuscular volume (MCV) of erythrocytes differentiates iron deficiency anemia from megaloblastic. MCV values <80 dL correspond to microcytic anemia (hypochromic, each red blood cell is reduced and the cells are smaller than normal like, is characteristic of iron-deficiency) and MCV > 100 dL correspond to megaloblastic anemia (macrocytic, red cells are larger than normal, is characteristic of folate or vitamin B12 deficiencies [215, 289].

In the pregnancy, the iron deficiency is the most common cause of anemia among pregnant women. Pregnant women are among the most vulnerable groups to develop iron deficiency and anemia due to the increase in iron needs during pregnancy [289].

The evaluation of the hemoglobin concentration in the blood is the recommended method to diagnose anemia during pregnancy. As this concentration is influenced by gestational hemodilution, specific cutoff points should be used for pregnancy. This method is relatively easy and inexpensive and can be done with capillary or venous blood. However, isolated measurement does not determine the cause of anemia, although hemoglobin concentration is used as a proxy indicator of iron deficiency and iron deficiency anemia ([289, 294], Table 8.4).

In 2020, WHO [294] began to recommend the assessment of serum or plasma ferritin to identify the status of iron, as this parameter correlates with total body iron stores and serves to identify iron deficiency and iron overload in the body (Table 8.4). The evaluation of ferritin can be performed together with the evaluation of hemoglobin to identify anemia [294]. Physiological changes in pregnancy, such as expansion of blood volume, blood composition and inflammation, may make it difficult to define the single cutoff point for the diagnosis of iron deficiency during pregnancy according to the concentration of ferritin. With this, the measures of inflammation, C-reactive protein (CRP) or α-1 acid glycoprotein (AGP), and additional indices of iron such as the soluble transferrin receptor are analyzed together [294].

Some studies show that in communities where anemia is prevalent among pregnant women, vitamin A deficiency should also be investigated [159, 193, 269, 289].

Findings suggest that nutritional intervention to improve the nutritional status of vitamin A in deficient populations also results in a reduction in anemia. Supplementation with vitamin A or beta-carotene reduced the risk of anemia by 19% during pregnancy [269], and the increase in mean hemoglobin concentration during pregnancy was also demonstrated after vitamin A supplementation [269].

Management [149, 215, 289, 296, 297]

- Stimulate the consumption of food sources of iron (Table 8.7).
- Encourage the consumption of foods fortified with iron and folic acid, taking care not to encourage excessive consumption of fortified flours and products made with them, to avoid excessive weight gain.
- Stimulate the consumption of fruits rich in vitamin C with meals with sources of nonheme iron (vegetable), lunch, and dinner.
- Discourage the consumption of coffee, tea, mate, soda, milk and dairy products, soy drinks and foods rich in fiber (bran or whole foods) with lunch and dinner.
- Encourage adherence to the use of the iron supplementation scheme recommended by the prenatal team.
- Investigate parasites.
- Investigate gestational night blindness (Table 8.5) in all prenatal consultations, to assess the nutritional status of vitamin A.

Hypertensive Disorders of Pregnancy (HDP)

The hypertensive disorders of pregnancy (HDP) are among the main causes of maternal mortality [292] representing 14% of maternal deaths worldwide. In the classification adopted by the ACOG [14], the stages are as follows: preeclampsia/eclampsia (which stand out as the main causes of obstetric and perinatal mortality and morbidity), chronic hypertension, preeclampsia superimposed upon chronic hypertension, and gestational hypertension.

Diagnostic criteria for preeclampsia according to ACOG [14] are as follows: systolic blood pressure ≥140 mm Hg or diastolic blood pressure ≥90 mm Hg, on two occasions at least 4 hours apart, after 20 weeks of gestation in a woman with a previously normal blood pressure; or systolic blood pressure ≥160 mm Hg or diastolic blood pressure ≥110 mm Hg (severe hypertension), and proteinuria (≥300 mg/24 h urine collection), or protein/creatinine ratio ≥ 0.3 mg/dL or dipstick reading = 2 + (used only if other quantitative methods are not available).

Or in the absence of proteinuria, preeclampsia is diagnosed as hypertension with thrombocytopenia (platelet count <100,000 × 10^9/L), or renal insufficiency (serum creatinine concentrations >1.1 mg/dL), or impaired liver function (elevated blood concentrations of liver transaminases to twice normal concentration), or pulmonary edema.

The gestational hypertension is diagnosed after 20 weeks of gestation in a woman with a previously normal blood pressure [14]. The chronic hypertension is diagnosed before pregnancy or up to 20 weeks of pregnancy [188]. The preeclampsia is superimposed when developed upon chronic hypertension, and eclampsia is the convulsive manifestation of the HDP [14]. The most severe cases of preeclampsia are characterized by hemolysis, elevated liver enzymes, and very low platelet count, called HELLP syndrome, and are associated with increased rates of maternal morbidity and mortality [14].

Most maternal deaths from HDP are preventable through adequate prevention and treatment; prenatal care should be provided by a trained prenatal team and adequate resources. Adequate and early prevention and treatment of HDP is part of the recommended strategies for achieving the Sustainable Development Goals by 2030 [296].

It has been estimated that preeclampsia complicates 2–8% of pregnancies globally [14] and HDP is associated with low birth weight (birth weight <2.5 kg), asphyxia, fetal death, intrauterine growth restriction, premature and surgical delivery, fetal distress, and longer hospitalization of newborns. In addition, pregnant women who develop preeclampsia are at increased risk of future cardiovascular diseases [254] in addition to changes in the lipid profile. The highest concentrations of VLDL-cholesterol and triglycerides are positively correlated with proteinuria [157].

Rezende et al. [221] described that the prevalence of preeclampsia in pregnant women attended at a public maternity and school in Rio de Janeiro, Brazil, among all pregnant women attended at the unit in the period 2011–2012, was 6.7% (n = 301). Preeclampsia was associated with higher rates of prematurity and fetal death, especially among cases that occurred before the 34th–37th gestational week. Higher rates of small to gestational age were associated with cases that occurred before the 37th–42nd gestational week [221].

The women most at risk for developing HDP are those with risk factors such as nulliparity, multifetal gestations, preeclampsia in a previous pregnancy, chronic hypertension pregestational, DM, GDM, thrombophilia, systemic lupus erythematosus, prepregnancy BMI >30, antiphospholipid antibody syndrome, maternal age 35 years or older, kidney disease, assisted reproductive technology, obstructive sleep apnea, nulliparity, ethnic groups (afro-descendants), low socioeconomic status, dyslipidemia, history of early cardiovascular disease, family history of HDP [14, 302, 305].

In view of the impact of HDP on the health of the mother–child binomial, screening for women at risk should occur in the prenatal period as early as possible, preferably in the first trimester of pregnancy [14, 186].

In HDP, there are multisystemic alterations such as inflammatory reaction, endothelial dysfunction with increased platelet aggregation, and tissue hypoxia in target organs (kidneys, liver, brain, lung, heart, eyes, uterus, and placenta). These changes cause the appearance of clinical manifestations of pre-eclampsia impairing fetal development, such as possible growth restriction, fetal distress, and oligohydramnios. [14, 186].

Several researchers have tested nutritional interventions using food and nutritional supplements of single or combined nutrients to prevent preeclampsia in the past 30 years; however, the evidence available to date is insufficient to demonstrate the effectiveness of the interventions. Among the studied nutrients, vitamins C, D, E and folic acid, calcium, calcium and *n*-6, magnesium, fish oil, garlic supplementation, or sodium restriction are important [14]. WHO [296] has been reviewing the evidence about calcium supplementation in the prevention of HDP, and based on meta-analyses, WHO has recommended calcium supplementation for pregnant women with low dietary intake (<900 mg/day) [295–297]. The recommended dose is a daily supplementation of 1.5–2.0 g of oral elemental calcium, which is initiated from the first prenatal consultation [295, 296].

Among these dietary approaches, the DASH diet (Dietary Approaches to Stop Hypertension) has been recommended as a nonmedication strategy for the prevention and treatment of hypertension in adults, individuals with obesity or DM, and pregnant women with GDM [20, 25, 28–31, 34, 45, 83, 89, 141].

Management [236, 295–297]

- For nutritional assessment, follow the same procedures suggested for healthy pregnant women.
- Program gestational weight gain according to the pregestational BMI (Table 8.1). The restriction of gestational weight gain does not prevent HDP.

Nutritional recommendations for HDP cases:

- Energy: suitable for the recommended gestational weight gain (Table 8.6).
- Macronutrients: adequate diet in proteins, carbohydrates and lipids (Table 8.6), with reduced amount of saturated fat, trans, and cholesterol.
- Micronutrients: adequate diet in vitamins and minerals (Table 8.7).

- Normal sodium diet (up to 5 g/day), avoiding foods rich in sodium, such as processed and ultra-processed foods. Sodium restriction does not prevent HDP and may be associated with increased edema and is not indicated [295, 297].
- In cases of pregestational chronic hypertension, the diet should have low sodium, with an intake <2.4 g/day [188].
- Calcium supplementation should be prescribed when dietary intake is <900 mg/day (see section Use of Supplements During Pregnancy, [112, 113, 295–297]).
- Recommend increasing water and fluid intake.
- Recommend the consumption of food sources of n3 fatty acids: anchovies, carp, herring, mackerel, salmon, sardines and sturgeon, two to three servings of fish/week.
- Encourage the consumption of natural spices, fruits, vegetables, dairy products with less fat content, and fresh or minimally processed foods (Table 8.3).
- Adjust the consistency of the diet according to the acceptance of the pregnant woman, especially in the most severe cases of eclampsia and HELLP syndrome.
- Smoking and alcohol consumption should be discouraged [188].

Diabetes Mellitus in Pregnancy

DM is an important health problem that has reached alarming levels today, as, according to estimates by the International Diabetes Federation [135], 463 million people worldwide have the disease and by 2045 that number should reach 700 million [135]. It is estimated that hyperglycemia in pregnancy affects approximately one in six pregnancies [135].

During pregnancy, DM cases are classified as GDM (diabetes diagnosed in the second or third trimester of pregnancy that was not clearly overt diabetes prior to gestation), Type 1 diabetes (DM1, due to autoimmune β-cell destruction, usually leading to absolute insulin deficiency), Type 2 diabetes (DM2, due to a progressive loss of adequate β-cell insulin secretion frequently on the background of insulin resistance) and specific types of diabetes due to other causes (e.g., monogenic diabetes syndromes, diseases of the exocrine pancreas, and drug- or chemical-induced diabetes [18].

Cases of DM during pregnancy should be identified as early as possible and treated by a specialized multidisciplinary team to minimize the negative repercussions for the mother–child binomial [18]. Maternal hyperglycemia in the early gestation periods, embryonic period (4–8 weeks of gestation, [148]), can affect fetal development and can increase the chance of fetal anomalies (especially in the cardiovascular and nervous systems – NTD). Other negative repercussions are spontaneous abortion, fetal demise, macrosomy (birth weight >4.0 kg in term pregnancies or weight above the 90th percentile for gestational age), neonatal hypoglycemia, hyperbilirubinemia, and neonatal respiratory distress syndrome [18].

In addition, it has been described that DM in pregnancy can increase the risk of obesity, hypertension and DM2 in the offspring later in life [16]. Inadequate glycemic control increases the chance of complications from DM, such as retinopathy and nephropathy, in addition to the greater chance of preeclampsia [18, 47].

In Gestational Diabetes Mellitus (GDM), there is a change in insulin sensitivity due to the physiological adjustments of pregnancy, accompanied by an ineffective pancreatic counter-response, usually detected in the second half of pregnancy. The resulting hyperglycemia interferes with fetal growth by increasing the chance of fetal macrosomia (birth weight > 4.0 kg), neonatal hypoglycemia, in addition to obesity and slower psychomotor development in the children of these pregnant women [18, 47]. Women with DMG are at an increased risk of progressing to DM 2 in the future [18, 47].

Currently, there is no consensus on the best strategy for screening and diagnosing GDM (Table 8.4). The prevalence of GDM will vary depending on the diagnostic method adopted. The ADA [16, 18] recommends two diagnostic methods, the "one-step" 75-g OGTT derived from the International Association of Diabetes and Pregnancy Study Groups [134] criteria, or the older "two-step" approach with a 50-g (nonfasting) screen followed by a 100-g OGTT for those who screen positive [18]. And WHO [297] recommends screening for the diagnosis of GDM at any time during pregnancy, and indicates 75 g OGTT (Table 8.4).

To minimize the risk of developing DM2 after pregnancy, the ADA [18] recommends postpartum nutritional monitoring for women with GDM, with strategies to reduce excess weight.

In view of the increased risk of obstetric and perinatal morbidity and mortality, for pregnant women with DM with inadequate glycemic control, the ADA [18] emphasizes that women and adolescents of reproductive age are informed about pregnancy planning. The goal for the conception phase is glycated hemoglobin up to 6.5% (48 mmol/mol), as it is associated with a lower risk of fetal abnormalities [18].

The care with food in DM has a prominent role in the treatment and preparation of women for conception. Women with well-controlled illness have the same chances of conceiving a child as healthy as the general population, as long as some preconceptional care is taken and throughout pregnancy [18].

Management

Preconception: the care of women with DM must begin in the preconception phase. ADA [18] recommends the prescription of folic acid supplement (400μg); advice on moderate caffeine consumption; advise against the use of cigarettes, marijuana, and alcohol; counseling on the risks of obesity in pregnancy and specialized nutritional monitoring for weight loss in cases of overweight and obesity; meal planning to achieve glycemic goals before conception; correction of nutritional deficiencies; healthy lifestyle recommendations with regular moderate exercise; guidance to avoid hyperthermia (in hot tubs) and adequate sleep.

Objective of nutritional care for pregnant women with DM and DMG: to achieve glycemic goals, to promote adequate maternal weight gain according to the pregestational BMI and to prevent unfavorable fetal and neonatal obstetric outcomes and complications of DM and comorbidities.

- Ideally, prenatal care should be performed by a specialized multidisciplinary team.
- Nutritional monitoring should be done by a nutritionist, with a calendar of 5–6 consultations (individual and in groups) during the entire pregnancy, with an interval between consultations of 15 days between the first and the second and the following, it can be a 30-day interval [202].

The glycemic goals in pregnancy recommended by the ADA [18] for women with GDM and DM1 or DM2 are as follows:

- Fasting glucose <95 mg/dL (5.3 mmol/L).
- Either 1-hour postprandial glucose <140 mg/dL (7.8 mmol/L) or 2-hour postprandial glucose <120 mg/dL (6.7 mmol/L).

The goals must be achieved without significant hypoglycemia, so less strict control may be necessary to prevent hypoglycemia and care must be individualized. The goal of glycated hemoglobin (A1C) is 6% (42 mmol/mol) in the pregnancy of women with preexisting DM, without significant hypoglycemia [18].

- For nutritional assessment, follow the same procedures for healthy pregnant women.
- Program gestational weight gain according to the pregestational BMI (Table 8.1). The restriction of gestational weight gain is not recommended for pregnant women with DM or DMG [18].
- Nutritional recommendations: estimate nutritional recommendations considering BMI, maternal age, lifestyle and physical activity performed, recommended gestational weight gain, socioeconomic conditions, eating habits and clinical conditions of the pregnant woman, following the same procedures for healthy pregnant women (Table 8.6).
- The calculation of the daily TEV should be individualized and the distribution of macronutrients should be recommended according to Table 8.6. The recommendations for vitamins and minerals should reach the DRI (Table 8.7). Nutritional deficiencies must be addressed.
- The method of nutritional guidance to be adopted must be combined with the pregnant woman, aiming at greater adherence to the diet plan. The most adopted in practice are the energy distribution of macronutrients per meal, and carbohydrate count. Both methods are well accepted in practice and can offer good results, when the pregnant woman is accompanied by a specialized health team, including the nutritionist [18, 202, 252, 257].
- The diet should be divided throughout the day, respecting eating habits, adjusted to the pregnant woman's life routine, to avoid extreme variations in blood glucose. Five to six meals are recommended, including small snacks and supper. For pregnant women using insulin, meal times and doses should be agreed between the doctor and the nutritionist [47]. The insulin/carbohydrate ratio must be individualized [257].
- The energy distribution of macronutrients can vary according to each meal, with a smaller proportion of energy being suggested in small meals [19, 241]: break-

fast: 10–15%; snack: 5–10%; Lunch: 20–30%; Snack: 10–15%; Dinner: 20–30%; supper (snack before bedtime): 5–10%.

- The snack before bedtime (supper) is an important meal and should be adopted to prevent episodes of hypoglycemia among pregnant women who use insulin at night and must contain 25 g of carbohydrates, in addition to proteins or lipids [47].
- The choice of low glycemic index foods can bring benefits especially in the cases of GDM [95], such as reduced fasting and postprandial glycemia (2 hours), improved lipid profile and significant reduction in the need for insulin, however in practice it is difficult to adhere to for long periods. The glycemic index of a food is defined as the rate of increase in blood glucose 2 hours after eating a 50 g portion of this food relative to the same portion of the standard food (50 g white bread or glucose, [139, 251, 259]).
- Guide the pregnant woman and her family about the signs of recognition and treatment of hypoglycemia, especially in the first trimester for pregnant women with DM1 [18].
- The use of simple carbohydrates should be avoided, and should be replaced by complex carbohydrates [18]. The types of sweeteners considered safe, provided they are used in moderation are as follows: saccharin, cyclamate, aspartame, acesulfame-K, stevioside (stevia), sucralose, mannitol, thaumatin, maltitol, xylitol, erythritol [17, 182, 202, 257]. If the products containing sweeteners have to be used for a long period, the types of sweeteners should be utilized on a rotational basis and pregnant women should be advised to read the food labels. Consumption should be moderate, around up to 6 sachets or 15 drops a day [26, 202].
- Guide the reading of food labels to identify the sweeteners present in the food. Avoid foods containing sucrose, glucose, honey, glucose syrup, and fructose (as a sweetener, [202]).
- Encourage the intake of filtered water, at least 2 liters (from 6 to 8 glasses) per day, between meals, replacing sugary drinks, including fruit juices [18].
- Discourage the consumption of processed and ultra-processed foods, which are high-calorie, high-sodium foods. Stimulate the consumption of fresh and minimally processed foods, which are richer in complex carbohydrates and fibers (Table 8.3).
- Encourage the use of seeds (sunflower, sesame, flaxseed, and others) with fruit or yogurt; chestnuts, almonds, walnuts as small snacks [181, 183].
- The evaluation of capillary blood glucose monitoring with a glucometer, according to the scheme prescribed by the doctor, contributes to the adjustment of the diet.
- The key to success for good control of DM and GDM during pregnancy and better obstetric and perinatal results are monitoring of pregnant women by a trained multidisciplinary team and educating them with regard to DM and quality prenatal care.
- Table 8.8 summarizes the nutritional recommendations for pregnant women with DM and GDM.

Table 8.8 Nutritional recommendations for pregnant women with GDM and preexisting DM

TEV/ macronutrients, micronutrients	Recommendations	Comments
Total Energy Value (TEV)	Suitable for recommended weight gain, according to prepregnancy BMI	Estimated in the same way as for healthy pregnant women, considering the additional energy needed for programmed gestational weight gain (Table 8.1)
Carbohydrates	40–55% of TEV Carbohydrates: minimum 175 g Fibers: minimum 28 g/day Sucrose: <5% of the TEV (avoid use in cases of inadequate glycemic control and excessive weight gain) Prefer the use of sweeteners, avoid fructose as a sweetener	The percentage of carbohydrate must be estimated individually in order to promote adherence to the diet plan. The adoption of a lower percentage of carbohydrates, a reduction in saturated fatty acids and an increase in foods rich in monounsaturated fatty acids, may be a strategy for cases of difficult glycemic control Choosing low glycemic index foods, whole foods, rich in fiber can bring benefits, especially for GDM cases
Proteins	15–20% of TEV	Minimum intake of 71 g/day.
Lipids	30–40% of TEV	<10% saturated fat from TEV Free of trans fatty acids Prefer monounsaturated and polyunsaturated fat n-3: minimum of 2 servings of fish/week, except for fried preparations
Vitamins and minerals	Compliance with the DRI (Table 8.7)	Supplementation recommended for healthy pregnant women (folic acid, iron) The need for calcium supplementation should be assessed by the increased risk of HDP Nutritional deficiencies must be addressed

ADA [18], Filardi et al. [95], OPAS [202], SBD [257]
TEV total energy value, *BMI* body mass Index, *GDM* gestational diabetes mellitus, *HDP* hypertensive disorders of pregnancy, *DRI* dietary reference intake

Nutritional Aspects of Puerperium

The weeks after delivery are a critical period for maternal and child health, recognized as the "fourth trimester" of pregnancy [273]. Postpartum care must include physical, social, and psychological well-being aspects. However, the intense focus on women's health during prenatal care does not have follow-up after childbirth, which has motivated new proposals for structuring postpartum care, considering the need for continuity of comprehensive health care in this period [12].

Maternal health is essential for establishing and maintaining breastfeeding. Volume and composition of breast milk has a dynamic relationship with the mother's diet and nutritional status, with effect on children's health and development [84, 88]. However, it is important to consider that nutritional counseling cannot be isolated from environmental and psychosocial issues, such as a change in routine, sleep deprivation, tiredness, pain, body changes and body concerns, important health determinants related to motherhood [12].

Nutritional Assessment of Lactating Women

Nutritional assessment of lactating women includes anthropometric measures, biochemical markers, clinical evaluation, socioeconomic indicators, and dietary intake interview to identify possible nutritional deficiencies or eating habits that represent a risk to women and infants health, as well as monitoring and guiding safe weight loss. Breastfeeding support should be part of postpartum care with careful guidance in the mother's diet to produce milk in volume and composition suitable for child development, preserving maternal nutritional status [150].

The main limitation in the nutritional assessment of nursing mothers is the lack of specific guidelines to perform anthropometric measures and references for biochemical markers [196]. This is an important limitation, since physiological, emotional and behavioral factors characteristic of puerperium impact on dietary habits and nutritional status. Endocrine changes in the pregnancy-puerperal cycle promote an increase in appetite, influencing food intake and eating behavior [110]. Prolactin and oxytocin are hormones that play a central role in lactation and affect energy balance, lipolysis, and glycemic metabolism [39, 152]. Therefore, health providers need to consider several issues in nutritional care for lactating women.

Anthropometric Assessment

The increase in body weight and adiposity are physiological changes characteristic of the pregnancy-puerperal cycle, in order to ensure the proper fetus development [133]. However, excessive gestational weight gain and postpartum weight retention are strong predictors for obesity in future. The greater the weight gain during pregnancy, the greater the weight retention and the risk for obesity in future, so that anthropometric assessment and guidance for returning to pregestational weight are extremely important [43].

Six weeks after delivery, the weight retained in relation to the pregestational weight can be attributed to the remaining mass of fat acquired during pregnancy. The increase in breast tissue due to lactation should also be considered [133]. Postpartum weight retention is the difference between the current weight and the prepregnancy weight. Nutritional status can be defined by BMI (Table 8.1). It is recommended that the woman has her adequate weight at conception, gain weight within the indicated range during pregnancy and return to her pregestational weight within 12 months after delivery [260].

Weight loss in the postpartum period should be gradual, kept in safe ranges from 0.5 to 1 kg/month for women with normal weight or 2 kg/month for those who are overweight or obese, after the first month of lactation. No weight loss that leads women to low weight should be encouraged and these cases should be observed carefully to avoid compromising breastfeeding [128].

Although the breast milk production can be maintained in conditions of insufficient energy and nutritional intake through compensatory physiological mechanisms to guarantee the child's diet, such mechanisms can cause depletion of maternal reserves, which must be carefully evaluated [84]. On the other hand, maternal obesity can affect the performance of lactation due to hormonal issues – which interfere with lactogenesis, anatomical issues – which impair positioning and attachment of the baby to the breast, and emotional issues – which affect self-esteem by body shame [167]. So, signals of possible weight-related problems during lactation that need professional attention are [130]:

- Women with normal prepregnancy BMI: Weight loss in excess of 2 kg (4.5 lb)/month after the first month postpartum; weight falling below normal BMI; weight gain leading to overweight; preoccupation with weight combined with major fluctuations in weight (possible eating disorder).
- Women with prepregnancy low weight: Any weight loss after the weight returns to the prepregnancy weight; weight loss in excess of 2 kg/month after the first month postpartum.
- Women with prepregnancy overweight: weight loss in excess of 3 kg (6.5 lb)/month after the first month postpartum; postpartum weight gain.

Dietary Assessment

It is suggested to use a 24-hour food recall or a food frequency questionnaire at each appointment with a nutritionist to assess energy and macro and micronutrient intake, fluid intake, as well as meal locations, time and consumption patterns. The importance of maternal nutrition for child development is widespread in pregnancy and much less publicized in lactation, so a worrying decreasing consumption of healthy food from pregnancy to the postpartum period can be observed [138]. The intake of processed and ultra-processed foods (Table 8.3) should be evaluated, as they are related to obesity and associated morbidities [183]. As there is a frequent inadequacy in iron, vitamin A and calcium intake [231], source foods must be carefully evaluated for adequate guidance on diet improvement (Table 8.3).

Possible myths and cultural beliefs that cause unnecessary restrictions on the mother's diet need to be investigated and solved [143]. In cases of restrictions due to infant's food allergy, the necessary substitutions to guarantee the adequate nutritional supply must be provided, as well as the specific supplementation if necessary [85].

It is important to ask woman if she is on a diet to lose weight and where she has sought information to support her eating practices [143]. Currently, it is very common to adopt fad diets, widely available on the internet, especially in situations of body concerns, which can often occur in the postpartum period. This evaluation associated with anthropometric assessment should support recommendations that protect breastfeeding, since severe dietary restrictions, use of weight loss drugs, replacement of meals by drinks (shakes) and abrupt weight loss are factors that can impact the milk production and should be strongly advised against [130]. Thus, weight loss expectations, body image concerns and depressive symptoms are strong predictors for the development of eating disorders that deserve special attention, preferably in a multidisciplinary team [223].

Pica is an eating disorder characterized by persistent ingestion of substances that are not food, which deserves investigation in postpartum nutritional and medical appointments as it may compromise the woman's nutritional status or promote exposure to toxic agents. The types of pica most reported include the geophagia (eating of earth, clay, chalk, mud, or soil); amylophagia (eating of starch) or pagophagia (eating of ice/freezer frost). It is highly prevalent among pregnant and lactating women especially upon poor regions, lower educational attainment, and high rate of anemia. Women with anemia are 1.6 times more likely to have pica compared with women without anemia [93].

Clinical and Biochemical Evaluation

Clinical evaluation should consider obstetric history, pregnancy complications, delivery conditions, general postpartum health, and breastfeeding. Women are at increased risk of developing postpartum iron deficiency and anemia if they have iron deficiency in pregnancy, acute blood losses at delivery and/or if they practice diets that are low in bioavailable iron. Clinical symptoms and signs of anemia can be observed as tiredness, breathlessness, palpitations. Women who have anemia postpartum may be at greater risk of postpartum depression. Iron deficiency impairs mother–child interactions and may compromise the emotional bonds between mother and baby [180, 289]. In nonpregnant women hemoglobin levels <12 g/dl indicate anemia (11–11.9 g/dl mild anemia, 8–10.9 g/dl moderate anemia, < 8 g/dl severe anemia) [289], although at first week postpartum the suggested cutoff value is <11 g/dl (the cutoff value for anemia at delivery) in order to make a balance between women with low and high normal peripartum blood losses [180]. The WHO also recommends the use of serum ferritin concentrations for monitoring and evaluating iron status at individual level, the cutoff value is <15μ/L to detect iron deficiency in adult women [294].

The vitamin A deficiency can be investigated through the standardized interview for diagnosis of gestational night blindness (Table 8.5), validated by biochemical assessment of serum retinol levels [242] and indicated for application in nursing mothers [299]. Maternal vitamin A deficiency and anemia are significant public health problems in a context of social and environmental vulnerability and have been considered important determinants of poor maternal and child outcomes [193].

Women diagnosed with GDM should be tested at 4–12 weeks postpartum with a 75-g OGTT using nonpregnancy criteria for persistent diabetes (fasting plasma glucose ≥126 mg/dL or 2 hour plasma glucose ≥200 mg/dL) or prediabetes (fasting plasma glucose 110–125 mg/dL or 2 hour plasma glucose 140–199 mg/dL). The glycated hemoglobin test is not recommended for the postpartum evaluation of glucose levels because it may be yet impacted by pregnancy alterations and/or by blood loss at delivery. Women with GDM history should also be tested every 1–3 years by any recommended glycemic test (annual glycated hemoglobin test, annual fasting plasma glucose, or triennial 75-g OGTT using nonpregnant thresholds) because they are at increased risk for diabetes, estimated at 50–70% after 15–25 years. The insulin dose or oral drug requirement may be evaluated at postpartum in order to be adequate to hormonal fluctuations of delivery and lactation [18].

Postpartum hypertension represents a high risk to maternal health. Clinical assessment may identify new-onset or persistent hypertension from pregnancy, as systolic blood pressure ≥140 mmHg and/or diastolic blood pressure ≥90 mmHg or severe hypertension defined as systolic blood pressure ≥160 mmHg and/or diastolic blood pressure ≥110 mmHg, which represent high risk for maternal stroke and death. Although most cases of preeclampsia and eclampsia occur within the first 48 hours postpartum, the risk can be kept elevated in the 6 weeks following delivery and events can progress to chronic hypertension, therefore, monitoring blood pressure should be routine in postnatal appointments [218, 248]. Lactation can be a protective factor for postpartum hypertensive disorders [67].

Nutritional Requirements of Lactating Women

Energy requirements are increased from 500 to 670 kcal/day in the first 6 months and from 300 to 400 kcal/day between the seventh and twelfth month due to lactation, but it is dependent on rates of milk produced, maternal nutritional status and individual characteristics [96]. Fat stores accumulated during pregnancy may cover part of the energy requirements, so overweight women or those with postpartum weight retention may not need additional calories in the diet. All women should maintain a daily intake of at least 1800 calories during lactation to preserve milk production [130, 145, 163].

The main recommendations for energy, macronutrients, fibers, and liquids daily intake during lactation are given in Table 8.6. Among macronutrients, lipids show the greatest changes in concentration and sensitivity to maternal consumption in breast milk. The supply of essential polyunsaturated fatty acids (PUFAs) to the child is totally dependent on the breast milk during exclusive breastfeeding and partially on complementary breastfeeding. Due to the importance of long-chain omega-3 PUFAs, especially DHA, for the development of the central nervous system and visual acuity, guidance for fish consumption is important during lactation, as fish is the main dietary source of DHA [81]. However, fish with possible higher mercury content, such as swordfish, tuna, shark, king mackerel, and tilefish should be avoided [86]. Counseling on reducing the consumption of ultra-processed and fried foods which are rich in omega-6 PUFAs and improve consumption of DHA-rich foods or enriched foods can be a favorable strategy to favor the omega-6:omega-3 ratio since omega-6 is widely consumed in urbanized societies and w-3 little consumed [86, 98].

A substantial water loss via milk puts women at a high risk of dehydration. Increased thirst is a physiological protective reflex induced by osmoregulatory adaptations during lactation, so women should be aware of this sign and drink water whenever they feel thirsty [10]. However, half of women seem to not reach the requirement (3.8 l total fluids), which demonstrates that this recommendation needs to be further strengthened [35].

The main recommendations for micronutrients daily intake during lactation are summarized in Table 8.7 and are mostly based on the expected concentrations of vitamins and minerals in breast milk [124–127]. However, there is an intense current discussion regarding these recommendations due to the scientific-technological progress for analyzing the composition of human milk, the understanding of complex biological interactions, the changes in nutritional status and health profile of women in the last decades, and the need for larger samples for validation [9].

Despite limitations in studies, folate, calcium, iron, copper, and zinc are micronutrients that do not seem to have milk concentrations affected by maternal consumption. On the other hand, iodine, selenium, choline and vitamins A, D, E, K, B1, B2, B6, and B12 show variations in milk content due to mother's consumption [84]. An important evidence for nutritional care is that dietary intake and nutritional status prepregnancy and during pregnancy impact the composition of breast milk [88], reinforcing the importance of planning for a healthy pregnancy with nutritional counseling starting at preconception and extending to postpartum [309].

Interventions including both diet and physical activity are effective for postpartum weight loss [75, 82]. Dietary patterns like the american MyPyramid [64, 90], Mediterranean diet [263], and DASH diet [228, 229], as well as the energy restriction of 500 kcal/day [40, 69, 119] have already been successfully tested in interventions aimed at weight loss without impair breastfeeding. Future strategies may incorporate particular aspects of metabolism during lactation, optimizing nutritional recommendations [210].

Postpartum weight retention is a strong predictor for obesity in future. According to the Institute of Medicine [131, 132], half of women have a retention greater than 4.5 kg at 6 months postpartum, while for 25%, the retention is greater than 9 kg in the same period. Nutritional counseling about healthy losing weight to return to prepregnancy weight in up to a year postpartum and to achieve appropriate BMI is strongly recommended to prevent obesity and inadequate nutritional status in the next pregnancy [260].

Nutritional guidance for a balanced diet, healthy lifestyle, and weight maintenance in an appropriate range (BMI < 25 kg/m^2) is especially important in women with a history of GDM. It is a strategy of great impact in reducing risk for the development of DM2 and cardiometabolic diseases that represent a worse prognosis for women's health and for the next pregnancies outcomes [16, 18, 156].

Interventions show better results when conducted by nutritionists, compared with those performed by other health professionals [276]. Behavioral approaches to weight loss, such as mindfulness training and intuitive eating, seem promising to reduce postpartum weight retention. Women who use to eat to relieve unpleasant feelings are disconnected from physiological hunger and satiety, and behavioral approaches work on psychological aspects related to emotional eating [153, 279].

Nutrient supplementation in lactation

The current evidence does not support the use of multiple micronutrient supplementation during lactation to increase maternal and child health as a routine practice [1]. Nutrients in milk content are sensitive to maternal consumption, such as iodine, vitamin A, vitamin B12, vitamin D, and DHA have been the focus of research. Results indicate the need of an individualized and context-specific evaluation for supplements prescription, considering local health policies, access of fortified food, and nutritional status of the population [79, 84, 106, 191, 197, 199]. Iodine supplementation, for example, is recommended by WHO [291] in countries or regions where less than 90% of households use iodized salt, at a daily dose of 250μg for pregnant and lactating women [23], while the American Thyroid Association recommends daily supplementation of 150μg for all pregnant and lactating women [21].

The Scientific Advisory Committee on Nutrition does not consider sun exposure as a safe source to reach the daily vitamin D requirement, given the complexity of factors that affect its endogenous activation and the biological mechanisms of vitamin conversion, as well as seasonal variation in solar incidence. Few foods naturally contain vitamin D and in small amounts, so the use of supplements and fortified foods that provide 400 IU (10μg) daily should be encouraged [247]. The Endocrine Society [114] and the Brazilian Association of Nutrology [222] include lactating women in the risk group for hypovitaminosis D with a need for at least 600 IU daily of vitamin D and recognize that 1500–2000 IU daily may be necessary to maintain a blood level of 25-hydroxyvitamin D above 30 ng/ml [114].

It is worth mentioning the possible interindividual variability in response to nutrient supplementation and its actual availability in breast milk, as already reported for DHA, in which the effect on milk concentrations is limited by genetic characteristics of the mother [258]. Advances in the methods of analyzing breast milk composition and more robust research in the field will improve this knowledge [9].

WHO recommends iron supplementation, with or without folic acid, for 6–12 weeks after delivery to prevent maternal anemia in places where there is a prevalence of more than 20% of anemia during pregnancy, regardless of breastfeeding practice. The doses are the same practiced during pregnancy (30–60 mg of elemental iron and 400μg of folic acid). Upon diagnosis of anemia, doses may follow country-specific determinations or WHO recommendations of 120 mg of elemental iron and 400μg of folic acid, until hemoglobin concentrations are normalized [286]. Intravenous iron therapy can be considered as a treatment option for postpartum iron deficiency anemia [264].

Over the last few years, there has been a growing interest in the consumption of placenta after birth (placentophagy). Placenta encapsulation is the most common form of this practice as a process of placing it on pills after steaming and dehydration, offered by numerous companies. The supposed positive effects would be prevention of postpartum depression, improved mood and energy, improved milk supply, important micronutrients, and reduction of postpartum bleeding, but few studies have been conducted, and those available are often of poor quality. The evidence for positive effects of placentophagy in humans is either anecdotal or limited to self-reported surveys. To date, there is no scientific evidence for any clinical or nutritional benefit of human placentophagy and there is evidence for an actual risk of harm. Placenta capsules can be a source of infection by bacteria, viruses, and toxic substances and its use should be discouraged [92].

Next topics are current concerns to reach optimal nutritional care for pregnant and lactating women.

Chrononutrition: Effect on the Health of Pregnant and Postpartum Women

Currently, further the quantity and quality of food, the frequency and time of meals appear as important aspects of nutritional guidance. As the regulation of human metabolism is aligned with the day/night cycles (light/dark), sleep deprivation and late-night eating are considered disruptors of the circadian cycle [56]. During pregnancy, the maternal circadian cycle synchronizes with that of the fetus, so the rupture can cause damage to the health of both, including the fetal programming for greater risk of developing obesity and chronic diseases later in life [118]. During lactation, the increased melatonin levels present in breast milk at night synchronizes maternal circadian cycle with that of the baby [104].

Women who work in rotational shifts, fixed night shifts (11 pm–11 am), or long hours (over 40 hours per week) during pregnancy have an increased risk of preterm delivery, miscarriage, and an infant of low birthweight or small for gestational age [48]. Pregnant women who sleep less than 6.25 hours a day are almost three times more likely to develop gestational diabetes than those who have more sleep, which represents greater risk for type 2 diabetes and cardiometabolic diseases in future [219]. Higher energy intake at late-night during pregnancy may be related to greater weight retention at 18 months postpartum [164].

Short sleep duration, quite common during breastfeeding, is associated with weight retention and body adiposity in postpartum women. Sleeping less than 5 hours a day in the first year postpartum increases by two to three times the risk of weight retention greater than 5 kg and is associated with high body weight 3 years after delivery [301]. Black and Hispanic women with prepregnancy obesity and who slept less than 7 hours a day at 5 months postpartum showed weight gain at the end of the first year, unlike women with obesity who slept more than 7 hours or without obesity, who had weight loss. Sleep duration seems to have an independent association with weight loss or gain during first year postpartum [108].

Veganism and Vegetarianism During Pregnancy and Lactation

A diet that reduces or excludes animal-derived foods can be safely adopted in all stages of life, including pregnancy and lactation, as long as it is properly planned to meet the specific energy and nutrient requirements [176]. Proteins, calcium, iron, zinc, vitamin B12, vitamin D and omega-3 PUFAs are nutrients that may be critical in plant-based diets for pregnant and lactating women [5].

The Scientific Society for Vegetarian Nutrition has reviewed the available evidence for adequate nutritional guidance for vegan women during pregnancy and lactation and recommends adopting a diet with a wide variety of plant foods, including grains, legumes, vegetables, fruits, oils, nuts, and seeds, as well as complementary sources of DHA, vitamin B12, and vitamin D [37].

Protein intakes should be increased by 10% compared with the recommendation of the omnivorous pregnant or breastfeeding woman due to the lower digestibility and bioavailability of plant proteins. Additional servings of grains, legumes, soy products, nuts, and seeds may be needed [37].

Because omega-3 PUFAs from plant sources depend on rate-limited bioconversion into available DHA, pregnant and lactating women should supplement 200 mg/day of algal-derived DHA [37]. The nutritional status of vitamin D is dependent on sun exposure, with little contribution from food, except fortified ones. So, recommendations on supplements state a need for at least 600 IU daily and recognize that 1500–2000 IU daily may be necessary to maintain blood levels of 25-hydroxyvitamin D above 30 ng/ml in pregnant and lactating women, regardless of diet. Ideally, individual assessment should guide the supplementation and the need of high doses if women are vitamin D-deficient or insufficient [114, 222].

All vegan or vegetarian women of reproductive age should use supplements to reach the daily requirements of vitamin B12, since a sufficient amount cannot be found in plant foods. Optimal monitoring of B12 status includes dosage of serum homocysteine, methylmalonic acid, and holo-transcobalamin II, along with serum total vitamin B12. The usually recommended supplement doses for maintaining already normal B12 levels in pregnant and lactating women are 2μg, three times daily or 50μg in a single daily dose, which should be isolated from other micronutrients and preferably dissolved under the tongue or chewed slowly to increase the absorption. In cases of deficiency, specific schemes are indicated including injectable high doses [37].

Calcium, iron, and zinc can be obtained from dietary sources and fortified foods, as well as they can be favored by the use of appropriate dietary techniques, which can be guided by nutritionists [5, 37].

The macrobiotic diet, as well as other dietary patterns highly restricted in calories and nutrients are not safe for recommendation to pregnant and lactating women [5, 176].

DASH Diet: Health Benefits for Pregnant and Lactating Women

The DASH diet (*Dietary Approach to Stop Hypertension*) is the main nondrug treatment for reducing systemic blood pressure [58], also recommended for managing diabetes and preventing cardiovascular complications [16]. The DASH diet has a rich composition of fruits, vegetables, whole grains, nuts, seeds, and low fat dairy products, thus limiting the consumption of red meat, sweets, and foods rich in sodium [214].

Healthy women on a DASH diet at preconception may have the risk for preeclampsia reduced by up to 38%, comparing the highest with the lowest quintile of adherence to the diet [27]. In normotensive pregnant women, the DASH diet was associated with maintaining lower systolic and diastolic blood pressure throughout pregnancy [68]. Pregnant women with gestational or chronic hypertension on DASH diet for 12 weeks have the incidence of preeclampsia lower than pregnant women on a control diet (43.2% vs. 65.9%), and better outcomes of prematurity and low birth weight [140]. In pregnant women with GDM, the use of a DASH diet for 4 weeks resulted in better glycemic control, greater plasma antioxidant capacity, reduction in cesarean delivery and macrosomia compared with a control diet [29, 30].

The DASH diet was tested to reduce postpartum weight retention in a Brazilian pilot study, in which it was translated and adapted for nutritional counseling of low-income women at Primary Health Care [229]. After 3 months of intervention in monthly appointments with a nutritionist, women showed good adherence to the DASH diet and reduced postpartum weight retention, BMI, and waist circumference [228].

Early Life Programming

Intrauterine nutrition exposure exerts an effect on metabolic programming, with changes in body composition that can be determinant for health conditions and nutritional status throughout life. The risk for obesity, DM2 and cardiovascular diseases can be modulated early by nutritional factors [72, 172, 268].

Obesity and DM during pregnancy, intrauterine growth restriction, and extremes of birth weight are the factors associated with increased fat mass, reduced muscle mass, and decreased bone density, effects that can be present from childhood to adulthood [136].

Protein-energy malnutrition in pregnancy can change the expression pattern of the IGF-2 gene (insulin-like growth factor 2), which plays a central role in fetal metabolism. This change increases the risk for future obesity and is noticed in situations of intrauterine growth restriction [144]. The PPAR-gamma gene (peroxisome proliferator-activated receptor gamma) is the main regulator of adipogenesis and is overexpressed under energy–protein restriction or excessive weight gain during pregnancy, favoring hyperplasia, hypertrophy, and vascularization of fetal adipose tissue [57, 233]. Actually, both restricted diet and maternal overfeeding during pregnancy lead to changes in the expression of genes related to metabolism and the regulation of energy intake and expenditure at a central level, predisposing the individual to metabolic disorders throughout life [50].

The intake of specific nutrients during pregnancy can also modulate gene expression and modify fetal responses with long-term consequences. In this context, there are folic acid, vitamin B12, and vitamin B6, which act on the one carbon metabolism with a direct effect on genes methylation, activating or silencing gene expression. However, gene–nutrient interactions are complex and current evidence does not support specific recommendations for micronutrients that consider fetal programming, thus maintaining the nutritional recommendations already practiced for pregnant women [121].

As for macronutrients, lipids have the major potential of fetal modulation with long-term effect. Maternal diet excessive in lipids predisposes the offspring to obesity, dyslipidemia, insulin resistance, changes in endothelial function and hypertension [142]. The high consumption of saturated fatty acids during pregnancy lead to fetal dysbiosis, immune system impairment and negative behaviors in childhood [62]. On the other hand, the consumption of DHA promotes brain and visual development, offering neuroprotective effects and cognitive benefits [86].

It should be noted that the paternal nutritional status also has an impact on fetal programming. Male obesity in the reproductive age has been associated with a greater predisposition to overweight and chronic diseases in offspring. Consumption of a high-fat diet by the father before conception, as well as insulin resistance and other endocrine-metabolic characteristics related to excess body fat, imply a greater risk for metabolic syndrome in children [117, 282]. On the other hand, low protein paternal diet can modify epigenetic patterns in gametes that increase the risk for obesity and metabolic disorders in offspring [281].

The effects of maternal diet during lactation on metabolic programming are less explored compared with pregnancy. Supplementation with various doses of omega-3 PUFAs started during pregnancy or only postpartum does not present conclusive results about a possible benefit on risk for infant obesity and body composition. The same inconclusive results are observed for the effect of vitamin D supplementation and probiotics/symbiotics during lactation, with no evidence to support the effect of metabolic programming [78].

Maternal nutritional status has an important role in the composition of human milk and potential effect on the metabolic profile of children. Pregestational overweight and obesity are associated with an increase in pro-inflammatory and obesity-related fatty acids (saturated and omega-6) and insulin concentrations in breast milk assessed 2 weeks after delivery [88] and can be harmful to physical and cognitive development of children [76].

Insulin and leptin levels in the milk of overweight mothers may impair glucose metabolism as well as the regulation of hunger/satiety mechanisms and energy balance in breastfed children [173]. Even so, breastfeeding can reduce the odds for obesity by 13% [115] and to attenuate the effect of genetic predisposition to excess weight in adulthood [116]. In addition to the several benefits already well established in the literature, breastfeeding is recommended to all mothers, regardless of their nutritional status [278].

Further, the intrinsic interactions between diet, nutritional status, and maternal microbiome have been demonstrated as important factors for long-term health, an area of research that will certainly contribute to understanding the complex mechanisms involved in metabolic programming in the first years of life [49].

e-Health in Nutritional Counseling for Pregnant and Lactating Women

The use of information and communication technologies in health, called *e-Health*, has been widely disseminated in the last few decades and plays a strategic role in initiatives to improve the women's and children's health [300]. The interaction of pregnant women with health information through digital media motivated the concept of *e-pregnant*, placing women in a central role of engagement for decisions about their own care [249].

The use of mobile devices has demonstrated success in delivering information to improve nutrition and encourage the practice of physical exercises [6] and promote adherence to nutrients supplementation during pregnancy [232]. In women with gestational diabetes, interventions using technology (internet, smartphones, apps, and text message) to promote lifestyle changes, including diet, reduced gestational weight gain and improved glycemic control [154].

Postpartum women used to have low adherence to nutritional interventions, due to the motherhood attributions which distance them from health services. The use of technology is recommended to deliver nutritional information that encourage healthy eating and provide a return to prepregnancy weight [260].

The use of text messages, e-mail, internet, apps and/or social media sites associated with traditional nutritional counseling improves postpartum weight loss [213, 274]. Women report that this approach increases motivation [275], which is a good strategy to maintain better rates of adherence to follow-up in longitudinal research protocols that extend from pregnancy to the child's first years of life [53]. Initiatives to promote and support breastfeeding can also be adapted to the digital format and emerges as an important tool to increase maternal and child nutritional care [175].

Nutritional Counseling for Pregnant and Lactating Women

For pregnant women at habitual risk, it is recommended to be counseled by a nutritionist throughout the pregnancy, with a minimum schedule of four individual consultations or three group sessions, with concomitant initiation to that of prenatal care. For pregnant women with GDM or chronic diseases, the schedule should be extended to six consultations with the nutritionist during pregnancy, also starting concurrently with prenatal care. The number of visits should be adjusted as needed. Group sessions with a multidisciplinary team of health professionals are also important opportunities for educational actions on topics related to pregnancy including to clarify the pregnant women's doubts.

Pregnant and lactating women must be constantly advised on the importance of a healthy and balanced diet. Recommend at least three main meals (breakfast, lunch, and dinner) and two healthy snacks a day.

The consumption of nuts and seeds (sesame, flaxseed, and others) added to fruits or yoghurts can be stimulated as healthy snacks, as they are foods rich in energy, proteins, minerals, fibers, and fats with less atherogenic potential. Two to three daily servings of milk and dairy products need to be consumed to adequate calcium intake (or equivalent sources in women who do not consume dairy products).

Unprocessed and minimally processed foods should be the base of the diet. The consumption of ultra-processed foods, which are high energy-dense and high sodium content, is not recommended (Table 8.3).

Advice the use of vegetable oils in small amounts when tempering and cooking. Encourage the use of extra virgin olive oil (without heating) and natural spices, such as garlic, onions, fresh or dried herbs. Limit the consumption of added salt to a maximum of 5 g per day (1 coffee spoon/day) distributed in all meals.

WHO [297] warns that women with usual high daily intake of caffeine (more than 300 mg/day) should reduce their intake of foods rich in this substance during pregnancy, to avoid the risk of miscarriage and low birth weight newborns. There are no safe doses for the consumption of alcoholic beverages during pregnancy and lactation, and should be absolutely avoided.

WHO suggests that eating slowly, chewing the food well, and paying attention to food are important. Stressful and distracting environments, for example, the use of electronic devices during meals, can impair the perception of satiety leading to excessive consumption. Guide pregnant women to avoid lying down right after meals, in order to prevent gastroesophageal reflux. The daily intake of at least 2 liters (from 6 to 8 glasses) of filtered water should occur between meals.

Encourage purchase of food in places that offer a variety of fresh or minimally processed foods and prefer local vegetables and fruits of the season. This can be a family activity, as well as planning and preparing meals. Encourage and propose a critical evaluation of messages and advertisements about food published in the media. If it is necessary to have meals outside the home, prefer places that serve freshly made meals, avoiding fast-food restaurant chains.

References

1. Abe SK, Balogun OO, Ota E, Takahashi K, Mori R. Supplementation with multiple micronutrients for breastfeeding women for improving outcomes for the mother and baby. Cochrane Database Syst Rev. 2016;2:CD010647. https://doi.org/10.1002/14651858.CD010647.pub2.
2. Abrams B, Altman SL, Pickett KE. Pregnancy weight gain: still controversial. Am J Clin Nutr. 2000;71 Suppl 5:1233S–41S. https://doi.org/10.1093/ajcn/71.5.1233s.
3. Agarwal S, Kovilam O, Agrawal DK. Vitamin D and its impact on maternal-fetal outcomes in pregnancy: a critical review. Crit Rev Food Sci Nutr. 2018;58(5):755–69. https://doi.org/10.1080/10408398.2016.1220915.
4. Agência Nacional de Vigilância Sanitária (ANVISA). Memento Fitoterápico. Farmacopeia Brasileira. 2016. http://portal.anvisa.gov.br/documents/33832/2909630/Memento+Fitoterapico. Accessed 01 June 2020.
5. Agnoli C, Baroni L, Bertini I, Ciappellano S, Fabbri A, Papa M, et al. Position paper on vegetarian diets from the working group of the Italian Society of Human Nutrition. Nutr Metab Cardiovasc Dis. 2017;27(12):1037–52. https://doi.org/10.1016/j.numecd.2017.10.020.
6. Ainscough KM, O'Brien EC, Lindsay KL, Kennelly MA, O'Sullivan EJ, O'Brien OA. Nutrition, behavior change and physical activity outcomes from the PEARS RCT-an mHealth-supported, lifestyle intervention among pregnant women with overweight and obesity. Front Endocrinol (Lausanne). 2020;10:938. https://doi.org/10.3389/fendo.2019.00938.
7. Alizadeh L, Raoofi A, Salehi L, Ramzi M. Impact of maternal hemoglobin concentration on fetal outcomes in adolescent pregnant women. Iran Red Crescent Med J. 2014;16(8):e19670. https://doi.org/10.5812/ircmj.19670.
8. Allen LH. Anemia and iron deficiency: effects on pregnancy outcome. Am J Clin Nutr. 2000;71 Suppl 5:1280S–4S. https://doi.org/10.1093/ajcn/71.5.1280s.
9. Allen LH, Donohue JA, Dror DK. Limitations of the evidence base used to set recommended nutrient intakes for infants and lactating women. Adv Nutr. 2018;9 Suppl 1:295S–312S. https://doi.org/10.1093/advances/nmy019.
10. Amabebe E, Robert FO, Obika LFO. Osmoregulatory adaptations during lactation: thirst, arginine vasopressin and plasma osmolality responses. Niger J Physiol Sci. 2017;32(2):109–16.
11. American College of Obstetricians and Gynecologists (ACOG). ACOG Committee opinion no. 731: group prenatal care. Obstet Gynecol. 2018;131(3):e104–8. https://doi.org/10.1097/AOG.0000000000002529.
12. American College of Obstetricians and Gynecologists (ACOG). ACOG Committee opinion no. 736: optimizing postpartum care. Obstet Gynecol. 2018;131(5):e140–50. https://doi.org/10.1097/AOG.0000000000002633.
13. American College of Obstetricians and Gynecologists (ACOG). ACOG practice bulletin 189: nausea and vomiting of pregnancy. Obstet Gynecol. 2018;131(1):e15–30. https://doi.org/10.1097/AOG.0000000000002456.
14. American College of Obstetricians and Gynecologists (ACOG). ACOG practice bulletin 202: gestational hypertension and preeclampsia. Obstet Gynecol. 2019;133(1):e1–25. https://doi.org/10.1097/AOG.0000000000003018.
15. American College of Obstetricians and Gynecologists (ACOG). ACOG practice bulletin no. 187: neural tube defects. Obstet Gynecol. 2017;130(6):e279–90. https://doi.org/10.1097/AOG.0000000000002412.
16. American Diabetes Association (ADA). Cardiovascular disease and risk management: standards of medical care in diabetes-2020. Diabetes Care. 2020;43 Suppl 1:S111–34. https://doi.org/10.2337/dc20-S010.
17. American Diabetes Association (ADA). Standards of medical care in diabetes. Gestational diabetes mellitus. Diabetes Care. 2004;27 Suppl 1:S88–90. https://doi.org/10.2337/diacare.27.2007.S88.

18. American Diabetes Association (ADA). Management of diabetes in pregnancy: standards of medical care in diabetes-2020. Diabetes Care. 2020;43 Suppl 1:S183–92. https://doi.org/10.2337/dc20-S014.
19. American Diabetes Association (ADA). Gestational diabetes mellitus. Diabetes Care. 1995;18 Suppl 1:S24–5. https://doi.org/10.2337/diacare.18.1.S24.
20. American Diabetes Association (ADA). Cardiovascular disease and risk management: standards of medical care in diabetes-2019. Diabetes Care. 2019;42 Suppl 1:S103–23. https://doi.org/10.2337/dc19-S010.
21. American Thyroid Association. Iodine supplementation for pregnancy and lactation-United States and Canada: recommendations of the American Thyroid Association. Thyroid. 2006;16(10):949–51. https://doi.org/10.1089/thy.2006.16.949.
22. American Psychiatric Association. Diagnostic and statistical manual of mental disorders (DSM-5). 5th ed. Arlington: American Psychiatric Association; 2013.
23. Andersson M, de Benoist B, Delange F, Zupan J. Prevention and control of iodine deficiency in pregnant and lactating women and in children less than 2-years-old: conclusions and recommendations of the technical consultation. Public Health Nutr. 2007;10:1606–11. https://doi.org/10.1017/S1368980007361004.
24. Aouache R, Biquard L, Vaiman D, Miralles F. Oxidative stress in preeclampsia and placental diseases. Int J Mol Sci. 2018;19(5):E1496. https://doi.org/10.3390/ijms19051496.
25. Appel LJ, Brands MW, Daniels SR, Karanja N, Elmer PJ, Sacks FM, et al. Dietary approaches to prevent and treat hypertension: a scientific statement from the American Heart Association. Hypertension. 2006;47(2):296–308. https://doi.org/10.1161/01.HYP.0000202568.01167.B6.
26. Archibald AJ, Dolinsky VW, Azad MB. Early-life exposure to non-nutritive sweeteners and the developmental origins of childhood obesity: global evidence from human and rodent studies. Nutrients. 2018;10(2):E194. https://doi.org/10.3390/nu10020194.
27. Arvizu M, Stuart J, Rich-Edwards J, Gaskins A, Rosner B, Chavarro J. Adherence to pre-pregnancy DASH dietary pattern and diet recommendations from the American Heart Association and the risk of preeclampsia. Curr Dev Nutr. 2019;3 Suppl 1:nzz048. https://doi.org/10.1093/cdn/nzz048.OR35-06-19.
28. Asemi Z, Samimi M, Tabassi Z, Esmaillzadeh A. The effect of DASH diet on pregnancy outcomes in gestational diabetes: a randomized controlled clinical trial. Eur J Clin Nutr. 2014;68(4):490–5. https://doi.org/10.1038/ejcn.2013.296.
29. Asemi Z, Samimi M, Tabassi Z, Sabihi SS, Esmaillzadeh A. A randomized controlled clinical trial investigating the effect of DASH diet on insulin resistance, inflammation, and oxidative stress in gestational diabetes. Nutrition. 2013;29(4):619–24. https://doi.org/10.1016/j.nut.2012.11.020.
30. Asemi Z, Tabassi Z, Samimi M, Fahiminejad T, Esmaillzadeh A. Favourable effects of the Dietary Approaches to Stop Hypertension diet on glucose tolerance and lipid profiles in gestational diabetes: a randomised clinical trial. Br J Nutr. 2013;109(11):2024–30. https://doi.org/10.1017/S0007114512004242.
31. Associação Brasileira para o Estudo da Obesidade e da Síndrome Metabólica (ABESO). Diretrizes brasileiras de obesidade 2016. 2016. https://abeso.org.br/diretrizes/. Accessed 2 June 2020.
32. Atalah E, Castillo C, Castro R, Aldea A. Propuesta de un nuevo estándar de evaluación nutricional en embarazadas. Rev Med Chil. 1997;125(12):1429–36.
33. Ayeta AC, Cunha ACB, Heidelmann SP, Saunders C. Fatores nutricionais e psicológicos associados com a ocorrência de picamalácia em gestantes. Rev Bras Ginecol Obstet. 2015;37(12):571–7. https://doi.org/10.1590/S0100-720320150005419.
34. Azadbakht L, Mirmiran P, Esmaillzadeh A, Azizi T, Azizi F. Beneficial effects of a Dietary Approaches to Stop Hypertension eating plan on features of the metabolic syndrome. Diabetes Care. 2005;28(12):2823–31. https://doi.org/10.2337/diacare.28.12.2823.
35. Bardosono S, Morin C, Guelinckx I, Pohan R. Pregnant and breastfeeding women: drinking for two? Ann Nutr Metab. 2017;70(Suppl 1):13–7. https://doi.org/10.1159/000462998.

36. Barger MK. Maternal nutrition and perinatal outcomes. J Midwifery Womens Health. 2010;55(6):502–11. https://doi.org/10.1016/j.jmwh.2010.02.017.
37. Baroni L, Goggi S, Battaglino R, Berveglieri M, Fasan I, Filippin D, et al. Vegan nutrition for mothers and children: practical tools for healthcare providers. Nutrients. 2018;11(1):5. https://doi.org/10.3390/nu11010005.
38. Belizán JM, Villar J, Repke J. The relationship between calcium intake and pregnancy-induced hypertension: up-to-date evidence. Am J Obstet Gynecol. 1988;158(4):898–902. https://doi.org/10.1016/0002-9378(88)90091-9.
39. Bernard V, Young J, Binart N. Prolactin - a pleiotropic factor in health and disease. Nat Rev Endocrinol. 2019;15(6):356–65. https://doi.org/10.1038/s41574-019-0194-6.
40. Bertz F, Brekke H, Ellegård L, Rasmussen K, Wennergren M, Winkvist A. Diet and exercise weight-loss trial in lactating overweight and obese women. Am J Clin Nutr. 2012;96(4):698–705. https://doi.org/10.3945/ajcn.112.040196.
41. Blaner, W.S., 1998. Recent advances in understanding the molecular basis of vitamin A action. Newsletter, 2:3–6.
42. Bodnar LM, Siega-Riz AM, Simhan HN, Himes KP, Abrams B. Severe obesity, gestational weight gain, and adverse birth outcomes. Am J Clin Nutr. 2010;91(6):1642–8. https://doi.org/10.3945/ajcn.2009.29008.
43. Bogaerts A, de Baetselier E, Ameye L, Dilles T, Van Rompaey B, Devlieger R. Postpartum weight trajectories in overweight and lean women. Midwifery. 2017;49:134–41. https://doi.org/10.1016/j.midw.2016.08.010.
44. Brannon PM, Taylor CL. Iron supplementation during pregnancy and infancy: uncertainties and implications for research and policy. Nutrients. 2017;9(12):1327. https://doi.org/10.3390/nu9121327.
45. Bricarello LP, Poltronieri F, Fernandes R, Retondario A, de Moraes Trindade EBS, de Vasconcelos FAG. Effects of the Dietary Approach to Stop Hypertension (DASH) diet on blood pressure, overweight and obesity in adolescents: a systematic review. Clin Nutr ESPEN. 2018;28:1–11. https://doi.org/10.1016/j.clnesp.2018.09.003.
46. Brown JE, Murtaugh MA, Jacobs DR Jr, Margellos HC. Variation in newborn size according to pregnancy weight change by trimester. Am J Clin Nutr. 2002;76(1):205–9. https://doi.org/10.1093/ajcn/76.1.205.
47. Buzilco D, Zajdenverg L. Diabetes e gravidez. In: Milech A, Oliveira JEP, Zajdenverg L, Rodacki M, editors. Rotinas de Diagnóstico e Tratamento do Diabetes Mellitus. Rio de Janeiro: AC Farmacêutica; 2014. p. 585–602.
48. Cai C, Vandermeer B, Khurana R, Nerenberg K, Featherstone R, Sebastianski M, et al. The impact of occupational shift work and working hours during pregnancy on health outcomes: a systematic review and meta-analysis. Am J Obstet Gynecol. 2019;221(6):563–76. https://doi.org/10.1016/j.ajog.2019.06.051.
49. Calatayud M, Koren O, Collado MC. Maternal microbiome and metabolic health program microbiome development and health of the offspring. Trends Endocrinol Metab. 2019;30(10):735–44. https://doi.org/10.1016/j.tem.2019.07.021.
50. Candler T, Kühnen P, Prentice AM, Silver M. Epigenetic regulation of POMC; implications for nutritional programming, obesity and metabolic disease. Front Neuroendocrinol. 2019;54:100773. https://doi.org/10.1016/j.yfrne.2019.100773.
51. Cao C, O'Brien KO. Pregnancy and iron homeostasis: an update. Nutr Rev. 2013;71(1):35–51. https://doi.org/10.1111/j.1753-4887.2012.00550.x.
52. Caramaschi D, Sharp GC, Nohr EA, Berryman K, Lewis SJ, Davey Smith G, et al. Exploring a causal role of DNA methylation in the relationship between maternal vitamin B12 during pregnancy and child's IQ at age 8, cognitive performance and educational attainment: a two-step Mendelian randomization study. Hum Mol Genet. 2017;26(15):3001–13. https://doi.org/10.1093/hmg/ddx164.
53. Cardoso MA, Matijasevich A, Malta MB, Lourenco BH, Gimeno SGA, Ferreira UM, et al. Cohort profile: the maternal and child health and nutrition in acre, Brazil, birth

cohort study (MINA-Brazil). BMJ Open. 2020;10(2):e034513. https://doi.org/10.1136/bmjopen-2019-034513.
54. Centeno Tablante E, Pachón H, Guetterman HM, Finkelstein JL. Fortification of wheat and maize flour with folic acid for population health outcomes. Cochrane Database Syst Rev. 2019;7:CD012150. https://doi.org/10.1002/14651858.CD012150.pub2.
55. Chagas CB, Ramalho A, Padilha PC, Líbera BD, Saunders C. Reduction of vitamin a deficiency and anemia in pregnancy after implementing proposed prenatal nutritional assistance. Nutr Hosp. 2011;26(4):843–50. https://doi.org/10.3305/NH.2011.26.4.5053.
56. Challet E. The circadian regulation of food intake. Nat Rev Endocrinol. 2019;15(7):393–405. https://doi.org/10.1038/s41574-019-0210-x.
57. Chavan NR, Reynolds LJ, McQuerry K, Stromberg A, Pearson KJ, O'Brien JM. PPARG expression varies with excess gestational weight gain (GWG) in pregnancy: an important target in developmental programming. AJOG. 2018;218(1):S360. https://doi.org/10.1016/j.ajog.2017.11.131.
58. Chiavaroli L, Viguiliouk E, Nishi SK, Blanco Mejia S, Rahelić D, Kahleová H, et al. DASH dietary pattern and cardiometabolic outcomes: an umbrella review of systematic reviews and meta-analyses. Nutrients. 2019;11(2):E338. https://doi.org/10.3390/nu11020338.
59. Christian P, Katz J, Wu L, Kimbrough-Pradhan E, Khatry SK, LeClerq SC, et al. Risk factors for pregnancy-related mortality: a prospective study in rural Nepal. Public Health. 2008;122(2):161–72. https://doi.org/10.1016/j.puhe.2007.06.003.
60. Christian P, West KP Jr, Khatry SK, Kimbrough-Pradhan E, LeClerq SC, Katz J, et al. Night blindness during pregnancy and subsequent mortality among women in Nepal: effects of vitamin a and beta-carotene supplementation. Am J Epidemiol. 2000;152(6):542–7. https://doi.org/10.1093/aje/152.6.542.
61. Christian P, West KP Jr, Khatry SK, LeClerq SC, Kimbrough-Pradhan E, Katz J, et al. Maternal night blindness increases risk of mortality in the first 6 months of life among infants in Nepal. J Nutr. 2001;131(5):1510–2. https://doi.org/10.1093/jn/131.5.1510.
62. Chu DM, Meyer KM, Prince AL, Aagaard KM. Impact of maternal nutrition in pregnancy and lactation on offspring gut microbial composition and function. Gut Microbes. 2016;7(6):459–70. https://doi.org/10.1080/19490976.2016.1241357.
63. Chung EO, Mattah B, Hickey MD, Salmen CR, Milner EM, Bukusi EA, et al. Characteristics of pica behavior among mothers around Lake Victoria, Kenya: a cross-sectional study. Int J Environ Res Public Health. 2019;16(14):E2510. https://doi.org/10.3390/ijerph16142510.
64. Colleran HL, Lovelady CA. Use of MyPyramid menu planner for moms in a weight-loss intervention during lactation. J Acad Nutr Diet. 2012;112(4):553–8. https://doi.org/10.1016/j.jand.2011.12.004.
65. Cordina M, Bhatti S, Fernandez M, Syngelaki A, Nicolaides KH, Kametas NA. Association between maternal haemoglobin at 27-29weeks gestation and intrauterine growth restriction. Pregnancy Hypertens. 2015;5(4):339–45. https://doi.org/10.1016/j.preghy.2015.09.005.
66. Cornell A, McCoy C, Stampfel C, Bonzon E, Verbiest S. Creating new strategies to enhance postpartum health and wellness. Matern Child Health J. 2016;20(Suppl 1):39–42. https://doi.org/10.1007/s10995-016-2182-y.
67. Countouris ME, Schwarz EB, Rossiter BC, Althouse AD, Berlacher KL, Jeyabalan A, et al. Effects of lactation on postpartum blood pressure among women with gestational hypertension and preeclampsia. Am J Obstet Gynecol. 2016;215(2):241.e1–241.e2418. https://doi.org/10.1016/j.ajog.2016.02.046.
68. Courtney AU, O'Brien EC, Crowley RK, Geraghty AA, Brady MB, Kilbane MT. DASH (Dietary Approaches to Stop Hypertension) dietary pattern and maternal blood pressure in pregnancy. J Hum Nutr Diet. 2020; https://doi.org/10.1111/jhn.12744.
69. Craigie AM, Macleod M, Barton KL, Treweek S, Anderson AS, WeighWell T. Supporting postpartum weight loss in women living in deprived communities: design implications for a randomised control trial. Eur J Clin Nutr. 2011;65(8):952–8. https://doi.org/10.1038/ejcn.2011.56.

70. Crozier SR, Inskip HM, Godfrey KM, Cooper C, Robinson SM. Nausea and vomiting in early pregnancy: effects on food intake and diet quality. Matern Child Nutr. 2017;13(4):e12389. https://doi.org/10.1111/mcn.12389.
71. Cunha ACB, Patricio SF, Akerman LPF, Maynarde PS, Saunders C. Pica in the pregnancy and related psychological aspects. Temas psicol. 2017;25(2):613–30. https://doi.org/10.9788/TP2017.2-12En.
72. da Cunha AJLA, Leite AJM, de Almeida IS. The pediatrician's role in the first thousand days of the child: the pursuit of healthy nutrition and development. J Pediatr. 2015;91(6 Suppl 1):S44–51. https://doi.org/10.1016/j.jped.2015.07.002.
73. Çakmak BD, Türker ÜA, Öztaş S, Arık M, Üstünyurt E. The effect of first trimester hemoglobin levels on pregnancy outcomes. Turk J Obstet Gynecol. 2018;15(3):165–70. https://doi.org/10.4274/tjod.87269.
74. Dadon SB, Reifen R. Vitamin A and the epigenome. Crit Rev Food Sci Nutr. 2017;57(11):2404–11. https://doi.org/10.1080/10408398.2015.1060940.
75. Dalrymple KV, Flynn AC, Relph SA, O'Keeffe M, Poston L. Lifestyle interventions in overweight and obese pregnant or postpartum women for postpartum weight management: a systematic review of the literature. Nutrients. 2018;10(11):1704. https://doi.org/10.3390/nu10111704.
76. de la Garza PA, Martí Alemany A, Chisaguano AM, Montes Goyanes R, Castellote AI, Torres-Espínola FJ, et al. The effect of maternal obesity on breast milk fatty acids and its association with infant growth and cognition-the PREOBE follow-up. Nutrients. 2019;11(9):2154. https://doi.org/10.3390/nu11092154.
77. de Onis M, Onyango AW, Borghi E, Siyam A, Nishida C, Siekmann J. Development of a WHO growth reference for school-aged children and adolescents. Bull World Health Organ. 2007;85(9):660–7. https://doi.org/10.2471/blt.07.043497.
78. de Waard M, Brands B, Kouwenhoven SMP, Lerma JC, Crespo-Escobar P, Koletzko B, et al. Optimal nutrition in lactating women and its effect on later health of offspring: a systematic review of current evidence and recommendations (EarlyNutrition project). Crit Rev Food Sci Nutr. 2017;57(18):4003–16. https://doi.org/10.1080/10408398.2016.1158149.
79. Delgado-Noguera MF, Calvache JA, Bonfill Cosp X, Kotanidou EP, Galli-Tsinopoulou A. Supplementation with long chain polyunsaturated fatty acids (LCPUFA) to breastfeeding mothers for improving child growth and development. Cochrane Database Syst Rev. 2015;(7):CD007901. https://doi.org/10.1002/14651858.CD007901.pub3.
80. Della Líbera B, Ribeiro Baião M, Souza Santos MMA, Padilha P, Dutra Alves P, Saunders C. Adherence of pregnant women to dietary counseling and adequacy of total gestational weight gain. Nutr Hosp. 2011;26(1):79–85. https://doi.org/10.3305/NH.2011.26.1.4642.
81. Demmelmair H, Koletzko B. Lipids in human milk. Best Pract Res Clin Endocrinol Metab. 2018;32(1):57–68. https://doi.org/10.1016/j.beem.2017.11.002.
82. Dodd JM, Deussen AR, O'Brien CM, Schoenaker DAJM, Poprzeczny A, Gordon A, et al. Targeting the postpartum period to promote weight loss: a systematic review and meta-analysis. Nutr Rev. 2018;76(8):639–54. https://doi.org/10.1093/nutrit/nuy024.
83. Drehmer M, Odegaard AO, Schmidt MI, Duncan BB, Cardoso LO, Matos SMA, et al. Brazilian dietary patterns and the dietary approaches to stop hypertension (DASH) diet-relationship with metabolic syndrome and newly diagnosed diabetes in the ELSA-Brasil study. Diabetol Metab Syndr. 2017;9:13. https://doi.org/10.1186/s13098-017-0211-7.
84. Dror DK, Allen LH. Overview of nutrients in human milk. Adv Nutr. 2018;9 Suppl 1:278S–94S. https://doi.org/10.1093/advances/nmy022.
85. Dupont C, Chouraqui JP, Linglart A, Bocquet A, Darmaun D, Feillet F, et al. Nutritional management of cow's milk allergy in children: an update. Arch Pediatr. 2018;25(3):236–43. https://doi.org/10.1016/j.arcped.2018.01.007.
86. Echeverría F, Valenzuela R, Catalina Hernandez-Rodas M, Valenzuela A. Docosahexaenoic acid (DHA), a fundamental fatty acid for the brain: new dietary sources. Prostaglandins Leukot Essent Fatty Acids. 2017;124:1–10. https://doi.org/10.1016/j.plefa.2017.08.001.
87. Egorova O, Myte R, Schneede J, Hägglöf B, Bölte S, Domellöf E, et al. Maternal blood folate status during early pregnancy and occurrence of autism spectrum disorder in off-

spring: a study of 62 serum biomarkers. Mol Autism. 2020;11(1):7. https://doi.org/10.1186/s13229-020-0315-z.
88. Ellsworth L, Perng W, Harman E, Das A, Pennathur S, Gregg B. Impact of maternal overweight and obesity on milk composition and infant growth. Matern Child Nutr. 2020; https://doi.org/10.1111/mcn.12979.
89. Esmaillzadeh A, Azadbakht L. Different kinds of vegetable oils in relation to individual cardiovascular risk factors among Iranian women. Br J Nutr. 2011;105(6):919–27. https://doi.org/10.1017/S0007114510004423.
90. Falciglia G, Piazza J, Ollberding NJ, Spiess L, Morrow A. A theory-based dietary intervention for overweight, postpartum mothers and their children improves maternal vegetable intake. Open J Obstet Gynecol. 2017;7(7):679. https://doi.org/10.4236/ojog.2017.77068.
91. Fardet A. Minimally processed foods are more satiating and less hyperglycemic than ultra-processed foods: a preliminary study with 98 ready-to-eat foods. Food Funct. 2016;7(5):2338–46. https://doi.org/10.1039/c6fo00107f.
92. Farr A, Chervenak FA, McCullough LB, Baergen RN, Grünebaum A. Human placentophagy: a review. Am J Obstet Gynecol. 2018;218(4):401.e1–401.e11. https://doi.org/10.1016/j.ajog.2017.08.016.
93. Fawcett EJ, Fawcett JM, Mazmanian D. A meta-analysis of the worldwide prevalence of pica during pregnancy and the postpartum period. Int J Gynaecol Obstet. 2016;133(3):277–83. https://doi.org/10.1016/j.ijgo.2015.10.012.
94. Feghali MN, Catov JM, Zantow E, Mission J, Caritis SN, Scifres CM. Timing of gestational weight gain and adverse perinatal outcomes in overweight and obese women. Obstet Gynecol. 2019;133(5):962–70. https://doi.org/10.1097/AOG.0000000000003234.
95. Filardi T, Panimolle F, Crescioli C, Lenzi A, Morano S. Gestational diabetes mellitus: the impact of carbohydrate quality in diet. Nutrients. 2019;11(7):E1549. https://doi.org/10.3390/nu11071549.
96. Food and Agriculture Organization (FAO); World Health Organization (WHO); United Nations University (UNU). Human energy requirements. Report of a Joint FAO/WHO/UNU Expert Consultation. 2004. http://www.fao.org/3/a-y5686e.pdf. Accessed 02 June 2020.
97. Food and Agriculture Organization (FAO), World Health Organization (WHO). Scientific update on carbohydrates in human nutrition: conclusions. Eur J Clin Nutr. 2007;61 Suppl 1:S132–7. https://doi.org/10.1038/sj.ejcn.1602943.
98. Food and Agriculture Organization (FAO). Fats and fatty acids in human nutrition: report of an expert consultation. 2010. http://www.fao.org/nutrition/requirements. Accessed 22 Feb 2020.
99. García-Mantrana I, Selma-Royo M, González S, Parra-Llorca A, Martínez-Costa C, Collado MC. Distinct maternal microbiota clusters are associated with diet during pregnancy: impact on neonatal microbiota and infant growth during the first 18 months of life. Gut Microbes. 2020; https://doi.org/10.1080/19490976.2020.1730294.
100. Georgieff MK. Iron deficiency in pregnancy. Am J Obstet Gynecol. 2020; https://doi.org/10.1016/j.ajog.2020.03.006.
101. Goldstein RF, Abell SK, Ranasinha S, Misso M, Boyle JA, Black MH, et al. Association of gestational weight gain with maternal and infant outcomes: a systematic review and meta-analysis. JAMA. 2017;317(21):2207–25. https://doi.org/10.1001/jama.2017.3635.
102. Gomes MM, Saunders C, Ramalho A, Accioly E. Serum vitamin A in mothers and newborns in the city of Rio de Janeiro. Int J Food Sci Nutr. 2009;60(4):282–92. https://doi.org/10.1080/09637480701752210.
103. Goran MI, Plows JF, Ventura EE. Effects of consuming sugars and alternative sweeteners during pregnancy on maternal and child health: evidence for a secondhand sugar effect. Proc Nutr Soc. 2019;78(3):262–71. https://doi.org/10.1017/S002966511800263X.
104. Hahn-Holbrook J, Saxbe D, Bixby C, Steele C, Glynn L. Human milk as "chrononutrition": implications for child health and development. Pediatr Res. 2019;85(7):936–42. https://doi.org/10.1038/s41390-019-0368-x.

105. HAPO Study Cooperative Research Group, Metzger BE, Lowe LP, Dyer AR, Trimble ER, Chaovarindr U, et al. Hyperglycemia and adverse pregnancy outcomes. N Engl J Med. 2008;358(19):1991–2002. https://doi.org/10.1056/NEJMoa0707943.
106. Harding KB, Peña-Rosas JP, Webster AC, Yap CM, Payne BA, Ota E, et al. Iodine supplementation for women during the preconception, pregnancy and postpartum period. Cochrane Database Syst Rev. 2017;3(3):CD011761. https://doi.org/10.1002/14651858.CD011761.pub2.
107. Hemsing N, Greaves L, Poole N. Preconception health care interventions: a scoping review. Sex Reprod Healthc. 2017;14:24–32. https://doi.org/10.1016/j.srhc.2017.08.004.
108. Herring SJ, Yu D, Spaeth A, Pien G, Darden N, Riis V, et al. Influence of sleep duration on postpartum weight change in black and Hispanic women. Obesity (Silver Spring). 2019;27(2):295–303. https://doi.org/10.1002/oby.22364.
109. Hill C, Guarner F, Reid G, Gibson GR, Merenstein DJ, Pot B, et al. Expert consensus document. The International Scientific Association for Probiotics and Prebiotics consensus statement on the scope and appropriate use of the term probiotic. Nat Rev Gastroenterol Hepatol. 2014;11(8):506–14. https://doi.org/10.1038/nrgastro.2014.66.
110. Hirschberg AL. Sex hormones, appetite and eating behaviour in women. Maturitas. 2012;71(3):248–56. https://doi.org/10.1016/j.maturitas.2011.12.016.
111. Hofmeyr GJ, Lawrie TA, Atallah AN, Duley L, Torloni MR. Calcium supplementation during pregnancy for preventing hypertensive disorders and related problems. Cochrane Database Syst Rev. 2014;(6):CD001059. https://doi.org/10.1002/14651858.CD001059.pub4.
112. Hofmeyr GJ, Manyame S, Medley N, Williams MJ. Calcium supplementation commencing before or early in pregnancy, for preventing hypertensive disorders of pregnancy. Cochrane Database Syst Rev. 2019;9(9):CD011192. https://doi.org/10.1002/14651858.CD011192.pub3.
113. Hofmeyr GJ, Lawrie TA, Atallah AN, Torloni MR. Calcium supplementation during pregnancy for preventing hypertensive disorders and related problems. Cochrane Database Syst Rev. 2018;10(10):CD001059. https://doi.org/10.1002/14651858.CD001059.pub5.
114. Holick MF, Binkley NC, Bischoff-Ferrari HA, Gordon CM, Hanley DA, Heaney RP, et al. Evaluation, treatment, and prevention of vitamin D deficiency: an Endocrine Society clinical practice guideline. J Clin Endocrinol Metab. 2011;96(7):1911–30. https://doi.org/10.1210/jc.2011-0385.
115. Horta BL, Loret de Mola C, Victora CG. Long-term consequences of breastfeeding on cholesterol, obesity, systolic blood pressure and type 2 diabetes: a systematic review and meta-analysis. Acta Paediatr. 2015;104(467):30–7. https://doi.org/10.1111/apa.13133.
116. Horta BL, Victora CG, França GVA, Hartwig FP, Ong KK, Rolfe EL, et al. Breastfeeding moderates FTO related adiposity: a birth cohort study with 30 years of follow-up. Sci Rep. 2018;8(1):2530. https://doi.org/10.1038/s41598-018-20939-4.
117. Houfflyn S, Matthys C, Soubry A. Male obesity: epigenetic origin and effects in sperm and offspring. Curr Mol Biol Rep. 2017;3(4):288–96. https://doi.org/10.1007/s40610-017-0083-5.
118. Hsu CN, Tain YL. Light and circadian signaling pathway in pregnancy: programming of adult health and disease. Int J Mol Sci. 2020;21(6):E2232. https://doi.org/10.3390/ijms21062232.
119. Huseinovic E, Bertz F, Leu Agelii M, Hellebö Johansson E, Winkvist A, Brekke HK. Effectiveness of a weight loss intervention in postpartum women: results from a randomized controlled trial in primary health care. Am J Clin Nutr. 2016;104(2):362–70. https://doi.org/10.3945/ajcn.116.135673.
120. Hytten FL, Leitch I. The physiology of human pregnancy. 2nd ed. Oxford: Blackwell; 1971.
121. Ideraabdullah FY, Zeisel SH. Dietary modulation of the epigenome. Physiol Rev. 2018;98(2):667–95. https://doi.org/10.1152/physrev.00010.2017.
122. Institute of Medicine (IOM). Dietary reference intakes for calcium and vitamin D. 2011. https://www.nap.edu/read/13050. Accessed 22 Feb 2020.
123. Institute of Medicine (IOM). Dietary reference intakes for energy, carbohydrate, fiber, fat, fatty acids, cholesterol, protein, and amino acids. 2005. https://www.nap.edu/read/10490. Accessed 22 Feb 2020.

124. Institute of Medicine (IOM). Dietary reference intakes for thiamin, riboflavin, niacin, vitamin B6, folate, vitamin B12, pantothenic acid, biotin, and choline. 1998. https://www.nap.edu/read/6015. Accessed 22 Feb 2020.
125. Institute of Medicine (IOM). Dietary reference intakes for vitamin A, vitamin K, arsenic, boron, chromium, copper, iodine, iron, manganese, molybdenum, nickel, silicon, vanadium, and zinc. 2001. https://www.nap.edu/read/10026. Accessed 22 Feb 2020.
126. Institute of Medicine (IOM). Dietary reference intakes for vitamin C, vitamin E, selenium, and carotenoids. 2000. https://www.nap.edu/read/9810. Accessed 22 Feb 2020.
127. Institute of Medicine (IOM). Dietary Reference Intakes for Calcium and Vitamin D. Washington (DC): National Academies Press; 2010. https://www.nap.edu/collection/57/dietary-reference-intakes. Accessed 22 Feb 2020.
128. Institute of Medicine (IOM). Nutrition during lactation. 1991. https://www.nap.edu/catalog/1577. Accessed 28 May 2020.
129. Institute of Medicine (IOM). Nutrition during pregnancy. 1990. https://www.nap.edu/read/1451. Accessed 02 June 2020.
130. Institute of Medicine (IOM). Nutrition during pregnancy and lactation: an implementation guide. 1992. http://www.nap.edu/catalog/1984. Accessed 22 Feb 2020.
131. Institute of Medicine (IOM); National Research Council. Implementing guidelines on weight gain and pregnancy. 2013. https://www.nap.edu/catalog/18292. Accessed 02 June 2020.
132. Institute of Medicine (IOM); National Research Council. Leveraging action to support dissemination of the pregnancy weight gain guidelines: Workshop summary. 2013. https://www.nap.edu/catalog/18410. Accessed 02 June 2020.
133. Institute of Medicine (IOM); National Research Council. Weight gain during pregnancy: reexamining the guidelines. 2009. https://www.nap.edu/catalog/12584. Accessed 02 June 2020.
134. International Association of Diabetes and Pregnancy Study Groups Consensus Panel, Metzger BE, Gabbe SG, Persson B, Buchanan TA, Catalano PA, et al. International Association of Diabetes and Pregnancy Study Groups recommendations on the diagnosis and classification of hyperglycemia in pregnancy. Diabetes Care. 2010;33(3):676–82. https://doi.org/10.2337/dc09-1848.
135. International Diabetes Federation (IDF). Diabetes Atlas. 2019. http://www.diabetesatlas.org. Accessed 02 June 2020.
136. Isganaitis E. Developmental programming of body composition: update on evidence and mechanisms. Curr Diab Rep. 2019;19(8):60. https://doi.org/10.1007/s11892-019-1170-1.
137. Izadi V, Tehrani H, Haghighatdoost F, Dehghan A, Surkan PJ, Azadbakht L. Adherence to the DASH and Mediterranean diets is associated with decreased risk for gestational diabetes mellitus. Nutrition. 2016;32(10):1092–6. https://doi.org/10.1016/j.nut.2016.03.006.
138. Jardí C, Aparicio E, Bedmar C, Aranda N, Abajo S, March G, et al. Food consumption during pregnancy and post-partum. ECLIPSES study. Nutrients. 2019;11(10):2447. https://doi.org/10.3390/nu11102447.
139. Jenkins DJ, Wolever TM, Taylor RH, Barker H, Fielden H, Baldwin JM, et al. Glycemic index of foods: a physiological basis for carbohydrate exchange. Am J Clin Nutr. 1981;34(3):362–6. https://doi.org/10.1093/ajcn/34.3.362.
140. Jiang F, Li Y, Xu P, Li J, Chen X, Yu H, et al. The efficacy of the Dietary Approaches to Stop Hypertension diet with respect to improving pregnancy outcomes in women with hypertensive disorders. J Hum Nutr Diet. 2019;32(6):713–8. https://doi.org/10.1111/jhn.12654.
141. Karanja NM, Obarzanek E, Lin PH, McCullough ML, Phillips KM, Swain JF, et al. Descriptive characteristics of the dietary patterns used in the Dietary Approaches to Stop Hypertension Trial. DASH Collaborative Research Group. J Am Diet Assoc. 1999;99 Suppl 8:S19–27. https://doi.org/10.1016/s0002-8223(99)00412-5.
142. Kereliuk SM, Brawerman GM, Dolinsky VW. Maternal macronutrient consumption and the developmental origins of metabolic disease in the offspring. Int J Mol Sci. 2017;18(7):1451. https://doi.org/10.3390/ijms18071451.
143. Kidd M, Hnatiuk M, Barber J, Woolgar MJ, Mackay MP. "Something is wrong with your milk": qualitative study of maternal dietary restriction and beliefs about infant colic. Can Fam Physician. 2019;65(3):204–11.

144. Kitsiou-Tzeli S, Tzetis M. Maternal epigenetics and fetal and neonatal growth. Curr Opin Endocrinol Diabetes Obes. 2017;24(1):43–6. https://doi.org/10.1097/MED.0000000000000305.
145. Kolasa KM, Firnhaber G, Haven K. Diet for a healthy lactating woman. Clin Obstet Gynecol. 2015;58(4):893–901. https://doi.org/10.1097/GRF.0000000000000144.
146. Koletzko B, Godfrey KM, Poston L, Szajewska H, van Goudoever JB, de Waard M, et al. Nutrition during pregnancy, lactation and early childhood and its implications for maternal and Long-term child health: the early nutrition project recommendations. Ann Nutr Metab. 2019;74(2):93–106. https://doi.org/10.1159/000496471.
147. Kuang L, Jiang Y. Effect of probiotic supplementation in pregnant women: a meta-analysis of randomised controlled trials. Br J Nutr. 2020;123(8):870–80. https://doi.org/10.1017/S0007114519003374.
148. Kulay L Jr, Quntini MP, Mathias CV, Nakamura UM, Braga A. Uso de medicamentos. In: Montenegro CAB, Rezende Filho J, editors. Rezende Obstetrícia. Rio de Janeiro: Guanabara Koogan; 2017. p. 744–54.
149. Lacerda EMA. Deficiência de Ferro no grupo Materno-infantil. In: Accioly E, Saunders C, Lacerda EMA, editors. Nutrição em Obstetrícia e Pediatria. 2nd ed. Rio de Janeiro: Cultura Médica/Guanabara Koogan; 2012. p. 39–56.
150. Lacerda EMA, Saunders C. Nutrição da Nutriz. In: Accioly E, Saunders C, Lacerda EMA, editors. Nutrição em Obstetrícia e Pediatria. 2nd ed. Rio de Janeiro: Cultura Médica/Guanabara Koogan; 2012. p. 231–42.
151. Lai JS, Mohamad Ayob MN, Cai S, Quah PL, Gluckman PD, Shek LP, et al. Maternal plasma vitamin B12 concentrations during pregnancy and infant cognitive outcomes at 2 years of age. Br J Nutr. 2019;121(11):1303–12. https://doi.org/10.1017/S0007114519000746.
152. Lawson EA. The effects of oxytocin on eating behaviour and metabolism in humans. Nat Rev Endocrinol. 2017;13(12):700–9. https://doi.org/10.1038/nrendo.2017.115.
153. Leahy K, Berlin KS, Banks GG, Bachman J. The relationship between intuitive eating and postpartum weight loss. Matern Child Health J. 2017;21(8):1591–7. https://doi.org/10.1007/s10995-017-2281-4.
154. Li SY, Ouyang YQ, Qiao J, Shen Q. Technology-supported lifestyle interventions to improve maternal-fetal outcomes in women with gestational diabetes mellitus: a meta-analysis. Midwifery. 2020;85:102689. https://doi.org/10.1016/j.midw.2020.102689.
155. Líbera BD, Baião MR, Barros DC, Santos MMAS, Araújo RG, Saunders C. Prenatal nutritional care improved perinatal outcome of pregnant women in the context of primary health care. J Food Nutr Res. 2017;5(9):689–96. https://doi.org/10.12691/jfnr-5-9-9.
156. Lim S, Versace VL, O'Reilly S, Janus E, Dunbar J. Weight change and cardiometabolic outcomes in postpartum women with history of gestational diabetes. Nutrients. 2019;11(4):922. https://doi.org/10.3390/nu11040922.
157. Lima VJ, Andrade CR, Ruschi GE, Sass N. Serum lipid levels in pregnancies complicated by preeclampsia. Sao Paulo Med J. 2011;129(2):73–6. https://doi.org/10.1590/S1516-31802011000200004.
158. Lin L, Zhang L, Li C, Gai Z, Li Y. Vitamin D and vitamin D receptor: new insights in the treatment of hypertension. Curr Protein Pept Sci. 2019;20(10):984–95. https://doi.org/10.2174/1389203720666190807130504.
159. Lopes RE, Ramos KS, Bressani CC, Arruda IL, Souza AI. Prevalência de anemia e hipovitaminose A em puérperas do Centro de Atenção à Mulher do Instituto Materno Infantil Prof. Fernando Figueira, IMIP: um estudo piloto. Rev Bras Saude Mater Infant. 2006;6 Suppl 1:s638. https://doi.org/10.1590/S1519-38292006000500009.
160. López LB, Ortega SCR, de Pita Martín PML. Polipica durante el embarazo: geofagia asociada al consumo de tiza y pagofagia a la ingesta de jabón. Rev Chil Nutr. 2007;34(3):228–31. https://doi.org/10.4067/S0717-75182007000300006.
161. Louzada ML, Baraldi LG, Steele EM, Martins AP, Canella DS, Moubarac JC, et al. Consumption of ultra-processed foods and obesity in Brazilian adolescents and adults. Prev Med. 2015;81:9–15. https://doi.org/10.1016/j.ypmed.2015.07.018.

162. Louzada MLC, Martins APB, Canella DS, Baraldi LG, Levy RBI, Claro RM, et al. Impacto de alimentos ultraprocessados sobre o teor de micronutrientes da dieta no Brasil. Rev Saúde Pública. 2015;49:45. https://doi.org/10.1590/S0034-8910.2015049006211.
163. Lovelady C. Balancing exercise and food intake with lactation to promote post-partum weight loss. Proc Nutr Soc. 2011;70(2):181–4. https://doi.org/10.1017/S002966511100005X.
164. Loy SL, Cheung YB, Colega MT, Chia A, Han CY, Godfrey KM, et al. Associations of circadian eating pattern and diet quality with substantial postpartum weight retention. Nutrients. 2019;11(11):2686. https://doi.org/10.3390/nu11112686.
165. Luke B. Nutrition and multiple gestation. Semin Perinatol. 2005;29(5):349–54. https://doi.org/10.1053/j.semperi.2005.08.004.
166. Lumish RA, Young SL, Lee S, Cooper E, Pressman E, Guillet R, et al. Gestational iron deficiency is associated with pica behaviors in adolescents. J Nutr. 2014;144(10):1533–9. https://doi.org/10.3945/jn.114.192070.
167. Marchi J, Berg M, Dencker A, Olander EK, Begley C. Risks associated with obesity in pregnancy, for the mother and baby: a systematic review of reviews. Obes Rev. 2015;16(8):621–38. https://doi.org/10.1111/obr.12288.
168. Martens PJ, Gysemans C, Verstuyf A, Mathieu AC. Vitamin D's effect on immune function. Nutrients. 2020;12(5):E1248. https://doi.org/10.3390/nu12051248.
169. Mason JB, Shrimpton R, Saldanha LS, Ramakrishnan U, Victora CG, Girard AW, et al. The first 500 days of life: policies to support maternal nutrition. Glob Health Action. 2014;7:23623. https://doi.org/10.3402/gha.v7.23623.
170. Masulli M, Vitacolonna E, Fraticelli F, Della Pepa G, Mannucci E, Monami M. Effects of probiotic supplementation during pregnancy on metabolic outcomes: a systematic review and meta-analysis of randomized controlled trials. Diabetes Res Clin Pract. 2020;162:108111. https://doi.org/10.1016/j.diabres.2020.108111.
171. Mayne PE, Burne THJ. Vitamin D in synaptic plasticity, cognitive function, and neuropsychiatric illness. Trends Neurosci. 2019;42(4):293–306. https://doi.org/10.1016/j.tins.2019.01.003.
172. Mayneris-Perxachs J, Swann JR. Metabolic phenotyping of malnutrition during the first 1000 days of life. Eur J Nutr. 2019;58(3):909–30. https://doi.org/10.1007/s00394-018-1679-0.
173. Mazzocchi A, Giannì ML, Morniroli D, Leone L, Roggero P, Agostoni C, et al. Hormones in breast milk and effect on infants' growth: a systematic review. Nutrients. 2019;11(8):1845. https://doi.org/10.3390/nu11081845.
174. McCauley ME, van den Broek N, Dou L, Othman M. Vitamin A supplementation during pregnancy for maternal and newborn outcomes. Cochrane Database Syst Rev. 2015;2015(10):CD008666. https://doi.org/10.1002/14651858.CD008666.pub3.
175. Meedya S, Win K, Yeatman H, Fahy K, Walton K, Burgess L, et al. Developing and testing a mobile application for breastfeeding support: the Milky Way application. Women Birth. 2020; https://doi.org/10.1016/j.wombi.2020.02.006.
176. Melina V, Craig W, Levin S. Position of the academy of nutrition and dietetics: vegetarian diets. J Acad Nutr Diet. 2016;116(12):1970–80. https://doi.org/10.1016/j.jand.2016.09.025.
177. Middleton P, Gomersall JC, Gould JF, Shepherd E, Olsen SF, Makrides M. Omega-3 fatty acid addition during pregnancy. Cochrane Database Syst Rev. 2018;11:CD003402. https://doi.org/10.1002/14651858.CD003402.pub3.
178. Milman N. Dietary iron intake in pregnant women in Europe: a review of 24 studies from 14 countries in the period 1991-2014. J Nutr Metab. 2020;2020:7102190. https://doi.org/10.1155/2020/7102190.
179. Milman N. Oral iron prophylaxis in pregnancy: not too little and not TooMuch! J Pregnancy. 2012;2012:514345. https://doi.org/10.1155/2012/514345.
180. Milman N. Postpartum anemia I: definition, prevalence, causes, and consequences. Ann Hematol. 2011;90(11):1247–53. https://doi.org/10.1007/s00277-011-1279-z.

181. Ministério da Saúde (MS). Guia alimentar para a população brasileira. 2014. https://bvsms.saude.gov.br/bvs/publicacoes/guia_alimentar_populacao_brasileira_2ed.pdf. Accessed 02 June 2020.
182. Ministério da Saúde (MS). Agência Nacional de Vigilância Sanitária. Diretoria Colegiada. Resolução da Diretoria Colegiada - RDC n° 239. Estabelece os aditivos alimentares e coadjuvantes de tecnologia autorizados para uso em suplementos alimentares. Diário Oficial da União; 2018.
183. Monteiro CA, Cannon G, Lawrence M, Costa Louzada ML, Machado P. Ultra-processed foods, diet quality, and health using the NOVA classification system. FAO: Rome; 2019.
184. Monteiro CA, Cannon G, Moubarac JC, Levy RB, Louzada MLC, Jaime PC. The UN Decade of Nutrition, the NOVA food classification and the trouble with ultra-processing. Public Health Nutr. 2018;21(1):5–17. https://doi.org/10.1017/S1368980017000234.
185. Montenegro CAB, Bornia RG, Pesce RRP, Cardoso FFO, Guimarães T. Assistência Pré-natal. In: Montenegro CAB, Rezende Filho J, editors. Rezende Obstetrícia. Rio de Janeiro: Guanabara Koogan; 2017. p. 153–62.
186. Montenegro CAB, Burlá M, Rezende Filho J. Toxemia Gravídica. Pré-eclâmpsia. Eclâmpsia. In: Montenegro CAB, Rezende Filho J, editors. Rezende Obstetrícia. Rio de Janeiro: Guanabara Koogan; 2017. p. 278–93.
187. Montenegro CAB, Rezende FJ. Hiperêmese Gravídica. In: Montenegro CAB, Rezende Filho J, editors. Rezende Obstetrícia. Rio de Janeiro: Guanabara Koogan; 2017. p. 274–6.
188. Montenegro CAB, Rezende FJ. Hipertensão Crônica. In: Montenegro CAB, Rezende Filho J, editors. Rezende Obstetrícia. Rio de Janeiro: Guanabara Koogan; 2017. p. 491–4.
189. Montenegro CAB, Rezende FJ. Modificações do organismo materno. In: Montenegro CAB, Rezende Filho J, editors. Rezende Obstetrícia. Rio de Janeiro: Guanabara Koogan; 2017. p. 80–97.
190. Mousa A, Naqash A, Lim S. Macronutrient and micronutrient intake during pregnancy: an overview of recent evidence. Nutrients. 2019;11(2):E443. https://doi.org/10.3390/nu11020443.
191. Nazeri P, Kabir A, Dalili H, Mirmiran P, Azizi F. Breast-milk iodine concentrations and iodine levels of infants according to the iodine status of the country of residence: a systematic review and meta-analysis. Thyroid. 2018;28(1):124–38. https://doi.org/10.1089/thy.2017.0403.
192. Neves PAR, Castro MC, Oliveira CVR, Malta MB, Lourenço BH, Cardoso MA, et al. Effect of Vitamin A status during pregnancy on maternal anemia and newborn birth weight: results from a cohort study in the Western Brazilian Amazon. Eur J Nutr. 2020;59(1):45–56. https://doi.org/10.1007/s00394-018-1880-1.
193. Neves PAR, Lourenço BH, Pincelli A, Malta MB, Souza RM, Ferreira MU, et al. High prevalence of gestational night blindness and maternal anemia in a population-based survey of Brazilian Amazonian postpartum women. PLoS One. 2019;14(7):e0219203. https://doi.org/10.1371/journal.pone.0219203.
194. Neves PAR, Ramalho A, Padilha PC, Saunders C. The role of prenatal nutrition assistance on the prevalence of night blindness in pregnant adults. Nutr Hosp. 2014;29(5):1132–40. https://doi.org/10.3305/nh.2014.29.5.7241.
195. Nicolaides KH. A model for a new pyramid of prenatal care based on the 11 to 13 weeks' assessment. Prenat Diagn. 2011;31(1):3–6. https://doi.org/10.1002/pd.2685.
196. Nogueira JL, Saunders C, Leal MC. Anthropometric methods used in the evaluation of the postpartum weight retention: a systematic review. Cien Saude Colet. 2015;20(2):407–20. https://doi.org/10.1590/1413-81232015202.08112013.
197. O'Callaghan KM, Taghivand M, Zuchniak A, Onoyovwi A, Korsiak J, Leung M, et al. Vitamin D in breastfed infants: systematic review of alternatives to daily supplementation. Adv Nutr. 2020;11(1):144–59. https://doi.org/10.1093/advances/nmz098.
198. Oh C, Keats EC, Bhutta ZA. Vitamin and mineral supplementation during pregnancy on maternal, birth, child health and development outcomes in low- and middle-income countries:

a systematic review and meta-analysis. Nutrients. 2020;12(2):491. https://doi.org/10.3390/nu12020491.

199. Oliveira JM, Allert R, East CE. Vitamin A supplementation for postpartum women. Cochrane Database Syst Rev. 2016;3:CD005944. https://doi.org/10.1002/14651858.CD005944.pub3.
200. Organização Mundial da Saúde (OMS). Diretriz: Suplementação de vitamina A em gestantes. 2013. https://apps.who.int/iris/bitstream/handle/10665/44625/9789248501784 _por.pdf?sequence=31. Accessed 02 June 2020.
201. Organização Mundial da Saúde (OMS). Vitamina "A" na gestação e lactação: recomendações e relatório de uma consultoria. 2001. http://bvsms.saude.gov.br/bvs/publicacoes/vitaminaa_gestacao_lactacao_relatorio_consultoria.pdf. Accessed 02 June 2020.
202. Organização Pan-Americana da Saúde (OPAS); Ministério da Saúde; Federação Brasileira das Associações de Ginecologia e Obstetrícia; Sociedade Brasileira de Diabetes. Tratamento do diabetes mellitus gestacional no Brasil. 2019. https://www.diabetes.org.br/profissionais/images/pdf/Consenso_Brasileiro_Manejo_DMG_2019.pdf. Accessed 02 June 2020.
203. Padilha PC, Accioly E, Chagas C, Portela E, Silva CL, Saunders C. Birth weight variation according to maternal characteristics and gestational weight gain in Brazilian women. Nutr Hosp. 2009;24(2):207–12.
204. Padilha PC, Oliveira LM, Neves EQC, Ghedini AC, Costa T, Saunders C. Evaluation of efficacy and effectiveness of prenatal nutritional care on perinatal outcome of pregnant women; Rio de Janeiro, Brazil. Nutr Hosp. 2015;32(2):845–54. https://doi.org/10.3305/nh.2015.32.2.9045.
205. Palacios C, Kostiuk LK, Peña-Rosas JP. Vitamin D supplementation for women during pregnancy. Cochrane Database Syst Rev. 2019;7:CD008873. https://doi.org/10.1002/14651858.CD008873.pub4.
206. Pan American Health Organization (PAHO). Ultra-processed food and drink products in Latin America: sales, sources, nutrient profiles and policy implications. 2019. https://iris.paho.org/handle/10665.2/51094. Accessed 02 June 2020.
207. Pan J, Pan Q, Chen Y, Zhang H, Zheng X. Efficacy of probiotic supplement for gestational diabetes mellitus: a systematic review and meta-analysis. J Matern Fetal Neonatal Med. 2019;32(2):317–23. https://doi.org/10.1080/14767058.2017.1376318.
208. Peña-Rosas JP, De-Regil LM, Garcia-Casal MN, Dowswell T. Daily oral iron supplementation during pregnancy. Cochrane Database Syst Rev. 2015;7:CD004736. https://doi.org/10.1002/14651858.CD004736.pub5.
209. Peppard L, Oh KM, Gallo S, Milligan R. Risk of depression in pregnant women with low-normal serum Vitamin B12. Res Nurs Health. 2019;42(4):264–72. https://doi.org/10.1002/nur.21951.
210. Pereira LCR, Elliott SA, McCargar LJ, Bell RC, Vu K, Bell G, et al. The influence of energy metabolism on postpartum weight retention. Am J Clin Nutr. 2019;109(6):1588–99. https://doi.org/10.1093/ajcn/nqy389.
211. Petersen JM, Parker SE, Crider KS, Tinker SC, Mitchell AA, Werler MM. One-carbon cofactor intake and risk of neural tube defects among women who meet folic acid recommendations: a multicenter case-control study. Am J Epidemiol. 2019;188(6):1136–43. https://doi.org/10.1093/aje/kwz040.
212. Petry N, Jallow B, Sawo Y, Darboe MK, Barrow S, Sarr A, et al. Micronutrient deficiencies, nutritional status and the determinants of anemia in children 0-59 months of age and non-pregnant women of reproductive age in the Gambia. Nutrients. 2019;11(10):2275. https://doi.org/10.3390/nu11102275.
213. Phelan S, Hagobian T, Brannen A, Hatley KE, Schaffner A, Muñoz-Christian K, et al. Effect of an internet-based program on weight loss for low-income postpartum women: a randomized clinical trial. JAMA. 2017;317(23):2381–91. https://doi.org/10.1001/jama.2017.7119.
214. Phillips KM, Stewart KK, Karanja NM, Windhauser MM, Champagne CM, Swain JF, et al. Validation of diet composition for the Dietary Approaches to Stop Hypertension trial. DASH

Collaborative Research Group. J Am Diet Assoc. 1999;99(8):S60–8. https://doi.org/10.1016/s0002-8223(99)00418-6.
215. Portugal RD, Montenegro CAB. Doenças Hematológicas. In: Montenegro CAB, Rezende Filho J, editors. Rezende Obstetrícia. Rio de Janeiro: Guanabara Koogan; 2017. p. 522–6.
216. Rahman MM, Abe SK, Rahman MS, Kanda M, Narita S, Bilano V, et al. Maternal anemia and risk of adverse birth and health outcomes in low- and middle-income countries: systematic review and meta-analysis. Am J Clin Nutr. 2016;103(2):495–504. https://doi.org/10.3945/ajcn.115.107896.
217. Randunu RS, Bertolo RF. The effects of maternal and postnatal dietary methyl nutrients on epigenetic changes that lead to non-communicable diseases in adulthood. Int J Mol Sci. 2020;21(9):E3290. https://doi.org/10.3390/ijms21093290.
218. Redman EK, Hauspurg A, Hubel CA, Roberts JM, Jeyabalan A. Clinical course, associated factors, and blood pressure profile of delayed-onset postpartum preeclampsia. Obstet Gynecol. 2019;134(5):995–1001. https://doi.org/10.1097/AOG.0000000000003508.
219. Reutrakul S, Anothaisintawee T, Herring SJ, Balserak BI, Marc I, Thakkinstian A. Short sleep duration and hyperglycemia in pregnancy: aggregate and individual patient data meta-analysis. Sleep Med Rev. 2018;40:31–42. https://doi.org/10.1016/j.smrv.2017.09.003.
220. Rezende J, Montenegro CAB. Obstetrícia fundamental. Rio de Janeiro: Guanabara Koogan; 1999.
221. Rezende KB, Bornia RG, Esteves AP, Cunha AJ, Amim JJ. Preeclampsia: prevalence and perinatal repercussions in a University Hospital in Rio de Janeiro, Brazil. Pregnancy Hypertens. 2016;6(4):253–5. https://doi.org/10.1016/j.preghy.2016.08.229.
222. Ribas Filho D, Nogueira de Almeida CA, Oliveira Filho AE. Current position on vitamin D in clinical practice: position of the Brazilian Association of Nutrology (Abran). Int J Nutrol. 2020;12:82–96. https://doi.org/10.1055/s-0040-1709661.
223. Rodgers RF, O'Flynn JL, Bourdeau A, Zimmerman E. A biopsychosocial model of body image, disordered eating, and breastfeeding among postpartum women. Appetite. 2018;126:163–8. https://doi.org/10.1016/j.appet.2018.04.007.
224. Rogne T, Tielemans MJ, Chong MF, Yajnik CS, Krishnaveni GV, Poston L, et al. Associations of maternal vitamin B12 concentration in pregnancy with the risks of preterm birth and low birth weight: a systematic review and meta-analysis of individual participant data. Am J Epidemiol. 2017;185(3):212–23. https://doi.org/10.1093/aje/kww212.
225. Rohatgi KW, Tinius RA, Cade WT, Steele EM, Cahill AG, Parra DC. Relationships between consumption of ultra-processed foods, gestational weight gain and neonatal outcomes in a sample of US pregnant women. PeerJ. 2017;5:e4091. https://doi.org/10.7717/peerj.4091.
226. Salazar-López ME, Vanin AA, Cazella SC, Levandowski DC. Feeding consequences of orphans after the mother's death: a study using text mining software. Cad Saúde Pública. 2020;36(3):e00189717. https://doi.org/10.1590/0102-311X00189717.
227. Sanjarimoghaddam F, Bahadori F, Bakhshimoghaddam F, Alizadeh M. Association between quality and quantity of dietary carbohydrate and pregnancy-induced hypertension: a case-control study. Clin Nutr ESPEN. 2019;33:158–63. https://doi.org/10.1016/j.clnesp.2019.06.001.
228. Santos KD, Moreira TM, Belfort GP, Silva CFMD, Padilha PC, Barros DC, et al. Adaptation of DASH diet (Dietary Approach to Stop Hypertension) for postpartum nutritional care at primary healthcare. Rev Bras Epidemiol. 2019;22:e190035. https://doi.org/10.1590/1980-549720190035.
229. Santos KD, Patrício PT, Lima TSV, Barros DC, Saunders C. A pilot intervention to reduce postpartum weight retention at primary health care in Brazil. Nutr Hosp. 2019;36(4):854–61. https://doi.org/10.20960/nh.02508.
230. Santos MMAS, Barros DC, Nogueira JL, Baião MR, Saunders C. Impact of an intervention nutrition program during prenatal on the weight of newborns from teenage mothers. Nutr Hosp. 2013;28(6):1943–50.

231. Santos QD, Sichieri R, Marchioni DML, Verly JE. Brazilian pregnant and lactating women do not change their food intake to meet nutritional goals. BMC Pregnancy Childbirth. 2014;14:186. https://doi.org/10.1186/1471-2393-14-186.
232. Saronga NJ, Burrows T, Collins CE, Ashman AM, Rollo ME. mHealth interventions targeting pregnancy intakes in low and lower-middle income countries: systematic review. Matern Child Nutr. 2019;15(2):e12777. https://doi.org/10.1111/mcn.12777.
233. Sarr O, Yang K, Regnault TR. In utero programming of later adiposity: the role of fetal growth restriction. J Pregnancy. 2012:134758. https://doi.org/10.1155/2012/134758.
234. Saunders C, Accioly E, Costa RSS, Lacerda EMA, Santos MMAS. Gestante adolescente. In: Accioly E, Saunders C, Lacerda EMA, editors. Nutrição em Obstetrícia e Pediatria. 2nd ed. Rio de Janeiro: Cultura Médica/Guanabara Koogan; 2012. p. 151–75.
235. Saunders C, Bessa TCD, Padilha PC. Assistência Nutricional Pré-natal. In: Accioly E, Saunders C, Lacerda EMA, editors. Nutrição em Obstetrícia e Pediatria. 2nd ed. Rio de Janeiro: Cultura Médica/Guanabara Koogan; 2012. p. 103–26.
236. Saunders C, Chagas CB. Síndromes Hipertensivas da Gravidez. In: Accioly E, Saunders C, Lacerda EMA, editors. Nutrição em Obstetrícia e Pediatria. 2nd ed. Rio de Janeiro: Cultura Médica/Guanabara Koogan; 2012. p. 177–94.
237. Saunders C, do Carmo Leal M, Gomes MM, Campos LF, dos Santos Silva BA, Thiapó de Lima AP, et al. Gestational nightblindness among women attending a public maternity hospital in Rio de Janeiro, Brazil. J Health Popul Nutr. 2004;22(4):348–56.
238. Saunders C, Leal Mdo C, Neves PA, Padilha Pde C, da Silva LB, Schilithz AO. Determinants of gestational night blindness in pregnant women from Rio de Janeiro, Brazil. Public Health Nutr. 2016;19(5):851–60. https://doi.org/10.1017/S1368980015001846.
239. Saunders C, Montenegro CAB. Uso de medicamentos. In: Montenegro CAB, Rezende Filho J, editors. Rezende Obstetrícia. Rio de Janeiro: Guanabara Koogan; 2017. p. 164–8.
240. Saunders C, Neves EQC, Accioly E. Recomendações Nutricionais na Gestação. In: Accioly E, Saunders C, Lacerda EMA, editors. Nutrição em Obstetrícia e Pediatria. 2nd ed. Rio de Janeiro: Cultura Médica/Guanabara Koogan; 2012. p. 127–50.
241. Saunders C, Padilha PC. Diabetes Melito na Gestação. In: Accioly E, Saunders C, Lacerda EMA, editors. Nutrição em Obstetrícia e Pediatria. 2nd ed. Rio de Janeiro: Cultura Médica/Guanabara Koogan; 2012. p. 195–212.
242. Saunders C, Ramalho RA, de Lima AP, Gomes MM, Campos LF, dos Santos Silva BA, et al. Association between gestational night blindness and serum retinol in mother/newborn pairs in the city of Rio de Janeiro, Brazil. Nutrition. 2005;21(4):456–61. https://doi.org/10.1016/j.nut.2004.07.015.
243. Saunders C, Padilha PC, Líbera BD, Nogueira JL, Oliveira LM, Astulla A. Picamalácia: epidemiologia e associação com complicações da gravidez. Rev Bras Ginecol Obstet. 2009;31(9):440–6. https://doi.org/10.1590/S0100-72032009000900004.
244. Saunders C, Schilithz AOC, Santos MMAS, Santana RBB, Gama SGN, Leal MC. Gestational night blindness in teenagers in Rio de Janeiro, Brazil. Adolesc Saude. 2018;15(4):53–64.
245. Say L, Chou D, Gemmill A, Tunçalp Ö, Moller AB, Daniels J, et al. Global causes of maternal death: a WHO systematic analysis. Lancet Glob Health. 2014;2(6):e323–33. https://doi.org/10.1016/S2214-109X(14)70227-X.
246. Schulze KJ, Mehra S, Shaikh S, Ali H, Shamim AA, Wu LS, et al. Antenatal multiple micronutrient supplementation compared to iron-folic acid affects micronutrient status but does not eliminate deficiencies in a randomized controlled trial among pregnant women of rural Bangladesh. J Nutr. 2019;149(7):1260–70. https://doi.org/10.1093/jn/nxz046.
247. Scientific Advisory Committee on Nutrition. Vitamin D and health. 2016. https://www.gov.uk/government/groups/scientific-advisory-committee-on-nutrition. Accessed 27 Feb 2020.
248. Sharma KJ, Kilpatrick SJ. Postpartum hypertension: etiology, diagnosis, and management. Obstet Gynecol Surv. 2017;72(4):248–52. https://doi.org/10.1097/OGX.0000000000000424.
249. Silva AB, Assumpção AMB, Andrade Filha IG, Regadas CT, Castro MC, Silva CRA, et al. Cross-cultural adaptation of the Zero Mothers Die (ZMD-App) in Brazil: contributing to

digital health with the approach on care centred for e-pregnant woman. Rev Bras Saude Mater Infant. 2019;19(4):751–62. https://doi.org/10.1590/1806-93042019000400002.
250. Silva C, Keating E, Pinto E. The impact of folic acid supplementation on gestational and long term health: critical temporal windows, benefits and risks. Porto Biomed J. 2017;2(6):315–32. https://doi.org/10.1016/j.pbj.2017.05.006.
251. Silva F. Índice Glicêmico e Carga glicêmica. In: Bosco S, Genro J, editors. Nutrigenética e Implicações na saúde humana. São Paulo: Atheneu; 2014. p. 101–17.
252. Silva LBG, Rosado EL, de Carvalho PP, Dias JR, Moreira TM, de Paula TP, de Barros DC, Saunders C. Food intake of women with gestational diabetes mellitus, in accordance with two methods of dietary guidance: a randomised controlled clinical trial. Br J Nutr. 2019;121(1):82–92. https://doi.org/10.1017/S0007114518001484.
253. Silva SOCD, Saunders C, Zajdenverg L, Moreira LN, Heidelmann SP, Pereira ACDS, et al. Predictive factors for birth weight of newborns of mothers with gestational diabetes mellitus. Diabetes Res Clin Pract. 2018;138:262–70. https://doi.org/10.1016/j.diabres.2018.01.032.
254. Silva ML, Galvão AC, Souza NL, Azevedo GD, Jerônimo SM, Araújo AC. Women with cardiovascular risk after preeclampsia: is there follow-up within the Unified Health System in Brazil? Rev Lat Am Enfermagem. 2014;22(1):93–9. https://doi.org/10.1590/0104-1169.3197.2389.
255. Simşek M, Naziroğlu M, Simşek H, Cay M, Aksakal M, Kumru S. Blood plasma levels of lipoperoxides, glutathione peroxidase, beta carotene, vitamin A and E in women with habitual abortion. Cell Biochem Funct. 1998;16(4):227–31.
256. Singh MD, Thomas P, Owens J, Hague W, Fenech M. Potential role of folate in pre-eclampsia. Nutr Rev. 2015;73(10):694–722. https://doi.org/10.1093/nutrit/nuv028.
257. Sociedade Brasileira de Diabetes (SBD). Diretrizes da Sociedade Brasileira de Diabetes 2019–2020. 2019. https://www.diabetes.org.br/profissionais/images/DIRETRIZES-COMPLETA-2019-2020.pdf. Accessed 02 June 2020.
258. Sosa-Castillo E, Rodríguez-Cruz M, Moltó-Puigmartí C. Genomics of lactation: role of nutrigenomics and nutrigenetics in the fatty acid composition of human milk. Br J Nutr. 2017;118(3):161–8. https://doi.org/10.1017/S0007114517001854.
259. Souto D, Rosado E. Contagem de Carboidratos no Diabetes Melito - Abordagem Teórica e Prática. Rio de Janeiro: Rubio; 2018.
260. Stang J, Huffman LG. Position of the academy of nutrition and dietetics: obesity, reproduction, and pregnancy outcomes. J Acad Nutr Diet. 2016;116(4):677–91. https://doi.org/10.1016/j.jand.2016.01.008.
261. Stangret A, Wnuk A, Szewczyk G, Pyzlak M, Szukiewicz D. Maternal hemoglobin concentration and hematocrit values may affect fetus development by influencing placental angiogenesis. J Matern Fetal Neonatal Med. 2017;30(2):199–204. https://doi.org/10.3109/14767058.2016.1168395.
262. Steele EM, Juul F, Neri D, Rauber F, Monteiro CA. Dietary share of ultra-processed foods and metabolic syndrome in the US adult population. Prev Med. 2019;125:40–8. https://doi.org/10.1016/j.ypmed.2019.05.004.
263. Stendell-Hollis NR, Thompson PA, West JL, Wertheim BC, Thomson CA. A comparison of Mediterranean-style and MyPyramid diets on weight loss and inflammatory biomarkers in postpartum breastfeeding women. J Womens Health (Larchmt). 2013;22(1):48–57. https://doi.org/10.1089/jwh.2012.3707.
264. Sultan P, Bampoe S, Shah R, Guo N, Estes J, Stave C, et al. Oral vs intravenous iron therapy for postpartum anemia: a systematic review and meta-analysis. Am J Obstet Gynecol. 2019;221(1):19–29.e3. https://doi.org/10.1016/j.ajog.2018.12.016.
265. Suzuki S, Igarashi M, Yamashita E, Satomi M. Ptyalism gravidarum. N Am J Med Sci. 2009;1(6):303–4.
266. Tabela Brasileira de Composição de Alimentos (TBCA). Universidade de São Paulo (USP). Food Research Center (FoRC). Versão 7.0. 2019. http://www.fcf.usp.br/tbca. Accessed 22 May 2020.

267. Taylor BL, Woodfall GE, Sheedy KE, O'Riley ML, Rainbow KA, Bramwell EL. Effect of probiotics on metabolic outcomes in pregnant women with gestational diabetes: a systematic review and meta-analysis of randomized controlled trials. Nutrients. 2017;9(5):E461. https://doi.org/10.3390/nu9050461.
268. The Lancet. Executive summary of the lancet maternal and child nutrition series. 2013. https://www.thelancet.com/series/maternal-and-child-nutrition. Accessed 21 Apr 2020.
269. Thorne-Lyman AL, Fawzi WW. Vitamin A and carotenoids during pregnancy and maternal, neonatal and infant health outcomes: a systematic review and meta-analysis. Paediatr Perinat Epidemiol. 2012;26 Suppl 1(1):36–54. https://doi.org/10.1111/j.1365-3016.2012.01284.x.
270. Tielsch JM, Rahmathullah L, Katz J, Thulasiraj RD, Coles C, Sheeladevi S, et al. Maternal night blindness during pregnancy is associated with low birthweight, morbidity, and poor growth in South India. J Nutr. 2008;138(4):787–92. https://doi.org/10.1093/jn/138.4.787.
271. Tobias DK, Zhang C, Chavarro J, Bowers K, Rich-Edwards J, Rosner B, et al. Prepregnancy adherence to dietary patterns and lower risk of gestational diabetes mellitus. Am J Clin Nutr. 2012;96(2):289–95. https://doi.org/10.3945/ajcn.111.028266.
272. Tojal A, Neves C, Veiga H, Ferreira S, Rodrigues I, Martel F, et al. Perigestational high folic acid: impact on offspring's peripheral metabolic response. Food Funct. 2019;10(11):7216–26. https://doi.org/10.1039/c9fo01807g.
273. Tully KP, Stuebe AM, Verbiest SB. The fourth trimester: a critical transition period with unmet maternal health needs. Am J Obstet Gynecol. 2017;217(1):37–41. https://doi.org/10.1016/j.ajog.2017.03.032.
274. van der Pligt P, Ball K, Hesketh KD, Crawford D, Teychenne M, Campbell K. The views of first time mothers completing an intervention to reduce postpartum weight retention: a qualitative evaluation of the mums OnLiNE study. Midwifery. 2018;56:23–8. https://doi.org/10.1016/j.midw.2017.09.013.
275. van der Pligt P, Ball K, Hesketh KD, Teychenne M, Crawford D, Morgan PJ, et al. A pilot intervention to reduce postpartum weight retention and central adiposity in first-time mothers: results from the mums OnLiNE (Online, Lifestyle, Nutrition & Exercise) study. J Hum Nutr Diet. 2018;31(3):314–28. https://doi.org/10.1111/jhn.12521.
276. van der Pligt P, Willcox J, Hesketh KD, Ball K, Wilkinson S, Crawford D, et al. Systematic review of lifestyle interventions to limit postpartum weight retention: implications for future opportunities to prevent maternal overweight and obesity following childbirth. Obes Rev. 2013;14(10):792–805. https://doi.org/10.1111/obr.12053.
277. van der Pligt P, Willcox J, Szymlek-Gay EA, Murray E, Worsley A, Daly RM. Associations of maternal vitamin D deficiency with pregnancy and neonatal complications in developing countries: a systematic review. Nutrients. 2018;10(5):E640. https://doi.org/10.3390/nu10050640.
278. Victora CG, Bahl R, Barros AJ, França GV, Horton S, Krasevec J, et al. Breastfeeding in the 21st century: epidemiology, mechanisms, and lifelong effect. Lancet. 2016;387(10017):475–90. https://doi.org/10.1016/S0140-6736(15)01024-7.
279. Vieten C, Laraia BA, Kristeller J, Adler N, Coleman-Phox K, Bush NR, et al. The mindful moms training: development of a mindfulness-based intervention to reduce stress and overeating during pregnancy. BMC Pregnancy Childbirth. 2018;18(1):201. https://doi.org/10.1186/s12884-018-1757-6.
280. Villar J, Repke JT. Calcium supplementation during pregnancy may reduce preterm delivery in high risk populations. Am J Obstet Gyn. 1990;163(4):1124–31. https://doi.org/10.1016/0002-9378(90)90669-x.
281. Watkins AJ, Dias I, Tsuro H, Allen D, Emes RD, Moreton J, et al. Paternal diet programs offspring health through sperm- and seminal plasma-specific pathways in mice. Proc Natl Acad Sci U S A. 2018;115(40):10064–9. https://doi.org/10.1073/pnas.1806333115.
282. Wei Y, Yang CR, Wei YP, Zhao ZA, Hou Y, Schatten H, et al. Paternally induced transgenerational inheritance of susceptibility to diabetes in mammals. Proc Natl Acad Sci U S A. 2014;111(5):1873–8. https://doi.org/10.1073/pnas.1321195111.

283. World Health Organization (WHO). Global nutrition policy review 2016–2017: country progress in creating enabling policy environments for promoting healthy diets and nutrition. 2018. https://apps.who.int/iris/handle/10665/275990. Accessed 15 May 2020.
284. World Health Organization (WHO). Global prevalence of vitamin A deficiency in populations at risk 1995–2005. WHO Global Database on Vitamin A Deficiency. 2009. https://www.who.int/nutrition/publications/micronutrients/vitamin_a_deficiency/9789241598019/en/. Accessed May 2020.
285. World Health Organization (WHO). Growth reference data for 5–19 years. BMI-for-age GIRLS 5 to 19 years (percentiles). 2007. http://www.who.int/growthref/. Accessed 02 June 2020.
286. World Health Organization (WHO). Guideline: iron supplementation in postpartum women. 2016. https://apps.who.int/iris/handle/10665/249242. Accessed 24 Feb 2020.
287. World Health Organization (WHO). WHO recommendations on antenatal care for a positive pregnancy experience. 2016b. https://www.who.int/publications-detail/9789241549912. Accessed 05 May 2020.
288. World Health Organization (WHO). Indicators for assessing Vitamin A Deficiency and their application in monitoring and evaluating intervention programmes. 1996. https://apps.who.int/iris/handle/10665/63064. Accessed 24 Feb 2020.
289. World Health Organization (WHO). Nutritional anaemias: tools for effective prevention and control. 2017. https://apps.who.int/iris/handle/10665/259425. Accessed 28 May 2020.
290. World Health Organization (WHO). Physical status: the use and interpretation of anthropometry. 1995. https://apps.who.int/iris/handle/10665/37003. Accessed 02 June 2020.
291. World Health Organization (WHO). Reaching optimal iodine nutrition in pregnant and lactating women and young children. 2007. https://www.who.int/who-documents-detail/WHO-statement-IDD-pregnantwomen-children. Accessed 05 May 2020.
292. World Health Organization (WHO). Trends in maternal mortality 2000 to 2017: estimates by WHO, UNICEF, UNFPA, World Bank Group and the United Nations Population Division: executive summary. 2019. https://apps.who.int/iris/handle/10665/327596. Accessed 02 June 2020.
293. World Health Organization (WHO).Weekly iron and folic acid supplementation as an anaemia-prevention strategy in women and adolescent girls: lessons learnt from implementation of programmes among non pregnant women of reproductive age. 2018. https://apps.who.int/iris/handle/10665/274581. Accessed 12 May 2020.
294. World Health Organization (WHO). WHO guideline on use of ferritin concentrations to assess iron status in individuals and populations. 2020. https://apps.who.int/iris/handle/10665/331505. Accessed 12 May 2020.
295. World Health Organization (WHO). WHO recommendation: Calcium supplementation during pregnancy for prevention of pre-eclampsia and its complications. 2018. https://apps.who.int/iris/handle/10665/277235. Accessed 02 June 2020.
296. World Health Organization (WHO). WHO recommendation on calcium supplementation before pregnancy for the prevention of pre-eclampsia and its complications. 2020. https://apps.who.int/iris/handle/10665/331787. Accessed 15 May 2020.
297. World Health Organization (WHO). WHO recommendations on antenatal care for a positive pregnancy experience. 2016. https://www.who.int/publications-detail/9789241549912. Accessed 05 May 2020.
298. World Health Organization (WHO). WHO technical report series n° 935. Protein and amino acid requirements in human nutrition: report of a joint FAO/WHO/UNU expert consultation. 2007. https://apps.who.int/iris/handle/10665/43411. Accessed 22 Feb 2020.
299. World Health Organization (WHO). Xerophthalmia and night blindness for the assessment of clinical vitamin A deficiency in individuals and populations. 2014. https://apps.who.int/iris/handle/10665/133705. Accessed 02 June 2020.

300. World Health Organization (WHO); International Telecommunication Union (ITU). eHealth and innovation in women's and children's health: a baseline review. 2014. https://www.who.int/goe/publications/baseline_fullreport/en/. Accessed 06 May 2020.
301. Xiao RS, Kroll-Desrosiers AR, Goldberg RJ, Pagoto SL, Person SD, Waring ME. The impact of sleep, stress, and depression on postpartum weight retention: a systematic review. J Psychosom Res. 2014;77(5):351–8. https://doi.org/10.1016/j.jpsychores.2014.09.016.
302. Yang Z, Phung H, Freebairn L, Sexton R, Raulli A, Kelly P. Contribution of maternal overweight and obesity to the occurrence of adverse pregnancy outcomes. Aust N Z J Obstet Gynaecol. 2019;59(3):367–74. https://doi.org/10.1111/ajo.12866.
303. Yaribeygi H, Maleki M, Sathyapalan T, Iranpanah H, Orafai HM, Jamialahmadi T, et al. The molecular mechanisms by which vitamin D improve glucose homeostasis: a mechanistic review. Life Sci. 2020;244:117305. https://doi.org/10.1016/j.lfs.2020.117305.
304. Yoshida T, Stern PH. How vitamin D works on bone. Endocrinol Metab Clin N Am. 2012;41(3):557–69. https://doi.org/10.1016/j.ecl.2012.04.003.
305. Yue CY, Ying CM. Epidemiological analysis of maternal lipid levels during the second trimester in pregnancy and the risk of adverse pregnancy outcome adjusted by pregnancy BMI. J Clin Lab Anal. 2018;32(8):e22568. https://doi.org/10.1002/jcla.22568.
306. Zhang J, Ma S, Wu S, Guo C, Long S, Tan H. Effects of probiotic supplement in pregnant women with gestational diabetes mellitus: a systematic review and meta-analysis of randomized controlled trials. J Diabetes Res. 2019;2019:5364730. https://doi.org/10.1155/2019/5364730.
307. Zhang R, Han S, Chen GC, Li ZN, Silva-Zolezzi I, Parés GV, et al. Effects of low-glycemic-index diets in pregnancy on maternal and newborn outcomes in pregnant women: a meta-analysis of randomized controlled trials. Eur J Nutr. 2018;57(1):167–77. https://doi.org/10.1007/s00394-016-1306-x.
308. Zhao W, Li X, Xia X, Gao Z, Han C. Iodine nutrition during pregnancy: past, present, and future. Biol Trace Elem Res. 2019;188(1):196–207. https://doi.org/10.1007/s12011-018-1502-z.
309. Zive MM, Rhee KE. Call to action: continuum of care for females of reproductive age to prevent obesity and ensure better health outcomes of offspring through nutrition. Clin Obstet Gynecol. 2014;57(3):446–55. https://doi.org/10.1097/GRF.0000000000000046.

Chapter 9
Physical Exercise During Pregnancy

Antonio Claudio Lucas da Nóbrega and Renata Rodrigues Teixeira de Castro

Introduction

In 1949, the US Children's Bureau issued a standard recommendation for pregnant women to limit physical activity due to the possibility of decreasing oxygen supply to the baby and other potential risks [1]. Therefore, according to this document, pregnant women should avoid sports participation but could continue to do housework, gardening, daily walks (up to 1 mile/day), and swim occasionally. These recommendations were sustained in most prenatal exercise programs of the 1970s and 1980s [2].

It is not only before 35 years later in 1985 that the American College of Obstetricians and Gynecologists (ACOG) issued the first guideline from medical specialists for prenatal physical activity [3]. This document was based mainly on the consensus opinion of a panel of obstetricians and advised against high-impact activities that could elicit heart rates greater than 140 beats/minute and core body temperature above 38°C (100.4°F). Since then, several studies have evaluated the safety of prenatal physical activity and maternal and fetal outcomes with neutral or beneficial findings for the mother and the baby. These findings guide current recommendations for prenatal physical activity, as we aim to show in this chapter.

A. C. L. da Nóbrega
Laboratório de Ciências do Exercício, Instituto Biomédico, Universidade Federal Fluminense, Niterói, RJ, Brazil
e-mail: anobrega@id.uff.br

R. R. T. de Castro (✉)
Department of Cardiology, Hospital Naval Marcílio Dias & School of Medicine, Iguaçu University, Rio de Janeiro, RJ, Brazil

© Springer Nature Switzerland AG 2022
R. A. Moreira de Sá, E. B. d. Fonseca (eds.), *Perinatology*,
https://doi.org/10.1007/978-3-030-83434-0_9

Principles of Exercise Prescription

The World Health Organization defines physical activity as any bodily movement produced by skeletal muscles that requires energy expenditure [4]. Regular physical activity reduces the risk of cardiovascular disease, hypertension, diabetes, and different types of cancer as breast and colon in the general population [5–10]. Regular physical activity has also positive effects on mental health and can delay the onset of dementia [11]. Finally, physical activity helps the maintenance of a healthy weight [12, 13]. Despite all the proven benefits of physical activity, global prevalence of insufficient physical activity is 27.5% [14] and physical inactivity represents the fourth leading risk factor for global mortality [4].

It is important to note the differences between physical activity and exercise. Physical activity includes any bodily movement and is done as part of playing, working, and doing house chore or recreational activities. A subgroup of physical activity is "exercise," which is a planned, structured, repetitive, and purposeful physical activity performed to improve or maintain physical fitness. Further, "sports" is an exercise subgroup performed under certain rules with the aim of competition and recreation (Fig. 9.1).

Concerning the overall health benefits with physical activity, there is a close dose–response relationship between underline physiological effects and energy expenditure regardless of isolated variations of the components of the exercise practice. In other words, no matter how, keep accumulating energy expenditure with body movements and the benefits will develop.

Given the undisputable health benefits of exercise, its prescription should follow specific principles to pursue the lowest risk/benefits ratio. The American College of Physicians recommends the **FITT-VP** principle of exercise prescription (Table 9.1), which employs **F**requency (how often), **I**ntensity (how hard), **T**ime (duration of exercise session), **T**ype (mode or kind of exercise), **V**olume (amount of exercise throughout a period of time), and **P**rogression (advancement) [15]. The FITT-VP principle should guide exercise prescription tailored to each individual, according to

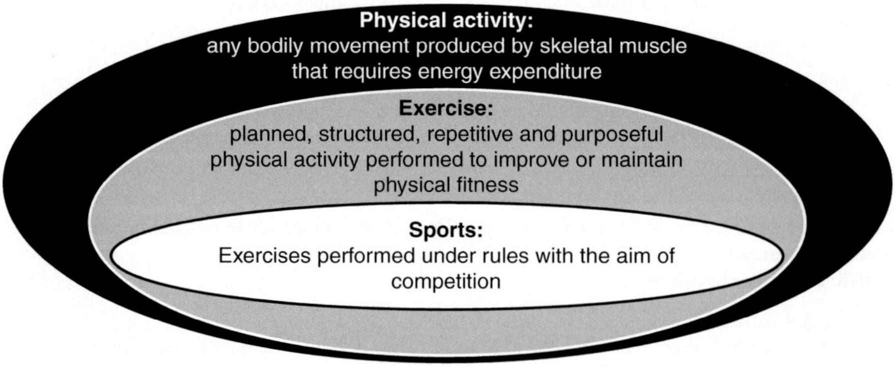

Fig. 9.1 The relationship between physical activity, exercise, and sport

Table 9.1 FITT-VP principles: basic components of exercise prescription

	Meaning	Description: example
F	Frequency	How often: times/week
I	Intensity	How hard: heart rate limits, speed, power
T	Time	Duration of exercise session: minutes/session
T	Type	Mode or kind of exercise: aerobic, strength training, flexibility
V	Volume	Amount of exercise: km/week
P	Progression	Advancement: increase in intensity or time/session

clinical and personal characteristics and scientific evidence of benefits and harm mitigation.

The American College of Sports Medicine (ACSM) recommends that all healthy adults aged 18–65 years old should participate in moderate intensity, aerobic physical activity for a minimum of 30 minutes on 5 days per week or vigorous intensity, aerobic activity for a minimum of 20 minutes on 3 days/week [15]. Also, every adult should perform activities that maintain or increase muscular strength and endurance at least twice a week [15].

Fetal and Maternal Anatomic and Physiologic Aspects of Exercise

Anatomic and physiologic aspects that are specific to pregnancy should be considered when prescribing exercise to pregnant women [16, 17]. Flores et al. [18] have recently published the first study that examined walking balance in pregnancy. They concluded that significant nonlinear changes in balance occur during pregnancy starting in the first trimester, even before significant weight gain is perceived. Thus, it is important for pregnant women to be advised about the risk of falling even while performing daily activities [18–20].

Pregnancy weight gain and the shift in the point of gravity result in progressive lordosis which increases the forces across joints and spine during weight-bearing exercise. Therefore, more than 60% of all pregnant women complains about low back pain [21]. Shiri et al. [22] published a meta-analysis including 2347 pregnant women and found a 9% risk reduction of low back pain with exercise. Another meta-analysis including 52,297 pregnant women did not prove the capacity of exercise to reduce this risk, but found that prenatal exercise decreased the severity of low back pain in pregnant women [23]. The antagonic results in both meta-analysis [22, 23] may be explained by the lack of details (FITT-VP) of prescribed exercise in the included studies. Considering the best available evidence, ACOG suggests that strengthening of back and abdominal muscles could minimize de risk of low back pain [16].

Pregnant women exhibit increased blood volume and resting heart rate, cardiac output, and reduced systemic vascular resistance. The acute cardiovascular responses to exercise are increased during pregnancy when compared to nonpregnancy [24–26]. While heart rate responses to exercise are increased in pregnant women, fetal heart rate demonstrates increases of only 10–30 beats per minute over the baseline [27, 28].

It is important to note that type of exercise and body upright position and other conditions such as exercise in the heat may decrease venous return and increase the risk of hypotension. Thus, Valsalva maneuver, certain yoga positions, and static supine exercise should be avoided [29]. In addition, pregnant women should avoid high heat and humidity, especially in the first trimester, as exposure to heat from hot tubes, sauna, or even fever has been associated with an increase in fetal neural tube defects [24–26]. Although exercise increase in core temperature is not so intense, pregnant women should wear loose-fitting clothing and stay well hydrated while exercising [16].

Exercise During Pregnancy

As regular exercise during pregnancy improves or maintains physical fitness, pregnant women should be encouraged to exercise. Also, women who exercised during pregnancy experienced reduction in gestational diabetes mellitus and preeclampsia [30–33]. A recent meta-analysis found no differences in cesarean section rates between usual care and telephone-delivered pelvic floor muscle training exercises [34]. Unfortunately, it has not been found other studies investigating the potential impact of regular exercise in preventing unnecessary cesarean sections.

Although regular physical exercise should be recommended to all pregnant women in the absence of contraindications (Table 9.2), it is important to warn women to terminate or not start exercise in the presence of vaginal bleeding, rest

Table 9.2 Relative and absolute contraindications for exercising during pregnancy [16]

Relative contraindications
Severe anemia
Poorly controlled clinical conditions such as maternal cardiac arrhythmia, hypertension, seizure disorder, hyperthyroidism
Heavy smoker
Chronic bronchitis
Poorly controlled type 1 diabetes mellitus
Extreme morbid obesity
Extreme underweight
History of extremely sedentary lifestyle
Intrauterine growth restriction in current pregnancy
Orthopedic limitations
Absolute contraindications
Hemodynamically significant heart disease
Restrictive lung disease
Incompetent cervix/cerclage
Multiple gestation at risk of premature labor
Persistent second or third semester bleeding
Placenta previa after 26 weeks of gestation
Premature labor during current pregnancy
Ruptured membranes
Preeclampsia/pregnancy-induced hypertension

dyspnea, dizziness, headache, chest pain, muscle weakness, calf pain or swelling, and amniotic fluid leakage [16].

The ACSM suggests that previously sedentary pregnant women should be cleared by the PARmed-X [35] questionnaire before starting physical exercise. The PARmed-X was developed by the Canadian Society for exercise physiology and is a convenient checklist and prescription for use by health care providers to evaluate pregnant patients who want to enter a prenatal fitness program and for ongoing medical surveillance of exercising pregnant patients [35]. Regardless of pregnant women healthy status, some sports should be avoided during pregnancy: contact sports (as boxing, soccer, and basketball); activities with a high risk of falling (e.g., downhill snow skiing, water skiing, surfing, off-road cycling, gymnastics, and horseback riding); scuba and sky diving; hot yoga; and hot Pilates [17].

The ACSM exercise prescription recommendations for pregnant women are detailed in Table 9.3. There are different ways to prescribe exercise intensity. As shown in Table 9.3, ACSM recommends that exercise intensity should be defined by heart rate. Nevertheless, some authors postulate that heart rate responses may be blunted in pregnant women suggesting that the rate of perceived exertion would be more effective while monitoring exercise intensity in this population [3, 36].

The original rate of perceived exertion scale (Table 9.4), also known as the Borg scale [37] was set to run from 6 to 20 as a simple way to estimate heart rate. Multiplying the Borg score by 10 gives an approximate heart rate for a particular level of activity. A revised Borg scale runs from 0 to 10 (Table 9.4). When perceived exertion is used to prescribe exercise intensity, moderate activity should be prescribed to women with a body mass index below 25 kg/m^2 and women with higher body mass index should start with light exercise (Table 9.5).

Table 9.3 ACSM's aerobic exercise prescription for pregnant women

Body mass index	Frequency	Intensity: Age (years)	Intensity: Fitness level	Intensity: Exercise heart rate (beats/minute)	Time (exercise session/day of the week)
<25 kg/m^2	3–4 exercise days/week	< 20	All	140–155	10–15 minutes of warm-up +15 minutes of dynamic, rhythmic activities +10–15 minutes of cool-down
		20–29	Low	129–144	
			Active	135–150	
			Fit	145–160	
		30–39	Low	128–144	
			Active	130–145	
			Fit	140–156	
<25 kg/m^2	3–4 exercise days/week	20–29	All	102–124	10–15 minutes of warm-up +25 minutes of dynamic, rhythmic activities +10–15 minutes of cool-down
		30–39	All	101–120	

Progression should be gradual and start after the first trimester, from 15 minutes to 30–40 minutes/session

Table 9.4 Rate of perceived exertion: original Borg scale

Exercise intensity	Borg rating (6–20)
None	6
Very, very light	7–8
Very light	9–10
Fairly light	11–12
Somewhat hard	13–14
Hard	15–16
Very hard	17–18
Very, very hard	19–20

Table 9.5 Rate of perceived exertion: modified Borg scale

Exercise intensity	Modified Borg rating (0–10)
Nothing at all	0
Extremely weak/just noticeable	0.5
Very weak	1
Weak/light	2
Moderate	3–4
Strong/heavy	5–6
Very strong	7–8
Extremely strong	9–10

Competitive Athletes

Serena Williams won in 2017, her 23rd tennis Grand Slam title while in the first trimester of her pregnancy. Other athletes, including 18 Olympians, are known to have competed while expecting. Some of them only discovered pregnancy after the Olympic games, as the American diver Juno Stover-Irvin who won the Bronze Medal in 1952, while in the second trimester of pregnancy [38]. Nevertheless, diving and other contact sports should be avoided, but strenuous training can be safely maintained by athletes throughout pregnancy, until pregnancy body changes (weight gain and change in the center of gravity) impairs performance [17, 39].

Exercise in the Postpartum Period

Women frequently reduce their level of exercise training after childbirth, frequently leading to overweight and obesity [40–42]. Health care providers should encourage women to exercise in the postpartum period, promoting faster recovery to prepregnancy status and collaborating to lifelong health habits.

After delivery, regular exercise routine should be resumed as soon as medically safe. Women who had an uncomplicated pregnancy and vaginal delivery can usually begin exercising a few days after giving birth. Nevertheless, even in the absence of adverse events in pregnancy and partum, resumption of activities should be gradual, as women are detrained. The decision to resume exercise routine after a cesarean section, extensive vaginal repair or complicated pregnancies should be individualized, considering the balance between specific obstetric risk and the undesirable sedentary status.

Many women who are breastfeeding are concerned that exercise could affect the quality or volume of breast milk, impacting infant's growth. Despite the fact that both exercise and breastfeeding demand energy, exercise in the lactation period is safe and does not affect milk or child development [43, 44]. However, inadequate fluid or nutritional intake can impact milk production, and nursing women should be advised about that and encouraged to drink fluids regularly. As there is no set number of recommended volumes to drink throughout the day, they should be educated that clearer urine means better hydration. Thus, darker yellow urine indicates poor hydration and the need to increase fluid intake.

Women should consider breastfeeding or express milk to reserve before exercise in order to avoid discomfort of engorged breasts and preventing milk acidity secondary to lactic acid [16, 43, 44]. Breasts' stabilization and support during exercise can be achieved by wearing two bras or even an ace bandage that compresses breasts against the chest wall. Nipple abrasion often occurs and should be prevented by the use of cotton or silk bras or even sports nipple covers.

Conclusion

Regular exercise is safe and should be practiced by pregnant women to reduce the risk of adverse events in pregnancy and to improve the overall quality of life. Physicians should encourage all patients to exercise regularly and specialists should be able to prescribe safe and effective exercise to pregnant women, maximizing beneficial effects and reducing potential risks.

References

1. Federal Security Agency and Social Security Administration. (1949). Prenatal care. Children's Bureau Publication, Washington D.C. 25–26.
2. Downs DS, et al. Physical activity and pregnancy: past and present evidence and future recommendations. Res Q Exerc Sport. 2012;83(4):485–502.
3. American College of Obstetrics and Gynecology (ACOG) Technical Bulletin: Exercise During Pregnancy and the Postnatal Period. Washington, DC, USA: ACOG; 1985.
4. WHO. Global recommendations on physical activity for health. World Health Organization; 2010.

5. Kraus WE, et al. Physical activity, all-cause and cardiovascular mortality, and cardiovascular disease. Med Sci Sports Exerc. 2019;51(6):1270–81.
6. Lear SA, et al. The effect of physical activity on mortality and cardiovascular disease in 130 000 people from 17 high-income, middle-income, and low-income countries: the PURE study. Lancet. 2017;390(10113):2643–54.
7. Kannel WB, Sorlie P. Some health benefits of physical activity. The Framingham study. Arch Intern Med. 1979;139(8):857–61.
8. Colpani V, et al. Lifestyle factors, cardiovascular disease and all-cause mortality in middle-aged and elderly women: a systematic review and meta-analysis. Eur J Epidemiol. 2018;33(9):831–45.
9. Ross R, et al. Importance of assessing cardiorespiratory fitness in clinical practice: a case for fitness as a clinical vital sign: a scientific statement from the American Heart Association. Circulation. 2016;134(24):e653–99.
10. Warburton DER, Bredin SSD. Health benefits of physical activity: a systematic review of current systematic reviews. Curr Opin Cardiol. 2017;32(5):541–56.
11. Guure CB, et al. Impact of physical activity on cognitive decline, dementia, and its subtypes: meta-analysis of prospective studies. Biomed Res Int. 2017;2017:9016924.
12. Plotnikoff RC, et al. Effectiveness of interventions targeting physical activity, nutrition and healthy weight for university and college students: a systematic review and meta-analysis. Int J Behav Nutr Phys Act. 2015;12:45.
13. Swift DL, et al. The effects of exercise and physical activity on weight loss and maintenance. Prog Cardiovasc Dis. 2018;61(2):206–13.
14. Guthold R, et al. Worldwide trends in insufficient physical activity from 2001 to 2016: a pooled analysis of 358 population-based surveys with 1·9 million participants. Lancet Glob Health. 2018;6(10):e1077–86.
15. Garber CE, et al. American College of Sports Medicine position stand. Quantity and quality of exercise for developing and maintaining cardiorespiratory, musculoskeletal, and neuromotor fitness in apparently healthy adults: guidance for prescribing exercise. Med Sci Sports Exerc. 2011;43(7):1334–59.
16. Artal R, O'Toole M. Guidelines of the American College of Obstetricians and Gynecologists for exercise during pregnancy and the postpartum period. Br J Sports Med. 2003;37(1):6–12; discussion 12.
17. American College of Obstetricians and Gynecologists. Exercise during pregnancy and the postpartum period. Clin Obstet Gynecol. 2003;46(2):496–9.
18. Flores D, et al. Walking balance on a treadmill changes during pregnancy. Gait Posture. 2018;66:146–50.
19. Cakmak B, Ribeiro AP, Inanir A. Postural balance and the risk of falling during pregnancy. J Matern Fetal Neonatal Med. 2016;29(10):1623–5.
20. Inanir A, et al. Evaluation of postural equilibrium and fall risk during pregnancy. Gait Posture. 2014;39(4):1122–5.
21. Wang SM, et al. Low back pain during pregnancy: prevalence, risk factors, and outcomes. Obstet Gynecol. 2004;104(1):65–70.
22. Shiri R, Coggon D, Falah-Hassani K. Exercise for the prevention of low back and pelvic girdle pain in pregnancy: a meta-analysis of randomized controlled trials. Eur J Pain. 2018;22(1):19–27.
23. Davenport MH, et al. Exercise for the prevention and treatment of low back, pelvic girdle and lumbopelvic pain during pregnancy: a systematic review and meta-analysis. Br J Sports Med. 2019;53(2):90–8.
24. Auger N, et al. Elevated ambient temperatures and risk of neural tube defects. Occup Environ Med. 2017;74(5):315–20.
25. Dadvand P. Congenital anomalies: an under-evaluated risk of climate change. Occup Environ Med. 2017;74(5):313–4.
26. Milunsky A, et al. Maternal heat exposure and neural tube defects. JAMA. 1992;268(7):882–5.

27. Cooper KA, et al. Fetal heart rate and maternal cardiovascular and catecholamine responses to dynamic exercise. Aust N Z J Obstet Gynaecol. 1987;27(3):220–3.
28. Bgeginski R, Almada BP, Kruel LF. Fetal heart rate responses during maternal resistance exercise: a pilot study. Rev Bras Ginecol Obstet. 2015;37(3):133–9.
29. Clark SL, et al. Position change and central hemodynamic profile during normal third-trimester pregnancy and post partum. Am J Obstet Gynecol. 1991;164(3):883–7.
30. Asvanarunat E. Outcomes of gestational weight gain outside the Institute of Medicine Guidelines. J Med Assoc Thail. 2014;97(11):1119–25.
31. Allehdan SS, et al. Dietary and exercise interventions and glycemic control and maternal and newborn outcomes in women diagnosed with gestational diabetes: systematic review. Diabetes Metab Syndr. 2019;13(4):2775–84.
32. Ueno M, et al. Quantitative analysis of exercise among pregnant women with impaired glucose tolerance using pedometer data: an observational study. J Obstet Gynaecol Res. 2020;46(3):396–404.
33. Dempsey JC, Butler CL, Williams MA. No need for a pregnant pause: physical activity may reduce the occurrence of gestational diabetes mellitus and preeclampsia. Exerc Sport Sci Rev. 2005;33(3):141–9.
34. Chen I, et al. Non-clinical interventions for reducing unnecessary caesarean section. Cochrane Database Syst Rev. 2018;9:CD005528.
35. The Canadian Society for Exercise Physiology's, PARmed-X for pregnancy. 2002. http://www.csep.ca/cmfiles/publications/parq/parmed-xpreg.pdf.
36. McMurray RG, et al. Recent advances in understanding maternal and fetal responses to exercise. Med Sci Sports Exerc. 1993;25(12):1305–21.
37. Borg GA. Psychophysical bases of perceived exertion. Med Sci Sports Exerc. 1982;14(5):377–81.
38. Sports O. Olympians who competed while pregnant. [cited 2020 01/10/2020]; Available from: https://www.sports-reference.com/olympics/friv/lists.cgi?id=77.
39. Pivarnik JM, Szymanski LM, Conway MR. The elite athlete and strenuous exercise in pregnancy. Clin Obstet Gynecol. 2016;59(3):613–9.
40. Minig L, et al. Building the evidence base for postoperative and postpartum advice. Obstet Gynecol. 2009;114(4):892–900.
41. O'Toole ML, Sawicki MA, Artal R. Structured diet and physical activity prevent postpartum weight retention. J Womens Health (Larchmt). 2003;12(10):991–8.
42. Rauh K, et al. Lifestyle intervention to prevent excessive maternal weight gain: mother and infant follow-up at 12 months postpartum. BMC Pregnancy Childbirth. 2015;15:265.
43. Larson-Meyer DE. Effect of postpartum exercise on mothers and their offspring: a review of the literature. Obes Res. 2002;10(8):841–53.
44. Bane SM. Postpartum exercise and lactation. Clin Obstet Gynecol. 2015;58(4):885–92.

Chapter 10
Standards In Prenatal Care

Fernanda Campos da Silva and Gustavo Mourão Rodrigues

Principles of Prenatal Care

Ensuring a safe pregnancy and delivery is a major concern to the world. There is still much to be done to reduce maternal deaths, maternal near misses, prematurity, perinatal deaths, and other adverse outcomes. Prenatal care has a key role in promoting health. During regular visits to her caregiver, a woman and her family have the opportunity to learn about her condition and to be educated about the physiologic changes she will go through, how her baby is developing, and her role in pursuing wellness.

Ideally, women should be offered preconceptional counseling as discussed in Part 1 of this book. However, although in developed countries more women have access to preconceptional care, it is still uncommon to assist women before pregnancy. Women should plan their pregnancy so that it occurs in good health, especially for those with comorbid illnesses such as chronic hypertension or diabetes. Unfortunately, many times, prenatal care is the first contact of woman with the health care system. Practitioners should not miss the chance to identify possible unknown comorbidities or other threatening conditions to pregnancy. It is also important to encourage positive changes in lifestyle including nutrition, physical exercises, and avoiding smoking and alcohol.

Different women have different needs in relation to pregnancy and childbirth and require access to appropriate levels of care. The level of care determines whether the woman is at the right place, at the right time, with the right health professional for her clinical needs. Models of care should, as far as possible, provide a range of options at the same time as closely matching quality services to clinical needs [1]. The American College of Obstetrics and Gynecology enforces standard of care in

F. C. da Silva (✉) · G. M. Rodrigues
Department of Obstetrics, Universidade Federal do Estado do Rio de Janeiro (UNIRIO), Rio de Janeiro, RJ, Brazil

© Springer Nature Switzerland AG 2022

R. A. Moreira de Sá, E. B. d. Fonseca (eds.), *Perinatology*,
https://doi.org/10.1007/978-3-030-83434-0_10

levels, so that according to the pregnancy risk, the woman receives what is best for her and her baby [2].

The first antenatal visit should occur before 10 weeks of gestational age due to the high information needs in early pregnancy. In the first trimester, one can calculate gestational age and test for chromosomal anomalies for example. The percentage of women that have access to prenatal care in the first trimester is an indicator of quality of care in maternal health. Approximately, 75 percent of pregnant women in the United States initiated prenatal care in the first trimester [3]. However, important discrepancies are noted. Less than 50 percent of women in developing regions received early antenatal care versus over 80 percent in developed regions, and more than 4 of 5 women in the highest income group received early antenatal care versus 1 of 4 women in the lowest income group [4].

Effective models of antenatal care focus on the individual woman's needs and preferences. Women, their partners, and their families should be treated with sympathy, respect, and dignity. Their views, beliefs, and values in relation to her care and that of her baby should be sought and respected at all times. Good communication between healthcare professionals and women is essential. It should be supported by evidence-based information appropriate to the woman's needs. All information should also be accessible to women with additional needs such as physical, sensory, or learning disabilities [5].

Countries have different policies regarding who can provide prenatal care. It is generally provided by midwives, obstetrician-gynecologists, family medicine clinicians, and maternal-fetal medicine (MFM) subspecialists. The greater the anticipated risk for complications, the more specialized should be the caregiver. Midwives and family medicine clinicians generally provide prenatal care for women with low-risk pregnancies, while obstetrician-gynecologists and MFM clinicians manage high-risk, complicated pregnancies [6]. Women also benefit from a multidisciplinary team including non-medical experts such as nutritionists or psychologists, or other medical specialists according to their comorbidities.

An alternative model is group prenatal care. It may be preferred in some practice setting, although individual care remains the standard. Participants with the same month of expected delivery receive the majority of their care in a group setting. The majority of the visit, which may last two hours, involves facilitated group discussion, education, and skills building to address explicit learning objectives in prenatal care, childbirth preparation, and postpartum and parenting roles. Additional studies are needed to compare outcomes. It seems to do no harm and appears to result in at least equivalent obstetric outcomes and high levels of patient satisfaction compared with traditional prenatal care [7].

First Prenatal Visit

Appropriate history, physical examination, and laboratory studies can help identify pregnant women at increased risk of medical complications, pregnancy complications, or fetal abnormalities. Early identification of these women gives the provider an opportunity to discuss these issues and their management with the patient and, in some cases, offer interventions to prevent or minimize the risk of an adverse outcome.

History

At the first prenatal visit, it is important that the practitioner undertakes a complete personal history, detailing woman's psychosocial, medical, obstetric, and family history. This information can be used to start an obstetric record that will document her prenatal, intrapartum, and postpartum course. A formal record helps to ensure complete and systematic documentation of the pregnancy and often may be used for risk-assessment planning.

Key elements in woman's history to be explored in the first prenatal visit:

- Personal and demographic information
- Personal medical history, including immunizations; risk assessment for heritable disorders and substance use; infection history/exposure; and teratogen exposure
- Past surgical history
- Menstrual and gynecologic history
- Family medical history
- Current pregnancy (planned, unplanned, wishes to proceed with or terminate the pregnancy)
- Obstetric (previous experience of pregnancy and birth)
- Infant feeding experiences
- Nutrition and physical activity
- Smoking, alcohol, and other substance misuse
- Expectations, partner/family involvement, cultural and spiritual issues, concerns, knowledge, pregnancy, birth, breastfeeding, and infant feeding options
- Factors that may affect the pregnancy or birth (e.g., female genital mutilation/cutting)
- Psychosocial factors affecting the woman's emotional health and well-being
- The woman's support networks and information needs
- Obstetric (previous experience of pregnancy and birth)

A family history that suggests a heritable disorder affecting the fetus could be a known or suspected genetic disease, multiple malformations, multiple miscarriages, recurrence of the same or similar disorders, intellectual disability, autism spectrum disorder, and consanguinity. In addition, a poor outcome in a previous pregnancy increases the risk of a poor outcome in the next pregnancy. A previous preterm or small-for-gestational-age birth is associated with an increased risk of stillbirth in a subsequent pregnancy, and the smaller and more preterm the previous infant, the higher the risk of stillbirth in the subsequent pregnancy [8]. In addition, mothers who had a previous stillbirth were more likely to have preterm or small for gestational age infants in the subsequent pregnancy.

Psychosocial issues potentially affect the well-being of pregnancy. It should be identified and discussed with the patient whether the pregnancy was planned or unintended and whether there are potential barriers to care such as communication, transportation, child care issues, economic constraints, or work schedule. Women should also be screened for depression and anxiety at least once during the perinatal period using a standardized, validated tool [9]. This is an opportunity to provide information and, if indicated, make suggestions for possible changes or referral.

Violence against women, by her intimate partner or not, verbal, physical, or sexual, is a frequent event, often hidden by the women suffering the attacks. Clinicians should routinely assess all pregnant women for past or current exposure to these behaviors [10, 11]. Possible signs of abuse are bruising, improbable injury, depression, late prenatal care (presentation in the late second or the third trimester), missed prenatal visits, and appointments cancelled on short notice. Counseling and intervention can reduce intimate partner violence and improve pregnancy outcome [12].

Calculation of Gestational Age and Estimated Date of Delivery

Methods used to assess gestational age include known date of ovulation, date of the last menstrual period (LMP), and diagnostic ultrasound. Ultrasound alone is more accurate than a "certain" menstrual date for determining gestational age in the first and second trimesters (≤23 weeks) in spontaneous conceptions, and it is the best method for estimating the delivery date. In the absence of better assessment of gestational age, routine ultrasound in the first or second trimester reduces inductions for post-term pregnancies. Ideally, every pregnant woman should be offered a first-trimester dating ultrasound; however, if the availability of obstetrical ultrasound is limited, it is reasonable to use a second-trimester scan to assess gestational age [13].

Physical Examination

Blood pressure, weight, and height should be recorded as part of the examination. High blood pressure in the first trimester points to undiagnosed chronic hypertension. Calculating body mass index (BMI) facilitates counseling about the appropriate amount of weight gain over the course of pregnancy. Underweight women are expected to gain more weight in pregnancy as opposed to obese women, who should gain less weight. Both groups have specific risks in pregnancy.

A complete physical examination should be performed, with special attention to uterine size and shape and evaluation of the adnexa. Pain during examination of the adnexa may point to ectopic pregnancy. When the uterine size on physical examination differs from that predicted by menstrual dating, sonographic assessment is indicated. Uterine fibroids, uterine malposition (e.g., retroverted uterus), multiple gestation, and incorrect menstrual date are causes of discrepancy between uterine size and estimated gestational age. The fetal heart can usually be heard by 12 weeks of gestation using a hand-held Doppler ultrasound device.

Ultrasound Examination

Ultrasound examination in the first trimester is the preferred method to calculate gestational age and the estimated date of delivery as discussed before. It is particularly important when menses are irregular, the last menstrual period is unknown or uncertain, in patients who conceive while taking oral contraceptive pills, and when the uterine size is discordant with menstrual dates. Also, it can lead to earlier detection of clinically unsuspected fetal malformations (including aneuploidies) and earlier detection of multiple pregnancy [14]. An accurate gestational age is essential later in pregnancy when growth charts are needed for the diagnosis of a small or large for gestational age fetus.

Although detection of fetal anomalies in the first trimester is limited by the small size of the fetus and ongoing fetal development, ultrasound technology is rapidly progressing and assessment of fetal anatomy in the first trimester is becoming more widely available. There is considerable heterogeneity among studies, and sonographic equipment and expertise improved over the years, but the findings affirm both the potential benefits and limitations of the first trimester fetal anatomic survey. Women will need a second trimester survey to provide a more reliable assessment of fetal anatomy [13].

Screening and Testing for Genetic Abnormalities

All women should be offered a screening test for genetic abnormalities regardless of maternal age. They should understand the difference between a screening test and diagnostic test. Couples need to understand what is and is not being screened for, the interpretation of screen positive and negative results, the possibility of false positive and negative results, possible follow-up invasive or noninvasive testing, and possible reproductive choices.

Screening tests will identify fetuses at high risk of aneuploidy. Either assessment of cell-free DNA and/or assessment of ultrasound and maternal serum levels biochemical markers are acceptable. Please refer to Chap. 5 for more information.

Diagnostic testing involves performing genetic studies on samples obtained by an invasive procedure, typically chorionic villus biopsy or amniocentesis, to identify fetuses who are aneuploid. The method will be chosen according to gestational age.

Laboratory Tests

Laboratory tests are an essential part of prenatal care. They should add information to the assessment of risk or on diagnosing conditions important to the well-being of the ongoing pregnancy. There are standard tests recommended to all pregnant women and specific tests that should be offered to women at risk for a condition identified in the patient's history and/or physical examination. In this manner, different populations may require different tests, according to the prevalence of a given disease in that population.

Standard laboratory tests in prenatal care include the following:

- ABO and Rh type and antibody screen
- Hematocrit, hemoglobin, and mean corpuscular volume
- Rubella
- Urine culture
- Cervical cancer screening
- Human immunodeficiency virus
- Hepatitis B virus
- Syphilis
- Fasting glucose

RhD-negative women without alloantibodies are at risk to develop alloimmunization and should receive prophylactic anti(D)-immune globulin at 28 weeks and when clinically indicated. RhD-positive or -negative women who have a positive antibody screen may be at risk for hemolytic disease of the fetus and newborn in offspring.

Anemia is defined by a hemoglobin level <11 g/dL (hematocrit <33 percent) in the first trimester, and 10.5 g/dL after that. The most common cause of anemia is iron deficiency, but vitamin B12 deficiency, folate deficiency, or hemoglobinopathies should be considered [15].

Serologic screening for rubella immunity is performed unless the woman is known to be immune by previous serologic testing. Once documentation of immunity to rubella as a result of infection or immunization has been obtained, repeat testing is unnecessary. If non-immune, she should be counseled to avoid exposure to individuals with rubella and receive postpartum immunization. The rubella vaccine is a live vaccine and thus contraindicated during pregnancy.

Routine urine culture is recommended because pregnant women with untreated asymptomatic bacteriuria are at high risk of developing pyelonephritis and at modestly increased risk for preterm birth, and rapid tests for bacteriuria do not have adequate sensitivity and specificity.

The frequency of cervical cancer screening is not influenced by pregnancy, but management of an abnormal test is different for pregnant women.

Universal human immunodeficiency virus (HIV) testing of pregnant women early in each pregnancy allows her to be counseled about prevention of transmission to or identification of infected partners, but most important, the appropriate maternal medical management can be initiated to avoid perinatal transmission.

Maternal and congenital syphilis is a major concern, especially in developing countries. Strategies for the diagnosis of syphilis depend on its prevalence. Protocols may include the use of both nontreponemal and treponemal tests. Either test can be used as the initial screening test depending on the availability. Confirmatory testing is interesting due to the potential for a false-positive screening test result, although countries with high prevalence of the disease suggest treatment after a positive screening test [16].

All pregnant women are tested for the hepatitis B surface antigen (HBsAg), regardless of previous vaccination status, because prevaccination screening to exclude acute or chronic hepatitis B virus (HBV) infection is not commonly performed. Women who carry the HBsAg can transmit HBV to the fetus, typically during delivery. Immunization of the newborn within 12 hours of delivery can reduce the risk of HBV transmission by more than 95 percent. Mothers without evidence of prior HBV infection or exposure (negative for anti-HBs and anti-HBc) should be vaccinated.

In the first trimester of pregnancy screening for diabetes aims to diagnose overt diabetes, women with unknown diabetes before pregnancy. Both the American Diabetes Association (ADA) [17] and ACOG suggest early pregnancy testing for undiagnosed type 2 diabetes in women with risk factors [18].

Risk factors for overt diabetes, besides body mass index (BMI) $\geq$25 kg/m^2 ($\geq$23 kg/m^2 in Asian Americans), include the following:

- Gestational diabetes mellitus in a previous pregnancy
- A1C $\geq$5.7 percent (39 mmol/mol), impaired glucose tolerance, or impaired fasting glucose on previous testing
- First-degree relative with diabetes
- High-risk race/ethnicity (e.g., African American, Latino, Native American, Asian American, Pacific Islander)
- History of cardiovascular disease
- Hypertension or on therapy for hypertension
- HDL cholesterol level <35 mg/dL (0.90 mmol/L) and/or a triglyceride level >250 mg/dL (2.82 mmol/L)
- Polycystic ovary syndrome
- Physical inactivity
- Other clinical condition associated with insulin resistance (e.g., severe obesity and acanthosis nigricans)

Overt diabetes is diagnosed at the initial prenatal visit if:

- Fasting plasma glucose $\geq$126 mg/dL (7.0 mmol/L)
- A1C $\geq$6.5 percent (48 mmol/mol) using a standardized assay
- Random plasma glucose $\geq$200 mg/dL (11.1 mmol/L) and classic symptoms of hyperglycemia

According to risk factors or previous diagnoses identified in the patient's history or physical examination, the practitioner should offer other laboratory tests.

Laboratory tests to be used and selective situations

- Chlamydia
- TSH (free T4)
- Measles
- Gonorrhea
- Hepatitis C
- Tuberculosis
- Toxoplasmosis
- Bacterial vaginosis
- *Trichomonas vaginalis*
- Herpes simplex virus
- Cytomegalovirus

Chlamydia prevalence is highly related to age and sexual behavior. The Centers for Disease Control and Prevention (CDC) recommends screening all pregnant women <25 years of age and those pregnant women ≥25 years of age with risk factors for sexually transmitted infection [19]. During prenatal care, the preferred approach is to test a specimen obtained from a swab of the endocervix or vagina, although urine testing appears to be as sensitive [19]. Treatment may reduce the risk of preterm birth, preterm rupture of membranes, and low birth weight [20].

Women with signs or symptoms of thyroid disease should have their thyroid-stimulating hormone (TSH) level measured. The TSH should be interpreted using population and trimester-specific TSH reference ranges for pregnant women, when available. If the TSH is abnormal, free or total T4 should be measured.

Screening for asymptomatic hypothyroidism is controversial. Professional societies such as ACOG [21], the Endocrine Society [22], and the American Thyroid Association [23] recommend targeted rather than universal screening in pregnant women. However, a targeted approach will miss as many as one-third of women with subclinical hypothyroidism. For this reason and concern that not treating these women may be associated with adverse pregnancy outcomes, some protocols have advocated universal screening for thyroid dysfunction in pregnant women or those attempting to become pregnant.

In areas of ongoing measles outbreaks, one could consider serologic testing for measles immunoglobulin G (IgG) in pregnant women without documented immunity to measles. Any of the standard serologic assays for measles-specific IgG may be used for laboratory documentation of measles. Women without documented evidence of immunity should be immunized postpartum, as MMR is a live vaccine.

Pregnant women with risk factors for gonorrhea or living in an area where the prevalence of *Neisseria gonorrhoeae* is high are screened for gonorrhea [19]. NAAT is the preferred test for the microbiologic diagnosis of *N. gonorrhoeae* because of its superior accuracy; a swab is used to collect a vaginal or endocervical specimen for testing. Pregnant women who test positive are treated immediately and retested in three months. Treatment may prevent neonatal infection.

Universal screening for hepatitis C infection is controversial. The Infectious Disease Society of America and the American Association for the Study of Liver

Diseases recommended universal hepatitis C screening in pregnancy [24]. Their arguments are that hepatitis C infection is increasing in women of childbearing age, risk-based screening is not consistently performed, and documentation of infection may affect pregnancy management. One should avoid, for example, chorionic villus sampling [25]. The counterpart is that the diagnosis does not affect treatment. Caesarian section does not seem to reduce the transmission rate and there is no viral therapy to be used in pregnancy. Still, breastfeeding is not contraindicated.

Women with suspicion for recent tuberculosis infection based on epidemiologic exposure or that have significant immunocompromise, such as HIV infection or profound immunosuppressive therapy, should be screened for tuberculosis in pregnancy [26].

Whether serological screening for toxoplasmosis should be universal is not clear. Countries with high prevalence of the disease tend to do universal screening. There is treatment to be offered during pregnancy and fetal diagnosis of toxoplasmosis is possible. Transmission is via environmental exposure (maternal ingestion of oocysts from consumption of contaminated soil or water or cat litter, which may contaminate fruit or vegetables and other unwashed handheld foods) and ingestion of undercooked or cured meat from infected animals [27].

Women with a history of prior preterm birth should be screened for bacterial vaginosis and treated, if positive, to lower the risk of recurrent preterm birth, but the benefits are controversial.

HIV infected women should be screened for *Trichomonas vaginalis* at the first prenatal visit and treated with metronidazole if infected [19]. Trichomoniasis in HIV-infected individuals is associated with an increased risk of vertical and horizontal transmission of HIV.

Serologic screening for herpes simplex virus has been proposed to identify women without herpes simplex virus (HSV). A negative test woman can take precautions to avoid acquiring an HSV infection and those with a past history of HSV can be offered suppressive antiviral therapy, examined carefully for lesions at the onset of labor, and offered cesarean delivery, if indicated [19].

Cytomegalovirus universal screening is controversial. Most organizations recommend against it. Universal screening supporters argue that knowing that her serology is negative for CMV antibodies and CMV counseling increase some women's motivation to practice good hygiene and thus decrease the risk of seroconversion during pregnancy. Testing pregnant women for CMV is indicated as part of the diagnostic evaluation of mononucleosis-like illnesses, when a fetal anomaly suggestive of congenital CMV infection is detected on prenatal ultrasound examination, or if the woman requests the test [28].

Timing and Frequency of Subsequent Visits

Following a thorough evaluation during the first prenatal visit, a plan should be made regarding subsequent consults. There is no consensus about optimal frequency or timing of visits. The National Institute of Health and Clinical Excellence (NICE) suggests 10 appointments for nulliparous women and 7 appointments for parous women, and each visit should have a specific purpose/goal [5]. Nulliparous woman, those with medical or fetal conditions or those with positive screening tests should be seen more frequently, while parous woman or those without risk factors could be seen on larger intervals.

Traditionally, women would be seen monthly during the first two trimesters, every two weeks from 28 to 36 weeks, then weekly. The purpose of this approach is to increase surveillance during the period that accounts for most of the complications. Recent publications suggest that, by increasing the number and accuracy of initial screening tests, women could be classified at low risk for pregnancy complications, and in this group, the number of medical visits could be substantially reduced [29].

Components of Subsequent Prenatal Visits

At each antenatal appointment, healthcare professionals should offer consistent information and clear explanations and should provide pregnant women with an opportunity to discuss issues and ask questions [5]. A common practice is to use initial prenatal visits to discuss physiologic changes of pregnancy and screening tests, and as pregnancy advances, discuss delivery and breastfeeding. Many aspects of delivery often require special attention, especially in nulliparous women. Signs and symptoms of labor, timing and route of delivery, and care of the newborn should be approached.

Routine prenatal examination includes maternal weight and blood pressure at all visits, fetal heart rate auscultation after 10–12 weeks with a Doppler monitor or after 20 weeks with a fetoscope, fundal height after 20 weeks, and fetal lie by 36 weeks [30].

It is essential to use proper technique when measuring blood pressure. Woman should be sitting with arm at heart level, after at least a few minutes of rest, and appropriate cuff should be used. Newly detected hypertension should prompt evaluation for preeclampsia.

Sinfisis fundal height measurement is a cheap and easy technique for screening fetal growth restriction. Despite inconclusive data [31], most national guidelines still recommend routine measurement [32].

Second Trimester

Mid trimester fetal scan should be offered between 18 and 22 weeks for all women [33]. At this time there is still good accuracy determining gestational age and allows detecting major congenital anomalies. It also provides opportunity to screen for short cervix and offer intervention. Despite some controversy regarding universal versus selective screening, it appears to be cost-effective [34].

Gestational diabetes mellitus screening is recommended after 24 weeks of gestation to reduce maternal and fetal complications [18].

A single antenatal dose of 300 micrograms of anti-D immunoglobulin at 28 weeks of gestation is recommended in Rh-negative women. Those with a Rh-positive newborn should receive additional dose after delivery. This practice is associated with less than a 0.2% rate of Rh alloimmunization [35].

Third Trimester

Hemoglobin concentration should be routinely measured at booking and at around 28 weeks' gestation. Anemia carries an increased risk for postpartum hemorrhage, depression, low birth weight, preterm birth, and higher risks of perinatal and neonatal mortality. Screening in the third trimester permits timely correction.

Maternal colonization by group B streptococcus (GBS) is associated with severe neonatal disease. Screening for GBS colonization should be carried between 36 and 37 weeks 6 days, obtaining swabs from the lower vagina and rectum. Universal screening protocols are associated with lower rates of early-onset group B streptococcal disease compared to risk-based protocols [36].

Repeat HIV testing before 36 weeks in pregnant women with initial negative anti-HIV tests known to be at high risk or in locations with elevated HIV incidence [37]. Women with unknown status should be screened during labor, delivery, or immediate postpartum period.

During the final weeks, pregnant women must be educated regarding labor, delivery, and postpartum. Details like route of delivery, timing, and pain control can be discussed during antenatal care. Patients with medical conditions, especially those who might require planned delivery, should receive special attention. Women identified as having breech presentation should be offered external cephalic version as a safe and effective method of decreasing caesarean section [38].

References

1. Australian Government Department of Health. Clinical practice guidelines: pregnancy care. 2019 Edition. Canberra: s.n.; 2018.
2. American Association of Birth Centers, Association of Women's Health, Obstetric and Neonatal Nurses, American College of Obstetricians and Gynecologists. Obstetric Care Consensus, Number 9: levels of maternal care. Am J Obstet Gynecol. 2019;221(6):B19–30.
3. U.S. Department of Health and Human Services, Health Resources and Services Administration, Maternal and Child Health Bureau. Child Health USA 2013. Rockville, Maryland: s.n.; 2013.
4. Moller AB, Petzold M, Chou D, Say L. Early antenatal care visit: a systematic analysis of regional and global levels and trends of coverage from 1990 to 2013. 2017;5:e977–e983.
5. National Institute for Health and Care Excellence (NICE). Antenatal care for uncomplicated pregnancies; 2019.

6. Hatem M, Sandall J, Devane D, Soltani H, Gates S. Midwife-led versus other models of care for childbearing women. [Online] Cochrane Database Syst Rev, 08 de october de 2008.
7. ACOG. ACOG Committee Opinion No. 731: group prenatal care. Obstet Gynecol. 2018;131(3):e104–8.
8. Malacova E, Regan A, Nassar N, Raynes-Greenow C, Leonard H, Srinivasjois R, et al. Risk of stillbirth, preterm delivery, and fetal growth restriction following exposure in a previous birth: systematic review and meta-analysis. BJOG. 2018;125(2):183–92.
9. ACOG Committee Opinion No. 757: screening for perinatal depression. Obstet Gynecol. 2018;132(5):e208–e212.
10. ACOG Committee Opinion No. 518: Intimate partner violence. Obstet Gynecol. 2012;119:412–7.
11. American College of Obstetricians and Gyenecologists. ACOG Committee opinion no. 554: reproductive and sexual coercion. Obstet Gynecol. 2013;121(2 Pt 1):411–5.
12. Kiely M, El-Mohandes AA, El-Khorazaty MN, Blake SM, Gantz MG. An integrated intervention to reduce intimate partner violence in pregnancy: a randomized controlled trial. Obstet Gynecol. 2010;115(2 Pt 1):273–83.
13. Butt K, Lim KI. Guideline No. 388-determination of gestational age by ultrasound. J Obstet Gynaecol Can. 2019;41(10):1497–507.
14. Karim JN, Roberts NW, Salomon LJ, Papageorghiou AT. Systematic review of first-trimester ultrasound screening for detection of fetal structural anomalies and factors that affect screening performance. Ultrasound Obstet Gynecol. 2017;50(4):429–41.
15. The WHO Reproductive Health Library. WHO recommendation on the method for diagnosing anaemia in pregnancy. WHO Reproductive Health Library. [Online] 2018. [Citado em: 05 de January de 2020.] https://extranet.who.int/rhl/topics/preconception-pregnancy-childbirth-and-postpartum-care/antenatal-care/who-recommendation-method-diagnosing-anaemia-pregnancy.
16. Brasil, Ministério da Saúde. Protocolo clínico e diretrizes terapêuticas para atenção integral às pessoas com infecções sexualmente transmisséveis; 2019.
17. American Diabetes Association. 2. Classification and diagnosis of diabetes: standards of medical care in diabetes-2019. Diabetes Care. 2019;42(Suppl 1):S13–28.
18. ACOG Practice Bulletin No. 190: Gestational Diabetes Mellitus. Committee on Practice Bulletins—Obstetrics. Obstet Gynecol. 2018;131(2):E49-e64.
19. Workowski KA, Bolan GA, Centers for Disease Control and Prevention. Sexually transmitted diseases treatment guidelines 2015. 2015, MMWR Recomm Rep, 64(RR-03), pp. 1–137.
20. Silva MJ, Florencio GL, Gabiatti JR, Amaral RL, Eleutério Junior J, Gonçalves AK. Perinatal morbidity and mortality associated with chlamydial infection: a meta-analysis study. Braz J Infect Dis. 2011;15(6):533–9.
21. Committee on Patient Safety and Quality Improvement, Committee on Professional Liability. ACOG Committee Opinion No. 381: subclinical hypothyroidism in pregnancy. Obstet Gynecol. 2007;110(4):959–60.
22. De Groot L, Abalovich M, Alexander EK, Amino N, Barbour L, Cobin RH, et al. Management of thyroid dysfunction during pregnancy and postpartum: an Endocrine Society clinical practice guideline. J Clin Endocrinol Metab. 2012;97(8):2543–65.
23. Alexander EK, Pearce EN, Brent GA, Brown RS, Chen H, Dosiou C. 2017 guidelines of the American Thyroid Association for the diagnosis and management of thyroid disease during pregnancy and the postpartum. Thyroid. 2017;27(3):315–89.
24. AASLD, IDSA. HCV in pregnancy. [Online] 06 de January de 2020. https://www.hcvguidelines.org/unique-populations/pregnancy.
25. Boudova S, Mark K, El-Kamary SS. Risk-based hepatitis C screening in pregnancy is less reliable than universal screening: a retrospective chart review. Open Forum Infect Dis. 2018;5(3):ofy043.
26. American Thoracic Society. Targeted tuberculin testing and treatment of latent tuberculosis infection. MMWR Recomm Rep. 2000;49(RR-6):1–51.

27. American College of Obstetricians and Gynecologists. Practice bulletin no. 151: cytomegalovirus, parvovirus B19, varicella zoster, and toxoplasmosis in pregnancy. Obstet Gynecol. 2015;125(6):1510–1525 Reaffirmed.
28. Society for Maternal-Fetal Medicine (SMFM), Hughes BL, Gyamfi-Bannerman C. Diagnosis and antenatal management of congenital cytomegalovirus infection. J Obstet Gynecol. 2016;214(6):B5–B11.
29. Nicolaides KH. Turning the pyramid of prenatal care. Fetal Diagn Ther. 2011;29(3):183–96.
30. Zolotor AJ, Carlough MC. Update on prenatal care. Am Fam Physician. 2014;89(3):199–208.
31. Robert Peter J, Ho JJ, Valliapan J, Sivasangari S. Symphysial fundal height (SFH) measurement in pregnancy for detecting abnormal fetal growth. Cochrane Database Syst Rev. 2015;(9):CD008136.
32. McCowan LM, Figueras F, Anderson NH. Evidence-based national guidelines for the management of suspected fetal growth restriction: comparison, consensus, and controversy. Am J Obstet Gynecol. 2018;218(2S):S855–68.
33. Salomon LJ, Alfirevic Z, Berghella V, Billardo C, Hernandez-Andrade E, Johnsen SL, et al. Practice guidelines for performance of the routine mid-trimester fetal ultrasound scan. Ultrasound Obstet Gynecol. 2011;37(1):116–26.
34. Einerson BD, Grobman WA, Miller ES. Cost-effectiveness of risk-based screening for cervical length to prevent preterm birth. Am J Obstet Gynecol. 2016;215(1):100.e1–100.e1007.
35. Committee on Practice Bulletins-Obstetrics. Practice Bulletin No. 181: Prevention of Rh D Alloimmunization. Obstet Gynecol. 2017;130(2):e57–70.
36. Hasperhoven GF, Al-Nasiry S, Bekker V, Villamor E, Kramer BWW. Universal screening versus risk-based protocols for antibiotic prophylaxis during childbirth to prevent early-onset Group B streptococcal disease: a systematic review and meta-analysis [published online ahead of print]. BJOG. 2020. https://doi.org/10.1111/1471-0528.16085.
37. Pollock L, Cohan D, Pecci CC, Mittal P. ACOG Committee Opinion No. 752: prenatal and perinatal human immunodeficiency virus testing. Obstet Gynecol. 2019;133(1):187.
38. American College of Obstetricians and Gynecologists, Society for Maternal-Fetal Medicine, Caughey AB, Cahill AG, Guise JM, Rouse DJ. Safe prevention of the primary cesarean delivery. Am J Obstet Gynecol. 2014;2010(3):179–93.

Chapter 11
Multiple Pregnancy

Carolina Carvalho Mocarzel and Ana Carla Zanchietta Nicolielo

Introduction

Multiple pregnancy is defined by the presence of two or more fetuses in the uterine cavity. Its incidence has been increasing mainly due to a later planning of motherhood and a greater use of assisted reproduction techniques [1, 2].

Twin pregnancies are associated with a high risk of perinatal mortality and morbidity. In 2009, the associated mortality rate was 12 per 1000 births of twins and 31 per 1000 births of triplets or multiples of higher order, as opposed to 5 per 1000 births of single pregnancies [2].

Preterm births occur in up to 60% of multiple pregnancies, contributing to an increased risk of neonatal mortality and morbidity [1]. The rate of such complications is inversely proportional to the gestational age at delivery. There is also an association with preterm iatrogenic delivery due to the prevalence of maternal and fetal complications, being higher in monochorionic pregnancies (Table 11.1).

C. C. Mocarzel (✉)
Department of Obstetrics, Hospital Federal dos Servidores do Estado,
Rio de Janeiro, Rio de Janeiro, Brazil

A. C. Z. Nicolielo
Maternidade Perinatal, Department of Obstetrícia,
Rio de Janeiro, Rio de Janeiro, Brazil

© Springer Nature Switzerland AG 2022
R. A. Moreira de Sá, E. B. d. Fonseca (eds.), *Perinatology*,
https://doi.org/10.1007/978-3-030-83434-0_11

Table 11.1 Risk factors for Mmultiple pregnancy

Risk factors	
Maternal age	The incidence of dizygotic twins increases with maternal age up to 37 years of age, and after this age, the rate starts to fall
Parity	The frequency of twin pregnancies is around 1.5% for primiparous women and approximately 3% for four pregnancies
Ethnicity	In white women, the dizygotic rate is 1/100 pregnancies, among black 1/80, and among Asian 1/155
Assisted reproduction technology	This technique is associated with higher chances of multiple pregnancies, but there is more and more control of the number of embryos transferred in each cycle in order to reduce the rates of multiple pregnancies. The transfer of blastocysts alone increases the risk of monochorionic pregnancies
Obesity	Patients with body mass index (BMI) of less than 20 kg/m^2 showed lower rates of dizygotic twin pregnancies compared to those with a BMI greater than 30 kg/m^2

Classification

Multiple pregnancies can be classified according to zygosity or chorionicity.

Dizygotic pregnancies result from the fertilization of more than one egg, each fertilized with one sperm. Thus, the embryos have different genetic material. Monozygotic embryos result from the fertilization of an egg by a sperm, originating an embryo that divides into two (or more) with identical genetic load.

The increase observed in the incidence of twin pregnancies is mainly due to a high incidence of dizygotic pregnancies. However, when blastocysts are transferred, assisted reproduction technology favors the occurrence of monozygotic pregnancies.

In dizygotic pregnancy, each embryo develops its own chorion and amnion, so they will always be dichorionic and diamniotic. In monozygotic pregnancies, chorionicity and amnionicity vary according to the moment when the division of the embryonic mass occurs. When the blastocyst division occurs within 72 hours, the pregnancy will be dichorionic and diamniotic. When division occurs between the 4th and 8th day after fertilization, differentiation of the cells that originate the corium has already occurred, resulting in diamniotic monochorionic pregnancy. In about 1% of the cases, the blastocyst division occurs between the 8th and 13th day after fertilization, when the chorionic plate and the amniotic sac have already formed, resulting in monoamniotic monochorionic pregnancies. Imperfect twinning results from the failure of the complete separation of the embryos and occurs when the process of division is later than the 13th day (Fig. 11.1).

Chorionicity should be determined as soon as possible and first trimester ultrasonography is a great ally in this process. The interval between 11 weeks and 13 weeks and 6 days allows evaluation through the thickness of the amniotic membrane at the placental insertion site (T sign or lambda sign) and the study of placental masses (Table 11.2) [2].

It is important to examine the dividing membrane carefully, because in dichorionic pregnancy, the twins are separated by a thick layer of fused chorionic membranes with two thin amniotic membranes, one on each side, giving the

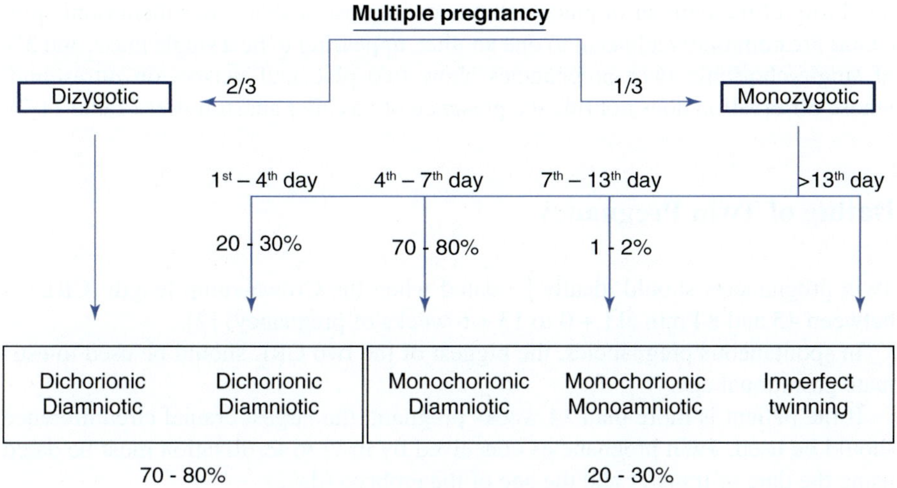

Fig. 11.1 Classification and incidence of multiple pregnancy

Table 11.2 Ultrasonographic findings of twin pregnancies according to gestational age

Ultrasound <11 weeks	AD: Two chorions, two vitelline vessels and two embryos. MD: Two amniotic sacs, single chorion, two embryos with two vitelline vessels MM: gestational sac, one vitelline vessel, two embryos in the same gestational sac, and absence of a membrane 8–10 weeks, the interfetal membrane may not be visible Diagnosis of amniocity only after 10 weeks
Ultrasound from 11 weeks to 13 weeks and 6 days	DC: presence of two placentas or fused placentas with a lambda sign MD: placenta with a T sign at the union of the amnion MM: single amniotic cavity
Ultrasound > 14 weeks:	Chorionicity is more clearly determined using the same ultrasound signals A combination of ultrasound characteristics, rather than one, would be more accurate, and the diagnosis of chorionicity may be uncertain. The lambda sign may disappear. The lambda sign is pathognomonic of DC pregnancy and is present until 15 weeks in all DC pregnancies, but by the 16th week, the sign is present in 97%, and in the 20th week, in 87% of the DC pregnancies Therefore, the absence of the lambda sign after 16 weeks is not an indication of MC. In case of doubt, the follow-up should be carried out as if it were a monochorionic pregnancy

appearance of a “full lambda” compared to only two thin amniotic layers (the T-signal) that separate the two fetuses in the monochorionic, diamniotic twin pregnancy (MCDA) [2].

In women assessed for the first time after 14 weeks of pregnancy, chorionicity is more accurately determined using the same ultrasound signals, by counting the layers of the interamniotic membrane and by observing fetus discordant in gender. The reliability of the number of placental masses is questionable, since dichorionic placentas are commonly adjacent to one another, appearing to be a single mass, and 3% of single-chorionic twin pregnancies show two placental masses on ultrasound, whose observation does not rule the presence of vascular anastomoses (Table 11.2).

Dating of Twin Pregnancy

Twin pregnancies should ideally be dated when the Crown-rump length (CRL) is between 45 and 84 mm (11 + 0 to 13 + 6 weeks of pregnancy) [2].

In spontaneous pregnancies, the biggest of the two CRL should be used to estimate gestational age.

If the patient is more than 14 weeks pregnant, the largest cranial circumference should be used. Twin pregnancies conceived by in vitro fertilization must be dated using the date of transfer and the age of the embryo (days).

A fetal crown-rump length greater than 10% (smaller fetal crown-rump length – bigger fetal crown-rump length × 100) is associated with increased adverse pregnancy outcomes in both MC and CD pregnancies (miscarriage, fetal death >24 weeks, birth weight discrepancy, premature birth, and malformations), although predictive value is low and clinical utility is limited [2].

Identification of Twins

It is importante the correct identification and description of the position of the fetuses (right, left, upper, lower) and the mapping the placental cord insertions as well as theirs relations to the placental margins and the membranes.

It is advisable to describe each twin using as many characteristics as possible so that another examiner can accurately identify them. For example, "twin A (female) is on the maternal right, with posterior placenta and insertion of the marginal umbilical cord." For pregnancies with weight discrepancies, the identification should be accompanied by a description such as "fetus A, potential receptor." It is important to recognize that identification is less accurate in MCMA pregnancies, particularly in the first trimester [2].

Chromosomal Abnormalities

Screening for aneuploidies in twin pregnancies should be performed as single pregnancies, preferably in the first trimester, using the combined first trimester test: maternal biochemistry (PAPP-A and b-hCG applying correction factor for each marker) and ultrasound (TN) between 11–13 weeks and 6 days (CCN: 45–84 mm). There are, however, some differences in the calculation of the combined risk in the first trimester that should be known [1, 2]:

- DC-twin: individual risk for each fetus for which the fetal nuchal translucency (NT) value is used (90% are dizygotic).
- MC-twin: single risk for both twins, for which the mean NT of both fetuses should be used. It is the first-choice screening and it has a trisomy 21 detection rate close to 90%, like detection in simple pregnancies, with a false-positive rate of 5–6%.
- Multifetal pregnancy (3 or + fetuses): maternal biochemistry is not applied and ultrasound screening (NT) with CRT between 45 and 84 mm associated with maternal age will be used.
- In the case of vanishing twin, if there is still a measurable fetal pole, only NT in combination with the maternal age should be used for the risk assessment.

Genetic counseling has no particularities when it comes to maternal age: advancing age increases both the prevalence of twin pregnancies and fetal aneuploidies. The indication of the invasive procedure for better study of the risks of genetic syndrome is done in the same way as in single pregnancies, however, in dichorionic pregnancies it is necessary to analyze material from both fetuses.

In theory, in MC pregnancies, a single puncture would be enough to make the diagnosis of genetic changes. However, although quite rare, post-meiotic nondisjunction of chromosomes can occur, and this would justify the puncture of the two amniotic cavities even in known MC pregnancies. In dichorionic diamniotic pregnancies, each fetus deserves a separate analysis (two punctures must be performed). If the option is chorionic villus biopsy, it should be performed near the insertion of the umbilical cord to confirm which fetus is being examined in each of the samples. It is worth mentioning that the highest defect detection rates in the first trimester by ultrasound are 40% [2].

The technique of choice is chorionic villus biopsy (CVB) – in the case of MC pregnancy, a single sample is enough and DC pregnancy requires a sample from both. In MC pregnancy, the discordance of NT, reversed a-wave in ductus venosus, or reflux of the tricuspid may be an early manifestation of second-stage treatment of hemodynamic disorders (TTTS). A 16-week sonographic re-assessment is then recommended to determine if it is TTTS or to confirm the suspicion of chromosomopathy (amniocentesis) [2].

The analysis of free DNA from cells and maternal blood to assess the risk of fetal aneuploidy is increasingly used in clinical practice. It has the potential to overlap many of these complex problems, as it has a much higher detection rate and a lower false-positive rate than the combined test. The weighted detection rate of trisomy 21 in single pregnancy was 99% for a false positive rate of 0.1%. The corresponding values for twin pregnancies were respectively 94.4% and 0% [1, 2].

Ultrasound Screening to Detect Structural Anomalies in Multiple Pregnancy

The risk of fetal anomaly is greater in twin pregnancies compared to one. The rate per fetus in dizygotic twins is probably the same as in single pregnancies but exhibits a twofold to threefold increase in monozygotic twins. The rate of major congenital anomaly, which normally affects only one twin, is about 1 in 25 dichorionic, 1 in 15 MCDA, and 1 in 6 monoamniotic twin pregnancies [2]. Therefore, screening for anomalies is an important factor in monochorionic twin pregnancy. Changes associated with twinning include neural tube defects, anterior abdominal wall defects, facial clefts, brain anomalies, heart malformation, and gastrointestinal anomalies. Echocardiographic screening is a routine exam in twin pregnancies. It is important to make the patient aware of the limitations of ultrasound screening, which vary according to the type of anomaly.

In 1–2% of twin pregnancies, there will be an anomaly present in only one fetus, leading to a difficult decision between the expectant conduct and the selective feticide of the affected twin. Even in monozygotic twinning, concordance for a structural anomaly occurs in less than 20% of cases [2].

Ultrasound in the Evaluation of Twin Pregnancy

The frequency of prenatal control and ultrasound evaluation will depend on the chorionicity of the pregnancy.

Uncomplicated dichorionic twin pregnancies should be assessed in the first trimester morphology at 11 weeks to 13 weeks and 6 days, second trimester morphology at 20 weeks to 22 weeks, and every 4 weeks thereafter. Complicated dichorionic pregnancies should be evaluated more often, depending on the intercurrent condition and its severity.

The evaluation of uncomplicated monochorionic twin pregnancies includes first trimester morphology with 11 weeks to 13 weeks and 6 days, every 2 weeks after the 16th week, in order to detect TTTS and TAPS in a timely manner and second trimester morphology with 20 weeks to 22 weeks. Complicated monochorionic pregnancies should be evaluated more frequently, depending on the intercurrent condition and its severity.

In each ultrasound assessment, the following should be assessed: fetal biometry, amniotic fluid volume, and umbilical artery Doppler (from 20 weeks of pregnancy in dichorionic and 16 weeks of monochorionic) for both fetuses. Discordance between the estimated fetal weight (EFW) must be calculated and documented in each exam. In monochorionic twin pregnancy, the peak-systolic velocity (PSV) of the middle cerebral artery (MCA) should be assessed after 16 weeks, in order to track the sequence polycythemia anemia (TAPS). In MCDA twins, the volume of the amniotic fluid (largest vertical pocket) should be assessed as a TTTS screening. The cervical length assessment should be performed in the second trimester morphology, in order to identify women at risk of premature delivery [2].

Screening for Premature Delivery

Measuring the length of the cervix is the preferred screening method for the risk of preterm birth in twin pregnancies. The cutoff point most used is 25 mm in the second trimester.

Progesterone use: Vaginal progesterone reduces the risk of premature birth and neonatal morbidity and mortality in patients with twin pregnancies and short cervix, without deleterious effects on the child's neurodevelopment. The recommended dosage ranges from 200 mg to 400 mg/day [1].

Bed rest, cervical pessaries, or oral tocolytics does not reduce the risk of preterm birth. Cerclage is not routinely indicated.

Maternal Complications

Maternal complications are more frequent than in single pregnancies and include complications during pregnancy, childbirth, and the puerperium. Maternal mortality is 2.5 times higher (Table 11.3).

Hypertensive Disorders and Preeclampsia

Hypertensive disorders occur in 5–10% of all single pregnancies and affect about 10–20% of twin pregnancies. These rates can be justified by a combination of factors such as advanced maternal age, parity, number of fetuses and, consequently, larger placental surface. Additionally, women who become pregnant through assisted reproduction technology face twice as many risks of preeclampsia as those with spontaneous twin pregnancies [1].

In addition to the higher incidence of preeclampsia in this population, severe and premature conditions (before 34 weeks) are also more frequent.

Table 11.3 Maternal complications in Mmultiple pregnancy

Maternal complications in twin pregnancy
Hyperemesis gravidarum (HG) Anemia Cholestasis Acute liver steatosis Hypertensive disorders
Gestational diabetes Acute lung edema
Premature labor
Placenta previa Placental abruption Thromboembolism Postpartum hemorrhage

Prevention of preeclampsia: Multiple pregnancy is considered a risk factor for preeclampsia (mainly late) and it is recommended to start a 150-mg dose of aspirin (taken at night) at between weeks 11 and 36 of gestational age if one or more of the following factors coexist: primigravida, age > 40 years, interval between pregnancies greater than 10 years, BMI > 35 kg/m^2 at the first doctor's appointment, and family history of preeclampsia [1].

Gestational Diabetes

The increased placental mass in twin pregnancies also increases the steroid hormones derived from the placenta, which can predispose to glucose intolerance. These pregnancies, in case of insulin therapy, require regimens like those of single pregnancies for adequate control of hyperglycemia.

Other Third Trimester Complications

Twin pregnancies are at increased risk for third trimester bleeding, such as placenta previa or placental abruption. These complications require hospitalization, maternal and fetal surveillance, and sometimes early delivery. Multiple pregnancies have an incidence of placenta previa of 40% more. Most cases of placenta previa require a caesarean delivery and increase the rates of bleeding, anemia, and the need for blood transfusion.

Besides, other complications may arise, such as gestational cholestasis, acute liver steatosis, and thromboembolism.

Fetal Complications

Premature Membranes Rupture (PMR) in One of the Twins

PMR diagnosis is performed in the same way as recommended for single pregnancies: clinical examination with visualization of amniotic fluid output through the cervical canal, assessment of vaginal pH (greater than 6.0), and arboriform crystallization of vaginal discharge.

There is no specific protocol for monitoring cases of twin pregnancies when one fetus has an intact pouch and the other has a ruptured pouch: the recommended management is similar for single pregnancies.

Table 11.4 Etiology of intrauterine growth restriction according to chorionicity

Dichorionic	Monochorionic
Research should include a detailed ultrasound to search for anomalies	Asymmetry of placental territories: in the same placental mass, different territories are responsible for the blood supply of each fetus. In this scenario, the existence of inequality of placental territories that nourish the fetuses may be the cause of an unequal growth pattern
Screening for viral infections (cytomegalovirus, rubella, and toxoplasmosis)	Blood transfusion between fetuses, which characterizes feto-fetal transfusion syndrome (FFTS) or the acardiac twin (TRAP sequence)
Velamentous cord insertion	Presence of velamentous cord insertion in the fetus with less growth
Genetic changes in one of the fetuses	Genetic changes

Intrauterine Growth Restriction (IUGR) Screening, Diagnosis, and Management

The curves applied to single pregnancies are also used to evaluate the growth pattern of twin pregnancies. It is extremely important to recognize that the growth rate of these fetuses tends to reduce after 32 weeks, as part of a phenomenon called intrauterine adaptation.

IUGR has been defined as a condition in which a fetus has a fetal-weight estimation (FWE) <10th percentile for gestational age and there is a mismatch of fetal weight above 25% between them. It is associated with a high risk of neurological impairment in both fetuses. If both twins have FWE <10th percentile, the fetuses should be called small for gestational age [2].

The FWE discordance is calculated using the following formula: [(weight of the largest fetus - weight of the smallest fetus) × 100]/weight of the largest fetus [2].

When diagnosing discordant growth among fetuses, the first step in investigation and management includes confirmation of chorionicity and gestational age and investigation of the etiology (Table 11.4).

Both diagnostic criteria, monitoring of fetal well-being, hospital admission criteria, pulmonary maturation, and resolution criteria are made following the management protocol for changes in fetal growth in a single pregnancy.

Particularity of Monochorionic Pregnancies

In monochorionic pregnancies there is a single placental mass that has distinct territories for nourishing each fetus. The presence of unequal placental territories is the main cause of selective intrauterine growth restriction (sIUGR) defined when there is a 25% difference between fetal weights.

Gratacós, in 2007, proposed a classification system for monochorionic pregnancies complicated by sIUGR based on the analysis of umbilical artery doppler: (1) type I: presence of persistent positive diastole, (2) type II: persistent zero or reverse diastole, and (3) type III: intermittent zero or reverse diastole [1, 2].

Type I Type I presents favorable perinatal results, with greater weight at birth and less weight discrepancy, expectant conduct and ultrasound monitoring with weekly Doppler, and biweekly biometrics. Resolution: worsening of AU Doppler. In general, delivery is at 36 weeks.

Type II Type II is associated with early placental insufficiency, with less placental territory and fewer anastomoses. Doppler changes in the venous duct and fetal biophysical profile are present in 90% of cases, with an average gestational age at delivery of 30 weeks and brain damage in 14% of the cases in the smallest twin. In this type, neurological damage is rare in the larger twin.

Type III Type III indicates the existence of a large arterio-arterial (AA) anastomoses. It represents a less predictable clinical evolution.

Type II and Type III still no ideal treatment. Consideration should be given to the possibility of selective feticide of the restricted fetus or laser until the 26th week. The moment of delivery is defined by the rigorous follow-up of the venous duct (fetal deterioration) performed, weekly, up to 26/28 weeks and, daily, thereafter. Delivery should be considered between 32 and 34 weeks, in the absence of other complications.

Death of One Twin

Monochorionic and dichorionic pregnancies may show the following complications in the event of death of one of the twins [2]:

1. Death of the other twin: 15% and 3%
2. Preterm delivery: 68% and 54%
3. Postnatal neurological injury of the surviving twin: 34% and 16%
4. Delay in neurodevelopment of the surviving twin: 26% and 2%

When a monochorionic twin dies during pregnancy, the surviving twin is at risk for potentially severe hypotension due to placental anastomoses. Consequently, there may be hypoperfusion in the brain and other organs, which can cause neurological damage or death in the other twin. Doppler flowmetry, especially middle cerebral artery peak systolic velocity (PVS-ACM), should be performed due to the risk of fetal anemia in the surviving twin [2].

Conservative treatment is the most appropriate approach. Immediate birth is generally not indicated because it cannot prevent neurological damage in the surviving fetus. When there are neurological sequelae, the injury is acutely established at the moment of the twin's death (Table 11.4).

Table 11.5 Death of one of the twins according to chorionicity

Dichorionic	Monochorionic
Good prognosis in both trimesters Prevalence of fetal death for the remainder, when death occurs in the second and third trimesters, is 2.5% Initial follow-up at short intervals that can later be spaced Childbirth can occur at 37 weeks in the absence of complications	More reserved prognosis Prevalence of fetal death for the remainder, when death occurs in the second and third trimesters, is 25% Important hypotension and ischemia in the surviving fetus Nuclear magnetic resonance imaging can be performed 4 weeks after fetal decease Delivery at 34 weeks old

If conservative treatment is chosen, fetal biometrics and umbilical artery Doppler flowmetry and ACM should be scheduled every 2 weeks, while delivery should be considered at 34 weeks. If PVS-ACM is normal in the first few days, fetal anemia is unlikely to occur later. Nuclear magnetic resonance image is recommended about 4 weeks after the death of the other twin in search of evidence of brain damage [2] (Table 11.5).

Exclusive Complications of Monochorionic Pregnancies

Monochorionic pregnancies have specific complications that are associated with the same placental mass nourishing the two fetuses.

- Fetal fetus transfusion syndrome (TTTS)
- Polycythemia anemia sequence (TAPS)
- Reverse arterial perfusion sequence (TRAP)
- Monoamniotic monochorionic (MCMA)
- Conjugated twins

Up to one-third of twin pregnancies are monochorionic. In almost all of them, the placenta contains vascular anastomoses that connect the two fetal circulations. Anastomoses can be arterial arteries (AA), veno-venous (VV), and venous arteries (VA). The AA and VV anastomoses have a bidirectional flow, whereas the AVs have a unidirectional flow and are those involved in cases of TTTS. The angioarchitecture of these vascular anastomoses determines the risk profile.

Twin-to-Twin Transfusion Syndrome (TTTS)

TTTS affects 10–15% of monochorionic twin pregnancies and is associated with increased perinatal mortality and morbidity. If left untreated, it leads to the death of one of the fetuses in up to 90% of cases, with morbidity rates in survivors higher than 50%. This is due to the presence of arteriovenous anastomoses, which are part of the placentas of monochorionic twins. However, under normal conditions, there is a balance of blood exchange between fetuses. Since these anastomoses have a unidirectional flow, there is an imbalance of blood transfusion in favor of one of the fetuses, should the TTTS be established. It is the angioarchitecture of these vascular anastomoses that determines the risk profile [1].

The diagnosis of TTTS requires the presence of a significant imbalance of amniotic fluid. The "donor" twin has a larger vertical pocket <2 cm (oligohydramnios) and the "recipient" has a larger vertical pocket >8 cm (polyhydramnios). Although not necessary for diagnosis, other ultrasound characteristics may be present in TTTS. They include discordant twin growth (usually 20%), restricted growth of the donor fetus, and abnormal insertions of the umbilical cord, particularly veiled insertions. When these factors are present, the complexity of the TTTS case increases [2].

Fetoscopic intervention with laser ablation significantly improves the prognosis and is possible with an early diagnosis. Laser treatment in these pregnancies results in 60–70% survival for both fetuses and 80–90% survival for at least one of them.

The presentation of TTTS is variable and does not always progress in a predictable manner. When managed expectantly, early-onset TTTS is associated with high mortality and morbidity.

The most accepted classification system was developed by Quintero. It should be noted that this classification has no correlation with the pregnancy outcomes and does not represent a chronological order of deterioration; for example, stage 1 can become stage 5 without going through stages 2, 3, and 4 and does not predict survival well after the treatment [2] (Table 11.6).

In monochorionic twin pregnancy, screening for TTTS should begin at the 16th week, with tests being repeated every 2 weeks thereafter.

The fetal echocardiogram may show changes at the time of diagnosis of TTTS. These changes mainly involve the recipient fetus, due to the cardiac remodeling that occurs due to the hypervolemic state, which can lead to hypertrophic cardiomyopathy and finally to cardiomegaly.

The procedure after the diagnosis of TTTS will depend on the gestational age, stage of the disease, the availability of resources and maternal manifestations. Ideally, these cases should always be referred to fetal medicine reference centers. Stages I and II have a better prognosis with an overall survival of 86%, while stages III and IV have an overall survival of 66%. Transvaginal measurement of the cervix less than 2.0 cm and gestational age below 18 weeks are signs of a worse prognosis [1] (Table 11.7).

Table 11.6 Quintero Staging

Quintero staging	Ultrasound findings
Quintero I	Presence of polyhydramnios (recipient) and oligohydramnios (donor)
Quintero II	Donor bladder not seen and recipient bladder enlarged
Quintero III	Presence of changes on Doppler
Quintero IV	Presence of fetal hydrops
Quintero V	Death of one fetus

Table 11.7 Conduct in TTTS cases in different settings (based on Multiple Pregnancy Management Advisor. Sao Paulo: Brazilian Federation of Gynecology and Obstetrics Associations; 2018)

Stage I and cervical length > 25 mm	Expectant management. Follow-up is weekly (Doppler ultrasound) to detect disease progression. Resolution of pregnancy between 36 and 37 weeks if the TTTS stage and symptoms remain stable
Stage I and gestational age between 16 and 26 weeks and cervical length ≤ 25 mm	Fetal laser ablation. Serial drainage of amniotic fluid indicated if laser is not available. Weekly Doppler ultrasound monitoring to detect abnormalities of amniotic fluid volume, in membranes and PVS-ACM, or in fetal growth. Pregnancy resolution will be 36–37 weeks of pregnancy, in the absence of further complications
Stage I with gestational age > 26 weeks and cervical length ≤ 25 mm	Serial drainage of amniotic fluid. Laser ablation in gestational age greater than 26 weeks is subject to several technical limitations. Weekly monitoring, with Doppler ultrasound, to detect abnormalities in the volume of the amniotic fluid, in the membranes and in PVS-ACM, or of the fetal growth. Pregnancy resolution will be between 36 and 37 weeks of pregnancy in the absence of complications that require earlier delivery
Stage II to IV between 16 and 26 weeks	Laser ablation of placental anastomoses
Stage II to IV after 26 weeks of pregnancy	Serial drainage of amniotic fluid. Doppler weekly follow-up to detect changes such as zero diastole or reversed diastole in the umbilical artery or reversed a-wave in ductus venosus in one or both fetuses that are indicative for the resolution of pregnancy. Pregnancy will be resolved at 34 weeks of pregnancy in the absence of complications that require earlier delivery
Stage V	If one fetus has died, the main concern for the other twin is death or neurological impairment due to shared placental circulation. The pregnancy will be full term in the absence of complications requiring early delivery

Currently, fetoscopy with laser ablation of placental anastomoses is considered the gold standard for the treatment of this disease. Laser ablation is the treatment of choice for TTTS in the Quintero II and higher stages.

If laser treatment is not available, serial amnioreduction is an acceptable alternative after 26 weeks of pregnancy.

According to the ISUOG manual (Practice Guidelines 2016) after laser treatment, the rate of TTTS recurrence is up to 14%, which probably occurs due to untreated anastomoses at the time of initial laser therapy. The risk of recurrence of TTTS and occurrence of TAPS is reduced by the use of the Solomon technique (equatorial technique where the laser is fired at placental anastomoses following the entire interface path between the membranes of the fetuses, isolating the territories) compared to the technique where the ablation is performed only at the points of the arteriovenous anastomoses identified during the procedure [2].

The main complications occur during surgery, especially the bleeding that can lead to the death of one or both fetuses. In the postoperative evolution, premature membrane rupture (PMR) occurs in 10–20% of cases. Maternal risks are rare and are related to uterine bleeding at the puncture site and infection.

In the case of the death of a fetus (post-laser), the image evaluation (magnetic resonance) of the brain of the surviving twin must be considered after 4 weeks and the assessment of neurological development must occur at 2 years of age.

The follow-up after the laser is performed consists of weekly Doppler ultrasonography and, after documentation of the resolution and well-being of the fetuses, it may be every two weeks. Treatment should result in normalization of the amniotic fluid within 14 days. Cardiac dysfunction in the recipient usually returns to normal in 1 month, while in the donor, this deficiency is temporary. Detailed assessment of the brain, heart, and limbs (due to the risk of amputation secondary to the formation of a thrombus or amniotic band) should be performed during these follow-up examinations. Problems with cardiac function and prenatal brain injuries may become evident only in the third trimester. Some fetal medicine centers offer 30-week fetal brain magnetic resonance imaging (MRI) to all survivors after laser treatment [1, 2].

However, 8% of all these twins, both recipients and donors, will have pulmonary artery stenosis at age 10 and 4% of survivors suffer antenatal brain damage.

Delivery at 34 weeks of pregnancy for persistent abnormalities and up to 37 weeks in those with complete resolution. According to the Manual of the Royal College of Obstetricians and Gynecologists (2016) on MC pregnancies, the recommendation to stop cases that evolve with TTTS should be between 34 + 0 and 36 + 6 weeks of pregnancy.

Polycythemia Anemia Sequence (TAPS)

The pathophysiology of the anemia-polycythemia sequence known as TAPS (*Twin Anemia-Polycythemia Sequence*) is the same as in TTTS, the presence of a pattern of placental vascular anastomoses that produces an unbalanced passage of blood from one twin to another due to the very small anastomoses (<1 mm) unidirectional arteriovenous (AV) types without the presence of arterio-arterial anastomoses (AA), allow a slow transfer of blood from the donor to the recipient, leading to a progressive discordance in hemoglobin levels. The recipient twin becomes polycythemic and the donor twin becomes anemic. The slowness of the process allows a hemodynamic compensation. This hypothesis explains the reason for the absence of discordance on the volume of the amniotic fluid. However, severe polycythemia can lead to fetal and placental thrombosis, while severe anemia can lead to fetal hydrops.

It presents in two forms:

- Spontaneous: affects approximately 5% in monochorionic pregnancies
- Post-treatment with laser ablation (complication): occurs in 13% of cases

Prenatal diagnosis is based on middle cerebral artery peak systolic velocity abnormalities (PSV-ACM: PVS-ACM > 1.5 multiples of the median (MoM) in the donor, suggesting fetal anemia and PVS-ACM < 1.0 MoM without receptor, suggesting polycythemia [1, 2].

Additional ultrasound findings in TAPS include differences in echogenicity and placental thickness, with a thick, shiny portion associated with the donor, and a thin, echolucent portion associated with the recipient. The “starry sky” appearance

Table 11.8 TAPS antenatal and postnatal staging

Phase	Prenatal	Difference in postnatal Hb between twins
1	PVS-ACM donor>1.5 MoM. PVS-ACM recipient <1.0 MoM No other signs of fetal impairment	Greater than 8 mg/dl
2	PVS-ACM donor>1.7 MoM. PVS-ACM recipient<0.8MoM. No other signs of fetal impairment	Greater than 11 mg/dl
3	Stage 1 or 2 and donor cardiac impairment (absent or reverse diastole umbilical artery, pulsating umbilical vein, IP venous duct, increased or reversed a-wave)	Greater than 14 mg/dl
4	Hydrops in the donor	Greater than 17 mg/dl
5	Death of one twin	Greater than 20 mg/dl

Adapted from Khalil et al. [2]
Hb hemoglobin, *PSV-ACM* peak systolic velocity of the middle cerebral artery, *PI* pulsatility index

of the liver seen in the twin with polycythemia is due to the decreased echogenicity of the hepatic parenchyma and the increased brightness of the portal venule walls [2].

The prenatal and postnatal staging classifications based on severity are summarized in Table 11.8.

The post-natal diagnosis of TAPS is based on the findings of chronic anemia (including reticulocytes) in the donor and polycythemia in the recipient. Diagnostic criteria include a difference in hemoglobin concentration between the twins greater than 8 g/dL and at least one between the reticulocyte count ratio greater than 1.7 or small vascular anastomoses (<1 mm in diameter) in the placenta [2].

Treatment options depend on the gestational age at the time of diagnosis, the choice of parents, the severity of the disease, and the technical feasibility for intrauterine therapy. Therefore, the management of twin pregnancies complicated by TAPS must be individualized.

The most frequent options include conservative treatment, early delivery, laser ablation, or intrauterine blood transfusion (IBT) for the anemic twin; combined intrauterine transfusion for the anemic twin; and partial exchange transfusion to dilute the blood of the polycythemic twin.

Reverse Arterial Perfusion Sequence (TRAP)

The occurrence of an acardiac twin is 1/35000 live births and represents approximately 1% of MC pregnancies [2].

It is characterized by the presence of a TRAP mass or an acardiac fetus perfused by an apparently normal twin (pump twin). The perfusion occurs in a retrograde way through arterio-arterial anastomoses, usually through a common site of insertion of the cords. This characteristic vascular arrangement predisposes to hyperdynamic circulation and progressive high-output heart failure in the pump twin (it is exposed to cardiac overload by promoting circulatory support for the cardiac fetus).

The blood supply coming from the umbilical artery is poor in oxygen, which leads to impairment in the development of the fetus that receives this blood. Consequently, there may be an absence of the head, heart, and upper limbs. Exceptionally, there is the formation of a rudimentary heart ("hemi-acardiac") [1].

The risk of death of the pump twin in the conservatively conducted TRAP sequence is up to 30% in the 18th gestational week [2].

The presence of AA anastomoses allows blood to be pumped from the normal twin to the acardiac twin without going through a capillary bed. The chances of survival of the twin who pumps the blood are increased through the use of minimally invasive techniques (for example, coagulation or ligation of the umbilical cord and photocoagulation of the anastomoses, as well as intrafetal methods), preferably, before 16 weeks of pregnancy.

Such a condition can be suspected as early as the first trimester when, in a monochorionic twin pregnancy, one of the fetuses does not show cardiac activity. Faced with this situation, most of the time it is believed to be simply the death of one of the fetuses. However, during an interrupted pregnancy that evolves to death, the dead fetus no longer grows, whereas in the TRAP sequence, the acardiac fetus increases in size over time. In the first months of pregnancy, slight changes in the development of one of the fetuses may be noticed. It should be noted that the identification of cardiac activity in both fetuses in the first trimester does not exclude the diagnosis.

Doppler velocimetry of the umbilical vessels showing reverse flow corroborates the diagnosis. In the case of more advanced pregnancies, the altered morphology facilitates the identification of the presence of the TRAP sequence.

In view of the high mortality rate with the expectant conduct in mono-chorionic pregnancies that follow a TRAP sequence, it is necessary to seek an intervention that improves the outcome of these cases.

TRAP sequence cases are carefully monitored by ultrasound to indicate intrauterine therapy if cardiac involvement is evident in the fetus pump or if there is an increase in perfusion and/or growth of the abnormal fetus [2]. Different minimally invasive techniques, such as umbilical cord coagulation, cord ligation and anastomotic photocoagulation, as well as intrafetal methods using laser in the acardiac fetus are performed to prevent the death of the morphologically normal fetus, also defined as fetal pump . The survival rate with these treatment modalities is approximately 80%.

Resolution of TRAP pregnancies between 34 and 36 weeks of pregnancy: The resolution within this range depends on the patient's clinical scenario and whether there are indications of impairment in the pump twin, which would lead to early delivery.

Monoamniotic Monochorionic Twinning (MCMA)

MCMA twin pregnancies represent roughly 1–2% of monochorionic twin pregnancies.

MCMA pregnancies almost always have cord interlacing when viewed using color Doppler. This finding does not consistently contribute to morbidity and mortality [1].

The rate of perinatal loss reported below 16 weeks of pregnancy reaches 50%. Most of the losses are attributable to fetal abnormalities and miscarriage. Conducting these pregnancies can be complex and should be performed in fetal medicine centers [2].

The incidence of TTTS and brain injury was 6% and 5%, respectively. The recommended time for delivery is 32–34 weeks of pregnancy.

Conjugated Twins

Imperfect twinning is very rare, occurring in about 1 in every 100,000 pregnancies (1% of monochorionic twin pregnancies). Conjugated twins are always twin MCMA pregnancies. Ultrasound diagnosis in the first trimester is currently common. A recent series of 14 cases from a single referral center reported that, after diagnosis, 20% of parents opted for interruption and 10% of fetuses died in the womb [2].

The classification of the conjugated twins depends on the fusion site.

They are classified as *cephalopagus, thoracopagus, omphalopagus, ischiopagus, parapagus, craniopagus, rachipagus, and pygopagus* [1].

Thoracoopagus is the most common form, in which the twins are face to face and have connections between the chest and abdomen, often sharing livers, hearts, and intestinal structures.

In ongoing pregnancies, detailed ultrasound assessment by an experienced professional (with or without MRI) is important in order to give as much detail as possible on the cardiovascular anatomy (and other systems) of the twins before delivery.

Although vaginal delivery of conjoined twins has been reported, there is a significant risk of obstructed delivery, dystocia, and uterine rupture, so cesarean delivery has become a consensual elective procedure.

Vaginal delivery can be attempted in the second trimester, especially for nonviable twins or for termination of pregnancy.

Childbirth During Twin Pregnancy

Labor and delivery during twin pregnancy have a higher incidence of perinatal complications, including premature labor, premature rupture of ovular membranes, uterine dyskinesias, positional dystocia, umbilical cord prolapse, placental abruption, uterine atony, postpartum hemorrhage, and intrauterine fetal death.

Table 11.9 Mode of delivery in Mmultiple pregnancy

Pregnancy ≥ 32 weeks or fetal weight > 1500 g	Cephalic – cephalic presentation: vaginal delivery in the absence of obstetric indications for cesarean delivery Cephalic presentation – non-cephalic: vaginal delivery with internal version and pelvic extraction of the second twin, depending on the experience of the care team and if the patient provides informed consent
Pregnancy < 32 weeks or estimated fetal weight < 1500 g	Both in cephalic: intention to deliver vaginally One or both non-cephalic: elective cesarean section (except in non-viable fetuses). In non-elective situations, one can individualize according to the obstetrician's criteria
Indications for cesarean section	First twin in non-cephalic presentation MC/MA twins Multiple pregnancies ≥3 fetuses Maternal, fetal, or placental pathology Second twin with weight >20% in relation to the first twin, especially in non-cephalic presentation Suspected alteration of fetal vitality, impossibility of correct monitoring of one or both fetuses during delivery

The gestational age of resolution of twin pregnancies varies according to chorionicity, amnionicity and, obviously, the complications during pregnancy.

- DC/DA: 38 + 0 to 38 + 6 weeks of pregnancy
- MC/DA: 36 + 0 to 36 + 6 weeks of pregnancy
- MC/MA: 32–34 weeks
- Triplet: 32–34 weeks

The indication for a cesarean delivery in monoamniotic pregnancies is well established. Prolapse or folding of cords and collision of fetal parts are complications related to these pregnancies.

However, it should be considered that 30–40% of twin labor becomes an indication for emergency cesarean delivery. In a smaller number of cases, there may be a need for an emergency cesarean section for the second fetus, after vaginal delivery of the first. Consequently, during the follow-up of a twin pregnancy, it is important to have easy and fast access to the cesarean delivery room [1].

The decision to give birth through the careful evaluation of these variables aims at reducing perinatal and maternal risk and lower conversion rates for emergency surgical interventions. The factors considered of greatest relevance in choosing the mode of delivery are feasibility of fetuses and gestational age, presentation of fetuses, conceptus weight estimation, and parity (Table 11.9).

Multiple Pregnancy with Gestational Trophoblastic Disease

Gestational trophoblastic disease (GTD) encompasses a heterogeneous group of cell proliferation originating from the placental trophoblastic epithelium. The most common form of GTD is the hydatidiform mole and is the only benign condition;

the other forms are jointly called gestational trophoblastic neoplasia (GTN) and include the invasive mole, choriocarcinoma, trophoblastic tumor of placental site, and epithelioid trophoblastic tumor. GTD has a very efficient biological marker, chorionic gonadotropin (hCG), as there is a linear correlation between hCG titers, number of trophoblastic cells, and tumor size.

A form of clinical presentation of GDT is twin pregnancy with hydatidiform mole and coexisting fetus (GMHFC). This entity is rare, with an estimated incidence of 1 case for 20,000 to 100,000 pregnancies. In contrast to single hydatidiform moles, most cases in twin pregnancies correspond to complete hydatidiform moles, but the reason for this difference in incidence is unknown [3, 4].

In twins with homozygous hydatidiform mole and alleles identical to normal co-twin, there is a probable fertilization of an oocyte by a sperm with duplication of the paternal genetic load, forming a triploid zygote. The triploid zygote would undergo diploidization, which may result in two situations: (1) Triploid division with formation of haploid, diploid, and triploid cells. If the triploid cells are eliminated and the paternal haploid cells undergo endoreduplication, biparental diploid and androgenetic diploid lines would remain. (2) Triploid division into two biparental diploid cells and one androgenetic diploid blastomere. In homozygous hydatidiform moles with alleles other than co-twinning, they must be generated from a triploid zygote formed by the fertilization of an oocyte by two sperms. This zygote would undergo diploidization and the division would occur as previously mentioned. In twins in which the hydatidiform mole is heterozygous with alleles different from the co-twin, the zygote initially formed would be tetraploid and then undergo diploidization and cleavage forming two cell lines: biparental diploid and androgenetic diploid. The formation of the tetraploid zygote can originate from the fertilization of an oocyte by three spermatozoa or by the fertilization of one oocyte by two spermatozoa (with a doubling of the genetic load of one of them) [3, 4].

In most cases, the diagnosis of GMHFC pregnancy is made by ultrasound, where you can observe multiple anechoic areas, adjacent to a normal echographic-looking placenta, associated with a fetus without morphological changes, which strongly suggests the diagnosis of multiple pregnancy with coexistence of complete mole and normal fetus. Differential diagnosis with mesenchymal dysplasia can be difficult. Mesenchymal dysplasia presents with placentomegaly with cystic areas, associated with fetal growth restriction and even fetal death; however, the levels of β-hCG in these patients are usually not elevated.

Several reports in the literature have associated GMHFC pregnancy with clinical complications typical of late hydatidiform moles more frequently than in single moles, leading to a higher risk of potentially fatal and near-miss complications. Obstetric complications have also been associated with GMHFC pregnancies, such as miscarriage, fetal death, and premature delivery. There are also reports in the literature of twin pregnancies that go with the complete mole, behaving like a placenta previa, and may even present placental accretism, making it difficult a differential diagnosis with the invasive mole.

References

1. Carvalho FH, Vela HW, Morais AL, Feitosa FE. Management of multiple pregnancies. Sao Paulo: Brazilian Federation of Gynecology and Obstetrics Associations (FEBRASGO); 2018. (Protocol FEBRASGO - Obstetrics, no. 37/National Commission Specialized in Fetal Medicine).
2. These Guidelines should be cited as: Khalil A, Rodgers M, Baschat A, Bhide A, Gratacos E, Hecher K, Kilby MD, Lewi L, Nicolaides KH, Oepkes D, Raine-Fenning N, Reed K, Salomon LJ, Sotiriadis A, Thilaganathan B, Ville Y. ISUOG Practice Guidelines: role of ultrasound in twin pregnancy. Ultrasound Obstet Gynecol. 2016;47:247–263.
3. Soper JT, Mutch DG, Schink JC, American College of Obstetricians and Gynecologists. Diagnosis and treatment of gestational trophoblastic disease: ACOG Practice Bulletin No. 53.
4. Lurain JR. Gestational trophoblastic disease I: epidemiology, pathology, clinical presentation and diagnosis of gestational trophoblastic disease, and management of hydatidiform mole.

Part III
Fetal Proceedings

Chapter 12
Ultrasound

Alberto Borges Peixoto and Edward Araujo Júnior

Introduction

Pregnancy management includes several measures and interventions aimed at maintaining maternal and fetal well-being. In recent times, progress in diagnostic technologies has facilitated early diagnosis of conditions affecting pregnant women and the fetus, thereby improving the quality of prenatal care. Ultrasonography has played an important role in the detection of fetal pathologies, as well as in the identification of women with high-risk pregnancies who present with conditions that directly or indirectly affect their well-being, as well as the development and well-being of the fetus and the newborn.

First-trimester ultrasonography is essential for the early evaluation of pregnancy. Owing to significant upgrades in ultrasound technology, high-quality, high-resolution ultrasonographic images can be obtained, which facilitate close monitoring of fetal development immediately after confirmation of embryonic viability (indicated by the appearance of a gestational sac within the uterine cavity and detection of cardiac activity). Ultrasonographic imaging also helps to determine the number of embryos, and chorionicity [1]. Between 6 and 8 weeks of gestation, it is

A. B. Peixoto
Department of Gynecology and Obstetrics, University of Uberaba (UNIUBE), Uberaba, Brazil

Department of Gynecology and Obstetrics, Federal University of Triângulo Mineiro (UFTM), Uberaba, Brazil

E. Araujo Júnior (✉)
Discipline of Fetal Medicine, Department of Obstetrics, Paulista School of Medicine –Federal University of São Paulo (EPM-UNIFESP), São Paulo, SP, Brazil

© Springer Nature Switzerland AG 2022

R. A. Moreira de Sá, E. B. d. Fonseca (eds.), *Perinatology*,
https://doi.org/10.1007/978-3-030-83434-0_12

possible to assess embryonic viability and accurately determine the location of the gestational sac, the number of fetuses, chorionicity, amnionicity, and gestational age by measuring the crown-rump length (CRL). Between 11 and 13 weeks and 6 days, in addition to the aforementioned data, it is possible to obtain the following information: risk of aneuploidy (based on assessment of first-trimester ultrasonographic markers) and the risk of maternal conditions such as preeclampsia. Moreover, detection of major fetal anomalies, fetal growth restriction (FGR), and premature birth is also possible [1–3].

Second-trimester ultrasonography should be performed by trained professionals and should preferably be offered to all pregnant women between 18 and 22 weeks [4]. The main objective of this examination is to perform detailed evaluation of fetal anatomy [4] in addition to evaluation of fetal biometrics, evaluation of the uteroplacental vascularization (based on uterine artery Doppler studies) [3], evaluation of amniotic fluid, and endovaginal measurement of the length of the uterine cervix [5].

Third-trimester ultrasonography enables assessment of fetal growth and well-being in singleton and twin pregnancies [4, 6].

In this chapter, we discuss the role of ultrasonography in maternal-fetal medicine with regard to guidelines to determine gestational age, monitor and manage first-trimester complications, determine chorionicity and fetal anomalies, as well as assess fetal growth.

Assessment of Pregnancy Viability, Determination of Gestational Age, and Chorionicity in Twin Pregnancies During the First Trimester of Pregnancy

Ultrasonography during early pregnancy is important for assessment of pregnancy viability, accurate determination of the gestational age, and determination of the number of fetuses and chorionicity in cases of twin pregnancies [1].

Routine ultrasonography is not indicated during early pregnancy. Ultrasonographic examination at 6–8 weeks is essential in women with clinical signs and symptoms or specific indications that warrant this evaluation [7]. It is recommended that the first ultrasonographic examination should be performed between 11 and 13 weeks of gestation to assess the viability of the pregnancy and to determine the gestational age, the number of fetuses and chorionicity, fetal anatomy, and the risks for chromosomal disorders [7, 8].

The Federal University of Triângulo Mineiro recommends the following criteria to perform ultrasonography between 6 and 8 weeks: vaginal bleeding and/or abdominal pain concomitant with a positive beta-human chorionic gonadotropin (ßhCG) test result, unknown or uncertain date of last menstrual period (LMP), risk factors for ectopic pregnancy (EP), assisted reproductive treatment, and nausea/vomiting or hyperemesis gravidarum.

Assessment of Pregnancy Viability

Early non-viable pregnancies represent approximately 2.8% of all pregnancies. Among the various etiologies contributing to early pregnancy loss, chromosomal abnormalities (accounting for 45–70% of cases of non-viable initial pregnancy) serve as the main etiological factor associated with this complication until 10–13 weeks [9].

The differential diagnoses that should be considered in women with vaginal bleeding and abdominal pain during the early stages of pregnancy include the following: viable early pregnancy, abortion, and EP. First-trimester bleeding could occur in women with an early viable or non-viable pregnancy. Therefore, the following terminology has been suggested to guide management in such cases [10]:

(a) Viable pregnancy: pregnancy that can result in the birth of a live newborn.
(b) Non-viable pregnancy: pregnancy that possibly will not result in the birth of a live newborn. EP and abortion are considered non-viable pregnancies.
(c) Early pregnancy of uncertain viability: pregnancy showing a gestational sac with an embryo without a heartbeat but without definitive signs of pregnancy failure.
(d) Early pregnancy of unknown location (PUL): pregnancy in which ßhCG testing shows positive results, but that is not identified on transvaginal ultrasonography (TVUS), topical intrauterine pregnancy, or EP.

Quantitative serum ßhCG measurement and TVUS are the main propaedeutic methods used to diagnose and treat complications associated with early pregnancies [10]. Correct interpretation of these test results is necessary to accurately diagnose EP, as well as to minimize complications attributable to misinterpretation of results of complementary examinations and misdiagnosis [11].

TVUS can identify the gestational sac at approximately 5 weeks of gestation, and serum ßhCG levels are usually 1000–2000 mUI/mL (discriminatory value) during this same period [12, 13]. The yolk sac is identified at approximately 5.5 weeks and confirms an embryonic pregnancy [14]. The embryo is visualized close to the yolk sac at 6 weeks of gestation (Fig. 12.1) [12]. The CRL is approximately 2 mm during this period [15, 16] and increases at the rate of approximately 1 mm/day in viable pregnancies [15, 16]. The embryonic heartbeat is detected when the CRL is approximately 2 mm [17]. However, in 5–10% of viable pregnancies, the heartbeat is not detected in embryos with CRL measuring 2–4 mm [18].

At approximately 6–8 weeks of gestation, it is important to accurately differentiate between early abortion and very early viable pregnancy in women in whom early ultrasonography detects an embryonic heartbeat [19]. A recent study suggests that a gestational sac with a mean diameter > 25 mm and CRL > 7 mm are associated with a low risk of a false-positive diagnosis of abortion [19]. In women in whom these measurements are below the cut-off values, ultrasonography should be repeated in 7–15 days to assess the growth of the gestational sac or embryo [10].

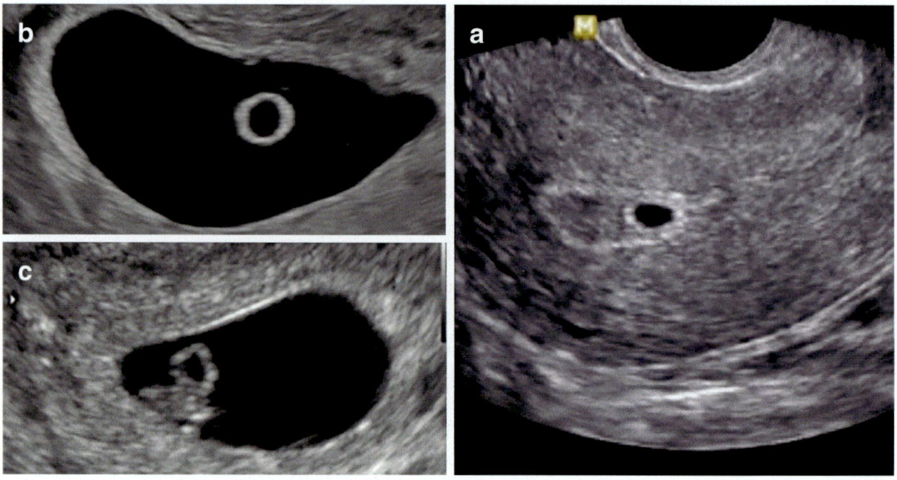

Fig. 12.1 (**a**) Transvaginal ultrasound at 5 weeks of gestation. (**b**) 5.5-week gestation, showing regular boundary gestational sac and normal-looking yolk sac. (**c**) 6-week gestation. Observe the presence of an embryo located close to the yolk sac

Early Pregnancy of Unknown Location

PUL is defined as pregnancy in a woman showing positive results on serum ßhCG testing but without topical intrauterine pregnancy or EP on TVUS. PUL outcomes include the following: intrauterine pregnancy (viable, non-viable, or early pregnancy with uncertain evolution), EP, failed PUL (PULF), or persistent PUL (PULP) [20–22].

Women with PULF show spontaneous resolution of pregnancy with negative results on serum ßhCG testing and a low risk of complications. Identification of the exact location of the pregnancy (topical or ectopic) is challenging in such cases [23].

PULP accounts for 2% of all cases of PUL and is associated with a high risk of complications [24, 25]. A spontaneous decline in serum ßhCG levels does not occur in PULP; usually a <15% increase is observed in the serum ßhCG level measured on three consecutive occasions at 48-hour intervals or this level tends to plateau. Additionally, an intrauterine or ectopic gestational sac is not visualized [22].

A series of flowcharts and guidelines have been proposed for the management of women with PUL [26–28]. However, in clinical practice, assessment of quantitative serum ßhCG levels is important to exclude the diagnosis of a viable topical pregnancy and for treatment decision-making.

Isolated assessment and a single quantitative serum ßhCG level measurement cannot differentiate between viable intrauterine pregnancy, fetal death, abortion, and EP [11, 29, 30]. Serial assessment of serum ßhCG levels and its correlation with TVUS findings and serum progesterone levels is necessary. Serum ßhCG levels increase from 53% to 66% within 48 hours in viable intrauterine pregnancies [31, 32]. Notably, a <53% elevation in serum ßhCG levels within 48 hours and the absence of an intrauterine gestational sac on TVUS lead to a high index of clinical suspicion for early pregnancy loss or EP [31, 32].

Currently, the discriminatory serum ßhCG level (which is considered along with the identification of a gestational sac on TVUS for accurate diagnosis) is 1000–2000 mUI/mL [12, 13]. Notably, serum ßhCG values within discriminatory levels are insufficient to accurately diagnose a viable intrauterine pregnancy. Absence of a gestational sac on ultrasonography in a woman with serum ßhCG levels greater than the discriminatory value could be attributed to the following factors: higher prevalence of twin pregnancies being observed currently, examiner's inexperience, uterine leiomyomas, use of low-resolution ultrasonography devices, and nonstandardized techniques used by the laboratory for serum ßhCG level analysis [33, 34]. Serum ßhCG levels are higher in twin pregnancies than those observed in singleton pregnancies for the same gestational age [10]. Some studies have reported identification of an embryo with a detectable heartbeat on ultrasonographic follow-up after an initial examination failed to identify a gestational sac in patients with serum ßhCG levels >2000 mUI/mL [35–37] or >3000 mUI/mL [35, 36]. A previous study performed in women with clinical signs suggestive of EP determined the best serum ßhCG cut-off value necessary for the identification of a gestational sac on TVUS [37]. For serum ßhCG values of 3510 mUI/mL, 2000 mUI/mL, and 1000 mUI/mL, the probability of visualizing the gestational sac in patients with PUL was 99%, 91.2%, and 80.9%, respectively [37].

Serum ßhCG levels undergo wide fluctuations in patients with EP, and usually, the pattern of serum ßhCG elevation in this category of patients does not follow the pattern observed in viable intrauterine pregnancies. Therefore, TVUS is indicated in patients with clinical suspicion of EP, even in those with serum ßhCG levels <1000 mIU/mL [10].

A study performed in patients diagnosed with PUL who showed serum ßhCG levels of 2000–3000 mUI/mL reported 19 EP and 38 non-viable intrauterine pregnancies for each viable intrauterine pregnancy in the study group [10]. Therefore, treatment with methotrexate or surgical intervention is contraindicated to avoid the risk of interrupting a viable intrauterine pregnancy in such cases. In addition, in hemodynamically stable patients, serial measurement of serum ßhCG levels over 48 hours can provide important information for diagnosis and decision-making [11, 38].

Diagnosis of non-viable intrauterine gestation is possible but unlikely in hemodynamically stable patients with serum ßhCG levels ≥3000 mUI/mL who show lack of evidence suggesting intrauterine pregnancy and normal adnexa on TVUS. The best option in these patients is to measure the serum ßhCG level at least once in 48 hours [10]. Patients with serum ßhCG levels ≥3500 mUI/mL associated with an increase of >53% in 48 hours and TVUS-proven absence of intrauterine gestational sac show a high likelihood of EP [21].

Expectant monitoring is recommended in clinically stable patients diagnosed with PUL in whom a reduction in serum ßhCG levels occurs after 48 hours because early pregnancy loss cannot be ruled out in such cases. Moreover, methotrexate use is contraindicated in cases of early pregnancy loss [39]. Treatment success rates did not differ between patients receiving methotrexate and expectant monitoring among women with suspected EP showing serum ßhCG levels ≤2000 mUI/mL [39].

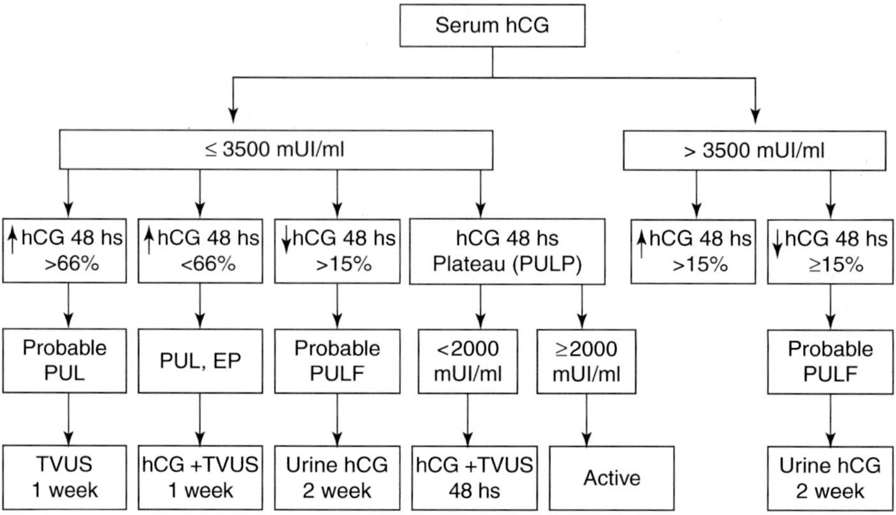

Fig. 12.2 Flowchart of the Hospital das Clínicas of the University of São Paulo (USP) for the prenatal care of women with pregnancy of unknow location (PUL). EP ectopic pregnancy, TVUS transvaginal ultrasound

Estimation of serum progesterone levels is used in conjunction with serum ßhCG measurement to monitor patients with PUL. Progesterone levels <5 ng/mL, >20 ng/mL, and 5–20 ng/mL are associated with a high risk for non-viable pregnancy, viable intrauterine pregnancy, and EP, respectively. A serum progesterone level ≤10 ng/mL is a significant predictor of PULF and can differentiate between PUL and PULF [40].

There is lack of consensus regarding the optimal management of PUL, and several protocols are described in clinical practice. The Hospital das Clínicas, University of São Paulo, has published a flowchart that outlines the management of PUL (Fig. 12.2) [22]. According to this guideline, expectant monitoring can be continued until serum ßhCG values are elevated to 3500 mUI/mL, after which it is recommended that serum ßhCG measurement should be performed every 48 hours along with TVUS. Active intervention includes manual vacuum aspiration or the administration of methotrexate (50 mg/m^2) depending on the diagnosis [22].

Determination of Gestational Age

Ultrasonography is useful for the calculation of gestational age; a study has shown that approximately 30% of women who received prenatal care were unaware of or uncertain regarding the date of their LMP [19].

Ultrasonographic estimation of gestational age is performed by measuring the mean diameter of the gestational sac (MSD) and the CRL. The MSD is calculated

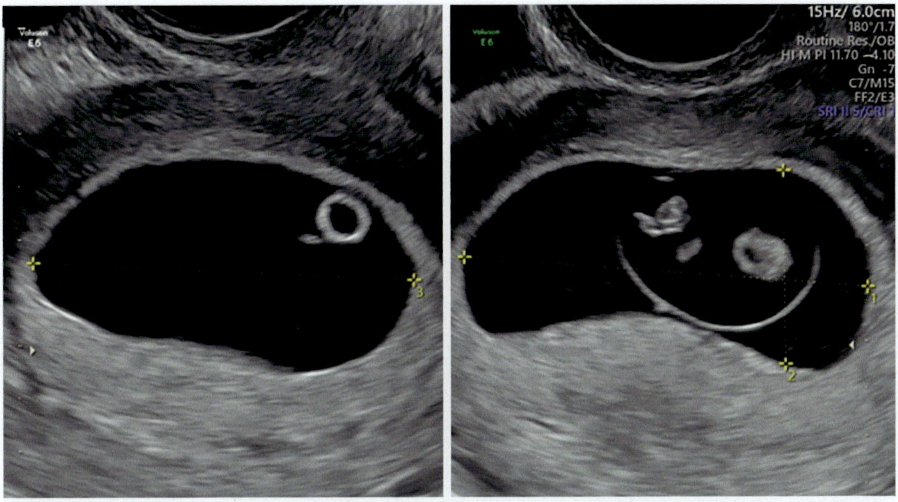

Fig. 12.3 Transvaginal ultrasound image showing the measurement of mean diameter of the gestational sac (MSD). To determine the MSD, the three orthogonal planes of the gestational sac are measured. MSD = 32.7 mm (MSD = 42.1 × 20.4 × 35.5 mm/3)

as the arithmetic mean of the 3 orthogonal planes (longitudinal, anteroposterior, transverse) of the anechoic portion of the gestational sac (Fig. 12.3). It is recommended that the MSD should be used to calculate gestational age only in women in whom the embryonic pole cannot be visualized.

CRL measurement is the most accurate and recommended parameter to determine gestational age considering the significant variability in the prediction of gestational age using the MSD and other techniques [7, 41, 42]. CRL measurement should preferably be performed between 10 and 13 weeks and 6 days for accurate determination of gestational age. For CRL measurement via the abdominal or transvaginal route, the fetus must be in a neutral position; hyperflexion or hyperextension should be avoided; the ultrasonography device screen should be horizontally oriented; and the vertex of the skull and the mid-point between the apices of the buttocks should be clearly visible. The image must be magnified to ensure that the fetus occupies nearly the entire screen (Fig. 12.4). To ensure standardization, the angle between the plane of the calipers and the direction of the sound beam should be 90° [7]. The examiner must carefully follow the steps described to ensure accurate calculation of gestational age. Incorrect measurements can lead to overestimation of gestational age, usually when CRL measurement is performed in a hyperextended fetus, or underestimation of gestational age, usually when the CRL measurement is performed in a hyperflexed fetus. Moreover, incorrect CRL measurements can affect optimal management of pregnancies, can lead to inaccuracies in estimating the risk of aneuploidy, or can result in inaccurate diagnosis of fetal growth deviations and calculation of the probable date of delivery [42].

Obtaining appropriate images with embryos in the neutral position is challenging at a very early gestational age (6–9 weeks) (Fig. 12.5). During this stage of the

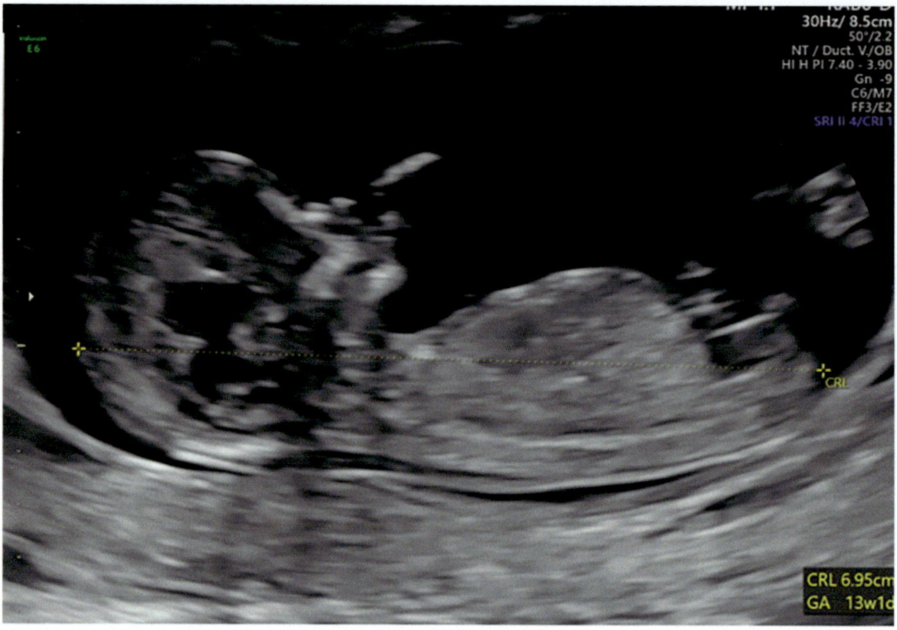

Fig. 12.4 Technique for measuring the measurement of the crown-rump length (CRL). Observe the fetus in a neutral position and the line between the calipers at an angle of 90° with the direction of the sound beam

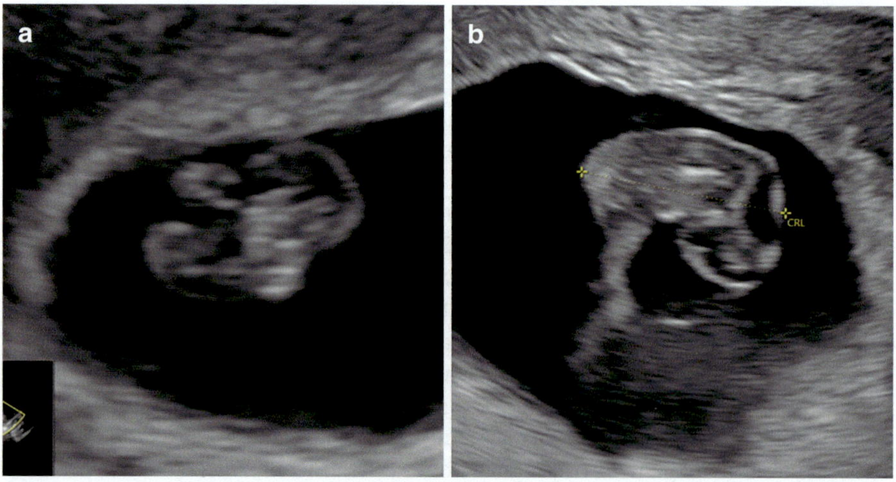

Fig. 12.5 (**a**) Image obtained by transvaginal ultrasound of an embryo at 6 weeks and 2 days. Observe the hyperflexion attitude of the embryonic pole, preventing an adequate measurement of the crown-rump length (CRL). (**b**) Image obtained by transvaginal ultrasonography of an embryo of 7 weeks and 6 days. Observe the CRL measurement between the buttock and cervical region

pregnancy, embryos are typically hyperflexed; therefore, using a buttock neck instead of a buttock head to measure CRL leads to underestimation of gestational age. In some cases, the cephalic and caudal poles are indistinguishable, contributing to overestimation of the gestational age [7]. When the gestational age is calculated using ultrasonography in very early pregnancies (particularly before 8 weeks of gestation), the gestational age should be recalculated between 10 and 13 weeks and 6 days and should not be recalculated during subsequent examinations.

The accuracy of ultrasonography for gestational age determination is low in cases where CRL > 84 mm (approximately 14 weeks of gestation). In such cases, other ultrasonographic parameters should be used to calculate gestational age [42]; head circumference (HC) measurement can be used to calculate gestational age because the accuracy of this parameter is greater than that associated with biparietal diameter (BPD) measurement [43].

Twin Pregnancies

Twin pregnancies are detected in 3% of first-trimester ultrasonographic examination [44]. Chorionicity determination is important because perinatal complications are more common in monochorionic vs. dichorionic twin pregnancies, thereby altering the clinical and ultrasonographic management during the prenatal period [45]. In monochorionic pregnancies, most pregnancy losses occur between the first and third trimesters and are primarily attributable to twin-to-twin transfusion syndrome, selective growth restriction, and discordant fetal anomalies [46–48].

During the first trimester of gestation, the lambda signal (present in dichorionic pregnancies) and the T signal (present in monochorionic pregnancies) show high reproducibility and accuracy [49]; these features are significantly lower during the second trimester [50] (Fig. 12.6).

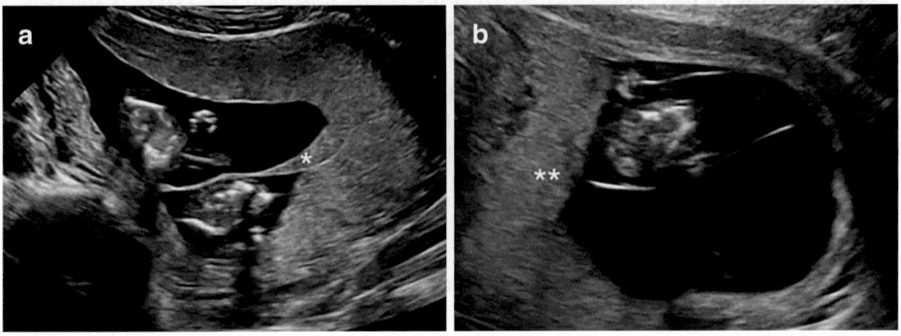

Fig. 12.6 Image of twin pregnancies during the first trimester of pregnancy. (**a**) Dichorionic twin pregnancy showing the Lambda sign (*). (**b**) Monochorionic twin pregnancy showing the T sign (**)

Ultrasonographic Determination of Fetal Anomalies

Detection of Fetal Anomalies During the First Trimester

Advances in ultrasonographic imaging technology and improved training of professionals have enabled accurate diagnosis of fetal malformations at an early gestational age. Some studies have reported that the detection rate of fetal abnormalities during the first trimester ranges from 31% to 45.3% [51–53]. However, the sensitivity of ultrasonography in the detection of fetal anomalies during the first trimester is lower if the detection rate of minor anomalies is also considered [54]. A retrospective single tertiary center study performed by Dulgheroff et al. [54] reported that the sensitivity of ultrasonography for the detection of fetal anomalies during the first trimester was 14.06%. The examiner's experience, resolution of the ultrasonographic devices, gestational age at the time of the ultrasonography, fetal movements, and inability to completely assess fetal anatomy may influence detection of fetal anomalies during the first trimester. Studies have reported that TVUS performed during the first trimester improved the assessment of fetal structures and the rate of detection of fetal structural anomalies [55, 56].

Based on the possibility of detection during the first trimester, fetal anomalies can be classified into three groups as follows [57]:

(a) Anomalies that are always detectable: anencephaly, body stalk anomaly, omphalocele, gastroschisis, megabexiga, and holoprosencephaly
(b) Anomalies that may potentially be detected: spina bifida, facial cleft, polydactyly, renal agenesis
(c) Anomalies that are never detected: microcephaly and corpus callosum agenesis

Evaluation of the following structures is necessary for complete evaluation of fetal anatomy between 11 and 13 weeks and 6 days [7]: head (presence, skull structures, cerebral sickle, choroid plexus) (Fig. 12.7a), neck (appearance, measurement of nuchal translucency) (Fig. 12.7b), face (eyes, lens, nasal bone, fetal profile, mandible, lips) (Fig. 12.7c, d), spine (bone and skin integrity) (Fig. 12.8), heart (symmetry of the four cardiac chambers and the cardiac rhythm) (Fig. 12.9), abdomen (stomach, kidneys and bladder), chest (lung symmetry, presence of masses and/or effusions) (Fig. 12.10a–c), abdominal wall (presence of defects in the abdominal wall) (Fig. 12.11), extremities (presence of upper and lower limbs, hands, and feet) (Fig. 12.12), and the number of umbilical cord vessels (Fig. 12.13).

Detection of Fetal Anomalies During the Second Trimester

Second-trimester ultrasonography is a screening test that should be offered to all pregnant women who receive prenatal care. The timing of the ultrasonographic examination depends on the indications for the imaging and the availability of local

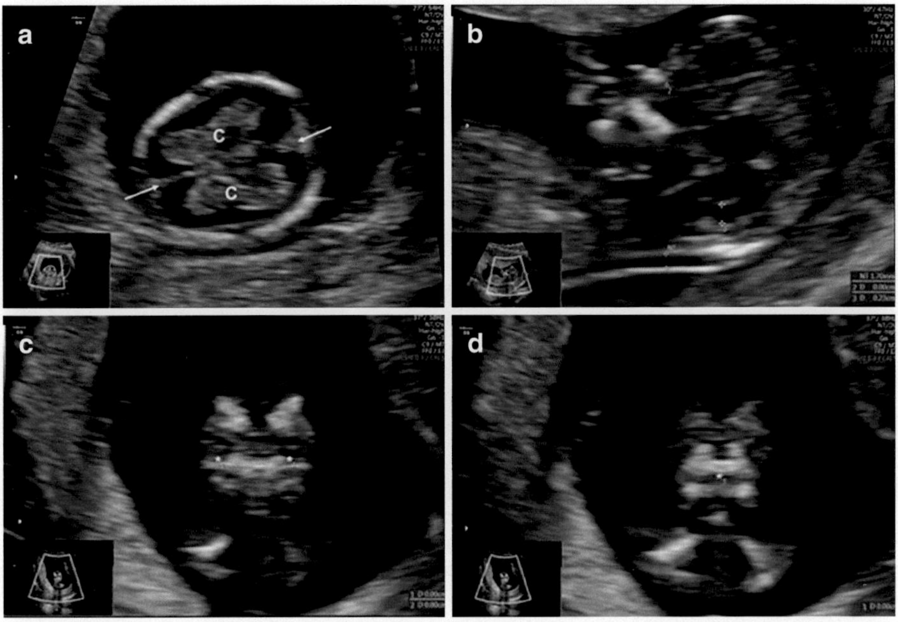

Fig. 12.7 (**a**) Fetal head: choroid plexuses (c), sickle (arrows). (**b**) Nuchal translucency. (**c**) eyes (*). (**d**) palate (*)

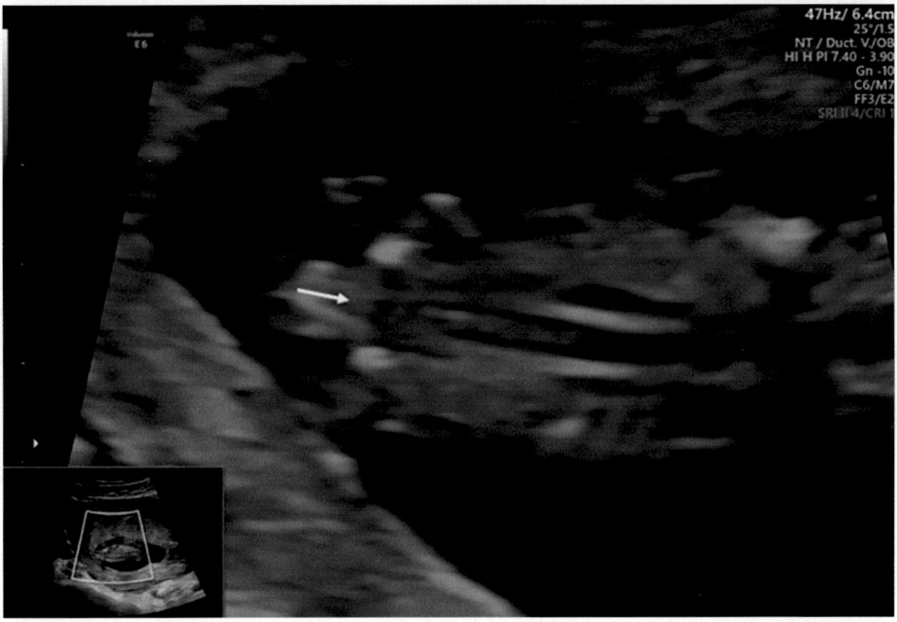

Fig. 12.8 Sagittal view of the fetal spine showing alignment and integrity of the vertebral processes (arrow)

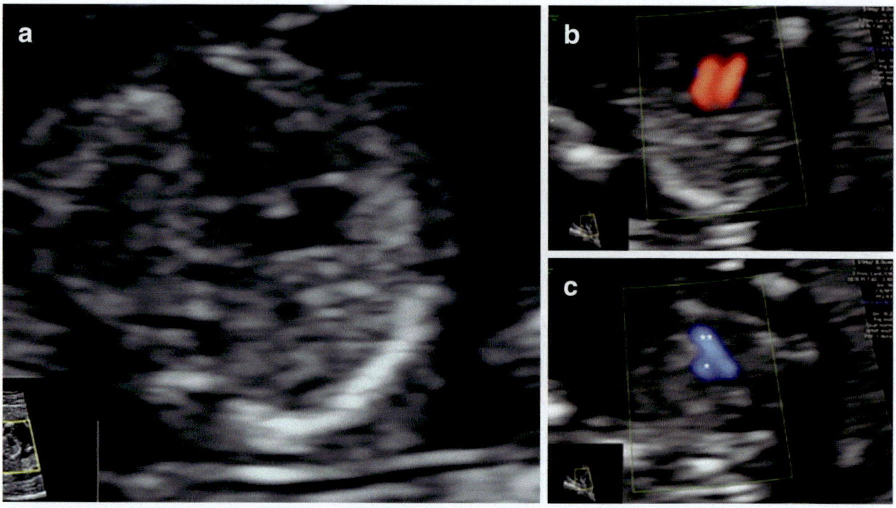

Fig. 12.9 (**a**) Four-chamber view of the fetal heart showing size and symmetries between the preserved chambers. (**b**) HD flow Doppler demonstrating diastolic flow (red) and (**c**) systolic flow through the aorta (*) and pulmonary (**) arteries

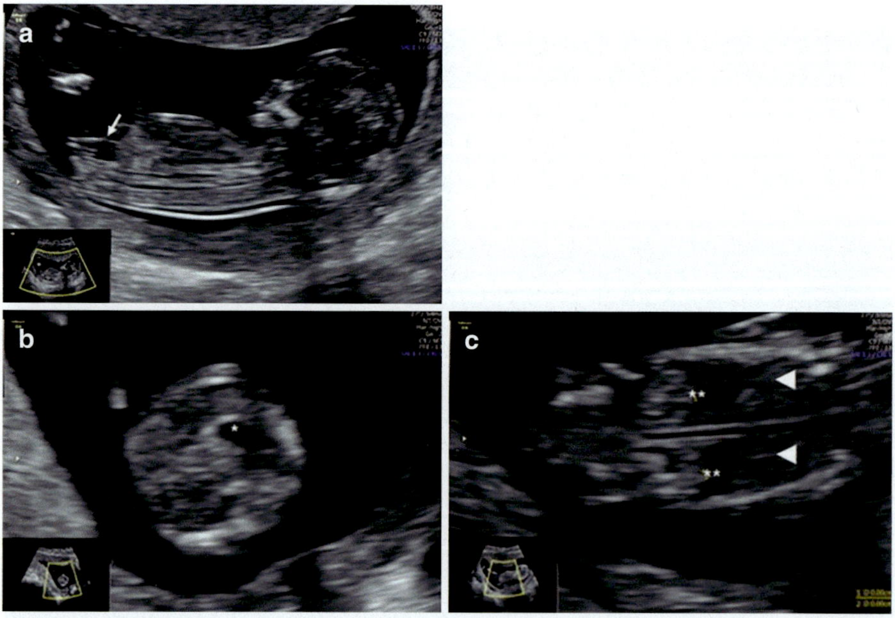

Fig. 12.10 (**a**) Sagittal view of the fetus showing bladder (arrow) with fullness and normal dimensions. (**b**) Axial view of the abdomen showing the stomach (*). (**c**) Sagittal section of the abdomen and chest showing kidneys (**) and lungs (arrowhead)

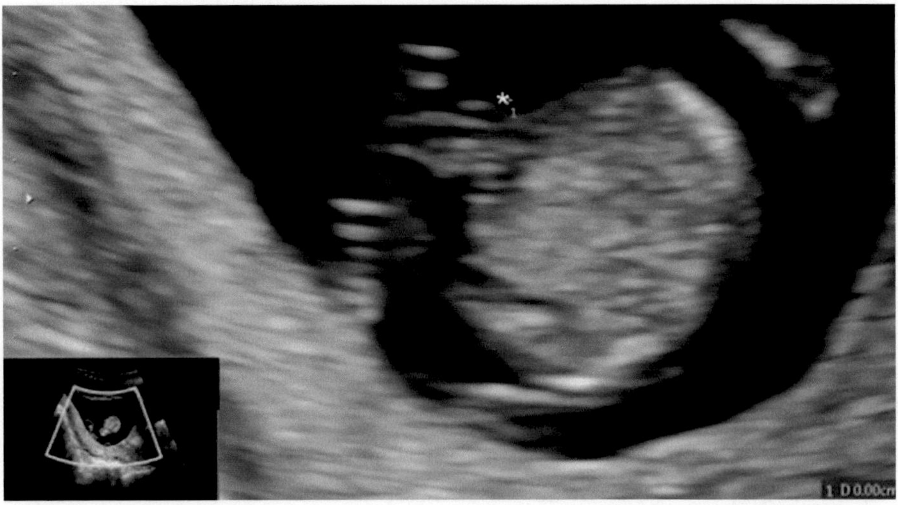

Fig. 12.11 Axial view of the fetal abdomen showing entry of the umbilical cord. Note the integrity of the abdominal wall

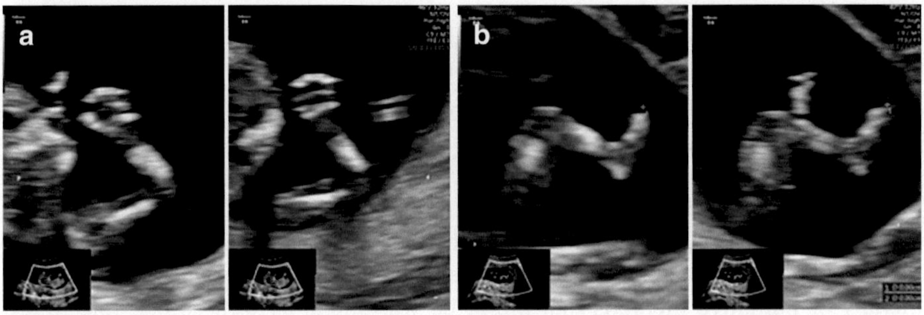

Fig. 12.12 (**a**) Sagittal view of the fetus showing two upper limbs and (**b**) two lower limbs

facilities. According to the International Society of Ultrasound in Obstetrics and Gynccology (ISUOG), the ideal time to perform the second-trimester ultrasonographic examination is between 18 and 22 weeks [4]. The Fetal Medicine Foundation recommends that the examination be performed between 20 and 22 weeks [58]. In Brazil, second-trimester ultrasonography is usually performed between 20 and 24 weeks of gestation, and the detection rate of fetal anomalies varies from 15% to 85.3% [54, 58]. The primary objective of second-trimester ultrasonographic screening is to identify preventable conditions and those that could be treated using intra- or extrauterine interventions, thereby reducing perinatal morbidity and mortality [58].

In utero diagnosis of fetal abnormalities is possible in 2–5% of cases [54, 58–61] with a neonatal mortality rate of 20–30% [62, 63]. The introduction of the fetal anomaly screening policy during the second trimester improves the detection of structural fetal defects; however, fetal anomaly screening is not necessarily

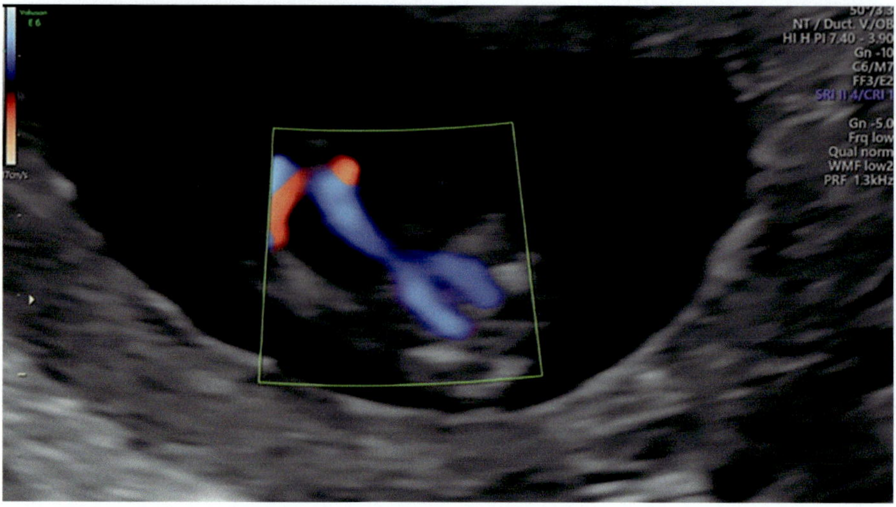

Fig. 12.13 Axial view of the fetal abdomen showing the exit of the two umbilical arteries

associated with reduced mortality and morbidity rates, which are dependent on an interplay between several factors. Mortality rates are associated with examiner expertise, the detection rate of fetal anomalies, and the implementation of public health policies that permit the termination of pregnancy in cases of fetal malformations [62].

According to the National Institute of Clinical Excellence of the United Kingdom, early detection of fetal abnormalities enables decision-making regarding couples' reproductive future and prepares the prospective parents for intrauterine or postnatal therapy or palliative methods that might be warranted, as well as possible future limitations in the newborn. It also aids in decision-making regarding the termination of pregnancy (in countries where this is permitted by the law), pregnancy management, and the hospital chosen for delivery [64].

The ISUOG [4] recommends that fetal anatomy assessment performed during the second trimester should include evaluation of the following parameters:

(a) Head: integrity of the skull, cavum septum pellucidum, cerebral sickle, thalamus, cerebral ventricles, cerebellum, and the cisterna magna (Fig. 12.14)
(b) Face: orbits, fetal profile, mouth and integrity of the upper lip, and alveolar portion of the palate (Fig. 12.15)
(c) Neck and spine: absence of masses and absence of signs indicating defects of fusion of the spinal elements and masses (axial and sagittal views) (Fig. 12.16)
(d) Heart and thorax: appearance, shape, and size of the thorax and lungs, cardiac activity, position of the heart, the four cardiac chambers, outlets of the right and left ventricles, absence of signs indicating congenital diaphragmatic hernia (Figs. 12.17 and 12.18)

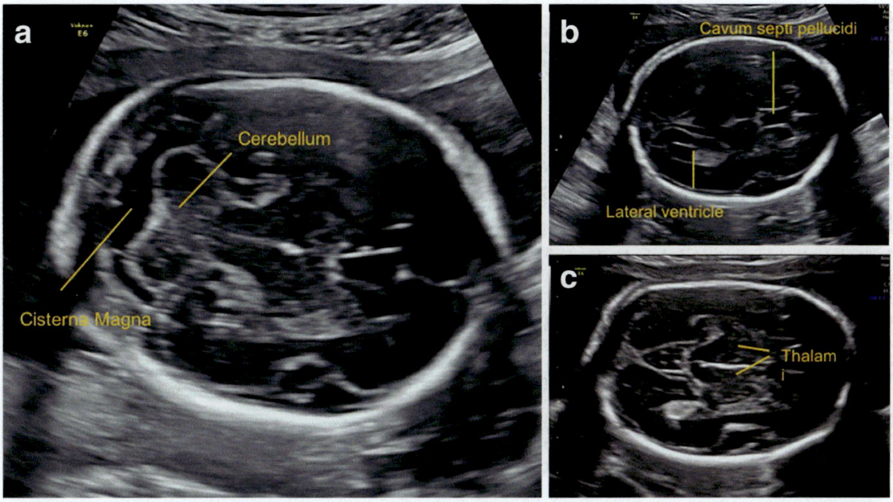

Fig. 12.14 Axial views of the fetal head showing (**a**) transthalamic, (**b**) transventricular, and (**c**) transcerebellar planes

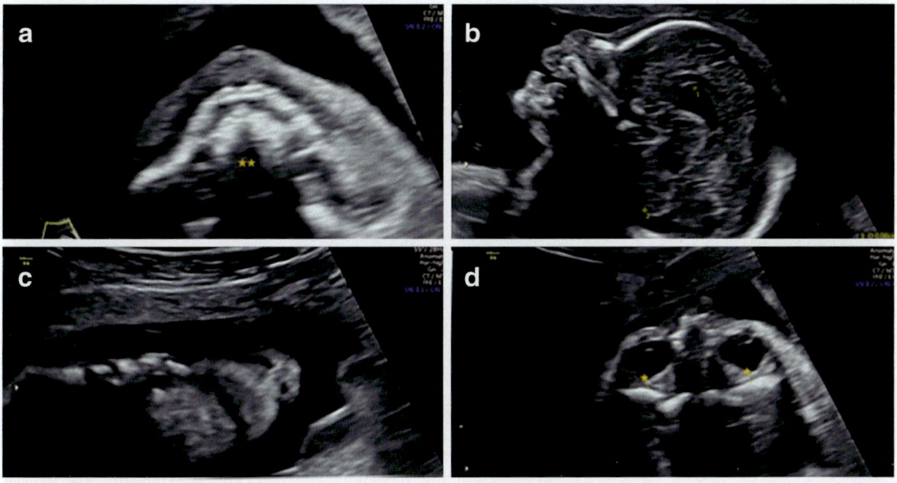

Fig. 12.15 Ultrasound images of the fetal face. (**a**) Alveolar portion of the palate (**); (**b**) fetal profile; (**c**) coronal section showing integrity of the lips; (**d**) orbits (*)

(e) Abdomen: position of the stomach, absence of intestinal dilatation, identification of both kidneys, location, and appearance of the umbilical cord insertion in the integrity of abdominal wall (Fig. 12.19)
(f) Skeleton: presence of arms and hands, relationship between upper and lower limbs and extremities (Fig. 12.20)

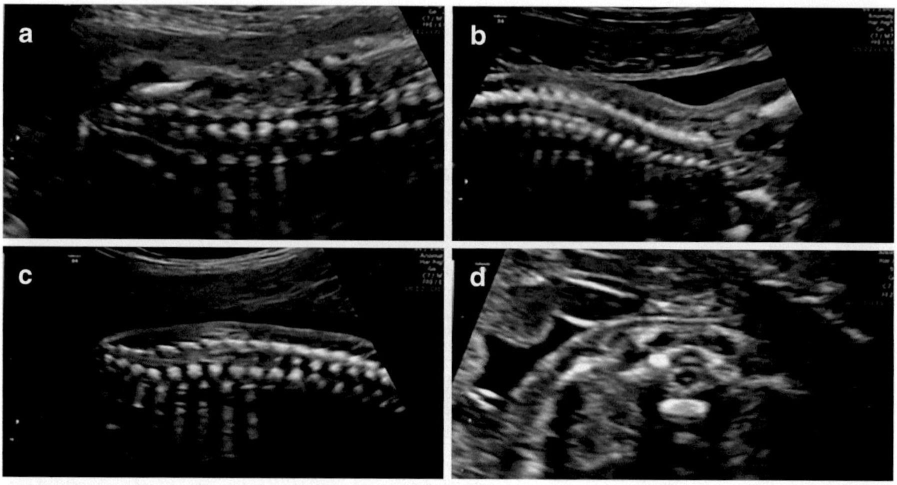

Fig. 12.16 Ultrasound images of the fetal spine. (**a**) Coronal view of the spine; (**b**) sagittal view of the cervical spine, showing absence of cervical masses; (**c**) sagittal view of the lumbar and sacral spine, showing integrity of the vertebral and skin processes; (**d**) axial view of the lumbar spine

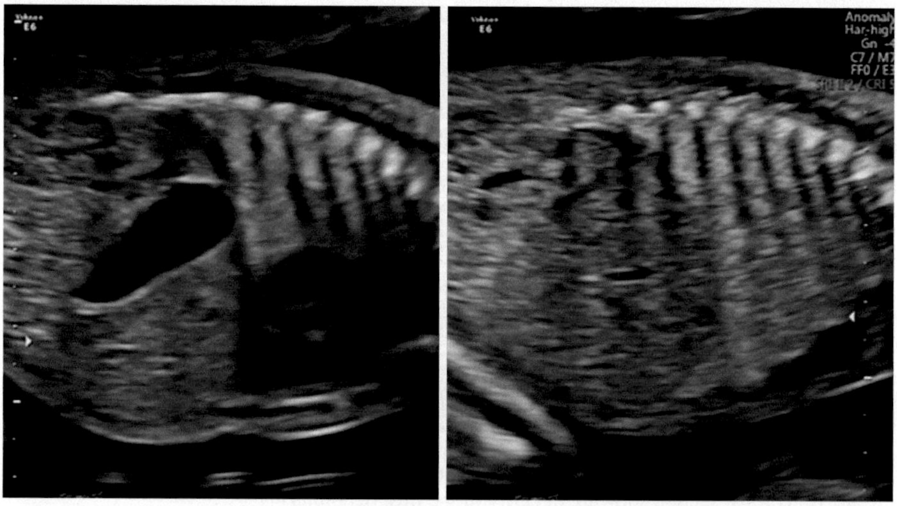

Fig. 12.17 Ultrasound image showing a sagittal view of fetal chest. Observe the integrity of the diaphragm and positioning of the stomach (*) located in the abdomen, just below the diaphragmatic line

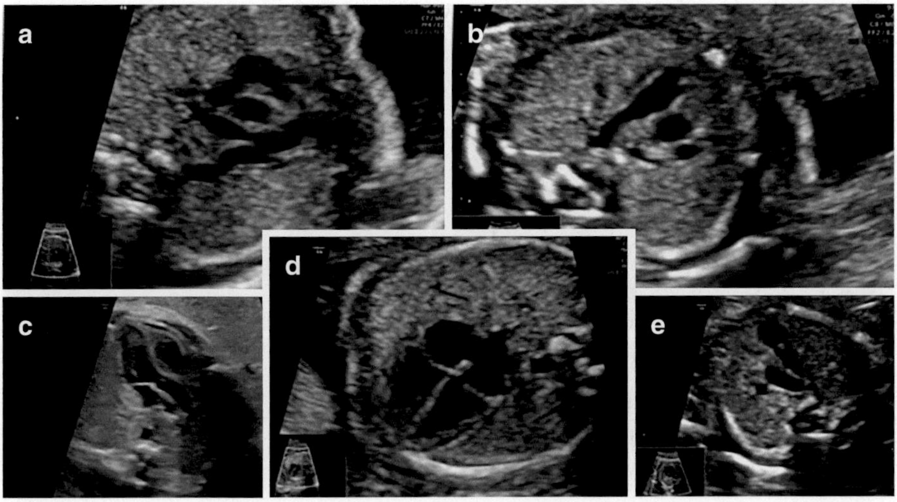

Fig. 12.18 Ultrasound evaluation of the fetal heart. (**a**) Right ventricular outflow tract; (**b**) three-vessel view; (**c**) left ventricular outflow tract; (**d**) four-chamber view; (**d**) threevessel and tracheal view

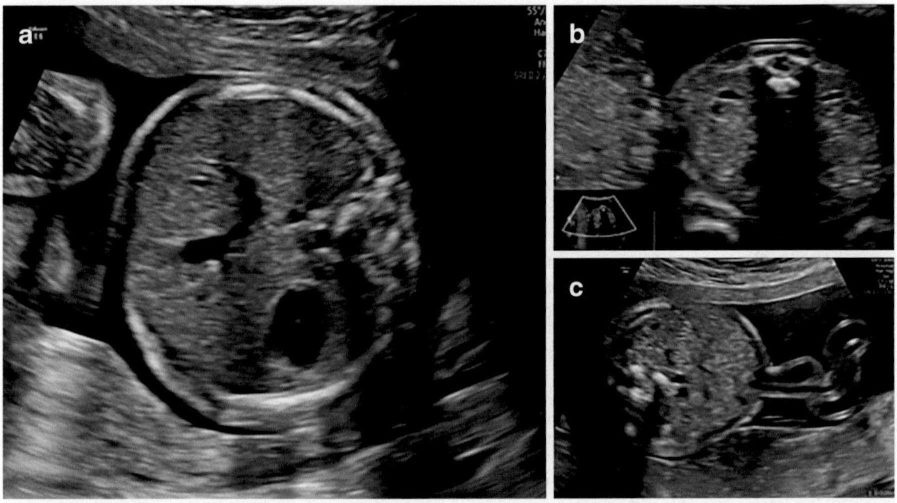

Fig. 12.19 Ultrasound images of the fetal abdomen and abdominal wall. (**a**) Axial view of the abdomen, showing a stomach located to the left of the fetus; (**b**) axial view of the abdomen showing the presence of the two kidneys located laterally to the fetal spine; (**c**) axial view of the abdomen at the level of the insertion of the umbilical cord into the abdominal wall

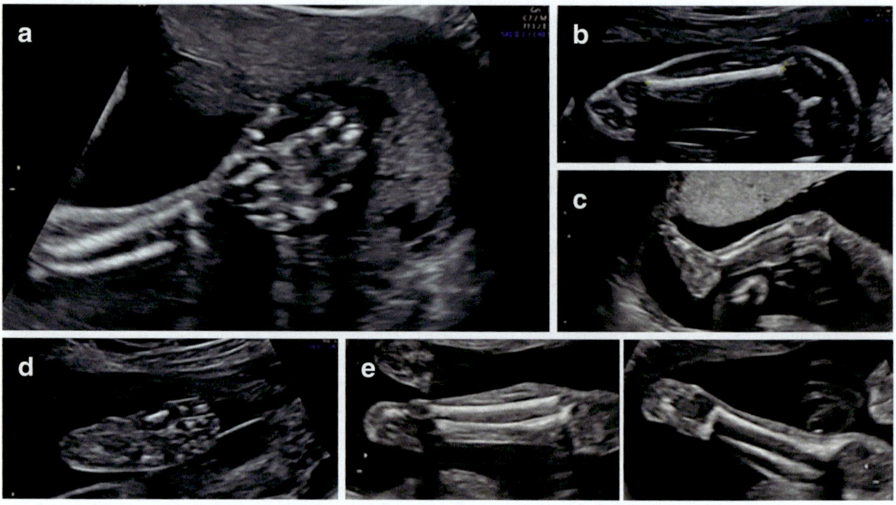

Fig. 12.20 Ultrasound images of the fetal upper and lower limbsFetal upper and lower limbs. (**a**) Hand, radio, and ulna; (**b**) femur; (**c**) sagittal view showing normal alignment between leg and foot; (**d**) coronal view of the foot print (**e**) coronal view of the right and left leg showing tibia and fibula

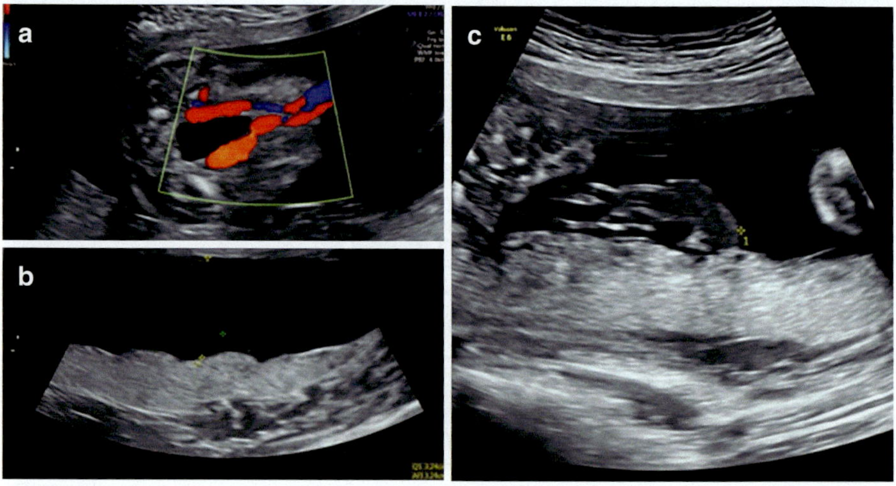

Fig. 12.21 (**a**) Ultrasound image of the fetal umbilical cord atbladder level using color Doppler; (**b**) measurement of the amniotic fluid volume; (**c**) umbilical cord at level of placenta insertion

(g) Placenta and amniotic fluid: quantification of amniotic fluid, placental position, absence of placental masses, placental invasion into the myometrium, umbilical cord insertion into the placenta, and presence of placental accessory lobes (Fig. 12.21)
(h) Umbilical cord: number of umbilical cord vessels (Fig. 12.21)
(i) External genitalia: evidence indicating the sex (male or female) (Fig. 12.22)

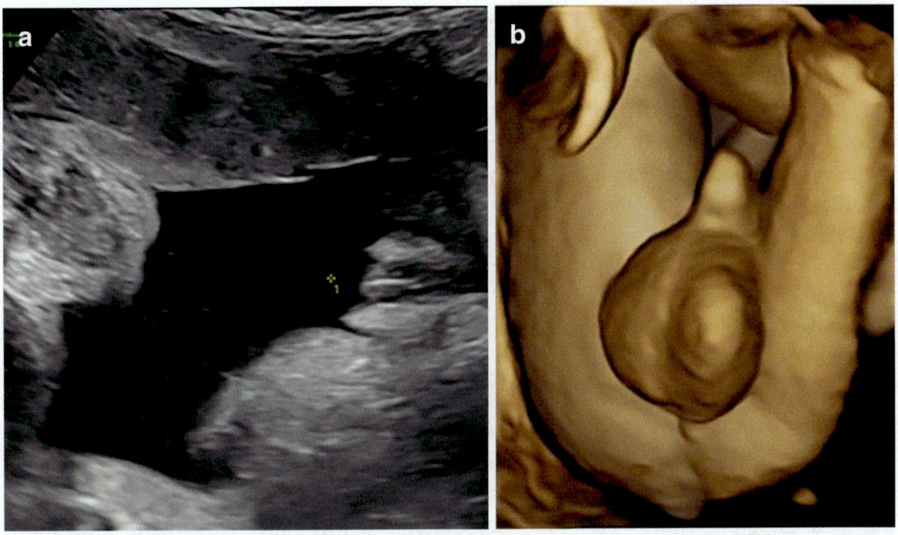

Fig. 12.22 Ultrasound image of the fetal external genitalia. (**a**) Two-dimensional image showing female external genitalia; (**b**) three-dimensional image in the rendering mode showing the male external genitalia

Assessment of Fetal Growth

As previously described in this chapter, accurate calculation of the gestational age is essential for appropriate evaluation of fetal growth.

Fetal growth evaluation should be based on CRL measurement before 14 weeks of gestation. After 14 weeks of gestation, the following measurements are used for fetal growth evaluation: BPD, HC, abdominal circumference (AC), and femur length (FL) [4, 6, 7].

Fetal biometry can be performed through the abdominal or transvaginal route. It is important to magnify the images and correctly identify the reference points for all measurements, in addition to correct placement and position of the calipers to reduce variability between measurements [4, 6]. Measurements of HC and AC can be performed using the ellipse tool or the two-diameter method with an out-out positioning of calipers [65].

Standardized measurements (based on strict quality criteria) are necessary to ensure accurate fetal biometry.

Biparietal Diameter

The biparietal diameter (BPD) is the maximum diameter of a cross-section of the fetal skull measured at the level of the parietal bones. According to ISUOG guidelines, the BPD can be measured in the thalamic plane [4] or in a transventricular plane. The advantage of using the transventricular plane to measure HC is that all three measurements (BPD, HC, and assessment of the ventricular atrium) can be performed using the same section. Calipers should be placed on the widest part of the skull perpendicular to the midline echo. Caliper positioning techniques include an outer-to-outer edge or outer-to-inner edge placement. The appropriate reference table must be used based on the technique used, for accurate interpretation of measurements [58].

Head Circumference

HC is measured in the same plane as that used for BPD measurement. Depending on the ultrasonography device and the operator's experience, HC can be measured by placing an ellipse tool directly around the outside of the skull bone or by measuring the BPD and occipitofrontal diameter (OFD). The calipers should be placed in the off-off position. HC is calculated using the following formula: $HC = 1.62 \times (BPD + OFD)$ [4].

Abdominal Circumference

The following reference points are used to obtain an appropriate plane for AC measurement: cross-section of the fetal abdomen (the cross-sectional area should be as circular as possible), the umbilical vein at the level of the portal sinus, and the visualized stomach bubble and the kidneys should not be visible.

Calipers should be positioned on the outer surface of the skin in the form of an ellipse or a two-diameter method should be used. The anteroposterior diameter of the abdomen (APAD) is measured from the skin covering the spine to the anterior abdominal wall. The transverse abdominal diameter (TAD) is perpendicular to the APAD, at the part corresponding to the widest AC. Measurement of both diameters requires the off-off positioning of calipers. AC is calculated using dedicated software or by applying the following formula: $AC = 1.57 \times (APAD + TAD)$ [4].

Femur Length

To measure the FL, an insonation angle of $<30°$ must be maintained in the horizontal plane with adequate visualization of both ends of the diaphysis, as well as visualization of the soft tissue in addition to the two extremities of the femur (Fig. 12.23).

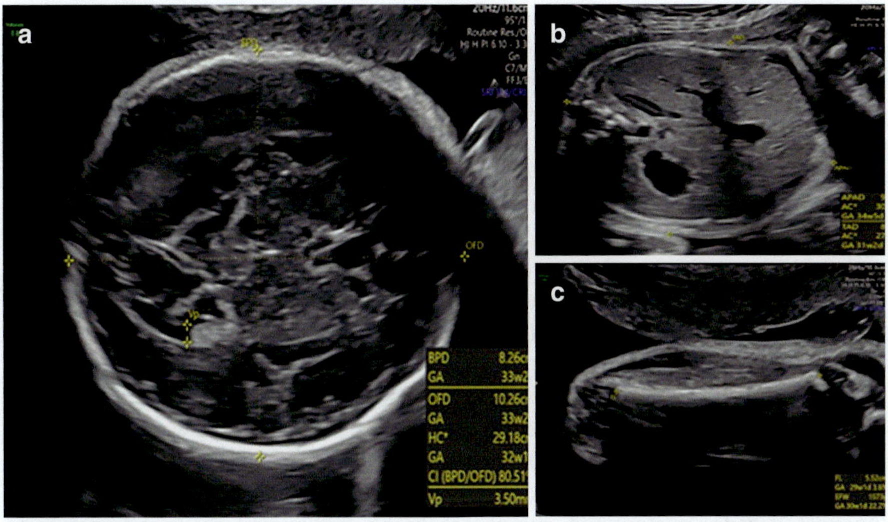

Fig. 12.23 Standard fetal biometry: ultrasound measurements of biparietal diameter (BPD) and head circumference (HC) (**a**), abdominal circumference (AC) (**b**), and femur length (FL) (**c**). In this example, the calipers are placed on the outer edges of the skull to measure BPD (**a**)

Estimated Fetal Weight

The estimated fetal weight (EFW) is calculated using mathematical formulas that incorporate BPD, HC, AC, and FL measurements as variables. The Hadlock formula utilizes these aforementioned parameters and is the commonest and most reliable method to calculate the EFW [66].

Although the EFW assists in monitoring fetal growth, this parameter is associated with an error that could be as high as 10–15% [67]. This margin of error can be attributed to the fact that the parameters used in this formula are multiplied in the equations and also to intra- and interobserver variability in measurements [68]. The margin of error is higher in small-for-gestational-age (SGA) and large-for-gestational-age fetuses. Technical difficulties in assessing even a single biometric parameter can also interfere with accurate calculation of the EFW. Most formulas used to calculate the EFW utilize AC measurement as a variable; AC measurement is often associated with technical difficulties [6].

Fetal Growth Assessment

Fetal growth is a dynamic process, and serial measurements are necessary at regular 2–3 week intervals to confirm normal and abnormal patterns. Normal fetal growth is defined by BDP, HC, AC, FL, and EFW measurements to confirm that these remain within normal limits for gestational age, based on reference charts [68–70]. Various references curves describing different percentiles for the same measurement are available for the estimation of fetal biometric parameters; these differences are attributable to diverse methodological approaches used in generating these curves [71–73]. Previous studies have reported retrospectively generated reference curves that describe the distribution of fetal biometric parameter measurement in a given population over a specific time period [66, 74, 75]. In contrast, other studies have reported prospectively generated fetal growth curves that describe fetal growth under ideal conditions. Prospective curves provide reference intervals that are expected for healthy pregnant women [67]. Furthermore, such reference curves facilitate continued assessment of growth during intrauterine and postnatal life [6].

Maternal characteristics, such as maternal weight at the first prenatal consultation, height, parity, ethnicity, as well as fetal characteristics including birth weight of previous newborns and fetal sex, affect fetal growth and birth weight. However, population-based growth curves do not consider these variables. Customized curves are used to adjust the ideal EFW considering the aforementioned factors [76]. Over the past decade, customized curves are being recognized as an alternative to population-based reference curves [77–80].

Clinicians must be aware that biometric measurements below or above the limits of normality do not always indicate fetal impairment. Using population-based reference curves, it has been observed that approximately 50% of fetuses with birth weight less than the 10th percentile for gestational age are constitutionally small but are categorized as normal. Gardosi et al. [76] reported that based on customized growth curves, the incidence of SGA fetuses is reportedly low, and this method doubles the detection of FGR by 20–50%. Identification of pregnancies complicated by FGR enables appropriate and timely intervention and improves perinatal outcomes, particularly by reducing the rates of stillbirths. The same principle is applicable to macrosomia in cases in which the fetus shows above-normal growth capacity, and the EFW is greater than the 90th percentile for gestational age based on the personalized growth curve.

The use of customized curves is relevant in areas comprising a diverse population with regard to height, parity, and/or ethnicity. Customized curves can more effectively identify fetuses at risk of perinatal complications such as FGR. In contrast, a recent prospective study reported no benefit associated with a personalized approach to population graphics [81].

Serial longitudinal ultrasonographic examinations can assess fetal growth. Serial examinations enable evaluation of the fetal growth rate by modifying the weight percentile or the Z-score [82]. Some studies have reported that reduced growth velocity during the third trimester is associated with an increased risk of adverse perinatal outcomes [81, 83, 84]. Caradeux et al. [85] prospectively investigated 2696 women with low-risk pregnancies and reported that compared with cross-sectional assessment, the longitudinal assessment of fetal growth from the second to the third trimester showed low predictive capacity for SGA and late-onset FGR; these results were in contrast to those reported by prior studies. Another recent prospective study investigated whether assessing growth velocity in combination with

Doppler evaluation improves the rate of prediction of adverse perinatal outcomes in fetuses with suspected SGA. These authors observed that the longitudinal evaluation of fetal growth did not independently predict adverse perinatal outcomes when used in combination with Doppler evaluation in fetuses with suspected SGA. Therefore, currently, the role of growth velocity as a predictor of adverse perinatal outcomes in fetuses weighing less than the 10th percentile for gestational age remains unclear.

Conclusion

Currently, obstetric ultrasonography is an important component of the best practices followed in maternal-fetal medicine. In addition to assessing pregnancy viability, the first-trimester examination assists with the management of patients with abnormalities. Chorionicity determination and interpretation of the lambda and T signals are important to schedule prenatal monitoring in women with twin pregnancies. Ultrasonography provides high spatial resolution, and the greater details provided by ultrasonographic images enable early diagnosis of fetal anomalies and subsequent optimization of management of fetal malformations during pregnancy and in the neonatal period. The correct application of fetal biometry is important for the management of fetal growth and to identify growth deviations throughout pregnancy.

References

1. Salomon LJ, Alfirevic Z, Bilardo CM, Chalouhi GE, Ghi T, Kagan KO, et al. ISUOG practice guidelines: performance of first-trimester fetal ultrasound scan. Ultrasound Obstet Gynecol. 2013;41(1):102–13.
2. Nicolaides KH. Turning the pyramid of prenatal care. Fetal Diagn Ther. 2011;29(3):183–96.
3. Sotiriadis A, Hernandez-Andrade E, da Silva CF, Ghi T, Glanc P, Khalil A, et al. ISUOG practice guidelines: role of ultrasound in screening for and follow-up of pre-eclampsia. Ultrasound Obstet Gynecol. 2019;53(1):7–22.
4. Salomon LJ, Alfirevic Z, Berghella V, Bilardo C, Hernandez-Andrade E, Johnsen SL, et al. Practice guidelines for performance of the routine mid-trimester fetal ultrasound scan. Ultrasound Obstet Gynecol. 2011;37(1):116–26.
5. Figo Working Group On Best Practice In Maternal-Fetal Medicine, International Federation of Gynecology and Obstetrics. Best practice in maternal-fetal medicine. Int J Gynaecol Obstet. 2015;128(1):80–2.
6. Salomon LJ, Alfirevic Z, da Silva CF, Deter RL, Figueras F, Ghi T, et al. ISUOG practice guidelines: ultrasound assessment of fetal biometry and growth. Ultrasound Obstet Gynecol. 2019;53(6):715–23.
7. Salomon LJ, Alfirevic Z, Bilardo CM, Chalouhi GE, Ghi T, Kagan KO, et al. ISUOG practice guidelines: performance of first-trimester fetal ultrasound scan. Ultrasound Obstet Gynecol. 2013;41(1):102–13.
8. Whitworth M, Bricker L, Neilson JP, Dowswell T. Ultrasound for fetal assessment in early pregnancy. Cochrane Database Syst Rev. 2010;(4):CD007058.

9. Pandya PP, Snijders RJ, Psara N, Hilbert L, Nicolaides KH. The prevalence of non-viable pregnancy at 10–13 weeks of gestation. Ultrasound Obstet Gynecol. 1996;7(3):170–3.
10. Doubilet PM, Benson CB, Bourne T, Blaivas M, Barnhart KT, Benacerraf BR, et al. Diagnostic criteria for nonviable pregnancy early in the first trimester. N Engl J Med. 2013;369(15):1443–51.
11. Barnhart KT. Early pregnancy failure: beware of the pitfalls of modern management. Fertil Steril. 2012;98(5):1061–5.
12. Bree RL, Edwards M, Böhm-Vélez M, Beyler S, Roberts J, Mendelson EB. Transvaginal sonography in the evaluation of normal early pregnancy: correlation with HCG level. AJR Am J Roentgenol. 1989;153(1):75–9.
13. Bateman BG, Nunley WC, Kolp LA, Kitchin JD, Felder R. Vaginal sonography findings and hCG dynamics of early intrauterine and tubal pregnancies. Obstet Gynecol. 1990;75(3 Pt 1):421–7.
14. Goldstein I, Zimmer EA, Tamir A, Peretz BA, Paldi E. Evaluation of normal gestational sac growth: appearance of embryonic heartbeat and embryo body movements using the transvaginal technique. Obstet Gynecol. 1991;77(6):885–8.
15. Bottomley C, Bourne T. Dating and growth in the first trimester. Best Pract Res Clin Obstet Gynaecol. 2009;23(4):439–52.
16. Bottomley C, Van Belle V, Mukri F, Kirk E, Van Huffel S, Timmerman D, et al. The optimal timing of an ultrasound scan to assess the location and viability of an early pregnancy. Hum Reprod. 2009;24(8):1811–7.
17. Goldstein SR. Significance of cardiac activity on endovaginal ultrasound in very early embryos. Obstet Gynecol. 1992;80(4):670–2.
18. Brown DL, Emerson DS, Felker RE, Cartier MS, Smith WC. Diagnosis of early embryonic demise by endovaginal sonography. J Ultrasound Med. 1990;9(11):631–6.
19. Abdallah Y, Daemen A, Kirk E, Pexsters A, Naji O, Stalder C, et al. Limitations of current definitions of miscarriage using mean gestational sac diameter and crown-rump length measurements: a multicenter observational study. Ultrasound Obstet Gynecol. 2011;38(5):497–502.
20. Centers for Disease Control and Prevention (CDC), Ectopic pregnancy-United States, 1990–1992. MMWR Morb Mortal Wkly Rep. 1995;44(3):46–8.
21. Scibetta EW, Han CS. Ultrasound in early pregnancy: viability, unknown locations, and ectopic pregnancies. Obstet Gynecol Clin North Am. 2019;46(4):783–95.
22. Pereira PP, Cabar FR, Gomez Ú, Francisco RPV. Pregnancy of unknown location. Clinics (Sao Paulo). 2019;74:e1111.
23. Kirk E, Bottomley C, Bourne T. Diagnosing ectopic pregnancy and current concepts in the management of pregnancy of unknown location. Hum Reprod Update. 2014;20(2):250–61.
24. Reid S, Condous G. Is there a need to definitively diagnose the location of a pregnancy of unknown location? The case for "no". Fertil Steril. 2012;98(5):1085–90.
25. Barnhart K, van Mello NM, Bourne T, Kirk E, Van Calster B, Bottomley C, et al. Pregnancy of unknown location: a consensus statement of nomenclature, definitions, and outcome. Fertil Steril. 2011;95(3):857–66.
26. Condous G, Van Calster B, Kirk E, Haider Z, Timmerman D, Van Huffel S, et al. Clinical information does not improve the performance of mathematical models in predicting the outcome of pregnancies of unknown location. Fertil Steril. 2007;88(3):572–80.
27. Condous G, Van Calster B, Kirk E, Haider Z, Timmerman D, Van Huffel S, et al. Prediction of ectopic pregnancy in women with a pregnancy of unknown location. Ultrasound Obstet Gynecol. 2007;29(6):680–7.
28. Kirk E, Condous G, Van Calster B, Van Huffel S, Timmerman D, Bourne T. Rationalizing the follow-up of pregnancies of unknown location. Hum Reprod. 2007;22(6):1744–50.
29. Barnhart KT. Clinical practice. Ectopic pregnancy. N Engl J Med. 2009;361(4):379–87.
30. Barnhart KT, Guo W, Cary MS, Morse CB, Chung K, Takacs P, et al. Differences in serum human chorionic gonadotropin rise in early pregnancy by race and value at presentation. Obstet Gynecol. 2016;128(3):504–11.

31. Seeber BE, Barnhart KT. Suspected ectopic pregnancy. Obstet Gynecol. 2006;107(2 Pt 1):399–413.
32. Mol BW, van der Veen F, Bossuyt PM. Symptom-free women at increased risk of ectopic pregnancy: should we screen? Acta Obstet Gynecol Scand. 2002;81(7):661–72.
33. Mausner Geffen E, Slywotzky C, Bennett G. Pitfalls and tips in the diagnosis of ectopic pregnancy. Abdom Radiol (NY). 2017;42(5):1524–42.
34. Ko JK, Cheung VY. Time to revisit the human chorionic gonadotropin discriminatory level in the management of pregnancy of unknown location. J Ultrasound Med. 2014;33(3):465–71.
35. Doubilet PM, Benson CB. Further evidence against the reliability of the human chorionic gonadotropin discriminatory level. J Ultrasound Med. 2011;30(12):1637–42.
36. Mehta TS, Levine D, Beckwith B. Treatment of ectopic pregnancy: is a human chorionic gonadotropin level of 2,000 mIU/mL a reasonable threshold? Radiology. 1997;205(2):569–73.
37. Connolly A, Ryan DH, Stuebe AM, Wolfe HM. Reevaluation of discriminatory and threshold levels for serum β-hCG in early pregnancy. Obstet Gynecol. 2013;121(1):65–70.
38. Bignardi T, Condous G, Alhamdan D, Kirk E, Van Calster B, Van Huffel S, et al. The hCG ratio can predict the ultimate viability of the intrauterine pregnancies of uncertain viability in the pregnancy of unknown location population. Hum Reprod. 2008;23(9):1964–7.
39. van Mello NM, Mol F, Verhoeve HR, van Wely M, Adriaanse AH, Boss EA, et al. Methotrexate or expectant management in women with an ectopic pregnancy or pregnancy of unknown location and low serum hCG concentrations? A randomized comparison. Hum Reprod. 2013;28(1):60–7.
40. Cordina M, Schramm-Gajraj K, Ross JA, Lautman K, Jurkovic D. Introduction of a single visit protocol in the management of selected patients with pregnancy of unknown location: a prospective study. BJOG. 2011;118(6):693–7.
41. Oh JS, Wright G, Coulam CB. Gestational sac diameter in very early pregnancy as a predictor of fetal outcome. Ultrasound Obstet Gynecol. 2002;20(3):267–9.
42. Committee on Obstetric Practice, the American Institute of Ultrasound in Medicine, the Society for Maternal-Fetal Medicine. Committee Opinion No 700: methods for estimating the due date. Obstet Gynecol. 2017;129(5):e150–e4.
43. Loughna P, Chitty L, Evans T, Chudleigh T. Fetal size and dating: charts recommended for clinical obstetric practice. Ultrasound. 2009;17:161–7.
44. Platt LD. First-trimester risk assessment: twin gestations. Semin Perinatol. 2005;29(4):258–62.
45. Khalil A, Rodgers M, Baschat A, Bhide A, Gratacos E, Hecher K, et al. ISUOG practice guidelines: role of ultrasound in twin pregnancy. Ultrasound Obstet Gynecol. 2016;47(2):247–63.
46. Sebire NJ, D'Ercole C, Hughes K, Carvalho M, Nicolaides KH. Increased nuchal translucency thickness at 10–14 weeks of gestation as a predictor of severe twin-to-twin transfusion syndrome. Ultrasound Obstet Gynecol. 1997;10(2):86–9.
47. Sebire NJ, Snijders RJ, Hughes K, Sepulveda W, Nicolaides KH. The hidden mortality of monochorionic twin pregnancies. Br J Obstet Gynaecol. 1997;104(10):1203–7.
48. Napolitano R, Thilaganathan B. Late termination of pregnancy and foetal reduction for foetal anomaly. Best Pract Res Clin Obstet Gynaecol. 2010;24(4):529–37.
49. Dias T, Arcangeli T, Bhide A, Napolitano R, Mahsud-Dornan S, Thilaganathan B. First-trimester ultrasound determination of chorionicity in twin pregnancy. Ultrasound Obstet Gynecol. 2011;38(5):530–2.
50. Bracero LA, Byrne DW. Ultrasound determination of chorionicity and perinatal outcome in twin pregnancies using dividing membrane thickness. Gynecol Obstet Invest. 2003;55(1):50–7.
51. Carvalho MH, Brizot ML, Lopes LM, Chiba CH, Miyadahira S, Zugaib M. Detection of fetal structural abnormalities at the 11–14 week ultrasound scan. Prenat Diagn. 2002;22(1):1–4.
52. Syngelaki A, Chelemen T, Dagklis T, Allan L, Nicolaides KH. Challenges in the diagnosis of fetal non-chromosomal abnormalities at 11–13 weeks. Prenat Diagn. 2011;31(1):90–102.
53. Kenkhuis MJA, Bakker M, Bardi F, Fontanella F, Bakker MK, Fleurke-Rozema JH, et al. Effectiveness of 12–13-week scan for early diagnosis of fetal congenital anomalies in the cell-free DNA era. Ultrasound Obstet Gynecol. 2018;51(4):463–9.

54. Dulgheroff FF, Peixoto AB, Petrini CG, Caldas TMRD, Ramos DR, Magalhães FO, et al. Fetal structural anomalies diagnosed during the first, second and third trimesters of pregnancy using ultrasonography: a retrospective cohort study. Sao Paulo Med J. 2019;137(5):391–400.
55. Ebrashy A, El Kateb A, Momtaz M, El Sheikhah A, Aboulghar MM, Ibrahim M, et al. 13–14-week fetal anatomy scan: a 5-year prospective study. Ultrasound Obstet Gynecol. 2010;35(3):292–6.
56. Chen M, Lee CP, Lam YH, Tang RY, Chan BC, Wong SF, et al. Comparison of nuchal and detailed morphology ultrasound examinations in early pregnancy for fetal structural abnormality screening: a randomized controlled trial. Ultrasound Obstet Gynecol. 2008;31(2):136–46.
57. Napolitano R, Papageorghiou AT. First-trimester detection of fetal anomalies. In: Coady AM, Bower S, editors. Twining's textbook of fetal abnormalities. Edinburgh: Churchill Livingstone; 2015. p. 1–30.
58. To M, Pereira S. Routine fetal anomaly scan. In: Coady AM, Bower S, editors. Twining's textbook of fetal abnormalities. Edinburgh: Churchill Livingstone; 2015. p. 60–80.
59. Sallout B, Obedat N, Shakeel F, Mansoor A, Walker M, Al-Badr A. Prevalence of major congenital anomalies at King Fahad Medical City in Saudi Arabia: a tertiary care centre-based study. Ann Saudi Med. 2015;35(5):343–51.
60. Parker SE, Mai CT, Canfield MA, Rickard R, Wang Y, Meyer RE, et al. Updated National Birth Prevalence estimates for selected birth defects in the United States, 2004–2006. Birth Defects Res A Clin Mol Teratol. 2010;88(12):1008–16.
61. Dolk H, Loane M, Garne E. The prevalence of congenital anomalies in Europe. Adv Exp Med Biol. 2010;686:349–64.
62. Bricker L, Garcia J, Henderson J, Mugford M, Neilson J, Roberts T, et al. Ultrasound screening in pregnancy: a systematic review of the clinical effectiveness, cost-effectiveness and women's views. Health Technol Assess. 2000;4(16):i–vi, 1–193.
63. Kalter H. Five-decade international trends in the relation of perinatal mortality and congenital malformations: stillbirth and neonatal death compared. Int J Epidemiol. 1991;20(1):173–9.
64. Sanapo L, Moon-Grady AJ, Donofrio MT. Perinatal and delivery management of infants with congenital heart disease. Clin Perinatol. 2016;43(1):55–71.
65. Napolitano R, Donadono V, Ohuma EO, Knight CL, Wanyonyi SZ, Kemp B, et al. Scientific basis for standardization of fetal head measurements by ultrasound: a reproducibility study. Ultrasound Obstet Gynecol. 2016;48(1):80–5.
66. Hadlock FP, Harrist RB, Sharman RS, Deter RL, Park SK. Estimation of fetal weight with the use of head, body, and femur measurements--a prospective study. Am J Obstet Gynecol. 1985;151(3):333–7.
67. Papageorghiou AT, Ohuma EO, Altman DG, Todros T, Cheikh Ismail L, Lambert A, et al. International standards for fetal growth based on serial ultrasound measurements: the Fetal Growth Longitudinal Study of the INTERGROWTH-21st project. Lancet. 2014;384(9946):869–79.
68. Dudley NJ. A systematic review of the ultrasound estimation of fetal weight. Ultrasound Obstet Gynecol. 2005;25(1):80–9.
69. Mongelli M, Ek S, Tambyrajia R. Screening for fetal growth restriction: a mathematical model of the effect of time interval and ultrasound error. Obstet Gynecol. 1998;92(6):908–12.
70. Johnsen SL, Rasmussen S, Wilsgaard T, Sollien R, Kiserud T. Longitudinal reference ranges for estimated fetal weight. Acta Obstet Gynecol Scand. 2006;85(3):286–97.
71. Napolitano R, Dhami J, Ohuma EO, Ioannou C, Conde-Agudelo A, Kennedy SH, et al. Pregnancy dating by fetal crown-rump length: a systematic review of charts. BJOG. 2014;121(5):556–65.
72. Ioannou C, Talbot K, Ohuma E, Sarris I, Villar J, Conde-Agudelo A, et al. Systematic review of methodology used in ultrasound studies aimed at creating charts of fetal size. BJOG. 2012;119(12):1425–39.
73. Nicolaides KH, Wright D, Syngelaki A, Wright A, Akolekar R. Fetal Medicine Foundation fetal and neonatal population weight charts. Ultrasound Obstet Gynecol. 2018;52(1):44–51.

74. Peixoto AB, da Cunha Caldas TMR, Dulgheroff FF, Martins WP, Araujo JE. Fetal biometric parameters: reference charts for a non-selected risk population from Uberaba, Brazil. J Ultrason. 2017;17(68):23–9.
75. Araujo Júnior E, Martins Santana EF, Martins WP, Júnior JE, Ruano R, Pires CR, et al. Reference charts of fetal biometric parameters in 31,476 Brazilian singleton pregnancies. J Ultrasound Med. 2014;33(7):1185–91.
76. Gardosi J, Chang A, Kalyan B, Sahota D, Symonds EM. Customised antenatal growth charts. Lancet. 1992;339(8788):283–7.
77. Gardosi J, Francis A. Adverse pregnancy outcome and association with small for gestational age birthweight by customized and population-based percentiles. Am J Obstet Gynecol. 2009;201(1):28.e1–8.
78. Kiserud T, Johnsen SL. Biometric assessment. Best Pract Res Clin Obstet Gynaecol. 2009;23(6):819–31.
79. Buck Louis GM, Grewal J, Albert PS, Sciscione A, Wing DA, Grobman WA, et al. Racial/ethnic standards for fetal growth: the NICHD Fetal Growth Studies. Am J Obstet Gynecol. 2015;213(4):449.e1–e41.
80. Chiossi G, Pedroza C, Costantine MM, Truong VTT, Gargano G, Saade GR. Customized vs population-based growth charts to identify neonates at risk of adverse outcome: systematic review and Bayesian meta-analysis of observational studies. Ultrasound Obstet Gynecol. 2017;50(2):156–66.
81. Sovio U, White IR, Dacey A, Pasupathy D, Smith GCS. Screening for fetal growth restriction with universal third trimester ultrasonography in nulliparous women in the Pregnancy Outcome Prediction (POP) study: a prospective cohort study. Lancet. 2015;386(10008):2089–97.
82. Royston P, Altman DG. Design and analysis of longitudinal studies of fetal size. Ultrasound Obstet Gynecol. 1995;6(5):307–12.
83. Owen P, Donnet ML, Ogston SA, Christie AD, Howie PW, Patel NB. Standards for ultrasound fetal growth velocity. Br J Obstet Gynaecol. 1996;103(1):60–9.
84. MacDonald TM, Hui L, Tong S, Robinson AJ, Dane KM, Middleton AL, et al. Reduced growth velocity across the third trimester is associated with placental insufficiency in fetuses born at a normal birthweight: a prospective cohort study. BMC Med. 2017;15(1):164.
85. Caradeux J, Eixarch E, Mazarico E, Basuki TR, Gratacós E, Figueras F. Second- to third-trimester longitudinal growth assessment for prediction of small-for-gestational age and late fetal growth restriction. Ultrasound Obstet Gynecol. 2018;51(2):219–24.

Chapter 13
Clinical Use of 3D Sonography

Asim Kurjak and Lara Spalldi Barišić

Background

Our growing understanding of detailed embryology, prenatal physiologic and pathologic changes, detailed fetal structural and functional development are all made possible by extraordinary medical innovations and diagnostic technology. Ultrasonography is definitely one of them. **Nowadays, perinatal medicine would be unthinkable without sonography**.

During embryonic, fetal, and neonatal period, ultrasonography is the imaging modality of choice for many reasons: it is safe and has no ionizing radiation, it is fast and non-invasive, it is an operator-friendly diagnostic tool that has a potential of dynamic display of images of targeted regions, it is cost-efficient and has exceptional quality of acquired information [1, 2].

State-of-the-art medicine requires cutting-edge technology such as three-dimensional ultrasound (3D US) and dedicated, skilled physicians who embrace and implement innovations in order to improve the quality of patients' life. Generally, the idea is to find the fine balance between the benefits and limitations of the diagnostic possibilities and address ethical issues that can arise [2].

The fundamental goal of any fetal ultrasound examination is to obtain the most reliable diagnostic information that will aid in the optimization of prenatal care and in the achievement of best outcomes for both mother and fetus [2]. Fetal ultrasound examination usually begins with two-dimensional (2D) ultrasound (as the gold standard) and can be supplemented by 3D or four-dimensional

A. Kurjak
Sarajevo School of Science and Technology, Sarajevo, Bosnia and Herzegovina

Department of Obstetrics and Gynecology, School of Medicine, University of Zagreb, Zagreb, Croatia

L. Spalldi Barišić (✉)
Fetal and Maternal Medicine, Private Clinic Veritas, Zagreb, Croatia

© Springer Nature Switzerland AG 2022

R. A. Moreira de Sá, E. B. d. Fonseca (eds.), *Perinatology*,
https://doi.org/10.1007/978-3-030-83434-0_13

ultrasound (4D US)-specific imaging modality of choice to enhance the diagnostic accuracy of particular area.

Since the first introduction by Baba and colleagues [3, 4], nearly three decades ago, 3D US underwent revolutionary transformation and became a highly valuable diagnostic tool in perinatal medicine. Evolution in transducers and data processors implemented in ultrasound technology were followed by impressive diagnostic and imaging advances published in many papers [2–18]. All of these was followed globaly and demonstrated by top specialists and experts in the field at the serie of World Congresses of 3D Ultrasound in Obstetrics and Gynaecology started in 1997. in Mainz (Germany), followed in 1999. in Las Vegas (U.S.A) and most recently held in 2019. in Dubrovnik (Croatia).

2D Ultrasound imaging can not be really compared with 3D imaging. Each technique has its own benefits and limitations, and combination of the two empowers the operator to enrich the diagnostic information. Benefits of 3D US are evident in enhanced visualization of the surface and display of targeted structures from various perspectives and in different modes. All the data can be additionally stored and acquired volumes can be improved and rendered for offline analysis. Higher resolution and realistic display in three dimensions made the counseling of the parents much easier. Those advances made the 3D ultrasound technology extremely valuable and popular.

Three-dimensional ultrasound in neonates is mainly used for neurosonography and heart assessment. As reported, 3D US has many benefits as a powerful diagnostic tool, but somehow it is still underutilized in neonatal period, owing partly to restricted availability, challenges with dynamic assessment, as well as missing a dedicated pediatric transducers [19, 20].

Terminology

A wide variety of terms have been used in 3D/4D ultrasound imaging. Here we list some [21].

Cinematic rate at or above 25 Hz (imaging frames or volumes/second, fps or vps); this is because human eye and brain hold the visual perception for approximately 1/25th of second (set as standard cinematic rate) [21, 22].

Real-time 3D imaging 3D ultrasound system is capable of providing an imaging volume at cinematic rate (i.e., at or above 25 Hz or imaging volumes/second, vps) and virtually as they are acquired [21–23].

4D ultrasound imaging is equal to dynamic 3D ultrasound imaging (not necessarily equal to real-time 3D; for more details, see gating necessity) [22, 23].

Frame rate number of 2D images (frames) acquired by cross-sectional imaging per second (time). Measuring unit: frames per second (fps or Hz). Should be preferably used when referring to 2D imaging [21].

Volume rate number of the volumes acquired by 3D/4D system per second (time). Measuring unit: volumes per second (vps or Hz). Should be used when referring to (matrix-array) real-time 3D scanning or reconstructed volume rate by motion-gated 4D imaging/spatiotemporal image correlation (STIC) [21–23].

Matrix-array transducer technology progressed from 256 to 512 elements in the tip of the probe and was run at 2.5–3.5 MHz in the 1990s [21–23], then upgraded to 3600 elements in 2000s [24, 25], then to 6000–8000 elements in 2010s [26], and now has approximately 10,000 elements. For real-time 2D imaging, frame rate can be as high as 150 fps (Hz), but for reconstructed 4D imaging, it is usually 10–40 vps (Hz). Volume rate during real-time 3D scanning can be 20–30 vps (Hz) with reasonable imaging volume size and can be increased up to 60 vps for STIC [21, 22].

Region of interest (ROI) refers to imaging plane size correctly used in 2D scanning [21, 22].

Volume of interest (VOI) refers to imaging volume size correctly used in 3D/4D scanning [21, 22].

Imaging volume size indication of whether or not VOI can include entirety of or just part of VOI.

Online in terms of 3D ultrasond imaging, online indicates that acquired data and processing are done fast (within few seconds or few minutes), in real-time and images are displayed on the same acquisition system where data was acquired, while patient is still there [22].

Offline in terms of 3D imaging, offline indicates that post-processing and displaying images need more time, and this can be done even on separate system where 3D data can be reloaded (like personal computer with, for example, ViewPoint®, GE Healthcare) [22]. This does not require the presence of patient. With offline post-processing, it is possible to reload the data from the system memory and use it for additional measurements, counseling, expert consultation, scientific research, and clinical teaching purposes.

Safety

Prenatal sonography seems to be safe for clinical use. To our knowledge and to date, there has been no independently confirmed research to indicate differently. Fetal exposure to ultrasound should be according to the ALARA principle (As Low as Reasonably Achievable), meaning minimal time and lowest acoustic output power should be used to acquire diagnostic data [27]. Biological effects are being continuously studied and accordingly manufacturers have to comply with the safety regulations [8–12].* Even though there is no evidence of risk, the operator has to ensure optimal usage. Advantages of 3D imaging as well as potential limitations have to be explained to the patient.

3D Transducers

Three-dimensional ultrasound imaging basically consists of three phases: acquisition, reconstruction, and visualization. In order to realize good real-time 3D images for clinical application, with the possibility of different rendering options, it is essential to have high computational power for processing, optimal quality and rate of data acquisition, as well as speed and accuracy of volume reconstruction algorithms [13, 14].

During prenatal period, acquisition of 3D US data can be obtained either with transabdominal or with transvaginal transducers. Transvaginal approach is preferably used for early pregnancies, sonoembryology, fetal neurosonography, and for assessment of cervix and adjacent or low-lying placenta. Transabdominal approach is mainly reserved for fetal assessment in second and third trimesters of pregnancy and in neonatal period. Besides the differences in scanning approach, there are two main types of 3D US probes.

Mechanical 3D transducers: These house convex array transducer that swivels back and forth continuously for fast acquisition of 2D frames needed for reconstruction into 3D volumes. The new-generation transducers produce high-quality, very realistic 3D images almost instantly. Acquisition of volume and necessary reconstruction time is very short which makes it suitable for clinical practice [13].

Matrix-array transducers are completely electronic, designed with several thousands of elements functionally organized on a two-dimensional matrix array that can be activated at the same time to provide real-time 3D images even in the most challenging diagnostic US examination with fast-moving objects such as heart [13, 22]. This technology allows real-time 3D rendering of moving structures with supreme temporal resolution and is progressively used in fetal and neonatal echocardiography. As mentioned earlier, matrix-array transducer requires tremendous computational power that makes it costly and less available compared to mechanical 3D transducers [13, 14, 22].

Acquiring the Volume

Skilled operator is aware of difficulties, strive to avoid all obstacles, and select ideal acoustic window to acquire best quality 3D volumes of targeted area. This is not always easy considering the dynamic of fetal movements and bone shadowing that can interfere with quality of imaging structures due to artifacts [15, 18, 28]. Technological advancements require continued education of the operator with the aim to optimally utilize all diagnostic potentials [29].

High-frequency and high-resolution 3D transvaginal transducers made real difference and revolutionary turn point in first trimester diagnostic imaging [29–47]. Detection of fetal abnormalities with 3D US is widely demonstrated [1, 2, 6, 7, 15, 29–62]. With different 3D US display modes, very detailed and realistic visualization of early embryonic period and during fetal period onward is now reality. Three-dimensional US imaging has several advantages over 2D imaging that will be presented in this chapter.

Clinical Use of 3D Ultrasound and Rendering Options for Detection of Fetal Anomalies

First several weeks of pregnancy are crucial for normal development of rapidly growing embryo. This intriguing and mysterious period of embryonic life is now partly revealed due to amazing technological advances in ultrasound systems. Stunning ultrasound images can leave no one indifferent, neither physician nor parents. Three-dimensional US imaging opens up countless diagnostic options.

With different 3D US display modes, real-time, detailed, vivid, and almost photographic visualization of embryonic and fetal life has now become a reality.

Sonoembryology is the term introduced in 1990s by Timor-Trish et al. [50], referring to an organ-oriented approach of studying embryonic development and morphological characteristics compared to Carnegie embryonic stages (numbered 1–23), only this time in vivo by using ultrasound with high-frequency transvaginal probe [60]. Embryonic period lasts from fertilization until the full 8 weeks. Sonographically, we count embryonic and fetal life according to the date of last menstrual period (LMP) which starts two weeks before the conception. So strictly, sonoembryologic timeline is from the second to the tenth (2nd-10th) week according to the LMP. Many authors published their data on 2D and 3D sonoembryology [50–63].

Since that time (1990s), ultrasound systems and transducers became more advanced and 3D technology brought a new additional dimension in sonoembryology (Fig. 13.1), such as vivid images of embryos in (near) real-time scanning, including embrional movements and display of blood circulation. The timeline of brain and any other organ development could be obtained to provide reference images that can be compared for possible developmental anomalies [51, 52, 54–57, 59–63]. In the recent publication by Kim*, an ultrasonographic evaluation of embryonic cardiac development was presented [60]. Pooh introduced a new field called fetal sono-ophthalmology studied by 3D HDlive Silhouette and flow ultrasound [55, 62].

Main benefits are achieved in the multiplanar mode. Simultaneous projection of all three perpendicular sectional planes called A, B, and C and 3D reconstruction of

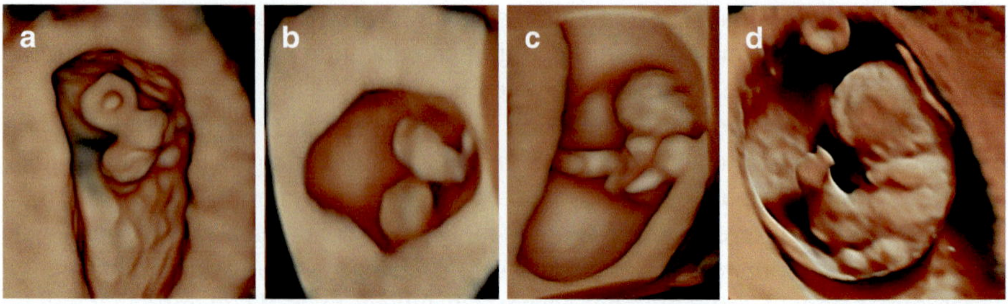

Fig. 13.1 (**a–d**) Images of 3D US HDlive rendering. Sonoembryology. (**a**), embryo at 6 gw, (**b**), embryo at 7gw, (**c**), embryo at 8gw, (**d**), embryo at 9gw. Notice all the details of yolk sac (getting smaller) and growing embryo (from small grain in (**a**), until embryo with clear display of the head, body arms, and legs in image (**d**))

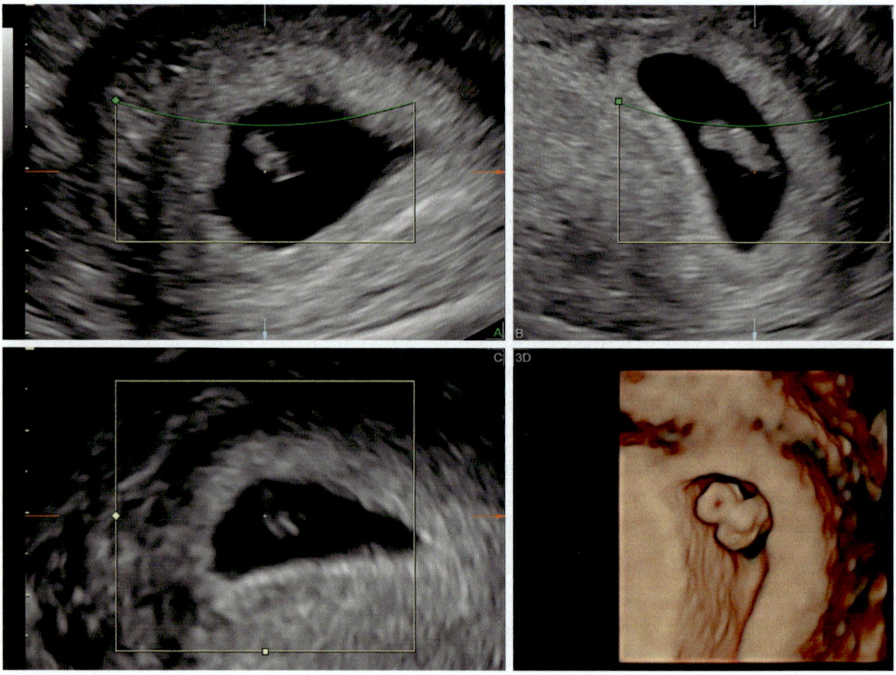

Fig. 13.2 3D Multiplanar view ABC, 3D reconstructed HDlive surface image. Fetus and yolk sac at 6 + 4 gw

the structures that are not visible otherwise are shown in Figs. 13.2 and 13.3. Getting the right sectional planes require some knowledge and skills to keep the orientation in the architecture (fetal anatomy) in order to navigate smoothly to the regions of special interest. There are several tools in multiplanar mode to achieve the navigation through the 3D volumes [34]. Operator can move the reference dot in any of the activated planes and the other two planes adjust accordingly. The three planes are

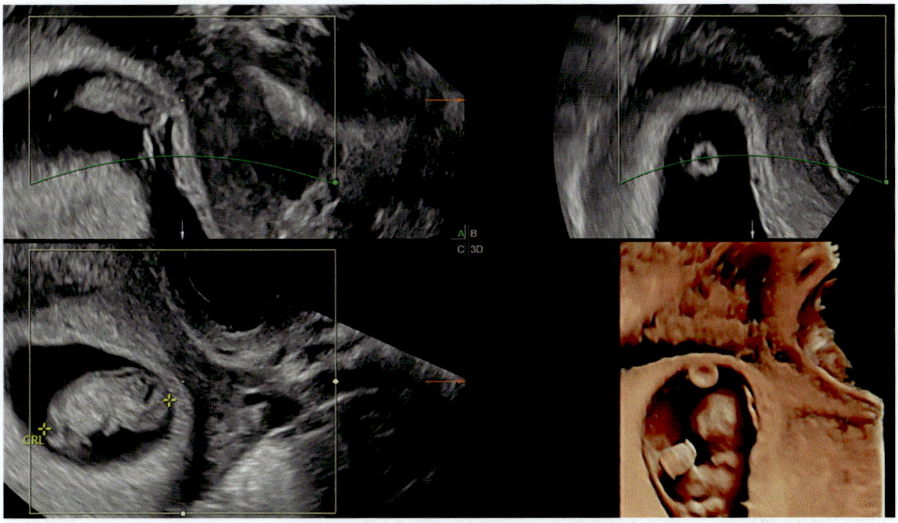

Fig. 13.3 3D Multiplanar view ABC, 3D reconstructed HDlive surface image. Fetus and yolk sac at 9 + 3 gw

intersecting in the reference dot which is orientation point and can be dynamically shifted to the targeted point. Further manipulation by rotation in either of three axes (x, y, z) automatically corrects the other two and allows the operator to adjust the position and the section of the embryo or fetus in ideal plane for measurements or assessment of targeted structures. Scrolling through the 3D volume allows translation and displays parallel images to the original plane [34]. Volume rendering can be obtained in surface, transparency, or volume calculation modes.

The mid-saggital view is essential for detailed fetal evaluation and accurate calculations in first trimester ultrasound screening. It can be obtained by navigation through the 3D multiplanar display [30, 32] (Figs. 13.3 and 13.4). The median and paramedian planes are mainly assessed for exclusion of fetal face and brain anomalies. In the end of first trimester, abnormalities of fetal face and profile such as retrognathia, flat or abnormal facial profile, significant cleft lip and palate, frontal bossing and abdominal wall defects should be excluded [29, 33]. In the second trimester, more structures are recognizable for evaluation such as corpus callosum and other midline structures [64, 65]. The axial and coronal planes are ideal for evaluation of symmetry of paired structures (left versus right) in the body such as choroid plexuses, brain ventricles, eyes, kidneys [33].

Surface rendering mode is yet another powerful tool with the incredible ability to show fetal surface and with the potential to discover abnormalities. However, to acquire high-quality data, prerequisite is substantial amount of amniotic fluid, also called "amniotic pocket" in front of the targeted structure [33]. For more emphasis and even better diagnostic accuracy, different 3D dynamic depth rendering tools and shadowing effects through the moving light source could be used in the real-time

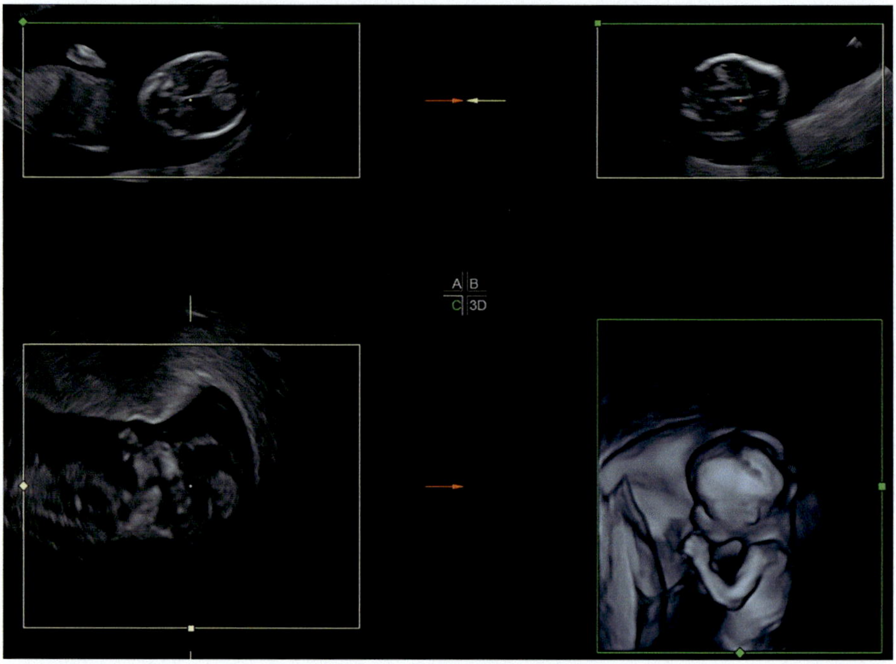

Fig. 13.4 Multiplanar imaging (**A**–**C**) and rendered 3D surface imaging from the acquired volume (VOI). Fetus at 12 gw

online and offline analyses of stored volume datasets. The electronic scalpel or so-called Magicut tool is handy option in editing and improving the visualization of the hidden structures (Fig. 13.5) when other adjacent objects obscure the view. It can be used to remove unwanted objects in different size and depth. This option is often used to clearly visualize fetal face and exclude the anomalies after removing imaging parts of umbilical cord, placenta, or limbs that are blocking the view [34].

Tomographic ultrasound imaging (TUI) or multislice ultrasound imaging presents multiple parallel planes of selected area in computer tomographic (CT) fashion. Operator is free to select the number of slices and the distance between the parallel slices (in millimeters). In the prenatal period, it is widely used for evaluation of any organ or specific selected area. Occasionally, it is used for assessment of embryo, twins (Fig. 13.6), fetal brain, fetal face, anomalies like cleft lip/ palate, orbits, size, and extent of any anomaly.

OmniView is a rendering tool that corrects the curved or irregular shapes of the structures in the way that can be viewed at the same plane. It is frequently used in combination with volume contrasting imaging (VCI), which makes it a powerful tool for imaging of fetal brain, spine, facial clefts. VCI allows the operator to select a slice thickness ranging from 1 to 20 mm. This tool can assist in enhancement of contrast resolution and visualization of the rendered structure with accuracy in any plane.

Inversion mode is a helpful rendering technique that transforms anechoic structures like cysts, fluid-filled structures like brain ventricles, multicystic kidneys, and ovarian cysts to hyperechoic structures in order to be clearly depicted.

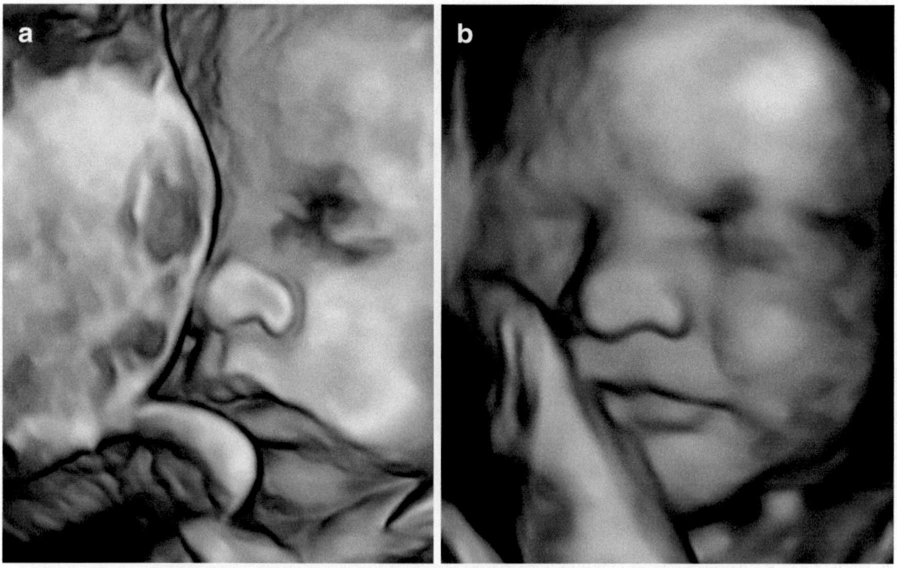

Fig. 13.5 3D surface rendering of the fetal face. In image (**a**), placental tissue is covering half of the face. In image (**b**), with the Magicut, placental tissue is removed, image is rotated, and clear view of fetal face is displayed

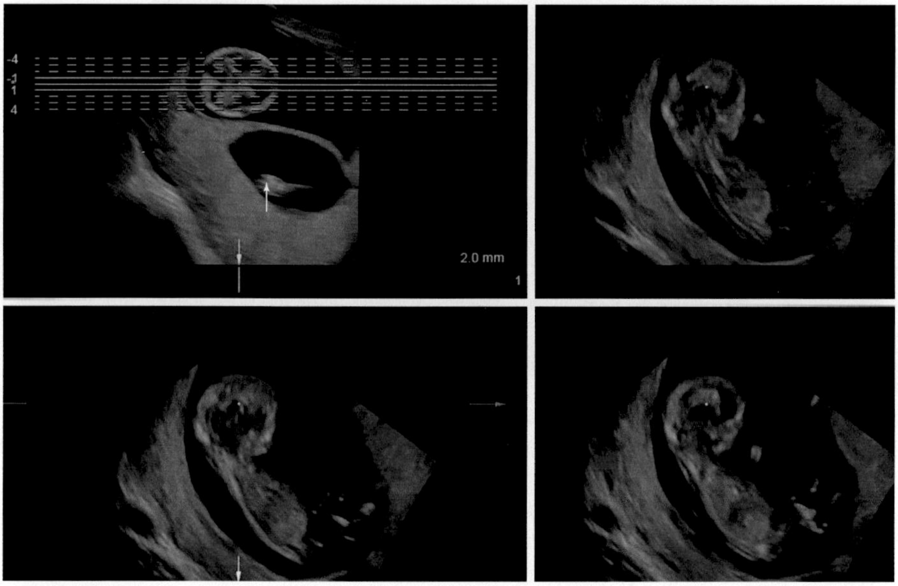

Fig. 13.6 3D TUI US imaging of fetus at 12 gw. Selection of slices is 2 mm from the axial view, getting mid-sagittal and parasagittal slices. In the reference (first) image, notice below the TUI selection of the vital fetus there is another gestational sac with "vanishing twin" (yellow arrow)

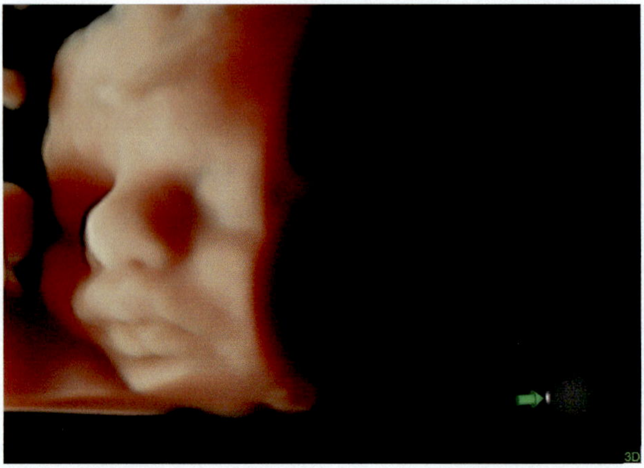

Fig. 13.7 3D US HDlive imaging of the fetal face, side view. The green arrow is showing the direction of the artificial light that can be adjusted from any angle

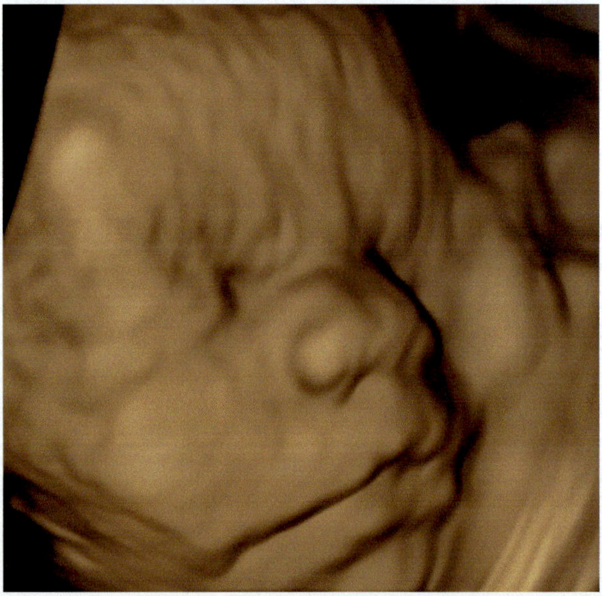

Fig. 13.8 3D surface imaging of the fetal face at 30 gestational weeks (gw). Notice "saddle nose"

Three-dimensional High Definition live (3D HDlive) surface ultrasound imaging mode allows fine tuning in the manner of illumination of targeted structure. Shadowing effects are used to highlight the important clinical details and delineate normal from abnormal structures [43, 47]. This tool is particularly useful in the assessment of fetal face [41–44] (Fig. 13.7). Implementation of different shades of skin-like color refines the presentation and gives stunning impression of a live fetus [43–49].

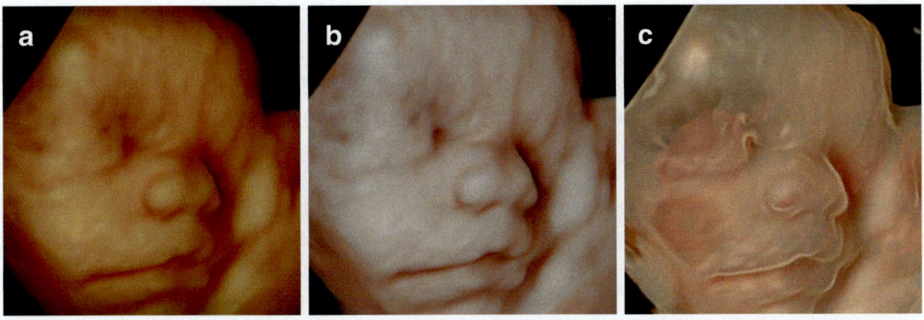

Fig. 13.9 3D HDlive different surface rendering of the fetal face at 30 gw (the same fetus as in Fig.13.5) in (**a–c**) images. (**a**, **b**), 3D surface rendering with different light shadows and different skin-like color tones; (**c**), HDlive Silhouette rendering of the same image. Notice the "saddle nose"

HDlive rendering can be efficiently used during entire course of pregnancy [41–44]. 3D/4D HDlive technology can be helpful in detecting fetal anomalies (Figs. 13.8 and 13.9) and syndromes in early and midtrimester scans as suggested in several studies [2, 36, 41, 65–72]. Nearly natural images of detailed brain architecture are displayed especially of those area surrounded by cerebrospinal fluid, such as the choroid plexuses or ganglionic eminences [67].

HDlive silhouette imaging application was launched several years ago (2014) and found its clinical significance in simultaneously displaying the inner morphology across the outer surface in a transparent manner. This is helpful in revealing the accurate location and volume of inner structures that could not be clearly seen otherwise (no matter being hyperechoic or hypoechoic) [54, 55]. In order to realize optimal display of the region or organ of interest, the operator can regulate the percentage of transparency (Fig. 13.9) (HDlive silhouette) by parallel manipulation of threshold and gain. This technique has proved to be helpful in the diagnosis of embryonic and fetal CNS abnormalities, pleural effusion, multicystic kidney, and many more anomalies [62].

HDlive flow application is an innovative technology that can be used to generate a 3D imaging of fetal, umbilical, and placental blood vessels and add more spatial resolution to a standard angiogram [46, 48].

With the simultaneous use of both techniques, HDlive flow and Silhouette, one can track the precise position of any vascular structure within the organs and discover the path and direction of the vascular flow. These two novel applications enabled the visualization of intracorporeal vascularity and assessment of structures like premature forebrain, midbrain, and hindbrain, as well as flow in the brain vessels [43]. The most recent application of these HDlive flow and Silhouette technologies are reported in the clinical assessment of fetal hepatic hemangioma [48] and fetal heart evaluation [49]. Several authors reported a shift of antenatally detected fetal anomalies and syndromes from the 2nd to the 1st trimester of pregnancy [42, 43, 46, 66].

The latest ultrasound software innovation is **HDlive studio** application where multiple light sources (up to three) can be adjusted and used to intensify the 3D

Table 13.1 Abnormalities and syndromes detected by operator with 3D US in the embryonic and early fetal period

Abnormalities	Syndromes (Sy)/multiple anomalies
Large/ hydropic yolk sac (> 5 mm before 7 weeks) Hyperechoic small yolk sac	Trisomy 21 (down) sy
Cystic hygroma	Trisomy 13 (Patau) sy
Umbilical cord cyst (true or pseudo)	Trisomy 18 (Edwards) sy
Acrania/anencephaly	Amniotic band sy
Holoprosencephaly	Pierre Robin Sy
Proboscis	Meckel-Gruber sy
Scoliosis	Turner sy (45,X0)
Spina bifida (NTD)/myelomeningocele	Body stalk anomaly
Encephalocele	Prune belly sy
Omphalocele	Achondrogenesis
Pleural effusion	
Single umbilical artery (SUA)	
Hyperechoic bowel	
Gastroschisis	
Multicystic dysplastic kidney (MCDK) Megabladder	
Cleft lip/palate	
Flat faces	
Retrognathia/micrognathia	
Vanishing twin phenomenon	
Limb abnormalities/wrist contractures/clubfoot	

NTD Neural tube defect

impression [34]. Major abnormalities that can be diagnosed by 3D US in the embryonic and early fetal life are listed in Table 13.1.

Clinical Evaluation of Embryonic and Early Fetal Period

Large or hydropic yolk sac is one of the ominous signs of fetal demise [36]. If the size is 5 mm or more before the 7th week of gestation, there is strong association with spontaneous abortion [36, 68].

Fetal neural tube defects (NTD) can be visualised with the use of 3D surface rendering mode, but OmniView and TUI can be very helpful and improve aquired information with additional details about the exact location and extent of the anomaly. HDlive and silhouette mode can be used for the assessment of *meningomyelocele and encephalocele* content [36]. Anencephaly is an NTD with the absence of cranial vault and exposure of the brain tissue to the amniotic fluid (Fig. 13.10).

Cystic hygroma are cystic structures found usually on the back or on the side neck area and are associated with Turner syndrome in 75% of the cases [69]. With

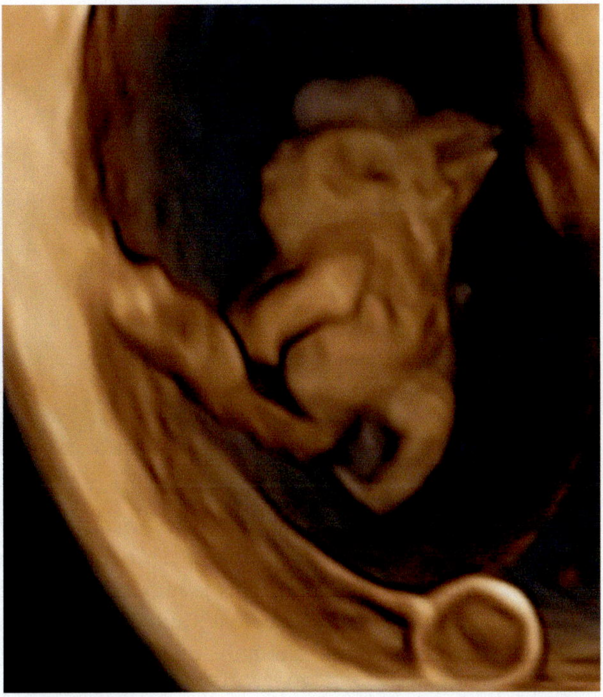

Fig. 13.10 3D dynamic surface imaging of anencephalic embryo. Notice missing skull bones and brain tissue exposed to the amniotic fluid

3D US multiplanar sections, there is good visualization of content of the cystic structure and differentiation with meningocele or hemangiomas. Hemangiomas can be excluded with the additional assessment of color Doppler [62, 63]. Very detailed visualization of cystic hygroma with presence of tiny septations within the cystic structure is accomplished with high percentage of transparency (silhouette) in HDlive Silhouette mode [36, 43, 46, 58].

Early bilateral pleural effusion is associated with fetal demise within one to two weeks. There is association with Turner syndrome. With 3D multiplanar mode and TUI in coronal and axial sections, pleural effusion is clearly evident [36].

Holoprosencephaly is an early embryonic brain malformation where the prosencephalon (forebrain) fails to separate (completely or partially) into two hemispheres. With the brain anomalies, there are also corresponding face anomalies (such as cyclopia, microphthalmia, ethmocephaly, proboscis, facial midline clefts), and severity of the one relates to the severity of the other. There are four types of holoprosencephaly: alobar, semi-lobar, lobar, and middle interhemispheric variant, the last one being least severe [70]. Sonographic appearance of the facial anomalies is best displayed with the 3D surface mode and additionally HDlive mode. 3D US volumes of facial clefts could be rendered in multiplanar mode. Correct diagnosis and determination of degree of brain separation (type of holoprosencephaly) in left and right hemispheres and observation of extent of the facial clefts are best obtained with TUI [36]. Holoprosencephaly is common forebrain anomaly with an incidence of 1 in 1298 fetuses [70] and is

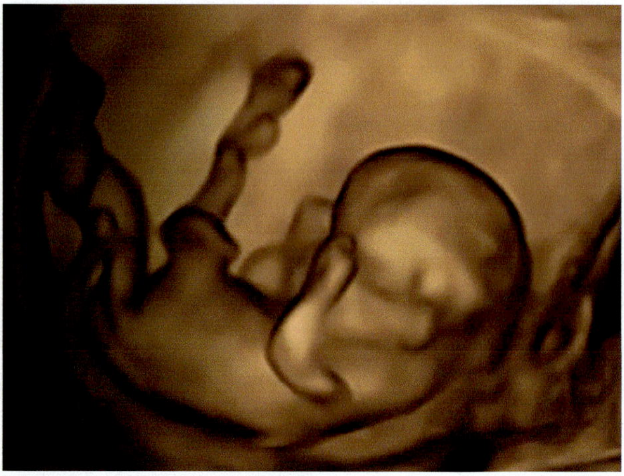

Fig. 13.11 3D US surface rendering of the fetus at 12gw. Notice omphalocele

associated with 40–60% of the cases with trisomy 13 (Patau syndrome), sometimes with trisomy 18 (Edwards syndrome) [71], but one should be aware that sometimes there is normal karyotype [36]. This is important when counseling the parents about the possible results of invasive (e.g., amniocentesis) or non-invasive prenatal test (NIPT). When there is one anomaly, one should always look carefully and exclude associated anomalies [2, 6, 29, 36, 37, 42, 44, 47, 63, 66].

Omphalocele presents ventral abdominal wall defect. In contrast to an physiological umbilical herniation that resolve spontaneously, omphalocele persist after the end of 11th week of gestation (Fig. 13.11). Defect in the abdominal wall is placed centrally and internal organs (intestine, liver, stomach) covered with the protective membrane protrude through the opening. The severity of the anomaly and the prognosis depend on the content of the sac (e.g., whether with or without liver and stomach) and the presence of associated anomalies [73]. Omphalocele is often associated with chromosomal abnormalities and karyotyping is required. Around one-third of the people born with omphalocele have a *Beckwith-Wiedemann (BWS) syndrome* [74–77]. Abdominal wall defects become very obvious when displayed by 3D US surface rendering mode. There is clear distinction made between omphalocele and gastroschisis, presence or absence of the covering membrane, and/or the protruding organs within the sac.

Gastroschisis is a ventral abdominal wall defect, paracentrally localized and usually to the right of the umbilical cord, through which the large and small intestines bulge out. There is no membrane covering the exposed organs in gastroschisis [77].

Single umbilical artery (SUA) represents one artery along the bladder wall instead of two, one on each side of the bladder wall. It is occasionally seen in aneuploidy, like *Edwards syndrome* (trisomy 18), accompanied with other fetal anomalies and some urogenital abnormalities [78].

Vanishing twin syndrome can be clearly visualized and differentiated from the hematoma. 3D surface rendering displays the content of the vanishing amniotic sac (Fig. 13.12). The surviving twin has more risk for cerebral palsy (CP) [2, 79–84]. Prenatal neurological assessment with the 4D US and KANET is adviced [2].

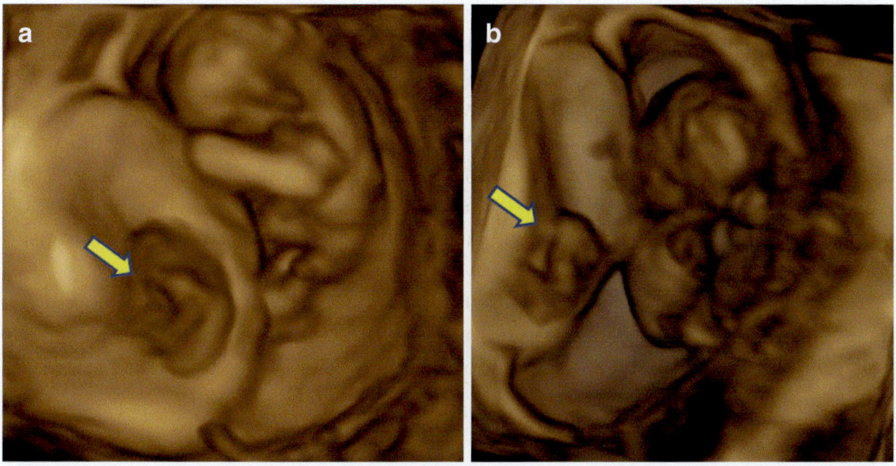

Fig. 13.12 3D surface images of two twin pregnancies (**a**, **b**), both dichorionic diamniotic gestation (DCDA). Vanishing twin phenomenon with demise of one twin (arrow)

Fig. 13.13 3D US surface imaging of the fetal profile at 34 gw. Notice frontal bossing and saddle nose in the case of achondroplasia

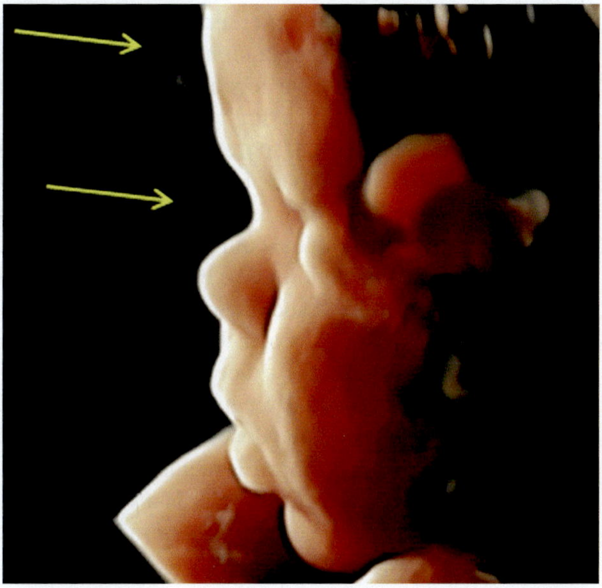

Postnatal follow-up should be performed at least until the 2nd-3rd year of life to be able to exclude the CP (for additional information and references, see section about KANET).

Low set ears and micrognathia in fetuses are sometimes associated with aneuploidies and many syndromes but have sometimes normal karyotype.

Frontal bossing can be seen in fetuses with achondroplasia (Fig. 13.13) or some syndromes such as Russell-Silver syndrome. Frontal bossing can be also seen in familial genetic diseases [29, 30, 36, 73].

Placental mesenchymal displasia (PMD) has similar sonographic appearance as partial molar pregnancy [83, 84]. It is a rare placental anomaly featured by placentomegaly and grapelike vesicles mimicking molar pregnancy [84]. As distinguished from molar pregnancies, PMD mostly features a normal fetus. There is association with BWS, preterm delivery, intrauterine growth restriction (IUGR), preeclampsia, and intrauterine fetal death (IUFD) [36, 83–85].

Scoliosis, also seen in body stalk anomaly, is best visualized with the maximum mode (for bone structure), OmniView, and 3D surface and 3D HDlive mode. Exact location could be assessed with TUI [36].

Ectopic Pregnancy

Ectopic pregnancy (EP) is one of the major contributors to maternal morbidity and mortality. Prompt diagnosis of EP remains challenging. Despite all technological improvements, there is still high number of delayed diagnosis. This might be partly due to unavailable ultrasound equipment, unavailable transvaginal US probe, diversity of presentations, different locations of EP, obese patient, and less experienced physicians. Accountable for rising incidence of EP are increasing number of pelvic inflammatory diseases (PID), more infertility cases, rising usage and availability of assisted reproductive techniques (ART), constantly growing popularity, and demand for cesarean section [86]. With regard to the location of ectopic pregnancy, in 95% of the cases, it will be found in the course of fallopian tube. Other sites of EP are ovaries, broad ligament, cervix, abdominal cavity, myometrium, uterine cornu, and scar [87]. Tubal EP can be visualized and diagnosed with 2D US and color Doppler (transvaginal approach). Three-dimensional US can give some additional information about surrounding anatomy and the exact location. Where 3D US really matters is in the cases of interstitial or angular pregnancy and special cases of cervix or scar EP [86, 87]. This last two have high incidence of maternal morbidity and mortality. Cervix EP leads to severe blood loss. Scar EP requires prompt intervention due to high risk for uterus rupture [87]. 3D power Doppler is a valuable tool in the assessment of vascularity and follow-up of the conservative or medicamentous treatments of EP [87].

Fetal Face Assessment

Cleft Lip and Palate (CLP)

Paramedian cleft lip (CL) and paramedian cleft palate (CP) or joined together paramedian cleftlip and palate (CLP) uni- or bilateral (Fig. 13.14) are the most common fetal facial anomalies. CLPs are one of the most frequent fetal anomalies [73].

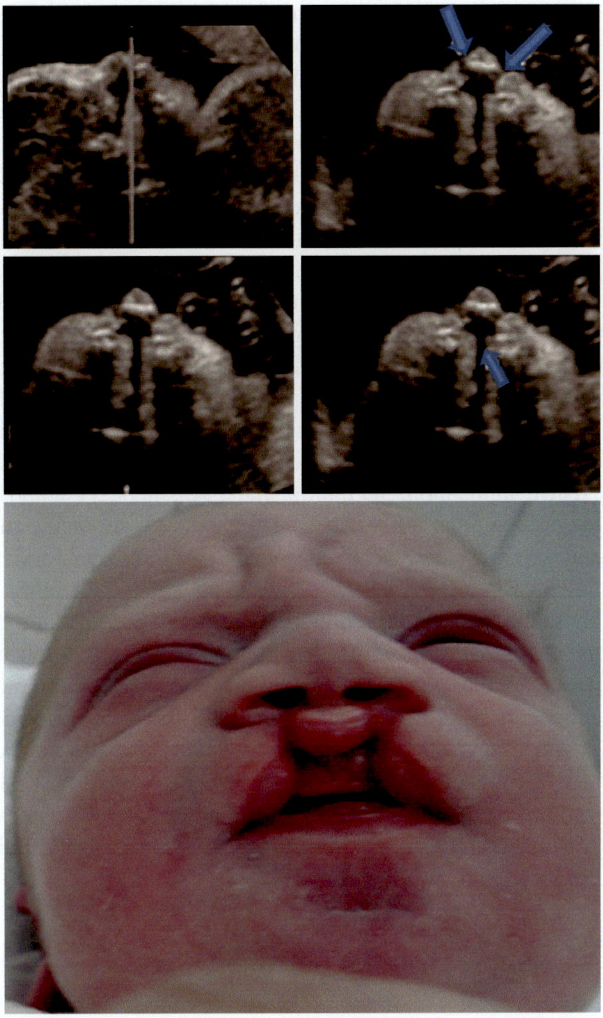

Fig. 13.14 Above is 3D TUI US axial view of fetal head. Notice the gaps in the lips and palatum (arrows). Image under is the neonate postpartum

These anomalies appear between the 8th and 9th week of embryonic development. The hard palate and the upper lip have different embryonical origin. Important separating landmark for anterior and posterior cleft anomalies is junction of primary and secondary palate located at the incisive foramen [73, 88]. Accordingly, lack of adequate fusion of medial nasal segments with the maxillary swelling on the same side results in cleft lip and cleft of primary palate. Failed midline fusion of palate shelves results in clefts of secondary palate [73, 88]. Visualization and distinction between the two are possible with the use of 3D US and modes such as TUI as demonstrated by Pooh et al. [36].

Anterior CLP can be uni- or bilateral and includes cleft lip and cleft lip with alveolus. Posterior cleft palate is midline or paramedian [73]. Surgical repair of isolated CLP (less than 50% of cases) has excellent prognosis and good postoperative results. Unfortunately, high number of fetuses with CLP have other anomalies that jeopardize the fetal outcome. Majority of these are associated with chromosomal or other genetic abnormalities and can be joined in syndrome [2, 73].

Facial clefts are found in 50% of fetuses with *Van der Woude (VdW) syndrome* that has autosomal dominant inheritance. This accounts for nearly 2% of all cases of CLP [73].

During assessment of fetal face with conventional 2D ultrasound, small defects like unilateral CL can be easily missed. Assessment with 3D US surface rendering is superior method to detect this kind of subtle defects that can be trigger to look for other associated anomalies [2, 29]. In general, if the symmetry of facial appearance is not disturbed, like in fetuses with bilateral CL, anomaly can be missed [37]. Asymmetric defects or the one that changes the appearance of fetal profile are most likely to be detected [29]. Bilateral complete CL and CP have the protrusion of the inner maxillary segment under the nose (Fig. 13.14), which is unexpected and uncommon mass when observing a fetal profile [73]. With 3D US surface rendering mode, operator is able to display every detail of the face and can provide almost photographic images with the HDlive application. 3D multiplanar assessment, VCI, and TUI multislice imaging, particularly in axial plane, are valuable tools for surveying the exact location (Fig. 13.14) and the extent and interference with surrounding anatomical structures [37].

Facial midline clefts are always severe and one should look for associated brain anomalies [37]. As previously mentioned, severity of the one reflects the severity of the other. Midline clefts are typically part of holoprosencephaly sequence with gross facial appearance (cyclopia, proboscis, midline facial cleft to a diverse extent, cebocephaly, arhinia, microphthalmia, flat nose) [72, 73].

Midline clefts and holoprosencephaly are anomalies that are frequently associated with the syndromes such as *Patau (trisomy 13)* and *Edwards (trisomy 18) syndrome*. Even though trisomy 13 is most frequently associated syndrome, as many as 75% of the fetuses with holoprosencephaly have normal karyotype [37, 73, 74].

Mandibular Anomalies

Mandibular anomalies such as agnathia, micrognathia, and retrognathia (Fig. 13.15) have been frequently described as isolated anomaly, part of multiple anomalies, or more heterogeneous fetal syndrome (*Treacher Collins, Turner, Pierre Robin sequence, Trisomies 13,18, 21*) [71, 73].

First indications can be made by fetal 2D US assessment in sagittal plane where impression of abnormal fetal profile can be made. Advanced 3D US with different surface applications are helpful in realistic imaging of fetal face and profile that can elucidate the presence of these abnormalities and other facial dysmorphism [2, 29]. Facial dysmorphism is an important part of the phenotype of many syndromes [2, 29, 71, 73].

Three-dimensional US multiplanar imaging is helpful when rendering ideal plane for measurements. Rotten et al. [89] provided normative data for diagnosis of micro-/retrognathia. There are many studies that evaluated mandibular and maxillar size and position in relation to the other facial landmarks [89–95].

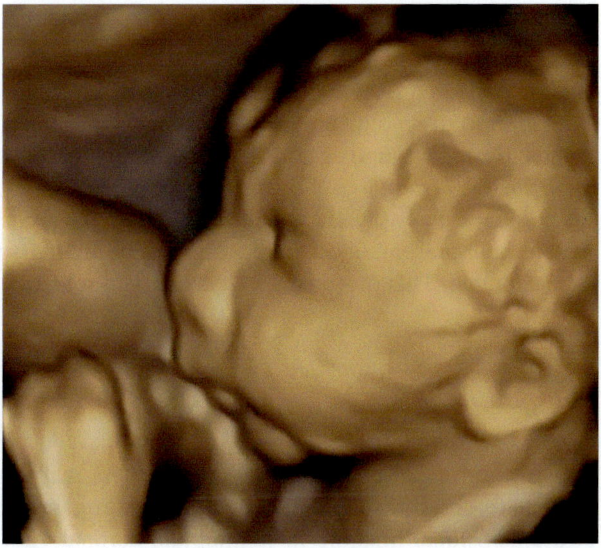

Fig. 13.15 3D US surface rendering, fetal profile at 30gw, retrognathia, and low-set ears and other anomalies (colpocephaly, AGCC, etc.)

Measurement of the frontomaxillary facial (FMF) angle and mandibulomaxillary facial (MMF) angle provides an objective way of evaluating the position of the maxilla with respect to the fetal forehead and could be used for early diagnosis of micrognathia and/or retrognathia [90, 91].

The measurements could be obtained with 2D US. However, getting the exact plane for measurement could be difficult and time-consuming while waiting for fetus to get in the right position. Acquiring the volume and rendering in 3D multiplanar mode take only few seconds to get exact mid-sagittal plane regardless of actual fetal position in utero. *Pierre-Robin sequence* (PRS) is defined by a triad of orofacial anomalies including retrognathia, glossoptosis, and posterior median soft CP [96]. An osseous defect of the mandible is rarely found. Mandibular hypoplasia is an initial defect that takes place early in gestation between the 7th and 11th week of gestation. It cause the chain reaction and forces the tongue to stay high up in the oral cavity which subsequently interrupts the fusion of the posterior soft palate [73, 88]. Several authors reported that diagnosis could be made with 3D US in the first trimester fetal assessment [37, 42, 96, 97].

Pooh et al. [37, 42, 44] used 3D US images and illustratively presented mandibular hypoplasia and slow jaw development in a cases of PRS during pregnancy. Vivid presentation of serial 3D scans clearly revealed the improvement and progress of mandibular growth [37]. Mandibular catch-up growth occurs during the first year of life and the adjustment of facial appearance and profile can be expected between the 3rd and 6th year of life [96–98]. Isolated PRS is found only in 50% of cases and the other half is usually part of a malformation syndrome. The clinical manifestation and the fetal prognosis depend on the existence and severity of associated anomalies [73].

Macroglossia

Macroglossia is an anomaly characterized by abnormal enlargement of the tongue in relation to the mouth size and can be diagnosed prenatally by 2D and 3D ultrasounds. It can be found as an isolated finding or associated with syndromes such as *Beckwith-Wiedemann syndrome or Down syndrome* [73, 88]. 2D imaging in sagittal and coronal views as well as additional 3D surface rendering of the fetal face reveals an abnormal presentation where a big protruding mass through the mouth happens to be a tongue. This protrusion is secondary to macroglossia [73].

Epignathus

This is a rare form of oropharyngeal teratoma that arises from oral cavity (upper jaw, palate, and sphenoid bone) and is protruding through the fetal mouth [99, 100]. Two-dimensional imaging in sagittal and coronal views indicate an unusual mass (which is not the tongue) coming out of the fetal mouth that prevents it from closing its mouth. 3D surface rendering of the fetal face discloses a gross fetal facial appearance with solid tumor coming out of the fetal mouth. With the additional TUI imaging in axial and sagittal views, precise origin of the tumor can be detected. Exact volume of the tumor could be calculated by virtual organ computer-aided analysis (VOCAL) of 3D US imaging or semi-automated sonography-based automated volume count (SonoAVC) [37].

When the volume of the tumor is acquired with the power Doppler (PD), VOCAL is applied to outline the volume of the tumor, which can be further rendered in glass-body or angio mode to illustrate the overall vascularity of the tumor. Another possibility is to use 3D HDlive Silhouette and flow to visualize the vascularity of the tumor.

This is a life-threatening condition leading to high mortality (from 80 up to 100%) at the time of delivery. Prenatal diagnosis and multidisciplinary approach (obstetrician, neonatologist, pediatric oral and maxillofacial surgeon, and anesthesiologist) to problem-solving are crucial in prompt and adequate postnatal management in order to secure the airway and resect the tumor [100].

Facial Dysmorphism and Syndromes

Facial dysmorphism commonly arises from a mixture of migration disorders and inadequate formation of facial mesenchyme, occasionally associated with disorders of the first and second branchial arches [101]. The nature of these anomalies is diverse.

Majority of mandibular anomalies are due to the first branchial arch developmental errors, various chromosomal disorders (*DiGeorge syndrome*), collagenopathies, or teratogenic agent exposure such as alcohol (*fetal alcohol syndrome, FAC*) [73]. In the study of 115 patient with PRS, as expected, 54% had isolated PRS [98]. The others included *syndromes* such as *Stickler (18%), velocardiofacial syndrome (7%), Treacher Collins syndrome (TCS) (5%), facial and hemifacial microsomia* (3%), and other defined (3.5%) and undefined disorders (9%) [98].

Goldenhar syndrome (GS) also referred to as oculo-auriculo-vertebral (OAV) syndrome is the combination of abnormalities owned to developmental disorders of 1st and 2nd branchial arch [73].

Malformations can be diagnosed prenatally by 3D US and demonstrated as asymmetric appearance of the fetal face [2, 29] and the body. The first sonographic clue for the detection of anomalies that are combined in GS can be detection of asymmetry of the face due to hemifacial microsomia or just small periauricular skin tag.

Mostly, poorly developed one side of the body includes unilateral craniofacial hypoplasias (70%), brain anomalies (cerebellar hemisphere hypoplasia) – right side more occasionally affected than left side, eye anomalies (micro/anophtalmia), low-set ears with malformation, skin tags around the ear, kidney anomalies (hydronephrosis), and vertebral anomalies [102–104].

Wang et al. [105] analyzed data from a large congenital birth defects registry in Spain and found possible indications that poorly controlled maternal diabetes interferes with cephalic neural crest cell migration, causing this GS syndrome.

Micrognathia and Low-Set Ears

Micrognathia and low-set ears (Fig. 13.15) are frequent combination of anomalies found in many syndromes (trisomies 13,18,21, GS, etc.). Bilateral symmetric hypoplasia of the face and preauricular tags in combination with micrognathia may be part of *Treacher Collins syndrome (TCS), Nager, or* Miller syndrome [73].

TCS is bilateral, symmetrical, otomandibular dysplasia often associated with downward slanting of the palpebral fissures. Cranioskeletal hypoplasia is a consequence of inadequate number of neural crest cells due to neuroepithelial progenitor cell death and occurs in early embryonic period between 4th and 8th weeks of gestation [97, 106, 107]. Prenatal diagnosis of TCS is highly relevant because due to distorted anatomy, tongue may obstruct the airways and lead to neonatal death [108]. First indications of the suspected TCS syndrome could be made by 2D US when noticing fetal facial dysmorphism and polyhydramnios [108]. Detailed facial features can be clearly displayed by 3D US surface mode and HDlive tools. Presence or exclusion of other anomalies of the head, neck, or limbs could be done by additional survey with 3D multiplanar or multislice imaging [2, 37].

Cranial Sutures/Head Shape

Cranial bones and sutures can be easily viewed in surface and maximum mode by 3D US (Figs. 13.16, 13.17, and 13.18) during whole pregnancy. Craniosynostosis is an anomaly where cranial sutures close prematurely, and depending on which sutures are involved, there is specific deviation in head shape. There are several syndromes featuring primarily cranyosinostosis such as *Apert, Carpenter,Crouzon Pfeiffer, Saethre-Chotzen,* and *Antley-Bixler syndromes* [73].

Very specific distinction in *Apert syndrome* in contrast to other craniosynostosis syndromes is specific finding of limb abnormalities called "mitten-like hands/feet" (syndactyly of the 2nd, 3rd, and 4th finger/toe in combination with a broad thumb/toe). A case of a prenatally detected fetus with Apert syndrome assessed by 3D US was published by Pooh et al. [37]. Illustrative correlation and amazing similarities between prenatal 3D US images and postnatal appearance had been made [37, 44].

Faro and colleagues [109] monitored the ossification process and development of cranial (frontal) bones and sutures (Fig. 13.19) in 16 fetuses during the 9th–34th week of gestation. At the initial stage frontal bones appear as tiny bilateral ossification centers and develop gradually to form metopic suture which normally begins to fuse at 32nd week of pregnancy. There are four different patterns of abnormal closure of metopic suture (V, Y, U shape and additional bone in between) identified by Choui et al. [110]. They also found that additional bone between the metopic suture is found mostly when holoprosencephaly or abnormalities of the corpus callosum were present, while patterns like V, Y, or U shape are mainly found in fetuses with facial anomalies involving the orbits, nasal bones, lip/palate, and mandible [109].

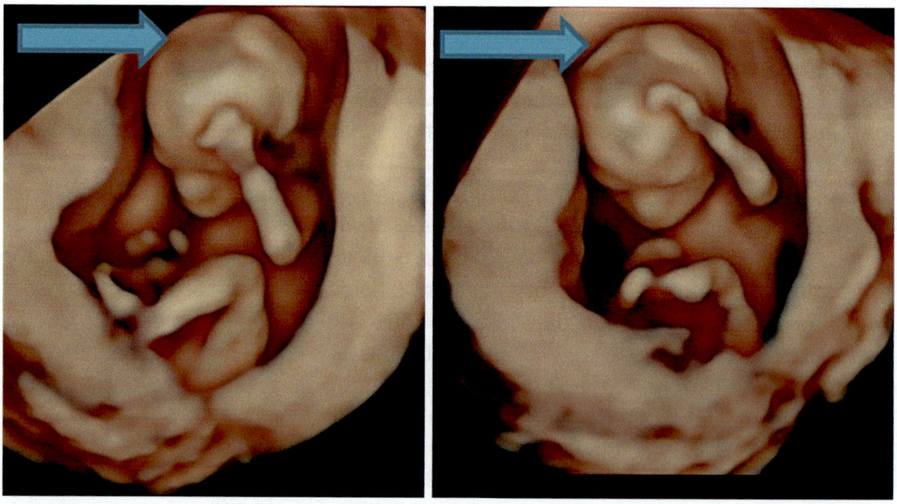

Fig. 13.16 3D HDlive surface imaging of fetus at 15gw. Notice the cranial sutures and anterior fontanel (arrows)

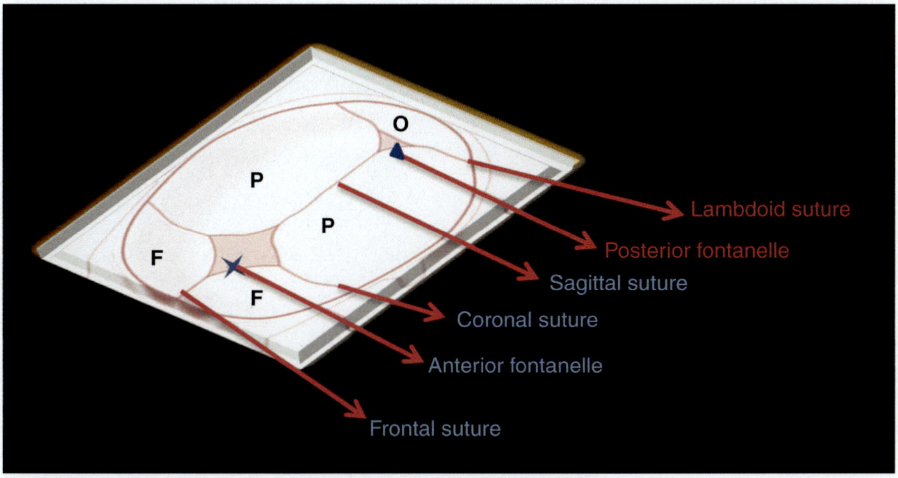

Fig. 13.17 Schematics image of fetal cranial bones, sutures, and fontanelles from superior view. F frontal, P parietal, C occipital bone. The ones marked with the blue color are visible in Figs. 13.16 and 13.18

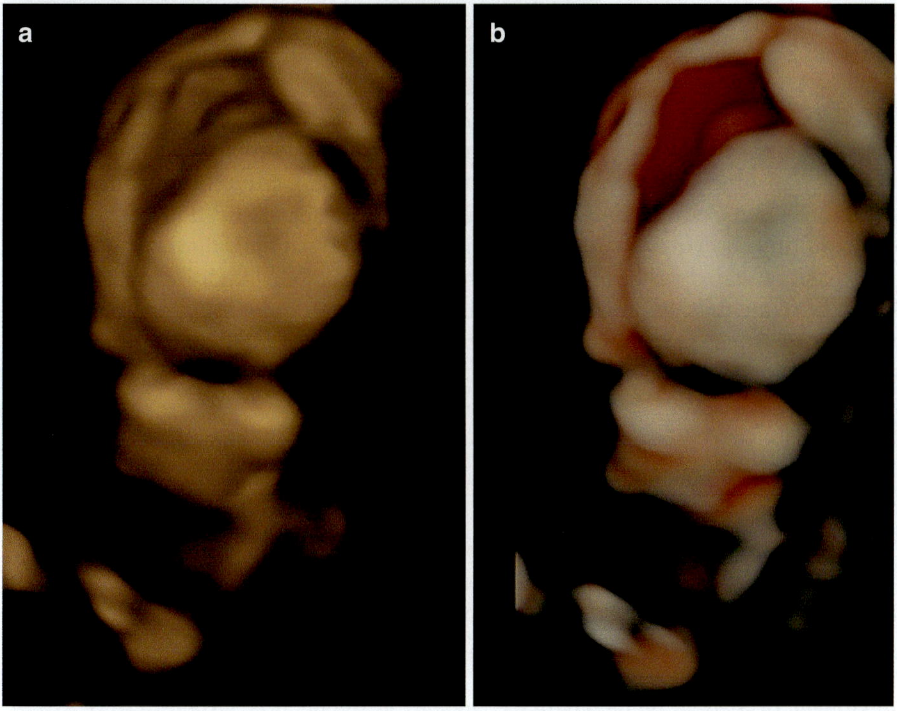

Fig. 13.18 Fetal cranial sutures, bones, and anterior fontanelles at 18 gw; right semi profile, view from above. (**a**), 3D skeleton mode; (**b**), 3D surface HDlive mode. Notice the anterior fontanelle

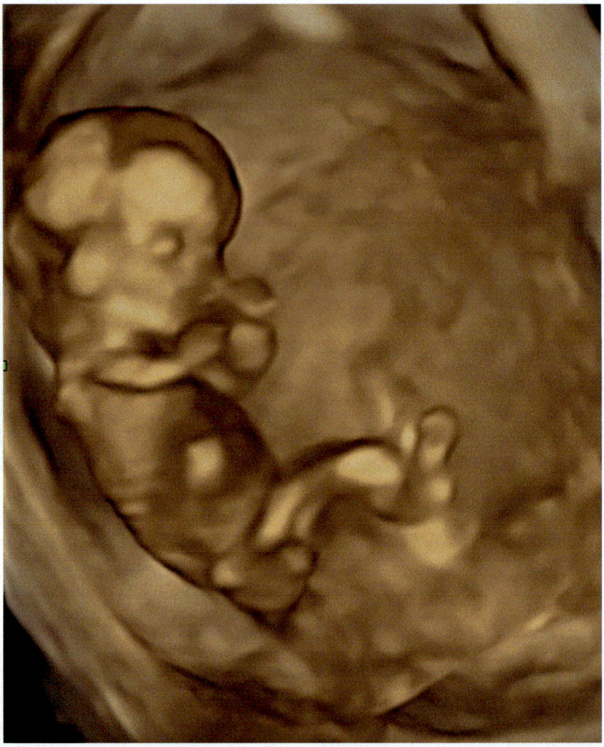

Fig. 13.19 3D skeleton rendering of the fetus at 13 gw. Notice the clear depiction of growing frontal and parietal bones. Wide gap on the top of the skull is anterior fontanelle

Abnormal head shapes are also seen in trisomy 18 with strawberry-like shape, open neural tube defect with lemon-shaped head, and different *craniosynostosis* syndromes like *Crouzon and Pfeiffer* with cloverleaf-shaped head [37, 73].

Acquiring the volume with 3D US is best in mid-sagittal plane of multiplanar mode and rendered further in maximum or skeleton mode. Additional adjustments could be made with the fine tuning in different axis, use of transparent mode, conventional surface or HDlive for surface rendering, and adjustment of color and shade modifications.

Brain and CNS

Three-dimensional US is highly valuable in the assessment of fetal brain and the rest of the CNS (Figs. 13.20, 13.21, and 13.22). Essential volume data to evaluate important midline structures of the brain are best obtained in sagittal plane. Structures such as corpus callosum (CC) and cavum septi pellucidi (CSP) can be observed when rendering adjustments are made in multiplanar display mode to ideal view of median plane where CC appears as hypoechoic structure [65].

Extensive morphologic survey could be done. Additional assessment with OmniView allows display of any plane in the volume. Thick slice display compresses the images of several slices together (thickness is adjustable) to accentuate the borders of CC or any other structure [65].

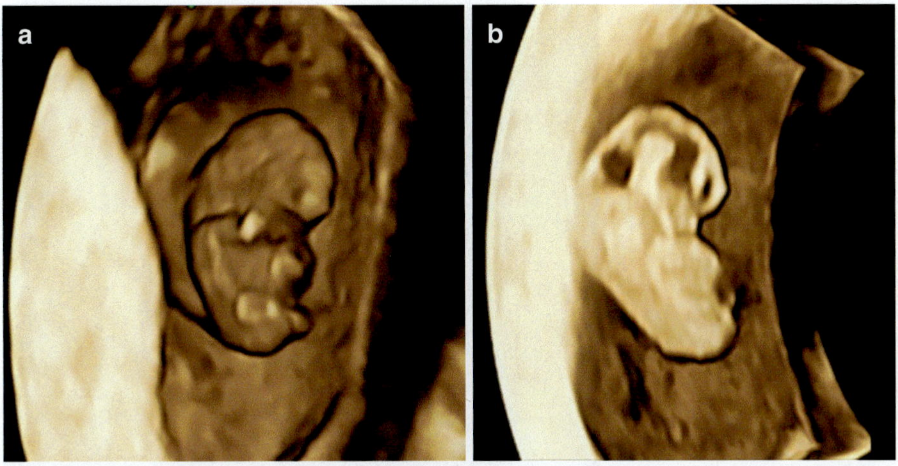

Fig. 13.20 (**a**) 3D surface imaging of the embryo at the 8 + 4gw. (**b**), same image, parasagittal view withe the visualization of the brain vesicles

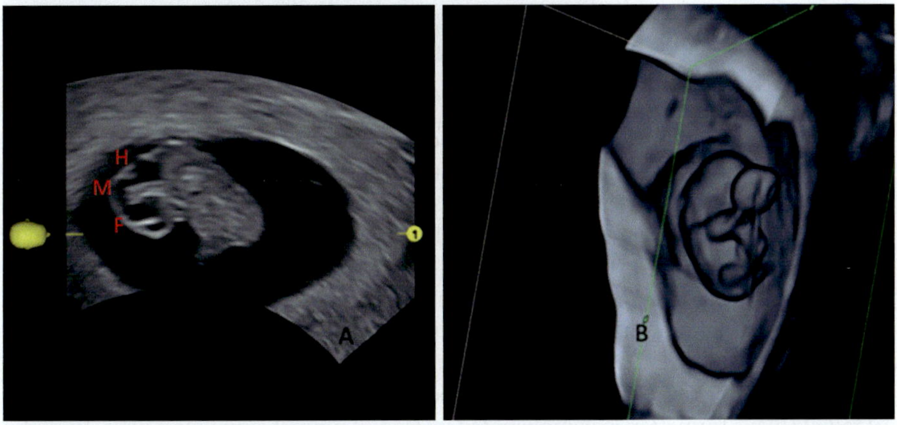

Fig. 13.21 3D OmniView: (**a**), parasagittal view of the embryo at 8 gw, notice the clear depiction of brain vesicles. (**b**), 3D surface rendering of the fetus and the yolk sac becomes visible. F Forebrain (prosencephalon), M Midbrain (mesencephalon), H Hindbrain (rhombencephalon)

Detailed morphology of the brain and CNS can be obtained with 3D TUI display mode for visualization of multiple parallel slices (adjustable for thickness in mm and number of slices) in CT-like fashion throughout whole volume of any targeted area. The selection of targeted midline structures in axial plane will result in TUI display in sagittal planes where CC can be visualized [37, 64, 65].

Existence of CSP indicates the existence of CC. However, absence of CSP does not necessarily imply the absence of CC [111]. For example in isolated Septo-Optic Dysplasia (SOD) it is possible to have a normal, thin or absent CC [111, 112]. From embryological and anatomical point of view, CC and CSP are linked together [113]. They develop from the commissural plate [114] between 12th and 18th gestational weeks [111]. The presence of CSP should be confirmed with US assessment around

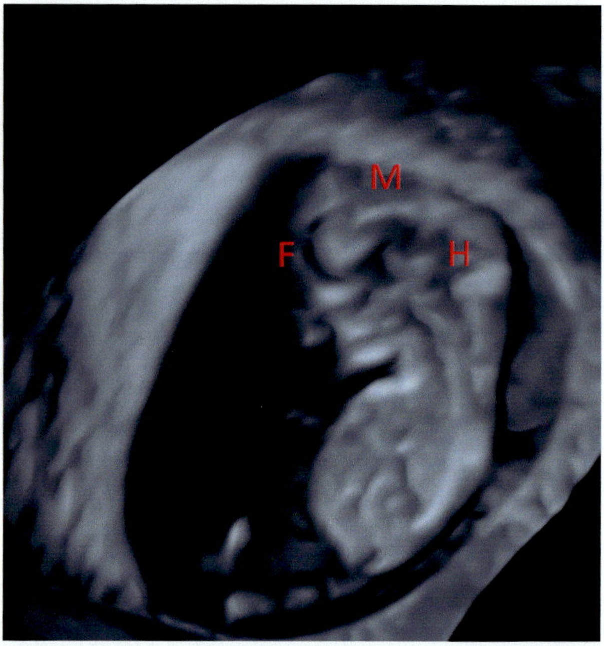

Fig. 13.22 3D surface dynamic imaging, clear view of the brain vesicles. F Forebrain (prosencephalon), M Midbrain (mesencephalon), H Hindbrain (rhombencephalon)

20th week of gestation when the so-called fetal "anomaly scan" is performed. If CSP is not initially found, fetal assessment should be repeated in week or two, and if necessary, additional neurosonography is advised.

The CSP is a significant indicator for normal fetal CNS development and absence of the CSP is never a normal finding [115]. Additionally, absence of the CSP is rarely an isolated finding. In conclusion, the presence of the CSP basically suggests normal development of the central forebrain, thereby excluding many complex malformations [111, 116].

Agenesis of the CC (AOCC) can be suspected when in the mid-sagittal section typical radial sulcus formation is demonstrated instead of normal cingulate sulcus. With the additional vascular assessment (Fig. 13.23) of angio-architecture by 3D power Doppler and glass body application, lack of the callosomarginal artery as the largest branch of the pericallosal artery becomes evident and indicates the absence of CC [37].

Fetal cranial posterior fossa architecture with organs like vermis can be appropriately visualized and precisely measured with 3D US [117]. Additionally, if anomaly is suspected, 3D US tools such as TUI, VOCAL, or HDlive Silhouette flow can be applied.

Several features of 3D US can be applied for accurate survey of fetal spine (surface rendering/ HDlive Silhouette, skeleton/ maximum mode, OmniView, TUI, etc.) (Figs. 13.24 and 13.25) The best is to acquire the volume of entire length of the spine in skeleton mode, where curved line is used to follow the curvature of the spine ideally with the anterior fetal spine position [118, 119]. Posterior and multiplanar view are used to track the position of conus medullaris [119].

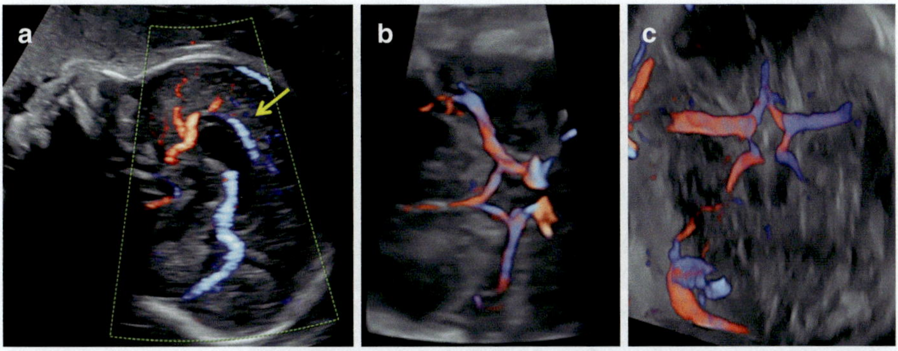

Fig. 13.23 Images of fetal brain circulation. (**a**), sagittal view with color Doppler and visualization of arteria pericallosa (arrow). (**b**, **c**), 3D STIC glass body, axial view, fetal brain circulation. Circle of Willis

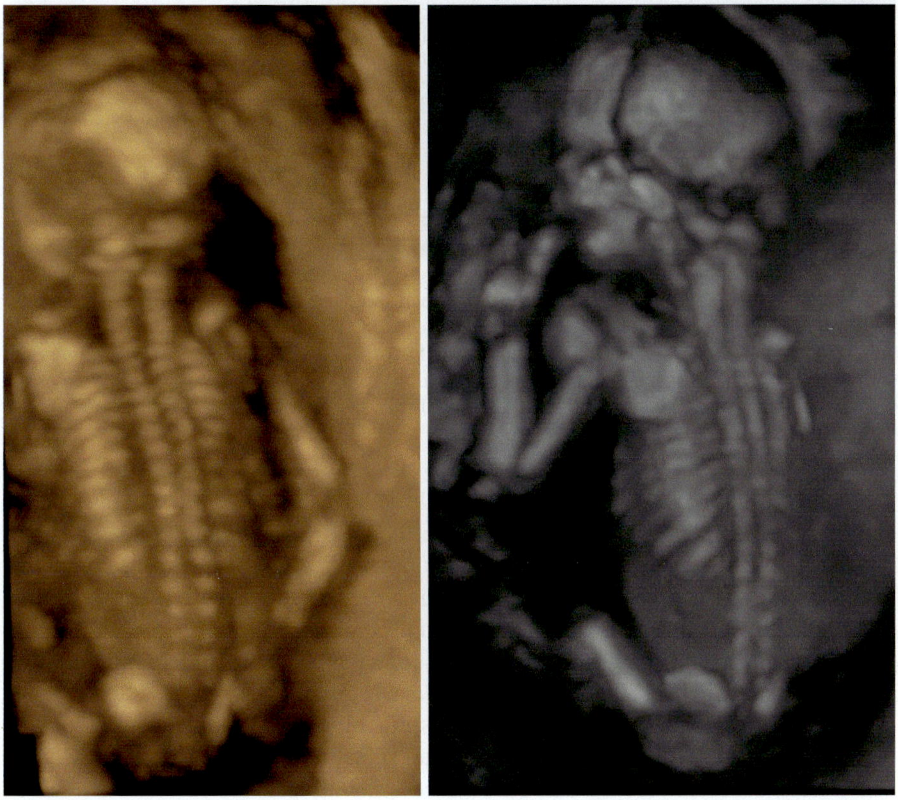

Fig. 13.24 First image in 3D US skeleton rendering mode. Second image in 3D max. Skeleton mode: fetal skeleton at 16gw from the head until the sacrum is displayed completely. Notice detaild visualization of cranial bones from the posterior and side view, spine, ribs, scapulae, arms, pelvic bones, and femur

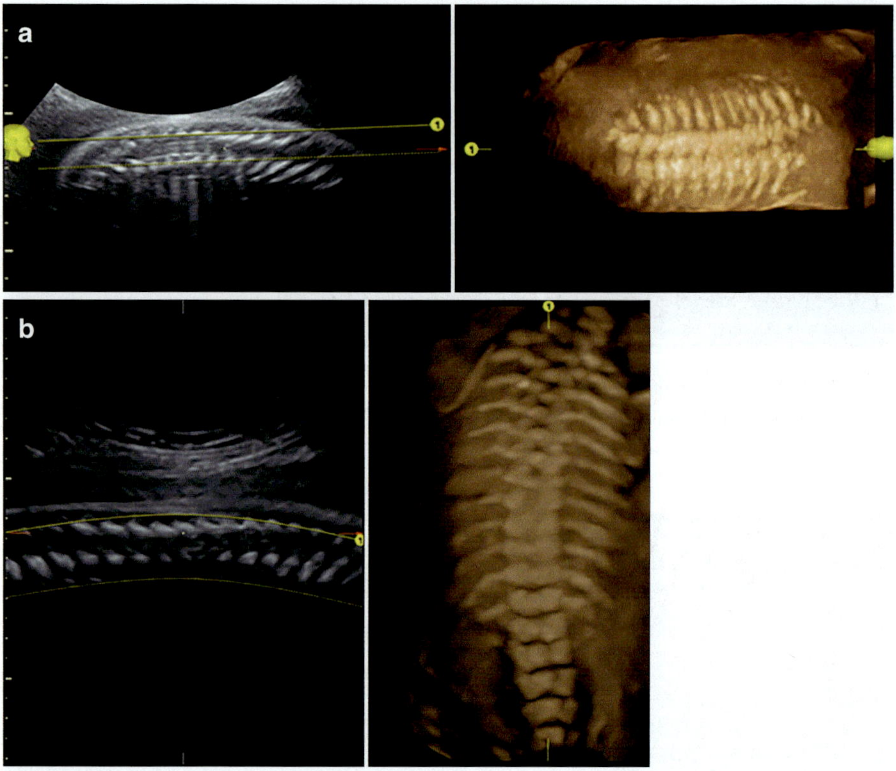

Fig. 13.25 (**a**, **b**). 3D OmniView rendering of the fetal spine in 3D skeleton application rendering. Fetal spine (2D image) is anteriorly positioned, ideal for 3D imaging. Notice curved spine, but straight line of OmniView selection (**a**), missing end parts of the spine. Notice curved OmnieView selection (**b**) on the 2D image and better visualization of 3D skeleton of the ventral view of the spine, and ribs form the cervical part until the sacral part

OmniView and multiplanar display are additional tools to show the images of the curved spine or the ribs in this regard. Rendering in surface or HDlive can give good impression on the symmetry and malformations like vertebral fusion anomalies, scoliosis, or any other anomaly that can be displayed vividly at certain level. HDlive Silhouette has the power to visualize also ventral part of the spine due to different levels of transparency (silhouette) used in imaging. Segmentational spine assessment is possible in 3D TUI (Fig. 13.26) mode in sagittal and axial views. Anomalies such as hemivertebrae, butterfly vertebrae, spina bifida, and sacral agenesis can be clearly displayed and outlined [58, 119]. Fetal spina bifida was suspected by 2D US and clearly demonstrated by 3D US surface imaging as early as the 9th week of gestation by Pooh et al. [56, 118].

The main advantage of multiplanar mode, besides getting the exact planes, is possibility to explore the anatomy simultaneously in all three orthogonal planes and switch to or adjust either of them at any point with automatic adjustment in other two. Modern 3D US devices are equipped with automatic presets in different applications that ideally display certain structures like CC.

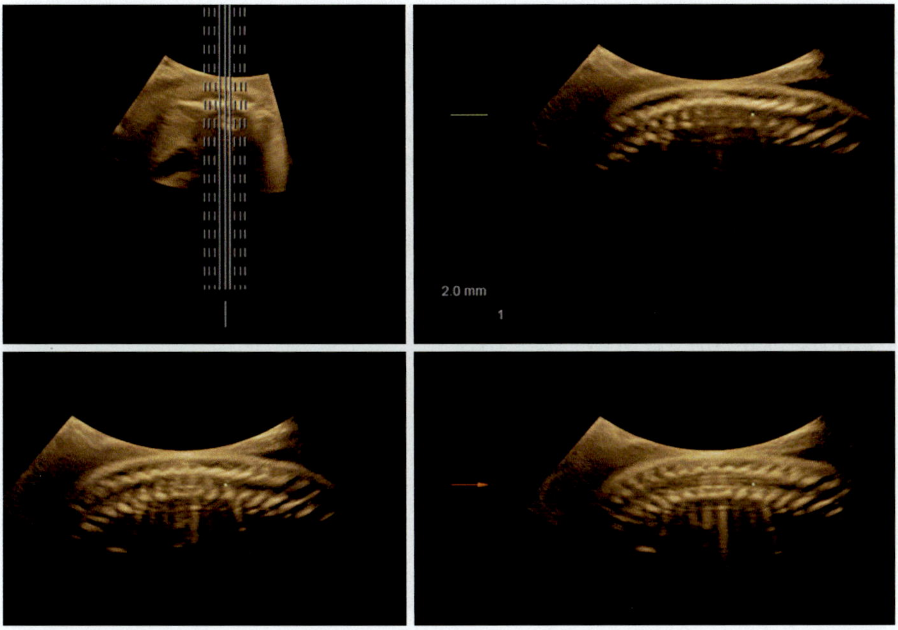

Fig. 13.26 3D TUI imaging of the fetal spine

Fetal Heart

Three-dimensional and four-dimensional US have amazingly improved over the last few decades. Introduction of *real time (RT 3D) with a matrix-array probe*, *motion-gated 3D US* imaging, is one of these remarkable technological accomplishments where fetal echocardiography booked the most benefits [120].

Novel cardiac assessment that was increasingly utilized in clinical practice is indirect motion-gated offline scanning mode, also called spatiotemporal image correlation (STIC). Acquisition of the volume in VOI is done automatically over several seconds (7.5–15 sec.) in an approximate 150 fps. Depending on fetal size, the sweep angle should be 20° (in 1st and 2nd trimesters) and −40° (3rd trimester) [120].

In 2003, Gonçalves et al. [121] have first reported the use of 3D STIC applications for fetal heart (Figs. 13.27 and 13.28) assessment. This novel application has undergone further improvements in the last decade, and besides the initially seen advantages like offline volume analysis, aid in diagnosis of congenital heart disease (CHD), and modality for medical teaching and training, [120, 121] there are some additional advantages seen over the time. They are: reduction in examination time, simplicity in acquiring unlimited number of conventional and non-conventional planes, heart morphology that can be assessed in surface mode with cine loop, possibility of digitally storing of all data for use in later/distant analysis, possibility of remote diagnosis, and aid in counseling the parents and multidisciplinary approach with pediatric cardiologists and surgeons [120–123]. The STIC application enables spatial assessment of the heart volume and structures (intraventricular septum, atrioventricular valves) and basic great vessels outflow tracts. The site and the extent of

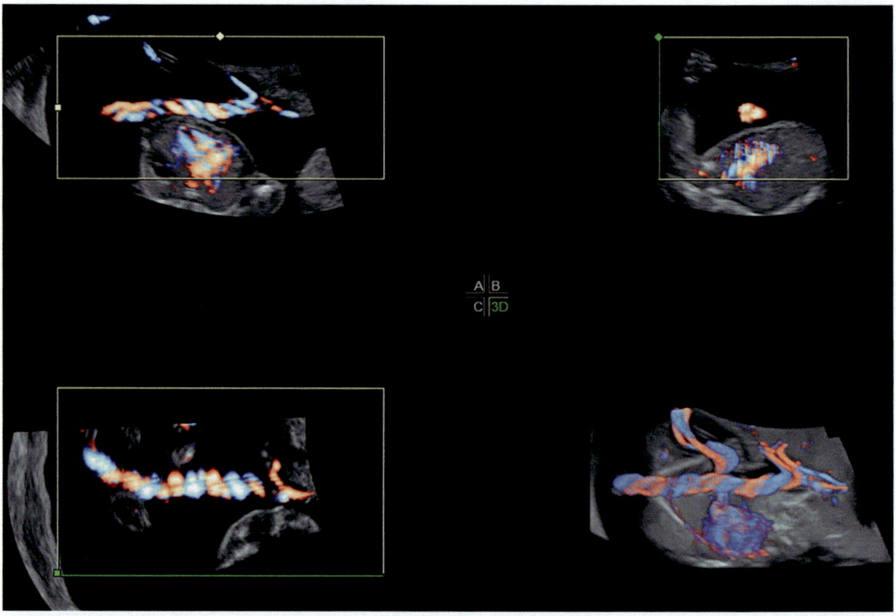

Fig. 13.27 Multiplanar view of the fetal heart and umbilical cord insertion. 3D reconstruction in STIC and glass-body imaging

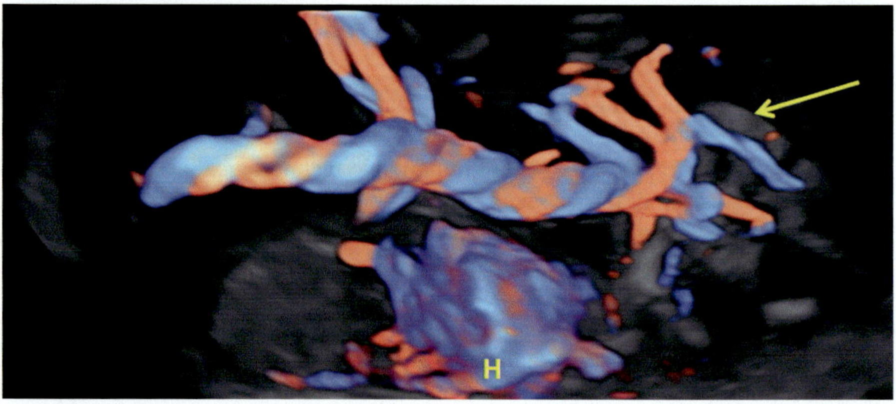

Fig. 13.28 Detailed display of 3D STIC, glass-body image of fetal heart (H) and umbilical cord insertion into placenta (arrow)

defects are outlined. More detailed fetal echocardiography by 3D/4D US available scanning modes and accompanied series of images is published by Yagel et al. [120].

The combination of **STIC with VOCAL** allows ventricular volume calculation, abnormal mass measurements, and ventricular and interventricular septum analysis. Another combination of **STIC and TUI** was proposed by Espinoza and colleagues [124] in order to standardize the fetal echocardiography and get targeted views in one panel. Veronese et al. [125] recently published the results of a prospective research of the Fetal Intelligent Navigation Echocardiography (FINE) application in order to obtain standard fetal echocardiography views. Authors concluded that FINE applied to STIC volumes can successfully produce 9 standard fetal echocardiography views (in 96–100%) in the 2nd and 3rd trimesters of pregnancies and this indicates that FINE can be used as a possible method of screening for CHD. Clinical application of STIC with FINE was demonstrated in specific case of fetal dextrocardia and situs solitus with complex congenital heart disease published recently, in which the FINE application was helpful in the detection of multiple abnormalities and defining complex anatomic relationships [126].

Clinical Use of 3D/4D US in Functional Studies of the Fetus

The introduction of 3D/4D ultrasound technologies revealed many clinical diagnostic possibilities (Table 13.2) in prenatal medicine. Due to increasing computational power of processing and acquiring data of **3D/4D ultrasound** systems, **dynamic**

Table 13.2 3D US display modes and clinical application in prenatal period

3D US display modes/tools	Application in antenatal period
Multiplanar mode	Early pregnancy, brain, face, palate, spine
Surface mode	Early pregnancy, face, abdominal wall, spine, hands/feet, sutures
TUI (multislice)	Early pregnancy, brain, face, orbits, palate, abdomen, any structure/organ
OmniView/VCI	CNS, palate, extremities
Volume rendering Vocal, SonoAVC	Fetal organs, placenta, cystic/solid structures
HDlive surface rendering HDlive Silhouette HDlive studio	Early pregnancy, face, orbits, abdominal wall, fetal organs, spine, hands/feet, cystic structures
3D color Doppler 3D bidirectional power Doppler Glass-body rendering or angio mode	Heart, umbilical cord, placenta, fetal solid tumors
HDlive Silhouette and flow	Brain, heart, umbilical cord, placenta, hemangioma
Magicut	Cutting out (electronically) and deleting artifacts and interfering objects
Inversion mode	Brain ventricles, cystic structures, multicystic kidneys, ovarian cysts
Transparent mode	Cranial sutures, bones, ossification, vessels, cystic structures
Maximum mode	Bones, calcifications, cranial sutures
Minimum mode	Brain ventricles, multicystic kidneys, diaphragmatic hernia, hydrothorax, heart, vessels, cystic structures
STIC Real-time algorithms	Heart, cardiac gating
4D US	Fetal movements, facial expressions, fetal organ function KANET

3D US three-dimensional ultrasound, *TUI* tomographic ultrasound imaging, *VCI* volume contrast imaging, *VOCAL* virtual organ computer-aided analysis, *SonoAVC* sonography-based automated volume count, *HD* high definition, *STIC* spatio-temporal image correlation, *4D US* four-dimensional ultrasound, *KANET* Kurjak antenatal neurodevelopmental test

3D US images (4D) can now be displayed in near- or real-time (not necessarily equal to real-time 3D, see earlier text about gating necessity) at the moment of scanning. 4D ultrasound systems have amazing image quality. Different 4D modes and applications (surface rendering, HDlive, HDlive Silhouette, HDlive studio, etc.) can be used to improve the visibility of the target structure and improve the certainty of diagnosis.

In comparison with 2D US, 4D US offers many benefits with regard to visualization of fetal face, grimacing, swallowing, mouthing, yawning, eye-blinking, and breathing movements and reveals dynamic movements of the body and the limbs. Evaluation of the structural and functional development can be followed throughout the whole pregnancy. Starting from the 5th–6th week of gestation details of gestational sac, the embryo and yolk sac can be visualized. (Figs. 13.29, 13.30, and 13.31). The first embryonic movements are noticed around 7th–8th gestational weeks and can be best acquired with the use of transvaginal (high-frequency) 3D/4D probe.

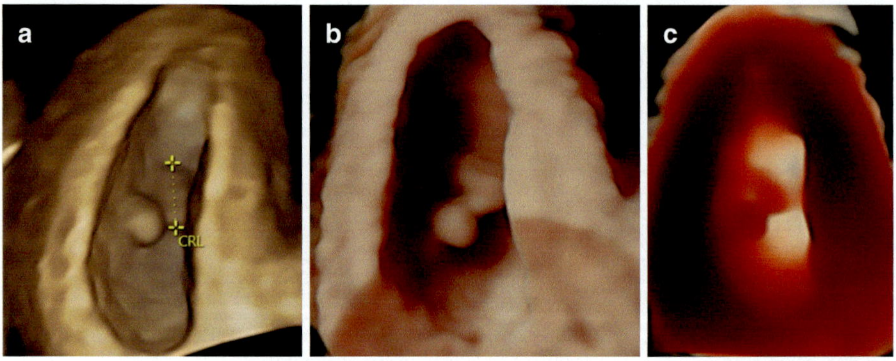

Fig. 13.29 (**a**) 3D surface imaging obtained by transvaginal 3D/4D probe; (**b**, **c**), HDlive imaging. Different illumination techniques. Notice clear view of embryo at 6 + 0 gw and yolk sac. (**c**), virtual light is placed behind the embryo

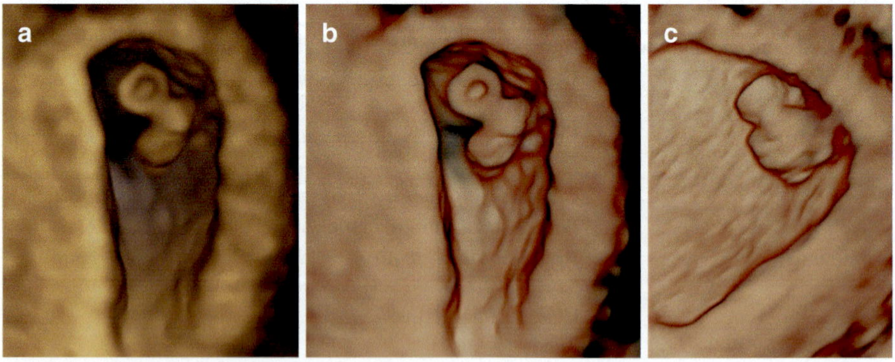

Fig. 13.30 (**a**) 3D surface imaging; (**b**, **c**), HDlive imaging. Different depth and axis of rendering techniques. Notice clear view of embryo at 6 + 5 gw and yolk sac

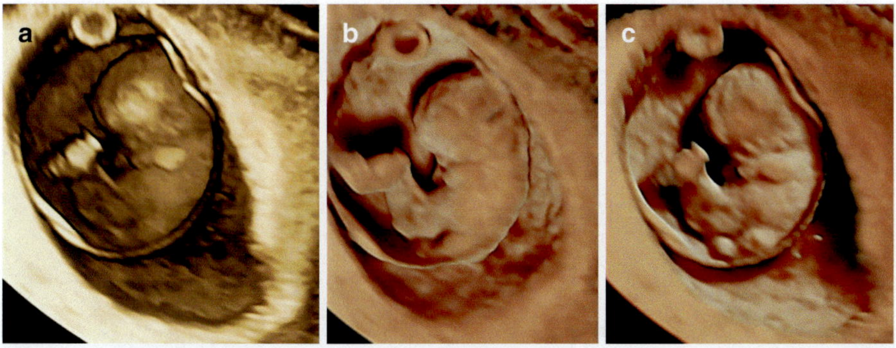

Fig. 13.31 (**a**) 3D surface imaging; (**b**, **c**), HDlive imaging. 3D dynamic imaging. Notice clear view of embryo with all body parts (head, body, limbs) at 9 gw, yolk sac, and umbilical cord

Assessment of Fetal Behavior

Fetal behavior can be described as any fetal action or reaction noted either by the mother or with the more objective method, such as sonography [127]. Combining the data of fetal dynamic and morphological studies revealed that fetal behavior reflects the activity of the fetal CNS [128–130]. Accordingly, it was assumed that the assessment of fetal behavior in different periods of gestation could give the opportunity to differentiate normal from abnormal brain development and enable early diagnosis of various structural or functional abnormalities [131–136]. The real breakthrough in the understanding of fetal behavior was achieved by introduction of 4D US technology and will be presented in this chapter.

Evaluation of the fetal neurobehavior remains a big challenge in perinatal medicine. Technological improvement in 3D/4D US offered the opportunity to explore the fetal anatomy with precise details and to observe the fetal behavior in real time [137–139].

The fetal central nervous system (CNS) has very well-defined path, and developmental steps are reflected accordingly by the fetal behavior corresponding with each week of pregnancy. Due to use of 4D US, we came to better understanding on which fetal movements or behavioral patterns are normal or abnormal in correspondence to timeline of pregnancy [140]. Unpredictable factors or events can occur at any point of this growth timeline and can influence very sensitive and delicate course of fetal brain development and maturation. During 1st trimester, there is increasing frequency of various fetal movement patterns. In the 2nd half of pregnancy, there is organization of fetal movement patterns and increase in complexity of movements. The existence of a full range of facial expressions (Figs. 13.32, 13.33, and 13.34) is seen in the 2nd and 3rd trimesters [133–169, 171, 172].

If there is evident structural damage, most of the time it can be detected by fetal US examination, but even if there is no visual damage of CNS, neurological damage and impairments can still exist. These damages are often diagnosed sometime after birth and possibly wrongly attributed to intrapartum or even postpartum events [141, 142].

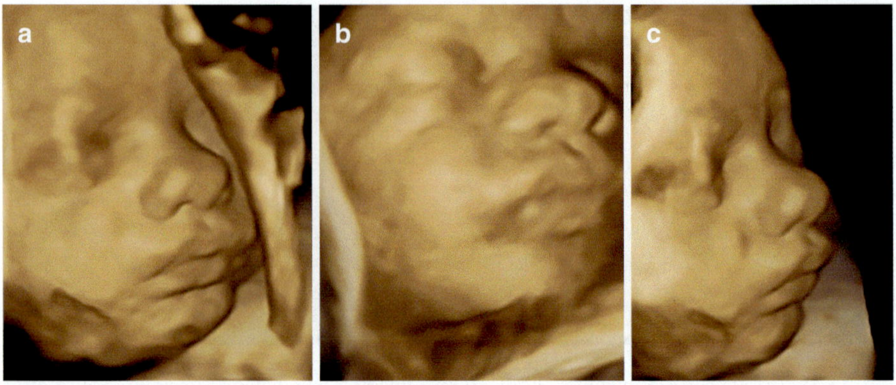

Fig. 13.32 Fetal face and profile. 3D US surface imaging. (**a**), fetal arm in front of the face; (**b**, **c**), adjustment of render axis to view profile and lips after removal of fetal arm with Magicut

Fig. 13.33 Fetal profile, 3D surface rendering

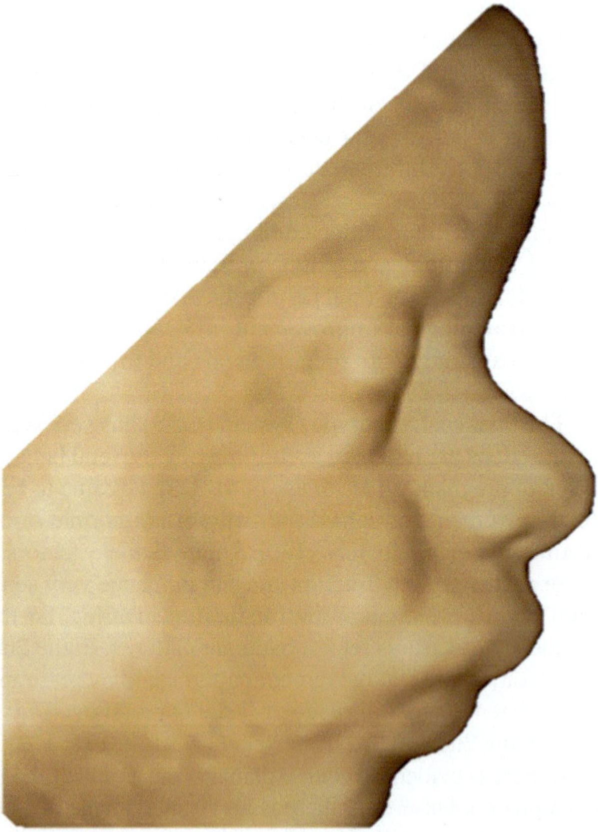

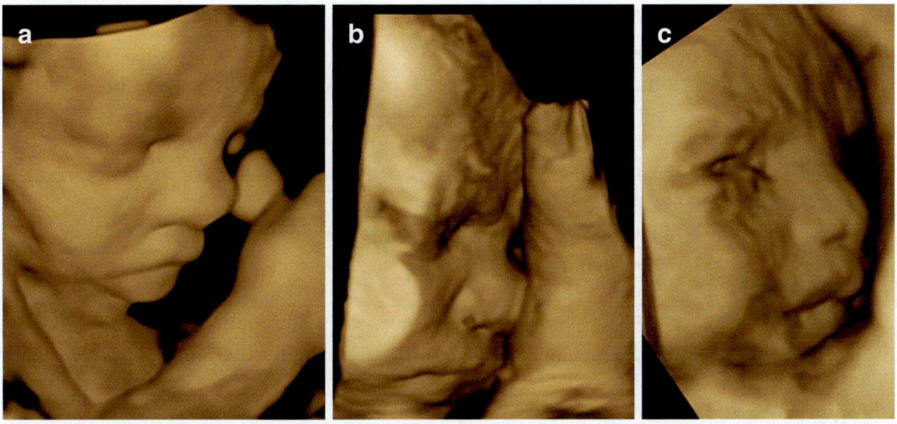

Fig. 13.34 Fetal face and profile 3D US surface imaging at 30gw. (**a**), Same fetus is sleeping; (**b**) grimace on the fetal face and frowning; (**c**), fetus is awake with open eyes

Functional Studies

Evaluation of fetal behavior is particularly important in the later stages of gestation, from the third trimester of pregnancy onward in order to verify the fetal well-being, central nervous system (CNS) maturation, and integrity.

A much needed assessment of fetal neurobehavior was finally available in 2008. The test is named **Kurjak Antenatal Neurological Test (KANET)** [133]. The KANET is based on prenatal fetal assessment by 4D sonography (Table 13.3). With the KANET, it is possible to determine several functional aspects and separate fetuses with normal, borderline, or abnormal neurobehavior that are at high risk for developing neurological impairments [133–136]. Scoring list is published in several papers [136, 162] and KANET scoring table is presented in Table 13.4. Various studies, several multicenter researches, and two consensuses have been conducted (with application of KANET), all of which showed over the time KANET value in the assessment of fetal behavior and fetal facial expressions during pregnancy [133–169, 171, 172].

A multicenter study, designed to assess the clinical features and value of KANET where it can be applied and to evaluate the clinical outcomes of these fetuses postnatally, was published recently [142]. KANET was used among random pregnancies, in specific patient groups such as low- and high-risk pregnancies and in pregnancies complicated by DM or GDM. In one study, the fetal acoustic stimulation was applied during KANET to evaluate its advantages. When KANET was applied in high- and low-risk pregnancies, more abnormal and borderline cases were observed in the high-risk group. Clinical use of 3D/4D US in the study of fetal neurobehavior in twins in all three trimesters of pregnancy was described in detail in the work of Kurjak et al. [144] (Figs. 13.35, 13.36, 13.37, and 13.38).

Table 13.3 Instruction for performing KANET

Instructions for performing KANET test:
Gestational age to perform KANET: Third trimester of pregnancy, from 28 weeks of gestation onwards.
The duration of KANET should be between 15–20 minutes
Preferably performed in a slightly (15%) right (or left) lateral-tilt position to reduce inferior vena cava compression by the gravid uterus.
At periods that the fetus is awake, if not awake – Repeat the test in 30 min or the next day
If score is abnormal or borderline, repeat the test every 2 weeks until delivery + do additional Doppler assessment
The learning curve for KANET test is very reasonable, cca. 80 test performed
Clinicians who apply KANET should have **adequate training and experience** in low- and high-risk pregnancies.
Inter-observer and intra-observer variability has to be documented.
Recommendation regarding the ultrasound machines is to have good resolution and quality for 4D scanning with the **frame rate of at least 24 volumes/s.**
2-year postnatal follow-up should be available and documented for all fetuses in order to draw safe conclusions.

Table 13.4 KANET scoring

Total score	Interpretation
0–5	Abnormal
6–9	Borderline
10–16	Normal

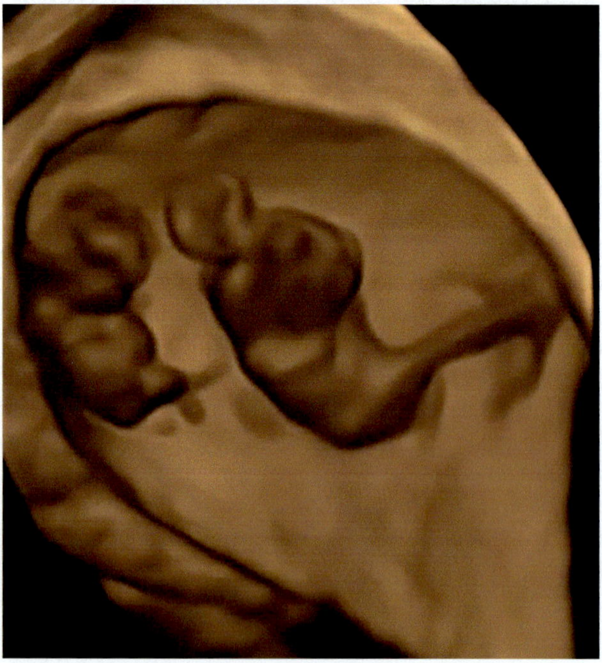

Fig. 13.35 3D US surface rendering of the MCMA twins at 9 gw

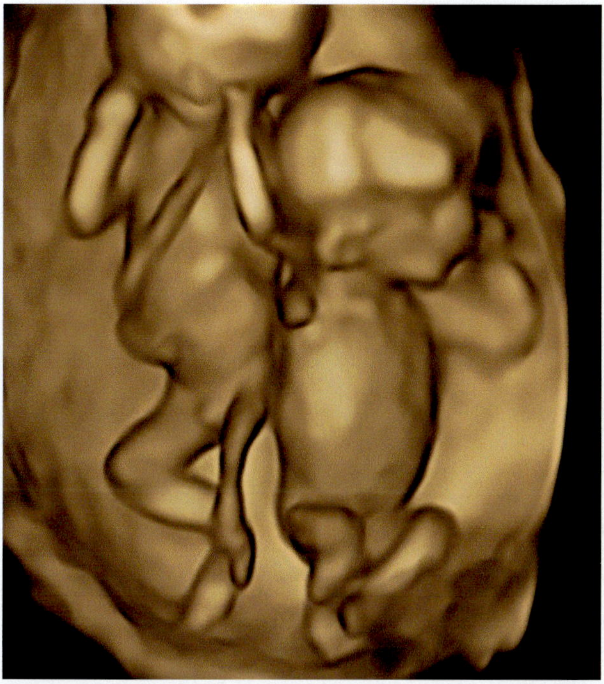

Fig. 13.36 3D US surface rendering of the MCMA twins at 14 gw

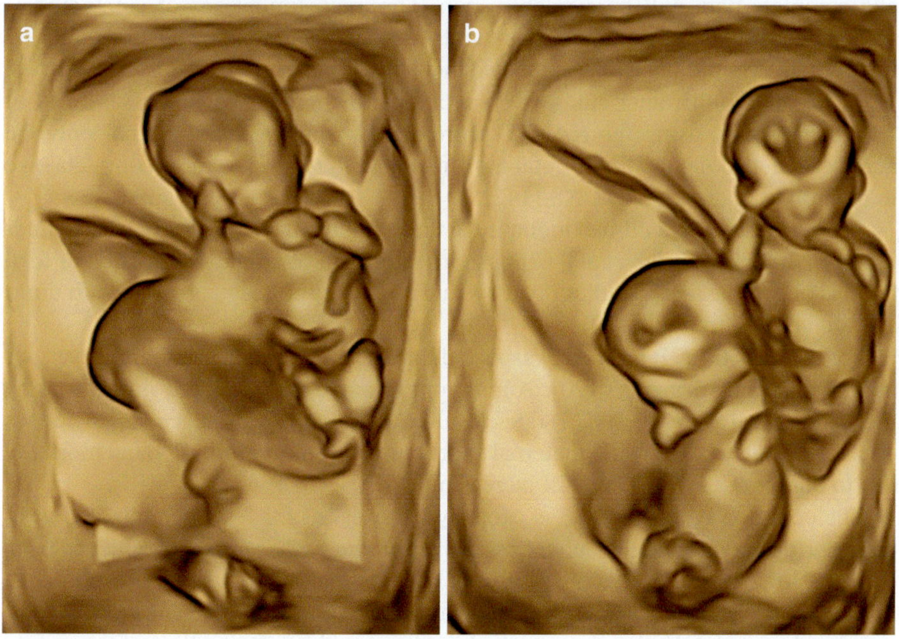

Fig. 13.37 3D surface imaging of DCDA Gemini at 12 gw. (**a**), unclear view of the lower fetus; (**b**), after rotation and adjustment in axis, and removal of ventrally laying tissue with Magicut, the clear view of both Gemini

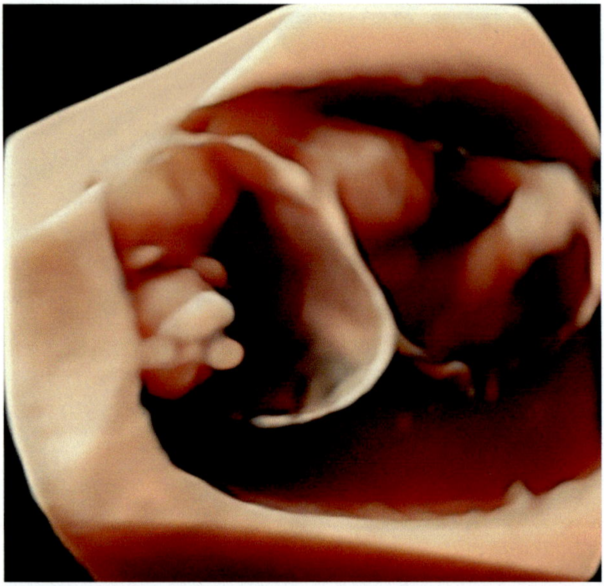

Fig. 13.38 3D HDlive image of MCDA twins at 10 gw

Apart from abnormal cases, with the respect to the scoring, it was clear that all fetuses with borderline scores had to be followed more closely in the postnatal period [142, 168]. As authors indicated, follow-up of most studies is still ongoing and complete data will be available soon. The main limitations of some studies could be the fact that the number of patients was small and that the postnatal follow-up is not always the same and even available in the more rural parts of the countries. However, this multicenter study offers a complete approach for the assessment of fetal behavior by using the KANET score and by simply observing not only the quantity but also the quality of fetal movements with respect to increasing fetal age in relation to maturation of CNS [142].

The potential of 4D ultrasonography in the assessment of fetal awareness is studied from 2005 by Kurjak et al. [171]. An investigation of cognitive function of fetal brain is one of the latest studies done by Kurjak and his colleagues and new findings are still coming to light [172].

For a longer time, it has been suspected that there is a prenatal origin for various neurological impairments [170]. An attempt to solve this problem in the past by increasing cesarean section (CS) rates resulted in the same prevalence and incidence of cerebral palsy (CP), while maternal short- and long-term morbidity and mortality due to higher rates of CS are still increasing [170].

The common belief that CP is exclusively reserved for fetal hypoxia and ischemia during and around the delivery was overthrown as there is clear evidence from epidemiological studies that the origins of CPs are mainly prior to labor (more than 90%) [170]. This is apparent from the data presented on the prevalence of CP compared with cesarean birth rates over the last 50 years [170]. Regardless of the sixfold increase in CS birth, worldwide CP rates did not change at all, and the prevalence

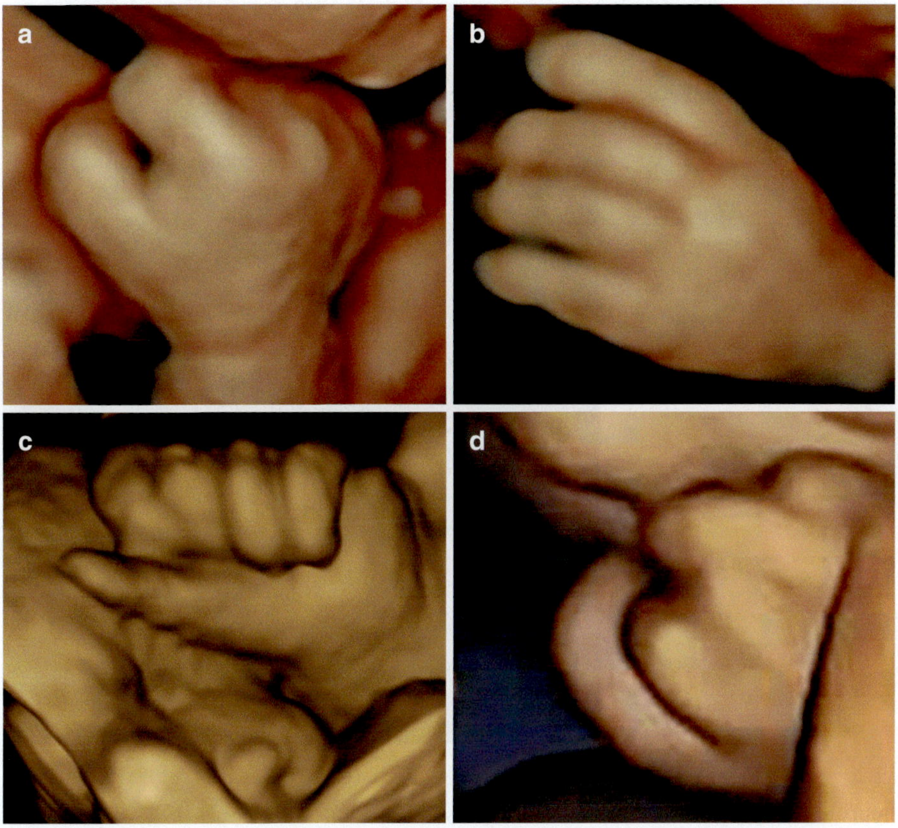

Fig. 13.39 Fetal hand. (**a**), fist; (**b**), open hand; (**c**), closed hand with thumb outside; all normal findings. (**d**), overlapping of fingers and thumb clenched inside, also called "neurological thumb", abnormal finding

remained stable at about 2–2.5/1000 births. This elucidates once again that CP has little to do with the mode of delivery. Recent genetic studies link sporadic cases of CP with the genetic mutations [170].

Now more than ever before, there is a need to find the way to detect these fetuses at risk for neurodevelopmental impairments as early as possible. A major concern is that delay in the diagnosis made sometimes many months and years after the birth limits the possibilities of adequate intervention. KANET is the first method that uses 4D US for the prenatal evaluation of the fetus in a similar way a neonate is evaluated after the birth [142, 168] (Fig. 13.39a–c).

Even though the initial injury that induces brain damage by definition does not aggravate through lifetime, the effects of CP manifest differently throughout the lifespan [173–177]. The high prevalence of CP along with the high percentage of children surviving into adulthood, no cure, and not known course of CP over the lifetime make this condition extremely relevant for clinical practice [170]. An attempt to use 4D US and KANET aiming to contribute to the prenatal detection of these fetuses which could be at higher risk for the development of CP, ASD, or other

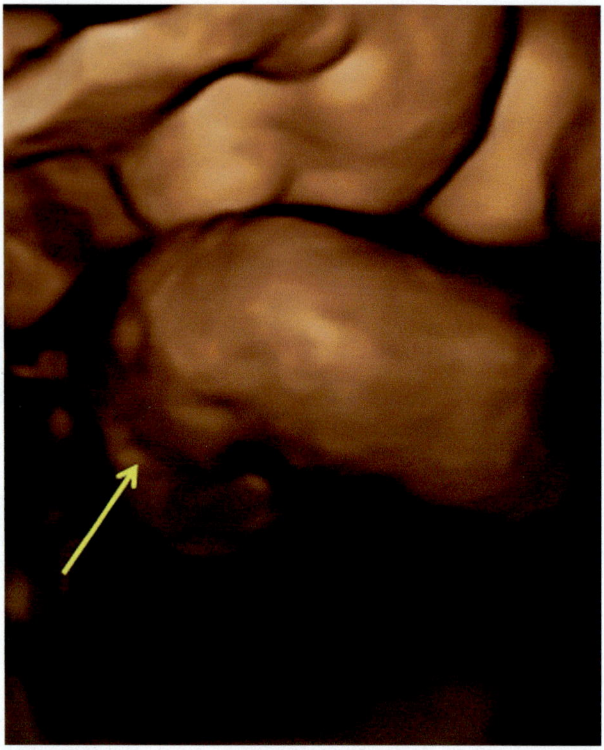

Fig. 13.40 3D surface rendering of the fetal forearm and hand in the forced, abnormal position. Clue for some neurological impairments!

neurological impairments becomes highly relevant as well [142] (Figs. 13.39d and 13.40). The latest state-of-the-art 4D US imaging is far advanced, empowering the clinicians in their precision and efficiency in making a successful diagnosis [142].

Maternal Bonding

Unique process of building relationship and attaching and growing positive maternal feelings toward the fetus and the pregnancy is called maternal-fetal bonding**.** This natural phenomenon gradually develops over the course of pregnancy and culminates right after the child is born [178].

During the years, there has been a range of approaches to promote the development of positive relationships and to observe and assess parent-fetus attachment. The crucial moment was introduction of fetal assessment with the use of ultrasound [179, 180]. Use of Doppler to hear fetal heartbeat and visual presentation by ultrasound imaging was like nothing else before. However, the most remarkable effect was noticed with the introduction of 3D and 4D US imaging in practice with the dynamic imaging of the fetus (real-time imaging) and especially detailed and vivid display of fetal faces (Figs. 13.41, 13.42, 13.43, 13.44, and 13.45). Ji and colleagues

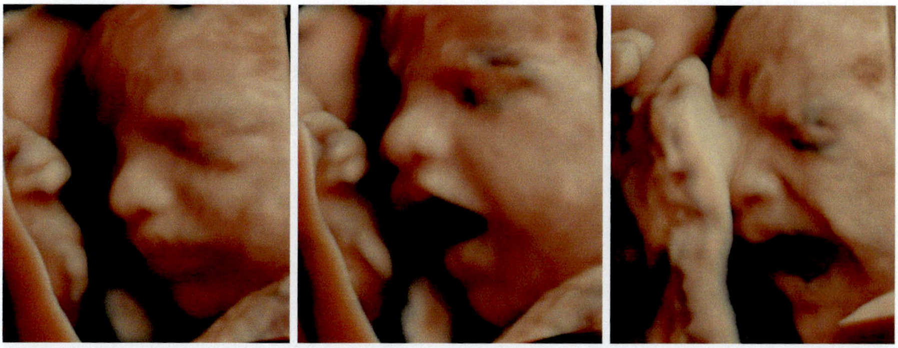

Fig. 13.41 3D/4D HDlive image of fetal face at 31 gw during KANET assessment. Image sequence of fetal yawning clerly displayed by 3D US

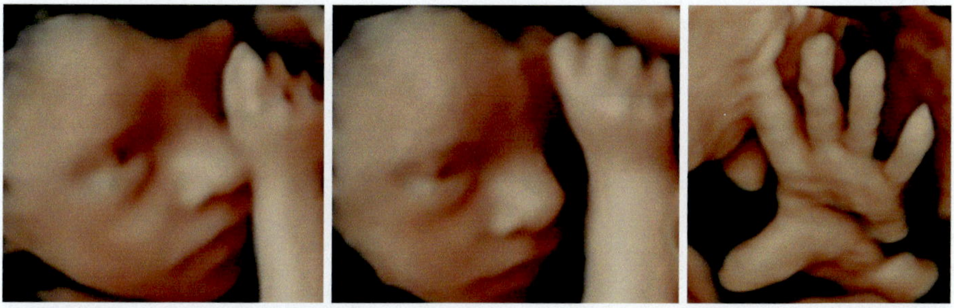

Fig. 13.42 3D/4D HDlive rendering of the fetal face and hand during KANET assessment. Fetus is awake. Notice open eyes

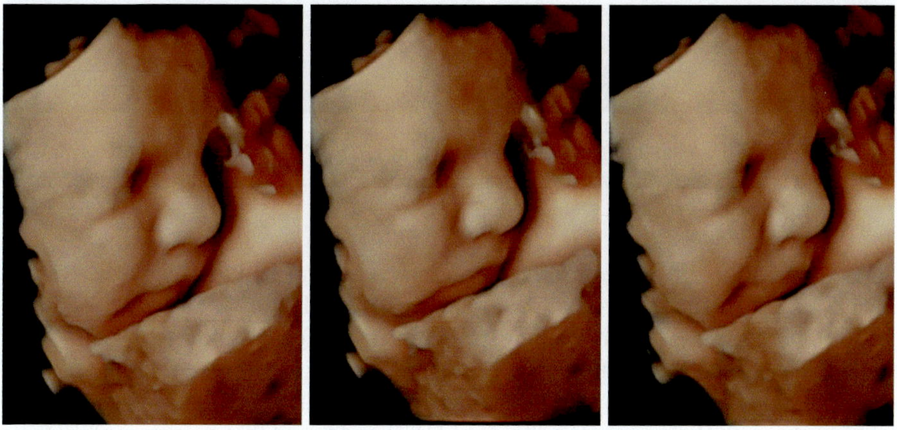

Fig. 13.43 3D/4D HDlive rendering of the fetal face during KANET assessment. Notice smile

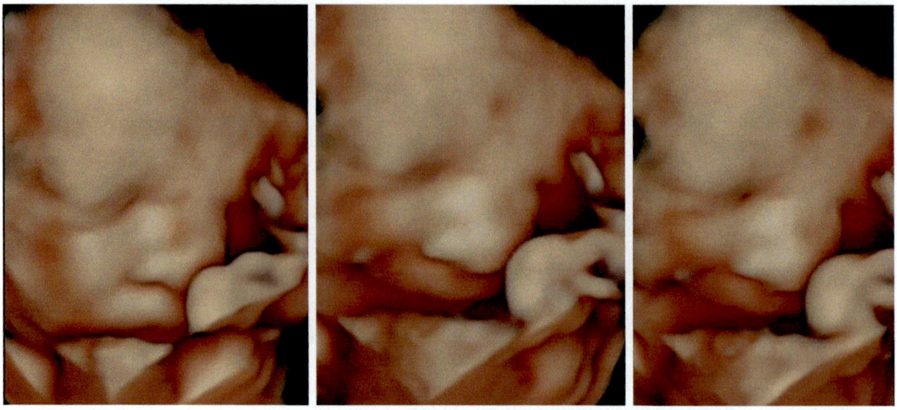

Fig. 13.44 3D HDlive rendering of the fetal face during KANET assessment. Notice smile

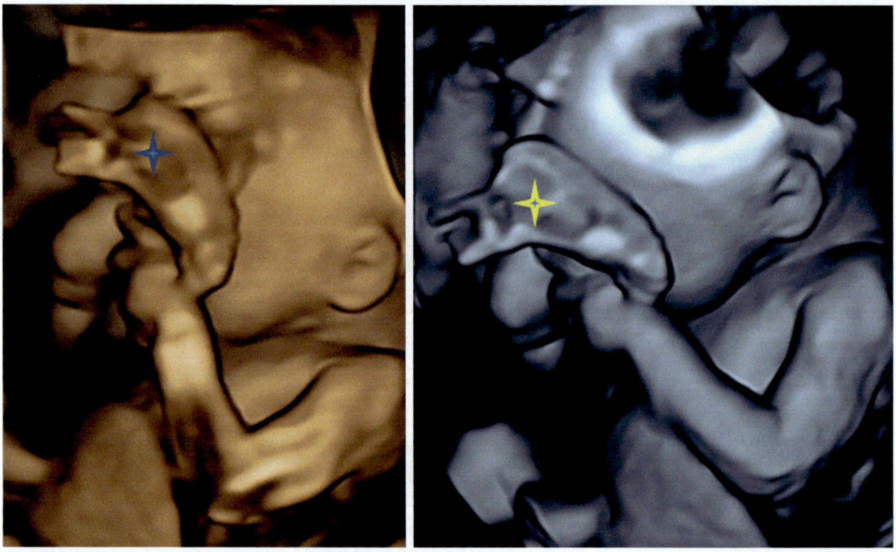

Fig. 13.45 3D surface rendering of the fetal face during KANET assessment of the MCMA twins. Notice foot (star) of one twin kicking in the face of another twin

[179] studied the difference in impact on maternal-fetal bonding between 2D and 3D US imaging. The majority of the mothers expressed their feeling of 'closer relationship with the baby' after being exposed to US images of their fetus, and slight superiority was booked in the 3D US group. These results were confirmed also by other studies that followed [181]. Parental- fetal bonding (both mother and father) was observed by Pretorius and colleagues [182] and found that parents modify their attitude regarding their fetus after experiencing 3D/4DUS. Mothers showed an

increase in bonding to their fetus after 3D/4DUS in more categories than fathers. Detailed review on majority of studies done on this subject was recently published by Rovner et al. [183].

In Summary

Ultrasound technology empowered with 3D/4D US imaging and diverse rendering options nowadays makes an essential and complementary part of diagnostic approach. It improves the physicians' ability and precision in diagnosing fetal anomalies in the prenatal period of life. Realistic images seem to have reassuring and in majority of cases positive effect on parental-fetal bonding .

We all strive to find the solution and prevent different disorders like CP, autism spectrum disorders, and other neurological impairments. Fetal antenatal neurological assessment with the 4D US and application of KANET seem to be helpful and make one of the steps toward the realization of this important aim. Special attention should be paid to doctors education and skill training on 2D, 3D, and 4D US to keep up with new emerging technology in order to benefit the most of it in difficult process of prenatal diagnosis and clinical decision-making [2, 29, 142]. Acquired volumes (3D/4D) can be also sent to a remote site for expert consultation for post-processing analysis.

A personalized approach to each fetus at high risk for any impairment is needed as well as a holistic approach to management and treatment [1, 2].

Global and multidisciplinary collaboration is essential to gain correct data, to see the impact, and to improve both prenatal assessment and postnatal monitoring for the purpose of reaching reasonable conclusions and maximal results [142, 168].

References

1. Kurjak A, Spalldi BL. Controversies on the beginning of human life. In: Kurajak A, Chervenak FA, editors. Donald school embryo as a person and as a patient. New Delhi: Jaypee Brothers Medical Publishers; 2019. p. 28–51.
2. Barišić LS, Kurjak A, Pooh RK. Three-dimensional sonography in fetal syndromes. In: Merz E, Kurjak A, editors. Donald school textbook current status of clinical use of 3D/4D ultrasound in obstetrics and gynecology. New Delhi: Jaypee Brothers Medical Publishers; 2020. p. 300–20.
3. Baba K, Okai T, Satoh K. Development of scan head position indicator for ultrasonic fetal three-dimensional reconstruction. JPN J Med Ultrasonics. 1986;13(Suppl. 1):121–2.
4. Baba K, Satoh K, Sakamoto S, et al. Development of an ultrasonic system for three-dimensional reconstruction of the fetus. J Perinat Med. 1989;17:19–24.
5. Kuo HC, Chang FM, Wu CH, et al. The primary application of three-dimensional ultrasonography in obstetrics. Am J Obstet Gynecol. 1992;166:880–6.
6. Merz E, Bahlmann F, Weber G. Volume scanning in the evaluation of fetal malformations: a new dimension in prenatal diagnosis. Ultrasound Obstet Gynecol. 1995;5:222–7.

7. Merz E, Bahlmann F, Weber G, Macchiella D. Three-dimensional ultrasonography in prenatal diagnosis. J Perinat Med. 1995;23:213–22.
8. Abramowicz JS, Kossoff G, Marsal K, Ter Haar G. Safety Statement, 2000 (reconfirmed 2003). International Society of Ultrasound in Obstetrics and Gynecology (ISUOG). Ultrasound Obstet Gynecol. 2003;21:100. SAFETY- ALARA.
9. Nelson T, Fowlkes J, Abramowicz J, Church C. Ultrasound biosafety considerations for the practicing sonographer and sinologist. Am Institute Ultrasound Med. 2009;28:139–50.
10. Maeda K, Kurjak A. The safe use of ultrasound in obstetrics and gynaecology. Donald School J Ultrasound Obstet Gynaecol. 2012;6(3):313–7.
11. Maeda K, Kurjak A. Diagnostic ultrasound safety. Donald School J Ultrasound Obstet Gynaecol. 2014;8(2):178–83.
12. Pooh RK, Maeda K, Kurjak A, Sen C, Ebrashy A, Adra A, Dayyabu AL, Wataganara T, de Sá RA, Stanojevic M. 3D/4D sonography - any safety problem. J Perinat Med. 2016;44(2):125–9.
13. Huang Q, Zeng Z. A review on real-time 3D ultrasound imaging technology. Biomed Res Int. 2017;2017:6027029.
14. Wang T, Wu J, Huang Q. Enhanced extended-field-of-view ultrasound for musculoskeletal tissues using parallel computing. Curr Med Imaging Rev. 2014;10(4):237–45.
15. Gonçalves LF. Three-dimensional ultrasound of the fetus: how does it help? Pediatr Radiol. 2016;46:177.
16. Tache V, Tarsa M, Romine L, et al. Three-dimensional obstetric ultrasound. Semin Ultrasound CT MR. 2008;29:147–55.
17. Lancellotti P, Zamorano JL, Habib G, Badano LP. The EACVI textbook of echocardiography. 2nd: Oxford University Press; 2016.
18. Nelson TR, Pretorius DH, Hull A, et al. Sources and impact of artifacts on clinical three-dimensional ultrasound imaging. Ultrasound Obstet Gynecol. 2000;16:374–83.
19. Riccabona M. Editorial review: pediatric 3D ultrasound. J Ultrason. 2014;14(56):5–20. https://doi.org/10.15557/JoU.2014.0001.
20. Stanojevic M, Hafner T, Kurjak A. Three-dimensional (3D) ultrasound--a useful imaging technique in the assessment of neonatal brain. J Perinat Med. 2002;30(1):74–83.
21. Smith SW, Trahey GE. von ramm OT. Two-dimensional arrays for medical ultrasound. Ultrason Imaging. 1992;14(3):213–33.
22. Deng J. Nomenclature of 3D and 4D Ultrasound in obstetrics, gynecology and fetal echocardiography. In: Merz E, Kurjak A, editors. Donald school textbook current status of clinical use of 3D/4D ultrasound in obstetrics and gynecology. New Delhi: Jaypee Brothers Medical Publishers; 2020. p. 61–74.
23. Houck RC, Cooke J, Gill EA. Three-dimensional echo: transition from theory to real-time, a technology now ready for prime time. Curr Probl Diagn Radiol. 2005;34(3):85–105.
24. Wang XF, Deng YB, Nanda NC, Deng J, Miller AP, Xie MX. Live three-dimensional echocardiography: imaging principles and clinical application. Echocardiography. 2003;20(7):593–604.
25. Chatterjee R, Deng J, Pellerin D, Todd-Pokropek A, Neild GH, Lees WR, Rodeck CH. Feasibility of dynamic 3-D color Doppler ultrasound for imaging penile vascular change in renal transplant patients with erectile dysfunction responding to sildenafil. Ultrasound Med Biol. 2008;34(6):885–91.
26. Carvalho JS, Allan LD, Chaoui R, Copel JA, DeVore GR, Hecher K, Lee W, Munoz H, Paladini D, Tutschek B, Yagel S. ISUOG practice guidelines (updated): sonographic screening examination of the fetal heart. Ultrasound Obstet Gynecol. 2013;41(3):348–59.
27. Abramowicz JS, Kossoff G, Marsal K, Ter Haar G. ISUOG Bioeffects and Safety Committee. Safety Statement, 2000 (reconfirmed 2003). International Society of Ultrasound in Obstetrics and Gynecology (ISUOG). Ultrasound Obstet Gynecol. 2003;21(1):100.
28. Miric Tesanic D, Merz E. Artifacts and pitfalls in 3D ultrasound. In: Merz E, Kurjak A, editors. Donald school textbook current status of clinical use of 3D/4D ultrasound in obstetrics and gynecology. New Delhi: Jaypee Brothers Medical Publishers; 2020. p. 218–24.

29. Spalldi Barišić L, Stanojević M, Kurjak A, Porović S, Gaber G. Diagnosis of fetal syndromes by three- and four-dimensional ultrasound: is there any improvement? J Perinat Med. 2017;45(6):651–65.
30. Benoit B, Chaoui R. Three-dimensional ultrasound with maximal mode rendering: a novel technique for the diagnosis of bilateral or unilateral absence or hypoplasia of nasal bones in second-trimester screening for Down syndrome. Ultrasound Obstet Gynecol. 2005;25(1):19–24.
31. Kurjak A, Miskovic B, Andonotopo W, Stanojevic M, Azumendi G, Vrcic H. How useful is 3D and 4D ultrasound in perinatal medicine? J Perinat Med. 2007;35(1):10–27.
32. Persico N, Molina F, Azumendi G, Fedele L, Nicolaides KH. Nasal bone assessment in fetuses with trisomy 21 at 16-24 weeks of gestation by three-dimensional ultrasound. Prenat Diagn. 2012;32(3):240–4.
33. Merz E, Pashaj S. Advantages of 3D ultrasound in the assessment of fetal abnormalities. J Perinat Med. 2017;45(6):643–50. https://doi.org/10.1515/jpm-2016-0379.
34. Chaoui R, Heling KS. 3D ultrasound in prenatal diagnosis: a practical approach. 2016. De Gruyter.
35. Pooh RK, Kurjak A. Novel application of three-dimensional HDlive imaging in prenatal diagnosis from the first trimester. J Perinat Med. 2015;43(2):147–58.
36. Pooh RK, Kurjak A. Donald school atlas of advanced ultrasound in obstetrics and gynecology. New Delhi: Jaypee Brothers Medical Publishers; 2015.
37. Bonilla-Musoles F, Raga F, Castillo JC, Bonilla F Jr, Climent MT, Caballero O. High definition real-time ultrasound (HDlive) of embryonic and fetal malformations before week 16. Donald School J Ultrasound Obstet Gynecol. 2013;7:1–8.
38. Kagan KO, Pintoffl K, Hoopmann M. First-trimester ultrasound images using HDlive. Ultrasound Obstet Gynecol. 2011;38:607.
39. Hata T. HDlive rendering image at 6 weeks of gestation. J Med Ultrason. 2013;40:495–6.
40. Hata T, Mashima M, Ito M, Uketa E, Mori N, Ishimura M. Three-dimensional HDlive rendering images of the fetal heart. Ultrasound Med Biol. 2013;39:1513–7.
41. Hanaoka U, Tanaka H, Koyano K, Uematsu R, Kanenishi K, Hata T. HDlive imaging of the face of fetuses with autosomal trisomies. J Med Ultrason. 2014;41:339–42.
42. Pooh RK, Kurjak A. 3D/4D sonography moved prenatal diagnosis of fetal anomalies from the second to the first trimester of pregnancy. J Matern Fetal Neonatal Med. 2012;25:433–55.
43. Pooh RK. Novel application of HDlive Silhouette and HDlive flow: clinical significance of the "see-through fashion" in prenatal diagnosis. Donald School J Ultrasound Obstet Gynecol. 2016;10:90–8.
44. Pooh RK, Kurjak A. Three-dimensional ultrasound in detection of fetal anomalies. Donald School J Ultrasound Obstet Gynecol. 2016;10:214–34.
45. Tonni G, Castigliano AP, Grisolia G, Lithuania M, Meagher S, Da Silva CF, et al. HDlive in early gestation. J Turk Ger Gynecol Assoc. 2016;17:110–9.
46. Pooh RK. Recent advances in 3D ultrasound, silhouette ultrasound, and sonoangiogram in fetal neurology. Donald School J Ultrasound Obstet Gynecol. 2016;10:193–200.
47. Barišić LS, Kurjak A, Pooh RK, Delić T, Stanojević M, Porović S. Antenatal detection of fetal syndromes by ultrasound: from a single piece to a complete puzzle. Donald School J Ultrasound Obstet Gynecol. 2016;10:63–77.
48. Tenkumo C, Hanaoka U, AboEllail MAM, Ishimura M, Morine M, Maeda K, Hata T. HDlive flow with HDlive silhouette mode in diagnosis of fetal hepatic hemangioma. Ultrasound Obstet Gynecol. 2017;49:540–5.
49. Hata T, Kanenishi K, Hanaoka U. HDlive flow silhouette mode for fetal heart. Donald School J Ultrasound Obstet Gynecol. 2019;13(1):10–22.
50. Timor-Tritsch IE, Peisner DB, Raju S. Sonoembryology: an organ-oriented approach using a high-frequency vaginal probe. J Clin Ultrasound. 1990;18:286–98.
51. Benoit B, Hafner T, Kurjak A, Kupesic S, Bekavac I, Bozek T. Three-dimensional sonoembryology. J Perinat Med. 2002;30(1):63–73.

52. Kurjak A, Pooh RK, Merce LT, Carrera JM, Salihagic-Kadic A, Andonotopo W. Structural and functional early human development assessed by three-dimensional and four-dimensional sonography. Fertil Steril. 2005;84(5):1285–99.
53. Blaas H-GK, Eik-Nes SH. Sonoembryology and early prenatal diagnosis of neural anomalies. Prenat Diagn. 2009;29(4):312–25.
54. Pooh RK. Sonoembryology by 3D HDlive silhouette ultrasound - what is added by the "see-through fashion"? J Perinat Med. 2016;44(2):139–48.
55. Pooh RK. A new field of 'fetal sono-ophthalmology' by 3D HDlive silhouette and flow. Donald School J Ultrasound Obstet Gynecol. 2015;9(3):221–2.
56. Pooh RK, Shiota K, Kurjak A. Imaging of the human embryo with magnetic resonance imaging microscopy and high-resolution transvaginal 3-dimensional sonography: human embryology in the 21st century. Am J Obstet Gynecol. 2011;204:77.
57. Hata T, Dai SY, Kanenishi K, Tanaka H. Three-dimensional volume-rendered imaging of embryonic brain vesicles using inversion mode. J Obstet Gynaecol Res. 2009;35:258–61. 31.
58. Pooh RK. Neurosonoembryology by three-dimensional ultrasound. Semin Fetal Neonatal Med. 2012;17:261–8.
59. Kim MS, Jeanty P, Turner C, Benoit B. Three-dimensional sonographic evaluations of embryonic brain development. J Ultrasound Med. 2008;27:119–24.
60. Kim JG. Ultrasonographic evaluation of embryonic cardiac development. In: Kurajak A, Chervenak FA, editors. Donald school embryo as a person and as a patient. New Delhi: Jaypee Brothers Medical Publishers; 2019. p. 105–16.
61. Wilson RD, Johnson MP. Congenital abdominal wall defects: an update. Fetal Diagn Ther. 2004;19(5):385–98.
62. Pooh RK. Sonoembryology. In: Kurajak A, Chervenak FA, editors. Donald school embryo as a person and as a patient. New Delhi: Jaypee Brothers Medical Publishers; 2019. p. 19–28.
63. Merz E, Pashaj S. Embryonic and early fetal abnormalities diagnosed with 3D US in the first trimester. In: Kurajak A, Chervenak FA, editors. Donald school embryo as a person and as a patient. New Delhi: Jaypee Brothers Medical Publishers; 2019. p. 51–65.
64. Merz E, Pashaj S. What is known about corpus callosum prenatally? Donald School J Ultrasound Obstet Gynecol. 2016;10:163–9.
65. Pashaj S, Merz E. Advantage of 3D US in exact diagnosis of normal and abnormal corpus callosum. Donald school textbook current status of clinical use of 3D/4D ultrasound in obstetrics and gynecology. In Merz E, Kurjak A (ed). New Delhi: Jaypee Brothers Medical Publishers 2020. 252–262.
66. Bonilla-Musoles F, Raga F, Castillo JC, Bonilla F Jr, Climent MT, Caballero O. High definition real-time ultrasound (HDlive) of embryonic and fetal malformations before week 16. Donald School J Ultrasound Obstet Gynecol. 2013;7:1–8.
67. Boitor-Borza D, Kovacs T, Stamatian F. Ganglionic eminence within the early developing brain visualized by 3D transvaginal ultrasound. Med Ultrason. 2015;17(3):289–94.
68. Tan S, Gülden Tangal N, Kanat-Pektas M, Sirin Özcan A, Levent Keskin H, Akgündüz G. Abnormal sonographic appearances of the yolk sac: which can be associated with adverse perinatal outcome? Med Ultrason. 2014;16(1):15–20.
69. Merz E. Transvaginal dertection of fetal anomalies. In: Merz E, Bahlmann F, editors. Ultrasound in obstetrics and gynecology. Stuttgart, New York: Thieme; 2005. p. 45–8.
70. Solomon BD, Gropman A, Muenke M. Holoprosencephaly overview. GeneReviews. 2013; http://www.ncbi.nlm.nih.gov/books/NBK1530/.
71. Kagan KO, Staboulidou I, Syngelaki A, Cruz J, Nicolaides KH. The 11–13-week scan: diagnosis and outcome of holoprosencephaly, exomphalos and megacystis. Ultrasound Obstet Gynecol. 2010;36(1):10–4.
72. Kruszka P, Muenke M. Syndromes associated with holoprosencephaly. Am J Med Genet C Semin Med Genet. 2018;178(2):229–37.
73. Benacerraf BR. Ultrasound of fetal syndromes. 2nd ed. London: Churchill Livingstone; 2008.

74. Brioude F, Kalish JM, Mussa A, Foster AC, Bliek J, Ferrero GB, et al. Clinical and molecular diagnosis, screening and management of Beckwith–Wiedemann syndrome: an international consensus statement. Nat Rev Endocrinol. 2018;14(4):229–49.
75. Wilkins-Haug L, Porter A, Hawley P, Benson CB. Isolated fetal omphalocele, Beckwith-Wiedemann syndrome, and assisted reproductive technologies. Birth Defects Res A Clin Mol Teratol. 2009;85(1):58–62.
76. Johnson JP, Beischel L, Schwanke C, Styren K, Crunk A, Schoof J, Elias AF. Overrepresentation of pregnancies conceived by artificial reproductive technology in prenatally identified fetuses with Beckwith-Wiedemann syndrome. J Assist Reprod Genet. 2018;35(6):985–92.
77. Wilson RD, Johnson MP. Congenital abdominal wall defects: an update. Fetal Diagn Ther. 2004;19(5):385–98.
78. Voskamp BJ, Fleurke-Rozema H, Oude-Rengerink K, Snijders RJ, Bilardo CM, Mol BW, et al. Relationship of isolated single umbilical artery to fetal growth, aneuploidy and perinatal mortality: systematic review and meta-analysis. Ultrasound Obstet Gynecol. 2013;42(6):622–8.
79. Pharoah PO, Cooke RW. A hypothesis for the aetiology of spastic cerebral palsy--the vanishing twin. Dev Med Child Neurol. 1997;39(5):292–6.
80. Blickstein I. Cerebral palsy in multifoetal pregnancies: facts and hypotheses. In: Chervenak FA, Kurjak A, editors. Fetal medicine: the clinical care of the fetus as a patient. London: Parthenon Publishing; 1999. p. 368–73.
81. Pharoah PO, Adi Y. Consequences of in-utero death in a twin pregnancy. Lancet. 2000;355:1597–602.
82. Monni MC, Iuculano A, Peddes C, Corda V, Monni G. Vanishing twin syndrome. In: Kurajak A, Chervenak FA, editors. Donald school embryo as a person and as a patient. New Delhi: Jaypee Brothers Medical Publishers; 2019. p. 121–31.
83. Jauniaux E, Nicolaides KH, Hustin J. Perinatal features associated with placental mesenchymal dysplasia. Placenta. 1997;18:701–6.
84. Parveen Z, Tongson-Ignacio JE, Frasier CR, Killeen JL, Thompson KS. Placental mesenchymal dysplasia. Arch Pathol Lab Med. 2007;131:131–7.
85. Umazume T, Kataoka S, Kamamuta K, et al. Placental mesenchymal dysplasia, a case of intrauterine sudden death of fetus with rupture of cirsoid periumbilical chorionic vessels. Diagn Pathol. 2011;6:38.
86. Honemeyer U. Three-dimensional ultrasound imaging in the diagnosis of ectopic pregnancy. In: Merz E, Kurajak A, editors. Donald school textbook current status of clinical use of 3D/4D ultrasound in obstetrics and gynecology. New Delhi: Jaypee Brothers Medical Publishers; 2020. p. 152–68.
87. Panchal S. Three-dimensional ultrasound in infertility and ectopic pregnancy. In: Merz E, Kurajak A, editors. Donald school textbook current status of clinical use of 3D/4D ultrasound in obstetrics and gynecology. New Delhi: Jaypee Brothers Medical Publishers; 2020. p. 225–51.
88. Jones KL. Smith's recognizable patterns of human malformation. 5th ed. Philadelphia: Elsevier Saunders; 1997.
89. Rotten D, Levaillant JM, Martinez H, Ducou Le Pointe H, Vicaut E. The fetal mandible: a 2D and 3D sonographic approach to the diagnosis of retrognathia and micrognathia. Ultrasound Obstet Gynecol. 2002;19:122–30.
90. Borenstein M, Persico N, Kaihura C, Sonek J, Nicolaides KH. Frontomaxillary facial angle in chromosomally normal fetuses at 11 + 0 to 13 + 6 weeks. Ultrasound Obstet Gynecol. 2007;30:737–41.
91. Borenstein M, Persico N, Strobl I, Sonek J, Nicolaides KH. Frontomaxillary and mandibulomaxillary facial angles at 11+0 to 13+6 weeks in fetuses with trisomy 18. Ultrasound Obstet Gynecol. 2007;30:928–33.
92. Zalel Y, Gindes L, Achiron R. The fetal mandible: an in utero sonographic evaluation between 11 and 31 weeks' gestation. Prenat Diagn. 2006;26:163–7.

93. Roelfsema NM, Hop WCJ, Wladimiroff JW. Three-dimensional sonographic determination of normal fetal mandibular and maxillary size during the second half of pregnancy. Ultrasound Obstet Gynecol. 2006;28:950–7.
94. Sonek J, Borenstein M, Dagklis T, Persico N, Nicolaides KH. Frontomaxillary facial angle in fetuses with trisomy 21 at 11–13(6) weeks. Am J Obstet Gynecol. 2007;196:271.e1–4.
95. Snijders RJM, Noble P, Sebire N, Souka A, Nicolaides KH. UK multicentre project on assessment of risk of trisomy 21 by maternal age and fetal nuchal translucency thickness at 10–14 weeks of gestation. Lancet. 1998;351:343–6.
96. Teoh M, Meagher S. First-trimester diagnosis of micrognathia as a presentation of Pierre Robin syndrome. Ultrasound Obstet Gynecol. 2003;21:616–8.
97. Tsai MY, Lan KC, Ou CY, Chen JH, Chang SY, Hsu TY. Assessment of the facial features and chin development of fetuses with use of serial three-dimensional sonography and the mandibular size monogram in a Chinese population. Am J Obstet Gynecol. 2004;190:541–6.
98. Evans AK, Rahbar R, Rogers GF, Mulliken JB, Volk MS. Robin sequence: a retrospective review of 115 patients. Int J Pediatr Otorhinolaryngol. 2006;70:973–80.
99. Too SC, Ahmad Sarji S, Yik S, Ramanujam TM. Malignant epignathus teratoma. Biomed Imaging Interv J. 2008;4:18.
100. Kumar SY, Shrikrishna U, Shetty J, Sitaram A. Epignathus with fetiform features. J Lab Physicians. 2011;3(1):56–8.
101. Johnson JM, Moonis G, Green GE, Carmody R, Burbank HN. Syndromes of the first and second branchial arches, part 2: syndromes. Am J Neuroradiol. 2011;32:230–7.
102. Castori M, Brancati F, Rinaldi R, Adami L, Mingarelli R, Grammatico P, et al. Antenatal presentation of the oculo-auriculo-vertebral spectrum (OAVS). Am J Med Genet A. 2006;140:1573–9.
103. Miller TD, Metry D. Multiple accessory tragi as a clue to the diagnosis of the oculo-auriculo-vertebral (Goldenhar) syndrome. J Am Acad Dermatol. 2004;50(2 Suppl):S11–3.
104. Martinelli P, Maurotti GM, Agangi A, Mazzarelli LL, Bifulco G, Paladini D. Prenatal diagnosis of hemifacial microsomia and ipsilateral cerebellar hypoplasia in a fetus with oculoauriculovertebral spectrum. Ultrasound Obstet Gynecol. 2004;24:199–201.
105. Wang R, Martinez-Frias ML, Graham JM Jr. Infants of diabetic mothers are at increased risk for the oculo-auriculo-vertebral sequence: a case-based and case-control approach. J Pediatr. 2002;141:611–7.
106. Paul A, Trainor PA, Dixon J, Dixon MJ. Treacher Collins syndrome: etiology, pathogenesis and prevention. Eur J Hum Genet. 2009;17:275–83.
107. Jones NC, Lynn ML, Gaudenz K, Sakai D, Aoto K, Rey JP, et al. Prevention of the neurocristopathy Treacher Collins syndrome through inhibition of p53 function. Nat Med. 2008;14:125–33.
108. Pereira DC, Bussamra LC, Araujo Júnior E, Drummond CL, Nardozza LM, Moron AF, et al. Prenatal diagnosis of Treacher-Collins syndrome using three-dimensional ultrasonography and differential diagnosis with other acrofacial dysostosis syndromes. Case Rep Obstet Gynecol. 2013;2013:203976.
109. Faro C, Benoit B, Wegrzyn P, Chaoui R, Nicolaides KH. Three-dimensional sonographic description of the fetal frontal bones and metopic suture. Ultrasound Obstet Gynecol. 2005;26(6):618–21.
110. Chaoui R, Levaillant JM, Benoit B, Faro C, Wegrzyn P, Nicolaides KH. Three-dimensional sonographic description of abnormal metopic suture in second- and third-trimester fetuses. Ultrasound Obstet Gynecol. 2005;26(7):761–4.
111. Winter TC, Kennedy AM, Byrne J, Woodward PJ. The cavum septi pellucidi: why is it important? J Ultrasound Med. 2010;29(3):427–44.
112. International Society of Ultrasound in Obstetrics and Gynecology Education Committee. Sonographic examination of the fetal central nervous system: guidelines for performing the "basic examination" and the "fetal neurosonogram.". Ultrasound Obstet Gynecol. 2007;29:109–16.

113. McGahan J, Pilu G, Nyberg D. Cerebral malformations. In: Nyberg D, McGahan J, Pretorius D, Pilu G, editors. Diagnostic imaging of fetal anomalies. Philadelphia: Lippincott Williams & Wilkins; 2003. p. 221–90.
114. Callen PW, Callen AL, Glenn OA, Toi A. Columns of the fornix, not to be mistaken for the cavum septi pellucidi on prenatal sonography. J Ultrasound Med. 2008;27:25–31.
115. Barkovich AJ, Norman D. Absence of the septum pellucidum: a useful sign in the diagnosis of congenital brain malformations. AJR Am J Roentgenol. 1989;152:353–60.
116. Filly RA, Cardoza JD, Goldstein RB, Barkovich AJ. Detection of fetal central nervous system anomalies: a practical level of effort for a routine sonogram. Radiology. 1989;172:403–8.
117. Esin S, Tarim E, Şen C. Three-dimensional ultrasonographic evaluation of the fetal posterior fossa. In: Merz E, Kurajak A, editors. Donald school textbook current status of clinical use of 3D/4D ultrasound in obstetrics and gynecology. New Delhi: Jaypee Brothers Medical Publishers; 2020. p. 296–9.
118. Pooh RK, Kurjak A. 3D and 4D sonography and magnetic resonance in the assessment of normal and abnormal CNS development: alternative or complementary. J Perinat Med. 2011;39(1):3–13.
119. Benoit B. The value of three-dimensional ultrasonography in the screening of the fetal skeleton. Childs Nerv Syst. 2003;19(7–8):403–9.
120. Yagel S, Cohen SM, Shapiro I, Messing B, Valsky DV. Three- and four dimensional ultrasound in fetal echocardiography: a new look at the fetal heart. In: Merz E, Kurjak A, editors. Donald school textbook current status of clinical use of 3D/4D ultrasound in obstetrics and gynecology. New Delhi: Jaypee Brothers Medical Publishers; 2020. p. 321–44.
121. Gonçalves LF, Lee W, Chaiworapongsa T, et al. Four-dimensional ultrasonography of the fetal heart with spatio-temporal image correlation. Am J Obstet Gynecol. 2003;189:1792–802.
122. Yagel S, Cohen SM, Shapiro I, Valsky DV. 3D and 4D ultrasound in fetal cardiac scanning: a new look at the fetal heart. Ultrasound Obstet Gynecol. 2007;29:81–95.
123. Gonçalves LF, Espinoza J, Romero R, Kusanovic JP, Swope B, Nien JK, Erez O, Soto E, Treadwell MC. Four-dimensional ultrasonography of the fetal heart using a novel Tomographic Ultrasound Imaging (TUI) display. J Perinat Med. 2006;34(1):39–55.
124. Espinoza J, Gonçalves LF, Lee W, Mazor M, Romero R. A novel method to improve prenatal diagnosis of abnormal systemic venous connections using three- and four-dimensional ultrasonography and 'inversion mode'. Ultrasound Obstet Gynecol. 2005;25(5):428–34.
125. Veronese P, Bogana G, Cerutti A, Yeo L, Romero R, Gervasi MT. A prospective study of the use of fetal intelligent navigation echocardiography (FINE) to obtain standard fetal echocardiography views. Fetal Diagn Ther. 2017;41(2):89–99.
126. Yeo L, Luewan S, Markush D, Gill N, Romero R. Prenatal diagnosis of dextrocardia with complex congenital heart disease using fetal intelligent navigation echocardiography (FINE) and a literature review. Fetal Diagn Ther. 2018;43(4):304–16.
127. Nijhuis JG. Neurobehavioral development of the fetal brain. In: Nijhuis JG, editor. Fetal behaviour: developmental and perinatal aspects. Oxford, UK: Oxford University Press; 1992. p. 489.
128. Nijhuis JG. Fetal behavior. Neurobiol Aging. 2003;24:41–6.
129. Prechtl HF. Qualitative changes of spontaneous movements in fetus and preterm infant are a marker of neurological dysfunction. Early Hum Dev. 1990;23(3):151–8.
130. De Vries JIP, Visser GHA, Prechtl HFR. The emergence of fetal behavior. Individual differencies and consistencies. Early Hum Dev. 1988;16:85–103.
131. Kurjak A, Carrera J, Medic M, Azumendi G, Andonotopo W, Stanojevic M. The antenatal development of fetal behavioral patterns assessed by four-dimensional sonography. J Matern Fetal Neonatal Med. 2005;17(6):401–16.
132. Kurjak A, Tikvica A, Stanojevic M, Miskovic B, Ahmed B, Azumendi G, Di Renzo GC. Assessment of fetal neurobehavior by 3D/4D ultrasound. J Matern Fetal Neonatal Med. 2008;21(10):675–84.

133. Kurjak A, Miskovic B, Stanojevic M, Amiel-Tison C, Ahmed B, Azumendi G, et al. New scoring system for fetal neurobehavior assessed by three- and four-dimensional sonography. J Perinat Med. 2008;36(1):73–81.
134. Stanojevic M, Antsaklis P, Kadic AS, Predojevic M, Vladareanu R, Vladareanu S, et al. Is kurjak antenatal neurodevelopmental test ready for routine clinical application? Bucharest consensus statement. Donald School J Ultrasound Obstet Gynecol. 2015;9:260–5.
135. Kurjak A, Abo-Yaqoub S, Stanojevic M, Yigiter AB, Vasilj O, Lebit D, et al. The potential of 4D sonography in the assessment of fetal neurobehavior – multicentric study in high-risk pregnancies. J Perinat Med. 2010;38:77–82.
136. Stanojevic M, Talic A, Miskovic B, et al. An attempt to standardize Kurjak's antenatal neurodevelopmental test: Osaka Consensus Statement. Donald School J Ultrasound Obstet Gynecol. 2011;5:317–29.
137. Yigiter AB, Kavak ZN. Normal standards of fetal behavior assessed by four-dimensional sonography. J Matern Fetal Neonatal Med. 2006;19:707–21.
138. Rees S, Harding R. Brain development during fetal life: influences of the intrauterine environment. Neurosci Lett. 2004;361:111–4.
139. Joseph R. Fetal brain and cognitive development. Dev Rev. 1999;20:81–98.
140. Kurjak A, Carrera JM, Stanojevic M, et al. The role of 4D sonography in the neurological assessment of early human development. Ultrasound Rev Obstet Gynecol. 2004;4:148–59.
141. Kurjak A, Antsaklis P. Four-dimensional ultrasound in functional studies of the fetus. In: Merz E, Kurajak A, editors. Donald school textbook current status of clinical use of 3D/4D ultrasound in obstetrics and gynecology. New Delhi: Jaypee Brothers Medical Publishers; 2020. p. 198–209.
142. Kurjak A, Spalldi Barišić L, Stanojević M, Antsaklis P, Panchal S, Honemeyer U, et al. Multicenter results on the clinical use of KANET. J Perinat Med. 2019;47(9):897–909.
143. Kurjak A, Stanojević M, Andonotopo W, Salihagic-Kadic A, Carrera JM, Azumendi G. Behavioral pattern continuity from prenatal to postnatal life – a study by four-dimensional (4D) ultrasonography. J Perinat Med. 2004;32:346–53.
144. Kurjak A, Stanojevic M, Andonotopo W, et al. Fetal behavior assessed in all three trimesters of normal pregnancy by four-dimensional ultrasonography. Croat Med J. 2005;46:772–80.
145. Stanojevic M, Kurjak A, Salihagic-Kadic A, et al. Neurobehavioral continuity from fetus to neonate. J Perinat Med. 2011;39:171–7.
146. Tomasovic S, Predojevic M. Four-dimensional ultrasound medical devices for recent advances on the etiology of cerebral palsy. Acta Inform Med. 2011;19:228–34. Vladareanu R, Lebit D, Constantinescu S. Ultrasound assessment of fetal neurobehavior in high-risk pregnancies. Donald School J Ultrasound Obstet Gynecol. 2012;6:132–47.
147. Honemeyer U, Talic A, Therwat A, Paulose I, Patidar R. The clinical value of KANET test in studying fetal neurobehavior in normal and at-risk pregnancies. J Perinat Med. 2013;41:187–97.
148. Kuno A, Akiyama M, Yamashiro C, Tanaka H, Yanagihara T, Hata T. Three-dimensional sonographic assessment of fetal behaviour in the early second trimester of pregnancy. J Ultrasound Med. 2001;20:1271–5.
149. Salihagic KA. Fetal neurology: the role of fetal stress. Donald School J Ultrasound Obstet Gynecol. 2015;9:30–9.
150. Hata T, Kanenishi J, Hanoka U, Uematsu R, Marumo G, Tanaka H. HDlive study of fetal development and behavior. Donald School J Ultrasound Obstet Gynecol. 2014;8:250–65.
151. Reynoso C, Crespo-Eguílaz N, Alcázar JL, Narbona J. Motor behavior of human fetuses during the second trimester of gestation: a longitudinal ultrasound study. An Pediatr (Barc). 2015;82:183–91.
152. Predojević M, Talić A, Stanojević M, Kurjak A, Salihagić KA. Assessment of motoric and hemodynamic parameters in growth restricted fetuses – case study. J Matern Fetal Neonatal Med. 2014;27:247–51.

153. Kurjak A, Talic A, Stanojevic M, Honemeyer U, Serra B, Prats P, et al. The study of fetal neurobehavior in twins in all three trimesters of pregnancy. J Matern Fetal Neonatal Med. 2013;26:1186–95.
154. Kurjak A, Talic A, Honemeyer U, Stanojevic M, Zalud I. Comparison between antenatal neurodevelopmental test and fetal Doppler in the assessment of fetal wellbeing. J Perinat Med. 2013;41:107–14.
155. Athanasiadis AP, Mikos T, Tambakoudis GP, Theodoridis TD, Papastergiou M, Assimakopoulos E, et al. Neurodevelopmental fetal assessment using KANET scoring system in low and high risk pregnancies. J Matern Fetal Neonatal Med. 2013;26:363–8.
156. Guimarães Filho HA, Araujo Júnior E, Mello Júnior CF, Nardozza LM, Moron AF. Assessment of fetal behavior using four-dimensional ultrasonography: current knowledge and perspectives. Rev Assoc Med Bras. 2013;59:507–13.
157. Kurjak A, Stanojević M, Predojević M, Laušin I, Salihagić KA. Neurobehavior in fetal life. Semin Fetal Neonatal Med. 2012;17:319–23.
158. Stanojevic M, Zaputovic S, Bosnjak AP. Continuity between fetal and neonatal neurobehavior. Semin Fetal Neonatal Med. 2012;17:324–9.
159. Kurjak A, Predojevic M, Stanojevic M, Kadic AS, Miskovic B, Badreldeen A, et al. Intrauterine growth restriction and cerebral palsy. Acta Inform Med. 2012;18:64–82.
160. Talic A, Kurjak A, Stanojevic M, Honemeyer U, Badreldeen A, DiRenzo GC. The assessment of fetal brain function in fetuses with ventrikulomegaly: the role of the KANET test. J Matern Fetal Neonatal Med. 2012;25:1267–72.
161. Talic A, Kurjak A, Ahmed B, Stanojevic M, Predojevic M, Kadic AS, et al. The potential of 4D sonography in the assessment of fetal behavior in high-risk pregnancies. J Matern Fetal Neonatal Med. 2011;24:948–54.
162. Kurjak A, Antsaklis P, Stanojević M, Vladareanu R, Vladareanu S, Moreira Neto R, et al. Multicentric studies of the fetal neurobehavior by KANET. J Perinat Med. 2017;45:717–27.
163. Miskovic B, Vasilj O, Stanojevic M, Ivanković D, Kerner M, Tikvica A. The comparison of fetal behavior in high risk and normal pregnancies assessed by four dimensional ultrasound. J Matern Fetal Neonatal Med. 2010;23:1461–7.
164. Honemeyer U, Kurjak A. The use of KANET test to assess fetal CNS function. First 100 cases. 10th World Congress of Perinatal Medicine 8–11 November 2011. Uruguay: Poster Presentation P. 209.
165. Abo-Yaqoub S, Kurjak A, Mohammed AB, Shadad A, Abdel-Maaboud M. The role of 4-D ultrasonography in prenatal assessment of fetal neurobehaviour and prediction of neurological outcome. J Matern Fetal Neonatal Med. 2012;25:231–6.
166. Hanaoka U, Hata T, Kanenishi K, AboEllail MAM, Uematsu R, Konishi Y, et al. Does ethnicity have an effect on fetal behavior? A comparison of Asian and Caucasian populations. J Perinat Med. 2016;44:217–21.
167. Hata T, Hanaoka U, AboEllail MAM, Uematsu R, Noguchi J, Kusaka T, et al. Is there a sex difference in fetal behavior? A comparison of the KANET test between male and female fetuses. J Perinat Med. 2016;44:585–8.
168. Antsaklis P, Porovic S, Daskalakis G, Kurjak A. 4D assessment of fetal brain function in diabetic patients. J Perinat Med. 2017;45:711–5.
169. Hata T, Kanenishi K, Mori N, Abo Ellail MAM, Hanaoka U, Koyano K, et al. Prediction of postnatal developmental disabilities using the antenatal fetal neurodevelopmental test: KANET assessment. J Perinat Med. 2018;47:77–81.
170. MacLennan AH, Thompson SC, Gecz J. Cerebral palsy: causes, pathways, and the role of genetic variants. Australian Collaborative Cerebral Palsy Research Group. Am J Obstet Gynecol. 2015;213:779–88.
171. Kurjak A, Stanojevic M, Azumendi G, Carrera JM. The potential of four-dimensional (4D) ultrasonography in the assessment of fetal awareness. J Perinat Med. 2005;33(1):46–53.

172. Kurjak A, Barišić LS, Stanojević M, Kadić AS, Porović S. Are we ready to investigate cognitive function of fetal brain? The role of advanced four-dimensional sonography. Donald School J Ultrasound Obstet Gynecol. 2016;10:116–24.
173. Haak P, Lenski M, Hidecker MJ, Li M, Paneth N. Cerebral palsy and aging. Dev Med Child Neurol. 2009;51:16–23.
174. Robinson EB, St Pourcain B, Anttila V, Kosmicki JA, Bulik-Sullivan B, Grove J, et al. Genetic risk for autism spectrum disorders and neuropsychiatric variation in the general population. Nat Genet. 2016;48:552–5.
175. Kunze A, Achilles A, Keiner S, Witte OW, Redecker C. Two distinct populations of double cortin-positive cells in the perilesional zone of cortical infarcts. BMC Neurosci. 2015;16:20.
176. Kunze A, Grass S, Witte OW, Yamaguchi M, Kempermann G, Redecker C. Proliferative response of distinct hippocampal progenitor cell populations after cortical infarcts in the adult brain. Neurobiol Dis. 2006;21:324–32.
177. Barker DJ. The developmental origins of chronic adult disease. Acta Paediatr Suppl. 2004;93:26–33.
178. Leckman JF, Feldman R, Swain JE, Eicher V, Thompson N, Mayes LC. Primary parental preoccupation: circuits, genes, and the crucial role of the environment. J Neural Transm (Vienna). 2004;111(7):753–71.
179. Ji E, Pretorius D, Newton R, Uyans K, Hull A, Hollenbach K, et al. Effects of ultrasound on maternal-fetal bonding: a comparison of 2D and 3D imaging. Ultrasound Obstet Gynecol. 2005;25:473–7.
180. Campbell S. Opinion. 4D and prenatal bonding: still more questions than answers. Ultrasound Obstet Gynecol. 2006;27:243–4.
181. de Jong-Pleij EA, Ribbert LS, Pistorius LR, Tromp E, Mulder EJ, Bilardo CM. Three-dimensional ultrasound and maternal bonding, a third trimester study and a review. Prenat Diagn. 2013;33(1):81–8.
182. Pretorius DH, Gattu S, Ji EK, Hollenbach K, Newton R, Hull A, Carmona S, D'Agostini D, et al. Preexamination and postexamination assessment of parental-fetal bonding in patients undergoing 3-/4-dimensional obstetric ultrasonography. J Ultrasound Med. 2006;25(11):1411–21.
183. Rovner LM, Horton KT, Perez MI, Pretorius DH. Three-dimensional ultrasoundand maternal bonding. In: Merz E, Kurajak A, editors. Donald school textbook current status of clinical use of 3D/4D ultrasound in obstetrics and gynecology. New Delhi: Jaypee Brothers Medical Publishers; 2020. p. 263–73.

Chapter 14
First-Trimester Ultrasonography

Fernando Maia Peixoto-Filho and Paulo Roberto Nassar de Carvalho

Introduction

Transvaginal ultrasound provides a dynamic view of embryonic development and ensures a detailed outline of the anatomical changes that occur in the first trimester of pregnancy [18]. Due to the proximity of the structures investigated by the transvaginal route, it is possible to use probes with higher frequencies, which determines the acquisition of image performance, and association with other biochemical s with higher resolution (Fig. 14.1). Confirmation of pregnancy by transvaginal ultrasound is only possible between 4 and 5 weeks of gestational age. Using the pelvic approach, the earliest possible diagnosis is later, between 5 and 6 weeks of gestation.

Main objectives of first-trimester ultrasound:

- Confirm pregnancy
- Location of the gestational sac
- Assessment of viability
- Detect signs of early pregnancy loss (Fig. 14.2)
- Define single or multiple pregnancy
- Define chorionicity in multiple (Figs. 14.3 and 14.4)
- Gestation dating
- Assess the normality of the embryo and gestational sac (before 10 weeks)
- Assess risk of aneuploidies and basic anatomy (after 11 weeks)

F. M. Peixoto-Filho (✉) · P. R. N. de Carvalho
Instituto Fernandes Figueira, Rio de Janeiro, Fundação Oswaldo Cruz –FIOCRUZ, Rio de Janeiro, Brazil

IETECS – Instituto de Estudos de Tecnologia em Saúde, Rio de Janeiro, Brazil

Grupo Perinatal, Rio de Janeiro, Brazil
e-mail: fernandomaia@ietecs.com.br; paulonassar@ietecs.com.br

© Springer Nature Switzerland AG 2022

R. A. Moreira de Sá, E. B. d. Fonseca (eds.), *Perinatology*,
https://doi.org/10.1007/978-3-030-83434-0_14

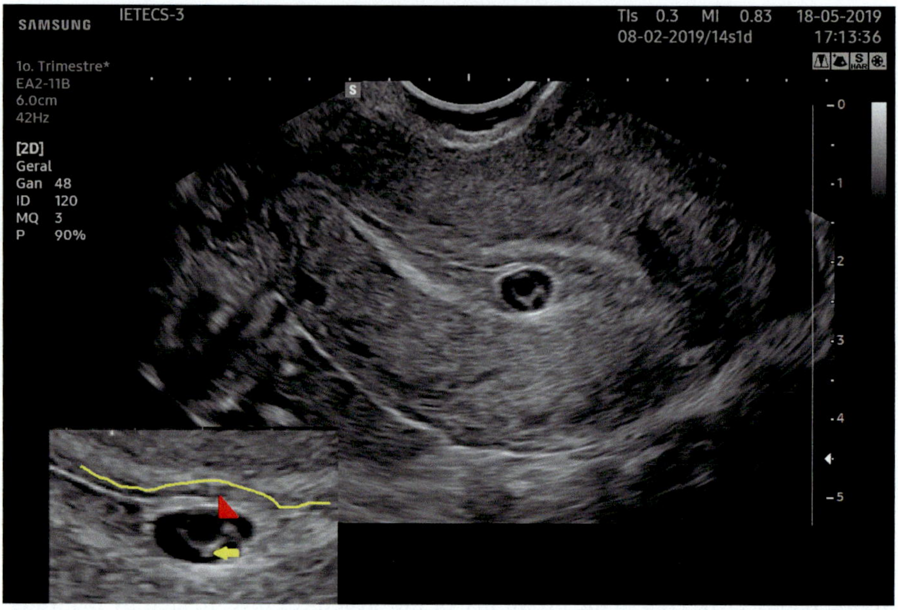

Fig. 14.1 Transvaginal scan demonstrating a gestational sac with eccentric location (yellow line in detail) and a collapsed uterine cavity visualized as a thin echogenic line. Observe the presence of a yolk sac (red arrow) and the embryo (yellow arrow) inside the gestational sac

First-Trimester Ultrasound Between 5 and 10 Weeks

At the end of the fourth week of gestation, the blastocyst cannot be identified on ultrasound yet, as it still measures 1 mm. The threshold size for visualizing the gestational sac transvaginally is 2–3 mm, which corresponds to 4 weeks and 1 day of gestational age (GA). The yolk sac is the first embryonic anatomical structure visible in the gestational sac transvaginally around the beginning of the fifth week of GA (Fig. 14.1). It is important to evaluate the shape, diameter, texture, and contour of the yolk sac.

Usually, the earliest evaluation of gestation subsequent to assisted fertilization or stimulated cycles is carried out between the sixth and seventh week, with the aim of confirming the presence of pregnancy, the number of embryos in evolution, gestational location (topical or ectopic), and prognosis. Crown-rump length (CRL) is the most reliable measure to determine the date of pregnancy in this period [14]. The gestational sac, the embryo, and the embryonic heart rate increase linearly with GA, with the heart rate peaking at 7–8 weeks.

At approximately the sixth week, a complex formed by the yolk sac and an embryo with a heartbeat can be observed within the gestational sac. The measurement of the embryo's crown-rump length provides an accurate determination of the GA. Cardiac activity has been demonstrated from the 37th day of GA [7]. Generally, the embryo is readily visible when it measures more than 5 mm, which corresponds to approximately 6 weeks and an embryonic heart rate (EHR) exceeding 90 bpm [21]. Occasionally, the embryo can be identified when the embryonic disc reaches 1–2 mm between the fifth and sixth weeks of gestation, and the embryo's cardiac activity can be perceived when the embryo reaches 4–5 mm (6 weeks).

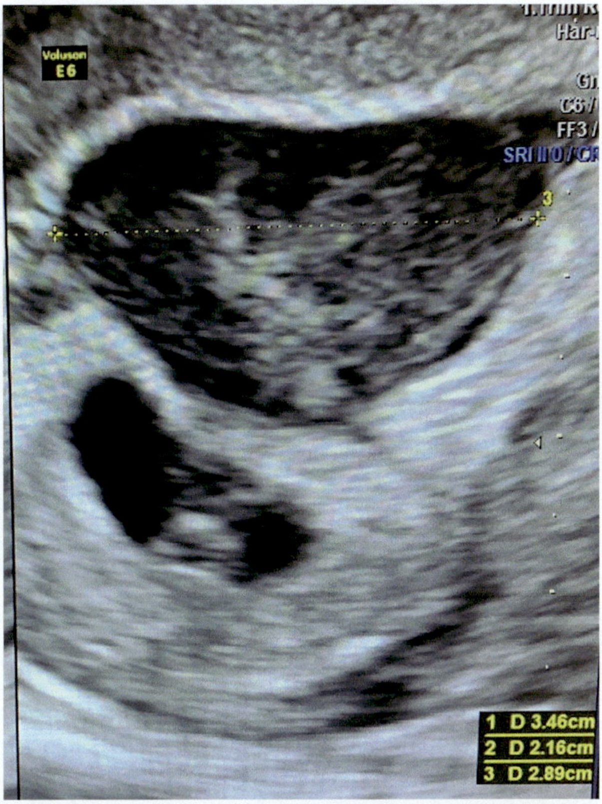

Fig. 14.2 Transvaginal scan of a 6 weeks gestation with a large subchorionic hematoma that appears as a large hypoechoic image adjacent to the gestational sac

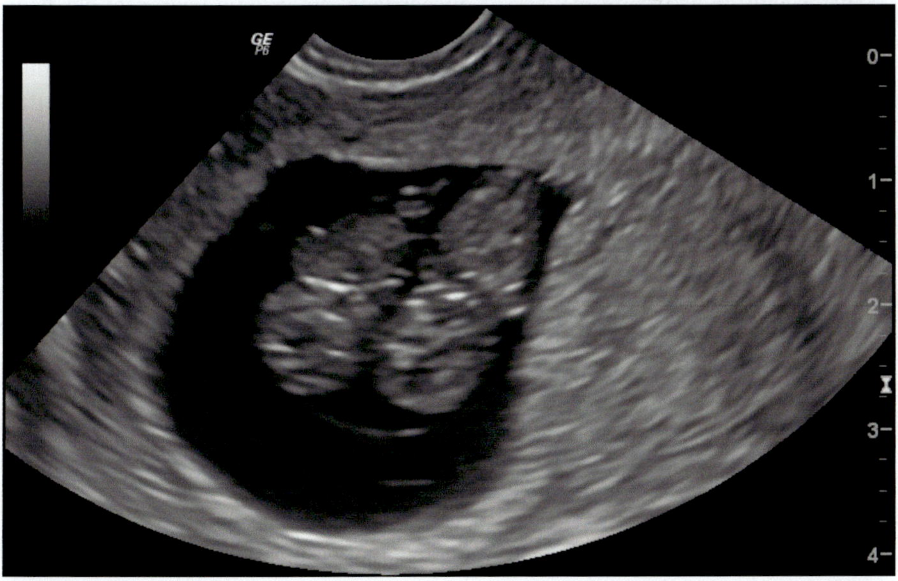

Fig. 14.3 Monochorionic–monoamniotic gestation at 8 weeks; there is only one gestational sac. Note the presence of a single amniotic sac, one yolk sac but two embryos. No separating membrane is observed

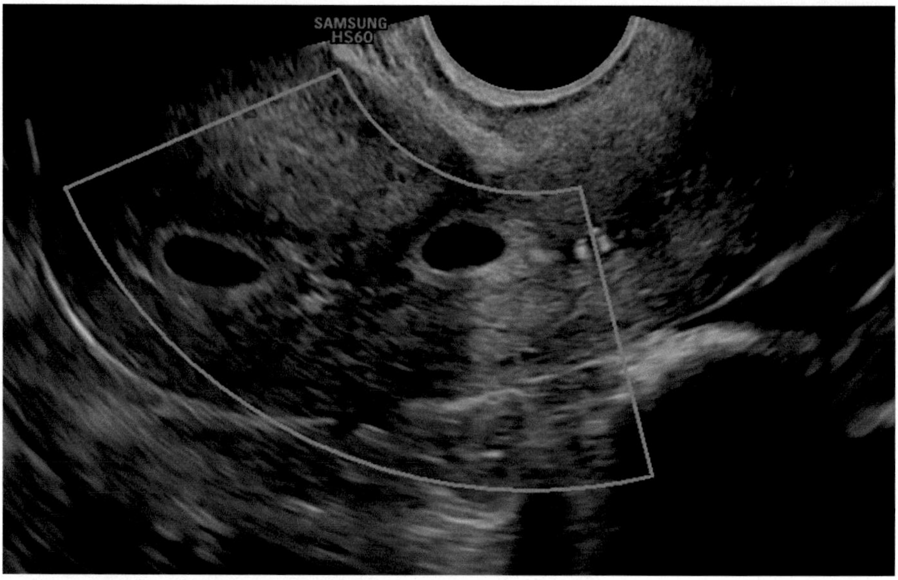

Fig. 14.4 Transvaginal ultrasound of a dichorionic diamniotic pregnancy at 5 weeks of gestation. Note two gestational sacs clearly separated

Changes and delays in the development of these parameters (gestational sac, yolk sac, CRL, and EHR) can be considered as predictors of poor prognosis in the evolution of the pregnancy. Heart rates below 85 bpm or declines in cardiac frequency over the course of a few days may indicate an increased risk of spontaneous abortion [19].

Historically in assessing the risk of miscarriage, embryonic heart rate has been the most valued single parameter for the analysis of prognosis of early pregnancies. Most studies of the evaluation of first-trimester pregnancies analyzed individual ultrasound morphological parameters separately as possible prognostic factors that indicate the occurrence of spontaneous abortion (Fig. 14.2). Combined analysis of these same parameters, however, revealed results of excellent reliability. These are presented as signs of certainty in Box 14.1, suspicious findings in Box 14.2, and sonographic signs of high risk for miscarriage in Box 14.3.

Box 14.1 Sonographic Findings Definitive for Failed Intrauterine Pregnancy

Definitive findings diagnostic of pregnancy failure

Crown-rump length of ≥7 mm and no heartbeat

Mean sac diameter of ≥25 mm and no embryo

Absence of embryo with heartbeat ≥2 weeks after a scan that showed a gestational sac without a yolk sac

Absence of embryo with heartbeat ≥11 days after a scan that showed a gestational sac with a yolk sac

Adapted from: Doubilet et al. [9]

Box 14.2 Findings Suspicious for, but Not Diagnostic of, Pregnancy Failure

Suspicious of pregnancy failure

Crown-rump length of <7 mm and no heartbeat

Mean sac diameter of 16–24 mm and no embryo

Absence of embryo with heartbeat 7–13 days after a scan that showed a gestational sac without a yolk sac

Absence of embryo with heartbeat 7–10 days after a scan that showed a gestational sac with a yolk sac

Absence of embryo ≥6 weeks after last menstrual period

Empty amnion (amnion seen adjacent to yolk sac, with no visible embryo)

Enlarged yolk sac (>7 mm)

Small gestational sac in relation to the size of the embryo (<5 mm difference between mean sac diameter and crown-rump length)

Adapted from: Doubilet et al. [9]

Box 14.3 Sonographic Signs of High Risk for Miscarriage

Slow embryonic heart rate—below 85 bpm

Large subchorionic hematoma at least two-thirds of the gestational sac

It is important to emphasize that approximately 1 in 150 live births has some type of chromosomal abnormality [1]. Chromosomal aberrations occur in two-thirds of miscarriages/with embryo death in unrecognized pregnancies, in half of clinical spontaneous abortions, and in 5% of stillbirths. Chromosomal abnormalities are more frequent in the setting of recurrent miscarriages and fetal structural abnormalities. Fetal Medicine Foundation guidelines recommend screening for aneuploidies using ultrasound at $11–13^{+6}$ weeks.

First-Trimester Ultrasound Between 11^{+0} and 13^{+6} Weeks

During the interval of $11^{+4}–13^{+6}$ weeks, the ideal time to perform the ultrasound exam is at 12 weeks, when combined first trimester tests offer the best diagnostic yields. At 11^{+0} weeks, the probability of diagnosing malformations is lower, and at 13 weeks, the results of the biochemical tests of the combined screening are less reliable.

Screening for Fetal Aneuploidy

Chromosomal abnormalities include aberrations in the number of chromosomes or their structure. The most common abnormality in the number of chromosomes is aneuploidy, in which there are one or more extra or missing chromosomes. It is also possible to have one or more extra complete sets of chromosomes (e.g., triploidy, tetraploidy). Mosaicism is an anomaly in the number of chromosomes, which consists that the abnormal number of chromosomes is not present in all cells.

Chromosomal abnormalities are observed at an approximate frequency of about six cases per 1000 births. Of these, chromosome 21 trisomy is the most frequent, with a prevalence ranging from 1:800 to 1:500 births depending on the age profile of the population considered. Other autosomal trisomies are much rarer, with a frequency of about one case of trisomy 18 (Edwards syndrome) for every 6500 births and one case of trisomy 13 (Patau syndrome) for every 12,500 births. Other frequent anomalies involve sex chromosomes, such as Turner's syndrome (X chromosome monosomy) and Klinefelter syndrome (47, XXY), in addition to triploidies [15].

The goal of screening programs is to estimate the specific risk of fetal aneuploidy for each pregnant woman according to her age and a variety of ultrasound and biochemical markers. Based on the adjusted individual risk, couples can then choose whether or not to use one of the invasive diagnostic tests, such as amniocentesis or chorionic villus sampling (CVS), which involve a small inherent risk of pregnancy loss [12]. The screening test or the test to detect aneuploidy should be offered to every woman in prenatal care, regardless of maternal age or other risk factors. Below we describe the main sonographic markers used in the first trimester. A more detailed discussion of their use, diagnostic performance, and association with other biochemical markers can be found in this chapter.

Screening Ultrasonographic Markers for Aneuploids in the First Trimester

Nucal Translucency

In the early 1990s, Nicolaides et al. proposed the ultrasound measurement of fetal nuchal translucency (NT), performed at the end of the first gestational trimester, as a screening method for fetal chromosomal changes [20]. Even today, it is considered the best isolated marker for predicting fetal aneuploidy. The literature brings together several prospective studies totaling more than 250,000 tested pregnancies that clearly demonstrate the increased risk of fetal aneuploidies with an increase in the NT. With a false-positive rate of 5%, the sensitivity of the method is around 75%–80%. In addition, increased NT is associated with a greater probability of fetal malformations, particularly cardiac, and rare genetic syndromes.

Other First-Trimester Ultrasound Markers

During the same ultrasound examination in which the measurement of NT is performed, it is possible to assess the presence of other markers of fetal aneuploidy, such as the nonvisualization of the nasal bone, increased pulsatility index (PI) in the venous duct, and tricuspid regurgitation. These additional markers are useful in reducing the overall false-positive rate.

Venous Duct

The venous duct is a vascular shunt that communicates the intrahepatic portion of the umbilical vein with the inferior vena cava. Through it, oxygenated blood is preferably directed to the right atrium. The sonogram of each cardiac cycle in this vessel is characterized by three moments: ventricular systole (S-wave), ventricular diastole (D-wave), and atrial contraction (A-wave). In the first trimester of pregnancy, increased PI in the venous duct and the occurrence of absent or reverse A-wave are considered markers of chromosomal abnormalities. In 2004, Toyama et al., studying the venous duct in 1217 cases in the 11–13 weeks of gestation period, observed a detection rate of 68.2% of chromosomal abnormalities with a false-positive rate of 6.4% [28].

Nasal Bone

Calcification of the nasal bone begins before the 11th week of pregnancy. During the ultrasound examination, it is possible to identify the nasal bone in a strict sagittal section similar to that used for the measurement of NT. It is a hyperechogenic linear structure located immediately below the skin line of the nose. Several studies have demonstrated that the nasal bone is not visualized between 11 and 13 weeks in about 60%–70% of fetuses with trisomy 21 while in less than 3% of normal fetuses.

Morphology Evaluation

Detailed examination of fetal anatomy during routine assessment at 11–14 weeks of gestation can detect approximately half of the major structural defects in low-risk pregnancies. The detection rate increases sharply between 13 and 14 weeks of gestation compared to 11 weeks of gestation, as well as by the use of the transvaginal approach [27].

Rossi in a meta-analysis [23] described the following rates of detection of fetal malformations in the first trimester.

- 100%—acrania, anencephaly, ectopia cordis, encephalocele
- 50–99%—hygroma cystic, double outflow tract right ventricle, Fallot tetralogy, gastroschisis, omphalocele, holoprosencephaly, left heart hypoplasia syndrome, limb reduction, megacystis, polydactyly, septal defects, transposition of large vessels, valve disease
- 1–49%—spina bifida, hydrocephalus, skeletal dysplasia, cleft palate, Dandy–Walker, coarctation of the aorta
- 0%—agenesis of the corpus callosum, bladder exstrophy, congenital adenomatoid malformation, cerebellar hypoplasia, duodenal atresia, hydronephrosis, renal agenesis, intestinal obstruction, extralobar sequestration

The evaluation of fetal morphology in the first trimester is very promising. However, the late development of several organs and systems and the late onset of a significant number of the principal anomalies, during the second and third trimesters, make it unlikely that ultrasound examination in the first trimester can supplant ultrasound in the second trimester in the routine morphological evaluation. The literature recommends this type of first- and also second-trimester investigation in high-risk patients. Patients with a history of risk for malformations or with abnormal findings in the first-trimester screening or with suspicious findings in the earliest exams between 6 and 10 weeks should ideally be evaluated transvaginally around 13 weeks, looking for abnormalities in organs and systems.

First-Trimester Cervical Measurement

The controversy regarding the value of the first-trimester transvaginal cervical measurement is associated with differences in the technique employed and other specific issues, typical of the first trimester. Currently, the most accepted practice is the same used during the second trimester [17], as described in detail in Chap. 15.

One of the main anatomical difficulties found during evaluation performed between 11 and 14 weeks is the differentiation between the lower segment of the uterus and internal orifice of the cervix. The presence of focal contractions in the lower segment also makes the examination more challenging, as they can transiently change the cervical shape, particularly the internal OS. The correct identification of endocervical canal by recognizing the mucosa instead of over-measuring the cervicoisthmic complex is an additional challenge encountered during transvaginal exams performed in the first trimester [26].

Gascón et al. measuring cervical canal length in 34 women between 11.0 and 13.6 weeks of gestation found 27 mm and 32 mm for the 10th percentile and the 50th percentile, respectively. These findings were shorter than older series [8]; these shorter cervical canal lengths can be attributed to the fact that Gascón et al. avoided the isthmus and obtained a more precise measure of the true cervix. The same study established that cervical length in the first trimester had good intraobserver and interobserver variability. The authors considered adequate training of paramount importance [11].

First-trimester evaluation exams historically have been made by group of well-trained experts, but many of these authors failed to prove a strong correlation of cervical length with prematurity and the need for progesterone, although some have found the clinical use of transvaginal cervical measurement during first trimester as a predictor of preterm birth or late miscarriage [3, 5, 24, 26].

The practitioner, who decides to include the cervical length measurement during the first-trimester examination, should be aware that, currently, no major national or professional obstetric society recommends this practice as a routine [25].

First-Trimester Uterine Artery Evaluation

Doppler velocimetry analysis during the first trimester is usually performed between 11.0 and 13.6 weeks of gestation, near the main branch of uterine arteries, either transabdominally or transvaginally [4, 16]. Usually, semiquantitative assessment of the velocity waveforms is commonly employed, with measurements, especially the pulsatility index, reported independently for the right and left uterine arteries, such as the presence or absence of notching. These measurements must be compared with appropriate reference ranges [13].

Some specific aspects of Doppler transvaginal insonation should be considered and are addressed, together with the transabdominal technique, in Box 14.4 [6]. Information about second-trimester technique is presented in Chap. 15.

Box 14.4 First-Trimester Uterine Artery Evaluation by Transvaginal Doppler Insonation

Transabdominal Technique

- Transabdominally, a midsagittal section of the uterus is achieved with cervical identification.
- An empty maternal bladder is recommended.
- The probe is then moved laterally searching the paracervical vascular plexus visualization.
- Color Doppler is used to identify the uterine artery which turns cranially to ascend to the uterine body.
- Measurements are taken at this point, before the division into the arcuate arteries.
- The same process is repeated on the contralateral side.

Transvaginal Technique

- The probe should be placed in the anterior vaginal fornix.
- The probe is moved laterally to visualize the paracervical vascular plexus and the same steps described for transabdominal technique (above) should be performed.
- The examiner should be aware to not insonate the cervicovaginal or arcuate arteries.
- Velocities over 50 cm/s are typical of uterine arteries, which can be used to differentiate this vessel from other local vessels.

It is important to note that Doppler velocimetry evaluation in the first trimester is rarely used as an isolated variable in preeclampsia (PE) prediction. In routine practice, these Doppler findings should be interpreted in the context of maternal family history, clinical features, mean arterial pressure, and serum levels of specific markers, such as pregnancy-associated plasma protein-A (PAAP-A) and placental growth factor (PLGF) [2, 10]. Recently, a large prospective first-trimester multicenter study (ASPRE), using an algorithm based on combined variables cited above, detected 76.6% of cases of preterm PE and 38.3% of term PE at a FPR of 10% [22].

In conclusion, it is possible to assign that first-trimester ultrasound examination is one of the most important exams performed during the whole gestation period. This early sonographic assessment can provide crucial obstetric information that, together with clinical features, can provide key help to evaluate the fetal risk of miscarriage, aneuploidy, and malformations.

References

1. ACOG. Practice bulletin no. 200: early pregnancy loss. Obstet Gynecol. 2018;132(5):e197–207.
2. Akolekar R, Syngelaki A, Sarquis R, et al. Prediction of early, intermediate and late pre-eclampsia from maternal factors, biophysical and biochemical markers at 11–13 weeks. Prenat Diagn. 2011;31(1):66–74.
3. Antsaklis P, Daskalakis G, Pilalis A, Papantoniou N, Mesogitis S, Antsaklis A. The role of cervical length measurement at 11-14 weeks for the prediction of preterm delivery. J Matern Fetal Neonatal Med. 2011;24:465–70.
4. Aquilina J, Barnett A, Thompson O, Harrington K. Comprehensive analysis of uterine artery flow velocity waveforms for the prediction of pre-eclampsia. Ultrasound Obstet Gynecol. 2000;16:163–70.
5. Berghella V, Talucci M, Desai A. Does transvaginal sonographic measurement of cervical length before 14 weeks predict preterm delivery in high-risk pregnancies? Ultrasound Obstet Gynecol. 2003;21:140–4.
6. Bhide A, Acharya G, Bilardo CM, Brezinka C, Cafici D, Hernandez-Andrade E, Kalache K, Kingdom J, Kiserud T, Lee W, Lees C, Leung KY, Malinger G, Mari G, Prefumo F, Sepulveda W, Trudinger B. Ultrasound Obstet Gynecol. 2013;41(2):233–9.
7. Britten S, Soenksen DM, Bustillo M, Coulam CB. Very early (24-56 days from last menstrual period) embryonic heart rate in normal pregnancies. Hum Reprod. 1994;9:2424–6.
8. Carvalho MHB, Bittar RE, Brizot ML, et al. Cervical length at 11–14 weeks' and 22–24 weeks' gestation evaluated by transvaginal sonography and gestational age at delivery. Ultrasound Obstet Gynecol. 2003;21(2):135–9.
9. Doubilet PM, Benson CB, Bourne T, Blaivas M, Society of Radiologists in Ultrasound Multispecialty Panel on Early First Trimester Diagnosis of Miscarriage and Exclusion of a Viable Intrauterine Pregnancy, Barnhart KT, Benacerraf BR, Brown DL, Filly RA, Fox JC, Goldstein SR, Kendall JL, Lyons EA, Porter MB, Pretorius DH, Timor-Tritsch IE. Diagnostic criteria for nonviable pregnancy early in the first trimester. N Engl J Med. 2013;369(15):1443–51.
10. Espinoza J, Romero R, Nien JK, et al. Identification of patients at risk for early onset and/or severe preeclampsia with the use of uterine artery Doppler velocimetry and placental growth factor. Am J Obstet Gynecol. 2007;196(4):326e1–13.
11. Gascón A, Goya M, Mendoza M, Gracia-Perez-Bonfils A, Higueras T, Calero I, Avilés M, Sánchez MA, Llurba E, Cabero L, Carreras E. Intraobserver and interobserver variabil-

ity in first-trimester transvaginal ultrasound cervical length. J Matern Fetal Neonatal Med. 2020;33(1):136–41.
12. Ghi T, Sotiriadis A, Calda P, Da Silva CF, Raine-Fenning N, Alfirevic Z, McGillivray G, International Society of Ultrasound in Obstetrics and Gynecology(ISUOG). ISUOG Practice Guidelines: invasive procedures for prenatal diagnosis. Ultrasound Obstet Gynecol. 2016;48(2):256–68.
13. Gómez O, Figueras F, Fernandez S, Bennasar M, Martínez JM, Puerto B, Gratacós E. Reference ranges for uterine artery mean pulsatility index at 11–41 weeks of gestation. Ultrasound Obstet Gynecol. 2008;32:128–32.
14. Hadlock FP, Shah YP, Kanon DJ, Lindsey JV. Fetal crown-rump length: reevaluation of relation to menstrual age (5-18 weeks) with high-resolution real-time US. Radiology. 1992;182(2):501–5.
15. Hook EB, Cross PK, Jackson L, Pergament E, Brambati B. Maternal age-specific rates of 47,+21 and other cytogenetic abnormalities diagnosed in the first trimester of pregnancy in chorionic villus biopsy specimens: comparison with rates expected from observations at amniocentesis. Am J Hum Genet. 1988;42(6):797–807.
16. Jurkovic D, Jauniaux E, Kurjak A, Hustin J, Campbell S, Nicolaides KH. Transvaginal colour Doppler assessment of the uteroplacental circulation in early pregnancy. Obstet Gynecol. 1991;77:365–9.
17. Kagan KO, Sonek J. How to measure cervical length. Ultrasound Obstet Gynecol. 2015;45(3):358–62.
18. Mei JY, Afshar Y, Platt LD. First-trimester ultrasound. Obstet Gynecol Clin N Am. 2019;46(4):829–52. https://doi.org/10.1016/j.ogc.2019.07.011.
19. Merchiers EH, Dhont M, De Sutter PA, Beghin CJ, Vandekerckhove DA. Predictive value of early embryonic cardiac activity for pregnancy outcome. Am J Obstet Gynecol. 1991;165:11–4.
20. Nicolaides KH, Azar G, Byrne D, Mansur C, Marks K. Fetal nuchal translucency: ultrasound screening for chromosomal defects in first trimester of pregnancy. BMJ. 1992;304(6831):867–9.
21. Rempen A. Diagnosis of viability in early pregnancy with vaginal sonography. J Ultrasound Med. 1990;9:711–6.
22. Rolnik DL, Wright D, Poon LCY, et al. ASPRE trial: performance of screening for preterm pre-eclampsia. Ultrasound Obstet Gynecol. 2017;50(4):492–5.
23. Rossi AC, Prefumo F. Accuracy of ultrasonography at 11-14 weeks of gestation for detection of fetal structural anomalies: a systematic review. Obstet Gynecol. 2013;122(6):1160–7.
24. Sanane's N, Schuller E, Gaudineau A, et al. What is predictive of preterm delivery in the first trimester: isthmus or cervical length? Prenat Diagn. 2013;33:894–8.
25. Society for Maternal-Fetal Medicine (SMFM), McIntosh J, Feltovich H, Berghella V, Manuck T. The role of routine cervical length screening in selected high- and low-risk women for preterm birth prevention. Am J Obstet Gynecol. 2016;215(3):B2–7.
26. Souka AP, Papastefanou I, Michalitsi V, et al. Cervical length changes from the first to second trimester of pregnancy, and prediction of preterm birth by first-trimester sonographic cervical measurement. J Ultrasound Med. 2011;30:997–1002.
27. Timor-Tritsch IE, Fuchs KM, Monteagudo A, D'Alton ME. Performing a fetal anatomy scan at the time of first-trimester screening. Obstet Gynecol. 2009;113(2 Pt 1):402–7.
28. Toyama JM, Brizot ML, Liao AW, Lopes LM, Nomura RM, Saldanha FA, Zugaib M. Ductus venosus blood flow assessment at 11 to 14 weeks of gestation and fetal outcome. Ultrasound Obstet Gynecol. 2004;23(4):341–5.

Chapter 15
Ultrasound in Second and Third Trimester: What Should Be Evaluated?

Victor Rocha de Castro Alves, Rafaela Cardoso Gil Pimentel, Augusto César Garcia Saab Benedeti, and Francisco Mauad Filho

Introduction

The second- and third-trimester obstetric ultrasound exam is an essential tool for prenatal care, being one of the mandatory complementary exams in obstetric routine. Its application is extremely important in the diagnosis of possible gestational anomalies and as an aid for certain clinical decisions. It must include the systematic evaluation of anatomy, biometrics, and fetal vitality, as well as the evaluation of the maternal pelvic organs that can be evidenced in each trimester [1].

Initially, the presence and quantity of fetuses in the uterine cavity must be determined, especially in patients without previous exams, since extra-uterine and twin pregnancies have particularities in the description and conduct. When the patient has provided previous exams information or has a reliable last menstrual period date, the gestacional age (GA) can be calculated for further comparisons and analysis [2].

In the initial screening, the observation of fetal statics is essential for directing the scan and determining the cardiac situs, in addition, to identify immediately the vitality through observation of the fetal and cardiac chambers movements. The situation is identified through the relation between the long fetal axis and the maternal long axis. When in agreement, the situation is longitudinal. When they are in a perpendicular position, it is considered transverse. Still, the fetus can be oblique to the maternal axis, being called oblique situation. The fetal presentation is recognized from the closest part of it body to the internal orifice of cervix, being classified as cephalic, pelvic/podalic and choric. The positioning, on the other hand, is due to

V. R. de Castro Alves · R. C. G. Pimentel · A. C. G. S. Benedeti · F. M. Filho (✉)
FATESA – Faculdade de Tecnologia em Saúde, Ribeirão Preto, SP, Brazil
e-mail: mauad@fatesa.edu.br

© Springer Nature Switzerland AG 2022

R. A. Moreira de Sá, E. B. d. Fonseca (eds.), *Perinatology*,
https://doi.org/10.1007/978-3-030-83434-0_15

Table 15.1 Fetopelvic Relationships

Fetal Posture						
Fetal lie	Longitudinal	Transverse	Oblique	–	–	–
Presentation	Cephalic	Pelvic	Choric	–	–	–
Position (dorsum)	Superior	Inferior	Right	Left	Anterior	Posterior

the relation between fetal dorsum and maternal anatomical planes, which may be superior, inferior, anterior, posterior, to the right or to the left. Fetal statics are summarized according to the table below (Table 15.1) [3].

Biometry and Fetal Anatomic Evaluation

Through fetal biometrics, anatomical evaluation is associated with the careful measurement of specific fetal structures, generating information and biometric parameters that assist in the evaluation of fetal growth and development and allow the tracking of any structural changes in the fetus [3].

Cephalic Pole

The anatomical evaluation of brain structures in a cross-sectional view of the fetal head at the level of the thalami is recommended and should be used to measure the biparietal diameter and head circumference, which must be performed with a 90° insonation angle with the midline to better structure demonstration. These structures are the falx cerebri, cavum septi pellucidi, and thalamus. Cerebellum and orbits should not be demonstrated in this plane [2].

The biparietal diameter (BPD) is classically measured by placing the cursors in the region with the largest lateral–lateral diameter of the skull, at an angle that is perpendicular to the midline, starting from the outer face of the bone board to the inner face of the contralateral board (Fig. 15.1). The cephalic index (CI) is a ratio between maximum width and extension of the cephalic pole and can be calculated to characterize the shape of the fetal skull (usual, brachycephaly, or dolichocephaly), being useful to validate the use of the BPD in the calculation of GA; besides this application, it can be also helpful in the evaluation of the fetal shape, as some are related to abnormal findings or genetic syndromes [4].

The head circumference (HC) can be calculated directly using an ellipse around the outer faces of the skull bone plate. It can also be calculated from biparietal diameter (BPD) and occipitofrontal diameter (OFD) measures, which can be done with the calipers placed in the external margin of the frontal and occipital bones, aligned with the cerebral sickle, using the formula: $HC = (BPD + OFD) \times 1.62$.

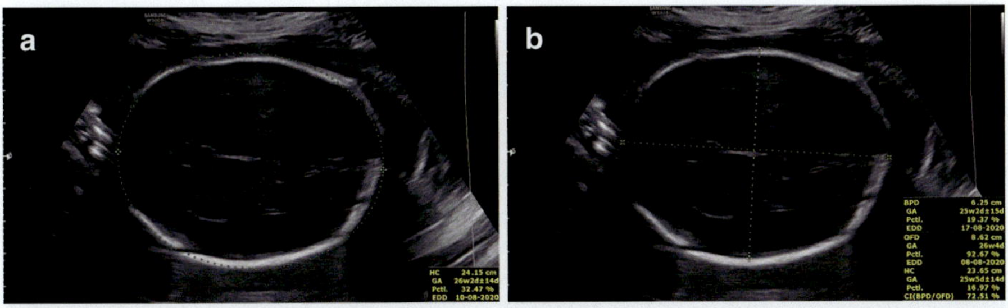

Fig. 15.1 Cephalic pole measured using ellipse (**a**) and calipers for BPD and OFD (**b**)

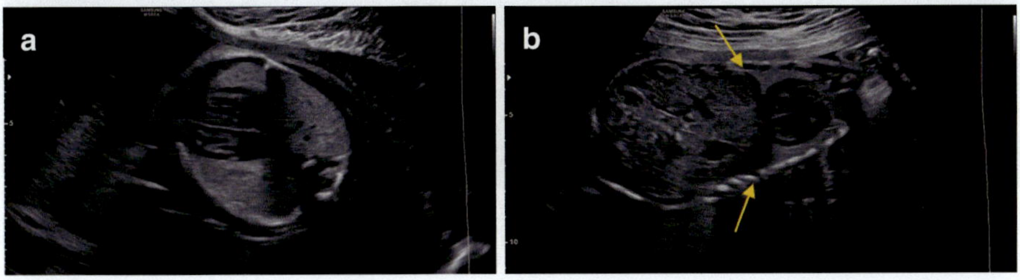

Fig. 15.2 Fetal thorax at four-chamber heart level (**a**). Note the lungs echogenicity and simetric heart chambers. Image (**b**) showing diaphragma line separating thorax and abdominal structures in coronal view (arrows)

Fetal Thorax

Normally seen in a round shape, with dimensions proportional to the abdomen, containing lungs with higher echogenicity compared to the liver and homogeneous echotexture. The fetal heart must be located predominantly at left hemithorax, same position as the stomach in the abdome (*situs solitus*), separated by diaphragma hipoechogenic lines, better shown in coronal and sagital planes (Fig. 15.2) [2].

The proper echographic evaluation of the thorax must be done in an axial symmetric plane, characterized by the presence of one single rib in the side of each hemithorax [1].

The basic cardiac exam is made at this level, visualizing the four chambers, in which a relative symmetry can be observed between them, associated with free valves movement and the complete cardiac cross identification. Heart sectional area must not be larger than one-third of thoracic area, with the apex rotated to approximately 45° to the left side. The heart rate (HR) can be measured by spectral Doppler (PW), being kept between 100 and 180 beats per minute (Fig. 15.3). Transitory variations of the frequency, during less than 2 minutes, may not be correspondent to rhythm alterations and are frequently detected during normal prenatal exams [5].

Cardiac abnormalities are the most frequent fetal conditions, however commonly underdiagnosed. The evaluation of the four chambers plane alone has a limited capacity of identifying those abnormalities, with a detection rate estimated between 30% and 48% [6].

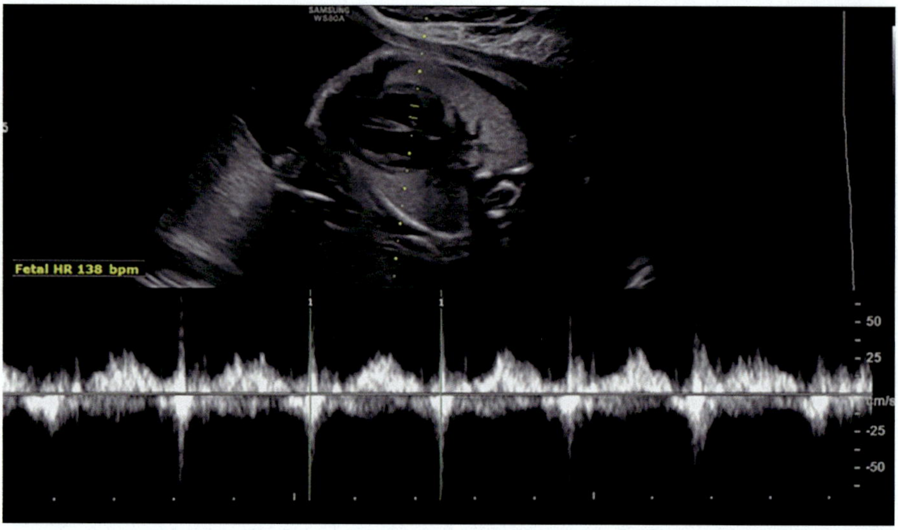

Fig. 15.3 Fetal heart rate measured in four chambers plane

Fetal Abdomen

The evaluation of fetal abdomen must be done in a very criterious way, once the abdominal circumference has a deep impact over the estimate fetal weight. Furthermore, it allows the identification of congenital malformations such as abdominal wall closure defect (gastroschisis and omphalocele), kidney abnormalities (hidronephrosis, cistic disease, posterior urethral valve), absent stomach, and more [1].

The proper image is shown in axial plane, featuring one rib at each side of the abdomen, containing the following structures: vertebral bones, stomach at the left side, and venous sinus at portal circulation level [1].

Calipers need to be positioned in the external limits of the abdomen skin, from specific reference points: passing through the middle of the vertebral bones toward the venous sinus (anteroposterior diameter—APD) and lateral-laterally, in the wider portions of the abdomen, perpendicular to the anterior measure (abdominal transverse diameter—ATD). The calculation of the abdominal circumference (AC) is made directly using the ellipse option or the formula: $AC = (APD + ATD) \times 1.57$ (Fig. 15.4) [2].

This image section should not contain kidneys and/or cardiac area, as well as the insertion of umbilical cord in the anterior abdominal wall. These structures must be examined individually in its proper planes. After the assessment of abdominal circumference, the integrity of the abdominal wall, the presence of the gallbladder and kidneys, and the appearance of the bowel must be verified (Fig. 15.5) [4].

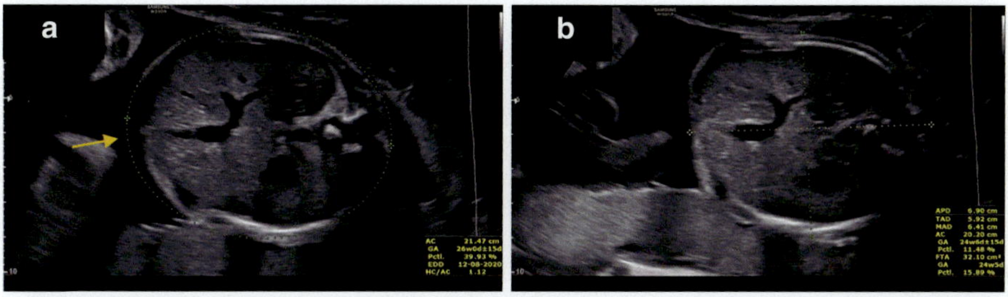

Fig. 15.4 Abdominal circumference (AC) made with ellipse surrounding the fetal skin (**a**) and with calculated by the acquisition of APD and TAD (**b**). Note that the calipers shall be placed at fetal skin limits, and lateral attenuation must be compensated (arrow)

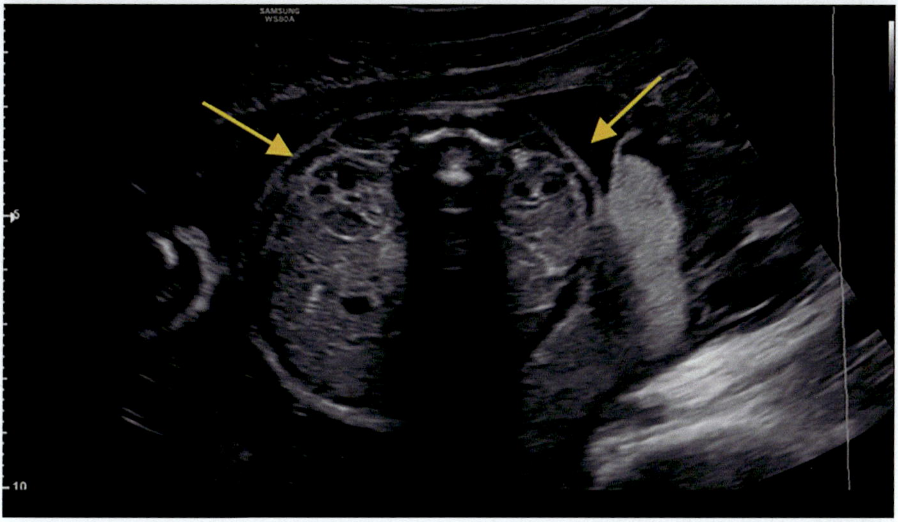

Fig. 15.5 Fetal kidneys (arrows) shown in a lower abdominal plane, better seen when fetal dorsum is placed anteriorly. The pelvis is poorly identified if normal. Also, the pyramids from parenchyma must not be mistaken by cistic lesions

Fetal Pelvis

The urinary bladder must be located in the interior of the pelvis, bordered by two vesical arteries, identified using color Doppler (CD). Difficulty to observe the urinary bladder inside the pelvis or the absence of one of the vesical arteries must be informed in the report, as it can be related to pathological findings (Fig. 15.6) [4].

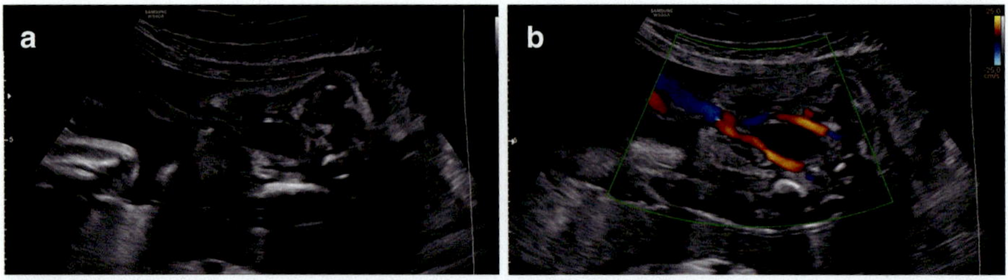

Fig. 15.6 Image (**a**) Vesical arteries and fluid-filled bladder in the fetal pelvic. Image (**b**) showing the use of color Doppler to identify and document perviety of the arteries

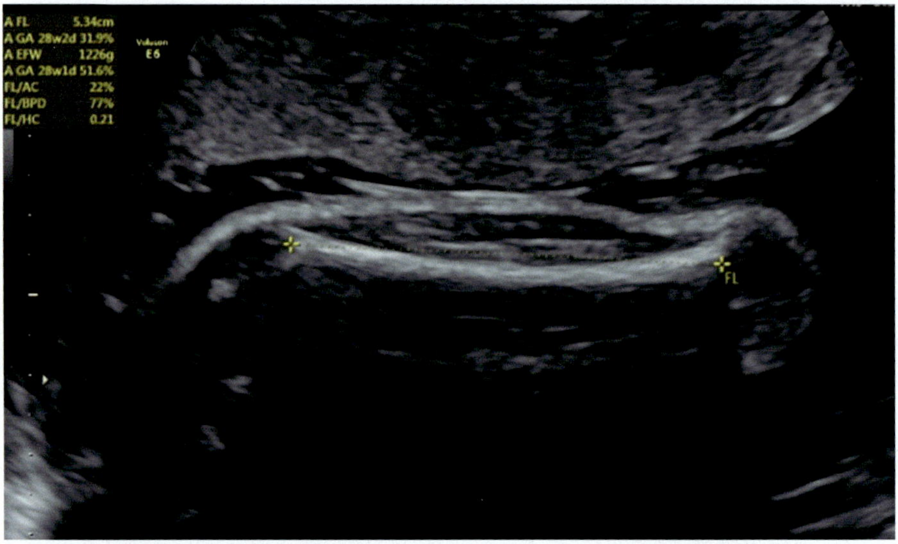

Fig. 15.7 Femur length measure

Fetal Limbs

All the limbs segments shall be evaluated, aiming to detect variations in number, shape, position, ossification, and dimensions. It is expected that with the progression of GA, some details like foot angle and number of the fingers might not be properly demonstrated, especially in the third trimester [2].

The femur measurement is done with the acquisition of its specific image, in coronal view, magnified (occupying more than half the image extension), in which the femur is found horizontalized in an ideal angle between 45° and 90° toward the insonation beam. Calipers should be positioned in the diaphysis ossified extremities, not including the distal epiphysis (Fig. 15.7) [3].

Other Structures

The routine obstetric exam from the second and third trimesters has no detailed morphologic assessment finality. Evaluation of fetal structures such as face, vertebral column, and genitalia are not mandatory but can provide important information, being encouraged in routine basic study [4].

Fetal Weight

Fetal biometry provides several parameters such as weight, estimate gestational age, cephalic index, among others, to allow a global evaluation and fetal evolution. Its realization and interpretation are an important part in the obstetric sonography practice [7].

In fetus with adequate establishment of GA (calculated by first-trimester screening or a reliable last period date), the measurements of biometric parameters and fetal weigh enable the detection of growth deviations for further control [8].

Although no consensus may be found in the literature, usually, fetus with adequate estimated fetal weight (AGA) are considered those between the percentile 10 and 95. Large fetus for gestational age (LGA) are the ones with a percentile above 95. Yet, fetus found between percentiles 3 and 10 are considered small for gestational age (SGA), and should be differentiated from constitutional small and growth-restricted fetus. This can be done based on Doppler fluxometric criteria and/or changes in biometric ratios [4].

Fetal weight or abdominal circumference under the third percentile can be considered an isolated criterion for fetal growth restriction diagnosis [2].

Others

Amniotic Fluid

The amount of amniotic fluid can be estimated in a subjective way, through careful observation by trained professional, or objectively, through measurements. Both ways present good results in obstetric routine. The main objective assessment is the semiquantitative analysis of the amniotic fluid index (AFI) and deepest vertical pocket (DVP) [9]. Both modalities include similar technical criteria: probe strictly vertical, without excessive compression of maternal abdominal wall. AFI is estimated by the sum of four different measures, one for each quadrant of uterine cavity, while the DVP uses only the biggest measure, observed in any region of the

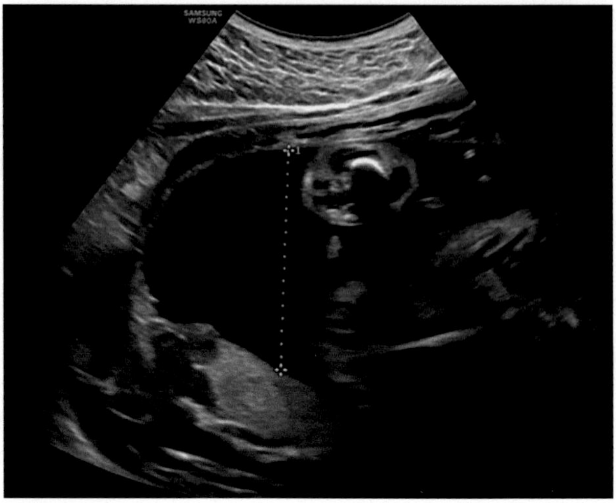

Fig. 15.8 Example of DVP measurement. For AFI, the gestational sac must be divided into four pockets and each will be measured and after summed for the result. Note that in both ways, fetal structures (limbs, cord) cannot be crossed by calipers

gestational sac (Fig. 15.8). Normal values are considered those between 5 and 25 cm for AFI and 2 and 8 cm for DVP. It is important to notice that DVP will be only be useful after 18 weeks, when the fetus starts to contribute more for the fluid production. AFI should not be measured under 24 weeks because of the simple fact that before this age usually there is no way to divide the cavity in four pockets [10].

Recent studies have not shown significative difference in accuracy amid methods and suggest a higher chance of over diagnostics, with higher rates of interventions and potential side effects with the use of AFI [11].

Variations in fluid quantity may suggest anatomic-functional alterations in the fetus and must be reported for further detailed assessment and follow-up [1].

Placenta

Placental description over ultrasonographic exam must include localization, echographic aspect, and its relationship toward internal cervical orifice (ICO). In general, the placenta must not reach or overlap the cervical orifice, maintaining a minimum distance of 2.0 cm from it, ideally. Otherwise, if the placental is closer than 2.0 cm, then a third trimestre reassessment by the transvaginal examination is recommended [12].

Abnormalities from the interface of the uterus walls and the placenta may indicate higher risk of placental acretism, particularly in patients with important risk factors, like previous uterine surgeries (cesarian delivery, myomectomy, curettage) and/or low placental implantation. Current evidence has implied that placental classification by degrees (Grannum 0, I, II, and III) presents poor correlation intra- and interobserver, beyond, offering few diagnostic and prognostic resources for clinical management (Fig. 15.9) [13].

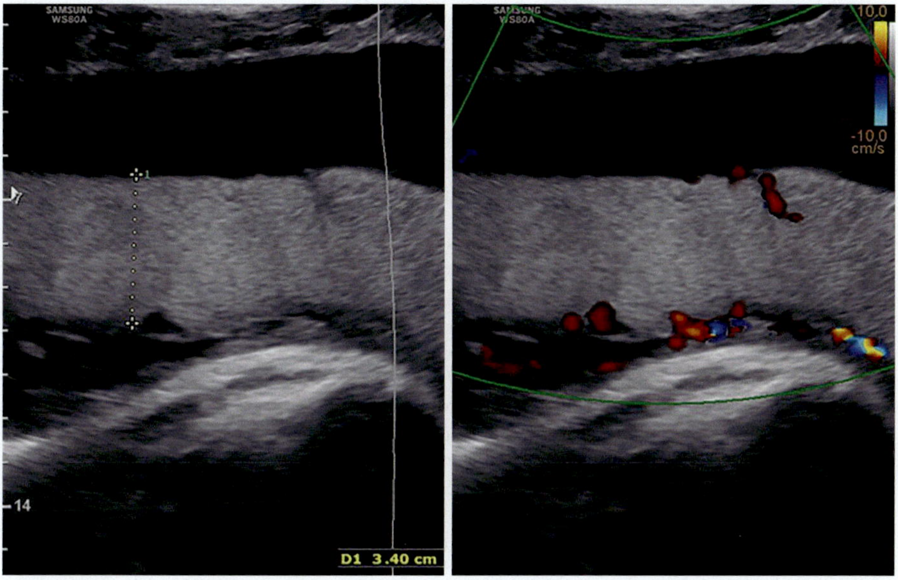

Fig. 15.9 Placental analysis with and without color Doppler, showing where to place calipers for measurement and myometrial flow

While there is no consensus over the measurement of placental thickness in obstetric sonographic routine, it may show relevance in the detection of several maternal-fetal alterations. Usually, it maintains a numeric relation with GA. When its thickness is above or under the expected for the GA, it might be related to the higher incidence of perinatal morbidity and mortality [14].

Cervix, Uterus, and Adnexa

Cervicometry is not recommended as routine obstetric evaluation, as there are no evidence supporting it. Benefits can be taken in premature labor prediction, when the assessment is made transvaginal, in morphologic study period [2].

The basic cervix evaluation transabdominally may use the bladder or amniotic fluid as acoustic window, conditioned by the image acquisition on a longitudinal plane in suprapubic area, aiming the complete visualization of endocervical canal among internal and external orifices of uterus cervix. Changes in the habitual morphology shall receive specific evaluation, transvaginal, to obtain better quality images with less interference from the bladder, fetal structures, and compression [12].

The screening of adnexal structures and myometrium can demonstrate significative alterations, especially those that may cause impact in delivery management or maternal health, such as large fibroids, ovarian mass, and c-section thinned myometrium scar [1].

References

1. Salomon LJ, Alfirevic Z, Berghella V, Bilardo C, Hernandez-Andrade E, Johnsen SL, Kalache K, Leung KY, Malinger G, Munoz H, Prefumo F, Toi A, Lee W, on behalf of the ISUOG Clinical Standards Committee. Practice guidelines for performance of the routine mid-trimester fetal ultrasound scan. Ultrasound Obstet Gynecol. 2011;37:116–26.
2. Mauad FF. Ultrassonografia em ginecologia e obstetrícia: guia prático. Rio de Janeiro: Revinter; 2010.
3. Breathnach FM, Fleming A, Malone FD. The second trimester genetic sonogram. Am J Med Genet C Semin Med Genet. 2007;145C:62–72.
4. American Institute of Ultrasound in Medicine. AIUM practice guideline for the performance of obstetric ultrasound examinations. J Ultrasound Med. 2013;32:1083–101.
5. International Society of Ultrasound in Obstetrics and Gynecology, Carvalho JS, Allan LD, Chaoui R, et al. ISUOG practice guidelines (updated): sonographic screening examination of the fetal heart. Ultrasound Obstet Gynecol. 2013;41:348–59.
6. Lopes L. Ecocardiografia fetal. 1st Ed. Rio de Janeiro - Brazil: Revinter; 2016.
7. Hadlock FP, Harrist RB, Sharman RS, Deter RL, Park SK. Estimation of fetal weight with the use of head, body, and femur measurements—a prospective study. Am J Obstet Gynecol. 1985;151:333–7.
8. Salomon LJ, Alfirevic Z, Da Silva CF, Deter RL, Figueras F, Ghi T, Glanc P, Khalil A, Lee W, Napolitano R, Papageorghiou A, Sotiriadis A, Stirnemann J, Toi A, Yeo G. ISUOG practice guidelines: ultrasound assessment of fetal biometry and growth. Ultrasound Obstet Gynecol. 2019;53:715–23.
9. Sekhon S, Rosenbloom JI, Doering M, Conner SN, Macones GA, Colditz GA, Tuuli MG, Carter EB. Diagnostic utility of maximum vertical pocket versus amniotic fluid index in assessing amniotic fluid volume for the prediction of adverse maternal and fetal outcomes: a systematic review and meta-analysis. J Matern Fetal Neonatal Med. 2019:1–10. https://doi.org/10.1080/14767058.2019.1691988. Online ahead of print.
10. Magann EF, Chauhan SP, Doherty DA, Magann MI, Morrison JC. The evidence for abandoning the amniotic fluid index in favor of the single deepest pocket. Am J Perinatol. 2007;24:549–55.
11. Rosati P, Guariglia L, Cavaliere AF, et al. A comparison between amniotic fluid index and the single deepest vertical pocket technique in predicting adverse outcome in prolonged pregnancy. J Prenat Med. 2015;9(1–2):12–5.
12. Pastore A. Ultrassonografia em ginecologia e obstetrícia. 1st ed. Editora Revinter; 2010.
13. Sau A, Seed P, Langford K. Intraobserver and interobserver variation in the sonographic grading of placental maturity. Ultrasound Obstet Gynecol. 2004;23:374–7.
14. Nagpal K, Mittal P, Grover SB. Role of ultrasonographic placental thickness in prediction of fetal outcome: a prospective Indian study. J Obstet Gynecol India. 2018;68:349–54. https://doi.org/10.1007/s13224-017-1038-8.

Chapter 16
Doppler Velocimetry

Cristos Pritsivelis, Jair Roberto da Silva Braga, and Jorge de Rezende-Filho

Doppler Flowmetry

Through the insonation of a blood vessel, a spectral wave is generated by ultrasonography in which indices that express peripheral vascular resistance are obtained. These indices have the advantage that they do not depend on the insonation angle, and the various points always refer to the enveloped wave (or wave casing) that expresses the maximum velocity. The indices most commonly used are the systole/diastole ratio (S/D), the resistance index (RI), and the pulsatile index (PI) (Fig. 16.1).

In obstetrics, Doppler applications include evaluation of placental circulation (uterine artery Doppler) and fetal vitality in the third trimester (Doppler of the umbilical artery, of the middle cerebral artery (MCA), and of the umbilical vein).

It is a pulsatile wave procedure, in which a single piezoelectric crystal emits and captures the sound waves. The detection of the frequency difference (ΔF) generated by the moving red blood cells can be obtained within any vessel area studied. The sample volume is electronically generated along the pulsatile sound beam and can be placed in the desired location within the vessel seen by two-dimensional (*duplex*) ultrasound.

The flow waveform speed indicates the maximum frequency of the enveloped wave, obtained through the cardiac cycle, showing one systolic and one diastolic peak (Fig. 16.2). The ratio between these peaks is independent of the insonation angle. The diastole flow velocity reflects the vessel resistance, so that the highest the flow velocity, the lowest the peripheral resistance.

C. Pritsivelis · J. R. da Silva Braga · J. de Rezende-Filho (✉)
Maternidade Escola da UFRJ, Universidade Federal do Rio de Janeiro,
Rio de Janeiro, RJ, Brazil
e-mail: cristos@me.ufrj.br; jairbraga@me.ufrj.br; rezendef@me.ufrj.br

© Springer Nature Switzerland AG 2022

R. A. Moreira de Sá, E. B. d. Fonseca (eds.), *Perinatology*,
https://doi.org/10.1007/978-3-030-83434-0_16

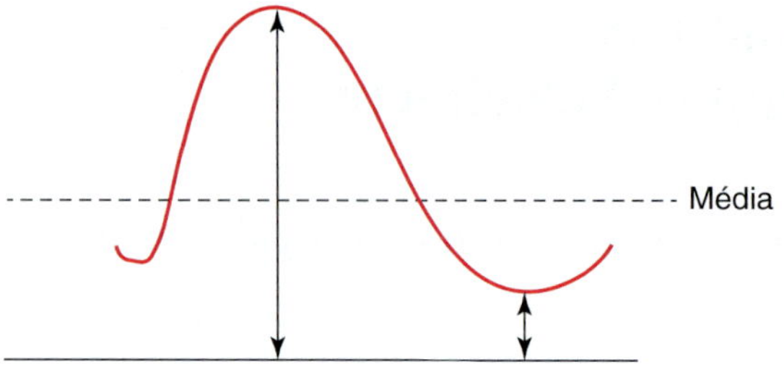

Fig. 16.1 Index formulas most commonly used in obstetric Doppler

$\frac{A}{B}$	A/B ratio	A = S B = D Relação A/B = S/D ratio
$\frac{A-B}{A}$	Resistance Index (RI)	A = S B = D indice de resistência = resistance index
$\frac{A-B}{\text{Média}}$	Pulsatility Index (PI)	A = S B = D média = mean indice pulsátil = pulsatile index

Investigations have been restricted particularly to the measurement of uterine artery flow velocities (uteroplacental circulation), umbilical artery flow (fetoplacental circulation), cerebral arteries, and of the venous Doppler (inferior vena cava, ductus venosus, umbilical vein).

The change in the flow velocity in the umbilical artery reflects, with extreme accuracy, the placental resistance (arterioles of the terminal villous system). The flowmetry procedure is the best method for evaluating the vitality in intrauterine growth restriction (IUGR) of placental origin.

Color Doppler

Also referred to as color flow Doppler or color mapping Doppler, this procedure displays blood flows in red and blue colors, in its various shades, depending on the direction of blood movement as it approaches or moves away from the transducer and the blood flow velocity. Very useful in fetal echocardiography, color Doppler also assists obstetric ultrasonography whenever it is important to characterize and localize blood flow (cord, placenta, fetal renal and cerebral circulation, gestational trophoblastic disease, fetal tumors, etc.).

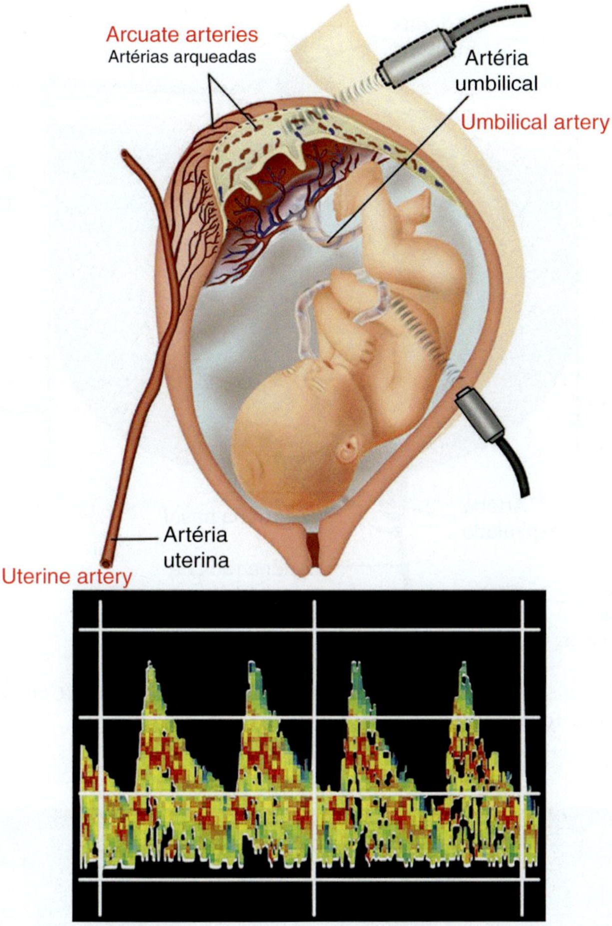

Fig. 16.2 Umbilical artery Doppler waveform. (Copyright © Editora Guanabara Koogan. Todos os direitos reservados)

Fetal Arterial Doppler

Umbilical Artery Doppler

In normal pregnancy, the umbilical circulation is characterized by increasingly low resistance, according to the evolution of pregnancy, as the vascular architecture of terminal villi develops (Fig. 16.3).

The umbilical artery Doppler, similarly to the aortic, can be divided into four categories (Fig. 16.4): normal, class I (decreased diastole), class II (diastole/zero), and class III (reverse diastole) [5].

Increased resistance is related to a reduction in the terminal villous vascular units, characterized by increased S/D ratio and pulsatile index (PI) [9]. When there is zero

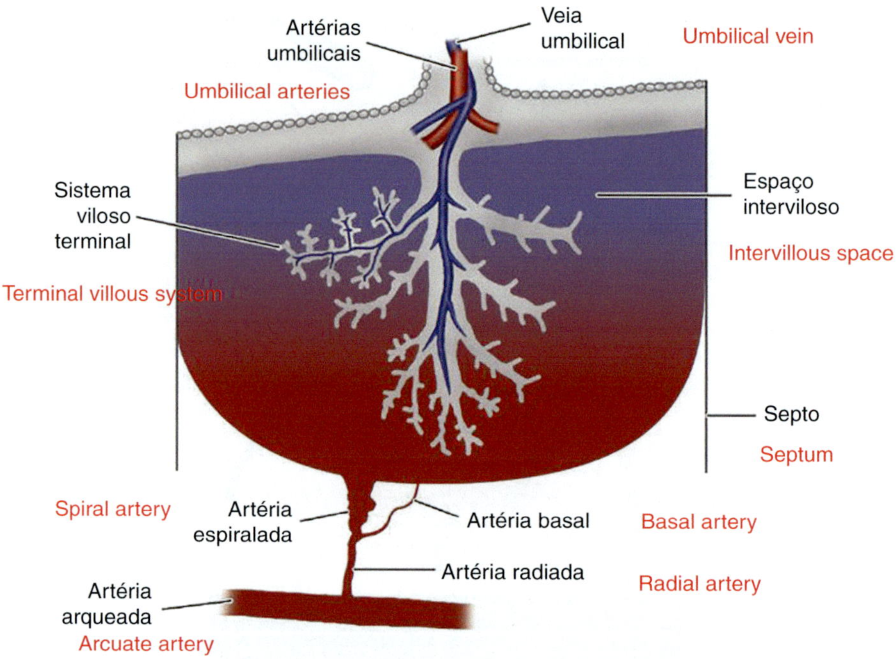

Fig. 16.3 Schematic representation of human placental circulation. (Copyright © Editora Guanabara Koogan. Todos os direitos reservados)

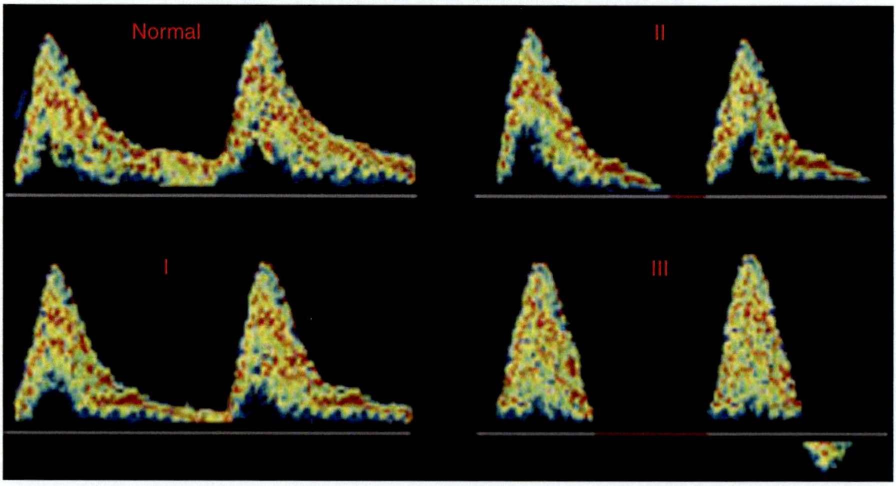

Fig. 16.4 Blood flow categories: normal flow, I (decreased diastole), II (zero diastole), and III (reverse diastole). (Copyright © Editora Guanabara Koogan. Todos os direitos reservados)

diastole in the umbilical artery Doppler, there is a 50% reduction in the function of the terminal villi, and in cases of reverse diastole, more than 70% are obstructed.

As a fetal vitality test, the umbilical artery Doppler was the only procedure that improved the perinatal mortality in randomized studies [1]. For this reason, it is the test of choice for assessing placental insufficiency in the IUGR from placental origin.

There are different flowmetry indexes obtained in different segments of the same umbilical artery. In the region near the placental insertion, the pulsatility and resistance indexes are lower than near the fetal abdominal insertion. The International Society for Ultrasound in Obstetrics and Gynecology (ISUOG) recommends that the evaluation should therefore be done in a cord-free loop [2].

Middle Cerebral Artery (MCA) Doppler

MCA is the most easily evaluated brain vessel. MCA is the largest branch of the Willis polygon that originates from the internal carotid and vertebral arteries. Willis polygon is visualized by axial section Doppler of the base of the fetal skull at the level of the thalamus and wings of the sphenoid bone. The best MCA insonation site for achievement of Doppler is in the proximal third, at its origin from the Willis polygon (Fig. 16.5—MCA).

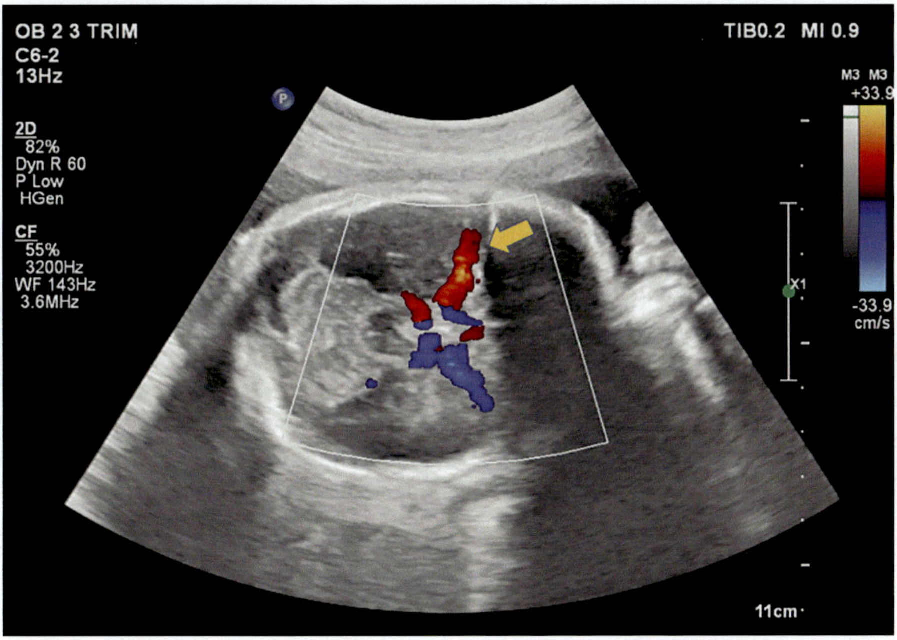

Fig. 16.5 Color Doppler identifying the Willis polygon with middle cerebral artery (arrow)

Fetal brain circulation has a higher impedance. With the development of fetal hypoxia, the redistribution of blood flow occurs in such a way that resistance in the middle cerebral artery (MCA) decreases and in the umbilical artery increases, due to the obliteration of the villous arterioles—the so-called brain-sparing effect or centralization [6, 10].

In cases of suspected fetal anemia, such as in cases of fetal hemolytic disease, it is important that the MCA insonation beam is parallel to the vessel, in an angle of 0° or, at most, 30°. In this way, it is possible to have more reliable measurements of speed. In fetal anemia, there is a decrease in serum hemoglobin, a decrease in blood viscosity, and an increase in cardiac work, with consequent increase in flow velocity. It is possible to evaluate the degree of fetal anemia through the systolic peak of the MCA velocity and, if necessary, indicate a possible treatment. When there is an increase above 1.50 multiples of the median (MoM) of the systolic velocity peak in at-risk fetuses, the sensitivity for detecting anemia is 100% [4].

Maternal Arterial Doppler

Uterine Artery Doppler

Uterine artery Doppler evaluates the resistance in the vessels that supply the placenta, reflecting the remodeling of the spiral arteries, that is impaired in preeclampsia, IUGR, abruptio placentae, and intrauterine fetal death. During pregnancy, there is an adaptation of the uterine circulation as a result of trophoblastic invasion, modifying the structure of the uterine spiral arteries, that become more dilated and less responsive to the autonomic nervous system. The purpose of this adaptation is to provide an increased blood flow to uterus and consequently the fetus, as pregnancy progresses [7].

The uterine artery Doppler is fully incorporated into ultrasonography from 20 to 24 weeks. The result is considered abnormal when the mean of the two uterine shows resistance index (RI) >0.58. The abnormal uterine Doppler is associated with an increased risk of preeclampsia and/or IUGR (4–8 times). In contrast, normal uterine Doppler has a negative predictive value of 99%, practically excluding these pregnancy complications.

The uterine artery Doppler in the first trimester (11–13 weeks) has been currently used for earlier preeclampsia prediction and thus better prevention.

The uterine artery can be evaluated by Doppler as soon as it crosses the hypogastric vessels before entering the uterus and dividing itself into the uterine and cervical branches (Fig. 16.6).

Currently, more attention has been given to the evaluation of the uterine arteries at the end of the second and third trimesters, especially in cases of intrauterine growth restriction [3] (Hernandez-Andrade et al. 2002).

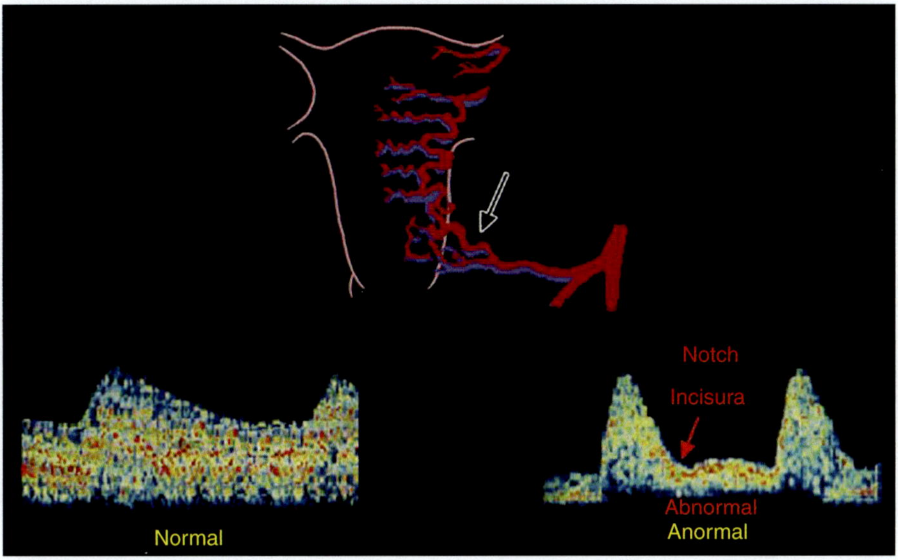

Fig. 16.6 Uterine artery Doppler after 24 weeks. (Copyright © Editora Guanabara Koogan. Todos os direitos reservados)

Fetal Venous Doppler

The venous system evaluation may better reflect the imminent impairment of fetal heart function and the need to terminate pregnancy. Deterioration of right ventricle contractility leads to its tricuspid dilatation and regurgitation (insufficiency), exacerbating the right atrial filling pressure and venous filling resistance. Such resistance is reflected in the venous duct that shows zero/reverse pattern during atrial contraction (A), a finding highly related to imminent fetal asphyxia (Fig. 16.7). Finally, the increase in systemic venous pressure determines the maximum dilation of the venous duct and direct transmission of the cardiac pulse to the umbilical vein, causing pulsation in this vessel. The pulsation in the umbilical vein is closely related to the terminal stage of the fetus.

The venous duct can be accessed through the transverse sections of the abdomen, in the same plane as the abdominal circumference measurement near the portal vein, or through the sagittal section, following the umbilical vein to the liver. The venous duct wave is biphasic, with the first phase corresponding to the ventricular systolic peak, the second phase to a diastolic peak, and a nadir during atrial contraction, with no reverse flow component after, known as the "A" wave. The absence of reverse flow in the venous duct may be the indirect result of the pressure gradient between the umbilical vein and the right atrium. Absent or reversed "A" wave can be resultant from reduced or reversed flow circulation during atrial systole, probably due to placental insufficiency and functional or anatomical changes of the fetal heart [8].

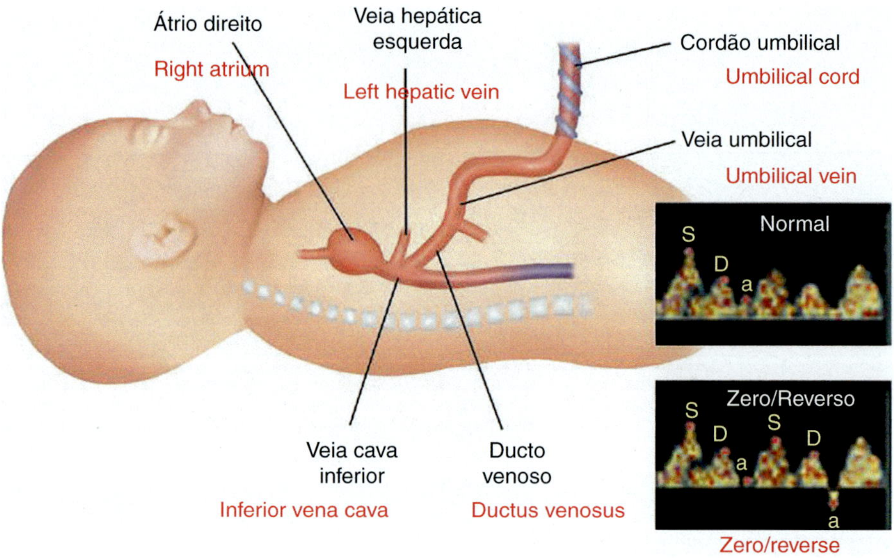

Fig. 16.7 Venous Doppler: Doppler of normal and abnormal venous duct. (Copyright © Editora Guanabara Koogan. Todos os direitos reservados)

References

1. Alfirevic Z, Stampalija T, Dowswell T. Fetal and umbilical Doppler ultrasound in high-risk pregnancies. Cochrane Database Syst Rev. 2017;6:CD007529.
2. Bhide A, Acharya G, Bilardo CM, et al. ISUOG practice guidelines: use of Doppler ultrasonography in obstetrics. Ultrasound Obstet Gynecol. 2013;41(2):233–9.
3. Figueras F, Gratacós E. Update on the diagnosis and classification of fetal growth restriction and proposal of a stage-based management protocol. Fetal Diagn Ther. 2014;36:86–98.
4. Hanif F, Drennan K, Mari G. Variable affecting the middle cerebral artery peak systolic velocity in anemic and IUGF fetuses. Am J Perinatol. 2007;24:501–5.
5. Laurin J, Marsal K, Persson PH, et al. Ultrasound measurement of fetal blood flow in predicting fetal outcome. BJOG. 1987;94(10):940–8.
6. Montenegro CAB, Rezende Filho J, Silva LGP. Centralização fetal. Femina. 1994;22:203.
7. Pijnenbog R, Bland JM, Robertson WB, et al. Uteroplacental arterial changes related to interstitial trophoblast migration in early pregnancy. Placenta. 1983;4:397.
8. Robertson WB, Brosens I, Dixon HG. Uteroplacental vascular pathology. Eur J Obstet Gynecol Reprod Biol. 1975;5:47.
9. Trudinger BJ, Stevens D, Connelly A, et al. Umbilical artery flow velocity waveforms and placental resistance: the effects of embolization of the umbilical circulation. Am J Obstet Gynecol. 1987;157:1443.
10. Wladimiroff JW, Tongue HM, Stewart PA. Doppler ultrasound assessment of cerebral blood flow in the human fetus. BJOG. 1986;93:471.

Chapter 17
Antepartum Cardiotography

Susana Santo and Diogo Ayres-De-Campos

Introduction

Cardiotocography (CTG), derived from the Greek terms "cardio" (heart) and "tokos" (uterine activity) [1], was introduced into clinical practice during the 1960s and is nowadays widely used in high-resource countries as a method of assessing fetal oxygenation during late pregnancy and labor. The physiological principles behind antepartum CTG are the same as those of intrapartum CTG, as are the main objectives of both, i.e., evaluation of ongoing fetal oxygenation. For these reasons, CTG interpretation is similar in both settings.

Fetal heart rate (FHR) is modulated by several stimuli. The central nervous system has a major influence on the FHR, mediated via the cardioregulatory center located in the brainstem. The efferent component of the autonomic nervous system has a major influence on FHR signals, with sympathetic impulses increasing their frequency and parasympathetic impulses having the opposite effect [2]. The input of sympathetic and parasympathetic systems creates a constant fluctuation of the FHR signal, known as variability [3]. These two components of the autonomic nervous system mature at different rates during intrauterine life. The sympathetic system matures faster and therefore preterm fetuses have a higher baseline. Later maturation of the parasympathetic system leads to a constant decrease in FHR baseline throughout gestation and post-term fetuses may present a baseline between 100 and 110 bpm [4].

The central nervous system is also responsible for the appearance of FHR accelerations, which are coincident with fetal movements and with the

S. Santo (✉) · D. Ayres-De-Campos
Departamento de Obstetrícia, Ginecologia e Medicina da Reprodução, Faculdade de Medicina da Universidade de Lisboa, Centro Hospitalar Universitário Lisboa Norte – Hospital de Santa Maria, Lisbon, Portugal

© Springer Nature Switzerland AG 2022

R. A. Moreira de Sá, E. B. d. Fonseca (eds.), *Perinatology*,
https://doi.org/10.1007/978-3-030-83434-0_17

occurrence of sleep-activity cycles. Fetal behavioral states refer to periods of deep sleep (no eye movements), alternating with periods of active sleep (rapid eye movements), and active wakefulness [5]. Constant transitions between different behavioral states are a sign of neurological responsiveness and of the absence of fetal hypoxia. These transitions usually become clearer after 32–34 weeks of gestation, as a consequence of central nervous system maturation [5]. Deep sleep can last up to 50 min [6] and is associated with borderline variability and very rare accelerations. Active sleep is the most frequent behavioral state and is represented by normal variability and a moderate number of accelerations. Active wakefulness is represented by normal variability and a high number of accelerations. Accelerations may be so frequent as to make baseline estimation difficult [4].

Uterine contractions are a hallmark of labor but may also occur irregularly before this period starts. Fetal head compression can stimulate intracranial baroreceptors and trigger a nervous reflex via the brainstem and parasympathetic pathways, leading to the appearance of early decelerations [2, 4]. These are not associated with fetal hypoxia [4].

Contractions can also cause umbilical cord compression, leading to the appearance of variable decelerations [7]. The pathophysiology behind these events is the occurrence of a temporary increase in blood pressure, stimulating baroreceptors located in central fetal vessels, and thus triggering a nervous reflex via the brainstem and parasympathetic pathways that lead to a drop in FHR. The response is very rapid, and a quick recovery of the baseline FHR is also observed [7, 4].

A sudden decrease in blood oxygen concentration activates chemoreceptors located in central fetal vessels, which stimulates a nervous reflex via the brainstem and parasympathetic pathways causing late decelerations of the FHR [3]. In comparison with baroreceptors, activation of chemoreceptors is associated with a slower response and time to recover the baseline FHR [4].

Reduced FRH variability is caused, among others, by central nervous system hypoxia, reducing both sympathetic and parasympathetic activity in the brainstem, and the resulting oscillations in FHR [4, 8].

As most CTG events occur in response to uterine contractions, efforts were made in the 1970s and 1980s to artificially stimulate uterine contractions during antepartum CTGs. Nipple stimulation and exogenous oxytocin were used for this purpose, in a technique that became known as the "contraction stress test" [9–11]. The time-consuming nature of the method, and the impossibility of standardizing the intensity and duration of contractions, led to its progressive abandonment. In contrast to the previous nomenclature, in some parts of the world, antepartum CTG without artificial stimulation of contractions became known as the "nonstress test," but this terminology has nowadays mostly been abandoned.

The aim of this chapter is to address the basic principles of antepartum CTG interpretation and to outline the management of normal and abnormal tracings.

Indications

Antepartum CTG is usually performed in clinical situations associated with an increased risk of fetal hypoxia. These conditions include prepregnancy diseases (e.g., systemic lupus erythematosus, antiphospholipid syndrome, diabetes mellitus, etc.), pregnancy-related diseases (preeclampsia, placental abruption, etc.), and fetal diseases (fetal growth restriction, congenital malformations, etc.), all of which are associated with an increased risk of adverse perinatal outcome [10].

Although it is more commonly performed during the third trimester, CTG can be acquired from around 25 weeks onward. The frequency of exams depends on the clinical situation, gestational age, interpretation of previous tracings, etc. The intervals of testing usually vary between three times a day and every week.

CTG Tracing Acquisition

All CTG monitors record FHR and uterine contraction signals. An audible FHR signal is available to help identify the ideal placement of the FHR sensor. The tracing itself may be printed on paper or displayed on a computer monitor. The horizontal scale for CTG registration is commonly called "paper speed," and the available options are 1, 2, or 3 cm/min. Paper speed has some impact on the detail of the information displayed but also on paper length, especially in settings where electronically storage is not available. In most countries, 1 cm/min is selected, but 3 cm/min is popular in countries like the USA and Japan. The vertical scale may also differ, varying from 20 to 30 bpm/cm. Paper scales used in each center should be the ones with which health care professionals are most familiar because patterns can look very distinct at different paper speeds. For example, variability may appear reduced at 3 cm/min for a health care professional familiar with the 1 cm/min scale [4].

A tracing should be identified from the start of acquisition, including mother's name, hospital identification number, date, and time. Modern machines automatically show the last two, but it is important to check that these parameters are correctly configured.

For antepartum CTGs, both FHR and uterine contraction signals must be acquired using noninvasive methods, i.e., external transducers placed on the maternal abdomen and fixed with elastic bands. External FHR monitoring uses a Doppler-ultrasound transducer that detects movement of fetal heart structures such as heart valves and interchamber septae. The acquired signal is processed using autocorrelation to guarantee an adequate tracing quality, and the result is an approximation to the real heart cycle [12]. Signal loss due to fetal movements, inadvertent recording of the maternal heart rate, inaccurate recording of fetal arrhythmias, and signal artifacts such as double and half-counting may all occur with this method [13].

Uterine contractility is recorded with an external tocodynameter placed on the uterine fundus, measuring the tensile strength of the uterine wall during contractions. The tocodynameter only allows an evaluation of the frequency of contractions [4]. Resting tone, duration, and intensity of the contractions can only be accurately assessed with invasive methods that are not applicable before labor. The uterine contraction signal may also be affected by incorrect placement of the transducer, inadequate tension applied to the elastic band, and maternal obesity.

Fetal movements are frequently integrated into the antepartum CTG. These can be recorded by the mother and signaled by pressing an event marker button or automatically extracted from the Doppler signal, using an algorithm that separates the low-frequency signals that correspond to fetal motor activity.

Some CTG monitors also acquire and record the maternal heart rate. This can be obtained by electrocardiography, pletismography, or a Doppler sensor placed within the tocodynamometer. Simultaneous recording of the FHR and maternal heart rate may be important to distinguish fetal from maternal signals.

Antepartum CTG should be performed in the lateral recumbent or half-sitting positions, thus avoiding aortocaval compression, which can reduce uterine blood flow and placental perfusion.

CTG Interpretation

The International Federation of Obstetrics and Gynecology (FIGO) recently updated their CTG interpretation guidelines, through a large consensus panel including 50 experts [1, 4, 14–16]. As referred before, the pathophysiology behind CTG features is the same, whether they occur in the antepartum or intrapartum periods, so the same concepts of CTG interpretation can be used in both periods.

Basic FHR Features

CTG interpretation requires the evaluation of four basic FHR features: baseline, variability, accelerations, and decelerations [4]. The combined evaluation of these features allows the classification of the CTG tracing into one of three categories: normal, suspicious, or pathological.

Baseline is the mean level of the most horizontal and less oscillatory FHR segments. It is estimated in 10-minute periods and expressed in beats per minute (bpm). Baseline values may vary between two periods of 10 min, but in antepartum CTGs, it is usually very stable. The baseline may be difficult to evaluate during the fetal behavioral state of active wakefulness, and review of previous segments or continued monitoring for longer time periods may be necessary in these situations. Normal baseline is defined as a value between 110 and 160 bpm (Fig. 17.1). It is important to consider gestational age in this equation, as preterm

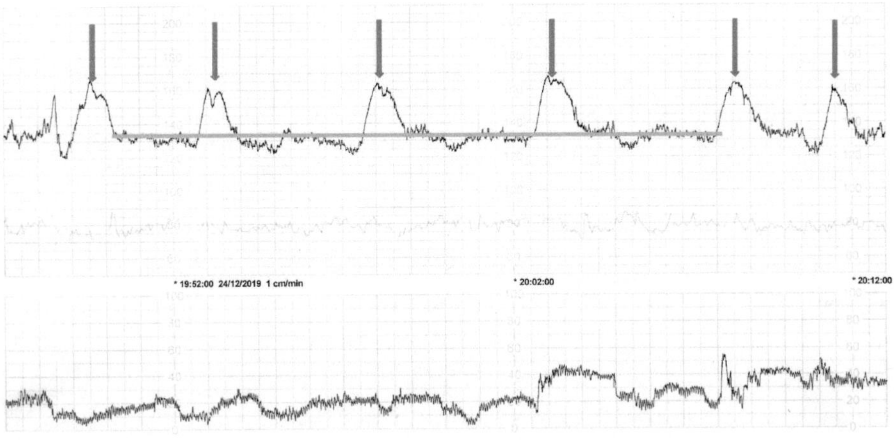

Fig. 17.1 Normal baseline (130 bpm); accelerations are identified with arrows

fetuses tend to have values toward the upper end of this range and post-term fetuses toward the lower end [4]. Tachycardia is defined as a baseline value above 160 bpm lasting more than 10 min. Maternal pyrexia is the most frequent cause, but it can also occur in the initial stages of a nonacute fetal hypoxemia, with the administration of beta-agonist drugs, parasympathetic blockers, and with fetal arrhythmias such as supraventricular tachycardia and atrial flutter [4]. Bradycardia is a baseline value below 110 bpm lasting more than 10 min. However, values between 100 and 110 bpm may occur in normal fetuses, especially in postdate pregnancies. Maternal hypothermia, administration of beta-blockers, and fetal arrhythmias such as atrial-ventricular block are other possible causes of bradycardia [4].

Variability refers to the fine oscillations in the FHR signal and is visually estimated as the average signal bandwidth amplitude in 1-minute segments. Normal variability is defined as a bandwidth amplitude between 5 and 25 bpm [4] (Fig. 17.2). Reduced variability is a bandwidth amplitude below 5 bpm for more than 50 min in baseline segments, or for more than 3 min during decelerations [4] (Fig. 17.3). There is a high degree of subjectivity in the visual evaluation of this parameter, and therefore careful re-evaluation or computer analysis is recommended in borderline situations. Reduced variability can occur in situations associated with central nervous system hypoxia that result in decreased autonomic system activity. It may also occur in fetuses with cerebral injury, infection, and administration of central nervous system depressants or parasympathetic blockers. During deep fetal sleep, variability is usually in the lower range of normality, but the bandwidth amplitude is seldom under 5 bpm. Increased variability, also known as the saltatory pattern, corresponds to a bandwidth exceeding 25 bpm for more than 30 min [4] (Fig. 17.4). The pathophysiology of this pattern is incompletely understood, but it has been described in the initial stages of subacute hypoxia and may be caused by fetal autonomic instability [17].

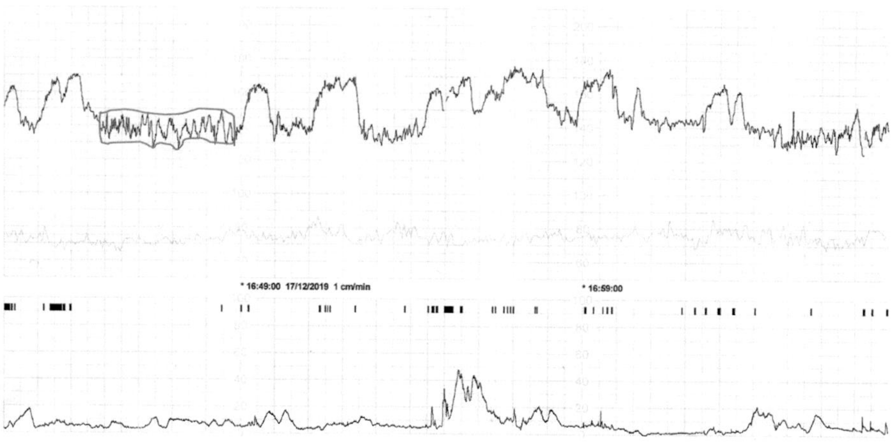

Fig. 17.2 Normal variability (5–25 bpm)

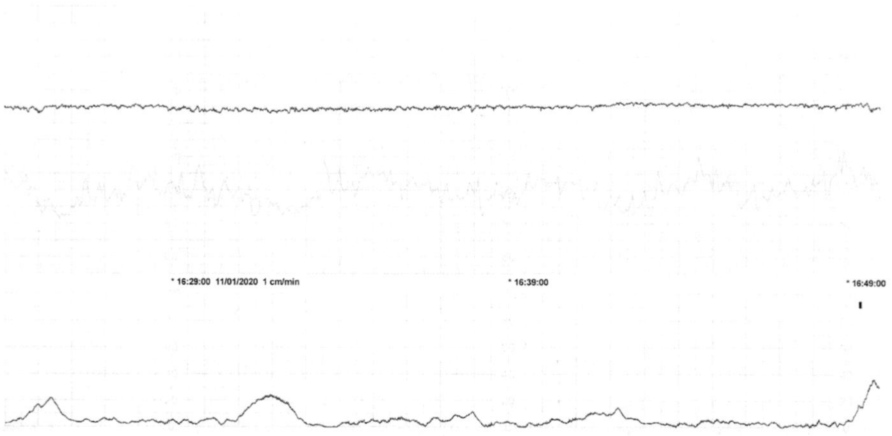

Fig. 17.3 Reduced variability (<5 bpm). To be clinically meaningful, the pattern needs to last for at least 50 min, and medication depressing the central nervous system needs to be ruled out

Accelerations are abrupt increases in FHR above the baseline, of more than 15 bpm in amplitude, and lasting more than 15 s but less than 10 min [4] (Fig. 17.1). Before 32 weeks of gestation, accelerations may be of slightly lower amplitude and duration. Accelerations usually coincide with fetal movements and are a sign of a neurologically responsive fetus that is not suffering from hypoxia.

Decelerations are abrupt decreases in FHR below the baseline with an amplitude of more than 15 bpm and a duration of more than 15 s. Decelerations may be classified as early, variable, late, or prolonged, mainly according to their shape and duration. They are usually associated with uterine contractions, and therefore are much less frequent in antepartum CTGs. Early decelerations are shallow, short-lasting, with normal variability within the deceleration, and coincident with

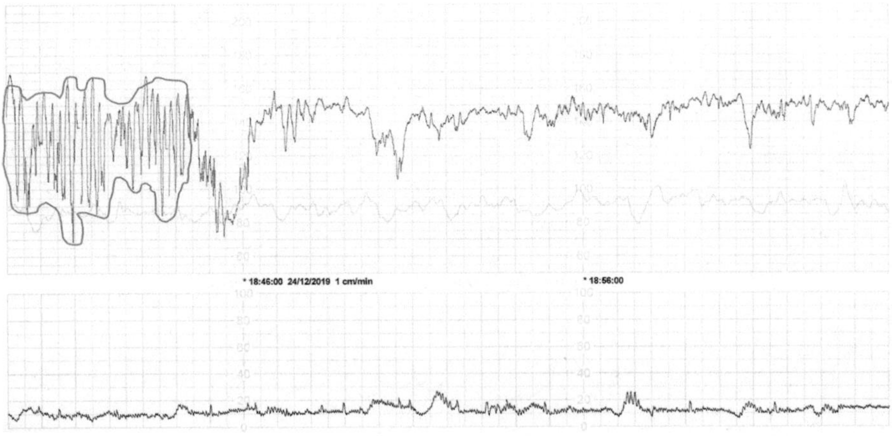

Fig. 17.4 Increased variability (>5 bpm). To be clinically meaningful, this pattern needs to last for at least 30 min

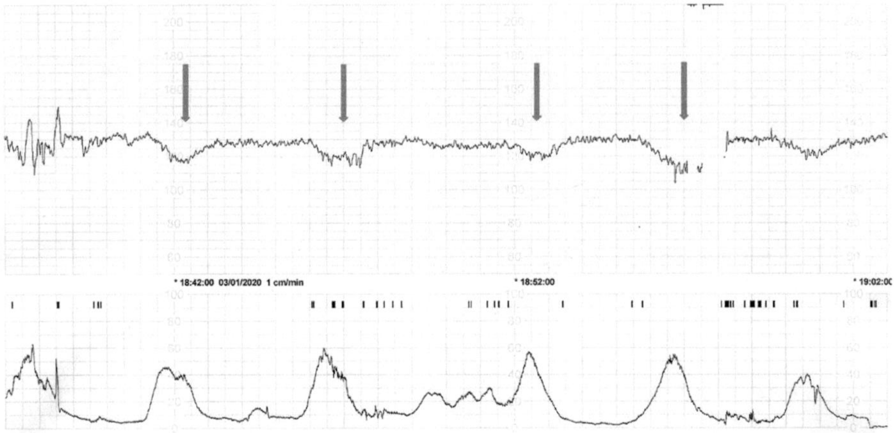

Fig. 17.5 Early decelerations (identified with arrows)

contractions (Fig. 17.5). It is believed that they are caused by fetal head compression and therefore do not indicate fetal hypoxia. Variable decelerations (V-shaped) exhibit a rapid drop (onset to nadir in less than 30 s), good variability within the deceleration, and rapid recovery to the baseline. They vary in size, shape, and relationship to uterine contractions (Fig. 17.6). They translate a baroreceptor-mediated response to increased arterial pressure, as occurs with umbilical cord compression, and are seldom associated with an important degree of hypoxia. Late decelerations (U-shaped or with reduced variability) have a gradual onset or a gradual return to the baseline (>30 s), or reduced variability within the deceleration. In the presence of a tracing with reduced variability and no accelerations, the definition of late decelerations also includes those with an amplitude of 10–15 bpm (Fig. 17.7). Late

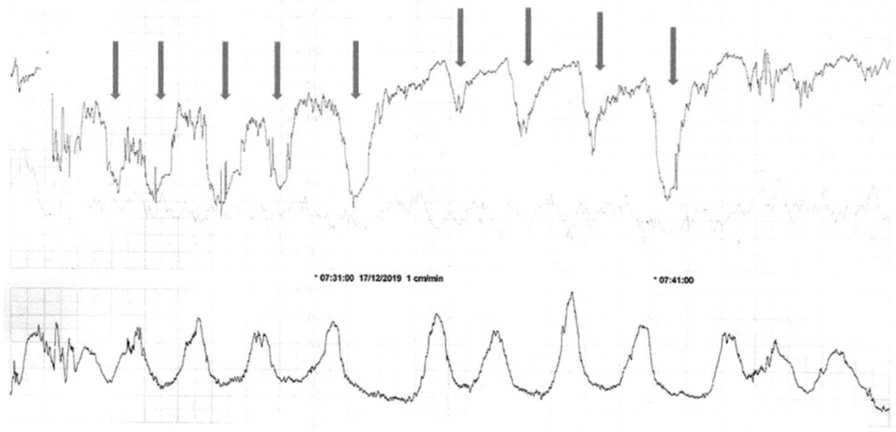

Fig. 17.6 Repetitive variable decelerations (identified with arrows)

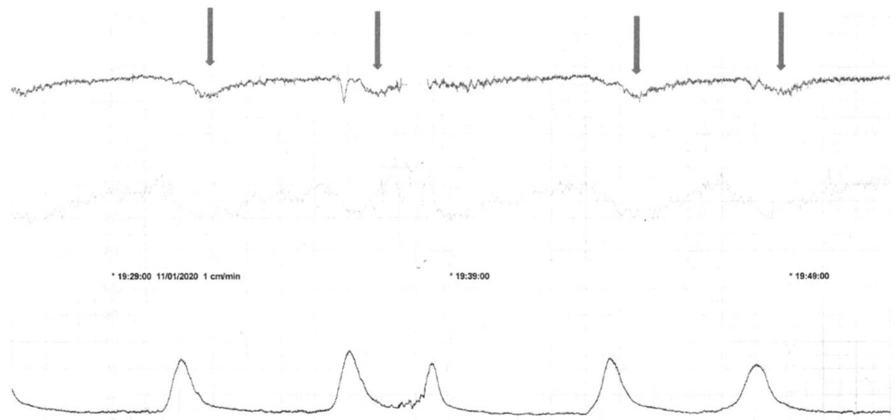

Fig. 17.7 Repetitive late decelerations (identified with arrows). In the context of a tracing with reduced variability and no accelerations, late decelerations only need to have 10 bpm of amplitude

decelerations start more than 20 s after the onset of a contraction, have a nadir after the acme, and return to the baseline after the end of the contraction. They are indicative of a chemoreceptor-mediated response to sudden fetal hypoxemia. Prolonged decelerations last more than 3 min and are very likely to include a chemoreceptor-mediated component, and thus to indicate some degree of hypoxemia (Fig. 17.8). When they exceed 5 min, FHR is maintained <80 bpm, and there is reduced variability within the deceleration, they are usually indicative of an episode of acute fetal hypoxemia and therefore require emergent intervention [4].

The sinusoidal pattern is regular, smooth, undulating signal, resembling a sine wave that lasts more than 30 min. The amplitude of this undulation is 5–15 bpm, and the frequency is 3–5 cycles per minute (Fig. 17.9). The pathophysiological basis for

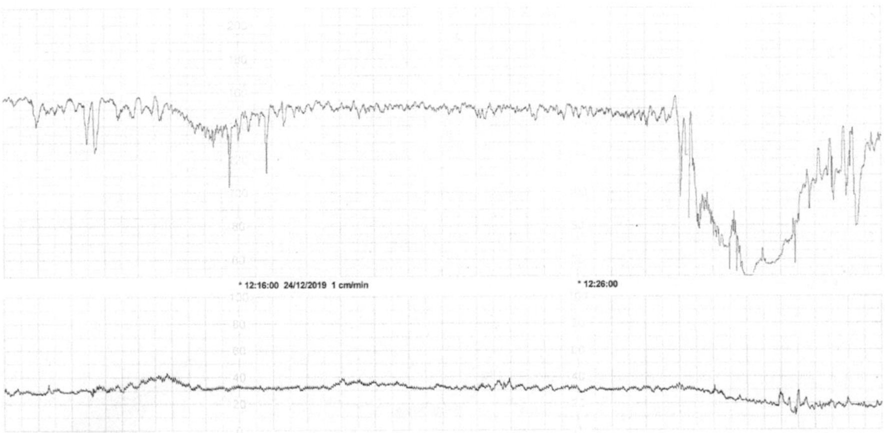

Fig. 17.8 A prolonged deceleration lasting around 4.5 min

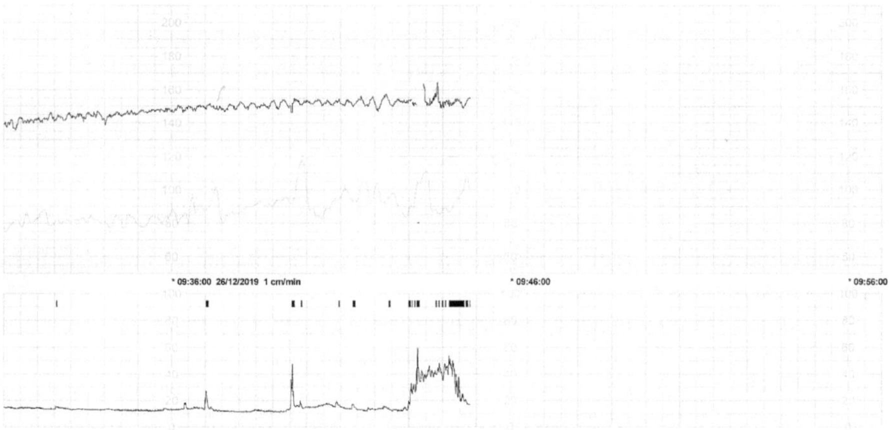

Fig. 17.9 A sinusoidal pattern. To be clinically meaningful, this pattern needs to last at least 30 min

the sinusoidal pattern is incompletely understood, but it is known to occur in association with severe fetal anemia (fetal-maternal hemorrhage, twin-to-twin transfusion syndrome, and ruptured vasa previa). Less frequently, it has been described in cases of acute fetal hypoxia, infection, or fetal malformations [4]. The *pseudosinusoidal pattern* resembles the sinusoidal pattern but has a more jagged "saw-tooth" appearance, rather than a smooth undulating form (Fig. 17.10). The duration seldom exceeds 30 min, and it is characterized by normal patterns before and after. This pattern has been described after analgesic administration to the mother and during periods of fetal sucking and other mouth movements. It is sometimes difficult to distinguish the pseudosinusoidal pattern from the true sinusoidal pattern, and the short duration of the former is the most important aspect that discriminates between the two [4].

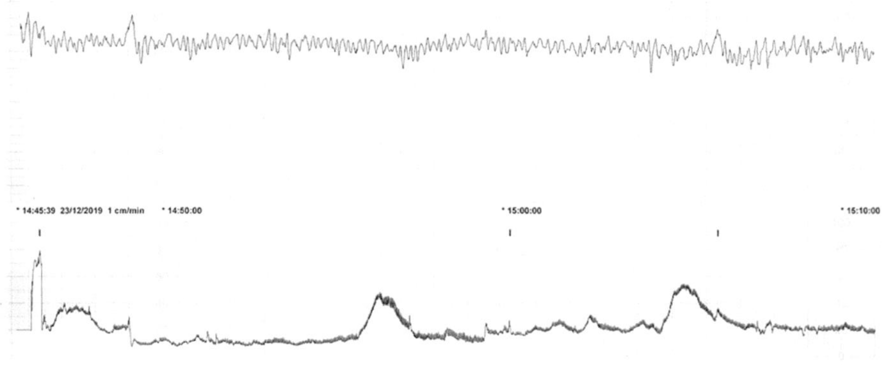

Fig. 17.10 A pseudosinusoidal pattern

Contractions are bell-shaped gradual increases in the uterine activity signal followed by roughly symmetric decreases, with 45–120 s in total duration [4].

Tracing Classification

Classification of CTG tracings requires a systematic evaluation of the basic FHR features described above (Table 17.1).

A *normal* CTG tracing has a normal baseline (110–160 bpm), normal variability (5–25 bpm), and no repetitive decelerations. In the antepartum period, accelerations also need to be present. It is important to emphasize that sporadic decelerations may occur in normal tracings and are usually early or variable in nature. A *suspicious* tracing lacks at least one characteristic of normality but has no pathological features. *Pathological* tracings have one or more of the flowing criteria: bradycardia (<100 bpm), reduced variability (<5 bpm for more than 50 min or for more than 3 min in decelerations), increased variability (>25 bpm for more than 30 min), repetitive late or prolonged decelerations (for more than 30 min; or for >20 min if variability is <5 bpm), prolonged deceleration with more than 5 min, or a sinusoidal pattern [4].

Antepartum CTGs have also been classified as reactive or nonreactive, according to the presence of accelerations within a given period [6, 18, 19]. Causes of nonreactive tracings include fetal sleep, hypoxia, prematurity, maternal smoking, fetal neurologic or cardiac abnormalities, or maternal ingestion of drugs. Vibroacoustic stimulation, using an artificial larynx placed on the maternal abdomen, has been used to distinguish between the state of deep sleep and fetal hypoxia, but this practice has largely been abandoned.

Table 17.1 CTG classification adapted from the 2015 FIGO guidelines [4]

	Normal	Suspicious	Pathological
Baseline	110–160bpm	Lacking at least one characteristic of normality, but with no pathological features	<100 bpm
Variability	5–25bpm		Reduced variability Increased variability Sinusoidal pattern
Decelerations	No repetitive* decelerations		Repetitive* late or prolonged decelerations for >30 min (or >20 min if reduced variability) Deceleration >5 min
Interpretation	No hypoxia/acidosis	Low probability of hypoxia/acidosis	High probability of hypoxia/acidosis

*Decelerations are repetitive when associated with > 50% contractions.

*Decelerations are repetitive when associated with >50% contractions

Clinical Management of Antepartum CTG

Because antepartum CTGs are easy to perform, noninvasive, have no contraindications, and are usually well-liked by women, they rapidly became part of routine care in high-resource countries. Although only few skills are needed for signal acquisition, extensive experience is required for interpretation. Gestational age, maternal medication, and other accompanying clinical information need to be taken into account for the interpretation of antepartum CTGs and for subsequent management. Fetal ultrasound and multivessel Doppler evaluation may add essential elements for the decision process.

A normal CTG excludes ongoing fetal hypoxia in the central organs, but the method cannot reliably determine whether this will occur in the near or long-term future. A suspicious tracing is unlikely to be associated with ongoing hypoxia in the central organs, but additional tests may be necessary to clarify the cause. Pathological tracings are frequently associated with ongoing fetal hypoxia in central organs and it is essential to clarify the underlying cause [4]. Reversible causes of fetal hypoxia (i.e., excessive uterine contractility, maternal supine position, hypotension) are frequently seen during labor but are rare events in the antepartum period. Irreversible conditions such as placental insufficiency or placental abruption are the most frequent causes of pathological CTGs in these settings. CTG changes appear late in the context of chronic placental insufficiency, as they translate hypoxia of central fetal organs, which are protected until late by the brain-sparing phenomenon.

Antepartum CTG provides valuable information on the oxygenation of the fetal brain and heart at a given moment in time, but the initial expectations that it can predict fetal "reserve" or what will occur in the next hours, days, or weeks are unrealistic. Fetal oxygenation may be quickly affected by acute and subacute events (placental abruption, uterine rupture, cord prolapse) that can follow a normal CTG. On the other hand, abnormal tracings may reflect different degrees of central hypoxia, and thus have a limited capacity to predict adverse outcomes, such as metabolic acidosis, low Apgar score, and neonatal intensive care unit admissions. A meta-analysis of six randomized controlled trials carried out in the 1980s and 1990s, comparing the use of antepartum CTGs with no use, showed no differences in perinatal mortality (RR 2.05, 95% confidence interval (CI) 0.95–4.42) or potentially preventable deaths (RR 2.46, 95% CI 0.96–6.30) [20]. Studies were clearly underpowered to evaluate these rare outcomes. Despite the limited scientific evidence, antepartum CTG continues to be extensively used in high-resource countries and is recommended by several international scientific societies for the surveillance of high-risk pregnancies [10, 11].

The complex nature of the FHR signal conditions a limited intra- and interobserver agreement in the evaluation of basic CTG features and in CTG classification [21–23]. Several human factors have also been appointed as important limitations of CTG analysis [24]. They are mainly related to the experience of health care professionals using the technology, and to the guidelines used for interpretation [25].

In modern days, antepartum CTG relies heavily on the evaluation of variability, and aspect that, on its own, may swerve the classification from normal to pathological. This is a difficult parameter to assess with the naked eye because constant changes in bandwidth are observed and there is much subjectivity in the evaluation of their amplitude. This limitation may be overcome by computer analysis of CTGs, which emerged in the 1080s and 1990s. The Dawes/Redman and SisPorto systems were the first to be developed for this purpose [26–28]. These systems incorporate complex mathematical algorithms that estimate the FHR baseline, quantify variability, and identify accelerations and decelerations. Using computer analysis, variability can be separated into short-term (oscillations between adjacent or near adjacent signals) and long-term variability (bandwidth values evaluated over the course of 1 min), providing additional information on the pathophysiological mechanisms of the central nervous system oxygenation.

Conclusions

CTG is one of the most adopted tools for antenatal fetal surveillance in high-resource countries. Antepartum and intrapartum CTG share the same pathophysiological mechanisms, so the same CTG interpretation guidelines can be used for both periods. Antepartum CTG should be used in conditions that carry a high-risk of fetal hypoxia. A normal CTG tracing excludes the occurrence of ongoing fetal hypoxia in central organs, but cannot evaluate the "fetal reserve" or predict hypoxic events occurring at a later time. Chronic placental insufficiency and placental abruption are the most frequent causes of pathological CTGs. These occur with ongoing hypoxia in central fetal organs, but may also be mimicked by deep sleep and by medication given to the mother. CTG changes appear late in the course of chronic placental insufficiency, as central organs are protected by the brain-sparing effect. Computer analysis of antepartum CTGs can provide a more reliable quantification of FHR variability, thus overcoming eyeball limitations in visual analysis and detecting changes that occur over the course of time. Tracing interpretation and subsequent clinical management requires expertise, needing to take into account other aspects of the clinical situation.

References

1. Ayres-de-Campos D, Arulkumaran S. Intrapartum Fetal monitoring expert consensus panel. FIGO consensus guidelines on intrapartum fetal monitoring: introduction. Int J Gynecol Obstet. 2015;131(1):3–4.
2. Gracia-Perez-Bonfils A, Chandraharan E. Physiology of Fetal heart rate control and types of intrapartum hypoxia. In: Chandraharan E, editor. Handbook of CTG interpretation: from patterns to physiology. United Kingdom: Cambridge University Press; 2017. p. 13–25.
3. Pinas A, Chandraharan E. Continuous cardiotocography during labour: analysis, classification and management. Best Pract Res Clin Obstet Gynaecol. 2016;30:33–47.
4. Ayres-De-Campos D, Spong CY, Chandraharan E. Intrapartum Fetal monitoring expert consensus panel. FIGO consensus guidelines on intrapartum fetal monitoring: cardiotocography. Int J Gynecol Obstet. 2015;131(1):13–24.
5. Suwanrath C, Suntharasaj T. Sleep-wake cycles in normal fetuses. Arch Gynecol Obstet. 2010;281(3):449–54.
6. Evertson LR, Gauthier RJ, Schifrin BS, Paul RH. Antepartum fetal heart rate testing. I. Evolution of the nonstress test. Am J Obstet Gynecol. 1979;133(1):29–33.
7. Ball RH, Parer JT. The physiologic mechanisms of variable decelerations. Am J Obstet Gynecol. 1992;166(6):1683–9.
8. Nelson K, Dambrosia J, Ting T, Grether J. Uncertain value of electronic fetal monitoring. N Engl J Med. 1996;334:613–8.
9. Ray M, Freeman R, Pine S, Hesselgesser R. Clinical experience with the oxytocin challenge test. Am J Obstet Gynecol. 1972;114(1):1–9.
10. Liston R, Sawchuck D, Young D, Brassard N, Campbell K, Davies G, et al. Fetal health surveillance: antepartum and intrapartum consensus guideline. J Obstet Gynaecol Canada. 2007;29(9):S3–4.
11. ACOG. Antepartum Fetal Surveillance. Obstet Gynecol. 2014;123(5):1118–32.
12. Carter M. Signal processing and display-cardiotocographs. Br J Obstet Gynaecol. 1993;100:21–3.
13. Stevenson H, Chandraharan E. Understanding the CTG. In: Chandraharan E, editor. Handbook of CTG interpretation: from patterns to physiology. United Kingdom: Cambridge University Press; 2017. p. 26–31.
14. Ayres-De-Campos D, Arulkumaran S. Intrapartum Fetal monitoring expert consensus panel. FIGO consensus guidelines on intrapartum fetal monitoring: physiology of fetal oxygenation and the main goals of intrapartum fetal monitoring. Int J Gynecol Obstet. 2015;131(1):5–8.
15. Visser GH, Ayres-De-Campos D. Intrapartum Fetal monitoring expert consensus panel. FIGO consensus guidelines on intrapartum fetal monitoring: adjunctive technologies. Int J Gynecol Obstet. 2015;131(1):25–9.
16. Lewis D, Downe S. Intrapartum Fetal monitoring expert consensus panel. FIGO consensus guidelines on intrapartum fetal monitoring: intermittent auscultation. Int J Gynecol Obstet. 2015;131(1):9–12.
17. Nunes I, Ayres-de-Campos D, Kwee A, Rosén KG. Prolonged saltatory fetal heart rate pattern leading to newborn metabolic acidosis. Clin Exp Obstet Gyn. 2014;41(5):507–11.
18. Brown R, Patrick J. The nonstress test: how long is enough? Am J Obstet {&} Gynecol. 1981;141(6):646–51.
19. Devoe LD, Castillo RA, Sherline DM. The nonstress test as a diagnostic test: a critical reappraisal. Am J Obstet Gynecol. 1985;152(8):1047–53.

20. Grivell RM, Alfirevic Z, Gyte GML DD. Antenatal cardiotocography for fetal assessment. Cochrane database Syst Rev. 2015;(9. Art. No.: CD007863).
21. Ayres-de-Campos D, Bernardes J, Marsal K, Nickelsen C, Makarainen L, Banfield P, et al. Can the reproducibility of fetal heart rate baseline estimation be improved? Eur J Obstet Gynecol Reprod Biol. 2004;112(1):49–54.
22. Ayres-de-Campos D, Bernardes J. Early, variable and late decelerations: can a consensus be reached in their identification? Int J Gynaecol Obstet. 1999;65(3):305–6.
23. Ayres-de-Campos D, Bernardes J, Costa-Pereira A, Pereira-Leite L. Inconsistencies in classification by experts of cardiotocograms and subsequent clinical decision. Br J Obstet Gynaecol. 1999;106(12):1307–10.
24. Santo S, Ayres-de-Campos D. Human factors affecting the interpretation of fetal heart rate tracings: an update. Curr Opin Obstet Gynecol. 2012;24(2):84–8.
25. Santo S, Ayres-de-Campos D, Costa-Santos C, Schnettler W, Ugwumadu A, Da Graça LM, et al. Agreement and accuracy using the FIGO, ACOG and NICE cardiotocography interpretation guidelines. Acta Obstet Gynecol Scand. 2017;96(2):166–75.
26. Dawes GS, Moulden M, Redman CWG. Improvements in computerized fetal heart rate analysis antepartum. J Perinat Med. 1996;
27. Bracero L, Roshanfekr D, Byrne D. Analysis of antepartum fetal heart rate tracing by physician and computer. J Matern Fetal Med. 2000;9(3):181–5.
28. Costa MA, Ayres-de-Campos D, Machado AP, Santos CC, Bernardes J. Comparison of a computer system evaluation of intrapartum cardiotocographic events and a consensus of clinicians. J Perinat Med. 2010;38(2):191–5.

Chapter 18
Evaluation of Fetal Pulmonary Maturity

Evaldo Trajano de Souza Silva Filho, Matheus Cabral L. Beleza, and Lucas Trigo

Introduction

The respiratory system is one of the last set of organs to achieve functional development in fetal life. For the past decades, pulmonary maturity has been considered a significant marker in neonatal respiratory morbidity prediction [1]. Gestational age (GA) is considered the strongest predictor of lung maturity, and preterm births are related to significant morbidity, mortality, and admission in the Neonatal Intensive Care Unit (NICU) [2]. These complications occurs often due to the difficulty of providing efficient oxygen support to an immature pulmonary system [1].

The neonatal respiratory morbidity (NRM), which includes respiratory distress syndrome (RDS) and transient tachypnea of the newborn (TTN), is the most common complication in preterm (<37 weeks) and early-term (<39 weeks) infants [3, 4]. While obstetric management of early-preterm fetuses is a consensus, the late-preterm period, from 34.0 to 36.6 weeks, has been constantly discussed [5]. Although closer to the term, the risk of the newborn developing NRM is still between 5% and 20% [2]. These numbers have supported further discussions regarding the proper classification of "term" and "preterm," and their own subclassification. Considering the not so small risk of pulmonary distress for the newborn, obstetricians may find themselves in a position in which they have to balance the pros and cons of a preterm delivery and the use of maternal corticosteroids, hoping to ensure a better maternal and fetal outcome [6–8].

The first fetal lung maturity (FLM) direct test was developed over 40 years ago. It was used to assess potential risk of NRM, and help to define a better delivery

E. T. de Souza Silva Filho · M. C. L. Beleza (✉)
Maternal-Fetal Medicine Department, NEXUS Institute, Brasília, Federal District, Brazil

L. Trigo
Maternal-Fetal Medicine Department, Fetal Medicine Research Center (BCNatal), Hospital Clinic and Hospital Sant Joan de Déu, University of Barcelona, Barcelona, Catalunya, Spain

© Springer Nature Switzerland AG 2022
R. A. Moreira de Sá, E. B. d. Fonseca (eds.), *Perinatology*,
https://doi.org/10.1007/978-3-030-83434-0_18

timing in complex obstetrical conditions. [9, 10]. However, in 2019, the ACOG guidelines stated that this procedure has no more utility in clinical management [11]. Historically, obstetricians used amniocentesis to document FLM via biochemical or biophysical testing [12].

FLM test purpose was well-intended, but it required an invasive procedure, thus, increasing the risks of infection and miscarriage. Therefore, in the last years, studies have explored the possibility of assessing FLM through ultrasound techniques, such as echogenic evaluation of the lung parenchyma and the pulmonary artery Doppler [13]. The adoption of a noninvasive test such as the ultrasound represents a safer diagnostic method with neither maternal nor neonatal adverse outcomes [6].

Although guidelines help obstetricians in preterm delivery management and in the usage of antenatal corticosteroids, there are some situations in which the path is not always clear. Especially in these cases where the benefits of a preterm birth are uncertain and/or the risk of NRM seems to be high, FLM assessment is more relevant for the clinical practice [14].

Fetal Lung Development

Fetal lung development is a complex and highly regulated process that begins about 3 weeks after conception and continues throughout childhood and young adulthood [15, 16]. It can be divided into five stages: embryonic, glandular (or pseudoglandular), canalicular, saccular (or terminal sac), and alveolar (Fig. 18.1).

During the embryonic period, from 22 to 26 days after conception, the lungs organogenesis starts as an outgrowth of the primitive foregut. At 34 days, it is

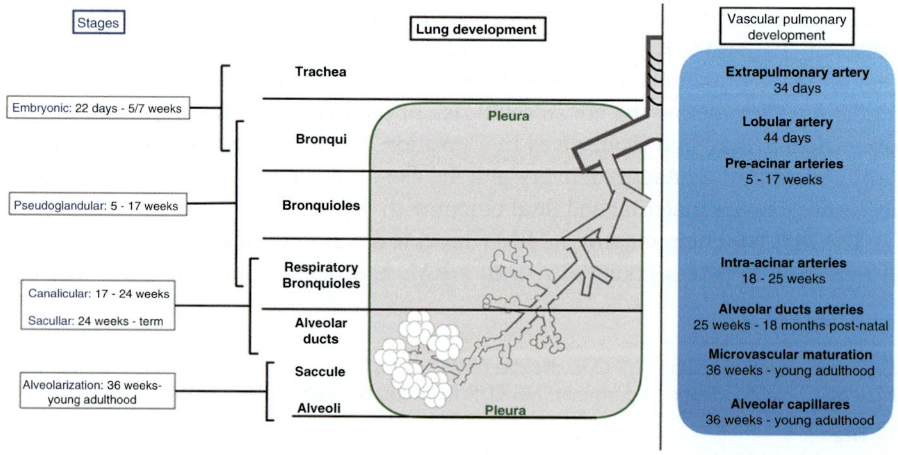

Fig. 18.1 Correlation of the stages of lung and vascular development. (Reproduced from Dr. Matheus Beleza)

divided into left and right sides that will later correspond to the major units of the lung, with more than 40 cell types [16].

The following phases refer to the proper lung development and are basically divided by morphological criteria. The inner surface of the lung is formed by two mechanisms: branching morphogenesis and septation (also called alveolarization). Since the lung development is dynamic and happens from the proximal region toward periphery, both lungs can present different regions' characteristics at the same time [16].

The glandular period occurs approximately from 5 to 17 weeks of pregnancy [16]. It consists basically on the formation of the "pulmonary tree," by the expansion of the bronchial airways and blood vessels that begin to develop in parallel [17]. From 17 to 24 weeks, the canalization caused by the fetal airways growth entitles the canalicular period [17]. This phase is characterized by the early bronchioles development and the differentiation and vascularization of the lungs epithelium [15].

The saccular period is considered one of the most important phases during the intrauterine pulmonary development. It starts around 24 weeks and extends into term. This stage is characterized by the arising of thin spherical sacs from the division of terminal bronchioles called alveoli. They form the respiratory lobules, known as the functional units of the lung. The alveoli are lined by types I and II pneumocytes and they are vascularized by an increasing net of capillaries, which will allow gas exchange after delivery due to their proximity [17, 16].

While type I pneumocytes are predominantly covering the alveolar surface, type II pneumocytes play two roles: being type I progenitor cells and producing surfactant [15]. The surfactant is a "surface-active" phospholipid released within the alveolar spaces as granular packages, known as lamellar bodies [18]. This substance is key for reducing the alveolar surface tension during breathing out, maintaining its stability and preventing it from collapse [17].

Among the surfactant compounds, the most important are lecithin (phosphatidylcholine) and phosphatidylglycerol, followed by phosphatidylinositol and sphingomyelin. Lecithin synthesis increases gradually after 28 weeks, peaking at 36 weeks. The phosphatidylinositol also appears at 28 weeks of gestation, but reaches its peak production between 32 and 35 weeks. Finally, the phosphatidylglycerol is the last phospholipid to be produced, only appearing in the surfactant at 36 weeks, and constantly increasing until birth [18]. As a result of intrauterine respiratory movements, these substances are present in the amniotic fluid cavity and can be detected in FLM tests [1, 19].

Finally, the last phase of pulmonary development occurs extrauterine and it is called alveolar period. During this period, which starts after birth and goes until young adulthood, the lungs maintain the ability of developing new alveoli. Their distal saccular walls subdivision form new alveoli, while double capillary network fuses into a single capillary system, resulting that each capillary is completely surrounded by gas exchange surfaces [16]. Therefore, the alveolar period consists of a continued septation (alveolarization) and microvascular maturation, with an increase of the gas exchange surface area [16].

All stages of lung development are complex and overlap with each other [16]. The better comprehension of fetal pulmonary system development and surfactant production is helpful to understand the evolution of tests performed for FLM [1].

Neonatal Respiratory Morbidity

After delivery, countless physiological changes happen to ensure proper pulmonary adaptation in extrauterine life. Pulmonary fluids reabsorption and alveoli gas exchange initiate after the first newborn gasp. Starting from that moment, the alveoli are filled with air and the vascular pressure decreases, allowing higher blood flow through the capillary system [20].

The NRM is usually related to the newborn incapacity of achieving adequate gas exchange at birth [20]. NRM clinical manifestations are associated with surfactant deficiency and poor anatomical development of the lungs, among other structures [8]. Thus, preterm infants are at greater risk for morbidity and mortality in comparison to term newborns; hence, neonatal survival improves with length of gestation [18, 21, 22].

NRM major causes are related to respiratory distress syndrome (RDS) and transient tachypnea of the newborn (TTN) [23], and they are both characterized by poor oxygenation and tachypnea. Other conditions may also be present in NRM cases and vary from hyperbilirubinemia, hypoglycemia, hypothermia, and feeding difficulty, to apnea, necrotizing enterocolitis, and infections or sepsis [3, 22, 24]. The correct early diagnosis will object to the best clinical management and help to improve each case prognosis, hopefully preventing long-term disability or death.

Respiratory Distress Syndrome

RDS, also called hyaline membrane disease, is the primary cause of neonatal death and disability observed in preterm infants [17, 20]. It affects up to 50% of babies who were born before 28 weeks and a third of those born before 32 weeks. About 42% of extremely low birthweight (<1500 g) babies have RDS and only less than 8% of infants born after 37 weeks are diagnosed with RDS, most of them delivered by cesarean section and from mothers diagnosed with diabetes [17, 20, 25].

The most common cause of RDS is the deficiency of surfactant, both qualitative and quantitative, observed in premature newborns [17]. When this deficiency is associated with a reduction of the pulmonary volume due to expiration, a higher surface tension is generated. As consequence, those infants may present atelectasis and other ventilatory disorders [17]. Pulmonary perfusion becomes unequal, some alveolar regions are unventilated, and the surfactant becomes inactivated by some inhibitors that were previously only present in the plasma. All these changes lead to acidosis, hypothermia, and hypoxia, reducing surfactant production, deteriorating the newborn clinical condition, and increasing their risk of chronic lung disease [17, 18].

RDS typical clinical manifestations are those for respiratory distress, including tachypnea, grunting, nasal flaring, and costal contraction [26]. The diagnosis is confirmed by a "ground glass" reticulogranular infiltrate pattern and air bronchograms in the chest radiography (Fig. 18.2) [4, 27] .

RDS prognosis depends on its severity, which has a direct relation with gestational age and birth weight. Almost 90% of RDS occurs in infants with low birthweight (<2500 g), and 95% in those below 37 weeks, with a mortality rate of 50% in those born under 1000 g, and 11% in those born over 2500 g [28].

Corticosteroids and surfactant administration have improved the prognosis of newborns with RDS and have been adhered in clinical recommendations worldwide [7]. Some frequent use in clinical practice is the antenatal corticosteroid therapy in a preterm delivery, aiming to improve the surfactant production and antioxidant system function. Also, surfactant administration is frequently adopted in preterm fetuses that will need tracheal intubation at birth, as a way to avoid RDS [20].

Despite the improvements in antepartum and postpartum therapies, RDS still plays a significant role in neonatal morbidity and mortality. This stresses the critical importance of RDS prevention and treatment in both fetal and newborn medicine [1, 18].

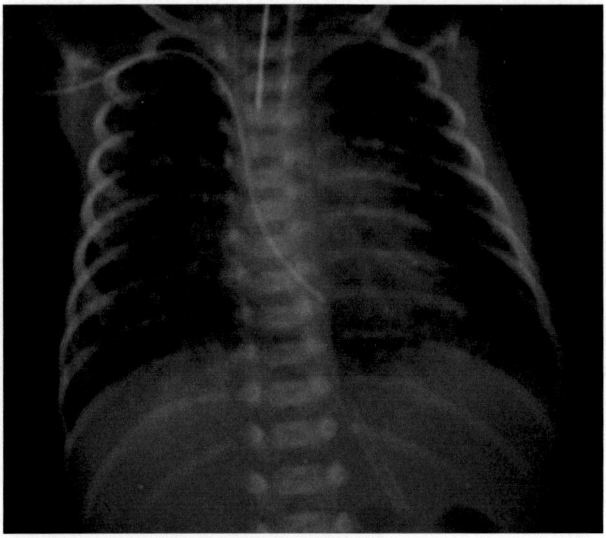

Fig. 18.2 Neonatal chest radiography for RDS: newborn with 26 + 3 weeks, intubated with RDS. *Radiography:* bilateral "ground glass" appearance of reticulogranular infiltrate and air bronchograms. (Parental consent obtained for publication). (Reproduced from Personal Archive Dra. Thaiana Beleza)

Transient Tachypnea of the Newborn

TTN is considered the main cause of neonatal respiratory morbidity in term infants [20, 29]. It is also called "wet lung" since the newborn lungs have a delayed resorption after birth [26, 30, 31]. TTN most important risk factor is the cesarean section delivery, especially before the beginning of spontaneous labor [30, 32]. The rise of maternal catecholamines during labor increases surfactant production and transepithelial sodium transport, promoting fluid reabsorption in the fetal lung. Hence, in cases where there is no labor stimulation, a decrease in the fetal pulmonary reabsorption is expected [32]. Other risk factors are maternal diabetes, maternal asthma, male sex, low birth weight, and macrosomia [33].

TTN diagnosis is challenging due to its resemblance with other respiratory complications such as RDS, pneumonia, and respiratory failure [4, 18]. Usually, TTN symptoms of respiratory distress initiate early after birth with isolated tachypnea, rare grunting, and minimal retraction. Chest infant radiography showing signs of increased perihilar interstitial marking, lungs hyperaeration, and prominent pulmonary vascular patterns helps to differentiate it from other diagnostic methods (Fig. 18.3) [14, 26, 27]. Although not always used, neonatal lung ultrasound can detect some findings that may also help in the correct diagnosis. Double lung point, disrupted pleural line, and partial or complete disappearance of A-lines seem to be related to a good positive prediction for TTN [26].

Most of TTN has mild distress symptoms and generally presents good prognosis with conservative management, using noninvasive respiratory care. TTN natural history is mostly of self-resolution, with the newborn showing clinical improvement and no need of oxygen supplementation within 72 h [20]. However, even though not usual, TTN can complicate with pulmonary hypertension and pneumothorax, which can demand a more intensive care with mechanical ventilation and prolonged hospitalization [29].

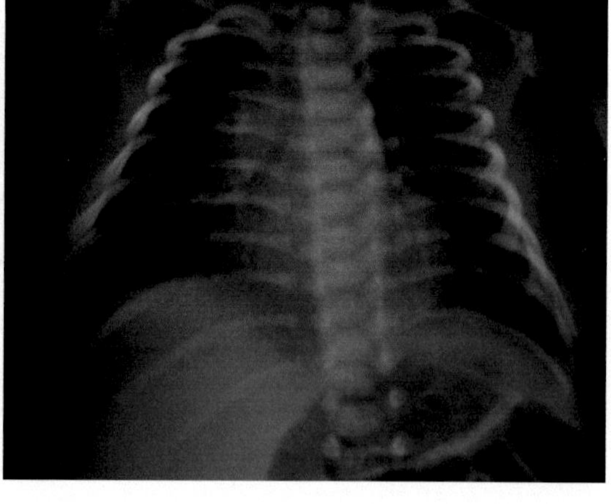

Fig. 18.3 Neonatal chest radiography for TTN: newborn with 34 + 1 weeks, symptoms of TTN. *Radiography:* "wet silhouette" around the heart, increased perihilar interstitial marking, lungs hyperaeration, and prominent pulmonary vascular patterns. (Parental consent obtained for publication.) (Reproduced from Personal Archive Dra. Thaiana Beleza)

TTN high prevalence and the possibility of evolving into pulmonary complications highlights the importance of this condition. Its diagnosis should always be considered in late-preterm and term deliveries, mostly in those cases delivered by an elective cesarean section [29].

Antenatal Corticosteroids

Antenatal corticosteroids administration in pregnant women between 24.0 and 33.6 weeks with a high risk of delivery is standard of care worldwide [5, 7]. It increases the production and release of surfactant and it accelerates FLM in preterm pregnancies, reducing the risks associated with prematurity [34]. Therefore, when correctly used, corticosteroids may reduce the incidence of RDS, intraventricular hemorrhage, infections, necrotizing enterocolitis, and neonatal intensive care unit, among others [17]. Considering these recognized benefits of corticosteroids administration, the question is if late-preterm fetuses would also benefit from it and if the benefits outweigh the risks [8].

While the use of corticosteroids can significantly decrease NRM, these infants long-term follow-up is still uncertain [8, 27, 35]. In short term, it can affect placental function and fetal growth and increase the risk of neonatal hypoglycemia [27, 36]. In the long term, it may be related to a higher vulnerability for stress-related physical and psychiatric disorders in childhood, due to hypothalamic–pituitary–adrenal axis change [37].

Antenatal corticoids main indication is the high probability of premature labor or birth within 7 days, from 24.0 to 33.6 weeks, regardless of the integrity of the amniotic membranes or the number of fetuses [38]. This includes a wide variety of conditions that requires special attention, such as preeclampsia, fetal malformations, abnormal placental implantation, placenta previa, fetal growth restriction, and others. Except in imminent delivery conditions or high risk of maternal or fetal death, tocolytics should be considered to optimize corticoids administration and to try to reduce the risk of prematurity [5, 38, 39].

The most studied corticosteroids for antenatal usage are two glucocorticoids: betamethasone and dexamethasone. Both can cross the placenta maintaining their activated form with similar biologic activity, without a high risk of immunosuppression in a short-term use. Betamethasone is the more frequently used due to a longer half-life. Preconized treatment of betamethasone consists of two intramuscular doses of 12 mg each, with a 24-h interval. Dexamethasone posology is four intramuscular doses of 6 mg each, with one dose every 12 h [5].

In clinical conditions where it is unlikely to have the time needed to administer all doses of antenatal corticosteroids, the first dose(s) should still be administered with a significant reduction in neonatal morbidity and mortality. However, there is no benefit in shortening the interval between doses [40, 41].

Antenatal corticosteroids effects are expected to last for 7 days. A rescue course of corticosteroids is indicated in those cases of possible delivery before 34 weeks and prior corticosteroids administration, when the first therapy was applied more than 2 weeks before [42, 43].

Once the recommendations are respected, it is unquestionable the important contribution of antenatal corticosteroids use. However, there are some unanswered questions remaining regarding its usage in some scenarios, and the FLM evaluation can adjoin information to avoid excessive and unnecessary fetal exposure to this therapy.

Fetal Lung Maturity Evaluation

FLM assessment has contributed significantly in NRM prediction. Initially focused in late-preterm and early-term fetuses, it aimed to advise obstetrical decision regarding antenatal corticosteroids administration and delivery [2, 44]. Further studies have also included early-preterm fetuses to analyze the neonatal respiratory outcomes prediction successfully [14].

FLM testing can be divided in direct and indirect measurements [1]. While the direct tests measure the concentration or surface-active effect of particular components of pulmonary development, the indirect tests rely on maternal and fetal information to infer the neonatal respiratory response after birth. To assess the indirect risk, variables as calculated gestation age, fetal weight, maternal risk factors and comorbidities, and ultrasound images can be used [1].

During fetal lungs development, phospholipids are released into the amniotic fluid due to fetal respiratory movements, and its concentration varies during pregnancy [1, 18]. Hence, to predict FLM, an amniocentesis should be performed to obtain samples for biochemical or biophysical testing. However, further data analysis showed that gestational age was the real variable playing the role in the NRM prediction. Therefore, although widely used throughout the years, this evaluation is no longer recommended [9, 10, 12]. Finally, since invasive procedures increase maternal and fetal risks, noninvasive techniques using obstetric ultrasound have been developed and improved in the last years [6, 14].

Direct Tests

Lecithin/Sphingomyelin Ratio

The lecithin/sphingomyelin ratio was the first widely accepted direct method for the assessment of fetal pulmonary status [1]. It is a biochemical test that evaluates through chromatography changes in the concentration of both phospholipids in amniotic fluid samples. A ratio close to 1.0 is expected until 33 weeks. In the next couple of weeks, lecithin (phosphatidylcholine) concentration raises significantly, while sphingomyelin remains stable, reaching a ratio of 2.0 around 35 weeks [1, 19].

Once the ratio achieves 2.0, FLM is considered adequate, and very few cases present NRM [1]. However, many aspects can interfere in the result of the test. The presence of blood or meconium in the amniotic fluid sample may falsely increase the ratio, and improper storage conditions, and bad timing management to run and interpret the tests may invalid the results [1].

Detection of Phosphatidylglycerol

The phosphatidylglycerol is one of the surfactant components and can be quantified weeks after the increase of lecithin concentration [45]. Since its release optimizes the phospholipids distribution over the alveolar surface, phosphatidylglycerol presence indicates more advanced pulmonary maturity. It is another thin-layer chromatography test that can be executed within the lecithin/sphingomyelin ratio or separately [1].

Conversely to the prior test, this evaluation is not influenced by physiologic contaminants, such as blood or meconium. Thus, vaginal samples from pregnancies with spontaneous rupture of membranes rupture can be used for analysis [1]. Unfortunately, phosphatidylglycerol late appearance during pregnancy is the main disadvantage when compared to the other direct methods [46].

Lamellar Body Count

Lamellar bodies are packages of surfactant produced by type II pneumocytes and excreted into alveolar space. There, the lamellar bodies disentangle and recover the alveolar layer. Some others lamellar bodies cross structures and pass to the amniotic fluid. Differently from the previous tests, the lamellar body count is a biophysical testing. Due to its similar size to platelets, they can be counted in most hematology analyzer equipment, which makes the test very convenient and affordable [18].

To be considered as a good FLM, the lamellar body count has to be over 50.000/μL, while values under 15.000/μL indicate immaturity and, hence, high risk of NRD. Values in the intermediate range usually request a different test to confirm the FLM [10, 18].

Surfactant/Albumin Ratio

The surfactant-to-albumin ratio uses fluorescence polarization to measure the concentration of surfactant and albumin in the amniotic fluid. It is another biochemical test that quantifies the competitive connection between albumin and the surfactant [47]. Polarization is considered high when the probe binds to albumin, and low when it binds to surfactant [1]. Unfortunately, both meconium and blood can interfere in the test.

Results are expressed in milligrams of surfactant per gram of albumin. Values greater or equal to 55 mg/g suggest pulmonary maturity, while values under 40 mg/g can be considered immature. Same as in the lamellar body count, intermediate levels are considered undetermined and a secondary test is encouraged to a correct diagnosis [47]. Although it was one of the most used FLM tests, both equipment and reagents were discontinued by the only vendor that manufactured it, limiting its utilization since 2011 [18].

Clements Test/Shake Test

Clements test was first described in 1972 based on the surfactant ability to develop and sustain a stable foam when mixed with ethanol [48]. It is a biophysical test, in which different dilutions of ethanol are mixed in a constant quantity of amniotic fluid. Through this test, it is possible to determine the surfactant concentration by its surface-active properties. When shaken, the sample of amniotic fluid and ethanol generates a stable ring of foam, demonstrating the presence of surfactant [1]. It is a quick test that only takes 15 min, and it is very affordable. Nevertheless, same as some previous tests, the Clement test is vulnerable to the presence of blood and meconium in the sample.

Foam stability index (FSI) is a functional measurement of the Clemens test. It uses several tubes containing progressive greater amounts of 95% ethanol to try to quantify the presence of surfactant over different concentrations [9]. Maturity is indicated when the foam stability persists in a cut-off ethanol dilution greater or equal to 0.47 [49].

Indirect Tests

Another possibility of assessing FLM is through indirect methods that propose a noninvasive diagnosis combining fetal and maternal characteristics [14]. In the last decade, fetal ultrasound acquisition and computer image processing have improved dramatically, creating innovative ways of fetal development evaluation. Regarding FLM, the pulmonary artery Doppler study and the quantitative texture analysis of the lungs are powerful techniques that have gained space in clinical practice [14, 50].

Pulmonary Artery Acceleration to Ejection Time

The pulmonary artery acceleration to ejection time (PATET) ratio is a noninvasive method that uses pulmonary artery Doppler parameters to predict FLM [23, 50]. As the lungs develop, changes in the pulmonary vasculature occur, reducing pulmonary vascular resistance and increasing pulmonary blood flow [29]. Any disturbance in this dynamic process can directly change pulmonary tissue impedance, affecting pulmonary blood flow pattern, which can be detected by the ultrasound Doppler (Fig. 18.4). Thus, by measuring the resistance of the pulmonary artery, the Doppler index indirectly reflects the tissue impedance. Among pulmonary Doppler indexes, the PATET ratio has been proven to be a reliable choice as noninvasive method to assess impedance to flow and pulmonary tissue pressure [51], reflecting FLM (Figs. 18.5 and 18.6).

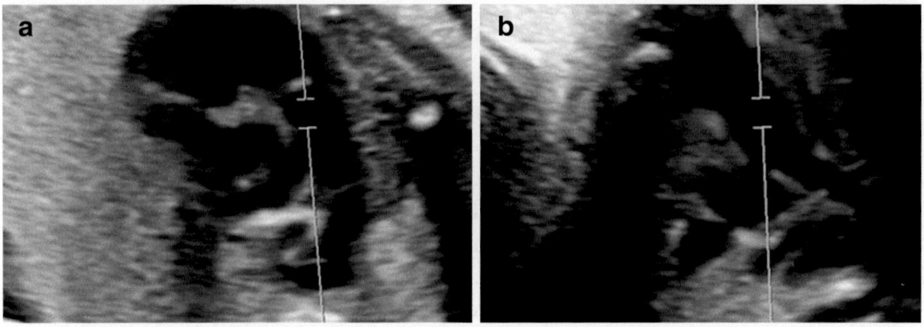

Fig. 18.4 Correct views to measure the PATET: the caliper is positioned in the area evaluated when obtaining the main pulmonary artery Doppler waveform. (**a**) Ductal arch view; (**b**) right outflow tract view. (Reproduced from Personal archive Dr. Evaldo Trajano)

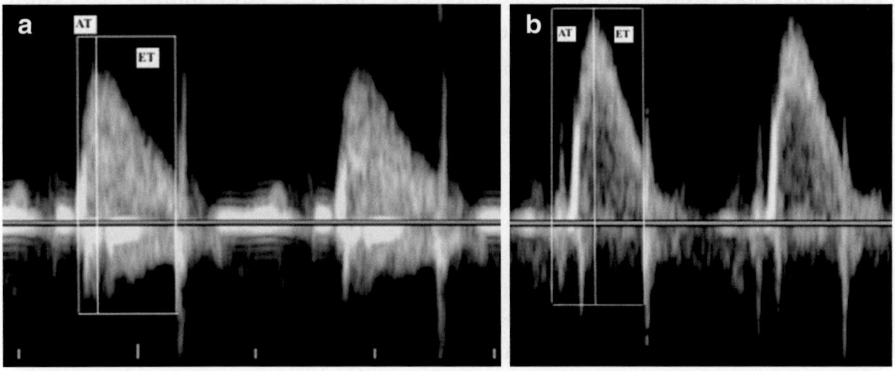

Fig. 18.5 Measurement of the acceleration (AT) and ejection time (ET) in the main pulmonary artery Doppler waveform. (**a**) Representation of an immature-type wave; (**b**) representation of a mature-type wave. (Reproduced from Personal archive Dr. Evaldo Trajano)

***PATET** = Acceleration time / Ejection time*

Fig. 18.6 PATET (Pulmonary artery acceleration time/ejection time ratio) value is obtained by the division of the main pulmonary artery Doppler acceleration time by its ejection time

Recent data supported PATET ratio as a useful marker to predict FLM. Although not very sensitive (73%) is highly specific (93%), with good predictive values (around 85% for both) [23, 50]. It has shown to be a very feasible procedure, stressing its applicability in clinical practice and a good alternative to amniocentesis and direct tests. Even though it is still under scientific consolidation, fetal PATET ratio seems to be a promising tool for FLM, and certainly more robust data are to be published [29, 50].

Ultrasound Lung Texture Analysis

Several approaches to pulmonary maturity analysis were developed among the last decades, varying from gray scale measurements, fetal breath movements, and the correlation with placental grade [52–54]. On account of technology evolution, due to machine learning trained algorithms, quantitative texture analysis allows to detect subtle tissue changes in both aspect and texture, not visible to the human eye [13].

In the last decade, a FLM software was launched showing similar performance to the direct tests [14, 55, 56]. It is currently called "Quantitative ultrasound fetal lung maturity analysis" (quantusFLM™) and it is based on the quantitative texture analysis of the fetal lungs. The software classifies the ultrasound image in low or high risk for NRM, taking also into consideration the gestational age from 28.0 to 39.0 weeks (Fig. 18.7). A large multicentric study has been published, showing an accuracy of 86.5% [14]. This noninvasive technique is easily introduced into the clinical routine and may add important information in the definition of the obstetrical conduct [13, 55]. Moreover, further studies are being developed to better understand the texture analysis in different subgroups of pregnant women.

Conclusion

It is possible to conclude the strong relation between FLM and neonatal pulmonary outcomes. Over the last decades, technological development has entailed on novel and less invasive testing. While initially focused in preterm fetuses, scientific research has been broadening FLM valuation to older fetuses, also with promising results. New advances are constantly being made in this subject, in order to improve obstetrical care of each case individually and to try to prevent NRM and prematurity.

Fetal Lung Maturity Test

quantus FLM
www.quantusFLM.com

Patient & Provider Information

PATIENT NAME: xxxxxxxxxx	CLINIC NAME: xxxxxxxxxx
PATIENT ID: **PULM 5**	REFERRING/ORDER CLINICIAN: xxxxxxxxxx
quantusFLM ID: **CEMEF-15909**	REPORT DATE: xxxxxxxxxx

Sample Information

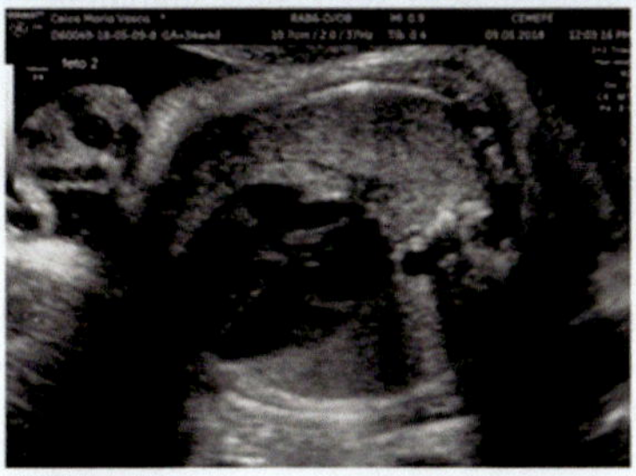

GESTATIONAL AGE:	**34 WEEKS 4 days**
US ACQUISITION DATE: (dd/mm/yyyy)	**09/05/2018**
REQUEST DATE. (dd/mm/yyyy hh:mm)	**09/05/2018 17:56**

Test Result from NRM

quantusFLM ID:

CEMEF-15909

RESULT:

Low risk

Baseline risk by gestational age:

17.7 %

Risk adjusted by quantusFLM(*):

11 %

NEONATAL RESPIRATORY MORBIDITY RISK

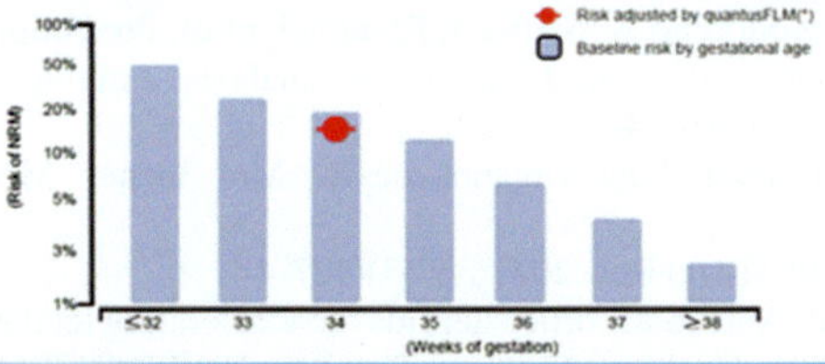

Authorized signer/s

TRANSMURAL BIOTECH

Technical responsible:
Álvaro Pérez Moreno

(*)The risk indicates the probability of Neonatal Respiratory Morbidity (NRM), which is defined as respiratory distress syndrome or transient tachypnea of the newborn, obtained by means of adjusting the baseline risk for gestational age by the positive or negative likelihood ratio obtained by the analysis of ultrasound fetal lung textures.

TEST DESCRIPTION
quantusFLM™ offers an automatic assessment of the Neonatal Respiratory Morbidity (NRM) risk using the quantitative texture analysis of a fetal lung image. Quality of image and acquisition is relevant and must be taken following product specifications (quantusFLM™ has been validated in singleton pregnancies from 28.0 to 39.0 weeks with maternal BMI<35 and no fetal structural or chromosomal abnormalities). quantusFLM™ is not intended as a final indication for delivery but as additional information to be considered in the management of the patient. NRM is defined as respiratory distress syndrome or transient tachypnea of the newborn.

quantusFLM™ Test is intended for clinical use and should not be regarded as investigational or for research. Present result has been obtained using quantusFLM 03.0. quantusFLM™ has been developed by Transmural Biotech, B65084675. C/Sabino Arana 38 1-1, 08028 Barcelona Spain. Under the previous of Law 15/1999 normative, we inform you that your data will be included in a data base owned by TransmuralBiotech, S.L. for its clinical treatment. You may exercise the rights of access, rectification, cancellation and opposition contacting us at info@transmuralbiotech.com

Fig. 18.7 Late-preterm fetus demonstrating a low risk of developing respiratory morbidity: 17.7% basal risk by gestational age, 11% of risk adjusted by quantusFLM™. (Reproduced from Personal archive Dr. Matheus Beleza)

References

1. ACOG educational bulletin. Assessment of fetal lung maturity. Number 230, November 1996. Committee on Educational Bulletins of the American College of Obstetricians and Gynecologists. Int J Gynaecol Obstet. 1997;56(2):191–8.
2. Sengupta S, Carrion V, Shelton J, Wynn RJ, Ryan RM, Singhal K, et al. Adverse neonatal outcomes associated with early-term birth. JAMA Pediatr. 2013;167(11):1053–9.
3. Teune MJ, Bakhuizen S, Gyamfi Bannerman C, Opmeer BC, van Kaam AH, van Wassenaer AG, et al. A systematic review of severe morbidity in infants born late preterm. Am J Obstet Gynecol. 2011;205(4):374.e1–9.
4. Hibbard JU, Wilkins I, Sun L, Gregory K, Haberman S, Hoffman M, et al. Respiratory morbidity in late preterm births. JAMA. 2010;304(4):419–25.
5. Committee Opinion No. 713: antenatal corticosteroid therapy for Fetal maturation. Obstet Gynecol. 2017;130(2):e102–e9.
6. Lopez Sanchez F, Delgado Sanchez E, Duyos Mateo I, Gonzalez Alvarez MC, Antolin Alvarado E, Bartha JL. Evaluation of Fetal lung maturity by quantitative analysis (quantusFLM) in women with gestational diabetes mellitus. Fetal Diagn Ther. 2019;45(5):345–52.
7. Jobe AH, Goldenberg RL. Antenatal corticosteroids: an assessment of anticipated benefits and potential risks. Am J Obstet Gynecol. 2018;219(1):62–74.
8. Saccone G, Berghella V. Antenatal corticosteroids for maturity of term or near term fetuses: systematic review and meta-analysis of randomized controlled trials. BMJ. 2016;355:i5044.
9. Gluck L, Kulovich MV, Borer RC Jr, Brenner PH, Anderson GG, Spellacy WN. Diagnosis of the respiratory distress syndrome by amniocentesis. Am J Obstet Gynecol. 1971;109(3):440–5.
10. Johnson LM, Johnson C, Karger AB. End of the line for fetal lung maturity testing. Clin Biochem. 2019;71:74–6.
11. Committee Opinion No ACOG. 764: medically indicated late-preterm and early-term deliveries. Obstet Gynecol. 2019;133(2):e151–e5.
12. Visconti KC, DeFranco E, Kamath-Rayne BD. Contemporary practice patterns in the use of amniocentesis for fetal lung maturity(). J Matern Fetal Neonatal Med. 2018;31(20):2729–36.
13. Bonet-Carne E, Palacio M, Cobo T, Perez-Moreno A, Lopez M, Piraquive JP, et al. Quantitative ultrasound texture analysis of fetal lungs to predict neonatal respiratory morbidity. Ultrasound Obstet Gynecol. 2015;45(4):427–33.
14. Palacio M, Bonet-Carne E, Cobo T, Perez-Moreno A, Sabria J, Richter J, et al. Prediction of neonatal respiratory morbidity by quantitative ultrasound lung texture analysis: a multicenter study. Am J Obstet Gynecol. 2017;217(2):196.e1–14.
15. Kaplan F. Molecular determinants of fetal lung organogenesis. Mol Genet Metab. 2000;71(1–2):321–41.
16. Schittny JC. Development of the lung. Cell Tissue Res. 2017;367(3):427–44.
17. Roberts D, Brown J, Medley N, Dalziel SR. Antenatal corticosteroids for accelerating fetal lung maturation for women at risk of preterm birth. Cochrane Database Syst Rev. 2017;3:Cd004454.
18. Yarbrough ML, Grenache DG, Gronowski AM. Fetal lung maturity testing: the end of an era. Biomark Med. 2014;8(4):509–15.
19. Verder H, Heiring C, Clark H, Sweet D, Jessen TE, Ebbesen F, et al. Rapid test for lung maturity, based on spectroscopy of gastric aspirate, predicted respiratory distress syndrome with high sensitivity. Acta Paediatr. 2017;106(3):430–7.
20. Gallacher DJ, Hart K, Kotecha S. Common respiratory conditions of the newborn. Breathe (Sheff). 2016;12(1):30–42.
21. Doyle LW. Outcome at 5 years of age of children 23 to 27 weeks' gestation: refining the prognosis. Pediatrics. 2001;108(1):134–41.
22. Ramachandrappa A, Rosenberg ES, Wagoner S, Jain L. Morbidity and mortality in late preterm infants with severe hypoxic respiratory failure on extra-corporeal membrane oxygenation. J Pediatr. 2011;159(2):192–8.e3.
23. Eraslan Sahin M, Col Madendag I, Sahin E, Madendag Y, Acmaz G, Bastug O, et al. Fetal pulmonary artery acceleration/ejection ratio for transient Tachypnea of the Newborn in

uncomplicated term small for gestational age Fetuses. Eur J Obstet Gynecol Reprod Biol. 2020;247:116–20.
24. Tita ATN, Jablonski KA, Bailit JL, Grobman WA, Wapner RJ, Reddy UM, et al. Neonatal outcomes of elective early-term births after demonstrated fetal lung maturity. Am J Obstet Gynecol. 2018;219(3):296.e1–e8.
25. Hintz SR, Van Meurs KP, Perritt R, Poole WK, Das A, Stevenson DK, et al. Neurodevelopmental outcomes of premature infants with severe respiratory failure enrolled in a randomized controlled trial of inhaled nitric oxide. J Pediatr. 2007;151(1):16–22. e1-3
26. Ibrahim M, Omran A, AbdAllah NB, Ibrahim M, El-Sharkawy S. Lung ultrasound in early diagnosis of neonatal transient tachypnea and its differentiation from other causes of neonatal respiratory distress. J Neonatal Perinatal Med. 2018;11(3):281–7.
27. Gyamfi-Bannerman C, Thom EA, Blackwell SC, Tita AT, Reddy UM, Saade GR, et al. Antenatal betamethasone for women at risk for late preterm delivery. N Engl J Med. 2016;374(14):1311–20.
28. Qian LL, Liu CQ, Guo YX, Jiang YJ, Ni LM, Xia SW, et al. Current status of neonatal acute respiratory disorders: a one-year prospective survey from a Chinese neonatal network. Chin Med J. 2010;123(20):2769–75.
29. Buke B, Akkaya H. A non-invasive method to rule out transient tachypnea of the newborn (TTN): fetal pulmonary artery acceleration to ejection time ratio. J Perinat Med. 2018;46(2):219–24.
30. Ramachandrappa A, Jain L. Elective cesarean section: its impact on neonatal respiratory outcome. Clin Perinatol. 2008;35(2):373–93, vii.
31. Guglani L, Lakshminrusimha S, Ryan RM. Transient tachypnea of the newborn. Pediatr Rev. 2008;29(11):e59–65.
32. Tutdibi E, Gries K, Bucheler M, Misselwitz B, Schlosser RL, Gortner L. Impact of labor on outcomes in transient tachypnea of the newborn: population-based study. Pediatrics. 2010;125(3):e577–83.
33. Dani C, Reali MF, Bertini G, Wiechmann L, Spagnolo A, Tangucci M, et al. Risk factors for the development of respiratory distress syndrome and transient tachypnoea in newborn infants. Italian Group of Neonatal Pneumology. Eur Respir J. 1999;14(1):155–9.
34. Zafman KB, Fox NS. Amniocentesis compared with antenatal corticosteroids prior to early term scheduled cesarean delivery. J Matern Fetal Neonatal Med. 2019;32(21):3571–6.
35. Srinivasjois R, Silva D. Antenatal steroid administration in medically uncomplicated pregnancy beyond 37 weeks of gestation for the prevention of neonatal morbidities prior to elective caesarean section: a systematic review and meta-analysis of randomised controlled trials. J Matern Fetal Neonatal Med. 2017;30(10):1151–7.
36. Eriksson L, Haglund B, Ewald U, Odlind V, Kieler H. Health consequences of prophylactic exposure to antenatal corticosteroids among children born late preterm or term. Acta Obstet Gynecol Scand. 2012;91(12):1415–21.
37. Alexander N, Rosenlocher F, Stalder T, Linke J, Distler W, Morgner J, et al. Impact of antenatal synthetic glucocorticoid exposure on endocrine stress reactivity in term-born children. J Clin Endocrinol Metab. 2012;97(10):3538–44.
38. Areia AL, Almeida MF, Braga AJC, Pereira NB, Macedo CVD, Nogueira-Silva C. Corticoterapia para maturação pulmonar fetal. Acta Obstétrica e Ginecológica Portuguesa. 2018;12:311–3.
39. Patel SS, Ludmir J. Drugs for the treatment and prevention of preterm labor. Clin Perinatol. 2019;46(2):159–72.
40. Antenatal corticosteroids revisited: repeat courses - National Institutes of Health Consensus Development Conference Statement, August 17–18, 2000. Obstet Gynecol. 2001;98(1):144–50.
41. No PB. 171: Management of Preterm Labor. Obstet Gynecol. 2016;128(4):e155–64.
42. Garite TJ, Kurtzman J, Maurel K, Clark R. Impact of a 'rescue course' of antenatal corticosteroids: a multicenter randomized placebo-controlled trial. Am J Obstet Gynecol. 2009;200(3):248.e1–9.
43. Peaceman AM, Bajaj K, Kumar P, Grobman WA. The interval between a single course of antenatal steroids and delivery and its association with neonatal outcomes. Am J Obstet Gynecol. 2005;193(3 Pt 2):1165–9.

44. Spong CY, Mercer BM, D'Alton M, Kilpatrick S, Blackwell S, Saade G. Timing of indicated late-preterm and early-term birth. Obstet Gynecol. 2011;118(2 Pt 1):323–33.
45. Hallman M, Kulovich M, Kirkpatrick E, Sugarman RG, Gluck L. Phosphatidylinositol and phosphatidylglycerol in amniotic fluid: indices of lung maturity. Am J Obstet Gynecol. 1976;125(5):613–7.
46. Lewis DF, Towers CV, Major CA, Asrat T, Nageotte MP, Freeman RK, et al. Use of Amniostat-FLM in detecting the presence of phosphatidylglycerol in vaginal pool samples in preterm premature rupture of membranes. Am J Obstet Gynecol. 1993;169(3):573–6.
47. Luo G, Norwitz ER. Revisiting amniocentesis for fetal lung maturity after 36 weeks' gestation. Rev Obstet Gynecol. 2008;1(2):61–8.
48. Clements JA, Platzker AC, Tierney DF, Hobel CJ, Creasy RK, Margolis AJ, et al. Assessment of the risk of the respiratory-distress syndrome by a rapid test for surfactant in amniotic fluid. N Engl J Med. 1972;286(20):1077–81.
49. Sher G, Statland BE, Freer DE. Clinical evaluation of the quantitative foam stability index test. Obstet Gynecol. 1980;55(5):617–20.
50. Schenone MH, Samson JE, Jenkins L, Suhag A, Mari G. Predicting fetal lung maturity using the fetal pulmonary artery Doppler wave acceleration/ejection time ratio. Fetal Diagn Ther. 2014;36(3):208–14.
51. Kitabatake A, Inoue M, Asao M, Masuyama T, Tanouchi J, Morita T, et al. Noninvasive evaluation of pulmonary hypertension by a pulsed Doppler technique. Circulation. 1983;68(2):302–9.
52. Harman CR, Manning FA, Stearns E, Morrison I. The correlation of ultrasonic placental grading and fetal pulmonary maturation in five hundred sixty-three pregnancies. Am J Obstet Gynecol. 1982;143(8):941–3.
53. Serizawa M, Maeda K. Noninvasive fetal lung maturity prediction based on ultrasonic gray level histogram width. Ultrasound Med Biol. 2010;36(12):1998–2003.
54. Cosmi EV, Anceschi MM, Cosmi E, Piazze JJ, La Torre R. Ultrasonographic patterns of fetal breathing movements in normal pregnancy. Int J Gynaecol Obstet. 2003;80(3):285–90.
55. Palacio M, Cobo T, Martinez-Terron M, Ratta GA, Bonet-Carne E, Amat-Roldan I, et al. Performance of an automatic quantitative ultrasound analysis of the fetal lung to predict fetal lung maturity. Am J Obstet Gynecol. 2012;207(6):504.e1–5.
56. Cobo T, Bonet-Carne E, Martinez-Terron M, Perez-Moreno A, Elias N, Luque J, et al. Feasibility and reproducibility of fetal lung texture analysis by automatic quantitative ultrasound analysis and correlation with gestational age. Fetal Diagn Ther. 2012;31(4):230–6.

Chapter 19
Fetal Surgery

Masami Yamamoto, Yves Ville, Fernando Javier Rojas Bravo, Viral Mahesh Pandya, Matthew A. Shanahan, and Michael W. Bebbington

Introduction

Fetal diseases affect the child before birth, and in some, their prenatal development is responsible for irreversible damage causing peri- or postnatal sequelae or death. This can be questioned in around 2% of all newborns. They are a major cause of mortality, and in some countries, they are more important than prematurity. The costs of the sequelae of fetal diseases are not clearly estimated, and they may be high due to their long duration.

The diseases that may be stabilized or cured in utero are not many, and they include twin-to-twin transfusion syndrome, myelomeningocele, congenital diaphragmatic hernia, low urinary tract obstruction, compressive pleural effusion or intrathoracic cystic masses, and perinatal anemia. Lethal diseases without therapeutic options are numerous although individually they are rare anomalies, including anencephaly, achondrogenesis, osteogenesis imperfecta type 2, highly lethal chromosomopathies, such as trisomy 18 and 13, Body-stalk syndrome, some forms of twins, bilateral renal agenesis, and Potter syndrome due to renal dysplasia, among others. In general, genetically based diseases, in which the correction of a malformation does not necessarily allow an improvement of the general condition, are not candidates for fetal therapy. Theoretically, fetal diseases candidates for therapy are those in which the long-term prognosis can recover following intervention.

M. Yamamoto (✉) · Y. Ville · V. M. Pandya
GHU Paris-Centre, Hôpital Necker-Enfants Malades, Paris, France

F. J. R. Bravo
Clínica Universidad de los Andes, Las Condes, Chile

M. A. Shanahan · M. W. Bebbington
Washington University School of Medicine in St. Louis, Louis, US

© Springer Nature Switzerland AG 2022

R. A. Moreira de Sá, E. B. d. Fonseca (eds.), *Perinatology*,
https://doi.org/10.1007/978-3-030-83434-0_19

Ethical Principles in Medicine

Fetal medicine raises several ethical dilemmas that must be faced by doctors, patients, and the society in general, especially in the context of the law governing prenatal diagnosis and its consequences in every country. The primary issue is that of autonomy, which is significantly impacted by the availability of termination of pregnancy for fetal malformation, the principle of benevolence, and the application of innovative treatments. Pregnant women and doctors could center their attention to the fetus, but this may be conflicting with other principles.

The principle of autonomy is one that allows patients to make decisions, previously informed by the treating doctors. The patient is required to be fully aware of the risks and benefits of the therapy, and freely willing to undergo treatment. It is inappropriate for doctors or family members to replace the pregnant woman in her ability to choose, because she will live through the risks and the benefits for herself and is also the sole representative of her fetus and its "rights" until it is born. It is therefore widely accepted that the woman's decision is sufficient to accept or decline fetal therapy. The women's autonomy is therefore the only challenge according to most countries' laws governing termination of pregnancy as a whole and especially in the context of fetal anomaly.

Fetal therapies are often innovative, and in their first attempts, they are therapeutic test based on the theoretical rationality of the desired success. These difficulties make the principle of benevolence unclear in fetal medicine. Many of the proposed therapies are the consequences of the poor prognosis of the natural history of the disease for which therapeutic possibilities are not previously demonstrated.

However, the uncertainty about the therapies is not absolute, but with the accumulation of experience, they consolidate and become the standard of care. This can already be said of some fetal therapies that have randomized studies that support their performance. In turn, the fetal treatment centers have the obligation to report their results periodically and keep registries with the aim of ascertaining long-term outcome. Statistics apply only to the centers that have responsively developed the therapies. There is a moral obligation to ensure competence through a learning curve that should be exposed to the patients and secured in order to minimize harm to the patient.

Finally, the principle of justice, which obliges to equate the possible benefits to the population, as well as resources for different health needs, also affects fetal medicine. Fetal pathology is uncommon, complex and expensive in general. It is not feasible to develop centers in all hospitals because none of them will have enough experience to provide the expected quality of care to the population. Therapeutic procedures require an accumulation of experience that ensures the results.

Therapeutic Innovation and Clinical Research

When a therapy is proposed to a patient, and this is not the standard of care, it can be confused with research. Some have proposed that innovative therapy should not be carried out without the approval of an ethics committee, however, it is clear that many of the therapies do not achieve the approval of a research ethics committee in time for the patient's need. Instead, clinical research aims to demonstrate the effectiveness of treatment. How to distinguish a therapy and a research is a common dilemma for a doctor. The therapeutic action seeks to cure the patient. The Belmont Report defines clinical research as an activity to test a hypothesis, obtain conclusions of generalizable clinical application and subsequently applicable. A nonstandard intervention, but offered as a treatment, aims to relieve or cure a disease in a patient. As noted, in clinical research, patients are not the objective of the benefit but to test the hypothesis. There may be patients benefited from clinical research, however, it is only a consequence of the research.

An investigation and a therapy may look similar but are different objectives of the same medical act. For this reason, a new and innovative therapy that is not looking to prove its effectiveness but to help the patient can be considered a therapy and not an investigation. The opposite can also happen, since a therapy can be considered an investigation when it has been carried out previously, periodically and constantly. This distinction, as well as the approval by the research committees, is the responsibility of the physician.

In the world, research based on existing surgical therapies has several references and one of them is the CORONIS [1] study. Their objective was to test different variations in the technique of cesarean section, and to assess whether they affected the results. The study allowed us to question whether the surgery performed around the world is similar or different, as well as if the variations have different results. Historically, a surgical technique is named after the inventor. There is no clear definition to distinguish slightly different surgeries from the completely new surgeries.

Innovative therapies can be considered advantageous by the institutions, because they seek recognition for innovation and this is a good motor for marketing.

After a first case, and in front of a clinical setting that proposes a therapy, a formal investigation is carried out with objectives and methods, occasionally in animal models and later in human models. The concepts of feasibility, safety and efficacy of therapy can only be demonstrated in larger series. When a clinical doubt is established about the merits of the intervention, a randomized study should be considered. This doubt is called "clinical equipoise," a state in which evidence do not satisfy all specialists and there is disagreement [2].

The question about therapy arises when there are three requirements: historical series show that the intervention has benefits, that the intervention has risks to the fetus and that the woman's morbidity is low or relatively low. Finally, researchers must define clear objectives to measure their results. The results must be presented in an academic environment to be able to be commented and evaluated in an appropriate way and thus turn them into a standard of care.

Sometimes, there is no place for a randomized study: when the pathology in question is extremely severe with mortality close to 100%. A research ethical board may justify conducting a pilot trial or even reject a randomized study because there is no alternative therapy.

Most Relevant Fetal Surgeries

Twin-to-twin transfusion syndrome is considered the first fetal disease that has a randomized study that supports surgery and became the first to be considered a standard of treatment [3]. Published in 2004, the study compared fetal surgery versus usual management and demonstrated the benefit of fetal surgery. Survival without neurological damage increased from 50% to 75%. This reopened the horizon of fetal surgery in the world after the first series of cases were shown in the 1990s. The first were Ville [4] and De Lia [5], concomitantly in different centers. The rationale for this therapy was that the disease left untreated had an adverse prognosis, and that the proposed therapy had a reasonable chance of success. This surgery consists of entering a 3 mm endoscope percutaneously through the abdominal wall and uterine wall, which allows the communicating vessels to be seen and coagulated in monochorionic twins. Having established a clinical equipoise, the French group tried to prove the benefit of therapy by organizing a randomized study in about 150 pregnancies with twin-to-twin transfusion syndrome between 18 and 26 weeks of gestational age. Following the publication, there were more than 1000 cases operated in the world in 3 years, which in turn demonstrates that the information obtained from the randomized study allowed the generalization of knowledge and application.

The simplicity of the inclusion criteria made it applicable as the indication of surgery until now, 15 years after. The only exception was that Quintero stage 1 (one) has been reevaluated as an indication of surgery. In turn, the surgery seemed so adequate internationally that no other randomized studies were repeated to confirm the benefit of the therapy. Furthermore, the following cohorts had similar results to the therapeutic arm of the trial.

Different was the course of fetal therapy for congenital diaphragmatic hernia. In San Francisco, Harrison published in 2003 [6] the first study of open and endoscopic surgery of tracheal occlusion in fetuses with congenital diaphragmatic hernia. The study showed results in which survival was similar between groups with fetal surgery versus usual management, 73% versus 77%. The authors decided not to continue with the prenatal intervention. The main criticism of this study was the selection of fetuses, in which a fairly high lung size (LHR less than 1.4) was accepted. This explained that the control group achieved excellent survival and annulled the chance to demonstrate any benefit. Subsequently, Ruano [7] published a randomized study conducted in Brazil including fetuses with much smaller lung size (LHR less than 1). The prenatal therapy showed a survival of 50% versus 5% in controls. This study refloated hopes to treat these fetuses. The Leuven group, which has largely developed the endoscopic technique, as well as many prognostic studies, is currently carrying out the TOTAL study, in its severe and moderate forms, which should draw conclusions (NCT00763737).

Myelomeningocele is the most common congenital disease of the central nervous system. Various estimates suggest a frequency of 3.4 cases per 1000 live births. About two-thirds of women who have this diagnosis prefer the option of terminating their pregnancy in countries where regulation allows. Myelomeningocele is caused by the lack of closure of the caudal neuroporus in the fourth week of pregnancy. This leads to severe complications depending on the damage of the cerebellum, the medulla at the defect and the affected peripheral nerves. This malformation can produce hydrocephalus, with cranial hypertension. A total of 80% of the children require a ventricular-peritoneal valve. Fetal surgery for this pathology was initiated by Brunner [8] endoscopically. The ethical justification for this surgery was questioned, because the disease does not produce fetal death, has maternal risks, and there was no evidence that the neurological prognosis improved due to a correction in the intrauterine period. It was the MOM study [9], which compared open (laparotomy) myelomeningocele closure surgery with standard postnatal surgery that showed the benefits of prenatal surgery. The reduction of the use of ventriculoperitoneal valve and the gait were improved. These results motivated many patients to accept the procedure. However, the maternal risks of open fetal surgery were important. The same MOM study reported 8% of uterine rupture in the current pregnancy, and Goodnight reported the risks for subsequent pregnancies, which was 10% of the uterine rupture with two fetal deaths among the five cases with rupture, all in the early third trimester when delivery was not yet planned. [10] These risks rapidly boosted the fetoscopic surgery, taking advantage of the experience on twin-to-twin transfusion syndrome and congenital diaphragmatic hernia. Kohl [11], Lapa [12], and Belfort [13] have developed endoscopic techniques with variations. A consortium keeps track of the cases operated in centers that have agreed to perform the surgery endoscopically [14].

Renal Agenesis

There is a recent report [15] of intrauterine treatment in a fetus with bilateral renal agenesis. This was a 34-year old pregnant woman referred at 23 weeks with the diagnosis of bilateral renal agenesis. The patient requested amnioinfusion to avoid pulmonary hypoplasia. At the time of diagnosis at 23 weeks, the fetus had anhydramnios, but the duration of the condition was unknown. The patient, informed that in the absence of interventions there was a high chance of death, requested serial amnioinfusion. The first amnioinfusion was performed at 24 weeks with the injection of 250 ml of saline solution. At the end of the procedure, 10 ml of indigo carmine was injected, which confirmed that there was no rupture of the membranes. A weekly amnioinfusion was performed until week 28. In each amnioinfusion, the objective was to obtain an amniotic fluid index of 10. The patient had ruptured membranes at week 28, evolved with labor and had a vaginal delivery of a newborn that weighted 1230 g. She presented a respiratory distress of prematurity with normal lung size. Peritoneum dialysis was performed hoping to be a candidate for renal transplantation at 12–24 months. At the end of the report, the authors acknowledge that a normal long-term result could not be guaranteed. However, this case showed that serial amnioinfusion may be an option. The public opinion of the United States called him the miracle child. Other authors have commented on the limitations of this case [16]. First, the case should not be considered a demonstration that all cases could be treated in the future. Long-term outcome of these children is unknown. The success of this case is highly dependent on dialysis and renal transplantation. If these two strategies were unavailable, the amnioinfusion would be useless.

Principles of in Utero Interventions

Since its inception, the International Fetal Medicine and Surgery Society (IFMSS) [17] published its guidelines for fetal therapy. The principles mentioned were the following:

1. The natural history of the disease must be known.
2. The condition must be severe, either in mortality or morbidity.
3. The intervention must have a rationality that allows to expect a favorable result, in reducing the consequences or lethality.

These approaches were delineated, because many possible interventions would be raised in the coming years, seeking the correction of a malformation. Many therapies have been tried to correct ventriculomegaly, gastroschisis, and hydrothorax without an adequate objective and results. In order to reduce inappropriate treatments, the IFMSS had declared its purposes, defining the indication of a fetal treatment is long and tedious. New therapies need to aim a correctable specific fetal condition, test on animals, pilot trials in humans and scale to larger prospective cohort or randomized trials.

The alternative to fetal therapy for many parents is termination of pregnancy. The burden of a disabled child is taken by the parents with some aid of the insurance companies. In this context, parents may opt for pregnancy termination, a legal alternative to a high cost and non-reassuring fetal therapy [18]. This depends on local regulations, as well as that of institutions and the conscience of professionals. In particular, professionals have a duty to commit to their principles, however, they cannot ignore and misinform patients regarding the alternatives existing in the country's medical practice. They should have the ability to report on all medical alternatives, including termination of pregnancy, if regulation allows.

The Fetus as a Patient

Unthought but true, the fetus is treated, although the mother is healthy, and this is occurring worldwide. The concept of a fetus as a patient was developed by McCullough and Chervenak [19]. Their vision is based on the viability of the fetus and the mother's decision as fundamental elements for any therapy or termination of pregnancy. The fetus can be considered as a patient when is defined by the mother as a candidate for therapy or to continue the pregnancy. According to the authors, the decision of the mother gives the character of a patient to the fetus, and from that moment, he becomes creditor of the principle of beneficence. From this decision, the treating doctors must balance the beneficence of the mother and the fetus for any therapy.

Fetal Anesthesia

Anesthesia for a pregnant patient itself is a challenging case from the anesthesiologist's viewpoint. During fetal surgery, the anesthesiologist is responsible for taking care of two or more patients simultaneously. When the homeostasis of these interconnected and highly sensitive systems needs to be maintained, use of the correct medication in the appropriate dosage at the right time becomes very essential. Appropriate patient screening and selection, along with a multidisciplinary team approach will reduce the incidences of perioperative complications. A well-planned and well-prepared anesthesia setup tailored to the requirement of the specific fetal surgery will aid in creating a safe environment for the unborn fetus. A stable mother and a stable fetus will be helpful in continuation of the pregnancy till term and in delivery of a healthy newborn.

Development of Fetal Pain Sensitivity

Assessment of pain perception in the fetus is difficult and controversial, due to the physical limitations in monitoring fetal response, and the ethics that are involved with any fetal procedures. Nociception is a fundamental neural function, and the ability of the fetus to perceive pain evolves as it passes through the different stages of growth and development of its neural system. The sensory innervation of the skin and formation of its corresponding connections within the spinal cord begins as early as 8 weeks of gestation. This is followed by the proliferation of neural tissue and formation of the cerebral cortex from tenth week onward. Differentiation into specific cell types – neurons, fibers, glia, etc. – begins at the 17th week. However, this neural development, differentiation and maturation is a very long and complex process, which continues till a long time beyond birth.

In order to understand the need for fetal anesthesia, it is necessary to understand the fetal response to pain perception, which is shown in Fig. 19.1.

Hence, it becomes essential to block this physiological pain response of the fetus in order to maintain the fetoplacental perfusion levels. However, the long-term implications of such anesthesia and analgesia on fetal neurodevelopment are still unclear.

The exact gestational age from when the fetus can feel pain is debatable. The thalamocortical connections are established around 26 weeks. However, starting from the 22nd week onward, there exists an abundance of cholinergic, thalamocortical, and cortico-cortical transient synaptic circuits. Hence, it can be safely assumed

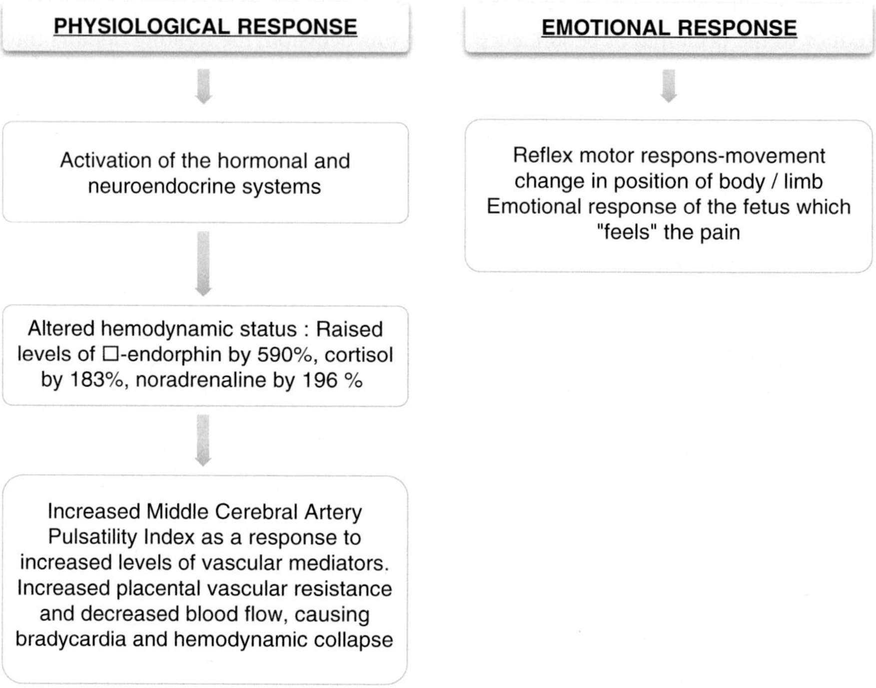

Fig. 19.1 Fetal response to noxious stimuli [20, 21]

that the fetus cannot feel pain before 22 weeks because of its immature neural system. By 26 weeks of gestation, the fetus has all the peripheral nervous system, the spinothalamic tracts, and the thalamocortical connections necessary to feel pain [22–24].

Anesthetic Agents and Monitoring of Fetus as a Patient

It is important to know how the fetus reacts differently to anesthetic medication, specifically from the perspective of hemodynamics. For example, sevoflurane has the potential to cause myocardial depression, and rarely ventricular and valvular dysfunction [25]. Moreover, some preclinical studies in animal embryos suggest that exposure to halogenates during fetal life can potentially cause neuronal apoptosis, and the damage is dose dependent. There is increasing evidence from rat and monkey infant animal models that anesthetic drugs like propofol, midazolam, etc. can have short- and long-term neurotoxic effects on the developing brain tissue [26, 27].

To minimize the cardiovascular and neurological side-effects, total intravenous anesthesia (TIVA) becomes a reasonable choice. At 26 weeks of gestation, the non-specific plasmatic esterase levels of the fetus are adequate to metabolize remifentanil, which is a potent synthetic opioid used in TIVA. In case the use of halogenates or propofol is essential, their neurotoxic effects can be attenuated to some extent by coadministration of the alpha-2 agonist dexmedetomidine. It acts as a synergic drug, so that adequate anesthesia can be achieved with a lower dose of the other drugs [28].

The principal purpose of fetal monitoring is to detect any variation in fetal perfusion and the subsequent impairment in oxygen delivery to fetal tissues. The method of fetal monitoring depends on the type of fetal procedure and usually starts from the preoperative assessment stage itself. Ultrasound and magnetic resonance imaging (MRI) are used preoperatively to document the baseline anatomy and pathophysiology of the fetus. During mid-gestation procedures, the simplest indicator of fetal well-being is the fetal heart rate measured by ultrasound. Because fetal heart rate is the most important determinant of cardiac output [29], fetal bradycardia is a strong indicator of fetal distress. Doppler blood flow assessment of the umbilical artery is also an option, where reversed or absent diastolic flow is considered a sign of placental insufficiency [30]. Another parameter which can be used to assess fetal hemodynamics is peak systolic and end-diastolic blood flow of the umbilical vessels. During ex utero intrapartum treatment (EXIT) procedure, a fetal echocardiography is performed every 3–5 minutes, and a fetal pulse oximeter is placed to check the fetal oxygen saturation; however, it has limitations [31].

Certain fetal surgeries need insufflation of the amniotic cavity with CO_2. Recent studies on fetal lamb models show that cold and dry CO_2 can cause hypercapnia, acidosis, hypotension, and fetal membrane inflammation. However, the use of humidified, warmed CO_2 mitigates these detrimental consequences. This can be explained by almost 40% reduction in the solubility of CO_2 by increasing the temperature. Additionally, humidification reduces the intrauterine partial pressure of CO_2 [32]. Because the fetal and placental hemodynamics are closely linked to the intrauterine pressure, it is recommended not to insufflate beyond 15 cmH_2O, and the minimum and maximum insufflation pressure should be recorded. Simultaneous, continuous monitoring of the duration of insufflation, maternal ventilation pressures, exhaled CO_2, and maternal hemodynamic parameters is essential. Fetal blood gas analysis is not recommended as a routine practice, because of the risk of fetal vasospasm or hemorrhage.

Maternal Anesthesia for Fetal Surgery

Detailed discussion of the physiological changes of pregnancy and its anesthetic implications are beyond the scope of this chapter. During pregnancy, a difficult airway can be frequently encountered because of the changes in body weight, enlargement of breasts, the relative shortness of the neck and swelling of the nasopharyngeal and laryngeal tissues. There is also an increase in oxygen consumption, which, combined with the lower residual capacity of the lungs, can lead to faster hypoxemia and hypoxia during the induction of anesthesia. Hemodynamically, there is an increase in about 40% in total circulating volume. Subsequently, cardiac output, heart rate and stroke volume are also increased, but the systemic vascular resistance and mean arterial pressure are diminished. Pregnancy is generally a state of hypercoagulability, increasing the propensity to have thromboembolic complications. These factors make a pregnant patient a high-risk case from the anesthesia point of view. Hence, whenever possible, it is safer to prefer regional or local anesthesia over general anesthesia.

A preoperative maternal evaluation should include a complete history of patient's comorbidities, with a special focus on cardiovascular and pulmonary disease, and any contraindications for the surgical procedure under consideration. Detailed notes need to be prepared regarding ongoing medications, previous surgeries or procedures, gynecological history, reactions to anesthesia, food or drug allergies, and habits like tobacco, alcohol, or any drugs. History-taking is complemented by a physical examination focused on difficult airway predictors, cardiovascular and pulmonary system assessment. Preoperative laboratory testing should include a complete blood count, crossmatch testing, and any other specifics depending on the patient's history and physical examination.

Selection of Route of Anesthesia

The first fetal surgery was performed in 1981, and since then, surgical as well as anesthetic techniques have evolved and become less invasive with lower risk to the mother and the fetus. The route of anesthesia greatly depends on the type of fetal surgery and the gestational age at which it is performed (Tables 19.1 and 19.2).

The anesthetist is an important member of the preoperative multidisciplinary assessment team which organizes and plans the fetal surgery. A recent retrospective analysis suggests that local anesthesia with monitored anesthesia care is preferred over regional anesthesia. Patients under local anesthesia have less need of vasoactive drugs and intravenous fluids for hemodynamic management [35]. This can lead to improved maternal, placental, and fetal perfusion and oxygen delivery. However, in such cases, it is important to have good communication with the patient, informing and preparing her beforehand for the minor pain and inconvenience that she might encounter during the procedure, for example, during administration of local anesthesia at the site for fetoscope insertion.

Maternal General Anesthesia for Fetal Procedures

Even if the surgery needs general anesthesia, it is preferred but not mandatory to place an epidural catheter for postoperative pain management. The patient is adequately pre-oxygenated. After administration of intravenous sedation, rapid sequence intubation is carried out so that chances of bronchial aspiration are minimized. Additional wide-bore intravenous cannula placement is done, and arterial cannula is placed for pressure monitoring if it is a part of the protocol. There is no

Table 19.1 A summary of the main anomalies amenable to fetal intervention as suggested by most common diseases

Disease	Procedure	Prognosis without/ or alternative therapy	Prognosis following fetal therapy	Evidence	Author
Twin-to-twin transfusion syndrome	Fetoscopic photocoagulation of placental anastomosis	50% survival	75% survival	Randomized control trial	Senat et al., 2003
Myelomeningocele	Hysterotomy and open closure of defect	80% of ventriculoperitoneal shunt. 20% of independent walk at 2 years	40% of ventriculoperitoneal shunt 40% of independent walk at 2 years	Randomized controlled trial	Adzick et al. 2011
Congenital diaphragmatic hernia	Fetoscopic tracheal occlusion in severe cases, with suspected lung hypoplasia	5% survival	50% survival	Randomized controlled trial	Ruano et al. 2015
Posterior urethral valves	Vesicoamniotic shunt	13% survival	53% survival	Randomized controlled trial, when compared as treated analysis	Morris et al. 2013
Hypoplastic left heart syndrome	Aortic valvuloplasty	26% survival	80% survival	Comparison of cohorts in registry	Moon Grady 2015
Twin reversed transfusion syndrome	Cord occlusion or fetoscopic photocoagulation of placental anastomosis	<50% survival	80% survival	Comparison of historic cohorts	Lewi 2006

Table 19.2 Indications for anesthesia in fetal surgery [33, 34]

Type of Surgery	Maternal anesthesia	Fetal anesthesia
Mid-gestation minimally invasive surgery on placenta or cord	Local anesthesia Regional anesthesia in selected cases (spinal/epidural)	Not indicated
Mid-gestation minimally invasive fetal surgery	Local anesthesia Regional anesthesia in selected cases (spinal/epidural)	Intramuscular opioid + muscle relaxant medication
Mid-gestation open fetal surgery	General anesthesia with intubation + tocolysis + optional post-operative epidural analgesia	Transplacental passage of maternal anesthetic medication + intramuscular opioid + muscle relaxant medication
EXIT procedures	General anesthesia or regional anesthesia (spinal/epidural) + tocolysis	Transplacental passage of maternal anesthetic medication + intramuscular opioid + muscle relaxant medication

evidence to support the use of PiCCO®, VIGILEO®, or any other specific device for invasive monitoring. Hemodynamics and airway should be under constant watch, and fluid infusion should be restricted to less than 750 milliliters due to the higher risk of developing pulmonary edema [31].

As discussed earlier, use of inhaled halogenates and propofol should be minimal because of the potential fetal neurotoxicity. A warning to this effect has been published by the Food and Drug Administration (FDA) (United States of America) [36]. As an alternative, supplementary dexmedetomidine can be used for dose reduction of the halogenates, along with intravenous non-GABA agonist agents such as opioids (fentanyl, remifentanil, etc.) for TIVA which are better tolerated by the fetus. Use of intravenous opioid medications in the mother, for example, remifentanil, has twofold benefits – better safety profile for mother as well as fetus and complimentary fetal sedation and quiescence [37]. This may lessen the need for fetal intramuscular anesthesia for short procedures like shunt placement.

Tocolysis is also an important component, specifically for open fetal surgeries where it is essential to maintain the fetoplacental perfusion. Inhalational anesthetic agents are potent tocolytics, but due to the above considerations, intravenous tocolytic agents like nitroglycerin, atosiban, smooth muscle relaxants, nifedipine, indomethacin, magnesium, etc. are preferred. Most of these agents have effects on maternal hemodynamics adversely, so special care should be given to the monitoring and treatment of the mean arterial pressure in order to ensure placental and fetal perfusion. Nitroglycerine can be used in repeated bolus administrations of 50–100 μg or a continuous infusion starting at 0.5–1 μg/kg/min. Atosiban can also be used before and after the procedure in the dose of 6.75 mg single dose or a continuous infusion at 3 mg/hr. [25, 38]

Maternal Local Anesthesia for Fetal Procedures

Minimally invasive fetal surgeries usually involve a single fetoscopic port for access to the uterine cavity. As there is minimal uterine manipulation involved, the target is to provide adequate local anesthesia and analgesia with monitored anesthesia. This is achieved by infiltration of the proposed port tract from skin up to the peritoneum. Plain lignocaine 2% is the most preferred medication because of its well-established fetomaternal safety profile. For procedures which may involve multiple entry ports or ports at a significant distance away from each other, regional anesthesia (spinal or epidural) provides superior patient comfort and pain control.

In some cases, anxiolysis or additional analgesia is required for the mother in order to facilitate the fetal procedure [39]. Light intravenous sedation is preferred in order to reduce the probability of maternal aspiration. Along with short-acting anxiolytics like midazolam, opioids like remifentanil are the medication of choice because of their low fetotoxic potential.

Fetal Intramuscular Anesthesia

Although fetal anesthesia can be achieved by the administration of intravenous or inhalational anesthetics to the mother, some surgeries require complete fetal anesthesia and immobilization. This can be achieved by blocking the motor response to pain or stimulus using intramuscular injection of anesthetic agent into the fetal thigh under ultrasound guidance.

Opioids that can be used are fentanyl in a dose of 5–20 μg/kg with or without atropine (20 μg/kg) to diminish the possible fetal bradycardia with its consequent hemodynamic collapse. Neuromuscular block can be achieved with pancuronium (0.2–0.3 mg/kg), atracurium (1 mg/kg), rocuronium (2 mg/kg), or vecuronium (0.1–0.3 mg/kg) [25, 40–42]. Because of its pharmacology, vecuronium has some advantages, specifically over pancuronium. Vecuronium has a more rapid clearance, shorter half-life, and minimal placental transfer. Compared to pancuronium, the fetal hemodynamic impact of vecuronium is much less, and there is less probability of fetal bradycardia with vecuronium use [43].

Open Fetal Surgery

With improvements in imaging technology and more ready access to prenatal imaging, our ability to diagnose major fetal malformations continues to increase. Understanding of the natural history of many malformations led to questions about the possibility to intervene during the prenatal period for those lesions that would otherwise be lethal. Interventions were intended to be lifesaving. The field of fetal surgery has evolved from these tenuous beginnings and with that evolution there has been a paradigm shift away from interventions solely as lifesaving procedures to interventions that can improve morbidity and alter the natural history of a disease. No longer strictly experimental, in utero surgery has become a standard of care for the management of several fetal malformations.

Fetal surgery myocardial is challenging. Not only are fetuses smaller than all other surgical patients, but the surgery has to be done with as little perturbation of the intrauterine environment. While improved instrumentation has allowed the development of less-invasive approaches to the treatment of some conditions, open fetal surgery remains the gold standard for the management of the most complex lesions. Surgery for these cases has to be performed through a uterine incision that both controls the fetal membranes and provides complete hemostasis, exposes the anatomy of interest, and yet is small enough not to compromise the integrity of the pregnancy. Essentially, we operate on our smallest, most delicate patients with the smallest surgical field to operate in.

Success has come from incorporating highly integrated multidisciplinary surgical teams. An open fetal surgery case involves specially trained physicians from maternal–fetal medicine, pediatric surgery, pediatric surgical subspecialties, and anesthesia teams from obstetrics to care for the mother and from pediatrics to provide for fetal considerations. Fetal cardiology supports sonographers who continuously monitor fetal cardiac status. A team from newborn medicine are also on hand in the event that delivery of the fetus becomes necessary. Each team is supported by specially trained OR staff, nurses, blood bank, and pharmacy. Managing the patient's care before surgery, during the initial postoperative recovery, and post discharge care requires an even larger team, adding nurse coordinators, social workers, sonographers, specialized labor and delivery nursing, and countless others. Open fetal surgery has been likened to a ballet with careful choreography under the watchful eye of the surgical team leader.

The overarching myocardial question with every patient is even if it is possible to operate on the fetus, is surgery the right thing to do? While an in-depth ethical examination of fetal surgery is beyond the scope of this review, there are obvious ethical questions that must be addressed. Does the patient really understand the risks of surgery and are they willing to accept them in exchange for the potential of benefit? Are we willing to accept significant maternal morbidity, and even potential mortality, to attempt surgery on a fetus with no guarantee of success or survival of the fetus? Fetal surgery is a unique discipline as with two separate patients with conflicting needs, and while the mother's well-being takes priority, the impact of any decision has an effect on both mother and fetus. The dichotomy of mother and fetus makes the application of the four standard ethical principles of autonomy, justice, beneficence, and non-maleficence much more complicated and requires a careful nuanced approach.

Open fetal surgery has serious inherent risks that all patients should be counseled on comprehensively prior to being offered any fetal intervention. First and foremost, patients should be counseled regarding the maternal risks of general anesthesia, laparotomy, and uterine hysterectomy. These include hemorrhage, infection, injury to surrounding organs, thromboembolic phenomenon, myocardial infarction, stroke, and even death. The hemodynamic changes of pregnancy along with the use of tocolytic medications and intravenous fluids, and maternal pulmonary edema is a well-recognized complication of fetal surgery [44]. The patient should also be counseled about the necessity for cesarean delivery for the current pregnancy and for all subsequent pregnancies due to increased risks for uterine dehiscence and rupture. The obstetrical risks of open fetal procedures include preterm labor and/or delivery, preterm premature rupture of membranes, intra-amniotic infection, uterine rupture at the hysterotomy site, and fetal demise. Patients should be explicitly counseled that at any point during the surgical intervention, the fetus may require immediate delivery, exposing the fetus to all of the myocardial complications of prematurity or may expire intraoperatively. Again, counseling is best achieved by the use of an interdisciplinary team with expertise in each facet of a patient's care.

Patients that elect to undergo fetal surgery also have a significant burden placed on them for the duration of the pregnancy. Bed rest is required for several weeks after an open surgery is performed with continued oral tocolytic therapy until delivery. At least weekly visits are required for ultrasound and prenatal care. They can reside no more than 30 minutes driving distance from the institution providing care and must have the ability to get to our facility at any time. For myocardial patients who live farther away or do not have ready access to transportation, relocation of the patient and at least one care giver is necessary.

As can been seen from these considerations, careful patient selection, both maternal and fetal, is key to the success of any fetal surgery.

Myelomeningocele

A myelomeningocele (MMC) is also known as open spina bifida or an open neural tube defect. This is a protrusion of the meninges and spinal cord fibers that results from a failure of fusion of the vertebral column. These lesions are covered only by a thin membrane without overlying dura, muscle, or skin. The natural history is that damage occurs to the unprotected developing neural tissue, leading to devastating neurologic damage affecting both motor and sensory nerve function to the lower extremities, bowel, and bladder. The vast majority of MMCs involve the lumbosacral spine, although lesions involving the thoracic and cervical spine are also observed. The vast majority of patients with MMC also have a concomitant Chiari II malformation, with caudal displacement of the cerebellum and brainstem into the upper spinal column. There is compression of the displaced tissues, obstruction of the fourth ventricle, and effacement of the cisterna magna [9, 45]. This leads to an obstruction in the normal flow of cerebrospinal fluid, resulting in the ventriculomegaly seen in a large majority of fetuses diagnosed with MMC. The Chiari II malformation with secondary hydrocephalus also results in impaired motor and cognitive function [45, 46].

In the United States, an MMC occurs in 3 per 10,000 children under the age of 18 [47]. The exact etiology of MMC is not well understood, but folic acid deficiency, exposure to folic acid antagonist medications and use of valproate are known risk factors. The failure of neurulation occurs very early in gestation but it has been hypothesized that the underlying nervous tissue is normal. It is the exposure of the developing neural tissue to amniotic fluid and the repetitive trauma associated with just remaining in utero that results in the observed damage to the developing nerves. This process is known as the "two hit hypothesis." [45, 48–50] This hypothesis provides the rationale for the concept that timely in utero closure of the defect affords an opportunity to prevent worsening neurological damage, thus altering the natural history of the disease.

The support for this concept was developed over many years of careful study. This involved not only the development of the surgical technique for open fetal surgery, but the development and testing of an animal model prior to applying the concept to human fetuses. These are well outlined in a series of papers from the Fetal Surgery group at the University of California in San Francisco. The first reported case of open fetal surgery for MMC in humans was published in the Lancet in 1998 [51]. A large cohort of patients undergoing open fetal surgery were assembled in several centers but the best described comes from the Fetal Surgery group at the Children's Hospital of Philadelphia. They published outcomes from an initial cohort, documenting reversal of hindbrain herniation, decreased need for shunting in the first year of life and improved motor function of up to 2 levels. They have continued to publish ongoing follow-up documenting subsequent neurologic and neurocognitive development [52–61]. This body of work formed the basis for the final stage of investigation, a randomized controlled trial.

The Management of Myelomeningocele Study (MOMS) was a randomized controlled trial evaluating in utero repair of MMC compared to postnatal repair, with the initial results published in 2012 [9]. Subsequent publications of obstetric and pediatric results for the entire cohort were forthcoming in 2016 and 2018, respectively [62, 63]. The primary outcome was a composite outcome comprised of fetal or neonatal death or the need for cerebrospinal fluid shunt at 12 months of age. The secondary outcome was motor function and mental development at 30 months of life. Assessment of outcomes was done in a blinded fashion with evaluators having no knowledge of the group to which the child was randomized. The trial was stopped early when a planned interim analysis showed a significant improvement in the efficacy of in utero repair compared to postnatal repair. Results for infant outcomes at 12 months are given in Table 19.3. Thirty-month outcomes are given in Tables 19.4 and 19.5.

The risk of maternal and obstetric complications continues to be part of the decision-making process for families. The maternal hysterotomy increases the risks for preterm labor, dehiscence of the incision, and membrane complications like preterm premature rupture of the membranes. Patients remain on activity restrictions and oral tocolytic therapy for the duration of their pregnancy. Delivery is by cesarean section at a goal of 37 weeks, requiring a second uterine incision. There is an increased risk for preterm delivery with a mean gestational age at delivery of

Table 19.3 MOMS Trial – infant outcomes at 12 months

	Prenatal Surgery (n=78)	Postnatal Surgery (n=80)	RR (95% CI)	P value
Primary Outcome (%)	**68**	**98**	**0.70(0.58-0.84)**	**<0.001**
Death	3	0		
Shunt criteria met	65	92		
Placement of shunt (%)	**40**	**82**	**0.48(0.36-0.640**	**<0.001**
Any hindbrain herniation (%)	**64**	**96**	**0.67(0.56-0.81)**	**<0.001**
None	36	4		
Mild	40	29		
Moderate	19	45		
Severe	6	22		

From Adzick et al. [9]

34 weeks. All subsequent pregnancies must be delivered by cesarean section with risks of dehiscence or rupture of the hysterotomy site [9, 64–66].

The results of the MOMS trial changed the paradigm for management of the fetus with a MMC. The American College of Obstetricians and Gynecologists issued a statement in 2017 and reaffirmed it in 2019 that said "[we] recommend that women with pregnancies complicated by fetal myelomeningocele who meet established criteria for in utero repair should be counseled in a nondirective fashion regarding all management options, including the possibility of open maternal–fetal surgery." [67] All patients should be offered the opportunity for open in utero repair if they are appropriate candidates with the criterion for selection being the same as were used in the MOMs trial [9]. This initial criterion for maternal body mass index (BMI) was 35 kg/m [2], although some centers are studying surgery in patients with a BMI up to 40 kg/m [2] [68].

The surgical procedure has been well described in the MOMS trial papers. Some modifications have been adopted, primarily in the administration of maternal anesthesia, to minimize fetal exposure to the inhaled anesthetic. Magnesium sulfate is given intravenously with the loading dose of 6 grams started just after the induction of maternal anesthesia and a maintenance dose of 4 g/hr. continued through the duration of the case. Many centers now do a two-layer closure of the MMC. After dissecting out the placode and dropping it back into the spinal canal, the dura is not sutured. Myofascial flaps are created and closed to provide a watertight seal, followed by closure of the skin. Some institutions use relaxing incisions on the fetal skin to achieve skin closure that is not under tension; others will use a collagen patch such as Duragen or Alloderm to achieve closure of the skin. There is no evidence to suggest one method to be superior to the other and both were employed during the MOMS trial, but further study is ongoing to define the optimal surgical technique for closure when a primary skin closure cannot be obtained.

Table 19.4 MOMS Trial – infant outcomes at 30 months

	Prenatal Sx N=87	Postnatal Sx N=88	P value
Primary outcome score	199.4±80.5	166.6±76.7	0.004
BMDI - MDI	89.5±14.0	86.2±18.4	0.22
Difference between anatomic level & functional level	-0.80±5.5	-1.56±4.7	0.002
Difference (%)			
≥ 2 levels better	26.4	11.4	0.005
1 level better	11.5	8.0	
no difference	26.4	21.6	
1 level worse	19.5	27.3	
≥ 2 levels worse	16.1	31.8	0.03

From Adzick et al. [9]

Table 19.5 Ambulation at 30 months

	Prenatal Surgery (N=87)	Postnatal Surgery (N=88)	Relative Risks	P value
Not Walking (%)	27.6	40.9		
Walking with orthotics/devices (%)	27.6	35.2		
Walking Independantly (%)	44.8	23.9	1.88 (1.21-2.92)	0.004

From Adzick et al. [9]

One of the other results from the MOMS trial was that the overall duration of surgery and the duration of the closure itself were important predictors of preterm PROM suggesting that experience in performing the procedure matters [9, 62]. A recent report, using a CUSUM technique, looked at how many cases it would take to achieve "competence" for a new group undertaking open fetal surgery for

MMC. Using data from published reports, they found that it would take 35 cases to achieve "competence." [69]

Open fetal surgery for MMC has, by virtue of its careful development and rigorous study, become the gold standard by which other approaches must be judged. The natural evolution of fetal surgical procedures is toward the development of less-invasive approaches. The best example is found in the current evaluation of percutaneous endoscopic placement of endotracheal balloons in the treatment of severe congenital diaphragmatic surgery. Efforts are underway to develop an endoscopic approach to closure of myelomeningoceles. While the arguments in favor of decreased maternal risks associated with an endoscopic approach are compelling, the fetal benefits have not yet been proven to match those achieved from open fetal surgery and they must be demonstrated with the same research rigor.

Sacrococcygeal Teratomas

Sacrococcygeal teratomas (SCTs) are found in approximately 1 out of every 27,000 pregnancies, making SCTs the most commonly observed neoplasm in fetuses [70]. There is a fourfold predilection toward females, for reasons that are not well understood [71]. SCTs are generally comprised of fully differentiated tissue representing all three embryologic layer (ectoderm, endoderm, and mesoderm). Some teratomas contain incompletely differentiated components which confers an elevated risk of malignancy [72]. Only approximately, 10% of SCTs are malignant [73]. Chromosomal abnormalities are not commonly observed in fetuses with SCTs.

Most fetal SCTs are diagnosed during the mid-trimester ultrasonographic anatomic survey as a mass observed near the fetal lumbar and/or sacral spine. The mass is typically a mixture of solid, cystic, and vascular components [72]. Other ultrasonographic evidence that suggests the presence of a tumor occur secondary to mass effect on other local tissues. These include bladder displacement or urinary tract obstruction with resultant fetal pyelectasis, or dilated bowel from a colonic and/or rectal obstruction. There is a significant risk for high-output heart failure as a result of the low resistance vascular nature of the tumor, thus fetal hydrops may be part of the initial presentation. SCTs are classified anatomically by the Altman Classification system originally described by the American Academy of Pediatrics (Surgical Section) in 1973 [74]. Type 1 is essentially entirely external (by definition there is a small internal component). Type 2 lesions are mostly external but have more of an intrapelvic component than Type 1. Type 3 lesions are primarily intrapelvic but do have a small external component. Type 4 lesions are entirely intrapelvic or intraabdominal. The majority of lesions diagnosed prenatally are Altman either type 1 or type 2 [44]. Fetal MRI and a baseline fetal echocardiogram are important additional investigations to assess the impact of the SCT. A careful search for additional anomalies is undertaken along with an amniocentesis to document a normal genetic status in anticipation that an open fetal resection may be considered in the future. Part of the antenatal counseling for families with a fetal SCT should include a multidisciplinary discussion of open fetal resection and the procedure-related risks to allow the family to have a greater understanding of what is involved before they are faced with actually making the decision to undergo open fetal surgery.

The perinatal mortality rate of SCTs diagnosed antenatally approaches 50% [75]. As may be expected, the larger the SCT the greater the risk for adverse outcomes. Tumor volume-to-fetal weight ratio can be helpful in prognostication [76–78], as a value of 0.12 (before 24 weeks) has been shown to confer a nearly fivefold increased risk for significant fetal morbidity and/or mortality [76]. Larger tumors with a significant vascular component can greatly increase the fetal cardiac output required for survival. Frequent monitoring of cardiac function and combined cardiac output is essential. Increased cardiac demand can lead to high-output cardiac failure in the fetus and the development of hydrops and ultimately may result in fetal demise.

Fetuses with a rapidly enlarging SCT and worsening cardiac function are the group for which in utero surgical intervention may prevent fetal demise. Timing of a surgical intervention prior to the development of hydrops is important. The first decision point regarding potential in utero surgery is the gestational age at which the cardiac dysfunction develops. Generally, if it develops at 28 weeks or beyond, a course of antenatal steroids is administered, and the fetus is delivered with intent to perform a postnatal resection of the tumor [44, 72, 75, 79]. If the fetus demonstrates cardiac compromise prior to 28 weeks, in utero surgery for resection or debulking of the tumor may be considered for carefully selected patients. The fetus should not have any other major abnormality that would impact survival, along with a normal karyotype obtained via amniocentesis prior to surgery.

The goal of open fetal surgery for fetal SCT is to reduce the tumor mass and not to completely resect the tumor. As such, only Type 1 and Type 2 lesions are amenable to open fetal surgery. Decreasing the tumor mass decreases the demand on the fetal cardiac system allowing it to compensate. Also, it usually is impossible to remove the entire tumor prenatally, given that all SCTs have an intrapelvic component. Limited published data regarding the outcomes of in utero SCT resection exist, but the published perinatal survival rate is 50% from a group of 12 published cases [80].

The surgical approach to open fetal resection of an SCT is similar to that for a MMC although, depending on the size of the mass, may require a larger hysterotomy. Deep maternal general anesthesia, preoperative and intraoperative tocolytic therapy, antibiotics, hemostatic hysterotomy, fetal paralytic medications, and careful monitoring of the fetal cardiac status during surgery are common components. Anticipation of fetal hemorrhage requires the establishment of means to provide fetal transfusion if necessary. The mass is brought into the hysterotomy in a fashion to maximize the tumor exposure . This usually means delivery of the legs through the hysterotomy. The external portion of the tumor is then resected. Once the tumor is resected, fetal hemostasis is confirmed, and the fetus is then placed back inside the amniotic cavity and uterine closure follows the same sequence as in an open MMC surgery. Postoperative care also follows the same careful protocol although additional monitoring is necessary as the tumor will continue to grow. The goal for delivery is usually between 36 and 37 weeks via cesarean section. Postnatal resection is then performed by pediatric surgery to resect the remaining portion of the tumor.

Congenital Pulmonary Airway Malformation

Congenital pulmonary airway malformations (CPAM, also referred to as congenital cystic adenomatoid malformation (CCAM)) are benign cystic lung masses comprised of pulmonary tissue that does not participate in alveolar gas exchange. They are classified by their appearance. Microcystic lesions appear echogenic and solid on ultrasound but are comprised of multiple small cysts. Macrocystic lesions are composed of larger cysts usually measuring more than 1 cm in diameter. Microcystic lesions account for about 75% of the total CPAMs. [81, 82] CPAMs are thought to develop sporadically without any known genetic predisposition or other identifiable risk factor. They are almost always unilateral and affect both lungs equally. Usually, only one lobe of the lung is involved. Their blood supply is pulmonary in origin.

Bronchopulmonary sequestrations (BPS) are another benign lung mass of pulmonary tissue that is not in communication with the bronchial tree. Their blood supply is systemic usually arising from the descending aorta. Overall, they tend to be smaller than CPAMs and hydrops is less likely [83–85]. Echogenic lung masses can also arise from other lung malformations such as congenital lobar emphysema or foregut duplication cysts but these are beyond the scope of this discussion. For the rest of this section, we will discuss CPAMs only, but in utero resection of a BPS can be considered if the same clinical situations arise.

CPAMs can grow at a rapid rate in the mid-trimester with a peak in growth usually occurring around 28 weeks' gestation [86]. The decreased growth rate or shrinking observed in the third trimester is not well understood. Approximately, 50% of the CPAMs noted antenatally will appear to "resolve" prior to delivery [87]. Visualization of most CPAM lesions depends on the persistence of the macrocysts or increased echogenicity from the multiple interfaces the cysts form along with differential water content of the tissues. In the third trimester, it is not uncommon for the microcystic lesions to become isoechoic with the normal lung tissue. At this point, the size of these lesions cannot be measured directly and must be inferred from the extent of mass effect on the cardiac position. Survival rates of fetuses diagnosed with CPAM are excellent with published rates over 90% [88]. Even if regression does not occur, the vast majority likely will either shrink or stop growing as the normal lung parenchyma grows, decreasing the size of mass relative to healthy lung [81, 85].

Large CPAMs cause a significant mass effect, displacing the heart and potentially altering cardiac function as well as compressing the developing normal lung surrounding the lesion. Cardiac dysfunction can result in the development of fetal hydrops. Hydrops results from mass effect causing mediastinal shifting with cardiac and vena cava compression, compromising blood return to the fetal heart. This results in cardiac compromise and ultimately cardiac failure. This is of greatest concern at previable gestational ages and is nearly universally fatal if fetal intervention is not performed [85]. Mediastinal shift can also compress the fetal esophagus, impeding swallowing and ultimately leading to polyhydramnios. Pulmonary hypoplasia may develop from compression of the normal developing lung. The mass occupies space in the fetal thorax that would otherwise allow normal lung parenchyma to expand [81].

The diagnosis of a CPAM is often made at the mid-trimester sonographic anatomical survey. Determination of the CPAM volume ratio (CVR) has important prognostic value. This is calculated from the formula for the volume of an ellipse, by multiplying the lesion's length, height, and width by a factor of 0.523. A CVR of >1.6 is associated with an increased risk for the development hydrops, the need for fetal surgical intervention, and neonatal respiratory distress, whereas a CVR of <0.91 predicts a good overall prognosis with low risk for needing prenatal intervention [88, 89].

The typical first-line therapy for a large CPAM at increased risk for developing hydrops is a course of intramuscular betamethasone, consisting of two 12 mg doses 24 hours apart. Steroids are most commonly used as an initial therapy with microcystic CPAMs as these lesions are not amenable to other minimally invasive therapies such as drainage or placement of a thoracoamniotic shunt, but can be considered in other situations. Betamethasone is effective at decreasing the size of the lesions, and may even resolve hydrops, although the data are limited regarding the efficacy of steroids in reversing or preventing hydrops [90–92]. Up to four courses of antenatal steroids can be administered.

Fetuses with a CPAM resulting in cardiac compromise or hydrops represent a select patient population for which in utero fetal intervention can prevent fetal demise. If the intervention results in the resolution of fetal hydrops, reported fetal survival rates exceed 90% [90]. If the gestational age is 32 weeks or beyond, delivery with possible ex utero intrapartum therapy (EXIT) should be considered. If the fetus is less than 32 weeks gestation, fetal intervention is a potential option. For a mass with larger cysts, fetal thoracentesis to drain the cystic spaces should be considered, although this is often a temporizing measure as the fluid often reaccumulates. Drainage makes it possible to calculate how much the CVR will decrease with drainage and to verify that the normal lung is capable of expansion. Amniotic fluid can also be sent for genetic studies. If the cystic fluid re-accumulates, then placement of a thoracoamniotic shunt has been shown to both decrease the size of the lesion and improve survival [93–95].

Open in utero CPAM resection is an option in fetuses less than 32 weeks with large microcystic lesions that have not responded to multiple courses of steroids and are at high risk for the development of hydrops. This has become an increasingly uncommon situation. Open fetal surgery for fetal lobectomy to resect a CPAM can be considered for patients who can give informed consent, have no other major fetal anomalies, and have normal fetal karyotype. As previously described, extensive preoperative multidisciplinary counseling is performed prior to consideration of any fetal surgical procedure. Patients with a placenta previa, a short cervical length, or history of preterm birth or other strong risk factors for a preterm birth are not offered open fetal surgery for lobectomy [81].

Open fetal surgery for a CPAM resection follows the same protocol as for other open fetal surgeries with deep general anesthesia, maternal laparotomy and hysterotomy. Two additional considerations are necessary. More of the fetus must be delivered through the incision to allow for the thoracotomy and resection and requires a larger incision. Fetal position and placental location may complicate the decision-making. Intravenous access to the fetus must be established to allow for transfusion as the mass is mobilized. With the thoracotomy and removal of the mass, compression of the heart is lessened. The circulating blood volume in the fetus often needs to be augmented as more filling volume is required once the mass is mobilized to prevent circulatory collapse. A pulse oximeter is applied to the fetal hand for closer monitoring of the fetal status and continuous ultrasound evaluation of the fetal heart is imperative to monitor cardiac filling as the mass is mobilized. Postoperative care also follows the usual protocols for open fetal surgeries. Postoperative imaging of the fetal chest will show a large effusion that gradually resolves as the remaining normal lung tissue expands. As with all open fetal surgeries, delivery is by cesarean section by 37 weeks.

Given the rarity of cases that require in utero resection and the advanced expertise required to perform these cases, there are limited data regarding the outcomes. Adzick et al. published a series of 13 cases where resections were performed with eight having complete resolution of the hydrops and neonatal survival [69].

Some fetuses with large CPAMs (CVR >1.6) with mediastinal shift never develop hydrops. The presence of the large intrathoracic mass can cause significant respiratory difficulty following delivery with the concern that it may not be possible to stabilize the newborn to allow for resection following delivery. These patients may be considered for an ex utero intrapartum therapy (EXIT) to delivery procedure [81, 86, 96, 97]. The EXIT approach allows resection of the mass prior to cutting of the umbilical cord, with the placental circulation providing a functional cardiothoracic bypass circuit. The preoperative and intraoperative procedure is similar to an open fetal resection described above with the additional consideration that the fetus will be delivered. Typically, the location for the uterine incision is in the lower uterine segment with the fetus in a vertex presentation and does require the use of the special stapling device to provide complete hemostasis for the duration of the procedure. Upon completion of the excision, a chest tube is placed and the fetus is intubated and ventilated. Once adequate oxygenation is achieved, the umbilical cord is clamped and cut, and the delivery is completed. Since agents have been used to provide maternal uterine relaxation during the EXIT procedure, there is an increased risk for maternal hemorrhage once the placenta is removed. Anticipating this, aggressive use of uterotonic medications is recommended. Typically, the uterine staples placed in the creation of the incision are removed prior to closure of the hysterotomy. Published outcomes from EXIT delivery for CPAM resection are excellent. One published series reported 21 of 23 neonates surviving the procedure [81].

Fetoscopy-Guided Procedures

In 1954, Westin published the first attempt to observe a live fetus under direct vision [98]. A hysteroscope was used and its objective was to visualize external malformations and obtain tissues for diagnostic purposes. However, with the development of high-resolution ultrasound equipment, the quality of the image obtained made it unnecessary to continue with fetoscopy. The diagnostic indication was delayed, and the invasive procedures were relegated to pathologies with therapy. The surgical needs required important adaptations. The optical fiber allowed to transport the image and bring light to cavities which were inaccessible to the doctor's vision. These endoscopes have diameters from 0.5 to 3 mm today, reaching 100,000 to 1 million pixels. In the first trimester, the procedure is called embryoscopy, and semirigid endoscopes of 1 mm in diameter are recommended. Embryoscopy performed under 12 weeks may be indicated for congenital malformations with external abnormalities and allows differential diagnosis. Local anesthesia is used, and trocars are inserted under ultrasound vision through the maternal abdomen, piercing skin and uterine wall. Fetoscopy is the name of the procedure from the second trimester of pregnancy and has various instruments of different diameter, up to 3 mm. The procedure can be performed under local anesthesia, but some indications need additional ports or uterine exteriorization, which requires regional or general anesthesia. The endoscopic procedure is unfamiliar to most obstetricians, however, due to the low frequency of the pathologies. It is therefore not appropriate that the procedure could be performed everywhere, from the point of view of public health and quality.

The instruments are now specifically manufactured for this surgery. A powerful light source, optic fiber camera, and recording system are required. The equipment must allow the intervention and complete review. The endoscopes used are 20–30 cm long with a diameter of 1–3 mm. A remote eyepiece is used to separate the light source and camera to be far from the operator's hand, to allow movements with greater precision without weight. There are specific instruments for anterior wall. The endoscopes are rigid, and in order to visualize the anterior wall, the placenta has to be visualized from the side in upward direction. There are two strategies for this: the curved scope, which produces an arc of 1/3 of circumference, and fiber deflector scope, which allows coagulation in the anterior wall. The entry of the endoscope requires the installation of a trocar that allows to pass through the uterine wall and move this endoscope to the surgical sites. A central venous catheter set of size 11 French, which can be inserted using the Seldinger technique, is enough for this purpose. This allows an access port for smooth and safe manipulation. A surgical port of these characteristics can be performed with local anesthesia that includes the skin, the maternal abdominal wall, and the uterine serosa. These are sensitive structures which, once anesthetized, can allow for a longer, easier surgery and avoid the use of regional or general anesthesia and their associated costs and risks. A minimally invasive procedure should consider all the associated maternal risks and not just the instrumentation diameters. In general, fetal surgeries even with a single port are considered surgeries and are performed in a ward using aseptic technique and under all hospital regulations.

Secondly, the entry site must be chosen correctly. The uterus is an ovoid cavity, in which the fetus and placenta can have any position and orientation, but their access is limited to the anterior wall. The exteriorization of the uterus, or the use of an accessory laparoscopy to enter the uterine posterior wall can facilitate the intervention in terms of the intrauterine visualization but complicates the intervention in terms of maternal risks. When the placenta is at an adequate distance and opposite to the site of entry into the uterus, easy access and successful placental surgery is most likely.

For this reason, fetoscopic surgery requires expert ultrasound support to review continuously the fetal orientation, placental location, trocar insertion, intrauterine bleeding, fetal heart rate monitoring, polyhydramnios and oligohydramnios and many more parameters. The positions of the trocars in the surgery must be defined in the pavilion, during the preparatory stage. Extreme care must be taken not to damage mesenteric or uterine vessels. Color Doppler imaging is useful in this step.

Once inside the amniotic cavity, it is important to keep the reference points for surgery: These are the horizon, the cord insertion, the fetal position and the placental limits. For a theoretical case of left side trocar insertion (from the patient's left), the fetoscopic image will be toward the right of the patient. In this setting, with the patient in supine position on the operation table, keeping the horizon of the image, the left in the screen will correspond to the caudal part of the uterine cavity. Occasionally, the amniotic fluid may be stained with blood and amniotic fluid replacement may be required or the procedure can be performed under continuous fluid irrigation. The use of gas to insufflate the amniotic cavity is a recent innovation and allows myelomeningocele repair.

The type of endoscopes needed for surgery depends on indication and the procedure needed to be performed. There are scopes with a 0.8 mm channel, which allows the passage of a laser fiber with a diameter of 400–600 μm. Scopes are available with a bipolar clamp mounted on the camera sheath or with a scissor for specific uses.

Complications of a single-port fetoscopy intervention are generally low, less than 5% of cases. The rupture of membranes occurs in less than 5% of cases. In fetoscopic surgery for myelomeningocele, which requires three or four trocars, the rupture rate of membranes exceeds 50% in some series.

Twin-to-Twin Transfusion Syndrome (TTTS)

Historically, the treatment was amniodrainage, and since 1995, fetoscopy has developed, becoming the standard [99, 100]. Fetoscopy treatment seeks to identify placental anastomoses and occlude them by laser photocoagulation. The demonstration of the benefit of fetoscopy and laser photocoagulation over serial amniodrainage was published in 2004, where survival at 6 months of age was 76% versus 51% [101].

The diagnosis of TTTS is made by ultrasound before 26 weeks of gestational age.

Polyhydramnios in the recipient twin, with a maximum vertical pocket of at least 8 cm or 10 cm, before or after 20 weeks, respectively (Figs. 19.2 and 19.3).

Oligohydramnios in the donor twin, defined as a vertical pocket less than 2cm at any gestational age.

The presence of a "stuck twin" or fixed fetus at the border of the amniotic sac, and the uterine wall, is due to extreme oligohydramnios. The presence of a "stuck twin" and polyhydramnios in the other twin is diagnostic of the disease.

By definition, all monochorionic twin pregnancies have fetal transfusion between twins due to the constant presence of anastomoses. Only some of them lead to the

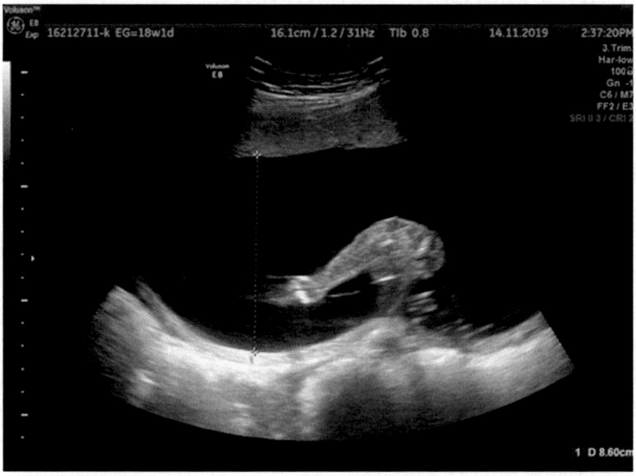

Fig. 19.2 Deepest vertical pouch of 8.6 cm is diagnostic of polyhydramnios before 20 weeks

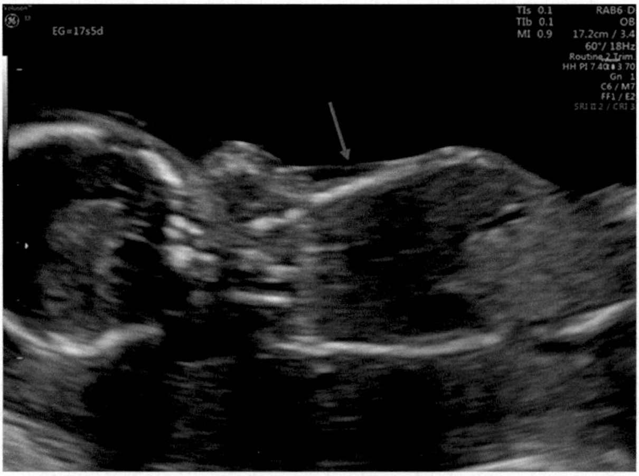

Fig. 19.3 Donor twin stuck with membranes attached to the body. Blue arrow shows the membrane

polyhydramnios/oligoamnios sequence, which has been named as severe fetal transfusion or "twin-to-twin transfusion syndrome" by the Eurofetus group. This severity criterion is associated with the indication of fetoscopy. Weight discordance of more than 20% or 25% is not a requisite. The presence of a visible bladder in the donor fetus does not rule out the diagnosis.

The Quintero classification was described in 1999 [102]. Stage one consists of amniotic fluid discordance, greater than 8 cm and less than 2 cm in the recipient and donor fetuses, respectively. After 20 weeks, the polyhydramnios criterion is >10 cm. In stage two, the donor fetus bladder should be empty during the whole examination. In stage three, there are Doppler abnormalities, either absent or reverse flow in the donor's umbilical artery, or absent or reverse flow in the recipient's venous ductus A wave. In stage four, hydrops in one of the fetuses is required. Stage five is characterized by the death of one or both twins; however, this stage is no longer indicative of fetal surgery.

Before the use of ultrasound and the possibility of antenatal diagnosis, TTTS was considered in newborns with 20% weight discordance and 5 g/dl in hemoglobin concentration. These criteria were good for neonatology but were discarded because it was not possible to demonstrate them antenatally by ultrasound. In addition, these criteria are used for surviving twins that were born alive and are not applicable in cases of double or individual fetal death, which were possibly more affected by severe fetal transfusion. With the development of ultrasound, new prenatal findings were needed. These were correlated with the adverse outcome and the polyhydramnios-oligoamnios sequence has been shown to have the highest mortality in obstetrics, approaching 90% in untreated cases.

Selective intrauterine growth restriction (growth discordance and abnormal umbilical Doppler) has been described as a new entity in monochorionic twin pregnancies [103]. There are cases of monochorionic pregnancies that develop anemia of one twin and polycythemia of the other, without polyhydramnios/oligohydramnios called TAPS (Twin Anemia Polycythemia Sequence). These scenarios support the theory that the vascular communications are variable in number and type, which can lead to different diseases [104].

The surgical technique to increase survival is a controversial issue. The most popular techniques are nonselective, selective, and Solomon [105, 106] The objective of these surgical techniques is to improve the results of the intervention, seeking a better survival and a lower probability of complications, such as fetal demise, TAPS, or recurrence of polyhydramnios-oligohydramnios. Nonselective technique is the coagulation of all crossing anastomoses at the membrane insertion. The selective technique seeks to preserve normal crossing vessels and coagulate only the identified anastomoses. The Solomon technique additionally traces a coagulation line along the placental surface, thus joining the coagulation points of the selective technique (Fig. 19.4 and Table 19.6). The latter allows reducing the occurrence of complications caused by persistent small anastomoses.

Cord Occlusion in TRAP and in Complicated Monochorionic Twins

Cord occlusion is an important procedure for monochorionic twin pregnancies. The vascular connections that exist between the fetuses precludes the use of intravascular medication, as they can pass to its co-twin. The surgical approaches can be a coagulation at the placenta, such as in TTTS, or cord occlusion with bipolar forceps [107]. Cord occlusion can be ultrasound guided with bipolar forceps, by radiofrequency, or by fetoscopy-guided bipolar forceps.

TRAP is an acronym for Twin Reversed Arterial Perfusion. It occurs in monochorionic twin pregnancies, in which a fetus has no cardiac activity, and is perfused by the healthy fetus, which delivers part of its cardiac output. The sick fetus has a weak blood circulation, with great deterioration of its upper body. In general, they are better developed in their lower body. The TRAP fetus does not have a normal postnatal life prognosis, but the healthy fetus has a high probability of a healthy and normal life after treatment in 80% of the cases. Cord coagulation by bipolar forceps or by radiofrequency are the preferred surgical approaches [108].

The indication of surgery depends on severity criteria since the spontaneous evolution allows the resolution of many cases. The proposed criteria are a TRAP twin larger than the healthy fetus with polyhydramnios, abnormal Doppler, or cardiomegaly. All these may be signs of cardiac overload. Cord occlusion will reduce this cardiac overload in the healthy twin.

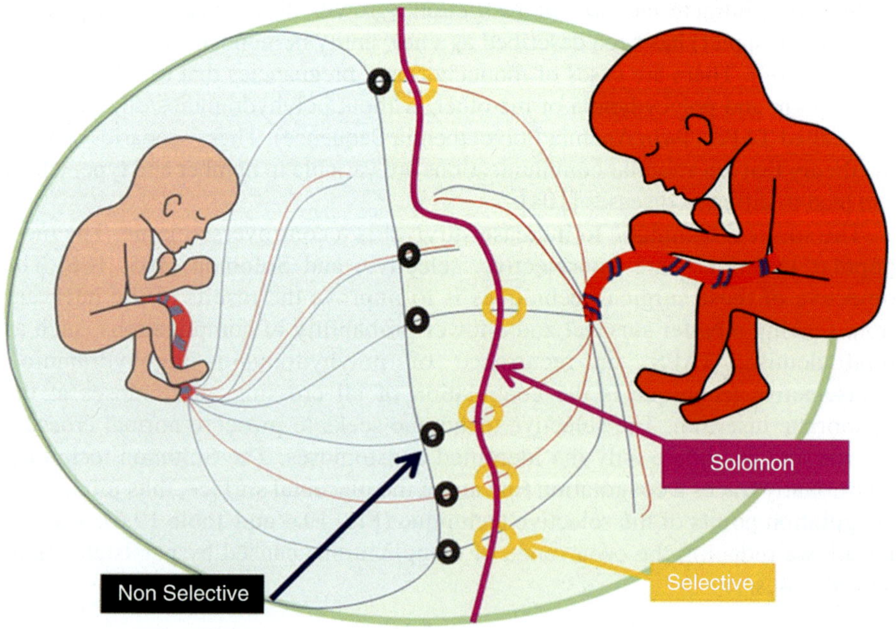

Fig. 19.4 Classical surgical approaches in TTTS

Table 19.6 Studies comparing the Solomon technique with the selective technique. Survival was similar in the only randomized controlled trial

	Solomon	Selective	Significance
Solomon trial (randomized controlled trial)	$n = 139$	$n = 135$	
TAPS	3%	16%	$p < 0.05$
Recurrence	1%	7%	$p < 0.05$
Double survivors	64%	60%	Not significant
One or both alive	87%	85%	Not significant
Ruano (comparative)	$n = 76$	$n = 26$	
TAPS	0%	8%	Not significant
Recurrence	0%	5%	Not significant
Double survivors	84%	46%	$p < 0.01$
One or both alive	88%	77%	Not significant

In the case of complicated monochorionic twins, this surgical technique can be applied to the cord of the affected fetus in order to protect the healthy fetus [109]. Complicated monochorionic twins can be defined differently by the centers. In most centers, pregnancies with severe malformation of one twin or growth restriction using abnormal Doppler have been considered for selective termination. The rationale under this procedure is the high risk of double death in monochorionic twins.

Congenital Diaphragmatic Hernia (CDH).

The prevalence of congenital diaphragmatic hernia is 1–4 per 10,000 births [110]. The defect in the diaphragm can be left-sided in 85% of cases, right in 13%, and bilateral in 2%. CDH can be isolated or associated with other anomalies, with the latter having an adverse prognosis. In its isolated form, CDH causes neonatal death in about 30%, due to respiratory distress associated with the anatomical defect and variable pulmonary hypoplasia. Pulmonary hypoplasia occurs as a result of impaired lung development from the embryonic period. The lung has a smaller size, altered vascularization, and is not able to perform oxygenation despite ventilatory support (Fig. 19.5).

On second trimester ultrasound, 60% of cases are diagnosed. The diagnosis is made by the deviation from the normal position of the thorax due to herniated viscera. Usually, the stomach, liver, or bowel loops can be seen in the thoracic cavity. Complementary exams, such as magnetic resonance imaging (MRI) and genetic studies are commonly performed, aiming to individualize the prognosis and to allow the couple to decide between expectant management or fetal intervention. The associated genetic or chromosomal pathologies are Trisomy 18, Trisomy 13, Trisomy 21, Fryns syndrome, Goldenhar, and Beckwith-Wiedemann, among others.

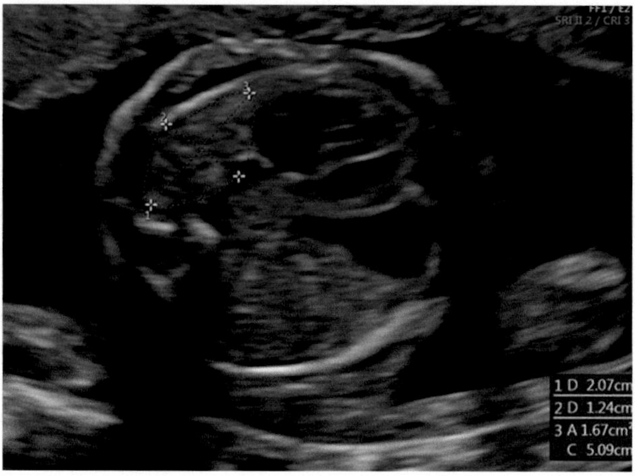

Fig. 19.5 Left CDH. The right lung is measured by longest diameter methods (1D x 2D) and by tracing method (3A). Generally, values obtained by the tracing method is 30% smaller than the longest diameter method

Prenatal Study of the Severity of CDH

Once associated abnormalities are ruled out, prenatal ultrasound is used to establish the severity of pulmonary hypoplasia. Through this, the size of the lung is measured, and the position of the liver is identified, both being predictors of survival. Pulmonary size is the most important factor in neonatal survival in isolated cases. Currently, the best method to quantify it is the head lung index (LHR) [111], which consists of ultrasonic measurement of the lung contralateral to the defect in a 2D transverse image at the level of the cardiac four chamber section. This must be corrected according to the gestational age, expressed as a percentage of what is expected (observed to expected; O/E LHR; calculator available at www.totaltrial.eu). For left diaphragmatic hernias, a contralateral lung size less than 25% O/E LHR has an adverse prognosis, with less than 10% survival, and is considered the indication for surgery. In the case of right hernias, 45% O/E LHR is considered an indictment of fetal surgery before 28 weeks [112].

Fetal Endoluminal Tracheal Occlusion (FETO)

The ability to identify fetuses with adverse prognosis has led to interventions. The tracheal occlusion by positioning a detachable balloon, prevents outflow of the pulmonary fluid that leads to an increase in pulmonary stretching and acceleration of its growth. The first randomized control trial, by open surgery, could not demonstrate the benefit of antenatal intervention [113], but the selection criteria was not appropriate. Fetoscopic occlusion (fetal endoluminal tracheal occlusion; FETO) is performed with local anesthesia for the mother and analgesia and intramuscular immobilization for the fetus. Through a 3.3 mm fetoscope, the uterine cavity and

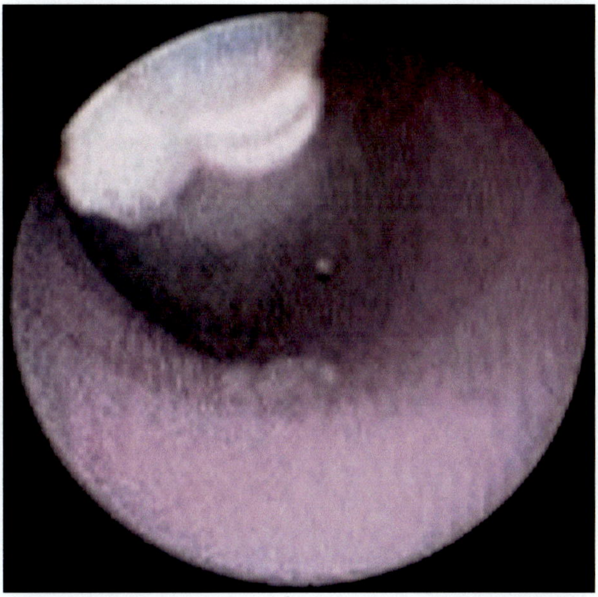

Fig. 19.6 Fetoscopic endotracheal view with the balloon in situ

fetal trachea are accessed, and a latex balloon is positioned under the vocal cords, thus occluding the trachea (Fig. 19.6).

In the report of 210 consecutive cases of severe CDH, this intervention was performed at 26–28 weeks of pregnancy. The most frequent complication was premature delivery as a result of premature rupture of membranes, which occurs within 3 weeks of performing the procedure in 16.7%, requiring hospitalization, antibiotic prophylaxis, and surveillance of signs of infection. The average gestational age at delivery was 35.3 weeks, being one in three deliveries before 34 weeks [114]. FETO needs a retrieval and is ideally performed in utero at 34 weeks by fetoscopy or ultrasound-guided puncture. In cases presenting in with imminent delivery before this date or of technical impossibility for the percutaneous removal of the balloon, it is removed at the time of a cesarean delivery by performing an Ex utero Intrapartum Therapy (EXIT) procedure, keeping the fetus in the placental circulation while the balloon is removed under direct laryngoscopic access. In rare cases, the balloon should be removed by postnatal laryngoscopy. In emergency situations, due to the proximity of the delivery, the withdrawal of the balloon should not be underestimated, since an unprepared or inexperienced team can cause tracheal damage or be unable to withdraw the balloon in time, leading to neonatal death.

FETO increases survival in severe cases of left CDH from 15% to 40%, following the results of the TOTAL trial [116]. The fetal therapy increases prematurity, and retrieval of the device from the fetal trachea needs specialized care. The therapy was effective in reducing the need of ECMO and increasing the survival without oxygen at six months of age. Instead, the moderate cases of left CDH did not show benefits, as survival was increased from 50% to 63%, without statistical significance [117]. Rupture of the membranes remained a main concern.

	Severe			Moderate		
	FETO	Control	RR	FETO	Control	RR
n	40	40		98	98	
Survival	16 (40%)	6(15%)	2.67 (1.22–6.11)	62 (63%)	49 (50%)	1.27 (0.99–1.63)
Surivival w/o oxygen at 6 months	9 (22%)	3(8%)	3 (096–9.76)	53(54%)	43 (44%)	1.23 (0.93–1.65)
Preterm rupture of the membranes (<37 s)	19 (48%)	4(11%)	4.51 (1.83–11.9)	43 (44%)	11 (12%)	3.79 (2.13–6.91)
GA at delivery (mean)	34.6	38.4		35.9	38.1	
Birthweight (meant)	2300	2768		2500	2945	
Need of ECMO	2(5%)	11 (29%)	0.18 (0.05–0.66)	20(21%)	19 (20%)	1.12 (0.97–1.31)

Myelomeningocele (MMC)

Myelomeningocele is a form of spina bifida, with a 10% risk of death in the initial years of life and a great rehabilitation burden in 100% of survivors. In addition to the morbidity and permanent sequelae, it has been reported that the long-term follow-up mortality of these children is 24%. Of the patients alive at 25 years of age, 80% had urinary retention, 30% needed spinal anchor release surgery, 90% needed a peritoneal bypass valve, and 30% developed latex allergy. Despite this, 80% were able to complete full school or university education [115]. Undoubtedly, the disease means a long and difficult road for the patients.

The Management of Meningomyelocele (MOM) Study

An important study published in 2011, the MOM Study Trial, evaluated the benefit of antenatal MMC repair before 26 weeks, compared to traditional surgery performed after birth [9]. Prenatal surgery allowed better reversal of cerebellar herniation and better autonomic gait at 2 years of age compared to postnatal surgery. There are maternal risks against prenatal surgery given that 35% of the cases underwent significant thinning of the uterus and partial or total dehiscence, which means risk of uterine rupture. Uterine rupture is a late complication of open fetal surgery; it can be associated with fetal death, maternal hemorrhage, hysterectomy, and sometimes, maternal death (Table 19.7).

Endoscopic Surgery

The endoscopic technique seeks to replicate the effect of open surgery, with less maternal damage. Endoscopic surgery has been developed by Drs. Kohl (Bonn) [118], Lapa Pedreira (Brazil), and recently by Belfort (Houston) [119, 120] (Fig. 19.7a and b). In the first two centers, the technique is similar. In Houston, it is performed with a laparotomy and with the direct insertion of the endoscopes in the mother's womb (Table 19.8). A recent publication of all groups of fetoscopic closure of myelomeningocele reported similar neurological outcome of that of open surgery, avoiding maternal risks. The reported rate of uterine rupture and dehiscense reach 20% in most reports. Kohl Lapa Pedreira Belfort FETOSCOPY CONSORTIUM

Table 19.7 Main findings of the MOM study that support performing surgery in the fetal period

	Open prenatal repair (MOM)	Postnatal repair	Significance
Number of cases	80	78	
Thinning, dehiscence or uterine rupture	36%	0%	
GA at delivery	34	37	$p < 0.001$
Delivery <30 weeks	13%	0%	
Delivery 30–34 weeks	66%	15%	
Neonatal or fetal demise	2	2	
Causes of demise	Prematurity 26 wks & 23 wks	Severe Chiari malformation	
Ventriculoperitoneal shunt	82%	40%	$p < 0.001$
Complete hindbrain herniation at 1 yr. of life	36%	4%	
Autonomous walk at 2 yrs. of life	42%	21%	$p = 0.01$
Baylor mental developmental index	89.7 ± 14	87.3 ± 18	Not significant

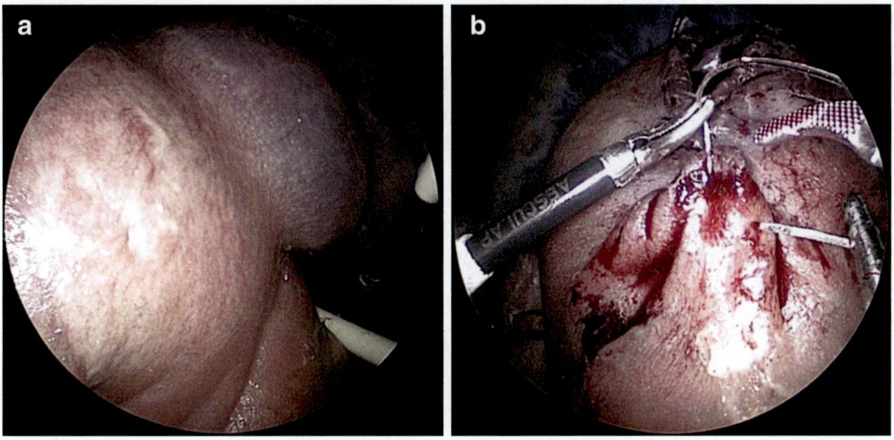

Fig. 19.7 (**a** and **b**) Fetoscopic views of a myelomeningocele repair at GA 26 weeks

Table 19.8 Main findings of the three studies for endoscopic surgery for fetal MMC [121]

	Kohl	Lapa Pedreira	Belfort	Fetoscopy consortium
Published	2014	2016	2017	2021
N	51	10	28	300
Non completed surgeries	0	1	6	15
Completed surgeries	51	9	22	285
GA at surgery	23 (21–29)	27 (25–28)	25 (22–26)	25.9 (22.7–31.6)
Mean operating time (range)	223	242	250	204 (72–458)
Mean GA at delivery	33	32	38	34
Deliveries under 30 weeks	11%	20%	5%	14%
Perinatal deaths	4	2	0	5
Ventriculoperitoneal shunt.	45%	40%	20%	43%

Published 2014 2016 2017 2021 N 51 10 28 300 non completed surgeries 0 1 6 15 Completed surgeries 51 9 22 285 GA at surgery 23 (21-29) 27 (25-28) 25 (22-26) 25.9 (22.7-31.6) Mean operating time (range) 223 242 250 204 (72-458) Mean GA at delivery 33 32 38 34 Deliveries under 30 weeks 11% 20% 5% 14% Perinatal deaths 4 2 0 5 Ventriculoperitoneal shunt. 45% 40% 20% 43% [121]. A recent publication of all groups of fetoscopic closure of myelomeningocele reported similar neurological outcome of that of open surgery, avoiding maternal risks. The reported rate of uterine rupture and dehiscense reach 20% in most reports.

Maternal Risks of Open MMC Repair

Open fetal surgery is a complex procedure, in which the medical risks may expose the mother to intensive care unit, blood transfusion and rarely maternal death. In the MOM trial ($n = 76$), in 25% of the cases, the wall of the uterus was found to be very thin, 9% with partial dehiscence and 1% with complete dehiscence in the index pregnancy. For the following pregnancies, out of 693 patients contacted prospectively, there were 77 subsequent pregnancies, with 10% of uterine rupture and 5% of fetal demise. These uterine ruptures occurred in early third trimester [122]. This suggests that open surgery has risks for both the index as well as any subsequent pregnancies.

Criteria for prenatal MMC repair

- Criteria for case selection (all necessary).
- Myelomeningocele with upper limit in L1 maximum.
- Arnold Chiari II.
- Gestational age <26 weeks.

Contraindication (surgery contraindicated if even one is fulfilled)

- Obesity: BMI >35 at the time of surgery.
- Severe fetal kyphosis.
- Associated fetal malformations.
- Suspicion of aneuploidy. In cases with increased risk, a normal karyotype or normal cfDNA test is considered sufficient to be a candidate.
- Multiple uterine surgeries, myomectomies, two or more previous cesarean sections.
- Suspicion of placenta accreta.
- Risk of premature delivery (cervical length <25 mm at 22 weeks).
- Risk of placental abruption (current bleeding in last 4 weeks, history in previous pregnancy).

Conclusions

Fetal surgery is a relatively new, blossoming field that has changed the long-term prognoses for fetuses with what were previously lethal conditions. Open fetal surgery has also now been shown to alter the natural history in pregnancies complicated by nonlethal conditions such as a myelomeningocele and is capable of improving life-long morbidity. While in utero repair is cutting-edge medicine, it is far from benign and carries serious maternal and fetal risks, both in the short- and long term. Fetal surgery should only be performed on patients who have undergone an exhaustive consent process and demonstrate understanding of the risks of fetal intervention. Open fetal procedures should be carried out by multidisciplinary teams of experts in maternal–fetal medicine, pediatric surgery, obstetric anesthesia, and neonatology in quaternary academic centers. Going forward, the field of fetal surgery is moving toward minimally invasive approaches to the procedures described above. As these techniques are developed, it is vital that the evaluation of the risks and benefits stays are compared to existing therapies in an equally rigorous fashion. Fetoscopy-guided procedures have greatly advanced in quality, instrument adaptations, and clinical applications. The intrauterine environment is more familiar to doctors and the population, being more acceptable and requested. Future indications may broaden the use. For the while, twin-to-twin transfusion syndrome, complicated monochorionic twin pregnancies, severe congenital diaphragmatic hernia, and myelomeningocele repair are the most accepted procedures.

Thorough patient selection and consent processes are essential to ensure that as we move forward, we continue to be guided by both evidence-based medicine and ethical principles to do our best for both patients.

References

1. The CORONIS Collaborative Group. Caesarean section surgical techniques (CORONIS): a fractional, factorial, unmasked, randomised controlled trial. Lancet. 2013;382:234–48.
2. Chervenak FA, McCullough LB, Birnbach DJ. Ethical issues in fetal surgery research. Best Pract Res Clin Anaesthesiol. 2004;18(2):221–30.
3. Senat MV, Deprest J, Boulvain M, et al. Endoscopic laser surgery vs serial amnioreduction for severe twin-to-twin transfusion syndrome. New Engl J Med. 2004;351:136–44.
4. Ville Y, Hyett J, Hecher K, Nicolaides K. Preliminary experience with endoscopic laser surgery for severe twin-twin transfusion syndrome. New Engl J Med. 1995;332:224–7.
5. De Lia J, Kuhlmann R, Harstad T, Cruikshank D. Fetoscopic laser ablation of placental vessels in severe previable twin-twin transfusion syndrome. Am J Obstet Gynecol. 1995;172(4):1202–11.
6. Harrison M, Keller R, Hawgood S, Kitterman J, Sandberg P, Farmer D, et al. A randomized trial of fetal endoscopic tracheal occlusion for severe fetal congenital diaphragmatic hernia. N Engl J Med. 2003;349(20):1916–24.
7. Ruano R, Yoshisaki CT, da Silva MM, Ceccon ME, Grasi MS, Tannuri U, et al. A randomized controlled trial of fetal endoscopic tracheal occlusion versus postnatal management of severe isolated congenital diaphragmatic hernia. Ultrasound Obstet Gynecol. 2012 Jan;39(1):20–7.
8. Bruner JP, Tulipan NE, Richards WO. Endoscopic coverage of fetal open myelomeningocele in utero. Am J Obstet Gynecol. 1997;176:256e7.
9. Adzick NS, Thom EA, Spong CY, et al. A randomized trial of prenatal versus postnatal repair of myelomeningocele. N Engl J Med. 2011;364:993e1004.
10. Goodnight WH, Bahtiyar O, Bennett KA, et al. Subsequent pregnancy outcomes after open maternal-fetal surgery for myelomeningocele. Am J Obstet Gynecol. 2019;220:494.e1–7.
11. Kohl T. Percutaneous minimally invasive fetoscopic surgery for spina bifida aperta. Part I: surgical technique and perioperative outcome. Ultrasound Obstet Gynecol. 2014;44:515–24.
12. Pedreira D, Zanon N, Nishikuni K, Moreira de Sa R, Acacio G, et al. Endoscopic surgery for the antenatal treatment of myelomeningocele: the CECAM trial. Am J Obstet Gynecol. 2016;214:111.e1–11.
13. Belfort M, Whitehead W, Shamshirsaz A, Bateni Z, Olutoye O, Olutoye O, et al. Fetoscopic open neural tube defect repair. Obstet Gynecol. 2017;129:734–43.
14. Sanz Cortes M, Lapa DA, Acacio GL, Belfort M, Carreras E, Maiz N, et al. Proceedings of the first annual meeting of the international Fetoscopic myelomeningocele repair consortium. Ultrasound Obstet Gynecol. 2019;53:855–63.
15. Bienstock J, Bisner M, Coleman F, Hueppchen N. Successful in utero intervention for bilateral renal agenesis. Obstet Gynecol. 2014;124(2):413–5.
16. Johnson A, Luks F. A cautionary note on new fetal interventions. Obstet Gynecol. 2014;124(2):411–2.
17. Jancelewicz T, Harrison M. A history of fetal surgery. Clin Perinatol. 2009;36:227–36.
18. Ville Y. Fetal therapy: practical ethical considerations. Prenat Diagn. 2011;31:621–7.
19. McCullough LB, Chervenak FA. Ethics in obstetrics and gynecology. 1st ed. New York: Oxford University Press; 1994.
20. Giannakoulopoulos X, Sepulveda W, Kourtis P, Glover V, Fisk NM. Fetal plasma cortisol and beta-endorphin response to intrauterine needling. Lancet Lond Engl. 1994;344:77–81.
21. White MC, Wolf AR. Pain and stress in the human fetus. Best Pract Res Clin Anaesthesiol. 2004;18:205–20.
22. Ring LE, Ginosar Y. Anesthesia for fetal surgery and fetal procedures. Clin Perinatol. 2019;46:801–16.
23. Hoagland MA, Chatterjee D. Anesthesia for fetal surgery. Pediatr Anesth. 2017;27:346–57.
24. Lee SJ, Ralston HJP, Drey EA, Partridge JC, Rosen MA. Fetal pain: a systematic multidisciplinary review of the evidence. JAMA. 2005;294:947–54.
25. Ferschl M, Ball R, Lee H, Rollins MD. Anesthesia for in utero repair of myelomeningocele. Anesthesiology. 2013;118:1211–23.

26. Young C, Jevtovic-Todorovic V, Qin Y-Q, Tenkova T, Wang H, Labruyere J, Olney JW. Potential of ketamine and midazolam, individually or in combination, to induce apoptotic neurodegeneration in the infant mouse brain. Br J Pharmacol. 2005;146:189–97.
27. Jevtovic-Todorovic V, Hartman RE, Izumi Y, Benshoff ND, Dikranian K, Zorumski CF, Olney JW, Wozniak DF. Early exposure to common anesthetic agents causes widespread neurodegeneration in the developing rat brain and persistent learning deficits. J Neurosci. 2003;23:876–82.
28. Shan Y, Yang F, Tang Z, Bi C, Sun S, Zhang Y, Liu H. Dexmedetomidine ameliorates the neurotoxicity of sevoflurane on the immature brain through the BMP/SMAD signaling pathway. Front Neurosci. 2018; https://doi.org/10.3389/fnins.2018.00964.
29. Rychik J. Fetal cardiovascular physiology. Pediatr Cardiol. 2004;25:201–9.
30. Vasconcelos RP, Brazil Frota Aragão JR, Costa Carvalho FH, Salani Mota RM, de Lucena Feitosa FE, Alencar Júnior CA. Differences in neonatal outcome in fetuses with absent versus reverse end-diastolic flow in umbilical artery Doppler. Fetal Diagn Ther. 2010;28:160–6.
31. Goodnight WH, Bahtiyar O, Bennett KA, et al. Subsequent pregnancy outcomes after open maternal-fetal surgery for myelomeningocele. Am J Obstet Gynecol. 2019;220:494.e1–7.
32. Amberg BJ, Hodges RJ, Kashyap AJ, Skinner SM, Rodgers KA, McGillick EV, Deprest JA, Hooper SB, Crossley KJ, DeKoninck PLJ. Physiological effects of partial amniotic carbon dioxide insufflation with cold, dry vs heated, humidified gas in a sheep model. Ultrasound Obstet Gynecol Off J Int Soc Ultrasound Obstet Gynecol. 2019;53:340–7.
33. Mavi J. Anesthesia for fetal intervention and surgery. In: Anesthesiol. Approach: Pract; 2018. p. 287–91.
34. van de Velde M, Buck FD. Fetal and maternal analgesia/anesthesia for fetal procedures. Fetal Diagn Ther. 2012;31:201–9.
35. Ferschl MB, Feiner J, Vu L, Smith D, Rollins MD. A comparison of spinal anesthesia versus monitored anesthesia care with local anesthesia in minimally invasive fetal surgery. Anesth Analg. 2020;130:409–15.
36. Olutoye OA, Baker BW, Belfort MA, Olutoye OO. Food and Drug Administration warning on anesthesia and brain development: implications for obstetric and fetal surgery. Am J Obstet Gynecol. 2018;218:98–102.
37. Van de Velde M, Van Schoubroeck D, Lewi LE, Marcus MAE, Jani JC, Missant C, Teunkens A, Deprest JA. Remifentanil for fetal immobilization and maternal sedation during fetoscopic surgery: a randomized, double-blind comparison with diazepam. Anesth Analg. 2005;101:251–8, table of contents.
38. Manrique S, Maiz N, García I, et al. Maternal anaesthesia in open and fetoscopic surgery of foetal open spinal neural tube defects: a retrospective cohort study. Eur J Anaesthesiol EJA. 2019;36:175–84.
39. Saxena KN. Anaesthesia for fetal surgeries. Indian J Anaesth. 2009;53:554.
40. De Braga AFA, Rousselet MS, Zambelli H, Sbragia L, Barini R. Anesthesia for intrauterine myelomeningocele correction: case report. Rev Bras Anestesiol. 2005;55:329–35.
41. Fan SZ, Huang FY, Lin SY, Wang YP, Hsieh FJ. Intrauterine neuromuscular blockade in fetus. Ma Zui Xue Za Zhi Anaesthesiol Sin. 1990;28:31–4.
42. Watson WJ, Atchison SR, Harlass FE. Comparison of pancuronium and vecuronium for fetal neuromuscular blockade during invasive procedures. J Matern Fetal Med. 1996;5:151–4.
43. Dailey PA, Fisher DM, Shnider SM, Baysinger CL, Shinohara Y, Miller RD, Abboud TK, Kim KC. Pharmacokinetics, placental transfer, and neonatal effects of vecuronium and pancuronium administered during cesarean section. Anesthesiology. 1984;60:569–74.
44. Adzick NS. Open fetal surgery for life-threatening fetal anomalies. Semin Fetal Neonatal Med. 2010;15(1):1–8. https://doi.org/10.1016/j.siny.2009.05.003.
45. Adzick NS. Fetal myelomeningocele: Natural history, pathophysiology, and in-utero intervention. 2010;15(1):9–14. https://doi.org/10.1016/j.siny.2009.05.002.
46. Oakeshott P, Hunt GM. Long-term outcome in open spina bifida. Br J Gen Pract. 2003;53(493):632–6.
47. Shin M, Besser LM, Siffel C, Kucik JE, Shaw GM, Lu C, Correa A. Prevalence of Spina bifida among children and adolescents in 10 regions in the United States. 2010;126(2):274–9. https://doi.org/10.1542/peds.2009-2084.

48. Hutchins GM, Meuli M, Meuli-Simmen C, Jordan MA, Heffez DS, Blakemore KJ. Acquired spinal cord injury in human fetuses with myelomeningocele. Pediatr Pathol Lab Med. 1996;16(5):701–12.
49. Meuli M, Meuli-Simmen C, Hutchins GM, Seller MJ, Harrison MR, Adzick NS. The spinal cord lesion in human fetuses with myelomeningocele: Implications for fetal surgery. 1997;32(3):448–52. https://doi.org/10.1016/s0022-3468(97)90603-5.
50. Kabagambe SK, Jensen GW, Chen YJ, Vanover MA, Farmer DL. Fetal surgery for myelomeningocele: a systematic review and Meta-analysis of outcomes in Fetoscopic versus open repair. Fetal Diagn Ther. 2018;43(3):161–74. https://doi.org/10.1159/000479505.
51. Adzick NS, Sutton LN, Crombleholme TM, Flake AW. Successful fetal surgery for spina bifida. Lancet. 1998;352(9141):1675–6. https://doi.org/10.1016/s0140-6736(98)00070-1.
52. Sutton LN, Adzick NS, Bilaniuk LT, Johnson MP, Crombleholme TM, Flake AW. Improvement in hindbrain herniation demonstrated by serial fetal magnetic resonance imaging following fetal surgery for myelomeningocele. JAMA. 1999;282(19):1826–31. https://doi.org/10.1001/jama.282.19.1826.
53. Johnson MP, Sutton LN, Rintoul N, Crombleholme TM, Flake AW, Howell LJ, Hedrick HL, Wilson RD, Adzick NS. Fetal myelomeningocele repair: short-term clinical outcomes. Am J Obstet Gynecol. 2003;189(2):482–7. https://doi.org/10.1067/S0002-9378(03)00295-3.
54. Johnson MP, Gerdes M, Rintoul N, Pasquariello P, Melchionni J, Sutton LN, Adzick NS. Maternal-fetal surgery for myelomeningocele: neurodevelopmental outcomes at 2 years of age. Am J Obstet Gynecol. 2006;194(4):1145–50. https://doi.org/10.1016/j.ajog.2006.01.072.
55. Danzer E, Johnson MP, Bebbington M, Simon EM, Wilson RD, Bilaniuk LT, Sutton LN, Adzick NS. Fetal head biometry assessed by fetal magnetic resonance imaging following in utero myelomeningocele repair. Fetal Diagn Ther. 2007;22(1):1–6. https://doi.org/10.1159/000095833.
56. Danzer E, Finkel RS, Rintoul NE, Bebbington MW, Schwartz ES, Zarnow DM, Adzick NS, Johnson MP. Reversal of hindbrain herniation after maternal-fetal surgery for myelomeningocele subsequently impacts on brain stem function. Neuropediatrics. 2008;39(6):359–62. https://doi.org/10.1055/s-0029-1202835.
57. Danzer E, Flake AW. In utero repair of myelomeningocele: rationale, initial clinical experience and a randomized controlled prospective clinical trial. Neuroembryology Aging. 2008;4(4):165–74. https://doi.org/10.1159/000118926.
58. Danzer E, Gerdes M, Bebbington MW, Zarnow DM, Adzick NS, Johnson MP. Preschool neurodevelopmental outcome of children following fetal myelomeningocele closure. Am J Obstet Gynecol. 2010;202(5):450.e451–9. https://doi.org/10.1016/j.ajog.2010.02.014.
59. Danzer E, Gerdes M, Bebbington MW, Koh J, Adzick SN, Johnson MP. Fetal myelomeningocele surgery: preschool functional status using the functional Independence measure for children (WeeFIM). Childs Nerv Syst. 2011;27(7):1083–8. https://doi.org/10.1007/s00381-011-1388-y.
60. Houtrow AJ, Burrows PK, Thom EA. Comparing neurodevelopmental outcomes at 30 months by presence of hydrocephalus and shunt status among children enrolled in the MOMS trial. J Pediatr Rehabil Med. 2018;11(4):227–35. https://doi.org/10.3233/prm-170481.
61. Houtrow AJ, Thom EA, Fletcher JM, Burrows PK, Adzick NS, Thomas NH, Brock JW, Cooper T, Lee H, Bilaniuk L, Glenn OA, Pruthi S, MacPherson C, Farmer DL, Johnson MP, Howell LJ, Gupta N, Walker WO. Prenatal repair of myelomeningocele and school-age functional outcomes. Pediatrics. 2020;145(2):e20191544. https://doi.org/10.1542/peds.2019-1544.
62. Johnson MP, Bennett KA, Rand L, Burrows PK, Thom EA, Howell LJ, Farrell JA, Dabrowiak ME, Brock JW, Farmer DL, Adzick NS. The management of myelomeningocele study: obstetrical outcomes and risk factors for obstetrical complications following prenatal surgery. Am J Obstet Gynecol. 2016;215(6):778.e771–9. https://doi.org/10.1016/j.ajog.2016.07.052.

63. Farmer DL, Thom EA, Brock JW, Burrows PK, Johnson MP, Howell LJ, Farrell JA, Gupta N, Adzick NS. The management of myelomeningocele study: full cohort 30-month pediatric outcomes. Am J Obstet Gynecol.2018:218(2); 256.e251–13. https://doi.org/10.1016/j.ajog.2017.12.001.
64. Moldenhauer JS, Soni S, Rintoul NE, Spinner SS, Khalek N, Martinez-Poyer J, Flake AW, Hedrick HL, Peranteau WH, Rendon N, Koh J, Howell LJ, Heuer GG, Sutton LN, Johnson MP, Adzick NS. Fetal myelomeningocele repair: the post-MOMS experience at the Children's Hospital of Philadelphia. Fetal Diagn Ther. 2015;37(3):235–40. https://doi.org/10.1159/000365353.
65. Moldenhauer JS, Adzick NS. Fetal surgery for myelomeningocele: after the Management of Myelomeningocele Study (MOMS). Semin Fetal Neonatal Med. 2017;22(6):360–6. https://doi.org/10.1016/j.siny.2017.08.004.
66. Heuer GG, Moldenhauer JS, Scott Adzick N. Prenatal surgery for myelomeningocele: review of the literature and future directions. Childs Nerv Syst. 2017;33(7):1149–55. https://doi.org/10.1007/s00381-017-3440-z.
67. Committee Opinion No. 720: maternal-fetal surgery for myelomeningocele. Obstet Gynecol. 2017:130(3);e164–7. https://doi.org/10.1097/aog.0000000000002303.
68. Hilton SA, Hodges MM, Dewberry LC, Handler M, Galan HL, Zaretsky MV, Behrendt N, Marwan AI, Liechty KW. MOMS plus: single-institution review of outcomes for extended BMI criteria for open fetal repair of myelomeningocele. Fetal Diagn Ther. 2019;46(6):411–4. https://doi.org/10.1159/000499484.
69. Joyeux L, De Bie F, Danzer E, Russo FM, Javaux A, Peralta CFA, De Salles AAF, Pastuszka A, Olejek A, Van Mieghem T, De Coppi P, Moldenhauer J, Whitehead WE, Belfort MA, Lapa DA, Acacio GL, Devlieger R, Hirose S, Farmer DL, Van Calenbergh F, Adzick NS, Johnson MP, Deprest J. Learning curves of open and endoscopic fetal spina bifida closure: a systematic review and meta-analysis. Ultrasound Obstet Gynecol. 2019. https://doi.org/10.1002/uog.20389.
70. Swamy R, Embleton N, Hale J. Sacrococcygeal teratoma over two decades: birth prevalence, prenatal diagnosis and clinical outcomes. Prenat Diagn. 2008;28(11):1048–51. https://doi.org/10.1002/pd.2122.
71. Lakhoo K. Neonatal teratomas. Early Hum Dev. 2010;86(10):643–7. https://doi.org/10.1016/j.earlhumdev.2010.08.016.
72. Peiró JL, Sbragia L, Scorletti F, Lim FY, Shaaban A. Management of fetal teratomas. 2016;32(7):635–47. https://doi.org/10.1007/s00383-016-3892-3.
73. Rescorla FJ, Sawin RS, Coran AG, Dillon PW, Azizkhan RG. Long-term outcome for infants and children with sacrococcygeal teratoma: a report from the childrens cancer group. J Pediatr Surg. 1998;33(2):171–6. https://doi.org/10.1016/s0022-3468(98)90426-2.
74. Peter Altman R, Randolph JG, Lilly JR. Sacrococcygeal teratoma: American Academy of Pediatrics surgical section survey—1973. J Pediatr Surg. 1974;9(3):389–98. https://doi.org/10.1016/s0022-3468(74)80297-6.
75. Wilson RD, Hedrick H, Flake AW, Johnson MP, Bebbington MW, Mann S, Rychik J, Liechty K, Adzick NS. Sacrococcygeal teratomas: prenatal surveillance, growth and pregnancy outcome. Fetal Diagnosis Therapy. 2009;25(1):15–20. https://doi.org/10.1159/000188056.
76. Shue E, Bolouri M, Jelin EB, Vu L, Bratton B, Cedars E, Yoke L, Byrne F, Hirose S, Feldstein V, Miniati D, Lee H. Tumor metrics and morphology predict poor prognosis in prenatally diagnosed sacrococcygeal teratoma: a 25-year experience at a single institution. 2013;48(6):1225–31. https://doi.org/10.1016/j.jpedsurg.2013.03.016.
77. Akinkuotu AC, Coleman A, Shue E, Sheikh F, Hirose S, Lim F-Y, Olutoye OO. Predictors of poor prognosis in prenatally diagnosed sacrococcygeal teratoma: a multiinstitutional review. J Pediatr Surg. 2015;50(5):771–4. https://doi.org/10.1016/j.jpedsurg.2015.02.034.
78. Sy ED, Filly RA, Cheong ML, Clifton MS, Cortes RA, Ohashi S, Takifuji K, Ventura DE, Grethel EJ, Wagner AJ, Gress EA, Ball RH, Lee H, Harrison MR. Prognostic role of tumor-

head volume ratio in fetal Sacrococcygeal Teratoma. Fetal Diagn Ther. 2009;26(2):75–80. https://doi.org/10.1159/000238113.
79. Roybal JL, Moldenhauer JS, Khalek N, Bebbington MW, Johnson MP, Hedrick HL, Adzick NS, Flake AW. Early delivery as an alternative management strategy for selected high-risk fetal sacrococcygeal teratomas. J Pediatr Surg. 2011;46(7):1325–32. https://doi.org/10.1016/j.jpedsurg.2010.10.020.
80. Van Mieghem T, Al-Ibrahim A, Deprest J, Lewi L, Langer JC, Baud D, O'Brien K, Beecroft R, Chaturvedi R, Jaeggi E, Fish J, Ryan G. Minimally invasive therapy for fetal sacrococcygeal teratoma: case series and systematic review of the literature. Ultrasound Obstet Gynecol. 2014;43(6):611–9. https://doi.org/10.1002/uog.13315.
81. Khalek N, Johnson MP. Management of prenatally diagnosed lung lesions. Semin Pediatr Surg. 2013;22(1):24–9. https://doi.org/10.1053/j.sempedsurg.2012.10.005.
82. Swarr DT, Peranteau WH, Pogoriler J, Frank DB, Adzick NS, Hedrick HL, Morley M, Zhou S, Morrisey EE. Novel molecular and phenotypic insights into congenital lung malformations. Am J Respir Crit Care Med. 2018;197(10):1328–39. https://doi.org/10.1164/rccm.201706-1243oc.
83. Azizkhan RG, Crombleholme TM. Congenital cystic lung disease: contemporary antenatal and postnatal management. Pediatr Surg Int. 2008;24(6):643–57. https://doi.org/10.1007/s00383-008-2139-3.
84. Adzick NS. Management of fetal lung lesions. Clin Perinatol. 2009:36(2);363–76, x. https://doi.org/10.1016/j.clp.2009.03.001.
85. Adzick NS, Harrison MR, Crombleholme TM, Flake AW, Howell LJ. Fetal lung lesions: management and outcome. Am J Obstet Gynecol. 1998;179(4):884–9. https://doi.org/10.1016/s0002-9378(98)70183-8.
86. Kunisaki SM, Fauza DO, Barnewolt CE, Estroff JA, Myers LB, Bulich LA, Wong G, Levine D, Wilkins-Haug LE, Benson CB, Jennings RW. Ex utero intrapartum treatment with placement on extracorporeal membrane oxygenation for fetal thoracic masses. 2007:42(2);420–5. https://doi.org/10.1016/j.jpedsurg.2006.10.035.
87. Cavoretto P, Molina F, Poggi S, Davenport M, Nicolaides KH. Prenatal diagnosis and outcome of echogenic fetal lung lesions. Ultrasound Obstet Gynecol. 2008;32(6):769–83. https://doi.org/10.1002/uog.6218.
88. Hellmund A, Berg C, Geipel A, Bludau M, Heydweiller A, Bachour H, Müller A, Müller A, Gembruch U. Prenatal diagnosis and evaluation of sonographic predictors for intervention and adverse outcome in congenital pulmonary airway malformation. PLoS One. 2016;11(3):e0150474. https://doi.org/10.1371/journal.pone.0150474.
89. Costanzo S, Flisetti C, Vella C, Rustico M, Fontana P, Lista G, Zirpoli S, Napolitano M, Riccipetitoni G. Pulmonary malformations: predictors of neonatal respiratory distress and early surgery. J Neonatal Surg. 2016;5(3):27. https://doi.org/10.21699/jns.v5i3.375.
90. Curran PF, Jelin EB, Rand L, Hirose S, Feldstein VA, Goldstein RB, Lee H. Prenatal steroids for microcystic congenital cystic adenomatoid malformations. J Pediatr Surg. 2010;45(1):145–50. https://doi.org/10.1016/j.jpedsurg.2009.10.025.
91. Derderian SC, Coleman AM, Jeanty C, Lim FY, Shaaban AM, Farrell JA, Hirose S, Mackenzie TC, Lee H. Favorable outcomes in high-risk congenital pulmonary airway malformations treated with multiple courses of maternal betamethasone. J Pediatr Surg. 2015;50(4):515–8. https://doi.org/10.1016/j.jpedsurg.2014.08.019.
92. Peranteau WH, Boelig MM, Khalek N, Moldenhauer JS, Martinez-Poyer J, Hedrick HL, Flake AW, Johnson MP, Adzick NS. Effect of single and multiple courses of maternal betamethasone on prenatal congenital lung lesion growth and fetal survival. J Pediatr Surg. 2016;51(1):28–32. https://doi.org/10.1016/j.jpedsurg.2015.10.018.
93. Mann, S., Wilson, R.D., Bebbington, M.W., Adzick, N.S., Johnson, M.P.: Antenatal diagnosis and management of congenital cystic adenomatoid malformation. 12(6), 477–481 (2007). doi:https://doi.org/10.1016/j.siny.2007.06.009
94. Wilson RD. In utero therapy for fetal thoracic abnormalities. Prenat Diagn. 2008;28(7):619–25. https://doi.org/10.1002/pd.1968.

95. Peranteau, W.H., Scott Adzick, N., Boelig, M.M., Alan W, F., Hedrick, H.L., Howell, L.J., Moldenhauer, J.S., Khalek, N., Martinez-Poyer, J., Johnson, M.P.: Thoracoamniotic shunts for the management of fetal lung lesions and pleural effusions: a single-institution review and predictors of survival in 75 cases. 50(2), 301–305 (2015). doi:https://doi.org/10.1016/j.jpedsurg.2014.11.019
96. Hedrick, H.L., Flake, A.W., Crombleholme, T.M., Howell, L.J., Johnson, M.P., Wilson, R.D., Adzick, N.S.: The ex utero intrapartum therapy procedure for high-risk fetal lung lesions. 40(6), 1038–1044 (2005). doi:https://doi.org/10.1016/j.jpedsurg.2005.03.024
97. Liechty KW. Ex-utero intrapartum therapy. Semin Fetal Neonatal Med. 2010;15(1):34–9. https://doi.org/10.1016/j.siny.2009.05.007.
98. Westin B. HYSTEROSCOPY IN EARLY PREGNANCY. Lancet. 1954;264:872.
99. Ville Y, Hyett J, Hecher K, Nicolaides K (2009) Preliminary Experience with Endoscopic Laser Surgery for Severe Twin–Twin Transfusion Syndrome. http://dx.doi.org/101056/NEJM199501263320404. https://doi.org/10.1056/NEJM199501263320404.
100. Lia JDD, Kuhlmann RS, Harstad TW, Cruikshank DP. Fetoscopic laser ablation of placental vessels in severe previable twin-twin transfusion syndrome. Am J Obstet Gynecol. 1995;172:1202–11.
101. Senat M-V, Deprest J, Boulvain M, Paupe A, Winer N, Ville Y. Endoscopic laser surgery versus serial Amnioreduction for severe twin-to-twin transfusion syndrome. N Engl J Med. 2004;351:136–44.
102. Quintero RA, Morales WJ, Allen MH, Bornick PW, Johnson PK, Kruger M. Staging of twin-twin transfusion syndrome. J Perinatol. 1999;19:550–5.
103. Gratacós E, Lewi L, Muñoz B, Acosta-Rojas R, Hernandez-Andrade E, Martinez JM, Carreras E, Deprest J. A classification system for selective intrauterine growth restriction in monochorionic pregnancies according to umbilical artery Doppler flow in the smaller twin. Ultrasound Obstet Gynecol. 2007;30:28–34.
104. Sananès N, Veujoz M, Severac F, et al. Evaluation of the utility of in utero treatment of twin Anemia-polycythemia sequence. Fetal Diagn Ther. 2015;38:170–8.
105. Slaghekke F, Lopriore E, Lewi L, et al. Fetoscopic laser coagulation of the vascular equator versus selective coagulation for twin-to-twin transfusion syndrome: an open-label randomised controlled trial. Lancet. 2014;383:2144–51.
106. Ruano R, Rodo C, Peiro JL, et al. Fetoscopic laser ablation of placental anastomoses in twin–twin transfusion syndrome using 'Solomon technique. Ultrasound Obstet Gynecol. 2013;42:434–9.
107. Yamamoto M, Barki G, Ville Y. Direct visual control on cord coagulation using a fetoscopy-guided bipolar forceps. Description of a new technique. Prenat Diagn. 2010;30:156–8.
108. Hecher K, Lewi L, Gratacos E, Huber A, Ville Y, Deprest J. Twin reversed arterial perfusion: fetoscopic laser coagulation of placental anastomoses or the umbilical cord. Ultrasound Obstet Gynecol. 2006;28:688–91.
109. Rossi AC, D'Addario V. Umbilical cord occlusion for selective feticide in complicated monochorionic twins: a systematic review of literature. Am J Obstet Gynecol. 2009;200:123–9.
110. Kotecha S, Barbato A, Bush A, et al. Congenital diaphragmatic hernia. Eur Respir J. 2012;39:820–9.
111. Metkus AP, Filly RA, Stringer MD, Harrison MR, Adzick NS. Sonographic predictors of survival in fetal diaphragmatic hernia. J Pediatr Surg. 1996;31:148–51. discussion 151-152
112. Jani J, Nicolaides KH, Keller RL, et al. Observed to expected lung area to head circumference ratio in the prediction of survival in fetuses with isolated diaphragmatic hernia. Ultrasound Obstet Gynecol Off J Int Soc Ultrasound Obstet Gynecol. 2007;30:67–71.
113. Harrison MR, Keller RL, Hawgood SB, Kitterman JA, Sandberg PL, Farmer DL, Lee H, Filly RA, Farrell JA, Albanese CT. A randomized trial of fetal endoscopic tracheal occlusion for severe fetal congenital diaphragmatic hernia. N Engl J Med. 2003;349:1916–24.
114. Jani JC, Nicolaides KH, Gratacós E, Valencia CM, Doné E, Martinez J-M, Gucciardo L, Cruz R, Deprest JA. Severe diaphragmatic hernia treated by fetal endoscopic tracheal occlusion. Ultrasound Obstet Gynecol. 2009;34:304–10.

115. Bowman RM, McLone DG, Grant JA, Tomita T, Ito JA. Spina bifida outcome: a 25-year prospective. Pediatr Neurosurg. 2001;34:114–20.
116. Deprest JA, Nicolaides KH, Benachi A, Gratacos E, Ryan G, Persico N. et al. Randomized Trial of Fetal Surgery for Severe Left Diaphragmatic HerniaN Engl J Med 2021;385:107-118. https://doi.org/10.1056/NEJMoa2027030.
117. Deprest JA, Benachi A, Gratacos E, Nicolaides KH, Berg C, Persico N et al. Randomized Trial of Fetal Surgery for Moderate Left Diaphragmatic Hernia. N Engl J Med 2021;385:119-129. https://doi.org/10.1056/NEJMoa2026983.
118. Kohl T. Percutaneous minimally invasive fetoscopic surgery for spina bifida aperta. Part I: surgical technique and perioperative outcome. Ultrasound Obstet Gynecol. 2014;44:515–24.
119. Pedreira DAL, Zanon N, Nishikuni K, de Sá RAM, Acacio GL, Chmait RH, Kontopoulos EV, Quintero RA. Endoscopic surgery for the antenatal treatment of myelomeningocele: the CECAM trial. Am J Obstet Gynecol. 2016;214:111.e1–111.e11.
120. Belfort M, Whitehead W, Shamshirsaz A, et al. Fetoscopic open neural tube defect repair: development and refinement of a two-port, carbon dioxide insufflation technique. Obstet Gynecol. 2017;129:734–43.
121. Sanz cortes M, Chmait RH, Lapa DA, Belfort MA, Carreras E, Miller JL et al. Experience of 300 cases of prenatal fetoscopic open spina bifida repair: Report of the International Fetoscopic Neural Tube Defect Repair Consortium., American Journal of Obstetrics and Gynecology (2021), https://doi.org/10.1016/j.ajog.2021.05.044.
122. Goodnight WH, Bahtiyar O, Bennett KA, et al. Subsequent pregnancy outcomes after open maternal-fetal surgery for myelomeningocele. Am J Obstet Gynecol. 2019;220:494.e1–7.

Part IV
Clinical Complications in Pregnancy: Diagnosis and Management

Chapter 20
Anemia in Pregnancy

Camila Luiza Meira Pucci and Lisandra Stein Bernardes

Definition

Anemia is defined by decreased concentration of erythrocytes or hemoglobin in the blood, below the level needed to maintain the physiological activities [16]. In pregnancy, it is characterized when the hemoglobin (Hgb) and hematocrit (Hct) are below the fifth percentile of a reference population of healthy pregnant women using iron supplementation, as recommended by the Centers for Disease Control and Prevention (CDC): Hgb (g/dL) and Hct (percentage) below 11 g/dL and 33%, respectively, in the first and third trimester; and below 10.5 g/dL and 32%, respectively, in the second trimester [2, 7].

Physiological Changes in Pregnancy

The normal values of hemoglobin and hematocrit are reduced in pregnancy when compared to nonpregnant female population due to physiologic volume expansion. This expansion has the function of supplying the increased metabolic demand of the uterine vascular system, providing nutrients and elements to the placenta and fetus,

C. L. M. Pucci (✉)
Department of Obstetrics and Gynecology, University of São Paulo, São Paulo, Brazil

Sepaco Hospital, São Paulo, Brazil

L. S. Bernardes
Department of Obstetrics and Gynecology, University of São Paulo, São Paulo, Brazil

Sepaco Hospital, São Paulo, Brazil

School of Medicine, Faculdade Israelita de Ciências da Saúde Albert Einstein, São Paulo, Brazil

© Springer Nature Switzerland AG 2022
R. A. Moreira de Sá, E. B. d. Fonseca (eds.), *Perinatology*,
https://doi.org/10.1007/978-3-030-83434-0_20

and protecting against the adverse effects of blood loss associated with childbirth. Blood volume begins to increase in the first trimester and occurs more intensely in the second trimester [7]. After 32–34 weeks of gestation, the volemia is increased by 40–45% the prenatal volume [17, 23]. Although the volume of erythrocytes increases considerably—about 450 mL [18]—the plasma increase is proportionally greater, resulting in hemodilution, which is reflected by a decrease in hemoglobin and hematocrit levels.

Since the production of erythrocytes is increased, there is also increased demand for elements required in its production such as iron and folic acid. The total iron content in adult women is about 2300 mg [2]. About 70% is found in hemoglobin and the remaining is present in the form of deposits, such as ferritin and hemosiderin [24]. A normal pregnancy requires approximately 1000 mg of additional iron, 300 mg for the fetus and placenta, 500 mg for erythrocyte expansion, and 200 mg that are eliminated through the intestine, urine, and skin [7]. The amount of iron ingested in the diet added to the iron mobilized from the reserves is not enough to cover this demand in the vast majority of pregnant women, especially in the second half of pregnancy [19]. The need for folic acid increases from 50 μg/day in nonpregnant women, to 400 μg/day during pregnancy [2].

Causes and Classification

Anemia can be classified by its pathophysiological mechanism, by the morphology of erythrocytes, and also by being hereditary or acquired.

(a) Pathophysiology: anemia can result from decreased red blood cell production, increased destruction, or blood loss [2], as shown in Table 20.1. Erythropoiesis can be impaired by the lack of elements necessary for the production of red blood cells, such as iron, folate, and vitamin B12, either by deficient intake or by malabsorption in the gastrointestinal tract. In addition, the lack or changes in hematopoietic tissue will also result in decreased production, as it occurs in bone marrow aplasias and in primary or secondary hematological neoplasms (metastases). Lack of stimulating factor, erythropoietin, is what leads to anemia in chronic kidney disease. Premature destruction of red blood cells in the periphery, or hemolysis, can occur due to intrinsic changes of the red cell or by extrinsic factors. Sickle cell anemia, thalassemia, hereditary spherocytosis, and sideroblastic anemia, as well as deficiencies in erythrocyte enzymes and nocturnal paroxysmal hemoglobinuria are pathologies that culminate in hemolysis due to a defect in the erythrocyte itself. Extrinsic factors that cause hemolysis are drugs, poisons and toxins, antibodies (autoimmune hemolysis), and microangiopathies. Anemia secondary to blood loss can occur in both acute and chronic bleeding.

(b) Morphology of erythrocytes: the morphology of erythrocytes also allows reasoning about the cause of anemia (see Table 20.2). Macrocytic anemias are

Table 20.1 Anemias classified based on pathophysiologic mechanism

Pathophysiologic classification		
Decreased red blood cell production (not increased reticulocytes)	Lack of essential elements in the production of red blood cells	Iron deficiency anemia
		B12 deficiency anemia (megaloblastic anemia)
		Folic acid deficiency anemia (megaloblastic anemia)
	Lack of hematopoietic tissue	Aplastic anemia
		Secondary (drugs, radiation, infection, bacterial toxins)
		Neoplasms (hematological or metastatic)
		Idiopathic
	Lack of stimulating factor (erytropoiethin)	Chronic kidney disease
Increased red blood cell destruction (increased reticulocytes)	Intrinsic changes of the red blood cell	Hemoglobinopathies: sickle cell anemia, thalassemias
		Sideroblastic anemia
		Paroxysmal nocturnal hemoglobinuria
		Membrane defects: hereditary spherocytosis
		Enzymatic defects
	Extrinsic factors	Autoimunne hemolytic anemia
		Microangiophathies
		Drugs, poison, toxins
Blood loss	Acute blood loss	
	Chronic blood loss	

those in which the mean corpuscular volume (MCV) is greater than 100 fL, and microcytic when the MCV is less than 80 fL. If the MCV is between 80 and 100 fL, anemia is considered normocytic. In the group of microcytic anemias are iron deficiency anemia, thalassemias, hereditary sideroblastic anemia, and long-standing chronic disease anemias—the first one presents reduced iron stores and anisocytosis (increased RDW). The classic example of macrocytic anemias is megaloblastic anemia, due to a lack of vitamin B12 and/or folate, which have the highest MCV values, between 110 and 140 fL. The other macrocytic anemias have MCV values usually between 100 and 110 fL and include aplastic anemia, myelodysplastic syndromes (including acquired sideroblastic anemia), anemia of alcoholism, as well as those in which there is peripheral destruction or loss of blood cells and bone marrow hyperproliferation in response, which is the case of hereditary (with the exception of thalassemias) and acquired hemolytic anemias, and anemia due to acute hemorrhage. Bone marrow hyperproliferation causes the immediate precursor of red blood cells, the reticulocyte, to be released into the bloodstream, which is larger in size. The causes of normocytic anemia are diverse: anemia of chronic disease, anemia of

Table 20.2 Anemias classified based on erythrocytes morphology

Morphologic classification		
Hypochromic/microcytic	Decreased iron stocks	Iron deficiency anemia
	Normal or increased iron stocks	Thalassemias
		Anemia of chronic disease
		Hereditary sideroblastic anemia
Normochromic/normocytic	Increased reticulocytes	Hemolytic anemia
		Acute bleeding anemia
	Not increased reticulocytes	Anemia of chronic disease
		Anemia of chronic kidney disease
		Anemia of endocrinopathies
		Early iron deficiency anemia
		Aplastic anemia
		Myelodysplastic syndromes
Macrocytic	Increased reticulocytes	Hemolytic anemia
		Acute bleeding anemia
	Not increased reticulocytes	Megaloblastic anemia
		Aplastic anemia
		Anemia of alcoholism
		Anemia of liver disease
		Acute myelodysplastic syndromes

chronic kidney disease, anemia of endocrinopathies (hypothyroidism and hypopituitarism), iron deficiency anemia in the initial stage, aplastic anemia, myelodysplastic syndromes, hemolytic anemias, hemorrhage anemia, among others. It is worth mentioning that normocytic anemias include conditions that will become microcytic or macrocytic anemias as the disease progresses.

Prevalence and Etiology

North American population studies estimate a prevalence of approximately 21% of anemia during pregnancy [3, 22], the most common cause being iron deficiency, occurring in 16% of pregnant women [22]. It is estimated that in low-income populations, iron deficiency anemia rates are 1.8% in the first trimester, 8.2% in the second trimester, and reach 27.4% in the third trimester [21]. In addition, the prevalence of anemia among black pregnant women (35.38 per 1000 women) is twice higher than in white (18.02 per 1000 women) [3]. Regardless of race, the population of pregnant teenagers was the one with the highest prevalence [3]. The second most common cause is acute blood loss, especially during childbirth [7].

Several surveys show that anemia in pregnancy is associated with an increased risk of low birth weight, preterm birth, and perinatal mortality [20, 21].

Clinical Features

An anemic condition in pregnancy may present with symptoms, or be suggested only through changes present in routine laboratory exams of prenatal care. That is because the clinical manifestations of an insidious onset of anemia are mixed with frequent complaints of pregnant women, which often have no pathological meaning, but are related to gestational state itself: fatigue and malaise, dyspnea, palpitations, exercise intolerance, dizziness, and decompensation of underlying diseases.

Some signs on physical examination may suggest the etiology of the anemia. Deficiency anemias can present glossitis and angular cheilitis; hemolytics may develop with jaundice; the presence of petechiae suggests thrombocytopenia, present in immune thrombocytopenic purpura, acute leukemia, and bone marrow aplasia.

Iron Deficiency Anemia

Iron deficiency anemia is defined as the decrease of iron stores in the body, leading to a state of inefficiency in the production of erythrocytes and a consequent drop in hemoglobin and hematocrit values below normal levels.

Screening is recommended for all pregnant women, with Hb and Htc (level C of evidence) [2]. Although these tests are not specific to assess iron deficiency, iron deficiency anemia is the first suspect in the face of the finding of anemia in pregnancy. The laboratory evaluation of the iron profile (shown in Table 20.3) complements the evaluation, and the serum ferritin level is the most sensitive and specific test for the diagnosis of iron deficiency anemia. Nonspecific symptoms of anemia, mentioned above, may be present, as well as specific symptoms of iron deficiency: perversions of appetite (desire to eat earth, ice, or starch), koilonychia, bluish sclera [10, 24]. In practice, the diagnosis of mild to moderate iron-deficiency anemia is sometimes presumptive, and it is possible to start therapy empirically before obtaining results of the iron tests [2].

The characteristic features of erythrocyte morphology are hypochromia and microcytosis, but these changes are less common in iron deficiency anemia in

Table 20.3 Iron profile

Test	Normal value
Plasma iron level	40–175 mcg/dL
Plasma total iron-binding capacity	216–400 mcg/dL
Transferrin saturation	16–60%
Serum ferritin level	>30 mcg/L
Free erythrocyte protoporphyrin level	<3 mcg/g

pregnant women [7] and, therefore, they can be normochromic and normocytic, especially in the early stages. This variation in the size of red blood cells causes an increase in the anisocytosis index (RDW), which is usually above 14%. This parameter helps in the differential diagnosis with thalassemia, also microcytic, but with normal RDW. Because it is hypoproliferative, the reticulocyte index in iron deficiency anemia is normal.

Serum iron is low (usually <30 mg/dL) and also ferritin, with levels below 10–15 mcg/L confirming the diagnosis of iron deficiency anemia [2, 7]. The total iron-binding capacity (TIBC), which indirectly represents the concentration of transferrin in the blood, is increased above 400 mcg/dL. This is because since transferrin is an iron-carrying protein, its production increases in response to its deficiency, in order to mobilize it from reserves. However, as iron stores are low, transferrin saturation is decreased (below 18%) [2]. Protoporphyrin, a protein that binds to iron in the synthesis of the heme of the hemoglobin molecule, can also be measured in its unbound form, the free erythrocyte protoporphyrin. Thus, it is increased in iron deficiency. The iron profile can also help in the differential diagnosis of microcytic anemia, as displayed in Table 20.4.

The preferred treatment is orally, with 120–200 mg of elemental iron per day, which can be divided into 3 or 4 doses [10, 24], available in sulfate, fumarate, or gluconate preparations. It is administered 1 h before meals and may be accompanied by vitamin C or orange juice, which enhances absorption [10]. Gastrointestinal side effects, such as nausea, vomiting, epigastric pain, and diarrhea are common [24]. In this situation, one can choose to take the tablets with the meal, improving tolerance, but with reduced absorption. In total, 7–10 days after starting treatment, reticulocytosis is observed, and Hb and Htc increase in subsequent weeks [2]. Therapy should be continued for 3 months after correction of anemia, ensuring the replacement of iron stores [24].

The lack of response after 4 weeks of treatment with oral iron indicates therapeutic failure [24], which can be secondary to incorrect etiological diagnosis or other coexisting anemia, poor treatment compliance, failure in absorption, and chronic blood loss greater than replacement [2].

Parenteral therapy is reserved for patients with severe oral intolerance, disabsorptive syndromes, or severe anemia [2]. Ferric sucrose is considered safer than iron dextrin, with lower rates of adverse reactions, such as anaphylaxis, hypotension, and shock [2, 7, 10, 24]. The emergence of low-grade fever, chills, nausea, and local pain

Table 20.4 Differential diagnosis of microcytic hypochromic anemia

Test	Iron deficiency anemia	Thalassemia	Anemia of chronic disease
Iron level	Decreased	Normal	Decreased
Total iron-binding capacity	Increased	Normal	Decreased
Ferritin level	Decreased	Normal	Increased
Iron/total iron-binding capacity	<18%	Normal	>18%

occurs up to 1.5% of the time [24], but it is self-limited and does not indicates discontinuation of treatment [10]. Despite occurring slower in oral therapy, the increase in Hb and Htc is equivalent between the two forms of administration [4, 7].

Red blood cell transfusion is rarely indicated and is reserved for cases in which there is coexisting hypovolemia due to acute blood loss [2]. Hemoglobin levels below 6 mg/dL are associated with changes in fetal vitality and fetal death, and therefore, in these cases, blood transfusion should be considered.

In pregnant women who do not have anemia, the World Health Organization recommends supplementation with 30–60 mg of elemental iron per day. This action decreases the prevalence of maternal anemia at delivery (level A of evidence) [2, 15]. Supplementation is maintained for up to 3 months after delivery. The exception is in patients with increased iron deposits, such as those with hemochromatosis and sickle cell anemia [2, 24].

Megaloblastic Anemia

It is the anemia caused by impairment in DNA synthesis, which is mediated by folic acid and vitamin B12 [7]. Thus, cell division is slowed, and as the cytoplasm keeps growing, cells become larger [10].

In pregnancy is most commonly caused by a lack of folic acid, since there is an increase in its demand [7] and intake is not always sufficient, requiring a diet rich in green leaves, vegetables, and proteins. Substances that interfere in the absorption and/or metabolism of folic acids, such as some anticonvulsants and alcohol, may precipitate or aggravate this condition. Vitamin B12 deficiency occurs mainly in the presence of conditions that hinder its absorption in the gastrointestinal tract: patients with partial or total gastrectomy, Crohn's disease, and pernicious anemia. Pernicious anemia, an autoimmune condition in which there is a reduction in gastric acid and intrinsic factor, both necessary for the absorption of B12, is rare before the age of 40 [7]. Pregnant women in a state of malnutrition or strict vegetarians are at risk of deficiency due to insufficient intake, since B12 is present in products of animal origin (meat, eggs, dairy products). Other causes include drugs that directly interfere with DNA synthesis, chemotherapy, and antiretroviral drugs, for example.

In addition to the general manifestations of anemia, patients with megaloblastic anemia may experience diarrhea and weight loss, since enterocytes are also affected by impaired DNA synthesis. As B12 is involved in the synthesis of the myelin sheath, its deficiency may also present neurological manifestations: extremity paresthesias, decreased deep sensitivity, loss of proprioception, ataxia, weakness and spasticity in the lower limbs, deep hyperreflexia, dementia, and psychosis.

In the blood count, there is macrocytosis, with MCV above 100 fL. It is usually pronounced in megaloblastic anemia, with values up to 140 fL [10]. MCV values above 115 fL are seen almost exclusively in this anemia [2]. On the other hand, MCV may be normal if there is a concomitant lack of iron [7, 10]. Severe cases may progress with leukopenia and/or thrombocytopenia [7, 24]. In the peripheral blood smear, the finding of hypersegmented neutrophils is virtually pathognomonic [10] and peripheral nucleated erythrocytes appear [7].

The diagnosis can be confirmed by the serum levels of folic acid and vitamin B12 below normal levels [2]. It is important to note that in pregnant women, normal values are lower than in the general population. When these tests are still in doubt, the measurement of serum or urinary methylmalonic acid can be used, increased only in the deficiency of B12, and considered the most accurate parameter for this diagnosis [10]. The erythrocyte folate dosage may also be used to confirm the deficiency of folic acid. Homocysteine, on the other hand, has increased levels in both deficiencies, but since it is not specific, it should be requested only when this suspicion exists. These biochemical tests replace bone marrow aspirate in most cases.

The distinction between B12 or folic acid deficiencies, or the confirmation of both concomitantly, is important because the inadvertent use of folates in B12 deficiency can partially correct hematological changes, but neurological manifestations can progress and, over time, become irreversible.

The treatment of folic acid deficiency is typically orally, with 1 mg of folic acid daily, in 1 serving, associated with a dietary intake of foods rich in folic acid [2]. It is recommended that 400 mcg/day of folic acid is used prophylactically for all patients in the periconceptional period, from 3 months before pregnancy to the end of the first trimester, in order to prevent defects in the fetal neural tube [7, 10, 24]. In those who use anticonvulsants, or who have had previous pregnancies with fetuses affected by neural tube defects, the dose should be increased to 4 mg/day [24].

In vitamin B12 deficiency, 1000 mcg of cyanocobalamin is indicated, intramuscularly, once a week for 4 weeks, followed by monthly administration [24]. Gastrectomized patients require prophylactic 1000 mcg monthly.

Response to treatment can be observed in 4–7 days with an increase in reticulocyte count, in addition to repair of leukopenia and thrombocytopenia, when present [7]. Anemia begins to improve after 10 days and completely regresses in 1–2 months.

Aplastic Anemia

It is rare in pregnancy, but severe: it is characterized by pancytopenia and bone marrow with marked hypocellularity [7, 10]. It can be triggered by drugs, infection, radiation, leukemia, immune disorders, and hereditary conditions, such as Fanconi anemia and Diamond–Blackfan syndrome [7, 9, 12].

The greatest risks are hemorrhagic complications and infections. Mortality during or after pregnancy reaches 50% of cases and is usually associated with these causes [25]. Outside of pregnancy, bone marrow transplantation is the first line treatment, with a survival rate of 70–80%. During pregnancy, however, there is controversy about this procedure, since prior immunosuppressive therapy is needed [24].

Management during pregnancy should include screening for infections and prompt treatment, as well as transfusion of blood components, when necessary. Hematocrit should be maintained at least 20% and vaginal delivery is preferable [25].

Acquired Hemolytic Anemias

Hemolysis can be triggered by several factors. Among nonhereditary factors, there are autoantibodies, drugs, and pregnancy itself.

In autoimmune hemolytic anemia, there is disproportionate production of antibodies that can be IgG or IgM. The direct and indirect Coombs' test are positive, and in the peripheral blood smear there is spherocytosis and reticulocytosis. It may be idiopathic or secondary to underlying diseases such as leukemias, lymphomas, inflammatory diseases, collagen diseases, infections, or also be triggered by certain drugs [7]. Treatment with glucocorticoids is usually effective, such as prednisone 1 mg/kg/day, or equivalent. Red blood cell transfusion is complicated due to circulating antibodies, and it is recommended to warm the bags to room temperature to reduce the action of cold agglutinins [7, 25].

Drug-induced hemolysis is usually mild to moderate and reverses with discontinuation of its use. Some examples of drugs are penicillins, cephalosporins, quinidine, rifampicin, and thiopental [25]. Glucocorticoids can also be used.

When severe hemolytic anemia appears unexpectedly in early pregnancy and improves within a few months after delivery, it is classified as induced by pregnancy. There is no evidence of an immune mechanism or erythrocyte defects. It can respond to glucocorticoids, and use should be continued until delivery [25].

Paroxysmal Nocturnal Hemoglobinuria

It is an acquired disorder of hematopoietic stem cells that affects all strains, arising from an abnormal colony of cells, similar to a neoplasm. Defective cells are susceptible to lysis by the complement system [7].

Hemolysis is triggered after transfusions, infections, or surgery, and the severity varies from mild to lethal. Hemoglobinuria is not necessarily nocturnal and occurs at irregular intervals. The rate of complications, such as thrombosis, Budd–Chiari syndrome, renal failure, and hypertension, reaches 40%. During pregnancy, its evolution is unpredictable, with complications in 75% and thrombosis in 50% of patients. The mortality rate is 10–20%. The use of prophylactic anticoagulation is recommended [7].

Hereditary Hemolytic Anemias

Comprises the group of diseases in which mutations of genes encoding hemoglobin, cytoskeleton, or erythrocyte enzymes result in changes in the morphology and/or function of red blood cells, resulting in their premature peripheral destruction.

Hemoglobinopathies

Hemoglobin is formed by four interconnected globin polypeptide chains, each connected to a heme molecule. Of these chains, two are of the alpha type, and the other two vary: beta (hemoglobin A), gamma (hemoglobin F), or delta (hemoglobin A2) [25].

Sickle Cell Diseases

The substitution of an amino acid (glutamic acid for valine) in the beta chain results in the formation of hemoglobin S [7]. Homozygosis for this condition results in sickle cell anemia, or SS hemoglobinopathy. Another similar mutation causes the replacement of glutamic acid for lysine, resulting in hemoglobin C [25]. Thus, it is possible to combine these mutations with each other (Hemoglobinopathy SC), and also with the mutation that results in Beta-thalassemia, leading to various possible genotypes and phenotypes of sickle cell diseases. In addition, heterozygosis for the formation of hemoglobin S results in the sickle cell trait, a condition in which the individual is hematologically normal, but can transmit the gene to his descendants.

The prevalence is highest in the Afro-descendant population, and it is estimated that 1 in 12 black Americans has the sickle cell trait and that approximately 1 in 600 newborns in this population has sickle cell anemia.

The diagnosis is made through hemoglobin electrophoresis. In addition, laboratory findings of pure sickle cell anemia will show a mild to moderate drop in hemoglobin and hematocrit, reticulocytosis, indirect hyperbilirubinemia, and an increase in LDH. MCV is usually normal or slightly increased due to reticulocytes in the peripheral circulation. The peripheral blood smear shows the irreversibly sickled cells (ISC), in the shape of an ellipse [10, 25].

Red blood cells containing hemoglobin S undergo sickling in situations of low oxygenation. Pregnant women are more susceptible to sickling crises, due to hypercoagulability, vascular stasis, and metabolic increase. Sickle cell anemia causes the most severe conditions during pregnancy [25].

The adhesion of red blood cells to the endothelium in the micro- and macrocirculation, with the formation of thrombi, vascular occlusion, ischemia, and tissue necrosis, causing severe pain in the affected organs, consists of sickling crises. A common site is the bone marrow, resulting in bone pain and possible complications, such as osteomyelitis and osteoporosis. When this phenomenon occurs in the pulmonary vascular territory, it can evolve with acute chest syndrome [25]. Infection is another precipitator of this condition, in 50% of cases [7]. Acute chest syndrome manifests with pleuritic chest pain, cough, fever, hypoxia, and pulmonary infiltrate, and it is the most severe complication, occurring in 1–6% of patients [25]. Mortality is around 3% [7] but reaches 50% in cases that develop with acute respiratory failure [25].

The morbidity of these patients is also due to the higher rates of preeclampsia and eclampsia; pyelonephritis, endometritis, and sepsis; placental abruption and increased need for cesarean sections [24, 25]. Pre-existing disorders, such as pulmonary hypertension, hypertrophic cardiomyopathy, and renal failure, may worsen [7]. Fetal morbidity is also significant, including abortion, growth restriction, prematurity, and perinatal death [24, 25]. Other types of exacerbation of the disease are aplastic, megaloblastic, hemolytic, and splenic sequestration crises.

Prenatal follow-up must be careful. Supplementation of folic acid 4 mg/day is necessary to supply increased hematopoiesis in these patients [1]. In the occurrence of pain, fever, and worsening of anemia, the hypothesis of sickle cell crisis should be considered only after other possible causes are excluded, such as ectopic pregnancy, placental abruption, pyelonephritis, and appendicitis [7].

In the sickling crisis, adequate intravenous hydration associated with opioid analgesia should be instituted [7, 24, 25]. If there is hypoxemia, oxygenation with a nasal cannula is indicated, in order to decrease sickling at the capillary level [25]. The investigation of underlying infectious processes—pneumonia and pyelonephritis being the most common—and the institution of antibiotic therapy when necessary are essential [7, 25]. Surveillance of fetal vitality is also necessary, since acute fetal distress may occur during the crisis [14, 25].

Blood transfusion does not decrease the intensity or duration of crises [7], but it has precise indications in some situations: a drop of 30% or more in baseline levels of hematocrit or hemoglobin [24], the presence of hemodynamic instability, acute chest syndrome, stroke, high output heart failure, multiple organ failure, symptomatic anemia, severe pain crisis refractory to treatment (longer than 10 days) and reticulocytopenia [14]. Prophylactic transfusions, on the other hand, show an important benefit in preventing vaso-occlusive episodes [7, 25], but randomized trials showed no difference in perinatal outcomes [7, 11] and there are still risks associated with multiple transfusions. Thus, routine prophylactic transfusions during pregnancy remain controversial [1], and the current consensus is that their use should be individualized, in patients with frequent episodes of vaso-occlusion and unfavorable obstetric outcomes [5, 7, 25].

Due to the high incidence of fetal growth restriction and perinatal mortality, serial fetal assessment [7] is necessary, with ultrasound to estimate fetal growth and amniotic fluid, cardiotocography, and Doppler velocimetry [25].

The mode of delivery is an obstetric indication, with no contraindication to vaginal delivery [25]. Patients should not be oversedated, and early epidural analgesia is ideal [7]. If the hematocrit is less than 20%, transfusion of red blood cells is indicated, taking care to avoid circulatory overload, and pulmonary edema [7, 25].

Due to the increase in thrombotic risk, it is important to remember that thrombotic prophylaxis with low molecular weight heparin is indicated during hospitalizations, either in the presence of pain crises or in the postpartum period [25].

The concern with the transmission of sickle cell disease to the fetus must exist in all pregnant women with the manifested disease (hemoglobinopathy SS, SC, and combinations with thalassemia) and in those with the sickle cell trait (heterozygotes for hemoglobin S). The partner of these patients should be investigated with hemoglobin electrophoresis for genetic counseling [24]. Antenatal diagnosis using villus biopsy, amniocentesis, or preimplantation genetic evaluation are also available [7].

Thalassemias

Mutations in genes that encode the production of hemoglobin molecules can impair the synthesis of one or more globin chains, resulting in ineffective erythropoiesis, hemolysis, and anemia in several degrees. The two main forms involve impaired production or instability of alpha chains, causing alpha-thalassemia, or beta chains, causing beta-thalassemia [7]. The incidence of these disorders during pregnancy is between 1:300 and 1:500 [8, 25].

Alpha-Thalassemia

There are four genes encoding alpha-globin. Thus, the clinical manifestation will depend on the possible genotypes resulting from the mutation in these genes.

In the deletion of the four genes, homozygous alpha-thalassemia occurs, in which the production of alpha chains is absent. This change is manifested in fetal life, as alpha chains are necessary for the formation of hemoglobin F (two alpha chains and two gamma chains), predominant in the fetus. Thus, tetramers of gamma hemoglobin, called Bart's hemoglobin, appear. This hemoglobin has high avidity for oxygen, preventing its distribution to tissues, leading to hypoxia, heart failure, fetal hydrops, and fetal or neonatal death, being incompatible with extra-uterine life. This condition is more prevalent in populations from Southeast Asia.

The deletion of three of the four genes results in hemoglobin H disease, which manifests with moderate to severe hemolytic anemia even in the neonatal period. Over the course of life, affected individuals may develop hepatosplenomegaly, cholelithiasis, growth failure, thrombosis, hemochromatosis, liver, and heart failure. Pregnant women in this condition are at risk of worsening anemia, and obstetric complications such as preeclampsia, abortions, premature birth, fetal growth restriction, and perinatal death [25].

The deletion of two genes is manifested by alpha-thalassemia minor, characterized by mild to moderate microcytic hypochromic anemia [7]. It often goes unnoticed and does not increase maternal gestational morbidity [25].

The deletion of a single gene is the condition of silent carrier, with no clinical manifestation, and has its importance in the genetic counseling of carrier couples [10].

Beta-Thalassemia

More than 150 mutations in the beta-globin gene have been described, which can result in damage to the production of the beta-globin chain or to instability of the alpha chain, leading to beta-thalassemia [7]. There is a decrease in the production of beta chains, and the excess of alpha chains causes damage to cell membranes.

Depending on the genotype and the resulting beta-globin production deficiency, which may be absent or decreased to varying degrees, we classify their subtypes into beta-thalassemia major (Cooley's anemia), beta-thalassemia intermedia, and beta-thalassemia minor. In all of them, there is increased production Hemoglobin A2.

Beta-thalassemia major is a serious and often fatal disorder [7]. In childhood, there is already intense hemolysis and severe anemia, which leads to delayed neuropsychomotor development, growth deficit, immunosuppression, hepatosplenomegaly, and the need for repeated blood transfusions. The latter leads to iron overload and transfusional hemochromatosis. Gonadotrophic hypogonadism is common, with resulting infertility [7] and there is the significant reduction in life expectancy. Thus, the occurrence of pregnancy in this condition is rare.

Intermediate and minor betas-thalassemias usually present with moderate to mild anemia, which can worsen during pregnancy [7]. The diagnosis should always be suspected in the presence of hypochromic microcytic anemia with serum ferritin in normal to high concentrations, especially in pregnant women descendants of Mediterranean populations [24]. There is a twofold increase in the risk of fetal growth restriction [25]. In patients with this diagnosis, hemoglobin electrophoresis of the partner is recommended for genetic counseling. Due to the variety of possible mutations, prenatal diagnosis is difficult, but it can be performed through invasive tests when the familial mutation is already known [7].

Spherocytosis

It is caused by inherited molecular defects in membrane proteins. They are usually autosomal dominant, but they can also be autosomal recessive or de novo mutations [7]. As a result, varying degrees of anemia and jaundice resulting from hemolysis develop. The diagnosis is confirmed by the presence of spherocytes in the peripheral blood smear, reticulocytosis, and increased osmotic fragility [7, 25]. Patients usually evolve well during pregnancy [25]. However, hemolytic crises with worsening anemia may occur [7].

Enzymatic Defects

Deficiency of erythrocyte enzymes in red blood cells that participate in the anaerobic glucose cycle can cause hereditary nonspherocytic anemia [25]. The two most important are the pyruvate kinase deficiency, autosomal recessive, and glucose-6-phosphate dehydrogenase (G6PD) deficiency, X-linked [7].

During pregnancy, infections or drugs can induce hemolysis in homozygous or heterozygous women for this condition, and anemia is usually episodic and improves after resolution of the condition that precipitated it [7].

Fetal Anemia

The main cause of fetal anemia is still Rh alloimmunization. This issue will be addressed in a specific chapter. Here are exposed other possible causes of fetal anemia.

In the suspicion of fetal anemia through the assessment of the peak systolic velocity of the medium cerebral artery by Doppler velocimetry (see Fig. 20.1), after the exclusion of alloimmunization, other tests can be performed. The screening for fetal alpha-thalassemia is performed with an assessment of the parents' VCM, which when less than <80 fL, suggests that they are carriers of the thalassemia trait. The diagnosis of alpha-thalassemia can be confirmed by checking for deletions or point mutations in the fetal DNA, and also by detecting Bart's hemoglobin in the fetal blood [13]. In the suspicion of fetal-maternal hemorrhage, the Kleihauer–Betke test, which consists of the detection of fetal erythrocytes in the maternal circulation, allows not only to confirm this diagnosis but also to estimate the volume of fetal blood loss and, therefore, to estimate the volume of blood to be transfused into the fetus [7].

The presence of anemia with signs of fetal hemorrhage, such as the visualization of heterogeneous intracranial mass, for example, leads to the suspicion of fetal coagulopathy [6]. Alloimmune thrombocytopenia, the most common cause of

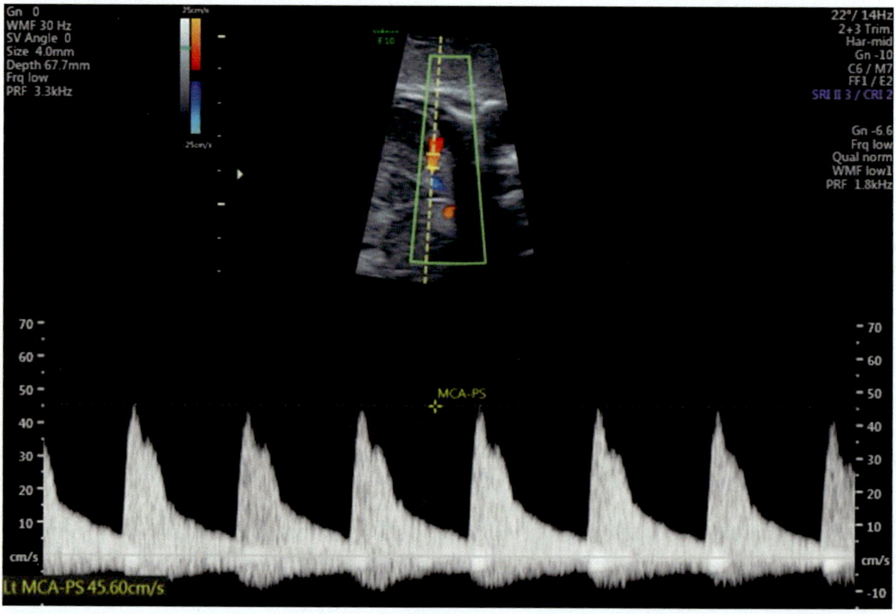

Fig. 20.1 Peak systolic velocity of the fetal medium cerebral artery by Doppler velocimetry

severe thrombocytopenia among term newborns [7], occurs due to the presence of maternal antibodies against the platelet antigen HPA1a, which can be measured in the maternal circulation. It occurs in the first pregnancy in 80% of cases, can manifest early (below 20 weeks), and has an 80% risk of recurrence, that's why is so important to make this diagnosis. In addition, the use of intravenous immunoglobulin may decrease its severity and the risk of intraventricular hemorrhage in those patients [6].

References

1. ACOG Practice Bulletin No. 78: Hemoglobinopathies in pregnancy. Obstet Gynecol. 2007;109(1):229–38.
2. ACOG Practice Bulletin No. 95: Anemia in Pregnancy. Obstet Gynecol. 2008;112(1):201–07.
3. Adebisi O, Strayhorn G. Anemia in pregnancy and race in the United States: blacks at risk. Fam Med. 2005;37:655–62.
4. Bhandal N, Russell R. Intravenous versus oral iron therapy for postpartum anemia. BJOG. 2006;113:1248–52.
5. Castro O, Hoque M, Brown B. Pulmonary hypertension in sickle cell disease: cardiac catheterization results and survival. Blood. 2003;101(4):1257–61.
6. Coady A, Bower S. Twining's textbook of fetal abnormalities. 3rd ed. London: Churchill Linvingstone; 2014.
7. Cunningham F. Williams obstetrics. 24th ed. New York: McGraw-Hill Education/ Medical; 2014.
8. Gehlbach D, Morgenstern I. Antenatal screening for thalassemia minor. Int J Gynecol Obstet. 1989;28(2):198.
9. Green A, Kupfer G. Fanconi anemia. Hematol Oncol Clin North Am. 2009;23(2):193.
10. Jameson J, Kasper D, Fauci A, Hauser S, Longo D, Loscalzo J. Harrison's principles of internal medicine. 20th ed. New York: McGrall-Hill; 2018.
11. Koshy M, Burd L, Wallace D, Moawad A, Baron J. Prophylactic red-cell transfusions in pregnant patients with sickle cell disease. N Engl J Med. 1988;319(22):1447–52.
12. Lipton J, Ellis S. Diamond-Blackfan anemia: diagnosis, treatment, and molecular pathogenesis. Hematol Oncol Clin North Am. 2009;23(2):261–82.
13. Norton M, Chauhan S, Dashe J. Society for Maternal-Fetal Medicine (SMFM) Clinical Guideline #7: nonimmune hydrops fetalis. Am J Obstet Gynecol. 2015;212(2):127–39.
14. Parrish M, Morrison J. Sickle cell crisis and pregnancy. Semin Perinatol. 2013;37(4):274–9.
15. Peña-Rosas J, Viteri F. Effects of routine oral iron supplementation with or without folic acid for women during pregnancy. Cochrane Database Syst Rev. 2006;(3):CD004736.
16. Perinatal. Manual de Perinatologia / Perinatal. Rio de Janeiro; 2012. p. 117–21.
17. Pritchard J. Changes in the blood volume during pregnancy and delivery. Anesthesiology. 1965;26(4):393–9.
18. Pritchard J, Adams R. Erythrocyte production and destruction during pregnancy. Am J Obstet Gynecol. 1960;79(4):750–7.
19. Pritchard J, Scott D. Iron demands during pregnancy. In: Hallberg L, Harwerth H, Vannotti A, editors. Iron deficiency-pathogenesis: clinical aspects and therapy. London: Academic Press; 1970. p. 173.
20. Rasmussen K. Is there a causal relationship between iron deficiency or iron-deficiency anemia and weight at birth, length of gestation and perinatal mortality? J Nutr. 2001;131(2):590S–603S.
21. Scholl T. Iron status during pregnancy: setting the stage for mother and infant. Am J Clin Nutr. 2005;81(5):1218S–22S.

22. Vandevijvere S, Amsalkhir S, Van Oyen H, Ines E, Moreno-Reyes R. Iron status and its determinants in a nationally representative sample of pregnant women. J Acad Nutr Diet. 2013;113(5):659–66.
23. Zeeman G, Cunningham F, Pritchard J. The magnitude of hemoconcentration with eclampsia. Hypertens Pregnancy. 2009;28(2):127–37.
24. Zugaib M, Bittar R, Francisco R. Protocolos assistenciais, clínica obstétrica, FMUSP. 5th ed. São Paulo: Atheneu; 2015. p. 155–9.
25. Zugaib M, Francisco R. Zugaib Obstetrícia. 4th ed. Barueri: Manole; 2019. p. 834–50.

Chapter 21
Chronic Hypertension in Pregnancy

Henri Augusto Korkes, Renato José Bauer, and Nelson Sass

Introduction

Hypertensive syndromes in pregnancy, along with hemorrhagic and infectious syndromes, are largely responsible for most maternal deaths worldwide [1]. Some factors contribute in special to the high rates of morbidity and mortality: lack of identification and adequate prevention of at-risk groups, poor-quality prenatal follow-up, delay in the diagnosis of complications, and adoption of effective measures for maternal protection, and finally, delay in adopting effective and safe obstetric measures for the care of these patients.

It is estimated that chronic arterial hypertension (CH) complicates about 6–8% of pregnancies [2], which can be aggravated by superimposed preeclampsia (PE) in 13–40% of cases [3, 4]. CH is defined when the systolic blood pressure (SBP) is greater or equal to 140 mmHg or the diastolic blood pressure (DBP) is greater or equal to 90 mmHg, or both, preceding pregnancy or identified before the 20th week of pregnancy or persisting beyond 12 weeks after the birth [3–5].

The correct diagnosis of CH depends on the quality of the blood pressure measurement. For this, some technical aspects need to be followed. The measure should be performed with the patient seated, with the back supported, applying the device on the right upper limb and keeping it elevated at the height of the heart. Although the left lateral position of the body is often adopted for resting the patient, for the correct measurement, it is preferable that she is seated.

H. A. Korkes · R. J. Bauer
Department of Obstetrics, Faculty of Medicine of Pontifical University of Sao Paulo, City of Sorocaba, SP, Brazil
e-mail: hakorkes@pucsp.br

N. Sass (✉)
Department of Obstetrics, Universidade Federal de São Paulo (Federal University of São Paulo) – UNIFESP, City of Sao Paulo, SP, Brazil

© Springer Nature Switzerland AG 2022

R. A. Moreira de Sá, E. B. d. Fonseca (eds.), *Perinatology*,
https://doi.org/10.1007/978-3-030-83434-0_21

The DBP should be considered the fifth Korotkoff sound, corresponding to the disappearance of the sound. Another important point is the use of cuffs suitable for the perimeter of the arm. International recommendations determine that cuffs 12–13 cm wide are ideal for arms with a circumference of 30 cm. If suitable cuffs are not available, use correction tables [6–8], such as Maxwell's [7] which is based on the measurement of the brachial circumference (Table 21.1).

Currently, the use of electronic devices has greatly facilitated the follow-up of these patients with regard to residential blood pressure measurement (MRPA), being an ally for the assessment of blood pressure control [9].

CH is classified as primary or essential in 90% and the rest being classified as secondary, that is, due to other pathologies [10] as pheochromocytoma, coarctation of the aorta, systemic lupus, scleroderma, and kidney problems such as glomerulonephritis and renal artery stenosis. It may also be related to endocrinopathies such as diabetes, hyperthyroidism, Cushing's disease, and primary hyperaldosteronism [10]. Secondary arterial hypertension should be considered in young women with difficult to control BP, which needs multiple hypotensive agents to control or patients with laboratory and clinical changes, such as hypokalemia, abdominal murmur, and proteinuria. Secondary hypertension presents a particularly high risk of adverse pregnancy outcomes [11].

CH is associated with adverse maternal and fetal outcomes including superimposed PE, HELLP syndrome, increased incidence of cesarean section, fetal growth restriction (FGR), placental abruption, and perinatal death. Thus, a special strategy for clinical follow-up and treatment must be applied in order to reduce maternal and perinatal risks.

Table 21.1 Correction factors for SBP and DBP according to the arm diameter for 13 cm cuffs, adapted from Maxwell et al. [7]

Arm circumference (cm)	SBP adjustment (mmHg)	DBP adjustment (mmHg)
20	+11	+7
22	+9	+6
24	+7	+4
26	+5	+3
28	+3	+2
30	0	0
32	−2	−1
34	−4	−3
36	−6	−4
38	−8	−6
40	−10	−7
42	−12	−9
44	−14	−10
46	−16	−11
48	−18	−13
50	−21	−14

Prenatal Care

In an ideal scenario, women with CH should be oriented toward ante-natal planning that includes weight control, change of drugs that can affect fetal development such as blockers of the angiotensin-converting enzyme or its receptors, best control of blood pressure, and reduction of risk factors such as smoking and diabetes mellitus.

During pregnancy, from the first consultation, many aspects are necessary to consider: diet, control of weight, stop smoking, physical activities, and adequacy of the hypotensive drugs, if necessary. For these patients, the number and interval of visits should be individualized.

Perinatal risks are proportional to the blood pressure level at early pregnancy. Mild CH (DBP < 100 mmHg), without other complications, can be followed up monthly for up to 28 weeks every 2 weeks up to 34 weeks and weekly thereafter. More serious cases will require more rigorous follow-up and more frequent returns.

When changes in antihypertensive drug doses are needed, weekly returns are recommended in order to observe the clinical response. Patients should be informed to seek emergency care in the face of symptoms like headache, dizziness, visual blurring, or uterine hypertonia [8, 10]. Patients who have suspected superimposed PE should be referred to a qualified service in order to receive effective management.

The renal function at the first consultation is recommended. This information will be useful during all follow-up, as well as in the differential diagnosis of possible superimposed PE. Other tests, such as electrocardiogram, echocardiogram, chest radiography, renal ultrasounds, among others, should be reserved for special cases. It should be noted that there is no acceptable reason for requesting routine laboratory tests for the diagnosis of PE before the 20th week.

Ultrasound evaluation should be rationalized and have the following objectives: to certify gestational age, to identify fetal anomalies, and monitoring fetal development, considering that CH, especially severe forms, can affect placental circulation and fetal development. Ideally, the first assessment should be scheduled between 11 and 14 weeks, when the accuracy of the method allows for certifying gestational age and assessing fetal morphology.

After the 24th week, the scheduling of ultrasounds should be individualized. The risk of CRF among pregnant women with CH can reach 40% and early detection could decrease the risk of fetal death by 20% [12, 13]. For suspected cases of FGR, the study of the umbilical and cerebral artery circulation through Doppler is indicated in order to identify the fetal adaptation to the circulatory difficulties of the placenta and progressive impairment of fetal vitality [10]. The Doppler assessment in these situations can reduce perinatal mortality by approximately 30% [14]. In cases of severe impairment, all methods of assessing fetal conditions should be used, such as the fetal biophysical profile and the Doppler of the uterine arteries, middle cerebral artery, and venous duct, thus supporting the most opportune moment for the anticipation of delivery.

Diagnosis of Superimposed PE

PE in these patients should always be considered clinical follow-up, after 20 weeks. The following situations suggest superimposed PE: (1) an increase in baseline BP levels; (2) proteinuria appears or worsens already detected in the first half of pregnancy; (3) occurrence of clinical and/or laboratory manifestations that characterize PE [19, 20].

Considering the various possibilities of clinical expression of PE, its diagnosis should be considered even without the presence and proteinuria in view of the following criteria: thrombocytopenia (<100,000/mm^3), the elevation of transaminases, elevation creatinine levels (>1.1 mg/dl), cardiac arrest or signs and symptoms in target organs such as headache, scotoma, or epigastric pain [3, 20]. The onset of placental insufficiency can also be associated with PE [20].

Prediction of PE

As a broad concept, prediction tests should be easy to access, low cost, high sensitivity, and mainly reproducible. Unfortunately, so far, there are no reliable models that meet these conditions to recommend in clinical practice [20, 21]. Therefore, maternal risks should be based on the clinical history and physical examination.

There is no evidence to recommend any biomarkers as a routine, given poor sensitivity and the costs of its incorporation, especially in low-income countries. Are included in this concept Doppler of uterine arteries in the first and second trimesters and blood markers as PAPP-A (pregnancy-associated plasma protein-A), ADAM-12 (disintegrin and metalloproteinase-12), PP-13 (Placental Protein-13), uric acid, leptin, homocysteine, sFlt-1 (Soluble fms-like tyrosine kinase-1) and PlGF (Placental Growth Factor) [20].

Currently, a close relationship between antiangiogenic factors and PE is admitted, especially among the antiangiogenic factors released by the placenta, sFlt-1 [21–24]. Apparently, the ratio sFLT-1/PLGF below 38 in patients with suspected PE can be useful to exclude the diagnosis of PE up to 1 week [25]; however, these tests are not recommended for prediction of PE in patients with CH.

Prevention of PE

Women with CH are at risk for superimposed PE. The best available evidence recommends two effective interventions to reduce the risks: acetylsalicylic acid (ASA) at doses of 100–150 mg/daily [15] and supplementation of 1.0 g /daily of calcium (Ca) for women with a poor diet in this nutrient [16].

The ASA should be administered during the night, ideally from the 12th week of gestation until delivery [8]. Regarding Ca, important trials showed a reduction of PE risk in pregnant women treated with Ca in women with a poor diet of this element [3, 17]. Many countries, such as Brazil, have a low intake of this micronutrient in their population [18]. In scenarios, routine Ca supplementation is strongly recommended, from the beginning of pregnancy until delivery [3, 8].

In addition, other risk factors should be considered for these patients: age over 40 years, nulliparity, family history of PE (mother, sister), previous history of PE, diabetes mellitus, twin pregnancy, obesity, and chronic kidney disease [3, 8].

Nonpharmacological Treatment of CH

Diet: Reduction of salt consumption does not result in better maternal or perinatal outcomes nor impact the risk of PE [26]. However, avoiding excess salt can help pressure control and less need for hypotensive drugs.

Physical Activity: Regular activities, weight control, and reduction of cardiovascular risk factors, such as smoking, are important recommendations for chronic hypertensive patients [5]. However, physical activities deserve monitoring by professionals in the corresponding areas [8]. There is no clear evidence that contraindicates light physical activities during pregnancy [27, 28]. Patients that practice physical activity on a regular basis should be encouraged to stay active, possibly with adjustments in the frequency and intensity of the exercises [28].

Pharmacological Treatment of CH

Antihypertensive Drugs: In patients with normal blood pressure levels, hypotensive drugs do not bring clear benefits [29]. It is currently recommended that drug therapy should be started when BP values reach 140 or 90 mmHg [20]. Regarding the goals for BP control, a controlled clinical trial [29] has tested two different control regimes: (1) tight (DBP up to 85 mmHg) and (2) less-tight (DBP up to 100 mmHg) and did not identify significant differences related to perinatal outcomes or superimposed PE between groups. However, patients in the tight group had lower risks of severe hypertension throughout pregnancy.

On the other hand, there is a consensus in the world literature that patients with severe hypertension need hypotensive drugs [29]. Hypertensive crises justify hospitalization for adequate treatment. Regardless of clinical symptoms, such conditions require the use of fast-acting antihypertensive drugs, preceded by magnesium sulfate [4].

The choice of antihypertensive drug is based on experience and familiarity, as well as its availability at the clinical scenario [20]. Table 21.2 shows the drugs most commonly used in clinical practice.

Table 21.2 Most common antihypertensive drugs for use in pregnancy

Drug	Action	Dosage
Methyldopa	Centrally acting α2 adrenergic agonists	250–2000 mg/day orally in three to four divided doses Commonly initiated at 250 mg, three doses, daily
Prazosin	α1peripheric blockers	Initial dose of 1.0 mg, once a day, for 7 days Increments of 1.0 mg/day each week until desired control Maximum 20 mg/day
Labetalol	Beta blockers	200–2400 mg/day orally in two to three divided doses Commonly initiated at 100–200 mg twice daily
Nifedipine	Calcium channel blocker	10–20 mg orally in two to three doses. Maximum 180 mg/day Extended-release 20–60 mg once daily. Maximum 120 mg/day
Hydrochlorothiazide	Diuretic	12.5–50.0 mg/daily, one dose

Methyldopa is a central adrenergic inhibitor with extensive clinical experience in obstetrics. No adverse effects or relevant fetal abnormalities have been reported, and this drug is the first choice in several countries [20, 30]. Methyldopa is metabolized to alpha-methylnorepinephrine, which replaces norepinephrine in the neurosecretory vesicles of the terminal adrenergic nerves. Centrally, it is resistant to degradation by monoamine oxidase, resulting in a decrease in sympathetic tone and systemic vascular resistance, associated with a small decrease in cardiac output. The pressure control is gradual, with effect in about 6–8 h, due to its indirect mechanism of action. Some adverse effects are described: reduced alertness, impaired sleep, tiredness or depression, and reduced salivation. It must be considered that about 5% of patients may have an increase in liver enzymes [30], which can induce a false interpretation of hepatic impairment due to PE.

Diuretics as thiazide are currently considered safe drugs for patients with CH, except in the lactation period. It is a common alternative in the clinical practice of clinicians and cardiologists. Therefore, for patients who already use these drugs and become pregnant, there are no reasons to stop it [8]. However, facing placental insufficiency with a reduction in the amniotic fluid volume or superimposed PE, diuretics should be interrupted [20]. When faced with emergency situations, such as cardiac arrest, acute lung edema, or renal function impairment, the diuretic of choice will be furosemide [20].

Regarding beta-blockers, some studies have reported a possible association with FGR [31], associated with metoprolol, pindolol, and oxprenolol. In addition, this class of drugs is often used to control conditions associated with CH such as migraine [32], thyrotoxic crisis [33], and heart diseases [34]. There are no acceptable medical reasons to stop these drugs during pregnancy considering their clinical benefits.

Among β-blockers, labetalol appears to be the most common option in pregnancy, although it is not available in all countries as Brazil. It is a good choice for a hypertensive emergency. Regarding the newborn effects, neonatal hypoglycemia is a common complication and can be more severe in newborns submitted to growth restriction due to placental insufficiency [30].

Hydralazine is a vasodilator acting by relaxing the arterial muscle wall in a direct way. Its use is widespread in clinical practice, especially in hypertensive emergencies. However, when used orally, it presents poor clinical expression as hypotensive.

Regarding calcium channel blockers, nifedipine is a good alternative for outpatient use and is also indicated for situations of hypertensive crisis [35–37]. There is no evidence to contraindicate the concomitant use of nifedipine and magnesium sulfate in situations of hypertensive emergency or severe PE [38]. Another option in this class of hypotensive drugs considered safe is amlodipine, alone or combined with other hypotensive agents.

A special warning should be directed to the use of drugs that act as inhibiting angiotensin-converting enzymes or blocking angiotensin II receptors. These drugs are associated with fetal abnormalities or fetal death. However, they are adequate alternatives during lactation [39].

Treatment of Hypertensive Crisis

Hypertensive emergencies are characterized by expressive blood pressure levels (SBP ≥ 160 mmHg or DBP ≥ 110 mmHg) that represent a high risk to severe damage at the central nervous system and even death [35]. Patients in hypertensive crisis need immediate and effective intervention. The aim of drug treatment is to reduce BP in order to preserve the mechanisms of self-control and avoid permanent damage to the brain [8]. This objective is achieved when SBP <150 mmHg and DBP <100 mmHg.

The first-line medications for a hypertensive crisis are hydralazine, nifedipine, and labetalol [35] (Table 21.3). Hydralazine and labetalol, both administered by IV

Table 21.3 Antihypertensive agents used for urgent blood pressure control in pregnancy

Drug	Dosage	Onset of action
Hydralazine	Starting dose 5 mg IV. Additional doses of 5 mg IV every 20–30 minutes until DBP <110 mmHg Every 6 h when pressure reduction is required, additional doses of 5.0 mg EV every 20–30 minutes until DBP <110 mmHg	10–20 minutes
Nifedipine	Starting dose 5 mg orally. Additional doses of 5 mg orally every 20–30 minutes until DBP <110 mmHg Every 6 h when pressure reduction is required, additional doses of 5.0 orally every 20–30 minutes until DBP <110 mmHg	5–10 minutes
Sodium Nitroprusside	Starting dose 0.25 μg/kg/min Additional doses of 0.25 μg/kg/min every 5 minutes until DBP <110 mmHg	Immediate
Labetalol	Starting dose 10–20 mg IV Additional doses of 20–80 mg IV. Maximum dose 300 mg Alternative dosage: 1–2 mg/minute, IV	1–2 minutes

route, are the most common alternatives in clinical practice. Nifedipine (VO) is considered effective but not as first-line drug [35]. Sodium nitroprusside is a good option in cases of hypertensive emergency associated with lung edema or heart failure [43].

A common dilemma in clinical practice is to define whether the hypertensive crisis is a single situation or superimposed PE is the main cause of this condition. To answer this question, it will be necessary to evaluate laboratory tests related to the investigation of the presence of PE. In addition, based on a clinical evaluation only, it will be decided by the administration of magnesium sulfate.

Obstetric Care

The decision related to the moment of birth in chronic hypertensive patients should consider some variables. Active conduct is indicated in case of complicating situations such as severe and persistent hypertension, need for multiple drugs for hypotension, secondary hypertension related to nephropathy and diabetes mellitus, superimposed PE, and fetal impairment due to placental damage.

For patients with mild hypertension without other complications, it is possible to wait for spontaneous birth. The mode of delivery will be an obstetric indication and the simple presence of CH does not justify cesarean section as a rule [44]. When inducing labor, special attention should be given to the use of oxytocin, since high doses can improve its antidiuretic effects, and there are risks of complications when cardiovascular or renal abnormalities are present [8]. The use of magnesium sulfate should not be considered a contraindication to carry out the necessary procedures for vaginal delivery [45].

Finally, all patients with CH should receive guidance on family planning. Contraceptive methods should be encouraged in this group. The World Health Organization recommends encouraging the insertion of the intrauterine device immediately after delivery or in the first 48 h after birth [46].

CH in the Puerperium

The first 72 h after birth require careful monitoring considering potential maternal risks of maternal complications as hypertensive crises, acute pulmonary edema, heart failure, renal dysfunction, and complications related to PE [40]. During this period, the behavior of blood pressure and laboratory tests deserves special attention from the healthcare team.

Some factors may interfere in this evolution, such as the mobilization of fluids from the extravascular space causing the increase of the blood pressure, as well as the inadequate management of pain in the postoperative period. Should be highlighted the impact of nonsteroid anti-inflammatory drugs in renal function and the rise of blood pressure related to ergotamine agents often used to control postpartum bleeding,

When lactation inhibition is indicated, the method of choice should be breast wrapping in view of the risks of acute events associated with the use of bromocriptine and cabergoline. In addition, these drugs can increase blood pressure levels and acute cardiocirculatory events such as brain hemorrhage and myocardial infarction [41].

There is no consensus related to the ideal regimen to control blood pressure or regarding hypotensive alternatives in this period. In the same way, as during pregnancy, the choice of the hypotensive agent will depend on clinical experience [42] and it is reasonable to recommend that blood pressure should be controlled at levels below 140 × 90 mmHg.

References

1. Say L, Chou D, Gemmill A, Tuncalp O, Moller A-B, Daniels J, et al. Global causes of maternal death: a WHO systematic analysis. Lancet Glob Health. 2014;2:e323–33.
2. Valdiviezo C, Garovic VD, Ouyang P. Preeclampsia and hypertensive disease in pregnancy: their contributions to cardiovascular risk. Clin Cardiol. 2012;35:160–5.
3. ACOG Practice Bulletin No. 202: Gestational hypertension and preeclampsia. Obstet Gynecol. 2019;133(1):e1–e25.
4. ACOG Practice Bulletin No. 203: Chronic hypertension in pregnancy. Obstet Gynecol. 2019;133(1):e26–e50.
5. Flack JM, Calhoun D, Schiffrin EL. The new ACC/AHA hypertension guidelines for the prevention, detection, evaluation, and management of high blood pressure in adults. Am J Hypertens. 2018;31:133–5.
6. Malachias M, Souza W, Plavnik F, Rodrigues C, Brandão A, Neves M, et al. 7a Diretriz Brasileira De Hipertensão Arterial. Arq Bras Cardiol Arq Bras Cardiol. 2016;107(3 Suppl.3):1–83.
7. Maxwell MH, Waks AU, Schroth PC, Karam M, Dornfeld LP. Error in blood-pressure measurement due to incorrect cuff size in obese patients. Lancet. 1982;2:33–6.
8. Ramos JGL, Sass N, Costa SHM. Preeclampsia. Rev Bras Ginecol Obstet. 2017;39(9):496–512.
9. Pavan MV, Saura GE, Korkes HA, Nascimento KM, Madeira Neto ND, Davila R, et al. Similarity between blood pressure values assessed by auscultatory method with mercury sphygmomanometer and automated oscillometric digital device. J Bras Nefrol. 2012;34:43–9.
10. Yoshizaki CT, Baptista FS, Osmundo Junior G de S, et al. Hipertensão Arterial Sistêmica, In: Zugaib M, Francisco RPV, organizadores. Obstetrícia Zugaib. 3ª ed. São Paulo: Editora Manole; 2016. p. 886–97.
11. Thorsteinsdottir B, Kane GC, Hogan MJ, Watson WJ, Grande JP, Garovic VD. Adverse outcomes of renovascular hypertension during pregnancy. Nat Clin Pract Nephrol. 2006;2(11):651–6.
12. Roman A. Hypertensive disorders. In: Maternal-fetal evidence based guidelines. 3rd ed. Boca Raton: CRC Press Taylor & Francis Group; 2017. p. 1–23.
13. Imdad A, Yakoob MY, Siddiqui S, Bhutta ZA. Screening and triage of intrauterine growth restriction (IUGR) in general population and high risk pregnancies: a systematic review with a focus on reduction of IUGR related stillbirths. BMC Public Health. 2011;11 Suppl 3:S1.
14. Alfirevic Z, Stampalija T, Gyte GM. Fetal and umbilical Doppler ultrasound in normal pregnancy. Cochrane Database Syst Rev. 2010;(8):CD001450.
15. Rolnik DL, Wright D, Poon LC, O'Gorman N, Syngelaki A, de Paco MC, et al. Aspirin versus placebo in pregnancies at high risk for preterm preeclampsia. N Engl J Med. 2017;377:613–22.

16. Hofmeyr GJ, Lawrie TA, Atallah AN, Duley L, Torloni MR. Calcium supplementation during pregnancy for preventing hypertensive disorders and related problems. Cochrane Database Syst Rev. 2014;(6):CD001059.
17. Milne F, Redman C, Walker J, et al. The pre-eclampsia community guideline (PRECOG): how to screen for and detect onset of pre-eclampsia in the community. BMJ. 2005;330:576–80.
18. IBGE. Instituto Brasileiro de Geografia e Estatística, Coordenação de Trabalho e Rendimento. Pesquisa de Orçamentos Familiares: 2008–2009. Análise do Consumo Alimentar Pessoal no Brasil [Internet]. Biblioteca do Ministerio do Planejamento, Orçamento e Gestão. 2011. 150 p. Available at: http://biblioteca.ibge.gov.br/visualizacao/livros/liv50063.pdf.
19. Tranquilli AL, Dekker G, Magee L, Roberts J, Sibai BM, Steyn W, et al. The classification, diagnosis and management of the hypertensive disorders of pregnancy: a revised statement from the ISSHP. Pregnancy Hypertens. 2014;4:97–104.
20. Peraçoli JC, Borges VT, Ramos JG, Cavalli RC, Costa SH, Oliveira LG, et al. Pré-eclâmpsia/eclâmpsia. Rev Bras Ginecol Obstet. 2019;41:318–32.
21. Ukah UV, De Silva DA, Payne B, Magee LA, Hutcheon JA, Brown H, et al. Prediction of adverse maternal outcomes from pre-eclampsia and other hypertensive disorders of pregnancy: a systematic review. Pregnancy Hypertens. 2018;11:115–23.
22. ACOG. 1. First-trimester risk assessment for early-onset preeclampsia. Committee Opinion No. 638. American College of Obstetricians and Gynecologists. Obstet Gynecol. 2015;126:e25–7.
23. Maynard SE, Min JY, Merchan J, Lim KH, Li J, Mondal S, et al. Excess placental soluble fms-like tyrosine kinase 1 (sFlt1) may contribute to endothelial dysfunction, hypertension, and proteinuria in preeclampsia. J Clin Invest. 2003;111:649–58.
24. Levine RJ, Maynard SE, Qian C, Lim KH, England LJ, Yu KF, et al. Circulating angiogenic factors and the risk of preeclampsia. N Engl J Med. 2004;350:672–83.
25. Zeisler H, Llurba E, Chantraine F, Vatish M, Staff AC, Sennstrom M, et al. Predictive value of the sFlt-1:PlGF ratio in women with suspected preeclampsia. N Engl J Med. 2016;374:13–22.
26. Duley L, Henderson-Smart D, Meher S. Altered dietary salt for preventing pre-eclampsia, and its complications. Cochrane Database Syst Rev. 2005;(4):CD005548.
27. Meher S, Abalos E, Carroli G. Bed rest with or without hospitalisation for hypertension during pregnancy. Cochrane Database Syst Rev. 2005;19(4):CD003514.
28. Martin CL, Brunner Huber LR. Physical activity and hypertensive complications during pregnancy: findings from 2004 to 2006 North Carolina Pregnancy Risk Assessment Monitoring System. Birth. 2010;37:202–10.
29. Magee LA, von Dadelszen P, Rey E, Ross S, Asztalos E, Murphy KE, et al. Less-tight versus tight control of hypertension in pregnancy. N Engl J Med. 2015;372:407–17.
30. Siqueira F, Moura TR, Silva SS, Peraçoli JC. Medicamentos anti-hipertensivos na gestação e puerpério. Com Ciências Saúde. 2011;22(1):55–68.
31. Tanaka K, Tanaka H, Kamiya C, Katsuragi S, Sawada M, Tsuritani M, et al. Beta-blockers and fetal growth restriction in pregnant women with cardiovascular disease. Circ J. 2016;80:2221–6.
32. Contag SA, Bushnell C. Contemporary management of migrainous disorders in pregnancy. Curr Opin Obstet Gynecol. 2010;22:437–45.
33. Alexander EK, Pearce EN, Brent GA, Brown RS, Chen H, Dosiou C, et al. 2017 guidelines of the American Thyroid Association for the diagnosis and management of thyroid disease during pregnancy and the postpartum. Thyroid. 2017;27:315–89.
34. Su C-Y, Lin H-C, Cheng H-C, Yen AM-F, Chen Y-H, Kao S. Pregnancy outcomes of anti-hypertensives for women with chronic hypertension: a population-based study. PLoS One. 2013;8:e53844.
35. Committee Opinion No. 623: Emergent therapy for acute-onset, severe hypertension during pregnancy and the postpartum period. Obstet Gynecol. 2015;125:521–5.
36. Shekhar S, Sharma C, Thakur S, Verma S. Oral nifedipine or intravenous labetalol for hypertensive emergency in pregnancy: a randomized controlled trial. Obstet Gynecol. 2013;122:1057–63.

37. Raheem IA, Saaid R, Omar SZ, Tan PC. Oral nifedipine versus intravenous labetalol for acute blood pressure control in hypertensive emergencies of pregnancy: a randomised trial. BJOG. 2012;119:78–85.
38. Magee LA, Miremadi S, Li J, Cheng C, Ensom MHH, Carleton B, et al. Therapy with both magnesium sulfate and nifedipine does not increase the risk of serious magnesium-related maternal side effects in women with preeclampsia. Am J Obstet Gynecol. 2005;193:153–63.
39. Korkes H, Oliveira LG, Berlinck L, Borges AF, Sampaio Goes F, Watanabe S, et al. Human fetal malformations associated with the use of angiotensin II receptor antagonist. Pregnancy Hypertens. 2012;2:314–5.
40. Kang E, Sugarman R, Ramadan H, Mueller A, Shahul S, Perdigao JL, et al. Prevalence, risk factors and associated complications of postpartum hypertension in rural Haiti. Pregnancy Hypertens. 2017;10:135–42.
41. AlSaad D, ElSalem S, Abdulrouf PV, Thomas B, Alsaad T, Ahmed A, AlHail M. A retrospective drug use evaluation of cabergoline for lactation inhibition at a tertiary care teaching hospital in Qatar. Ther Clin Risk Manag. 2016;12:155–60.
42. Ghuman N, Rheiner J, Tendler BE, White WB. Hypertension in the postpartum woman: clinical update for the hypertension specialist. J Clin Hypertens. 2009;11:726–33.
43. Sass N, Itamoto CH, Silva MP, Torloni MR, Atallah NA. Does sodium nitroprusside kill babies? A systematic review. Sao Paulo Med J. 2007;125(2):108–11.
44. David MLDC, Rahe PS, Campos VAP, Silva MLRB, Marques F, Dom Bosco KC, et al. [144-POS]: comparative analysis of vaginal delivery among pregnant women with chronic arterial hypertension and normotensive pregnant women. Pregnancy Hypertens. 2015;5(1):74–5.
45. Witlin AG, Friedman SA, Sibai BM. The effect of magnesium sulfate therapy on duration of labor in women with mild preeclampsia at term: a randomized, double-blind, placebo-controlled trial. Am J Obstet Gynecol. 1997;176(3):623–7.
46. Cameron S. Postabortal and postpartum contraception. Best Pract Res Clin Obs Gynaecol. 2014;28:871–80.

Chapter 22
Pregestational Diabetes Mellitus

Lenita Zajdenverg and Carlos Antonio Negrato

Introduction

Diabetes mellitus (DM) results from relative or absolute deficiency of insulin action, leading to hyperglycemia, and a metabolic risk profile related to the development of atherosclerosis and microvascular complications [1]. The prevalence of DM, especially type 2 (T2D), has been increasing significantly and is currently considered to be an epidemic in most industrialized countries. It is estimated that approximately 16% of live births come from women who had some form of hyperglycaemia in pregnancy. Of these, 8% are from women with diabetes diagnosed before pregnancy [2]. Continuous changes in lifestyle, high rates of urbanization, lipids and calories-rich diets, and a sedentary lifestyle are some factors related to the increased prevalence of obesity and DM [3].

Pregnancy in women with a previous diagnosis of type 1 (T1D) or T2D can be associated with several complications, both maternal and fetal. These complications are directly associated with maternal glycemic control from very early stages of pregnancy (organogenesis) and also throughout the entire pregnancy [4, 5].

The increase in the number of pregnancies complicated by DM is a reality that can be already observed in routine clinical practice in health centers that offer prenatal care, leading to an increasing need for training professionals to deal with the specificities of these high-risk pregnancies.

L. Zajdenverg (✉)
Internal Medicine Department, Diabetes Division, Hospital Universitário Clementino Fraga Filho, Universidade Federal do Rio de Janeiro, Rio de Janeiro, Brazil

C. A. Negrato
Medical school from Faculdade de Odontologia de Bauru (FOB), Universidade de São Paulo, Bauru, São Paulo, Brazil
e-mail: negrato@usp.br

© Springer Nature Switzerland AG 2022

R. A. Moreira de Sá, E. B. d. Fonseca (eds.), *Perinatology*,
https://doi.org/10.1007/978-3-030-83434-0_22

Classification of Diabetes Mellitus

The current classification of the type of pregestational diabetes was made based on the etiology of the metabolic dysfunction and some clinical characteristics can be useful to make the differential diagnosis (Table 22.1).

In a study conducted in the USA between 1994 and 2004, the occurrence of pregnancies complicated by pregestational diabetes was due to approximately 7% to T1D, 4.7% to T2D, and 3.6% to monogenetic diabetes (MODY) and other types [6].

Maternal Metabolism Adaptation Throughout Pregnancy

The fetus does not perform gluconeogenesis and has a constant requirement of energy supply, consequently, the demand for glucose is permanent even during periods of maternal fasting. The only energy sources for the fetus are glucose and amino acids, which cross the placenta by facilitated diffusion. Free fatty acids (FFA) are not able to cross the placental barrier. Thus, the glycemic levels of pregnant women,

Table 22.1 Etiological classification of pregestational diabetes mellitus—most frequent causes

	Etiopathogenesis	Clinical features
Type 1 (T1D)	Pancreatic beta-cell failure, usually immune-mediated, in genetically susceptible individuals	Tendency to ketoacidosis, insulin therapy is mandatory Association with other autoimmune pathologies can be observed
Type 2 (T2D)	Insulin resistance and impaired insulin secretion	Frequently associated with obesity and a positive family history of T2D In general, can be treated with oral antidiabetic drugs
Secondary	Pancreatic diseases (e.g., chronic pancreatitis, hemochromatosis, postpancreatectomy) Endocrinopathies (e.g., Cushing, pheochromocytoma)	Generally associated with signs or symptoms of the underlying pathologies
MODY (*maturity-onset diabetes of the young*)	Monogenetic Autosomal dominant	Several generations of the same family are commonly affected Diagnosis made before 25 years of age The use of insulin is not always necessary Glycosuria is not proportional to glycemia (MODY 3) Altered fasting glucose and normal or slightly elevated HbA1c (MODY 2)

during the fasting state, are approximately 15–20 mg/dL, lower than those observed outside pregnancy. Also, at the end of the first trimester, due to high estrogen levels, a transient increase in insulin sensitivity may occur, leading to an increased risk of maternal hypoglycemia, especially when nausea and vomiting are present [7].

From the second half of the gestational period, women's metabolism changes deeply. In the third trimester, peripheral insulin sensitivity falls between 40% and 60% when compared to the pregestational period and hepatic glucose production is found to be 30% higher than at the beginning of pregnancy. Lipolysis with greater availability of FFA also occurs [7].

Placental hormones, such as the placental lactogenic hormone (PLH) and the placental growth hormone (PGh), change maternal physiology and promote an environment with an increased insulin demand (Table 22.2). Due to its anti-insulin and lipolytic action, PLH has a fundamental role in metabolic changes. There is also a contribution of elevated levels of estrogens, progesterone, cortisol, and prolactin, making pregnancy a physiologic state of insulin resistance [8].

Pregnancy Affecting Diabetes and Its Complications

Diabetic Ketoacidosis

Hyperglycemia, metabolic acidosis, and ketosis characterize ketoacidosis [9]. The incidence of ketoacidosis during pregnancy varies from 0.5% to 10% and generally has serious consequences for the mother and the fetus [10]. It occurs predominantly in patients with T1D and may occur less frequently in those with T2D and gestational diabetes [10].

Ketoacidosis is a result of a relative or absolute deficiency of insulin secretion associated with increased secretion of counter-regulatory hormones such as cortisol, glucagon, and epinephrine, resulting in a hyperglycemic state, due to increased hepatic gluconeogenesis and decreased glucose utilization by the muscles. Consequently, there is an increase in lipolysis with increased levels of fatty acids in the circulation, which are oxidized, and lead to the formation of acetyl-coenzyme

Table 22.2 Congenital anomalies related to maternal diabetes

Caudal regression
Spina bifida, hydrocephalus, variable defects in the central nervous system
Anencephaly
Various cardiovascular anomalies
Anal/rectal atresia
Renal agenesis
Renal cyst
Ureter duplication
Situs inversus

A which is, in turn, converted into ketone bodies (β-hydroxy-butyrate and acetoacetate). An osmotic gradient occurs and consequently polyuria, dehydration, hypovolemia, osmotic diuresis, with consequent hyponatremia and intracellular potassium depletion [10–13].

The second and third trimesters are the periods when most cases of diabetic ketoacidosis occur, due to a significant decrease in insulin sensitivity with the need to increase insulin doses at approximately 50% [13]. The presence of infection, use of corticosteroids, undiagnosed diabetes, nonadherence to treatment, failures in the continuous subcutaneous insulin infusion (CSII) pump, use of sympathomimetic drugs, incoercible vomiting, and diabetic gastroparesis are precipitating factors for ketoacidosis in pregnancy [9–14].

The onset of diabetic ketoacidosis in pregnancy can be insidious, usually at lower glucose levels, and often progresses more quickly compared to nonpregnant women. Diabetic ketoacidosis in pregnancy can occur with not-so-high blood glucose levels and even in a state of euglycemia, due to increased ketogenesis, especially in late pregnancy [13, 14].

The most characteristic clinical presentation of ketoacidosis is the presence of abdominal pain, nausea, vomits, and altered conscience. Laboratory findings include low arterial pH (less than 7.3), low serum bicarbonate level (less than 15 mEq/L), high anion gap, and positive serum ketones [10, 15].

The treatment of diabetic ketoacidosis in pregnancy does not differ substantially from that performed outside pregnancy. Hydration and intravenous electrolyte replacement should be instituted as early as possible. Insulin therapy should be started after ensuring that the patient has an adequate rehydration. Initially, a bolus of 10–15 U of regular insulin EV or 0.2–0.4 U/kg is recommended and then intravenous infusion at 2–10 U/h should be offered [10].

During diabetic ketoacidosis, fetal heart rate may show minimal variability and late decelerations. This pattern usually disappears as the maternal condition improves and delivery should not be indicated in the presence of metabolic acidosis.

Ketoacidosis in pregnancy can be prevented by educating patients who, in case of blood glucose >200 mg/dL, mainly associated with the presence of precipitating factors, should intensify the number of self-monitoring of blood glucose, increase insulin doses, and ensure adequate intake of liquids.

Hypoglycemia

Hypoglycemia is a complication of pregnancy, found mainly in patients with T1D (about 18–40% of patients) [16], that occur more frequently during the dawn and in the first trimester [17]. Current guidelines have been recommending lower and lower blood glucose levels during pregnancy, which has led to an increased risk of severe hypoglycemia.

The production of counter-regulatory hormones such as cortisol, glucagon, and epinephrine is impaired in pregnancy [18]. Therefore, patients should perform daily and frequent self-monitoring of their blood glucose in order to detect asymptomatic hypoglycemia. Family members should be instructed to recognize the signs and symptoms of hypoglycemia as early as possible, and they must also know how to proceed and how to provide first aid, in order to avoid serious hypoglycemic crises [18].

The main risk factors leading to hypoglycemia are a previous history of hypoglycemia or poor adherence to treatment [18]. Efforts should be made to determine the underlying causes of hypoglycemia; adjustments to insulin doses must be made, verification of the insulin injection technique, time schedule for insulin administration, and insulin storage conditions. Patients with recurrent hypoglycemia episodes should be observed as to the possibility of being purposefully applying excessive doses of insulin, and in these cases, a psychiatric evaluation and follow-up are necessary [18]. The presence of adrenal insufficiency should be ruled out in pregnant women with T1D, especially in cases of recurrent hypoglycemia, hypotension, and nausea.

Blood glucose levels <60 mg/mL, in the presence or not of tremors, sweating, and tachycardia, should be treated immediately. Although in episodes of mild hypoglycemia, there is little maternal and/or fetal damage [19], those more severe and long-lasting cases can lead to coma or seizures. The increased frequency of maternal hypoglycemia has been linked to complications in the fetus such as increased abortion rates [6], as well as in animal models, when fetal growth restriction, increased neural tube defects, and changes in heart rhythm can be found [20].

Treatment of hypoglycemia varies according to the patient's state of consciousness. If she is conscious, 15–20 g of fast-absorbing carbohydrates should be offered orally (e.g., one tablespoon of sugar dissolved in 150 mL of water or 150 mL of orange juice). If the patient is unconscious or is in a hospital environment, an equivalent amount should be injected intravenously with hypertonic glucose (30–40 mL of 50% hypertonic glucose). In both situations, capillary blood glucose should be reevaluated 15 min after treatment and, if hypoglycemia persists, the therapy with glucose should be repeated. Once euglycemia is achieved, the patient should eat a snack to prevent its recurrence [21].

Diabetic Kidney Disease

Pregnancy leads to a 30–50% increase in kidney flow and in glomerular filtration and many pregnant women with diabetes kidney disease may initially show an improvement in creatinine clearance and worsening in proteinuria. From the third trimester on, due to an increase in peripheral vascular resistance, women with microangiopathy may progress with a decline in glomerular filtration rate, increased blood pressure levels, and finally preeclampsia [22, 23]. The assessment of creatinine clearance, the search for microalbuminuria and proteinuria in urine collected in a 24 h period should be performed in women with pregestational diabetes, ideally before pregnancy and every trimester [24]. Pregnant women with diabetic kidney disease are at increased risk of premature births, worsening of hypertension, and preeclampsia. The presence of diabetic kidney disease worsens the prognosis of pregnancy with a high risk of neonatal death, delayed intrauterine growth, and abortion [22, 25]. Pregnancy after kidney transplantation has a lower perinatal risk when compared to women undergoing dialysis.

Retinopathy

Diabetic retinopathy results from an insult to the microvasculature due directly or indirectly by the glucotoxic effect and by inflammatory and oxidative stress processes. Different stages of progression of retinal involvement in diabetes are recognized, from mild forms to the proliferative stage, characterized by the presence of vascular neoformation and risk of amaurosis due to vitreous hemorrhage or retinal detachment.

The risk of diabetic retinopathy progression during pregnancy is greater in women with long-standing diabetes and in those who have already had preproliferative and proliferative retinopathy preceding gestation [26]. Ideally, women with diabetes should be evaluated in the preconception stage and subsequently every 3 months during pregnancy [24]. The role of laser treatment in slowing the progression of diabetic retinopathy is well recognized as has been shown in the Diabetic Retinopathy Study [27] and in the Early Treatment Diabetic Retinopathy Study [28]. Laser treatment is indicated during pregnancy for women with severe retinopathy [27, 28]. The role of antivascular endothelial growth factor (VEGF) in pregnancy is still controversial. There are case reports suggesting that they may be involved in preeclampsia [29]. Transpelvic delivery should be contraindicated in these women due to the risk of vitreous hemorrhage and retinal detachment.

Neuropathy

The current prevalence of diabetic neuropathy is unknown due to the different criteria used to define the involvement of the nervous system in this population. Long-term diabetes, inadequate diabetes control, and alcoholism are some factors that increase the risk of developing neuropathy [30].

The presence of autonomic neuropathy can be especially important during pregnancy. In the first trimester, hyperemesis may be exacerbated in women with diabetic gastroparesis [31]. The presence of a neurogenic bladder increases the risk of urinary tract infections. The presence of cardiovascular system dysautonomy may increase the risk of arrhythmias and intolerance to physical exercises, in which case cesarean delivery under strict cardiac monitoring is indicated.

Atherosclerotic Cardiovascular Disease

Mortality due to atherosclerotic cardiovascular disease, compared to the nondiabetic population, is three to ten times higher in individuals with T1D and two times and four times higher in men and women with T2D, respectively [32, 33]. Women older than 30 years and who have other risk factors associated with nephropathy should undergo stress testing before conception [34].

The incidence of atherosclerotic cardiovascular disease in diabetic pregnant women has not been described. Cardiovascular evaluation is difficult to perform during pregnancy. Scintigraphy and angiography are contraindicated and exercise testing is limited in this period. Maternal mortality is high in women with atherosclerotic cardiovascular disease and in cases of strong clinical suspicion of acute coronary insufficiency, after maternal stabilization, termination of pregnancy is indicated [35].

Dyslipidemia

Lipid metabolism changes during pregnancy. A 50% increase in total and High-density lipoprotein (HDL) cholesterol and a 100% increase in triglycerides are found; also an increase in HDL cholesterol occurs during midpregnancy. These values return to baseline after pregnancy [36]. If the patient did not perform a lipid profile before pregnancy, it should be made at the initial visit since it helps to recognize those patients at increased risk of hypertriglyceridemia, mainly those with poor glycemic control and albuminuria [37].

Patients with T1D show similar lipid changes during pregnancy, with a less pronounced increase in HDL in midpregnancy [38].

Patients with T1D and albumiburia and retinopathy generally present higher cholesterol and triglycerides levels than those patients who do not have any complications [39].

Medical nutrition therapy should be provided and tailored to each individual patient; in general, they should be counseled to reduce saturated fat intake to <7% of the total caloric intake, to eliminate trans fat and if there is no contraindication, start a physical activity program. Patients with extremely high levels of triglycerides (>1000 mg/dL), which is rare in patients with T1D, can be prescribed with ômega 3 fatty acids in order to prevent pancreatitis [40].

Diabetes Affecting Pregnancy

Maternal Risks

The rate of indication for cesarean delivery is higher in pregnant women with pregestational diabetes compared to nondiabetic ones [41]. The increased incidence of polyhydramnios is associated with the risk of premature births. Preeclampsia is observed in 15–20% of pregnancies complicated by T1D without nephropathy and in approximately 50% with nephropathy [42].

Women with obesity and T2D are more likely to experience obstructive sleep apnea. The presence of apnea is associated with worse glycemic profiles and insulin resistance and the risk of gestational hypertension, preeclampsia, premature birth, and greater need for neonatal intensive care. It is recommended to look for the presence of obstructive sleep apnea in overweight or obese women planning pregnancy [43].

Fetal Risks

Observational studies show an increased risk of embryopathy, especially anencephaly, microcephaly, congenital heart disease, and caudal regression syndrome, directly proportional to elevations in HbA1c during the first 10 weeks of pregnancy [44, 45] (Table 22.2).

Other fetal complications that can occur in pregnancies complicated by diabetes are as follows.

- Macrosomia: it is related to fetal hyperinsulinemia, maternal obesity, genetic factors, among others, and is probably the most significant problem of pregnancy complicated by diabetes. It is defined as birth weight above 4 kg or above the 90th percentile for gestational age in term pregnancies and increases the risk of shoulder dystocia and brachial plexus injuries [46, 47].
- Intrauterine growth retardation: it can occur in more severe cases of diabetes in which there is a decrease in placental blood flow.
- Neonatal hypoglycemia: it is defined as glycemic values lower than 40 mg/dL in the first 5 h after delivery, maintaining up to 2–3 days of life. It results from fetal hyperinsulinemia due to maternal hyperglycemia and is mild and uncommon in pregnant women who remain euglycemic, especially during labor [48]. It can lead to seizures, coma, and brain damage if left untreated.
- Polycythemia and hyperviscosity: occur in 5–10% of the children of diabetic mothers and result from a potent stimulus for fetal erythropoiesis secondary to hyperglycemia. They can lead to renal vein thrombosis [49].
- Others: hypercalcemia, hyperbilirubinemia (due to hyperinsulinemia and hypoxemia), respiratory distress syndrome.

Future Risks to the Conceptus

Children born to mothers who had diabetes also have an increased future risk of having metabolic diseases, such as obesity, T2M, and metabolic syndrome. Maternal glucose freely crosses the placenta and, as a consequence, maternal hyperglycemia leads to intrauterine hyperglycemia, which leads to fetal hyperinsulinemia with implications for future fetus growth and metabolism [50].

Before Conception Care

The need for pregnancy planning in women of childbearing age who have diabetes should be addressed frequently, regardless of the presence or absence of sexual activity.

Ideally, women with diabetes should, when conceiving, have excellent glycemic control, evaluated through HbA1c levels, that should be measured by high-performance liquid chromatography (HPLC) or a methodology in line with the National Glycohemoglobin Standardization Program. Due to the high risk of developing fetuses with cardiac malformations, patients whose HbA1c are 10% above the reference value should be strongly discouraged from becoming pregnant until their blood glucose improves [51].

In addition, careful assessment of the risk of hypertension, retinopathy, nephropathy, and peripheral neuropathy is necessary.

In all women with T1D, the presence of thyroid dysfunction should be assessed dosing free T4, TSH, and antithyroperoxidase antibodies. The prevalence of autoimmune thyroid disease in women with T1D of childbearing age can be around 44% [52, 53]. Untreated hypothyroidism increases the risk of infertility and miscarriage [52, 53]. Patients with hypothyroidism and Hashimoto's disease should have their TSH levels measured every 4–6 weeks during pregnancy through the 30th week. Levothyroxine doses should be increased, usually between the 6th and 20th week of pregnancy. If a change in LT4 doses is made, a new measurement of serum TSH should be performed after 4 weeks. After delivery, levothyroxine doses should generally return to those used before the pregnancy.

Treatment of Pregnant Women with Pregestational Diabetes

Due to the complexity of the treatment of pregnant women with pregestational diabetes, it is ideal to refer the patient to a specialized center that offers a multidisciplinary team approach experienced in the management of pregnant women with diabetes [1].

Nutritional Therapy

Nutrition therapy must be individually tailored. Nutritional therapy is based on the assessment of weight at the beginning of pregnancy, gestational weight gain, eating habits, accessibility to food, regional dietary characteristics, and the pregnant's clinical, socioeconomic, and cultural conditions. The amount of calories prescribed should also be based on body mass index (BMI) and the frequency and intensity of physical exercise [54].

Gestational weight gain should be monitored at each visit. The adequacy of the weight gain is based on the pregestational BMI (Table 22.3) and adjustments in nutritional therapy must be made, mainly to avoid excessive weight gain and the consequent increased risk of developing large for gestational age babies [55].

During the gestation of women with pregestational diabetes, food intake should be controlled in order to ensure strict glycemic control and avoid excess or inadequate weight gain. Inadequate carbohydrate intake, which can lead to hunger and ketosis, should be avoided. To minimize the risk of diabetic ketoacidosis, women are advised to consume a daily minimum of 175 g of carbohydrates [1].

The doses and times of insulin administration must be appropriate to the content of nutrients provided at each meal. In general, it is necessary to split the food intake into three large and three small meals [56]. Dinner is a meal of great importance, especially for women who use neutral protamine Hagedorn (NPH) at night, and it must contain at least 25 g of complex carbohydrates, in addition to proteins or lipids, to avoid hypoglycemia during the night.

The carbohydrate counting technic is a widely recognized nutritional strategy for people with T1D. It helps to avoid hyper- and hypoglycemia, as it tries to combine the amount of carbohydrates consumed in the meal with the prandial dose of insulin and makes food options more flexible for a given patient [57]. As pregnancy progresses, there is an increase in insulin resistance, so adjustments in the relationship between the insulin dose and the amount of carbohydrates ingested are necessary [58].

Table 22.3 Weekly and total gestational weight gain ranges (kg) recommended until term, according to the pregestational body mass index (BMI) [54]

Pregestational BMI (kg/m^2)	Total weight gain (kg) until the 14th week	Weekly weight gain (kg) during 2° and 3° trimesters (from the 14th week on)	Total gestational weight gain (kg)
Low weight < 18.5	1.0–3.0	0.51 (0.44–0.58)	12.5–18.0
Adequate weight between 18.5 and 24.9	1.0–3.0	0.42 (0.35–0.50)	11.5–16.0
Overweight between 25.0 and 29.9	1.0–3.0	0.28 (0.23–0.33)	7.0–11.5
Obesity ≥ 30.0	0.2–2.0	0.22 (0.17–0.27)	5.0–9.0

Physical Activity

Exercise is an important adjuvant therapy in the treatment of diabetes during pregnancy. Physical activity is an effective method to increase peripheral insulin sensitivity in these women. Mild intensity activity can be indicated for previously sedentary pregnant women. Those who have previously practiced any kind of activity can do moderate-intensity exercises during pregnancy. Practice in overheated environments can lead to dehydration and should be avoided. Exercises that cause any impact should be done with caution to avoid osteoarticular injuries, which occur more frequently during pregnancy [59].

Glycemic response may differ depending on the intensity and duration of exercise. High-intensity activities cause greater release of counter-regulating hormones, which can lead to subtle elevations in blood glucose, while exercises of light to moderate intensity promote an immediate reduction in plasma glucose. In addition, longer physical activities are also associated with reduced plasma glucose [60]. Thus, in pregnant women using insulin, blood glucose response to exercise is highly variable based on the type of activity and time and requires monitoring of blood glucose and different insulin dose adjustments. Before conducting a physical activity session, it is necessary to assess the levels of glucose and ketones in the blood. The ideal time to start an exercise session is 2 h after the administration of fast-acting insulin or 8 and 10 h after the administration of the long-acting insulin [61].

The practice of physical exercises during pregnancy is contraindicated in cases of heart disease with hemodynamic impairment, restrictive lung disease, cervical incompetence or cerclage, multiple pregnancies with risk of premature delivery, persistent bleeding in the second and third trimesters, placenta previa after 26 weeks of gestation, premature aminiorrexis, and preeclampsia or uncontrolled systemic hypertension. Mild activity should be performed with great caution by pregnant women with morbid obesity, severe anemia (hemoglobin <10 mg/dL), smokers, or those with a history of spontaneous abortions and premature births [62].

Insulin

Insulin is the treatment of choice during pregnancy. The use of all oral hypoglycemic agents for the control of T2D should be avoided because data on the safety and efficacy of these drugs in pregnancy are scarce [24].

There are currently several types of available insulins. They can be classified as human (NPH and regular), that is, the molecule is identical to the insulin produced by the human pancreas, or insulin analogs (lispro, aspart, glulisine, glargine, detemir, and degludec) which are insulins with changes in their molecular arrangement that aim to modify its pharmacokinetics. In addition, insulins are classified according to their action profile as insulins with ultra-prolonged effect (Degludec, Glargine U300), prolonged (Glargine U100 and Detemir), intermediate (NPH), fast (regular), ultra-fast (lispro, aspart, glulisine), or faster (FIASP). There are also biphasic insulins that have a double, fast, and intermediate action profile (Table 22.4).

Some studies in pregnant women show that aspart and lispro insulin analogs promote better control of postprandial blood glucose with less hypoglycemia when compared to regular insulin [64, 65]. Regular, lispro, and aspart insulins are classified as category B. The ultrafast analog glulisine is classified as category C, due to the lack of studies in pregnant women.

The long-acting analog detemir is classified as category A for use in pregnancy. The use of insulin glargine is not recommended (C), although many previous reports show the safety of this insulin in pregnancy, there are no randomized controlled studies with this analog. The analog of ultra-prolonged action degludec is classified as category C, due to the lack of studies during pregnancy.

Insulin prescription must be individualized and frequent dose adjustments throughout pregnancy are commonly needed. Most of the time, multiple injections are necessary to avoid peaks of postprandial hyperglycemia in women with previous T1D or T2D, and adaptations throughout the gestation are necessary (Table 22.5).

The use of a continuous CSII is a therapeutic option during pregnancy. For the proper use of CSII, patients must be motivated and must understand the

Table 22.4 Most frequently used insulins, type of action, and FDA category for use in pregnancy [63]

Type of action		Action onset	Action peak	Duration	Category
Ultralent	Glargine 300 UI/mL	6 h	No	36 h	C
	Degludec	30–90 min	No	Up to 42 h	C
Long action	Glargine 100 UI/mL	2–4 h	No	20–24 h	C A
	Detemir	1–3 h	6–8 h	18–22 h	
Intermediate action	NPH	2–4 h	4–10 h	10–18 h	B
Rapid action	Regular	0.5–1 h	2–3 h	5–8 h	B
Ultrafast acting	Aspart	5–15 min	0.5–2 h	3–5 h	A
	Lispro	5–15 min	0.5–2 h	3–5 h	B
	Glulisine	5–15 min	0.5–2 h	3–5 h	C

Table 22.5 Particularities of insulin therapy during pregnancy [24]

In the first trimester of pregnancy, loss of glucose and gluconeogenesis substrates can lead to hypoglycemia. It is often necessary to reduce the current insulin dose by 10–20% in women with pregestational diabetes
On the 2nd and 3rd trimesters of pregnancy, there is a need to perform a gradual increase in insulin dose. Adjustments should be done weekly or every 15 days from the 30th week on
A reduction in the need for insulin, that is, occurrence of frequent episodes of hypoglycemia between 34th and 37th weeks is not expected in uncomplicated pregnancies and may indicate placental dysfunction or an increased risk of developing preeclampsia
The most commonly used regimens include NPH intermediate-acting insulin, two to three times a day, or a long-acting analog one to two times a day associated with preprandial administration of regular fast-acting insulin or ultra-fast analogs (lispro or aspart)
If corticosteroid therapy is indicated for tocolysis, the insulin dose should be increased by 30–50% and this dose should be maintained for up to 48 h after the last corticosteroid application [68]

carbohydrate count technic. Studies comparing CSII with multiple insulin doses during pregnancy did not find significant differences between both methods in gestational outcomes [66]. The potential benefits of the insulin pump include a decrease in the episodes of severe hypoglycemia, better glycemic control, and a more flexible lifestyle. Women with unstable T1D who are planning pregnancy can benefit from the use of CSII [67]. The potential disadvantages of CSII are the increased cost of the pump and its supplies and a risk of developing diabetic ketoacidosis when the system fails. Due to the risk of worsening glycemic control during the adaptation period, one should avoid starting therapy with CSII in the first trimester of pregnancy [24].

Glucose Monitoring and Goals

The goal of the treatment of diabetes in pregnancy is to achieve euglycemia without causing significant hypoglycemia. Patients should be encouraged to perform self-monitoring of blood glucose before and after meals, at bedtime and sporadically between 2 and 4 AM [24]. The use of continuous glucose monitoring (CGM) in real time may be indicated, especially in cases of pregnant women with high glycemic variability or in those at risk of asymptomatic hypoglycemia.

In 2017, a study compared women with T1D who were pregnant or planning to become pregnant and were using CGM to those who performed capillary blood glucose. Those patients on CGM spent more time on glycemic target and less time on hyperglycemia. Newborns had a lower incidence of large for gestational age babies, lower rates of hospitalizations in neonatal ICUs, less neonatal hypoglycemia, and shorter hospital stays, possibly because they were less exposed to maternal hyperglycemia [69].

Glycemic control during pregnancy is considered to be optimal when preprandial blood glucose values are between 65 and 95 mg/dL, with a peak of 1 h postprandial up to 140 mg/dL. In women at increased risk of hypoglycemia, these targets should be increased to a fasting blood glucose value of up to 99 mg/dL. The postprandial blood glucose values, 1 h after the start of meals are those that best reflect the values of the postprandial peaks assessed by CGM. The goals of glycemic control in pregnancy are shown in Table 22.6 [1]. During the night, glucose levels should not drop below 60 mg/dL. Ideally, average capillary glucose levels at dawn should be maintained at around 100 mg/dL [70].

In 2019, the International Consensus for the interpretation of CGM data in patients with diabetes was published, including data obtained during pregnancy

Table 22.6 Glycemic targets for pregestational diabetes [1]

Glycemic targetes for pregestational diabetes	Fasting mg/dL	1 h postprandial mg/dL	2 h postprandial mg/dL	Preprandial mg/dL	HbA1c
	60–100	<140	<120	60–100	<6%

Higher levels can be accepted when there is a risk for severe hypoglycemia

which suggested that for pregnant women with T1D who perform CGM, the ideal is to keep 70% of glucose measurements within the target (63–140 mg/dL), 25% above the target, 5% below the target, 4% below 63 mg/dL, and 1% below 54 mg/dL [71]. There is little data on CGM in pregnant women with T2D; a previous study has shown that pregnant women with T2D stay 1/3 of the time less in hyperglycemia than those with T1D and reach 90% of the time on target [72].

HbA1c should be evaluated every 4 weeks until reaching the target of 6.0%. HbA1C less than 6% in the second and third trimesters is associated with a lower risk of large for gestational age babies [47].

Management of Arterial Hypertension

As pregestational diabetes is considered a high-risk factor for the development of preeclampsia, it is indicated the prophylatic use of low-dose aspirin (81 mg/day). Ideally, aspirin should be started before the 16th week of pregnancy and maintained until delivery [24].

Management of hypertension should start before pregnancy. During pregnancy, antihypertensive drugs should be initiated to treat chronic hypertension, but not preeclampsia or gestational hypertension. Those patients that become pregnant in use of antihyperetensive drugs should change the drugs, they are using to drugs that are safe to be used during gestation. Each of the classes of antihypertensive pharmacologic agents has specific mechanisms of action by which they exert their antihypertensive effect. The most commonly used and safe first-line agents include labetalol, nifedipine, and methyldopa. Methyldopa shows noninferiority to labetalol in preventing adverse maternal and fetal outcomes [73]. Some drugs should be avoided such as atenolol, due to adverse fetal outcomes, mostly fetal apnea, bradycardia, and hypoglycemia with the former drug [74]. The safety of the use of diuretics during pregnancy is controversial and studies comparing thiazides with placebo in pregnancy have not shown a significant difference in preeclampsia, preterm births, or SGA [75]. ACE-Is and ARBs, when used during the second and third trimesters are associated with fetopathy [76]. When severe hypertension is present, nifedipine can be used [77].

Blood pressure goals for hypertensive patients and for those who are under antihypertensive therapy are a systolic blood pressure of 110–129 mmHg and a diastolic blood pressure of 65–79 mmHg [1, 78]. The targets for blood pressure for pregnant women with DM were defined based on data from nonpregnant women with diabetes and from pregnant women without diabetes.

When comparing tight blood pressure control (<140/90 mmHg) vs very tight control (<130/80 mmHg) in women without diabetes, the former group presented lower rates of severe hypertension, of hospitalizations, longer gestational age, and no difference in preterm birth and on birth weight [79]. However, blood pressure targets cannot be very stringent, since very low blood pressure levels have been associated with fetal growth restriction and higher rates of mortality [80].

A review of RCTs showed that a fall of around 50% in the development of severe hypertension and no better results in all other outcomes were related to the use of antihypertensive drugs in pregnancy [81].

Monitoring Fetal Well-Being

The screening for malformations should be carried out between the 18th and 20th weeks of pregnancy through a morphological ultrasound with special attention to the cardiac structures and the large fetal vessels.

Fetal echocardiography, when available, should be performed.

Fetal monitoring with nonstress tests and biophysical profiles should be performed at frequent intervals (usually once or twice a week) from the 32nd week of gestation or earlier in pregnant women with vascular complications [24].

Delivery

The American College of Obstetricians and Gynecologists recommends delivery at 39 0/7 weeks to 39 6/7 weeks of gestation in women without vascular complications and with well-controlled blood glucose values but recommends earlier delivery at 36 0/7–38 6/7 weeks if women have vascular complications or poor glycemic control [24].

Postpartum Care

Immediately after delivery, with the removal of the placenta, insulin sensitivity increases significantly. Insulin requirements in the immediate postpartum period are approximately 34% less than the nonpregnant period [82]. Insulin requirements decrease rapidly after delivery. It is recommended that in the first few days, the total insulin dose should be reduced to 1/3 or 1/2 of the dose before delivery. Women on continuous insulin infusion therapy should generally reduce the total insulin infusion rate by approximately 50% [24].

Breastfeeding

Besides strengthening maternal–fetal bonding, breastfeeding brings many benefits to the mother and to the infant. In patients with DM breastfeeding is beneficial due to an increase in insulin sensitivity and a faster rate of weight loss [83]. Data regarding the benefits of breastfeeding in protecting individuals at risk for T1D against the disease are conflicting. Some studies show that early exposure to cow's milk proteins increases the risk for T1D and others do not show this association [84]. A reduction in the rates of overweight in children who were breastfed has been also shown [85]. The rates of breastfeeding in women with T1D are lower than in the general population [86], generally due to higher rates of cesarian section found in this group and longer stay of the infants in the intensive care units, difficult latching, insufficient lactogenesis, and hypoglycemia.

Women on insulin therapy should be advised of the risk of hypoglycemia during and after breastfeeding. The amount of carbohydrates lost is variable (on average after 21 days of breastfeeding, each 100 mL of breast milk contains 7.4 g of carbohydrate). It is safe for lactating mothers using insulin, to ingest 10–15 g of extra carbohydrates with each breastfeeding [87].

The use of oral antidiabetic drugs in patients with T2D who were previously on sulfonylurea and metformin use and who are breastfeeding may be considered. Studies with a small sample show that the presence of sulfonylureas was not detected, and only minimal amounts of metformin were observed in breast milk. Hypoglycemia was not observed in exposed babies [88].

Patients treating dyslipidemia should not use their medication in this period since lipid-lowering drugs risks outweigh their benefits in this time frame.

Contraception

Guidance on family planning should be part of the routine consultation of women with diabetes of childbearing age. Unfortunately, more than two-thirds of women with diabetes from various countries start their pregnancies without any preconception counseling [89].

Several contraceptive methods are currently available and the choice must be made based on the safety, efficacy, convenience, and adaptation of the woman and/or the couple.

Long-acting reversible contraceptives (LARC) are not dependent on the patient's memory and are highly effective, which can make them a good choice for women with diabetes. The methods include intrauterine copper device (IUD), injectable contraceptives with only progestogen, subdermal implants with only progestogens, and combined vaginal ring. WHO assessed the eligibility criteria for different contraceptive methods for women with diabetes (Table 22.7) [90].

Intrauterine devices (IUDs) are safe, effective, and do not interfere with maternal metabolism [90].

If the oral contraceptive is the choice, the combined pill with low doses of estrogen and progestogen may be the best option, as well as the sequential pill with ≤35 μg of estrogen and a new progestagen (levonorgestrel, desogestrel, gestodene, or norgestimate) in low doses, but the risk of proatherogenic changes in the lipid profile must be considered. [90]

The use of hormonal methods is contraindicated in women with a higher risk of developing thromboembolic events. [90]

Table 22.7 WHO classification for the use of contraceptives by women with diabetes [90]

(a) Women without complications <20 years of diabetes and nonsmokers	
Class	Contraceptive
1	Copper IUD Barrier method
2	Combined hormonal contraceptives Hormonal contraceptives progesterone only IUD with levonorgestrel

(b) Women with vascular complications and >20 years of diabetes	
Class	Contraceptive
1	Copper IUD
2	Hormonal contraceptives progesterone only IUD with levonorgestrel
3	Depot medroxyprogesterone acetate; Norethisterone enanthate
3/4	Combined hormonal contraceptives

1: Without any restrictions
2: Can usually be indicated
3: Use of the method generally not recommended, unless other more appropriate methods are not available or are not acceptable
4: Contraindicated method.

Pills containing only progestogens are an alternative but there is a possibility of increased serum lipid levels, in addition to other adverse effects.

Barrier methods, such as a diaphragm with spermicide or a condom, have a high degree of failure. When the offspring is complete, permanent sterilization, if allowed, of patients with diabetes or their partners can be a convenient means of preventing an unplanned pregnancy, compared to other contraceptive methods. [90]

References

1. American Diabetes Association. Management of diabetes in pregnancy: standards of medical care in Diabetes-2020. Diabetes Care. 2020;43(Suppl 1):S183–S92.
2. International Diabetes Federation. IDF Atlas. 9th ed. Bruxelas: International Diabetes Federation; 2019. Available at: https://diabetesatlas.org/upload/resources/material/20200224_151105_IDFATLAS9e-final-web.pdf.
3. Animaw W, Seyoum Y. Increasing prevalence of diabetes mellitus in a developing country and its related factors. PLoS One. 2017;12(11):e0187670.
4. Pregnancy outcomes in the diabetes control and complications trial. The Diabetes Control Complications Trial Research Group. Am J Obstet Gynecol. 1996;174:1343–53.
5. Peterson C, Grosse SD, Li R, Sharma AJ, Razzaghi H, Herman WH, et al. Preventable health and cost burden of adverse birth outcomes associated with pregestational diabetes in the United States. Am J Obstet Gynecol. 2015;212:74.e1–9.
6. Albrecht SS, Kuklina EV, Bansil P, Jamieson DJ, Whiteman MK, Kourtis AP, et al. Diabetes trends among delivery hospitalizations in the U.S., 1994-2004. Diabetes Care. 2010;33(4):768–73.

7. Ryan EA. Hormones and insulin resistance during pregnancy. Lancet. 2003;362:1777–8.
8. Barbour L. New concepts in insulin resistance of pregnancy and gestational diabetes: long-term implications for mother and offspring. J Obstet Gynaecol. 2003;23(5):545–9.
9. Kitabchi AE, Umpierrez GE, Murphy MB, Kreisberg RA. Hyperglycemic crises in adult patients with diabetes: a consensus statement from the American Diabetes Association. Diabetes Care. 2006;29:2739–48.
10. Dalfrà MG, Burlina S, Sartore G, Lapolla A. Ketoacidosis in diabetic pregnancy. J Matern Fetal Neonatal Med. 2016;29(17):2889–95.
11. Foster DW, McGarry JD. The metabolic derangements and treatment of diabetic ketoacidosis. N Engl J Med. 1983;309:159–69.
12. Laffel L. Ketone bodies: a review of physiology, pathophysiology and application of monitoring to diabetes. Diabetes Metab Res Rev. 1999;15:412–26.
13. Khoo CM, Lee KO. Endocrine emergencies in pregnancy. Best Pract Res Clin Obstet Gynaecol. 2013;27(6):885–91.
14. Johnston DG, Alberti KG. Diabetic emergencies. Clin Endocrinol Metab. 1980;9:437–60.
15. Bryant SN, Herrera CL, Nelson DB, Cunningham FG. Diabetic ketoacidosis complicating pregnancy. J Neonatal Perinatal Med. 2017;10(1):17–3.
16. Vargas R, Repke JT, Ural SH. Type 1 diabetes mellitus and pregnancy. Rev Obstet Gynecol. 2010;3:92–100.
17. Howorka K, Pumprla J, Gabriel M, et al. Normalization of pregnancy outcome in pregestational diabetes through functional insulin treatment and modular out-patient education adapted for pregnancy. Diabet Med. 2001;18:965–72.
18. Sullivan SA, Goodier C. Endocrine emergencies. Obstet Gynecol Clin N Am. 2013;40(1):121–35.
19. Whiteman VE, Homko CJ, Reece EA. Management of hypoglycemia and diabetic ketoacidosis in pregnancy. Obstet Gynecol Clin N Am. 1996;23(1):88–107.
20. Smoak IW, Sadler TW. Embryopathic effects of short-term exposure to hypoglycemia in mouse embryos in vitro. Am J Obstet Gynecol. 1990;163:619–24.
21. ter Braak EW, Evers IM, Willem Erkelens D, Visser GH. Maternal hypoglycemia during pregnancy in type 1 diabetes: maternal and fetal consequences. Diabetes Metab Res Rev. 2002;18(2):96–105.
22. Young EC, Pires ML, Marques LP, de Oliveira JE, Zajdenverg L. Effects of pregnancy on the onset and progression of diabetic nephropathy and of diabetic nephropathy on pregnancy outcomes. Diabetes Metab Syndr. 2011;5:137–42.
23. Bramham K. Diabetic nephropathy and pregnancy. Semin Nephrol. 2017;37(4):362–9.
24. ACOG Practice Bulletin No. 201: Pregestational diabetes mellitus. Obstet Gynecol. 2018;132(6):e228–48.
25. Nielsen LR, Damm P, Mathiesen ER. Improved pregnancy outcome in type 1 diabetic women with microalbuminuria or diabetic nephropathy: effect of intensified antihypertensive therapy? Diabetes Care. 2009;32(1):38–44.
26. Diabetes Control and Complications Trial Research Group. Effect of pregnancy on microvascular complications in the diabetes control and complications trial. The Diabetes Control and Complications Trial Research Group. Diabetes Care. 2000;23(8):1084–91.
27. Rahman W, Rahman FZ, Yassin S, Al-Suleiman SA, Rahman J. Progression of retinopathy during pregnancy in type 1 diabetes mellitus. Clin Exp Ophthalmol. 2007;35(3):231–6.
28. Early photocoagulation for diabetic retinopathy. ETDRS report number 9. Early Treatment Diabetic Retinopathy Study Research Group. Ophthalmology. 1991;98(5 Suppl):766–85.
29. Errera MH, Kohly RP, da Cruz L. Pregnancy-associated retinal diseases and their management. Surv Ophthalmol. 2013;58(2):127–42.
30. Massey EW, Guidon AC. Peripheral neuropathies in pregnancy. Continuum (Minneap Minn). 2014;20(1 Neurology of Pregnancy):100–14.
31. Feldman AZ, Brown FM. Management of type 1 diabetes in pregnancy. Curr Diab Rep. 2016;16(8):76.

32. Huxley RR, Peters SA, Mishra GD, Woodward M. Risk of all cause mortality and vascular events in women versus men with type 1 diabetes: a systematic review and meta-analysis. Lancet Diabetes Endocrinol. 2015;3:198–06.
33. Wexler DJ, Grant RW, Meigs JB, Nathan DM, Cagliero E. Sex disparities in treatment of cardiac risk factors in patients with type 2 diabetes. Diabetes Care. 2005;28:514–20.
34. Hagay Z, Weissman A. Management of diabetic pregnancy complicated by coronary artery disease and neuropathy. Obstet Gynecol Clin N Am. 1996;23:205–20.
35. Pacheco LD, Saade GR, Hankins G. Acute myocardial infarction during pregnancy. Clin Obstet Gynecol. 2014;57(4):835–43.
36. Busaran A. Pregnancy-induced hyperlipoproteinemia: review of literature. Reprod Sci. 2009;16(5):431–7.
37. Nasioudis D, Doulaveris G, Kanninen TT. Dyslipidemia in pregnancy and maternal-fetal outcome. Minerva Ginecol. 2019;71(2):155–62.
38. Göbl CS, Handisurya A, Klein K, Bozkurt L, Luger A, Bancher-Todesca D, et al. Changes in serum lipid levels during pregnancy in type 1 and type 2 diabetic subjects. Diabetes Care. 2010;33(9):2071–3.
39. Basu A, Alaupovic P, Wu M, Jenkins AJ, Yu Y, Nankervis AJ, et al. Plasma lipoproteins and preeclampsia in women with type 1 diabetes: a prospective study. J Clin Endocrinol Metab. 2012;97(5):1752–62.
40. Blumer I, Hadar E, Hadden DR, Jovanovič L, Mestman JH, Murad MH, et al. Diabetes and pregnancy: an endocrine society clinical practice guideline. J Clin Endocrinol Metab. 2013;98(11):4227–49.
41. Lin SF, Kuo CF, Chiou MJ, Chang SH. Maternal and fetal outcomes of pregnant women with type 1 diabetes, a national population study. Oncotarget. 2017;8(46):80679–87.
42. Sibai BM, Caritis S, Hauth J, Lindheimer M, VanDorsten JP, MacPherson C, et al. Risks of preeclampsia and adverse neonatal outcomes among women with pregestational diabetes mellitus. National Institute of Child Health and Human Development Network of Maternal-Fetal Medicine Units. Am J Obstet Gynecol. 2000;182(2):364–9.
43. Farabi SS, Barbour LA, Heiss K, Hirsch NM, Dunn E, Hernandez TL. Obstructive sleep apnea is associated with altered glycemic patterns in pregnant women with obesity. J Clin Endocrinol Metab. 2019;104(7):2569–79.
44. Ray JG, O'Brien TE, Chan WS. Preconception care and the risk of congenital anomalies in the offspring of women with diabetes mellitus: a meta-analysis. QJM. 2001;94(8):435–44.
45. Agha MM, Glazier RH, Moineddin R, Booth G. Congenital abnormalities in newborns of women with pregestational diabetes: a time-trend analysis, 1994 to 2009. Birth Defects Res A Clin Mol Teratol. 2016;106(10):831–9.
46. Oral E, Cağdaş A, Gezer A, Kaleli S, Aydinli K, Oçer F. Perinatal and maternal outcomes of fetal macrosomia. Eur J Obstet Gynecol Reprod Biol. 2001;99(2):167–71.
47. Cyganek K, Skupien J, Katra B, Hebda-Szydlo A, Janas I, Trznadel-Morawska I, et al. Risk of macrosomy remains glucose-dependent in a cohort of women with pregestational type 1 diabetes and good glycemic control. Endocrine. 2017;55:447–55.
48. Thompson Branch A, Havranek T. Neonatal hypoglycemia. Pediatr Rev. 2017;38(4):147–57.
49. Sarkar S, Rosenkrantz TS. Neonatal polycythemia and hyperviscosity. Semin Fetal Neonatal Med. 2008;13(4):248–55.
50. Negrato CA, Montenegro RM Jr, Mattar R, Zajdenverg L, Francisco RP, Pereira BG, et al. Dysglycemias in pregnancy: from diagnosis to treatment. Brazilian consensus statement. Diabetol Metab Syndr. 2010;2:27.
51. Ludvigsson JF, Neovius M, Söderling J, Gudbjörnsdottir S, Svensson A, Franzén S, et al. Periconception glycaemic control in women with type 1 diabetes and risk of major birth defects: population based cohort study in Sweden. BMJ. 2018;362:k2638.
52. Korevaar TIM, Medici M, Visser TJ, Peeters RP. Thyroid disease in pregnancy: new insights in diagnosis and clinical management. Nat Rev Endocrinol. 2017;13(10):610–22.

53. Alexander EK, Pearce EN, Brent GA, Brown RS, Chen H, Dosiou C, et al. 2017 guidelines of the American Thyroid Association for the diagnosis and management of thyroid disease during pregnancy and the postpartum. Thyroid. 2017;27(3):315–89.
54. Institute of Medicine, National Research Council. Weight gainduring pregnancy: reexamining the guidelines. Washington, DC: The National Academies Press; 2013.
55. Siegel AM, Tita A, Biggio JR, Harper LM. Evaluating gestational weight gain recommendations in pregestational diabetes. Am J Obstet Gynecol. 2015;213(4):563.e1–563.e5635.
56. Roskjær AB, Andersen JR, Ronneby H, Damm P, Mathiesen ER. Dietary advices on carbohydrate intake for pregnant women with type 1 diabetes. J Matern Fetal Neonatal Med. 2015;28(2):229–33.
57. Dafne Study Group. Training in flexible, intensive insulin management to enable dietary freedom in people with type 1 diabetes: dose adjustment for normal eating (DAFNE) randomized controlled trial. BMJ. 2002;325(7367):746.
58. Zagury RL, Rodacki M, Mello de Oliveira L, Saunders C, de Carvalho PP, Zajdenverg L. Carbohydrate counting during pregnancy in women with type 1 diabetes: are there predictable changes that we should know? Ann Nutr Metab. 2017;70:140–6.
59. Di Biase N, Balducci S, Lencioni C, Bertolotto A, Tumminia A, Dodesini AR, et al. Review of general suggestions on physical activity to prevent and treat gestational and pre-existing diabetes during pregnancy and in postpartum. Nutr Metab Cardiovasc Dis. 2019;29(2):115–26.
60. Fahey AJ, Paramalingam N, Davey RJ, Davis EA, Jones TW, Fournier PA. The effect of a short sprint on postexercise whole-body glucose production and utilization rates in individuals with type 1 diabetes mellitus. J Clin Endocrinol Metab. 2012;97(11):4193–200.
61. Colberg SR, Sigal RJ, Yardley JE, Riddell MC, Dunstan DW, Dempsey PC, et al. Physical activity/exercise and diabetes: a position statement of the American Diabetes Association. Diabetes Care. 2016;39(11):2065–79.
62. ACOG Committee. Opinion no. 650: physical activity and exercise during pregnancy and the postpartum period. Obstet Gynecol. 2015;126(6):e135–42.
63. Blum AK. Insulin use in pregnancy: an update. Diabetes Spectr. 2016;29(2):92–7.
64. Durnwald CP, Landon MB. A comparison of lispro and regular insulin for the management of type 1 and type 2 diabetes in pregnancy. J Matern Fetal Neonatal Med. 2008;21(5):309–13.
65. Pettitt DJ, Ospina P, Howard C, Zisser H, Jovanovic L. Efficacy, safety and lack of immunogenicity of insulin aspart compared with regular human insulin for women with gestational diabetes mellitus. Diabet Med. 2007;24(10):1129–35.
66. Farrar D, Tuffnell DJ, West J, West HM. Continuous subcutaneous insulin infusion ver-sus multiple daily injections of insulin for pregnant women with diabetes. Cochrane Database Syst Rev. 2016;(6):CD005542.
67. Yeh HC, Brown TT, Maruthur N, Ranasinghe P, Berger Z, Suh YD, et al. Comparative effectiveness and safety of methods of insulin delivery and glucose monitoring for diabetes mellitus: a systematic review and meta-analysis. Ann Intern Med. 2012;157:336–47.
68. Rowe CW, Putt E, Brentnall O, Gebuehr A, Allabyrne J, Woods A, et al. An intravenous insulin protocol designed for pregnancy reduces neonatal hypoglycaemia following betamethasone administration in women with gestational diabetes. Diabet Med. 2019;36(2):228–36.
69. Feig DS, Donovan LE, Corcoy R, Murphy KE, Amiel AS, Hunt KF, et al. On behalf of the CONCEPTT CollaborativeGroup. Continuous glucose monitoring in pregnant women with type 1 diabetes (CONCEPTT): a multicenter international randomized controlled trial. Lancet. 2017;390:2347–59.
70. Gabbe SG, Graves CR. Management of diabetes mellitus complicating pregnancy. Obstet Gynecol. 2003;102:857–68.
71. Battelino T, Danne T, Bergenstal RM, Amiel SA, Beck R, Biester T, et al. Clinical targets for continuous glucose monitoring data interpretation: recommendations from the international consensus on time in range. Diabetes Care. 2019;42(8):1593-03.
72. Murphy HR, Rayman G, Duffield K, Lewis KS, Kelly S, Johal B, et al. Changes in the glycemic profiles of women with type 1 and type 2 diabetes during pregnancy. Diabetes Care. 2007;30(11):2785–91.

73. Magee LA, CHIPS Study Group, von Dadelszen P, Singer J, Lee T, Rey E, Ross S, et al. CHIPS Study Group. Do labetalol and methyldopa have different effects on pregnancy outcome? Analysis of data from the Control of Hypertension In pregnancy study (CHIPS) trial. BJOG. 2016;123(7):1143–51.
74. Butters L, Kennedy S, Rubin PC. Atenolol in essential hypertension during pregnancy. BMJ. 1990;301:587–9.
75. Churchill D, Beevers GD, Meher S, Rhodes C, et al. Diuretics for preventing pre-eclampsia. Cochrane Database Syst Rev. 2007;(1):CD004451.
76. Diav-Citrin O, Shechtman S, Halberstadt Y, Finkel-Pekarsky V, Wajnberg R, Arnon J, et al. Pregnancy outcome after in utero exposure to angiotensin converting enzyme inhibitors or angiotensin receptor blockers. Reprod Toxicol. 2011;31:540–5.
77. Duley L, Meher S, Jones L. Drugs for treatment of very high blood pressure during pregnancy. Cochrane Database Syst Rev. 2013;(7):CD001449.
78. Kitzmiller JL, Block JM, Brown FM, Catalano PM, Conway DL, Coustan DR, et al. Managing preexisting diabetes for pregnancy: summary of evidence and consensus recommendations for care. Diabetes Care. 2008;31:1060–79.
79. El Guindy AA, Nabhan AF. A randomized trial of tight vs. less tight control of mild essential and gestational hypertension in pregnancy. J Perinat Med. 2008;36:413–8.
80. von Dadelszen P, Magee LA. Fall in mean arterial pressure and fetal growth restriction in pregnancy hypertension: an updated metaregression analysis. J Obstet Gynaecol Can. 2002;24(12):941–5.
81. Abalos E, Duley L, Steyn DW. Antihypertensive drug therapy for mild to moderate hypertension during pregnancy. Cochrane Database Syst Rev. 2014;(6):2.
82. Roeder HA, Moore TR, Ramos GA. Changes in postpartum insulin requirements for patients with well-controlled type 1 diabetes. Am J Perinatol. 2016;33:683–7.
83. Riviello C, Mello G, Jovanovic LG. Breastfeeding and the basal insulin requirement in type 1 diabetic women. Endocrine Pract: Off J Am Coll Endocrinol Am Assoc Clin Endocrinol. 2009;15:187–93.
84. Knip M, Åkerblom HK, Becker D, Dosch HM, Dupre J, Fraser W et al. TRIGR Study Group. Hydrolyzed infant formula and early β-cell autoimmunity: a randomized clinical trial. JAMA. 2014;311(22):2279–87.
85. Hummel S, Pflüger M, Kreichauf S, Hummel M, Ziegler AG. Predictors of overweight during childhood in offspring of parents with type 1 diabetes. Diabetes Care. 2009;32(5):921–5.
86. Schoen S, Sichert-Hellert W, Hummel S, Ziegler AG, Kersting M. Breastfeeding duration in families with type 1 diabetes compared tonon-affected families: results from BABYDIAB and DONALDstudies in Germany. Breastfeed Med. 2008;3:171–5.
87. Achong N, Duncan EL, McIntyre HD, Callaway L. The physiological and glycaemic changes in breastfeeding women with type 1 diabetes mellitus. Diabetes Res Clin Pract. 2018;135:93–01.
88. Feig DS, Briggs GG, Koren G. Oral antidiabetic agents in pregnancy and lactation: a paradigm shift? Ann Pharmacother. 2007;41(7):1174–80.
89. Diabetes and Pregnancy Group, France. French multicentric survey of outcome of pregnancy in women with diabetes with pregestational diabetes. Diabetes Care. 2003;26:2990–3.
90. WHO Medical Eligibility Criteria for Contraceptive Use; Geneva: 2015. Available from: http://www.who.int/reproductivehealth/publications/family_planning/mec-wheel-5th/en/.

Chapter 23
Acquired Thrombophilia in Pregnancy

André Luiz Malavasi and Daniela Aires Moreira

Introduction

The thrombophilia are coagulation disorders represented by the predisposition for thrombotic events: deep vein thrombosis and pulmonary embolism.

The major acquired thrombophilia in pregnancy are antiphospholipid syndrome (APS) and hyperhomocysteinemia.

Antiphospholipid Syndrome (APS)

The APS is an important disease related to obstetric morbidity. Its diagnostic criteria are defined by International Society on Thrombosis and Haemostasis. The investigation for APS should not be performed in situations of increased risk for false-positive or false-negative results, such as pregnancy or puerperium, acute thrombosis, and use of anticoagulation. When the criteria are not fulfilled but the clinical judgment is strongly suggestive, the treatment can be performed, as long as the empiric character of the diagnosis is evident to the couple.

As described by Hughes in 1983, APS is characterized by a state of hypercoagulability mediated by thrombogenic autoantibodies that trigger venous and arterial

A. L. Malavasi
Pérola Byington Hospital, São Paulo, Brazil

Hospital do Servidor Público Municipal de São Paulo, São Paulo, Brazil

International Society on Thrombosis and Haemostasis, São Paulo, Brazil

D. A. Moreira (✉)
University of Medical Sciences, João Pessoa, Paraíba, Brazil

Maternal Fetal Medicine Group, Nova Diagnóstico por Imagem, João Pessoa, Brazil

© Springer Nature Switzerland AG 2022

R. A. Moreira de Sá, E. B. d. Fonseca (eds.), *Perinatology*,
https://doi.org/10.1007/978-3-030-83434-0_23

thromboembolic events, in addition to recurrent fetal losses. Pregnant women with APS have a higher incidence of miscarriage, fetal death, fetal growth restriction (FGR), severe and early forms of hypertensive disease specific to pregnancy, prematurity, and placental abruption [1–3].

The APS has strict and well-defined diagnostic criteria, which follow the standardization of the International Society on Thrombosis and Haemostasis. The diagnosis is established when there is the presence of at least one clinical criterion associated with at least one laboratory criterion (Fig. 23.1) [4].

Clinical Criteria

1. *Vascular Thrombosis: one or more episodes of arterial, venous, or small vessel thrombosis in any tissue or organ, except for superficial venous thrombosis. It should be confirmed by imaging or histopathological evidence. On the histopathological confirmation, thrombosis should be present without evidence of inflammation of the vessel wall* [4].
2. *Pregnancy Morbidity*
   - *One or more unexplained deaths of a morphologically normal fetus, documented by ultrasound or macroscopic examination, at ten or more weeks of gestation* [4].

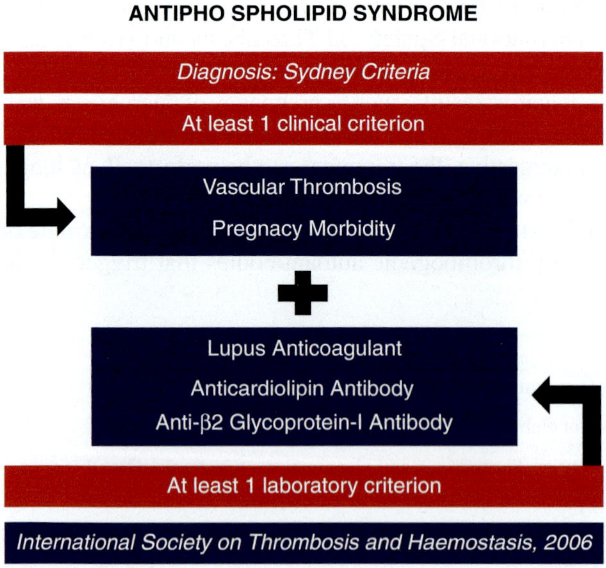

Fig. 23.1 Diagnosis of antiphospholipid syndrome

- *One or more premature births of a morphologically normal neonate before 34 weeks gestation because of severe preeclampsia, eclampsia, or placental insufficiency* [4].
- *Three or more consecutive spontaneous unexplained pregnancy losses before 10 weeks gestation, excluding maternal anatomical or hormonal causes and genetic alterations of the couple* [4].

Laboratory Criteria

1. *Lupus anticoagulant (LA) present in plasma, on two or more occasions at least 12 weeks apart, detected according to the guidelines of the International Society on Thrombosis and Haemostasis* [4].
2. *Anticardiolipin (aCL) antibody of IgG and/or IgM isotype in serum or plasma, present in moderate or high titer (>40 GPL or MPL units, or > the 99th percentile), on two or more occasions, at least 12 weeks apart, measured by a standardized ELISA* [4].
3. *Anti-β2 glycoprotein-I antibody of IgG and/or IgM isotype in serum or plasma (in titer > the 99th percentile), present on two or more occasions, at least 12 weeks apart, measured by a standardized ELISA* [4].

*The interval between the clinical event (vascular thrombosis or pregnancy morbidity) and the laboratory marker (LA, aCL, anti-β2-GPI) cannot be less than 12 weeks or more than 5 years [4].

Low titers of anticardiolipin antibody should be evaluated with caution, since 5% of normal pregnant women have antiphospholipid antibodies and, mostly, do not meet the criteria for APS, and most of these antibodies do not trend to thrombogenesis. Nonthrombogenic antiphospholipid antibodies can appear transiently and fleetingly after infections, traumas, thrombosis of other etiologies, use of medication, and even in relation to pregnancy itself [4].

When these antibodies are persistent and interfere with the function of phospholipids or phospholipid adhesion proteins, clotting regulation may be disturbed. The molecules that are usually involved or affected by the binding of antiphospholipid antibodies are β2-GPI, prostacyclin, protein C, annexin V, and tissue factor, which causes vascular or placental thrombosis, narrowing of the spiral arteries, intimal thickening, and fibrinoid necrosis of the placental bed [4].

Prenatal Care and Treatment

Patients with APS have an increased risk of thromboembolic events and early pregnancy loss and they should be advised to wear compression stockings throughout pregnancy, childbirth, and puerperium. They might also, whenever possible, plan pregnancies, starting the preconception use of aspirin 100 mg/day, which should be maintained throughout pregnancy [5]. The benefits of aspirin to patients with APS have not yet been confirmed in relation to other thrombophilia.

Women with a prior venous or arterial thrombosis and in use of oral anticoagulants should replace them with low molecular weight heparin (LMWH) as soon as pregnancy is confirmed. For those who plan to conceive and have regular menstrual cycles and access to a pregnancy test, as soon as there is a menstrual delay, they should choose the switch oral anticoagulants for heparin in full dose or 75% of this, when confirming pregnancy. On the other hand, in the case of patients with irregular cycles or difficulty in performing a pregnancy test, the change from oral anticoagulants to heparin can be done in the preconception period, and we must consider the cost and risk of heparin-induced thrombocytopenia and osteoporosis [5].

For the patients that do not make use of oral anticoagulants before pregnancy and prophylactic heparin is indicated, they should initiate its usage as soon as the transvaginal ultrasound of five to six weeks of gestational age confirms intrauterine viable pregnancy, with embryo cardiac activity [2].

For pregnant women with APS without a history of venous or arterial thrombosis, but with a previous history of obstetric morbidity (three early losses up to ten weeks or a late loss of ten weeks or more, severe pre-eclampsia or eclampsia, FGR, placental abruption, or placental insufficiency), the use of ASA (100 mg/day) in combination with a prophylactic dose of LMWH is indicated, that is, a single daily dose of enoxaparin (40 mg/day) or dalteparin (5000 U/day). Pregnant women with APS who do not respond positively to the association of AAS with LMWH may benefit from the use of hydroxychloroquine, gamma globulin, glucocorticoids, or plasmapheresis [6].

Heparins can cause immune thrombocytopenia (ITP), diagnosed by a platelet count below 100,000/mm [3] or by a 50% or more drop in the previous platelet count. ITP progresses with a paradoxical increase in the risk of thrombosis. This event, which occurs in less than 1% of pregnant women who use LMWH, motivates the accomplishment of control with a biweekly hemogram in the first month and then monthly for all patients who receive this medication [7].

Furthermore, heparins cause an increased risk of osteopenia and osteoporosis in pregnant women, with symptomatic vertebral fractures occurring in 0.5% of those women who use them for more than one month. To prevent this event, the recommendation is to increase the nutritional supply of calcium to 1.5 g/day with calcium carbonate supplementation [8].

Prenatal consultations should be monthly or every 2 weeks until the 20th week of pregnancy, changing to biweekly or weekly thereafter. Ultrasonography is requested at seven to eight weeks of gestational age, nuchal translucency ultrasound at the 12th week, and, subsequently, once a month [9].

Doppler velocimetry has a relevant role in the monitoring of pregnant women with thrombophilia, as it allows the evaluation of the placental vascular bed, which is the target of thrombosis. It must be started at nuchal translucency ultrasound exam from 11 to 13 weeks 6 days pregnancy, repeated around the 16th week, and followed every two to four weeks until 26 weeks of gestational age. If the Doppler values are normal, the exam will be repeated monthly from the 26th to the 34th week, but, if they are altered or there is a worsening of maternal clinical condition, it should be repeated at shorter intervals.

The use of LMWH during pregnancy, according to a systematic review of 64 studies that included 2777 pregnancies, reported a risk of severe bleeding in 0.43% of cases in the antepartum (95% CI: 0.22–0.75%), in 0.94% of the cases of postpartum hemorrhage (95% CI: 0.61–1.37%) and 0.61% of the cases of surgical wound hematoma (95% CI: 0.36–0.98%), with an overall risk of severe bleeding of 1.98% (95% CI: 1.50–2.57%) [10].

Management in Labor and Delivery

Aiming to enable the temporary discontinuation of the use of LMWH, delivery must be scheduled between 37 and 40 weeks. The use of ASA should be stopped one week before delivery and LMWH 12 hours before delivery if the dose is prophylactic or 24 hours before delivery if the dose is therapeutic, this approach will allow spinal or epidural anesthesia. The delivery route follows obstetric indications, and there is no contraindication for cervical ripening with prostaglandins or for induction of labor. In both vaginal delivery and cesarean sections, the patient should keep wearing compression stockings throughout the procedure.

Patients using heparin should be instructed not to administer the dose of the drug if they experience contractions or rupture of membranes and immediately go to their referral hospital.

Postpartum Care

In the puerperium, heparin should be reintroduced 6–8 hours after delivery (both vaginally and by caesarean section). The same is recommended for the reintroduction of ASA when its use is indicated. Early ambulation and the use of compression stockings should be encouraged [11, 12].

Hyperhomocysteinemia

Hyperhomocysteinemia is associated with a greater risk of venous and arterial thrombosis due to complex mechanisms that involve endothelial alterations, platelet functions, and fibrinolysis. Homocysteine is an intermediary product of the conversion of methionine into cysteine, which depends on the enzyme methylenetetrahydrofolate reductase (MTHFR). When MTHFR is deficient, homocysteine elevation may happen [13, 14].

The main defect of MTHFR is a punctual mutation (C677T), with the replacement of cytosine (C) with thymine (T) in the 677th nucleotide, which results in the substitution of alanine for valine, making MTHFR thermolabile and with lower enzymatic efficiency. It was later described as another alteration (A1298C), but there are no studies that connect it to unsatisfactory obstetric results [13].

Besides MTHFR, cystathionine β-synthetase (CBS) and B12 and B6 vitamins, as well as folic acid, are cofactors in the transformation of homocysteine in cysteine, and its deficiencies can also cause hyperhomocysteinemia [13–15].

Due to its frequent polymorphisms, MTHFR mutations should not be routinely tested. During pregnancy, homocysteine levels are considered normal if they measure up to 12 μmol/L. With levels from 15 to 30 μmol/L, it is considered moderate hyperhomocysteinemia; it is intermediate if levels vary from 31 to 100 μmol/L, and it is classified as severe if homocysteine levels are greater than 100 μmol/L [13–15].

The heterozygosis related to CBS is found in 0.3–1.4% of the population while heterozygosis related to MTHFR is found in about 11% of the individuals. Homozygosis related to these alterations, on the other hand, is rare, and it is associated with developmental delay, skeletal and neural tube defects, as well as thrombosis. However, it is the phenotype that results from these enzymatic defects, that is, hyperhomocysteinemia, that causes an increase in the risk of thromboembolism [16].

Folic acid, chemically named pteroylmonoglutamic acid, was initially described in 1945. Fifteen years before its discovery, the existence of a new hematopoietic factor in yeasts and liver extracts had already been described, which would have the ability to cure India's tropical macrocytic anemia. In 1941, to purify the extrinsic factor discovered in the liver capable of curing tropical India's macrocytic anemia—caused by vitamin B12 deficiency, another factor present in spinach leaves was obtained, which was not effective in the treatment of this kind of anemia, but it was responsible for stimulating the growth of *Streptococcus lactis*, and the nomenclature used for this unknown factor was folic acid, which derives from the Latin word *folium*—or simply leaf—due to its presence in predominantly leafy vegetables.

In the first half of the twentieth century, the synthesis of folic acid forms for the treatment of nutritional deficiencies and macrocytic anemia was identified, whereas in the second half of this century, the absorption and metabolism processes of this vitamin and its possible relation to other diseases such as cancer, cardiovascular diseases, and congenital malformations were discovered. Publications from the 1990s showed that the increased levels of homocysteine are associated with congenital neural tube defects, and in 1993, the American government started to recommend the adequate daily intake of folate to all women in fertile ages to reduce the risk of fetal malformations as spina bifida and other neural tube defects. The folates are present in almost every natural food of animal or vegetal origin, and they are mainly found in the form of polyglutamate. When the folates are oxidized, as, for instance, in the cooking of leafy vegetables, folate turns into folic acid. Folic acid's structure consists of the association of three important molecules: aminopterin, para-aminobenzoic acid (PABA), and glutamic acid [17–19].

Most of the folates naturally have a side chain of 3–11 peptide-linked glutamate residues. About 80% of the folate in food exists in the form of polyglutamate.

During gastrointestinal transport, polyglutamate is hydrolyzed to monoglutamate, reduced, and methylated. Folates, being predominantly polyglutamate, need to be hydrolyzed to monoglutamate to be absorbed in the small intestine. This process occurs at an optimal pH between 6 and 7; therefore, foods that alter the intestinal pH can cause an incomplete polyglutamate deconjugation and, consequently, a decrease in its bioavailability.

Folic acid, also known as the B9 vitamin, is water-soluble; it does not exist in a natural form and it has no biological activity, needing to be converted into dihydrofolate (DHF), tetrahydrofolate (THF), and finally, in methylfolate (MTHF), so this last one becomes biologically active. Folates act as coenzymes, mediating the transfer of carbon units and being able to act as receptors or donors of carbon units in a variety of critical reactions to the metabolism of nucleic acids and amino acids. They participate in two fundamental biological processes: They act as cofactors for the enzymes involved in the biosynthesis of ribonucleic acid (RNA) and deoxyribonucleic acid (DNA) and as a cofactor in the formation of methionine. Plasma folate is found mainly under the form of tetrahydrofolate; the main active form of the vitamin, which is a monoglutamate resulting from the reduction of pteroylglutamic acid (polyglutamate) from substitutions in positions 5 and 10 of the pteridine nucleus, this process being carried out in the liver [20].

From June 2002, the Brazilian Agency National Health Surveillance Agency (Anvisa) published in the Public Consultation no. 51, which became Resolution RDC no. 344 from December of the same year, the requirement to fortify wheat and corn flours and their by-products with folic acid, in which each 100 g of the product should provide a minimum amount of 150 mcg of the vitamin. Studies show that 70% of the cases of neural tube defects can be avoided with folic acid supplementation.

Folic acid is highly susceptible to oxidation, freezing, heating, and cooking with losses from 50% to 95% of the folate content on food during these processes. During the baking of bread made with laboratory enriched flour, there is a degradation of about 26% of the folic acid.

The foods with higher content of folates are greenery and vegetables, cereal, and fruits, whose values of folate vary between 20 and 160 μg/100 grams. In general, foods of animal origin have low levels of this vitamin, with the exception of the liver, which has higher concentrations.

The World Health Organization (WHO) has recognized in 2004 that the deficiencies of micronutrients are common among women in reproductive age, and that folate intake on the diet is insufficient in the general population, being unlikely that changes in eating patterns improve the state of serum folate concentration in the target populations.

Pregnant women with MTHFR enzyme mutation and hyperhomocysteinemia are at increased risk of recurrent fetal losses. A central feature of embryonic and fetal development is the generalized cell division, with folate playing a role in the synthesis of nucleic acids. During gestation, inadequate folate intake impairs cell division in the fetus and the placenta. Folate deficiency can occur because of low folate intake on diet or increased metabolic requirement for folate by specific genetic defects, like MTHFR mutation. During pregnancy, low concentrations of folate on nutrition and serum blood levels are associated with increased risks of premature childbirth, low weight at birth, and fetal growth retardation. A metabolic effect of folate deficiency is the elevation of blood serum homocysteine. Likewise, the presence of increased maternal concentrations of homocysteine has been associated with habitual spontaneous abortion and to pregnancy complications, like placental abruption and preeclampsia, which increases the risk of the pregnancy outcome and decreases the duration of pregnancy. The MTHFR mutation is related to an increased risk of autism, schizophrenia, heart disease, fetal neural tube defects, and colorectal cancer. Besides that, folate deficiency can cause glossitis, diarrhea, gastrointestinal injuries, and anemia.

The proper activity of the MTHFR enzyme is important for the conversion of 5,10-methylenetetrahydrofolate to 5-methyltetrahydrofolate (L-methylfolate), which is the main blood circulating folate. The L-methylfolate is involved in the recovery of homocysteine into methionine, with a decrease in homocysteine levels and the donation of methyl radicals, an essential step for the methylation of DNA strands, a process known as one-carbon metabolism. The lack of proper action of MTHFR in its two polymorphisms may cause hyperhomocysteinemia. There are two predominating MTHFR polymorphisms: C677T e A1298C. In general, 10% of the population is homozygous or compound heterozygous for these two polymorphisms.

Periconceptional use of supplements containing folic acid reduces the recurrence of neural tube defects. Intake of folate reduces the risks of pregnancy. Therefore, folate is a necessary vitamin in higher doses during pregnancy, playing an important role in preventing the formation of neural tube defects (anencephaly and spina bifida).

In addition to the prevention of neural tube defects, periconceptional supplementation with folic acid also appears to be beneficial in preventing congenital heart disease and cleft lip and it is possible that it also prevents premature birth. The mechanism by which folic acid prevents structural abnormalities in the fetus is not known, but it may involve regulating homocysteine metabolism.

Methylfolate is the biologically active form of folates, and, differently from folic acid, it is not toxic when ingested above the recommended dose. In addition, the use of methylfolate by pregnant women does not mask vitamin B12 deficiency. When administered orally, methylfolate reaches a serum level higher than the level reached by the intake of folic acid, even in women with MTHFR mutation.

However, because methylfolate is chemically volatile, it cannot undergo the process of cooking or freezing, which makes its usage as a food fortifier unfeasible. Remethylation of homocysteine in methionine requires, in addition to methylfolate, B6, and B12 vitamins. Excess of homocysteine is toxic and it is associated with thrombosis and cardiovascular events, abortion, preeclampsia, placental abruption, and FGR. Therefore, to work properly, methylation of DNA, or one-carbon metabolism, must rely on the organism's supply of methylfolate, B6, and B12 vitamins.

References

1. Hughes GRV. Hughes' syndrome: the antiphospholipid syndrome: a historical view. 1998. acesso accessed on em 23 Jul 2018. Disponível em Available at: http://www.lupus-support.org.uk/APS2.htm.
2. Di Prima FAF, et al. Antiphospholipid syndrome during pregnancy: the state of the art. J Prenat Med. 2011;5(2):41–53.
3. Galli M. Treatment of the antiphospholipid syndrome. Auto Immun Highlights. 2014;5(1):1–7.
4. Miyakis S, et al. International consensus statement on an update of the classification criteria for definite antiphospholipid syndrome (APS). J Thromb Haemost. 2006;4(2):295–306.
5. Montenegro CAB, et al. Rezende obstetrícia. 13th ed. Rio de Janeiro: Grupo Gen – Guanabara Koogan; 2017.
6. Del Papa N, et al. Management of antiphospholipid syndrome. Ther Adv Musculoskelet Dis. 2010;2(4):221–7.
7. Ahmed I, et al. Heparin induced thrombocytopenia: diagnosis and management update. Postgrad Med J. 2007;83(983):575–82.
8. Le Templier G, et al. Heparin-induced osteoporosis and pregnancy. Curr Opin Pulm Med. 2008;14(5):403–7.
9. Oliveira ALML, et al. Profilaxia de tromboembolismo venoso na gestação. J Vasc Bras. 2016;15(4):293–301.
10. Greer IA, et al. Low-molecular-weight heparins for thromboprophylaxis and treatment of venous thromboembolism in pregnancy: a systematic review of safety and efficacy. Blood. 2005;106(2):401–7.
11. Bates SM, et al. VTE, thrombophilia, antithrombotic therapy, and pregnancy: antithrombotic therapy and prevention of thrombosis, 9th ed: American College of Chest Physicians Evidence-Based Clinical Practice Guidelines. Chest. 2012;141(2 Suppl):e691S–736S.
12. Chan WS, et al. Venous thromboembolism and antithrombotic therapy in pregnancy. J Obstet Gynaecol Can. 2014;36(6):527–53.
13. Brustolin S, et al. Genetics of homocysteine metabolism and associated disorders. Braz J Med Biol Res. 2010;43(1):1–7.
14. U.S. National Library of Medicine (Genetics Home Reference). MTHFR gene: methylenetetrahydrofolate reductase. 2018. acesso accessed on em 23 Jul 2018. Available at Disponível em: https://ghr.nlm.nih.gov/gene/MTHFR.
15. Williams KT, et al. Homocysteine metabolism and its relation to health and disease. Biofactors. 2010;36(1):19–24.
16. Reitsma PH. Protein C deficiency: summary of the 1995 database update. Nucleic Acids Res. 1996;24(1):157–9.
17. Kim YI. Folate and colorectal cancer: an evidence-based critical review. Mol Nutr Food Res. 2007;51(3):267–92.
18. Koźmiński P, et al. Overview of dual-acting drug methotrexate in different neurological diseases, autoimmune pathologies and cancers. Int J Mol Sci. 2020;21(10):3483.
19. National Center for Biotechnology Information. PubChem Database. Folic acid, CID=135398658. acesso accessed on em 13 Jun 2020. Disponível em Available at: https://pubchem.ncbi.nlm.nih.gov/compound/Folic-acid.
20. Oregon State University. Folate. acesso acessed on em 13 Jun 2020. Disponível Available at em: https://lpi.oregonstate.edu/book/export/html/71.

Chapter 24
Hereditary Thrombophilia

Guilherme Ramires de Jesús, Flavia Cunha dos Santos, Marcela Ignacchiti Lacerda, Roger Abramino Levy, and Nilson Ramires de Jesús

During the pregnancy–puerperal cycle, the maternal organism undergoes several physiological changes. Among these are changes in blood coagulation, such as increased production of coagulation factors (I—fibrinogen, II—prothrombin, VII—proconvertin, VIII—antihemophilic factor A, X—Stuart, XII—Hageman), reduction in fibrinolytic activity leading to inhibition of fibrinolysis, and decreased activity of protein S [1]. Such changes cause a state of physiological hypercoagulability in pregnant women that can increase the chances of thrombotic events by five to ten times when compared with nonpregnant women of the same age group [2].

In addition, there are also pregnant women at risk for thromboembolic events in addition to intrinsic changes, such as those with thrombophilia, mechanical heart valve, recent events of arterial or venous thrombosis, pulmonary embolism, chronic atrial fibrillation, atrial enlargement, and stroke.

Thromboembolism is a major cause of maternal death, and in about 50% of cases of thrombosis in pregnancy, thrombophilia is identified [1]. Hereditary thrombophilias are described in Table 24.1.

Hereditary thrombophilias can be identified in approximately 10% of the Caucasian population and are responsible for about 50% of venous thromboembolic events during pregnancy, which makes the detection of these mutations relevant so that appropriate prophylactic measures are taken [3].

This group is composed of autosomal dominant genetic mutations that lead to a state of hypercoagulability, such as that of factor V Leiden (mFV) and the prothrombin gene mutation, in addition to deficiencies in natural anticoagulants such as proteins C and S and antithrombin. They can be divided, according to severity, into

G. R. de Jesús (✉) · F. C. dos Santos · M. I. Lacerda · N. R. de Jesús
Department of Obstetrics, Universidade do Estado do Rio de Janeiro, Rio de Janeiro, Rio de Janeiro, Brazil

R. A. Levy
Immunology and Inflammation, GlaxoSmithKline (GSK), Upper Providence, PA, USA

© Springer Nature Switzerland AG 2022

R. A. Moreira de Sá, E. B. d. Fonseca (eds.), *Perinatology*,
https://doi.org/10.1007/978-3-030-83434-0_24

Table 24.1 Hereditary thrombophilia

Hereditary	Factor V mutation (G1691A) Prothrombin gene mutation (G20210A) Protein S deficiency Protein C deficiency Antithrombin deficiency

low and high risk, which is essential to establish its thrombogenic potential and thromboprophylaxis during pregnancy, as will be discussed below.

Leiden's factor V is the most common cause of venous thromboembolism (VTE) in pregnancy, accounting for about 40–50% of cases. The mutation of the prothrombin gene and deficiencies in protein S, protein C, and antithrombin are responsible for most of the remaining cases.

Screening for hereditary thrombophilias is recommended if the patient has a history of thromboembolic event or a family history of a first-degree relative (parents, siblings) with thrombosis or hereditary high-risk thrombophilia, if the results of laboratory tests modify the clinical treatment.

The association between hereditary thrombophilia and uteroplacental thrombosis, fetal loss, preeclampsia, intrauterine growth restriction (IUGR), and placental abruption is still controversial and, therefore, screening is not recommended for these cases [2].

Factor V Mutation (G1691A)

Among hereditary thrombophilia, factor V mutation (heterozygous or homozygous form) is the most prevalent and found in 1–15% of the general population, with 5% of Caucasians (5.27%; 95% CI 4.42–6.22%), 21% of Latin Americans, 1.23% of African Americans, 0.45% of Asian Americans, and 1.25% of Americans being affected [4]. The mutation, which was described by the University of Leiden, the Netherlands, was also known by its name (Leiden's facto V). It occurs through the replacement of glutamine by arginine at position 506 of the factor V gene and results in the difficulty of its degradation by activated protein C, configuring the so-called resistance to activated protein C. Factor V, then, remains in the circulation, maintains its procoagulant action, and predisposes to thrombosis.

Mutation of the Prothrombin Gene (G20210A)

The G to A transition in the last 20,210 nucleotide (G20210A) of the 3′ nontranscribed region of the complementary DNA of the coagulation factor II (prothrombin) gene increases the stability of the prothrombin messenger RNA, thus resulting in elevated plasma levels of prothrombin. Individuals with heterozygous mutations have plasma levels of prothrombin approximately 30% higher than noncarriers [4]. It has a prevalence of 1–3% in the general population, with 3.6% of Caucasian Europeans, 3.5% of Hispanics, and 0–1.7% of African Americans being affected.

Protein S Deficiency

Protein S is a vitamin K-dependent glycoprotein that acts as a cofactor for protein C and is synthesized in the liver. Its deficiency is inherited in an autosomal dominant manner and has been described in several families that had recurrent thromboembolism. Homozygosity seems to be incompatible with human life, as well as in animal models. Protein S deficiency can manifest as a result of a quantitative reduction (less than 50% of the total S antigen, even less than the free S protein)—classic or type I deficiency, a qualitative reduction (normal free and total S protein, activity reduced functional S protein)—type II deficiency and reduced functional activity and low level of free protein S-type III deficiency. The prevalence in the general population is 0.03–1.3%.

Protein C Deficiency

Protein C is produced in the liver and is dependent on vitamin K, exerting its anticoagulant action after activation. The main effect of activated protein C is to inhibit the coagulation factors Va and VIIIa, an effect enhanced by protein S. Heterozygosis is transmitted in an autosomal dominant manner. Like Protein S deficiency, Protein C deficiency can be quantitative (more common) or qualitative. The peak incidence of thrombotic events is around 45 years, and 60% of patients with this deficiency will develop recurrent events. The prevalence in the general population is estimated at 0.2–1.5%, being more common among Asian or African descendants.

Antithrombin Deficiency

Antithrombin is an anticoagulant not dependent on vitamin K, which is one of the main inhibitors of thrombin and other coagulating factors, such as factors Xa and IXa. Antithrombin deficiency was the first hereditary thrombophilia identified and is transmitted in an autosomal dominant manner, with variable clinical penetrance and affecting both sexes equally. The deficiency can be quantitative, with a 50% reduction in the normal plasma value in the heterozygote, or qualitative, with a reduction in plasma functional activity. More than 250 different polymorphisms have been described, the majority of which are heterozygous. Analyzing only the quantitative deficiency, the prevalence of this deficiency varies between ½.000 and

1/5.000, but when functional analysis studies are included, the prevalence can reach 1 in 500 people. Approximately 60% of individuals with this deficiency will develop recurrent thrombotic episodes, starting between 15 and 35 years old [5]. The prevalence in the general population is 0.02–0.20%.

Polymorphisms of Methylenetetrahydrofolate Reductase (pMTHFR)

MTHFR is one of three enzymes involved in folic acid metabolism. In the liver cell, MTHFR reduces 5,10-methylenetetrahydrofolates to 5-methyltetrahydrofolates, which by remethylation converts homocysteine to methionine. The MTHFR gene is located on chromosome 1, position 1p36.3, and its mutation has an autosomal recessive characteristic. The homozygous mutation of MTHFR for the C677T and A1298C polymorphisms can be found in 10–16% and 4–6% of the European population, respectively. Likewise, heterozygous mutation is quite common, with a prevalence of up to 49% in asymptomatic populations being described. The presence of any MTHFR mutation, whether homozygous or heterozygous, does not increase the risk of venous thromboembolism or even of adverse pregnancy events, and the screening of these polymorphisms is therefore not recommended. Hyperomocysteinemia, which may be due to the homozygous polymorphism of MTHFR, does not appear to present a significant risk for VTE and should not be investigated routinely [2].

Other Thrombophilia

There are other thrombophilias described, such as alternative mutations in the factor V gene, a promoter mutation in the PAI-1 gene, protein Z deficiency, and mutations that increase activity in several coagulation factor genes. These appear to have a little independent risk of VTE but may increase the risk among patients with the mutations mentioned above. However, there is, to date, insufficient scientific evidence to recommend this screening, even in patients with VTE [2].

Venous Thromboembolic Disease

About 80% of thrombotic events that occur in the pregnancy–puerperal period are venous, with a prevalence of 0.5–2.0 per 1000 pregnant women. Physiological changes in the coagulation system during the pregnancy–puerperal cycle usually persist for 6–8 weeks after delivery and VTE is among the main causes of maternal mortality from nonobstetric causes in the world. Maternal death due to VTE can potentially be avoided in about 2/3 of women since, in most cases, we can identify risk factors and perform appropriate thromboprophylaxis. The odds ratio (OR) for the development of VTE during pregnancy is 34.4 and 26.36 in women with homozygous factor V mutation and homozygous prothrombin gene mutation, respectively [5].

In a systematic review and meta-analysis [6], it was described that pregnant women with hereditary thrombophilia have an absolute increased risk of VTE and in those with a positive family history of thrombosis, the risk is even greater. The authors concluded that thromboprophylaxis should be considered in all pregnant women with homozygous factor V mutation, regardless of family history, and in all those with antithrombin, protein C or S deficiency with a positive family history. Table 24.2 shows the prevalence of thrombophilia in the general population, the risks of VTE in women with and without a personal history of thrombosis and the probability of VTE during pregnancy, according to retrospective studies.

Obstetric Complications

Some observational studies, with a small number of cases, reported a positive association between hereditary thrombophilia and placenta-mediated obstetric complications—recurrent miscarriage, late fetal loss, IUGR, preeclampsia, and placental abruption. These trials are generally influenced by the small number of patients, by heterogeneous populations, by different definitions of early versus late loss, and by complications prior to pregnancy [7]. Current available evidence based on prospective studies, meta-analyses, and systematic reviews does not confirm this association, since the absolute risk is small and varies considerably between reports. Robertson et al. [5] analyzed 79 studies on the risk of obstetric complications in patients with thrombophilia and concluded that, despite a small increase in the

Table 24.2 Prevalence and risks of VTE from hereditary thrombophilia

Hereditary thrombophilia	Prevalence in population general (%)	VTE risk by pregnancy (no history) (%)	VTE risk by pregnancy (with history) (%)	Percent of all VTEs in pregnancy
Factor V (heterozygous)	1–15	0.5–3.1	10	40
Factor V (homozygous	<1	2.2–14.0	17	2
Prothrombin gene mutation (heterozygous)	2–5	0.4–2.6	>10	17
Prothrombin gene mutation (homozygous)	<1	2–4	>17	0.5
Heterozygous double factor V/prothrombin	0.01	4–8.2	>20	1–3
Antithrombin deficiency	0.02	0.2–11.6	40	1
Protein C deficiency	0.2–0.4	0.1–1.7	4–17	14
Protein S deficiency	0.03–0.13	0.3–6.6	0–22	3

Adapted from ACOG, 2018

relative risk, the absolute risk of complications is low and does not justify the clinical tracking of these changes. In addition, prospective studies evaluating the use of anticoagulants in patients with hereditary thrombophilia have not been able to prevent adverse pregnancy outcomes [8]. These inherited disorders likely have little impact on miscarriage or placental-mediated complications such as preeclampsia, with only modest effect on late-term loss. To date, there are no clinical trials with enough power to adequately determine the effect of inherited thrombophilia on these obstetric complications [9–11].

Screening for Hereditary Thrombophilia

In the general population, screening for hereditary thrombophilia is not recommended for the prevention of VTE due to the low frequency of symptomatic disease and the absence of long-term prophylaxis that is safe and cost-effective. Universal screening would require testing about 400,000 women to prevent one death from pulmonary embolism [12].

The most common situations for screening for hereditary thrombophilia are a personal history of VTE associated with a nonrecurring risk factor (fracture, surgery, prolonged immobilization) and a first-degree relative with a history of thrombotic event or diagnosis of high-risk thrombophilia (Table 24.3), although the American College of Obstetricians and Gynecologists (ACOG), in its latest update on hereditary thrombophilia and pregnancy [2], recommends screening all patients with any previous history of VTE.

Screening for hereditary thrombophilia in pregnant women with a previous adverse pregnancy outcome is not justified. The American College of Chest Physicians (ACCP, 2012), the ACOG (2018), and the Society of Obstetricians and Gynaecologists of Canada (SOGC, 2014) do not recommend screening for hereditary thrombophilia in women with a history of placental abruption, IUGR, preeclampsia, or recurrent pregnancy loss, due to the lack of evidence of association and/or effective therapeutic intervention.

Likewise, the investigation of hereditary thrombophilia in patients with a history of arterial thrombosis or failure after assisted reproduction therapy is not recommended.

Table 24.3 Recommendations for screening of hereditary thrombophilia

Yes	Women of reproductive age with a personal history of venous thrombosis associated or not with a risk factor nonrecurring (such as fracture of the femur, major surgery, prolonged immobilization) - Asymptomatic women (without previous deep venous thrombosis) planning a pregnancy that has a first-degree relative (parent or sibling) with VTE before age 50 or diagnosis of high-risk thrombophilia
No	Women with a history of recurrent or nonrecurring early fetal loss, premature detachment of placenta, fetal growth restriction, or preeclampsia Couples with failed IVF

In order to study the correlation of hereditary thrombophilia (low and high risk) with specific histopathological and/or placental immunohistochemical changes, Nacea et al. [15] analyzed the placenta of 90 women with a personal history of thrombotic and/or obstetric complications. Significant placental changes (fibrinoid necrosis, multiple thrombosis, hypoxia, and oxidative stress) were found predominantly in women with high-risk thrombophilia (homozygous factor V mutations and heterozygous factor V and prothrombin gene compounds). The authors suggest that this should be the first most cost-effective step in selecting patients who should be screened for high-risk hereditary thrombophilia.

In addition to selecting patients to be screened for, some factors must be considered when interpreting the tests. In normal pregnancy, there is a significant reduction in the levels of total and free protein S, an increase in factor VIII, and an increase in resistance to activated protein C. Another important fact is that anticoagulants can interfere in the interpretation of results since heparin reduces antithrombin levels and coumarin decreases the concentrations of proteins C and S. Considering these modifications, tests for investigating deficiencies in natural anticoagulants must be performed, if possible, some time away from any thrombotic event (at least 6 weeks) when the patient is not pregnant or postpartum (up to 12 weeks) and is not receiving anticoagulants or hormone therapy.

Recommendations for Screening

- All patients with a personal history of VTE associated or not with a nonrecurring risk factor (prolonged immobilization, major surgery, fractures), or first-degree relative with a history of thrombotic event and/or diagnosis of high-risk thrombophilia should be screened for hereditary thrombophilia.
- Patients with a personal history of VTE should also be investigated for antiphospholipid syndrome, which is an acquired thrombophilia, not discussed in this chapter.
- Evaluation of deficiency of antithrombin and proteins C and S in patients using anticoagulants is not recommended, as heparin may induce a decrease in antithrombin levels and warfarin reduces protein C and protein S, making it difficult to analyze the results.
- Protein S testing should not be performed during pregnancy, due to the physiological changes of this period. These changes can lead to increased resistance to activated protein C in first-generation coagulation assays due to increased levels of factor VIII and decreased levels of protein S.
- Patients with a history of obstetric complications should not be investigated for hereditary thrombophilia due to lack of evidence of association and/or effective therapeutic intervention.

Prophylaxis and Treatment of Thromboembolic Events

In comparison with individuals without a history of VTE, patients with previous events are at increased risk of future recurrent episodes. Thromboprophylaxis during pregnancy involves the use of long-term parenteral heparin, a treatment that has a high cost. Given the distribution of VTE in all three trimesters, antepartum prophylaxis, when indicated, should be performed early from the first trimester (Table 24.4). Anticoagulation can be started with both unfractionated heparin (UFH) and low molecular weight heparin (LMWH); however, the latter is the most recommended for use in pregnancy due to the better bioavailability, longer half-life, more predictable dose response, reduced risk of osteoporosis and thrombocytopenia, and less frequent doses [13].

New oral anticoagulants, direct thrombin inhibitors (dabigatran), and factor Xa inhibitors (rivaroxaban, apixaban, edoxaban, betrixaban) should be avoided during pregnancy and breastfeeding. There are few reports in the literature on the use of these anticoagulants in gestational period and, therefore, the human reproductive risk is unknown [16]. Studies with human placentas demonstrate the placental transfer of direct thrombin inhibitors and factor Xa inhibitors and these anticoagulants have also been detected in breast milk [17, 18]. In cases of heparin allergy or heparin-induced thrombocytopenia, fondaparinux (a synthetic pentasaccharide) is a therapeutic alternative [2, 19].

Patients with a previous history of VTE or who have an acute event during pregnancy should receive anticoagulation during pregnancy and the puerperium according to the recommendations, as shown in Table 24.4, regardless of the diagnosis of hereditary thrombophilia.

Patients with hereditary thrombophilia but without a personal history of VTE should receive prophylaxis according to the type of thrombophilia and family history of VTE.

Regarding the classification of hereditary thrombophilia by the type of risk (low or high) for VTE, there are differences between the studies and between the guidelines of several institutions [2, 6, 20]. ACOG [2] and RCOG [20] define as high-risk hereditary thrombophilias homozygous mutations of factor V and prothrombin

Table 24.4 Doses recommended for anticoagulation with heparin

Prophylactic	UFH: 5.000 U 12/12 h in the first quarter 7.500 U 12/12 h in the second quarter 10.000 U 12/12 h in the third quarter LMWH: Enoxaparin 40 mg/day; dalteparin 5.000 U/day
Intermediate	LMWH: Enoxaparin 40 mg 12/12 h; dalteparin 5.000 U 12/12 h
Therapy	UFH: application every 12 h until the aPTT ratio is extended 1.5–2.5 times the baseline LMWH: Enoxaparin 1 mg/kg/12 h; dalteparin 100 mg/kg/12 h

Adapted from Bates et al., 2012
UFH unfractionated heparin, *LMWH* low molecular weight heparin

gene, heterozygous compounds of factor V and prothrombin gene, and antithrombin deficiency, and classify as low-risk thrombophilia the isolated heterozygous mutations of factor V and prothrombin gene. Proteins C and S deficiencies are also classified as low risk by ACOG and high risk by RCOG. There is a consensus that, according to the estimated risks published in the literature, there is no support for the routine use of anticoagulants in those pregnant women with low-risk mutations such as isolated heterozygous factor V and prothrombin gene mutations. Management of deficiencies of proteins C and S should be evaluated and defined in accordance with the protocol followed in each institution, but most of the authors do not recommend anticoagulation for these patients. To classify hereditary thrombophilia according to risk, we suggest using the classification proposed by ACOG, 2018 (Table 24.5).

Recommendations for Prophylaxis and Treatment

To date, there is no consistent scientific evidence to support recommendations on prophylaxis and treatment of VTE during pregnancy. Most current protocols are based on estimated risk models and the opinions and experiences of specialists, such as cardiologists, hematologists, rheumatologists, and obstetricians. This lack of scientific evidence results in the absence of consensus among the main publications and reference guidelines that address this topic [2, 5, 12, 13, 20].

Thus, we chose to use these recommendations, adapted from ACOG 2018, for thromboprophylaxis of pregnancies complicated by hereditary thrombophilia:

- For patients with low-risk hereditary thrombophilia without previous VTE, it is recommended only clinical surveillance during pregnancy, without anticoagulant therapy. Postpartum surveillance without anticoagulant therapy or prophylactic anticoagulation could be considered if the patient has additional risk factors (obesity, cesarean section, prolonged immobilization).
- For patients with low-risk hereditary thrombophilia with a family history (first-degree relative) of VTE, it is recommended surveillance without anticoagulant therapy during pregnancy, but prophylactic anticoagulant therapy with LMWH/UFH can be considered. In postpartum, anticoagulation with prophylactic dose with LMWH/UFH is recommended.

Table 24.5 Hereditary thrombophilia

High risk	Factor V mutation-homozygous (G1691A) Prothrombin gene mutation-homozygous (G20210A) Heterozygous compounds from mutation Factor V and Prothrombin gene Antithrombin deficiency
Low risk	Protein S deficiency Protein C deficiency

Adapted ACOG, 2018

- For patients with low-risk hereditary thrombophilia with a single previous episode of VTE who are not receiving long-term anticoagulant therapy, prophylactic, or intermediate dose of anticoagulant therapy is recommended during pregnancy and postpartum period with LMWH/UFH.
- For patients with high-risk hereditary thrombophilia without previous VTE, surveillance without anticoagulant therapy is recommended. In postpartum, anticoagulation with prophylactic dose with LMWH/UFH is recommended.
- For patients with high-risk hereditary thrombophilia with a family history (first-degree relative) of VTE, prophylactic anticoagulant therapy with LMWH/UFH is recommended during pregnancy. Postpartum anticoagulation with prophylactic or intermediate dose with LMWH/UFH is recommended.
- For patients with high-risk hereditary thrombophilia with a single previous episode of VTE who are not receiving long-term anticoagulant therapy, intermediate or dose-adjusted anticoagulant therapy with LMWH/UFH is recommended during pregnancy and for 6 weeks after delivery. The dose in the postpartum period should always be equal to or greater than in the antepartum period.
- For patients with or without hereditary thrombophilia, with two or more episodes of VTE who are not receiving long-term anticoagulant therapy, intermediate or dose-adjusted anticoagulant therapy with LMWH/UFH is recommended during pregnancy and for 6 weeks after delivery. The dose in the postpartum period should always be equal to or greater than in the antepartum period.
- For patients with or without hereditary thrombophilia, with two or more episodes of VTE who are receiving long-term anticoagulant therapy, dose-adjusted anticoagulant therapy with LMWH/UFH is recommended during pregnancy and 6 weeks postpartum. It is also possible to return to long-term anticoagulation after delivery. Warfarin can be considered postpartum, based on the planned duration of therapy and patient's preference.

Key Points

The key points underlined about thrombophilia are as follows:

- Low molecular weight heparin is the most recommended anticoagulant than unfractionated heparin for use during pregnancy, due to its greater bioavailability, greater predictability of effect, and ease of administration.
- Women with a personal history of VTE or a first-degree family member with VTE should undergo screening tests for inherited thrombophilia and these tests should include the factor V mutation; mutation of prothrombin gene; and deficiencies of antithrombin, protein S, and protein C.
- The association between hereditary thrombophilia and adverse pregnancy outcomes is still controversial. Even if there is a small increase in risk, current evidence shows that treatment with anticoagulants for these patients is not able to prevent adverse results.
- Due to the lack of association between heterozygosity or homozygosity for the MTHFR C677T polymorphism and any negative results in pregnancy, including any increased risk of VTE, screening with MTHFR mutation analyzes, or fasting homocysteine levels, is not recommended.

- Universal screening for thrombophilia in pregnant women is not cost-effective or indicated due to the low incidence of VTE in pregnancy.
- Warfarin, low molecular weight heparin, and unfractionated heparin do not accumulate in breast milk and do not induce anticoagulant effect in the infant; therefore, these anticoagulants can be used in breastfeeding women.

Bibliography

1. Pierangeli SS, Leader B, Barilaro G, Willis R, Branch DW. Acquired and inherited thrombophilia disorders in pregnancy. Obstet Gynecol Clin N Am. 2011;38(2):271–95. x
2. ACOG Practice Bulletin No. 196 summary: thromboembolism in pregnancy. Obstet Gynecol. 2018;132(1):243–8. https://doi.org/10.1097/AOG.0000000000002707.
3. James AH, Jamison MG, Brancazio LR, Myers ER. Venous thromboembolism during pregnancy and the postpartum period: incidence, risk factors, and mortality. Am J Obstet Gynecol. 2006;194(5):1311–5.
4. Martinelli I, Legnani C, Bucciarelli P, Grandone E, Stefano V, Mannucci PM. Risk of pregnancy-related venous thrombosis in carriers of several inherited thrombophilia. Thromb Haemost. 2011;800:80.
5. Robertson L, Wu O, Langhorne P, Twaddle S, Clark P, Lowe GD, et al. Thrombophilia in pregnancy: a systematic review. Br J Haematol. 2006;132(2):171–96.
6. Croles FN, Nasserinejad K, Duvekot JJ, Kruip MHHA, Meijer K, Leebeek FWG. Pregnancy, thrombophilia and the risk of a first venous thrombosis: systematic review and bayesian meta-analysis. BMJ. 2017;359:J4452.
7. Kist WJ, Janssen NG, Kalk JJ, Hague WM, Dekker GA, de Vries JI. Thrombophilias and adverse pregnancy outcome a confounded problem. Thromb Haemost. 2008;99(1):77–85.
8. Tormene D, Grandone E, De Stefano V, et al. Obstetric complications and pregnancy-related venous thromboembolism: the effect of low-molecular-weight heparin on their prevention in carriers of factor V Leiden or prothrombin G20210A mutation. Thromb Haemost. 2012;107(3):477–84.
9. Bates SM. Management of pregnant women with thrombophilia or a history of venous thromboembolism. Hematology Am Soc Hematol Educ Program. 2007:143–50.
10. Leaf RK, Connors JM. The role of anticoagulants in the prevention of pregnancy complications. Clin Appl Thromb Hemost. 2017;23(2):116–23.
11. Fernández Arias M, Mazarico E, Gonzalez A, Muniesa M, Molinet C, Almeida L, Gómez Roig MD. Genetic risk assessment of thrombophilia in patients with adverse obstetric outcomes. PLoS One. 2019;14(2):e0211114.
12. American College of Obstetricians and Gynecologists. Antiphospholipid syndrome. ACOG Practice Bulletin No. 132. Obstet Gynecol. 2012;120:1514.
13. American College of Chest Physicians. VTE, thrombophilia, antithrombotic therapy, and pregnancy: Antithrombotic Therapy and Prevention of Thrombosis, 9th ed, ACCP Evidence-Based Clinical Practice Guidelines. Chest. 2012;141(Suppl 2):e691S.
14. Chan WS, Rey E, Kent NE, VTE in Pregnancy Guideline Working Group, Chan WS, Kent NE, Rey E, Corbett T, David M, Douglas MJ, Gibson PS, Magee L, Rodger M, Smith RE, Society of Obstetricians and Gynecologists of Canada. Venous thromboembolism and antithrombotic therapy in pregnancy. J Obstet Gynaecol Can. 2014;36(6):527–53.
15. Nacea JG, Rotaru I, Niculescu M, Stănescu R, Cernea N, Pătraşcu AM, Stoica LE, Tudorache Ş. Correlations between clinical and placental histopathological and immunohistochemical features in women with and without hereditary thrombophilia. Romanian J Morphol Embryol. 2019;60(1):195–203.

16. Bates SM, Middeldorp S, Rodger M, James AH, Greer I. Guidance for the treatment and prevention of obstetric-associated venous thromboembolism. J Thromb Thrombolysis. 2016;41:92–128.
17. Bapat P, Kedar R, Lubetsky A, Matlow JN, Aleksa K, Berger H, et al. Transfer of dabigatran and dabigatran etexilate mesylate across the dually perfused human placenta. Obstet Gynecol. 2014;123:1256–61.
18. Bapat P, Pinto LS, Lubetsky A, Aleksa K, Berger H, Koren G, et al. Examining the transplacental passage of apixaban using the dually perfused human placenta. J Thromb Haemost. 2016;14:1436–41.
19. De Carolis S, di Pasquo E, Rossi E, Del Sordo G, Buonomo A, Schiavino D, et al. Fondaparinux in pregnancy: could it be a safe option? A review of the literature. Thromb Res. 2015;135:1049–51.
20. Royal College of Obstetricians and Gynaecologists. Reducing the risk of venous thromboembolism during pregnancy and the puerperium. Green Top Guideline No. 37a. London (UK): RCOG; 2015.

Chapter 25
Gastrointestinal Disorders

Mario Julio Franco and Janaína Luz Narciso-Schiavon

Gastroesophageal Reflux in Pregnancy

Gastroesophageal reflux disease (GERD) affects more than 50% of pregnant women [1], with a negative impact on the quality of life in this group, and a significant impact on sleep [2]. It rarely represents an exacerbation of the preexisting disease. It typically begins during pregnancy, which becomes more frequent and more severe in the latter months of gestation and ceases soon after delivery [3, 4].

Possible Mechanisms of Disease

- *Lower Esophageal Sphincter (LES) Pressure*: Loss of intraabdominal portion of LES, decrease in resting LES tone—due to elevated serum levels of sex hormones [5, 6].
- *Mechanical Factors*: Increased abdominal pressure secondary to the enlarged gravid uterus.
- *Impaired Esophageal Clearance*: Slower wave velocity and lower amplitude of esophageal peristalsis [7].

Clinical Presentations

The most frequent GERD symptoms are heartburn, acid taste in the mouth, and regurgitation, with exacerbation of symptoms with food ingestion [1, 8].

M. J. Franco (✉) · J. L. Narciso-Schiavon
Florianópolis, SC, Brazil

© Springer Nature Switzerland AG 2022

R. A. Moreira de Sá, E. B. d. Fonseca (eds.), *Perinatology*,
https://doi.org/10.1007/978-3-030-83434-0_25

Complications of GERD during pregnancy are rare, due to its short duration, and include esophagitis, bleeding, and structure formation.

Diagnosis

Diagnosis of GERD during pregnancy is clinical based on typical symptoms.

Esophagogastroduodenoscopy (EGD) is the procedure of choice to evaluate intractable reflux symptoms or complications [9]. While many pregnant women have appropriate indications for endoscopy, fetal drug safety is a major consideration in the choice and dosage of endoscopic medications [10]. These are the medications habitually prescribed during EGD procedure, and their Food and Drug Administration (FDA) pregnancy risk categories are as follows:

Category B) Lidocaine, meperidine, naloxone, propofol.
Category C) Epinephrine, fentanyl, flumazenil, simethicone.
Category D) Diazepam, midazolam.

Lidocaine is frequently applied topically to the oropharynx before EGD. The pregnant patient who is administered topical lidocaine should be instructed to gargle and spit it out, to minimize systemic absorption.

Meperidine is rapidly transferred across the placenta. Meperidine should not be used in pregnant women prior to the labor period unless in the judgment of the physician the potential benefits outweigh the possible hazards. Nonetheless, meperidine is preferred over diazepam or midazolam as an EGD premedication during pregnancy.

Naloxone administration is appropriate for pregnant patients with serious signs of potential meperidine toxicity, such as respiratory depression, systemic hypotension, or unresponsiveness.

Propofol is now a preferred agent for sedation in some endoscopy centers. However, it is not recommended in the first and second trimesters due to lack of studies during this time.

Fentanyl may be used in low doses for EGD during pregnancy. Fentanyl is sometimes used as an alternative to meperidine during endoscopy because of a more rapid onset of action.

Flumazenil is sometimes used to reverse the effects of benzodiazepines administered during EGD; though the real safety of flumazenil during pregnancy is unknown.

Midazolam appears to be preferable to diazepam for endoscopy during pregnancy because of the potential association between diazepam and oral clefts and neonatal neurobehavioral abnormalities, although both have restricted use during endoscopy in pregnant patient.

Treatment

The major treatment for GERD, proton pump inhibitors (PPIs), cannot be administered during pregnancy. For this reason, a distinct approach is necessary for controlling the symptoms in this group of patients [1]. The recommended therapy for

GERD in pregnancy is a step-up algorithm beginning with lifestyle modifications, especially dietary measures, such as limiting oral intake within 3 hours of bedtime, increasing frequency and reducing the volume of meals, reducing dietary fat, and avoiding caffeine, chocolate, and mints are measures that have some effect in controlling the symptoms of gastroesophageal reflux. Alcohol and smoking should be discouraged.

Antacids are considered the first-line drug therapy due to their safety; only if severe symptoms persist, histamine$_2$-receptor antagonists (H_2RA) can be considered [11]. Despite their widespread use, H_2RA use may be associated with an increased risk of preterm birth [12].

These are H_2RA, FDA risk category B: Cimetidine, famotidine, nizatidine, and ranitidine.

PPIs are very potent suppressors of gastric acid and have made a major impact on the treatment and healing of severe peptic esophagitis. However, omeprazole is categorized as a class C drug by the FDA. A recent meta-analysis has suggested that PPI use is associated with an increased risk of congenital malformations [12], contradicting the previous belief that exposure to PPI therapy during pregnancy predisposes the fetus to minimal risk [13], and FDA category B for pantoprazole, rabeprazole, lansoprazole, and esomeprazole. In pregnancy, PPIs should be used as an exception, when patients with intensive erosive esophagitis do respond to a double dose of H_2RA.

Promotility agents may have a limited role to play in symptomatic GERD and could be added if acid suppression alone does not work. Read more about these agents on nausea and vomiting section.

Nausea and Vomiting (NV)

Nausea and vomiting (NV) are frequent symptoms during pregnancy, with a prevalence of 50% to 80%, especially in the first trimester. Symptoms are more common amongst weeks 6 to 15 of gestation and progressive recovery at around week 16 [14, 15]. By weeks 20 to 22, 90% of women will have resolved their symptoms [16, 14].

Due to its high frequency, NV are sometimes considered as "normal" part of pregnancy; however, they may affect the quality of life, contribute to depression, and stress family bonds [17].

First pregnancy, twin pregnancy, young age, low socio-cultural level, and overweight are considered risk factors for NV [18].

Hyperemesis gravidarum is a severe spectrum of NV, with prolonged and intractable symptoms, that may impair nutrition and cause dehydration, ketonuria, and/or electrolyte imbalance. Hyperemesis gravidarum is infrequent and affects 0.3% to 3.0% of pregnant women [19]. Women with multiple gestations, gestational trophoblastic disease, fetal aneuploidies, and hydrops fetalis are associated with higher rates of hyperemesis gravidarum [20].

Possible Mechanisms of Disease

The cause of NV is controversial and probably includes genetic, gastrointestinal, and hormonal changes possibly involving human chorionic gonadotropin (hCG), estrogen, progesterone, serotonin, and thyroid hormone [21]. Patients with hyperemesis gravidarum may present transient hyperthyroidism in 66–73% of cases. High hCG concentrations or hypersensitive thyrotropin receptors in the thyroid gland cause an increase in thyroid hormones. Routine thyroid function test is unnecessary unless patients exhibit clinical signs or symptoms of hyperthyroidism [22].

The relationship between hyperemesis gravidarum and *Helicobacter pylori* infection has been broadly investigated in pregnancy, and results are inconclusive. Even though some studies clearly indicate an increased seroprevalence of antibodies to *H. pylori* in symptomatic pregnant women, the findings have to be interpreted in the context of geography and socioeconomic status. *H. pylori* eradication could be pondered to relieve the symptoms in some intractable cases of hyperemesis gravidarum [23, 24].

Prognosis

NV in pregnancy have favorable prognosis: it is associated with good fetal outcomes and with lower rates of miscarriage in the first trimester. Unlike mild NV, hyperemesis gravidarum is a condition of noteworthy morbidity and can lead to adverse birth outcomes. Serious maternal complications of hyperemesis gravidarum are rare and consist of acute kidney injury, liver biochemistry abnormalities, splenic avulsion, esophageal rupture, pneumothorax, and Wernicke encephalopathy [17, 25].

Differential Diagnosis

It is important to keep in mind that NV in pregnancy can be secondary to other diseases, and differential diagnosis of gastrointestinal tract includes parasitosis, peptic ulcer disease, gastric cancer, pancreatitis, cholecystitis, and appendicitis. Conditions of the genitourinary tract that may present with NV include pyelonephritis, uremia, kidney stones, ovarian torsion, and degenerating uterine leiomyoma. Neurological disorders and psychological conditions might be considered as an alternative diagnosis. And acute fatty liver of pregnancy and preeclampsia must not be forgotten [21, 26].

When NV starts after the ninth week of gestation, abdominal pain, diarrhea, and/or fever should be investigated as these symptoms suggest other diseases than simply NV or hyperemesis gravidarum.

Once a different diagnosis is suspected, laboratory tests consist of hemogram, electrolytes, glycemia, creatinine, liver biochemical tests (including alanine aminotransferase, aspartate aminotransferase, gammaglutamyl transferase, alkaline phosphatases, bilirubins, and international normalized ratio), and urinalysis (both for infectious markers and ketones). If the patient does not have been submitted to a pelvic ultrasound before, it can be considered to rule out molar pregnancy and a multiple-gestation pregnancy [27–29].

Treatment

Lifestyle and dietary modifications are the main treatment for mild NV of pregnancy, despite the paucity of published evidence evolving these changes. Most women can be supported through their episodes without the use of antiemetics. Lifestyle changes include the avoidance of sensory stimuli (noise, odors, humidity, heat, and flickering lights), increased rest, not brushing teeth immediately after meals, and not lying down at least 2 hours after meals. Dietary modifications comprise eliminating iron-containing prenatal supplements, abstention of high-fat and spicy foods, frequent and small meals to avoid empty and full stomach, and maintain adequate hydration [25, 30].

Early treatment of NV of pregnancy is recommended to prevent progression to hyperemesis gravidarum [31]. Though medication may relieve the symptoms, it is important to recognize that the most important intervention is *fluid and electrolyte replacement*. It is the aggressive treatment of these disturbances that decrease mortality [26]. Intravenous hydration should be used for the patient who cannot tolerate oral liquids for a prolonged period or if clinical signs of dehydration are present. Dextrose and vitamins may be included in the therapy when prolonged NV is present, and thiamine could be administered before dextrose infusion to prevent Wernicke encephalopathy [32]. Enteral tube feeding (nasogastric or nasoduodenal) must be considered as the first-line treatment to provide nutritional support to the woman with hyperemesis gravidarum who is not responsive to medical therapy and cannot maintain her weight [31].

Pyridoxine (vitamin B_6) may be administered at a dose of 25 mg orally every 8 h for NV of pregnancy [33].

Acupuncture and Acupressure are great options for treating hyperemesis gravidarum [34].

Antiemetics are usually avoided in the first trimester. As with all medications, the potential risks, benefits, adverse effects, and costs should be evaluated in each case. Care should be exercised if multiple antiemetic medications are used simultaneously [31]. These are the most common antiemetics, and their respective FDA pregnancy risk categories are as follows:

Category B) Metoclopramide, ondansetron, dolasetron, and granisetron.

Category C) Domperidone, prochlorperazine, promethazine, and trimethobenzamide [10].

Metoclopramide is used as an antiemetic and is usually confined to the first trimester, but it is also used to enhance gastric emptying throughout pregnancy.

Ondansetron is used for hyperemesis gravidarum, but its safety has been recently questioned. In a recent meta-analysis and systematic review, ondansetron use during pregnancy was not associated with a significant increase in the rate of major or selected subgroups of malformations [35, 36].

Promethazine is a dopamine antagonist used as an antiemetic during pregnancy and adjunctive therapy for narcotics during labor. As it may cause dry mouth and drowsiness, so its use during the day might be impractical.

Diphenhydramine is an antihistamine drug frequently used and effective in controlling nausea and vomiting symptoms of pregnancy.

Domperidone is a dopamine antagonist used for short-term treatment of NV and for its prokinetic properties.

In refractory NV patients, a short course of *methylprednisolone* at 16 mg three times daily for 2 weeks may be an option [34, 37].

When a woman cannot tolerate liquids without vomiting and has not responded to outpatient management, *hospitalization* for evaluation and treatment of dehydration and electrolyte imbalance is recommended, and parenteral nutrition may be necessary [26, 31].

Inflammatory Bowel Disease (IBD)

The term IBD comprises two main clinical entities: ulcerative colitis and Crohn's disease [38].

Ulcerative Colitis

Ulcerative colitis is a chronic recurrent disease that is characterized by diffuse mucosal inflammation restricted to the colon. The disease affects primarily the rectum and involves continuously other parts of the colon.

Crohn's Disease

Crohn's disease is a chronic recurrent inflammatory disease, which may affect the whole alimentary canal, from the mouth to the anus. The inflammation is transmural with irregular distribution, alternating ulcerating lesions with healthy mucosa.

Prognosis

The majority of women with ulcerative colitis and Crohn's disease will proceed to have normal, full-term pregnancies, even though some of them present an adverse pregnancy outcome. A higher rate of preterm birth and low birth weight has been described when IBD is active at conception or during the course of the pregnancy. The best time to conceive is during IBD remission, as patients with inactive disease do very well. On the other hand, patients with active disease have poorer prognosis, principally those with Crohn's disease [39].

Ulcerative colitis tends to relapse more commonly in the first trimester, in a frequency similar to none pregnant population ~ 1/3. If patients have active disease by the time of conception, ulcerative colitis may exacerbate in approximately 45% and persist in approximately 26%. The active disease can reduce the chances of progressing with a normal term delivery unless step-up therapy is employed.

Inactive Crohn's disease will relapse in less than 1/3 of the pregnancies, usually in the third trimester and postpartum.

Higher fetal mortality is observed during severe exacerbations that require surgery or intensification of medical therapy.

Flares

Ulcerative colitis exacerbations are characterized by increased frequency of loose stools, rectal bleeding, abdominal pain, urgency, and may present fecal incontinence [40]. Patients with colonic Crohn's disease will have similar clinical picture during flares [41]. Patients with terminal ileal Crohn's disease ought to be enquired about symptoms of subacute small bowel obstruction such as abdominal pain, nausea, vomiting, weight loss, or failure to gain proper weight during pregnancy [42].

Treatment

The key priority during pregnancy is to sustain IBD in remission. A healthy mother tends to have an uncomplicated pregnancy and a healthy baby. Most IBD medications are safe to continue during pregnancy and postpartum and should be maintained [43]. Pregnant women tend to stop medications that have kept them in remission, in order to protect their babies. Nevertheless, it is fundamental for patients to maintain remission during pregnancy and in the postpartum period by strictly adhering to their medications [44].

These are the commonly prescribed medications for IBD during pregnancy, FDA pregnancy risk category:

Category B) Aminosalicylates (sulfasalazine, mesalamine, balsalazide), infliximab, adalimumab, metronidazole.
Category C) Corticosteroids, ciprofloxacin, cyclosporine, tacrolimus, olsalazine.
Category D) Azathioprine, 6-mercaptopurine. Methotrexate and thalidomide are contraindicated in pregnancy due to their teratogenic effects [45].

Aminosalicylates: Sulfasalazine is composed of 5-aminosalicylic acid and sulfapyridine. There is no indication to stop aminosalicylates during pregnancy because disease in remission may flare with discontinuation of the medication. Supplemental folic acid (1 mg twice daily) should be administered because sulfasalazine inhibits folate conjugase, interfering with folate absorption.

Corticosteroids: Steroids are very effective in inducing remission in active IBD. The ideal dose to maintain remission should be tapered to the lowest possible. It is controversial if corticosteroid use during the first trimester of pregnancy represents an increased risk of oral clefts in the newborn.

Azathioprine: Based on all available information, there are no clear data linking azathioprine or 6-mercaptopurine with fetal abnormalities, spontaneous abortions, or stillbirth, but the number of reported cases might not be enough to detect a small increase in baseline rates in the general population [46]. Despite this recent knowledge, it is still controversial if azathioprine should either be maintained or stopped when it is currently being used to maintain. Based on the substantial proficiency in transplant recipients and the body of evidence in IBD, the drugs are habitually continued during pregnancy to sustain remission. A flare of disease during pregnancy may be more detrimental to the neonatal outcome than any potential risk from the medication [[45], [47]].

Biologic Agents: Biologic medications for IBD include antitumor necrosis factor α (anti-TNF) medications, such as infliximab, adalimumab, certolizumab pegol, and golimumab; and an anti-integrin medication, such as natalizumab. It has been shown that anti-TNF medications do not increase the risk of pregnancy complications in comparison with thiopurines and with not taking IBD medications [48]. On the contrary, the use of thiopurines or anti-TNF agents is associated with fewer neonatal complications, which emphasizes the importance of maintaining disease remission in pregnant women with IBD [44]. Children born to mothers who have received infliximab, adalimumab, or golimumab after the 20th week of gestation cannot receive any live vaccinations during their first 6 months of life. As anti-TNF drugs cross the placenta, these newborns are immunosuppressed [49].

Vedolizumab is a monoclonal antibody that modulates gut lymphocyte trafficking and is increasingly used for moderate to severely active IBD. Current use of vedolizumab in pregnancy is limited to women with no other therapeutic options and is undertaken on a case by case basis [50]. Ustekinumab is a monoclonal antibody recently approved for use in moderate to severely active Crohn's disease. Data relating to ustekinumab in pregnancy for patients with IBD are extremely limited. The use of this agent in pregnancy is not currently recommended [50].

Antibiotics: Metronidazole and ciprofloxacin are the most frequently used antibiotics in IBD. Short courses of these drugs are most likely safe in pregnancy.

Mode of Delivery

Most women with inflammatory bowel disease should have a vaginal delivery and the mode of delivery must be determined by obstetric needs [51].

Finally, Table 25.1 shows current medications used in gastrointestinal diseases and their respective FDA risk categories.

Table 25.1 Food and Drug Administration (FDA) pregnancy risk categories of gastrointestinal medications

A	B	C	D	Contraindicated
Pyridoxine Thiamine	Adalimumab Aluminum hydroxide Balsalazide Certolizumab pegol Cimetidine Esomeprazole famotidine Golimumab infliximab Lansoprazole Lidocaine meperidine Magnesium hydroxide Metoclopramide Metronidazole Mesalamine Naloxone Nizatidine Pantoprazole Propofol Rabeprazole Ranitidine Sucralfate Sulfasalazine	Calcium carbonate Ciprofloxacin Corticosteroids cyclosporine Domperidone Epinephrine Fentanyl Flumazenil Hyoscyamine Loperamide Natalizumab Olsalazine Omeprazole Ondansetron Prednisone promethazine Simethicone Sodium bicarbonate Tacrolimus	6-mercaptopurine Azathioprine Diazepammidazolam	Methotrexatethalidomide

Food and Drug Administration. Federal Register 1980; 44:37434–67.
A—Appropriately designed studies in pregnant women have not demonstrated fetal risk.
B—No fetal risk in animal reproduction studies; no well-controlled studies in pregnant women OR adverse effect in animal studies, but studies in pregnant women failed to demonstrate fetal risk.
C—Animal reproduction studies show adverse fetal effects but no well-controlled studies in humans OR no animal reproduction studies and well-controlled studies in humans.
D—Evidence of human fetal risk in investigational or marketing experience or studies in humans.

References

1. Malfertheiner F, et al. A prospective longitudinal cohort study: evolution of GERD symptoms during the course of pregnancy. BMC Gastroenterol. 2012;12:131.
2. Malfertheiner F, et al. Impact of gastroesophageal reflux disease symptoms on the quality of life in pregnant women: a prospective study. Eur J Gastroenterol Hepatol. 29;892–6.
3. Barr W. Heartburn in pregnancy. J Obstet Gynecol Br Emp. 1958;65:1019–21.
4. Richter JE. Gastroesophageal reflux during pregnancy. Gastroenterol Clin N Am. 2003;32:235–61.
5. Nagler R, Spiro HM. Heartburn in late pregnancy: manometric studies of esophageal motor function. J Clin Invest. 1961;40:954–70.
6. Lind JF, Smith AM, McKiver DK, et al. Heartburn in pregnancy–a manometry study. CMAJ. 1968;98:571–4.
7. Ulmsten U, Sundstrom G. Esophageal manometry in pregnant and nonpregnant women. Am J Obstet Gynecol. 1978;132:260–4.
8. de Castro LP. Reflux esophagitis as the cause of heartburn in pregnancy. Am J Obstet Gynecol. 1967;98:1–10.
9. Capell MS. The safety and efficacy of gastrointestinal endoscopy during pregnancy. Gastroenterol Clin N Am. 1998;27:37–71.
10. American Gastroenterological Association Institute Technical Review on the Use of Gastrointestinal Medications in Pregnancy. Gastroenterology. 2006;131:283–311.
11. Lewis JH, Weingold AB. The use of gastrointestinal drugs during pregnancy and lactation. Am J Gastroenterol. 1985;80:912–23.
12. Li CM, Zhernakova A, Engstrand L, Wijmenga C, Brusselaers N. Systematic review with meta-analysis: the risks of proton pump inhibitors during pregnancy. Aliment Pharmacol Ther. 2020;51(4):410–20.
13. Majithia R, Johnson DA. Are proton pump inhibitors safe during pregnancy and lactation? Evidence to date Drugs. 2012;72(2):171–9.
14. O'Brien B, Zhou Q. Variables related to nausea and vomiting during pregnancy. Birth. 1995;22:93–100.
15. Boelig RC, Barton SJ, Saccone G, et al. Interventions for treating hyperemesis gravidarum: a Cochrane systematic review and meta-analysis. J Matern Fetal Neonatal Med. 2018;31(18):2492–505.
16. Nuangchamnong N, Niebyl J. Doxylamine succinate-pyridoxine hydrochloride (Diclegis) for the management of nausea and vomiting in pregnancy: an over- view. Int J Women's Health. 2014;6:401–9.
17. Bustos M, Venkataramanan R, Caritis S. Nausea and vomiting of pregnancy—what's new? Auton Neurosci. 2017;202:62–72.
18. Depue RH, Ross RK, Bernstein L, et al. Hypermemesis gravidarum in relation to estradiol levels, pregnancy outcome, and other maternal factors: a seroepidemiologic study. Am J Obstet Gynecol. 1987;156:1137.
19. Matthews A, Haas DM, O'Mathuna DP, et al. Interventions for nausea and vomit- ing in early pregnancy. Cochrane Database Syst Rev. 2015;9:CD007575.
20. Quinla JD, Hill DA. Nausea and vomiting of pregnancy. Am Fam Physician. 2003;68(1):121–8.
21. Pontius E, Vieth JT. Complications in early pregnancy. Emerg Med Clin North Am. 2019;37(2):219–37.
22. Malek NZH, Kalok A, Hanafiah ZA, Shah SA, Ismail NAM. Association of transient hyperthyroidism and severity of hyperemesis gravidarum. Horm Mol Biol Clin Investig. 2017;30(3).
23. Ng QX, Venkatanarayanan N, De Deyn MLZQ, Ho CYX, Mo Y, Yeo WS. A meta-analysis of the association between Helicobacter pylori (H. pylori) infection and hyperemesis gravidarum. Helicobacter. 2018;23(1).
24. Li L, Li L, Zhou X, Xiao S, Gu H, Zhang G. Helicobacter pylori infection is associated with an increased risk of hyperemesis Gravidarum: a Meta-analysis. Gastroenterol Res Pract. 2015;2015:278905.

25. Tian R, MacGibbon K, Martin B, et al. Analysis of pre- and post-pregnancy issues in women with hyperemesis gravidarum. Auton Neurosci. 2017;202:73–8.
26. Vanagunas A. Gastrointestinal complications in pregnancy. Glob Libr Women's Med. 2008;
27. Morgan SR, Long L, Johns J, et al. Are early pregnancy complications more com- Mon in women with hyperemesis gravidarum? J Obstet Gynaecol. 2017;37(3):355–7.
28. Niebyl JR. Clinical practice. Nausea and vomiting in pregnancy. N Engl J Med. 2010;363(16):1544–50.
29. Niemeijer MN, Grooten IJ, Vos N, et al. Diagnostic markers for hyperemesis gravidarum: a systematic review and metaanalysis. Am J Obstet Gynecol 2014;211(2):150 e1–15.
30. Anderka M, Mitchell AA, Louik C, et al. Medications used to treat nausea and vomiting of pregnancy and the risk of selected birth defects. Birth Defects Res A Clin Mol Teratol. 2012;94(1):22–30.
31. ACOG Practice Bulletin No. 189. Obstetrics & Gynecology. 2018:131(1);e15–e30.
32. Giugale LE, Young OM, Streitman DC. Iatrogenic Wernicke encephalopathy in a patient with severe hyper- emesis gravidarum. Obstet Gynecol. 2015;125:1150–2.
33. Sahakian V, Rouse D, Sipes S, et al. Vitamin B6 is effective therapy for nausea and vomiting of pregnancy: a randomized, double-blind placebo controlled study. Obstet Gynecol. 1991;78:33.
34. Sridharan K, Sivaramakrishnan G. Interventions for treating hyperemesis gravidarum: a network meta-analysis of randomized clinical trials. J Matern Fetal Neonatal Med. 2020;33(8):1405–11.
35. Kaplan YC, Richardson JL, Keskin-Arslan E, Erol-Coskun H, Kennedy D. Use of ondansetron during pregnancy and the risk of major congenital malformations: a systematic review and meta-analysis. Reprod Toxicol. 2019;86:1–13.
36. Lavecchia M, Chari R, Campbell S, Ross S. Ondansetron in pregnancy and the risk of congenital malformations: a systematic review. J Obstet Gynaecol Can. 2018;40(7):910–8.
37. Safari HR, Fassett MJ, Souter IC, Alsulyman OM, Goodwin TM. The efficacy of methylprednisolone in the treatment of hyperemesis gravidarum: a randomized, double-blind, controlled study. Am J Obstet Gynecol. 1998;179(4):921–4.
38. Ardizzone S, Bianchi PG. Inflammatory bowel disease: new insights into pathogenesis and treatment. J Intern Med. 2002;252(6):475–96.
39. Kane S. Inflammatory bowel disease in pregnancy. Gastroenterol Clin. 2003:32(1).
40. Magro F, Gionchetti P, Eliakim R, et al. Third European evidence-based consensus on diagnosis and management of ulcerative colitis. Part 1: definitions, diagnosis, extra-intestinal manifestations, pregnancy, cancer surveillance, surgery, and ileo-anal pouch disorders. J Crohns Colitis. 2017;11:649–70.
41. Gomollon F, Dignass A, Annese V, et al. 3rd European evidence-based consensus on the diagnosis and management of Crohn's disease 2016: part 1: diagnosis and medical management. J Crohns Colitis. 2017;11:3–25.
42. Bell SJ, Flanagan EK. Updates in the management of inflammatory bowel disease during pregnancy. Med J Aust. 2019;210(6):276–80.
43. Mahadevan U, McConnell RA, Chambers CD. Drug safety and risk of adverse outcomes for pregnant patients with inflammatory bowel disease. Gastroenterology. 2017;152:451–62.
44. Hashash JG, Kane S. Pregnancy and inflammatory bowel disease. Gastroenterol Hepatol (N Y). 2015;11(2):96–102.
45. Mahadevan U, Kane S. American gastroenterological association institute technical review on the use of gastrointestinal medications in pregnancy. Gastroenterology. 2006;131(1):283–311.
46. Natekar A, Pupco A, Bozzo P, Koren G. Safety of azathioprine use during pregnancy. Can Fam Physician. 2011;57(12):1401–2.
47. Gomes CF, Sousa M, Lourenço I, Martins D, Torres J. Gastrointestinal diseases during pregnancy: what does the gastroenterologist need to know? Ann Gastroenterol. 2018;31(4):385–94.
48. Casanova MJ, Chaparro M, Domènech E, et al. Safety of thiopurines and anti-TNF-α drugs during pregnancy in patients with inflammatory bowel disease. Am J Gastroenterol. 2013;108(3):433–40.

49. Zelinkova Z, van der Ent C, Bruin KF, Dutch Delta IBD Group, et al. Effects of discontinuing anti-tumor necrosis factor therapy during pregnancy on the course of inflammatory bowel disease and neonatal exposure. Clin Gastroenterol Hepatol. 2013;11(3):318–21.
50. Bell SJ, Flanagan EK. Updates in the management of inflammatory bowel disease during pregnancy. Med J Aust. 2019;210(6):276–80.
51. Nguyen GC, Seow CH, Maxwell C, et al. The Toronto consensus statements for the management of inflammatory bowel disease in pregnancy. Gastroenterology. 2016;150:734–57.

Chapter 26
Heart Disease during Pregnancy

D. P. Esteves and Juliana Silva Esteves

Introduction

Despite being considered a physiological event, fundamental in the preservation of the human species, pregnancy brings with it a fine threshold between physiological and pathological, throughout the gestational period, culminating in labor, expulsion of the fetus and puerperium. In this context, one of the organic systems most subjected to what we could call the physiological stress of pregnancy is the cardiovascular system.

Epidemiology

Exactly because of this physiological stress to which the heart is subjected during pregnancy, cardiovascular pathologies have great prevalence at this stage of a woman's life. Worldwide, the maternal mortality rate in 2015 was 216 maternal deaths/100,000 live births [1, 2].

In the United States of America, a report using data on nearly 3000 maternal deaths from 13 review committees, reported that more than 2/3 of the deaths were attributed to cardiovascular conditions [3].

In general, it is assumed that the prevalence of heart disease in pregnancy is between 1% and 4% worldwide, with an incidence in Brazil of around 4.2%, and cardiac death responsible for 20% of maternal deaths obstetric [4].

D. P. Esteves (✉)
Department of Cardiology, Pregnancy Heart Disease Sector, Hospital Federal dos Servidores do Estado, Rio de Janeiro, RJ, Brazil

J. S. Esteves
Maternal Fetal Medicine Unit, Hospital Federal Servidores do Estado, Rio de Janeiro, Brazil

© Springer Nature Switzerland AG 2022

R. A. Moreira de Sá, E. B. d. Fonseca (eds.), *Perinatology*,
https://doi.org/10.1007/978-3-030-83434-0_26

Hemodynamic Changes in Normal Pregnancy

The main hemodynamic changes related to pregnancy are the increase in cardiac output, the expansion of blood volume, and the reduction of peripheral resistance and systemic arterial pressure.

Systemic vasodilation starts around the fifth week and the systemic vascular resistance (SVR) progressively falls by 35% to 40%, reaching the nadir in the middle of the second trimester, while cardiac output (CO) begins to rise [5].

The reduction in SVR reaches a plateau in the middle of the second quarter and CO (cardiac output). continues to rise, now in a nonlinear manner. The CO reaches its peak at the beginning of the third trimester, the heart rate (HR) that rises during the whole pregnancy, reaches its maximum at the end of the third trimester with an average of 16 bpm above baseline [5].

The supine position reduces CO and Stroke volume and increases HR due to compression of the aorta and vena cava through the enlarged uterus. When placing the pregnant woman in the left lateral decubitus position, the uterus of the aorta and vena cava are deviated, increasing the blood flow to the heart and thus increasing the CD and the Stroke volume [5, 6].

In the intrapartum, the CO increases by 15% above the pre-labor values, at the beginning of this and 25% during the active phase. In the second stage, the CO increases around 50%. With epidural anesthesia, these CO variations are attenuated. Changing the supine position to the left side during delivery increases the CO,

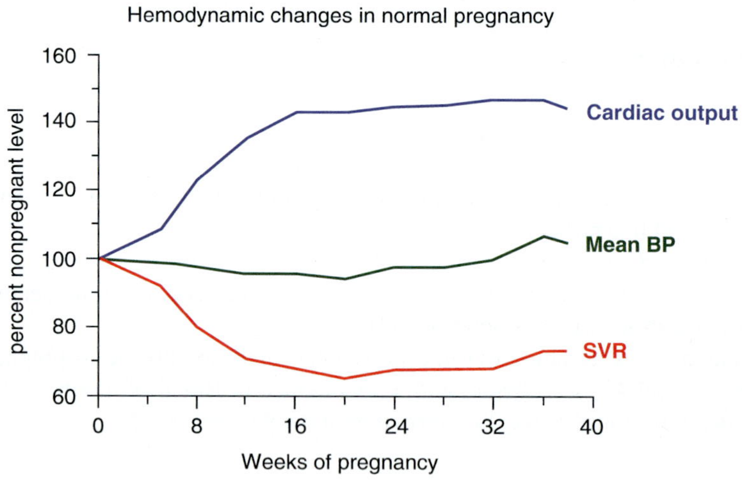

Fig. 26.1 Normal pregnancy is characterized by an increase in cardiac output, a reduction in systemic vascular resistance, and minimal change in mean blood pressure. These changes are associated with a 10 to 15 beat/min increase in heart rate. BP: blood pressure; SVR: systemic vascular resistance. (Reproduced with permission from: Foley MR. Maternal adaptations to pregnancy: Cardiovascular and hemodynamic changes. In: UptoDate, Post TW (Ed). UptoDate, Waltham, MA. (Accessed on 30 October 2020.) Copyright© 2020 UpToDate, Inc. For more information visit www.uptodate.com)

suggesting that during this period the CO is more dependent on the preload. After birth, HR and BP return to prepregnancy values and remain unchanged throughout the period [6].

Pharmacological Changes during Pregnancy

Pharmacokinetics in pregnancy is altered as a result of physiological changes that take place throughout gestation and the postpartum period. Delayed gastric emptying and motility, increased plasma volume and fat accumulation, increased volume of distribution (V_d), decreased albumin and plasma binding proteins, increased minute ventilation, and increased hepatic and renal clearance, all may affect drug distribution and clearance [8]. The sum of these changes commonly results in a reduced pharmacological effect of the drug; however, there are exceptions. The use of Cardiovascular medications during pregnancy requires knowledge of the physiological changes of pregnancy, which may alter the drug's properties, as well as the fetal effects of these medications. A multidisciplinary team should provide thoughtful and complete counseling to the pregnant woman with Cardiovascular disease regarding the risks and benefits of medication use. As per our understanding of pregnancy physiology, pharmacology, and the fetal and placental interactions continues to evolve, we will have an improved ability to treat maternal Cardiovascular conditions during pregnancy [9].

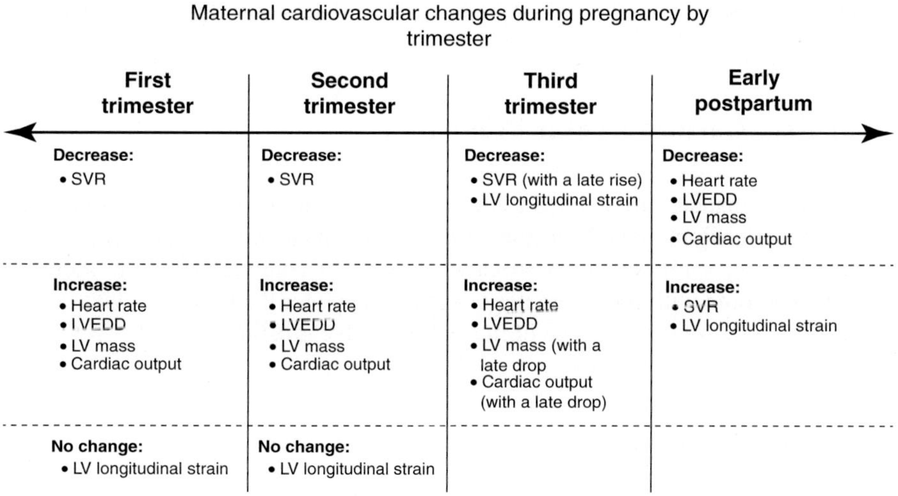

Fig. 26.2 Maternal cardiovascular changes during pregnancy. *SVR* systemic vascular resistance, *LV* left ventricular, *LVEDD* left ventricular end diastolic diameter. (Adapted from [7]. Reproduced with permission from: Foley MR. Maternal adaptations to pregnancy: Cardiovascular and hemodynamic changes. In: UptoDate, Post TW (Ed). UptoDate, Waltham, MA. (Accessed on 30 October 2020.) Copyright© 2020 UpToDate, Inc. For more information visit www.uptodate.com)

Increased Prevalence of Heart Disease in Pregnant Women

The evident increase in the prevalence of heart disease in pregnancy is due in part to the better approach of acquired and congenital heart diseases, to pregnancy at older ages, and a higher prevalence of obesity, arterial hypertension, and diabetes mellitus among women. In addition, many women are postponing childbearing until the fourth and fifth decades of life [10, 11]; with advancing maternal age, underlying medical conditions such as hypertension, diabetes, and hypercholesterolemia become more common and increase the incidence of acquired heart disease complicating pregnancy.

Predictors of Cardiac Events during Pregnancy

In the presence of a pregnant woman with some heart disease, the attending physician must observe the main factors that may predict the onset of adverse cardiac events during pregnancy. Those factors incude the presence of cardiac arrhythmias or a previous cardiac event such as heart failure (HF), transient ischemic attack (TIA), or stroke (stroke). Likewise, those patients in functional class above II of the New York Heart Association or who have cyanosis. In diseases with obstructions of the left heart, such as mitral and aortic valve stenosis, the mitral valve area less than 2 cm^2 as well as the aortic valve area less than 1.5 cm^2 or an left ventricular outflow tract gradient above 30 mmHg, are predictors of poor prognosis. Finally, the presence of systemic ventricular dysfunction is another major predictor of cardiac events during pregnancy.

High-Risk Cardiovascular Pregnancy

High-risk pregnancies are defined as those that occur in the presence of pulmonary arterial hypertension, dilated cardiomyopathy with an ejection fraction of less than 40%, following symptomatic obstructive lesions, in coarctation of the aorta, in Marfan syndrome with root diameter of the aorta greater than 40 mm, with cyanogenic lesions and in the presence of mechanical valve prostheses.

Pregnancy Risk Rating

The World Health Organization (WHO) classifies cardiovascular risk during pregnancy into four stages according to cardiac injury (Table 26.1).

Therefore, severe pulmonary arterial hypertension, severe ventricular dysfunction, dilatation of the aortic root above 4 cm, and severe obstructive lesions of the left heart are considered contraindications for pregnancy.

Table 26.1 Pregnancy risk rating (WHO)

Pregnancy risk rating	Cardiac injury
I—No detectable risk of mortality/minimal increase in maternal morbidity	Small pulmonary stenosis, simple corrected lesions (CIA CIV, PCA, anomalous pulmonary vein drainage)
II—Small risk of mortality/moderate increase in morbidity	Uncorrected CIA or CIV
II to III—Depends on the patient	Valvopathy/biological prosthesis, corrected Ao, Marfan syndrome without aortic dilation, bicuspid aortic valve with aorta 40 to 45 mm, mild ventricular dysfunction
III—Significant increase in the risk of mortality/significant morbidity/need for care by a specialized team	Mechanical prosthesis, Fontan circulation, uncorrected cyanogenic heart disease, Marfan with aorta 45 to 50 mm
IV—Pregnancy contraindicated	HAP/Eisenmenger, FE < 30%, NYHA III–IV, severe MS, severe symptomatic AS, Marfan syndrome with aorta >45 mm, v. bicuspid aortic with aorta >50 mm, severe Coa Ao.

IAC interatrial communication; *IVC* intraventricular communication; *PCA* patent ductus arteriosus; *Coa Ao* coarctation of the aorta; *PAH* pulmonary arterial hypertension; *EF* left ventricular ejection fraction; *NYHA* New York Heart Association functional classification; *MS* mital stenosis; *EA* aortic stenosis

Childbirth

Most patients can progress to vaginal delivery and, occasionally, the use of forceps in the second stage of delivery will be indicated.

Epidural analgesia is recommended for most cardiac patients, in order to reduce sympathetic stimulation and the consequent increase in O_2 consumption.

Epidural anesthesia is recommended because it produces fewer hemodynamic changes.

Cardiovascular indications for cesarean section would initially be restricted to the presence of aortic root dilation or aortic aneurysm, severe decompensated heart failure, a recent history of acute myocardial infarction, the presence of significant symptomatic aortic stenosis or the need for immediate valve replacement after delivery.

Anticoagulation

Pregnancy is a prothrombotic state with nearly a fivefold increased risk of VTE (venous thromboembolism), so choice of anticoagulant must balance maternal with fetal risk.

VKAs (vitamin K antagonists) are safest for the mother, and complications to the fetus, like fetal loss, embryopathy and bleeding, are dose dependent.

LMWH (low molecular weight heparin) requires frequent monitoring of anti-Xa levels, and despite therapeutics levels, thrombotic events may occur particularly in women with MHV.

Frequent monitoring of anticoagulation is essential.

Women should be converted to IV UFH (unfracionated heparin) prior to planned delivery to prevent life-threatening fetal bleeding, but some may require urgent delivery while taking VKAs, in which case cesarean delivery is recommended for fetal protection.

Finally, remember that the risk of maternal thrombosis remains elevated in postpartum period.

Recommendations Based on "Guidelines for Management of Cardiovascular Diseases During Pregnancy" ESC 2018

Cardiovascular Risk Assessment

Every cardiac woman of childbearing age must undergo an individual assessment based on cardiac pathology, ventricular and valve function, functional class, the presence of cyanosis, pulmonary arterial pressure level, among others.

The WHO modified risk classification is recommended (mWHO).

Women of moderate to high risk should receive preconception counseling and, if applicable, follow-up of the entire pregnancy, delivery and puerperium in a specialized center and by an experienced multidisciplinary team (pregnancy heart team).

Pregnancy and, consequently, infertility treatment are contraindicated in women in the mWHO IV class.

Percutaneous or surgical intervention, recommended before pregnancy in patients with mital stenosis (MS) and valve area <1.0 cm^2.

Attention in Monitoring Pregnancy, Childbirth, and the Puerperium

Every pregnant woman with congenital heart disease must undergo a fetal echocardiogram between the 19th and 22nd weeks of pregnancy.

Birth planning, detailing aspects of induction and monitoring of labor, the expulsive period and care in the immediate puerperium, should be done between the 20th and 30th weeks of pregnancy.

Labor induction should be considered in the 40th week of pregnancy, in cardiac patients.

The vaginal route is the first choice for most pregnant women with heart disease, and the indication for cesarean section is restricted to the following situations:

- Premature labor in a pregnant woman using oral anticoagulants.
- Presence of aggressive aortic pathology.
- Severe forms of pulmonary hypertension, including Eisenmenger syndrome.

Termination of pregnancy should be considered if there is a high risk of maternal morbidity and mortality and/or fetal abnormalities.

Special Situations

Pregnant women with mechanical valve prostheses have a high risk of morbidity and mortality (thrombosis and hemorrhage) and must be accompanied by a "pregnancy heart team."

The use of oral anticoagulant (warfarin) is recommended during the second and third trimesters, until the 36th week of pregnancy. In women using low doses of oral anticoagulant (warfarin <5 mg), this can be maintained throughout pregnancy, up to the 36th week, when it will be replaced by LMWH or UFH.

LMWH should be used when it is possible to monitor anti-Xa levels, with dose adjustment.

Women with peripartum cardiomyopathy or dilated cardiomyopathy should be advised about the risk of deteriorating their condition during pregnancy and the puerperium. New pregnancies should be discouraged if ejection fraction (EF) does not return to normal.

Pregnant women with long QT syndrome and catecholaminergic polymorphic VT should receive beta-blockers during pregnancy and childbirth.

Arterial Hypertension

Drug treatment is recommended for all pregnant women with BP ≥150/95 mmHg and> 140/90 mmHg in case of gestational hypertension (with or without proteinuria), gestational hypertension superimposed on pre-existing hypertension or hypertension with symptomatic or target organ damage.

Methyldopa, labetolol IV, and calcium channel blockers are recommended for the treatment of gestational hypertension.

References

1. Alkema L, Chou D, Hogan D, Sanquian Z, Moller AB, Gemmill A, et al. Global, regional, and national levels and trends in maternal mortality between 1990 and 2015, with scenario-based projections to 2030: a systematic analysis by the UN Maternal Mortality Estimation Inter-Agency Group. Lancet. 2016:387(1007);462–74.

2. World Health Organization. Maternal Mortality (internet). Maternal Mortality (September, 2019). Available from http://www.who.int/news-room/fact-sheets/detail/maternal-mortality.
3. Petersen EE, Davis NL, Goodman D, Cox S, Mayes N, Johnston E, et al. Vital signs: pregnancy-related deaths, United States, 2011-2015, and strategies for prevention, 13 states, 2013-2017. MMWR Morb Mortal Wkly Rep. 2019;68(18):423–9.
4. Sociedade Brasileira de Cardiologia. Diretriz da Sociedade Brasileira de Cardiologia para Gravidez na Mulher Portadora de Cardiopatia. Arq Bras Cardiol. 2009:93(6 supl.1);e110–78.
5. Meag VL, Cockcrof JR, Backx K, Shave R, Stöhr E. Cardiac output and related haemodynamics during pregnancy: a series of meta-analyses. Heart. 2016;102(7):518–26.
6. Chapman AB, Abraham WT, Zamudio S, Coffin C, Merouani A, Young D, et al. Temporal relationships between hormonal and hemodynamic changes in early human pregnancy. Kidney Int. 1998;54(6):2056–63.
7. Ashrafi R, Curtis SL. Heart disease and pregnancy. Cardiol Ther. 2017;6(2):157–73.
8. Pariente G, Leibson T, Carls A, Adams-Webber T, Ito S, Koren G. Pregnancy-associated changes in pharmacokinetics: a systematic review. PLoS Med. 2016:13(11);e1002160.
9. Halpern DG, Weinberg CR, Pinnelas R, Mehta-Lee S, Economy KE, Valente AM. Use of medication for cardiovascular disease during pregnancy: JACC state-of-the-art review. J Am Coll Card. 2019;73(4):457–76.
10. Fretts RC, Schmittdiel J, McLean FH, Usher RH, Goldman MB. Increased maternal age and the risk of fetal death. N Engl J Med. 1995;333(15):953–7.
11. Cunningham FG, Leveno KJ. Childbearing among older women--the message is cautiously optimistic. N Engl J Med 1995:333(15);1002–4.

Chapter 27
Thyroid Disorders

Luciana C. Cima, Mariane T. Tauile, Viviane P. Monteiro, and Isabela Bussade

Introduction

Many have suggested universally evaluating thyroid function in all women either before or during pregnancy. Given the complexity surrounding thyroid physiology and thyroid illness during pregnancy and the postpartum period, how and when to evaluate for thyroid dysfunction and how and if to treat thyroid illness during this period remain challenging. These physiological changes can happen seamlessly in healthy women, but thyroid dysfunction can occur in many pregnant women because of pathologic processes.

Placental human chorionic gonadotropin (hCG) stimulates thyroid hormone secretion, often decreasing maternal thyroid-stimulating hormone (TSH) concentrations, especially in early pregnancy. Increasingly, data suggest that antiperoxidase (TPO) positivity, especially hypothyroidism, adversely modulates the impact of maternal thyroid status on pregnancy and the developing fetus. Thyroid antibody positivity separately increases the risk of thyroid dysfunction following delivery and during the postpartum period.

Separate questions surround the optimal approach to the treatment of hypothyroidism and hyperthyroidism while lactating. Other special situations such as

L. C. Cima · M. T. Tauile
Perinatal/Rede D'or, Rio de Janeiro, RJ, Brazil

V. P. Monteiro (✉)
Instituto Fernandes Figueira / Fiocruz, Rio de Janeiro, RJ, Brazil

I. Bussade
Pontifícia Universidade Católica (PUC), Rio de Janeiro, RJ, Brazil
e-mail: isabelabussade@isabelabussade.com.br

© Springer Nature Switzerland AG 2022

R. A. Moreira de Sá, E. B. d. Fonseca (eds.), *Perinatology*,
https://doi.org/10.1007/978-3-030-83434-0_27

thyroid nodule, and treatment of thyroid illness in women undergoing assisted reproductive techniques (ART) were also addressed.

Screening all women either before or during pregnancy must take the cost, effectiveness, and practical nature of any such approach into account. Studies evaluating this question have not had conclusive findings to date. Further investigations should shed light on this difficult question.

Physiological Changes of the Thyroid Gland during Pregnancy

Many alterations occur during normal pregnancy, such as an increase in iodine excretion, increase in thyroid hormone production, increase in thyroxine binding proteins (TBG), and thyroid stimulatory effects of maternal hCG. Therefore, thyroid function tests change during pregnancy in women with a healthy thyroid gland [1, 2]. The thyroid is functioning normally if the TSH and FT4 remain in the trimester-specific normal ranges throughout pregnancy.

In the beginning of the first trimester TBG and total T4 (TT4) concentrations rise by week 7, and reach their peak at week 16 of gestation [3], and they remain elevated until birth. Human chorionic gonadotropin (HCG) directly stimulates the TSH receptor on the thyroid gland, resulting in an increase in hormone production, and consequently reduces TSH levels [2, 4]. These lower levels are well observed during the first trimester, and progressively rise throughout pregnancy [2]. In multiple pregnancies, the TSH limits are even lower due to higher hCG concentrations, when compared to singleton pregnancies [5].

Reference Range for Serum TSH in Pregnancy

Normal TSH reference values are reduced during pregnancy, in both its lower and upper limits. The lower reference can be reduced by approximately 0.4 mU/L, while the upper reference is reduced by 0.5 mU/L, which typically represents a TSH upper reference of 4.0 mU/L. Whenever possible a population-based curve for serum TSH should be used [6].

Iodine Requirements

Dietary intake of iodine should be higher during pregnancy since there is increased renal iodine excretion, fetal iodine requirements, and increased thyroid hormone production [7]. Women who already have an adequate intake of iodine before and during pregnancy, through consumption of iodized salt, usually present enough intrathyroidal iodine stores and therefore present no difficulty adapting to the higher demand for thyroid hormone during pregnancy [8]. However, women with severe iodine deficiency during pregnancy have increased rates of pregnancy loss, stillbirth, and increased perinatal an infant mortality [9]. Universal salt iodization is the most cost-effective way of delivering iodine to the population and reducing complications associated with iodine deficiency [10].

Thyroid Auto-Antibodies

Prevalence of thyroid peroxidase antibody (anti-TPO) or thyroglobulin antibody (anti-Tg) varies with ethnicity and age, and is present in 2% to 17% of pregnant women [11–19]. Euthyroid pregnant women who are anti-TPO or anti-Tg positive should have TSH level measured every 4 weeks until mid-pregnancy [6], since thyroid autoimmunity may be related to hypothyroidism [20].

Currently there is not enough evidence to support a direct relationship between the presence of thyroid antibodies and miscarriage, or preterm birth [6, 21].

Impact of Thyroid Disease upon Infertility and Assisted Reproduction

The risk of infertility in women with either overt hypothyroidism or hyperthyroidism is not well studied. Thus, despite imperfect data, the majority of evidence appears to support an association between overt thyroid dysfunction and an increased risk of infertility [6].

Among women presenting with infertility, TSH levels were highest among women with ovulatory dysfunction and unknown causes of infertility, and lower among those women with tubal infertility [24].

As for subclinical hypothyroidism, there is not enough evidence supporting any negative impact of the disease on fertility. Thus, insufficient data exist for recommending for or against routine LT4 therapy in subclinical hypothyroid, thyroid autoantibody–negative infertile women who are attempting conception but not undergoing assisted reproductive techniques (ART). There is little evidence suggesting that women with female-factor infertility are more likely to be anti-TPO positive, even if euthyroid [22]. Among women with polycystic ovarian syndrome (PCOS), the presence of thyroid antibodies has been associated with a worse response to treatment with clomiphene citrate [23]. Furthermore, the prevalence of antithyroid antibodies may be higher in women with PCOS [25].

As for treatment, administration of LT4 is recommended for infertile women with overt hypothyroidism who desire pregnancy. Insufficient evidence exists to determine if LT4 therapy improves fertility in thyroid autoantibody–positive euthyroid women who are attempting natural conception. Therefore, no recommendation can be made for LT4 therapy in this setting [6]. As for the subclinical hypothyroid women undergoing in vitro fertilization (IVF) or intracytoplasmic sperm injection (ICSI), LT4 should be administered, and the goal of treatment is to achieve a TSH concentration < 2.5 mU/L. Insufficient evidence exists to determine whether LT4 therapy improves the success of pregnancy following ART in anti-TPO euthyroid women. However, administration of LT4 to anti-TPO euthyroid women undergoing ART may be considered given its potential benefits in comparison to its minimal risk [6].

Thyroid Illness

Hypothyroidism

In the setting of pregnancy, maternal hypothyroidism is defined as a TSH concentration elevated beyond the upper limit of the pregnancy-specific reference range, which, if not available, an upper reference limit of 4.0 mU/L may be used. For most assays, this limit represents a reduction in the nonpregnant TSH upper reference limit of 0.5 mU/L. Isolated hypothyroxinemia is typically defined as a FT4 concentration in the lower 2.5th–fifth percentile of a given population in conjunction with a normal maternal TSH concentration.

Overt maternal hypothyroidism has consistently been shown to be associated with an increased risk of adverse pregnancy complications [26] as well as detrimental effects upon fetal neurocognitive development [27]. Such outcomes include increased risks of premature birth, low birth weight, pregnancy loss, and lower offspring Intelligence Quotient (IQ); thus demonstrating a clear association between the disease and serious risk to the maternal–fetal unit, therefore treatment of overt hypothyroidism is recommended during pregnancy.

Subclinical hypothyroidism is variably associated with an increased risk of adverse pregnancy outcomes in most studies, partly because separate studies use differing cutoffs to define an elevated TSH concentration.

Pregnant women with TSH concentrations >2.5 mU/L should be evaluated for anti-TPO status, since the presence of the antibody is relevant when considering treatment. LT4 therapy is not recommended for patients who are anti-TPO negative with a normal TSH. In this group of patients an ultrasound scan should be performed, since there are some findings that may suggest autoimmune disease, in which case treatment should be considered [28]. Isolated hypothyroxinemia should not be routinely treated in pregnancy. The recommended treatment of maternal hypothyroidism is administration of oral LT4. There are commercial presentations of the drug in varying doses, ranging from 25 to 200 mcg. The medication should be taken after overnight fasting, preferably 1 hour before breakfast [29]. The treatment should target a TSH value in the lower half of the trimester-specific reference range. When this is not available, it is reasonable to target maternal TSH concentrations below 2.5 mU/L [6].

Women with overt and subclinical hypothyroidism (treated or untreated) or those at risk for hypothyroidism (e.g., patients who are euthyroid but anti-TPO or anti-Tg positive, post-hemithyroidectomy, or treated with radioactive iodine) should be monitored with serum TSH measurement approximately every 4 weeks until mid-gestation and at least once near 30 weeks gestation.

Treated hypothyroid women of reproductive age should be counseled regarding the likelihood of increased demand for LT4 during pregnancy. For those who are planning pregnancy, serum TSH should be evaluated preconception, and LT4 doses adjusted to achieve TSH values between the lower reference limit and 2.5 mU/L.

Hypothyroid patients receiving LT4 treatment with a suspected or confirmed pregnancy should have their dose increased by 20%–30% [30]. One simple way of accomplishing this is to administer two additional tablets per week of the patient's current daily LT4 dosage.

After delivery, LT4 should be reduced to the patient's preconception dose. Additional thyroid function testing should be performed at approximately 6 weeks postpartum. Some women in whom LT4 is initiated during pregnancy may not require LT4 postpartum. Such women are candidates for discontinuing LT4, especially those using low doses (less or = 50 mcg). If LT4 is discontinued, serum TSH should be evaluated in approximately 6 weeks.

It is known that untreated (or under treated) hypothyroidism can adversely affect pregnancy. On the other hand, there is no data suggesting that women with adequately treated subclinical or overt hypothyroidism have an increased risk of any obstetrical complication. Consequently, there is no indication for any additional obstetric testing or surveillance in pregnancies of women with either subclinical or overt hypothyroidism who are being monitored and treated appropriately. An exception to this is women with Graves' disease (GD) effectively treated with ^{131}I ablation or surgical resection, who require TSH receptor antibody (TRAb) monitoring [6].

Hyperthyroidism

Thyrotoxicosis occurs when a person is exposed to supraphysiological amounts of thyroid hormones. Most cases of thyrotoxicosis are due to hyperthyroidism, and the most common cause in women of childbearing age is autoimmune Graves' disease (GD) occurring before pregnancy in 0.4–1.0% of women and in approximately 0.2% during pregnancy [31]. Less common non-autoimmune causes of hyperthyroidism in pregnancy include toxic multinodular goiter (Plummer's disease), subacute thyroiditis and toxic adenoma. Another possible cause of thyrotoxicosis is overtreatment with or inadequate intake of thyroid hormone.

More frequently than GD, gestational transient thyrotoxicosis can occur in the first half of pregnancy, and this condition is characterized by elevated FT4 and suppressed serum TSH, being diagnosed in about 1–3% of pregnancies. This frequency is secondary to elevated hCG levels [32, 33], being often associated with hyperemesis gravidarum. Other conditions associated with hCG-induced thyrotoxicosis include multiple gestation, hydatidiform mole, and choriocarcinoma [34, 35]. Serum hCG is usually higher in gestational transient thyrotoxicosis than in patients with GD, but overlap is considerable, and the clinical usefulness of such measurement is limited [36]. The management of women with gestational transient thyrotoxicosis depends on the severity of symptoms, and the approach should include supportive therapy, management of dehydration, and hospitalization if needed. Antithyroid drugs (ATD) are not recommended, though the use of b-blockers may be considered. Women already taking methimazole (MMI) and propylthiouracil (PTU) should be instructed to confirm potential pregnancy as soon as possible, and contact their caregiver immediately.

The biochemical diagnosis of hyperthyroidism is confirmed in the presence of a suppressed or undetectable serum TSH and elevated serum TT4/FT4, or T3. It is essential to diagnose the etiology of thyrotoxicosis in pregnant patients. In early pregnancy, the differential diagnosis in most cases is between GD and gestational transient thyrotoxicosis [32, 33]. In both situations, common clinical manifestations include palpitations, anxiety, tremor, and heat intolerance. A careful history and physical examination is essential in establishing the etiology. The findings of no prior history of thyroid disease, no stigmata of GD (goiter, orbitopathy), a self-limited mild disorder, and symptoms of emesis favor the diagnosis of gestational transient thyrotoxicosis.

If other causes for thyrotoxicosis are suspected, measurement of TRAb is indicated. If this is negative or thyroid nodules are suspected based on clinical examination, a thyroid ultrasound should be performed to evaluate nodularity.

For women with GD, pregnancy should be postponed until a stable euthyroid state is reached. Those seeking future pregnancy should be counseled regarding the complexity of disease management during gestation, including the association of birth defects with ATD use. Preconception counseling should review the risks and benefits of all treatment options, including ^{131}I ablation, surgical thyroidectomy, or ATD therapy, and the patient's desire to conceive.

Several studies have shown that obstetric and medical complications are directly related to control of maternal hyperthyroidism, and the duration of the euthyroid state throughout pregnancy [37–40]. When thyrotoxicosis is not adequately controlled, it can be associated with pregnancy loss, pregnancy-induced hypertension, prematurity, low birth weight, intrauterine growth restriction, stillbirth, thyroid storm, and maternal congestive heart failure [41]. Furthermore, some studies suggest fetal exposure to high levels of maternal thyroid hormone may lead the offspring to develop diseases such as seizure disorders and neurobehavioral disorders in later life [42].

Although ATD use in pregnancy is not recommended, in patients at high risk of developing thyrotoxicosis, use of antithyroid medication should be considered. Factors predicting high clinical risk include being currently hyperthyroid, or requirement of high doses of MMI or PTU for disease control. In such cases, PTU is recommended for the treatment of maternal hyperthyroidism through 16 weeks of pregnancy [6].

Thyroid stimulating antibodies, ATDs, and most maternal thyroid hormones can effectively cross the placental barrier. TRAb antibodies can stimulate the fetal thyroid gland, causing excess fetal production of thyroid hormone. Furthermore, if the mother is hyperthyroid from GD, the fetus will also be exposed to the hyperthyroxinemia produced by the mother's thyroid during gestation. Typically, fetal hyperthyroidism due to cross-placental passage of TRAb develops at or after week 20 of pregnancy [6].

It is important to note that all ATDs tend to be more potent in the fetus than in the mother. Thus, when the mother is made euthyroid, the fetus is often overtreated [43]. Therefore, in order to avoid an undesired fetal impact, the aim of treatment is to maintain maternal TT4/FT4 values at, or just above the pregnancy-specific upper limit of normal. These markers, along with TSH, should be monitored approximately every 4 weeks.

Women with previous or current GD have a higher risk for: fetal hyperthyroidism, neonatal hyperthyroidism, fetal hypothyroidism, neonatal hypothyroidism, and central hypothyroidism. The onset of these complications depends on several factors, such as poor control of hyperthyroidism throughout pregnancy inducing transient central hypothyroidism [44, 45]; excessive amounts of ATDs being responsible for fetal and neonatal hypothyroidism, even if the mother is biochemically euthyroid [46, 47]; and high levels of thyroid stimulating antibodies in the second half of pregnancy inducing fetal and neonatal hyperthyroidism [48–51]. The incidence of these complications range between 1% and 5% in all women with active or a past history of GD, and is associated with increased fetal/neonatal morbidity and mortality if unrecognized and untreated [52].

Fetal surveillance should be performed in women who have uncontrolled hyperthyroidism in the second half of pregnancy, and in women with high TRAb levels detected at any time during pregnancy (greater than 3 times the upper limit of normal). A consultation with an experienced obstetrician or maternal–fetal medicine specialist is recommended. Monitoring should include ultrasound to assess signs of potential fetal hyperthyroidism, such as fetal tachycardia (heart rate >170 bpm, persistent for over 10 min), intrauterine growth restriction, presence of fetal goiter (the earliest sonographic sign of fetal thyroid dysfunction), accelerated bone maturation, signs of congestive heart failure, and fetal hydrops [48, 53–55].

Thyroid Nodules

Patients who present with a thyroid nodule during pregnancy should be asked about family history of thyroid cancer, as well as personal history of cancer before 18 years of age which treatment involved head, neck, and/or cranial radiation and those exposed to ionizing radiation [56, 57]. Ultrasound is the most accurate tool for detecting and monitoring thyroid nodules. It can detect nodules features, growth and evaluates cervical lymph nodes [6]. Most women with thyroid cancer present with normal hormone levels, however, all women investigating a thyroid nodule should have TSH levels measured [58, 59]. In nonpregnant women, lower TSH values usually indicate a functioning nodule, which would further be evaluated with scintigraphy. Functioning nodules are rarely malignant, and therefore cytologic evaluation would not be indicated. In pregnant women, evaluation is limited since the lower TSH reference values are decreased, especially in the first trimester, and scintigraphy is contra-indicated during this period [6]. Fine needle aspiration (FNA) should be considered when nodules are >1 cm and ultrasound findings of suspicion are identified, such as hypoechoic nodules, with irregular borders and microcalcifications. FNA can be performed in any trimester, and is considered a safe diagnostic tool [60–69]. Even though survival rates do not change significantly when surgery is performed during gestation or postpartum in patients with thyroid cancer diagnosed during pregnancy [70–72] fine-needle aspiration is generally indicated to investigate newly detected nodules in pregnant patients with a nonsuppressed TSH. Cytologic benign nodules do not require special surveillance during pregnancy [6].

Postpartum Thyroiditis

Postpartum thyroiditis is an inflammatory autoimmune condition characterized by the occurrence of thyroid dysfunction, excluding GD, in the first postpartum year in women who were euthyroid prior to pregnancy [73]. In the classic form, which occurs in one quarter of cases, transient thyrotoxicosis is followed by transient hypothyroidism with a return to the euthyroid state by the end of the initial postpartum year [74]. This disease can also present as isolated thyrotoxicosis, in one quarter of cases, and isolated hypothyroidism, in one half.

The thyrotoxicosis phase can happen during the first postpartum year, but mostly in the first 2–6 months, and all cases resolve spontaneously. On the other hand, the hypothyroid phase can take place between 3 and 12 months postpartum and up to 20% of patients can become permanently hypothyroid.

Fetal and Neonatal Considerations

The fetal hypothalamic-pituitary-thyroid system develops mostly independently of maternal influence because the placenta regulates the passage of many substances to the fetus, under normal circumstances [6]. There is modest placental permeability for T4 [75], and this is particularly important for hypothyroid fetuses. This explains the normal or near-normal cognitive outcomes of newborns diagnosed with congenital hypothyroidism at birth and treated adequately [6].

Maternal autoantibodies (immunoglobulin G) can cross the placenta from mid-gestation onward [76]. Pregnant women with autoimmune thyroid disease can transmit the autoantibodies to TPO, Tg, and TSH receptor (TRAB) to the fetus, but only the latter can impact fetal thyroid function [77]. Hyperthyroidism usually develops in neonates born to mothers with high concentrations of TRAB, corresponding to 1–2% of mothers with Graves' disease (GD). This incidence is four times higher than that for transient neonatal hypothyroidism caused by the same antibody [78].

Maternal subclinical hypothyroidism during pregnancy is a risk factor for small for gestational age (SGA) neonate, and is associated with lower birthweight. By contrast, isolated hypothyroxinemia was associated with higher birthweight but not large for gestational age (LGA). Maternal TSH and FT4 concentrations were both inversely associated with birthweight, with the association of FT4 being most apparent during later pregnancy, whereas the association of TSH with birthweight was most apparent in women who were anti-TPO positive [79].

Thyroid Disease and Lactation

Uncontrolled hypothyroidism and hyperthyroidism can impact milk let-down and successful breastfeeding. Once other causes of unsuccessful lactation have been eliminated, TSH should be measured to assess thyroid disfunction since hypothyroidism can have a negative impact on breastfeeding. As for hyperthyroidism there is no recommendation for treatment since its impact on lactation is unknown.

A small amount of maternal thyroid hormone is present in the breast milk of lactating women, approximately 1% of the total daily requirement. Maternal transfer of thyroid hormone does not have a meaningful impact on the infant's thyroid hormone status [80]. PTU and MMI have also been detected in breast milk in small amounts, and their use is safe during lactation. It is recommended that these drugs should be used in the lowest effective dose since there have not been larger population studies yet [81]. The use of radioactive iodine is contraindicated during lactation [82].

Closing Remarks

The prevalence of thyroid disease, either anatomical or functional, is high in the general population, being markedly higher in women than men and showing a direct increasing rate with age. Therefore, we believe it is of vital importance that the obstetrician/primary care-taker should have adequate knowledge concerning its management, being able to refer the patient to a specialist when needed in order to preserve the maternal-fetal unit well-being. Women with medical history of infertility or recurrent gestational loss should have their thyrotropic axis adequately evaluated, for it can impact the course of future gestations. It is essential that this evaluation be a part of the initial workup for these patients. For pregnant women presenting with nodular disease, it is necessary to have an adequate suspicion level of high malignancy risk lesions in order to get to the diagnosis of neoplasia in a timely manner. As for diseases associated to glandular function it is imperative to fully understand the physiology and TSH levels behavior during pregnancy in order to correctly diagnose either hyperthyroidism or hypothyroidism, since overtreatment as well as insufficient treatment could present obstetric and fetal risk. In the postpartum period, considering the beginning of the lactation process, a new clinical scenario is presented and management of these diseases may need adjustment, such as suspension of LT4 administration in subclinical hypothyroid patients, as well as installment of antithyroid drugs in hyperthyroid patients.

References

1. van Raaij JM, Vermaat-Miedema SH, Schonk CM, Peek ME, Hautvast JG. Energy requirements of pregnancy in the Netherlands. Lancet. 1987;2:953–5.
2. Glinoer D. The regulation of thyroid function in pregnancy: pathways of endocrine adaptation from physiology to pathology. Endocr Rev. 1997;18:404–33.
3. Weeke J, Dybkjaer L, Granlie K, Eskjaer Jensen S, Kjaerulff E, Laurberg P, Magnusson B. A longitudinal study of serum TSH, and total and free iodothyronines during normal pregnancy. Acta Endocrinol. 1982;101:531.
4. Baloch Z, Carayon P, Conte-Devolx B, Demers LM, Feldt-Rasmussen U, Henry JF, LiVosli VA, Niccoli-Sire P, John R, Ruf J, Smyth PP, Spencer CA, Stockigt JR, Guidelines Committee, National Academy of Clinical Biochemistry. Laboratory medicine practice guidelines. Laboratory support for the diagnosis and monitoring of thyroid disease. Thyroid. 2003;13:3–126.
5. Sapin R, D'Herbomez M, Schlienger JL. Free thyroxine measured with equilibrium dialysis and nine immunoassays decreases in late pregnancy. Clin Lab. 2004;50:581–4.
6. Alexander E, Pearce E, Brent G, Brown R, Chen H, Dosiou C, Grobman W, Laurberg P, Lazarus J, Mandel J, Peeters R, Sullivan S. Guidelines of the American Thyroid Association for the diagnosis and Management of Thyroid Disease during Pregnancy and the postpartum. Thyroid. 2017;27(3):315–89.
7. Glinoer D. The importance of iodine nutrition during pregnancy. Public Health Nutr. 2007;10:1542–6.
8. Liberman CS, Pino SC, Fang SL, Braverman LE, Emerson CH. Circulating iodide concentrations during and after pregnancy. J Clin Endocrinol Metab. 1998;83:3545–9.
9. Delange FM, Dunn JT. Iodine deficiency. In: Braverman LE, Utiger RD, editors. Werner and Ingbar's the thyroid: a fundamental and clinical text. 9th ed. Philadelphia: Lippincott, Williams and Wilkins; 2005. p. 264–88.
10. Zimmermann MB. The effects of iodine deficiency in pregnancy and infancy. Paediatr Perinat Epidemiol. 2012;26(Suppl 1):108–17.
11. Moreno-Reyes R, Glinoer D, Van Oyen H, Vandevijvere S. High prevalence of thyroid disorders in pregnant women in a mildly iodine-deficient country: a population based study. J Clin Endocrinol Metab. 2013;98:3694–701.
12. Ashoor G, Maiz N, Rotas M, Jawdat F, Nicolaides KH. Maternal thyroid function at 11 to 13 weeks of gestation and subsequent fetal death. Thyroid. 2010;20:989–93.

13. Benhadi N, Wiersinga WM, Reitsma JB, Vrijkotte TG, van der Wal MF, Bonsel GJ. Ethnic differences in TSH but not in free T4 concentrations or TPO antibodies during pregnancy. Clin Endocrinol. 2007;66:765–70.
14. La'ulu SL, Roberts WL. Second-trimester reference intervals for thyroid tests: the role of ethnicity. Clin Chem. 2007;53:1658–64.
15. Abbassi-Ghanavati M, Casey BM, Spong CY, McIntire DD, Halvorson LM, Cunningham FG. Pregnancy outcomes in women with thyroid peroxidase antibodies. Obstet Gynecol. 2010;116(2 Pt 1):381–6.
16. Wasserman EE, Nelson K, Rose NR, Eaton W, Pillion JP, Seaberg E, Talor MV, Burek L, Duggan A, Yolken RH. Maternal thyroid autoantibodies during the third trimester and hearing deficits in children: an epidemiologic assessment. Am J Epidemiol. 2008;167:701–10.
17. Pearce EN, Oken E, Gillman MW, Lee SL, Magnani B, Platek D, Braverman LE. Association of first trimester thyroid function test values with thyroperoxidase antibody status, smoking, and multivitamin use. Endocr Pract. 2008;14:33–9.
18. Moleti M, Lo Presti VP, Mattina F, Mancuso A, De Vivo A, Giorgianni G, Di Bella B, Trimarchi F, Vermiglio F. Gestational thyroid function abnormalities in conditions of mild iodine deficiency: early screening versus continuous monitoring of maternal thyroid status. Eur J Endocrinol. 2009;160:611–7.
19. McElduff A, Morris J. Thyroid function tests and thyroid autoantibodies in an unselected population of women undergoing first trimester screening for aneuploidy. Aust N Z J Obstet Gynaecol. 2008;48:478–80.
20. Glinoer D, Riahi M, Grun JP, Kinthaert J. Risk of subclinical hypothyroidism in pregnant women with asymptomatic autoimmune thyroid disorders. J Clin EndocrinolMetab. 1994;79:197–204.
21. Netto LS, Coeli CM, Michmacher E, Da Costa AM, Nazar L, Galvão D, Buescu A, Vaisman M. Am J Reprod Immunol. 2004;52(5):312–6.
22. Poppe K, Glinoer D, Van Steirteghem A, Tournaye H, Devroey P, Schiettecatte J, Velkeniers B. Thyroid dysfunction and autoimmunity in infertile women. Thyroid. 2002;12:997–1001.
23. Ott J, Aust S, Kurz C, Nouri K, Wirth S, Huber JC, Mayerhofer K. Elevated antithyroid peroxidase antibodies indicating Hashimoto's thyroiditis are associated with the treatment response in infertile women with polycystic ovary syndrome. Fertil Steril. 2010;94:2895–7.
24. Arojoki M, Jokimaa V, Juuti A, Koskinen P, Irjala K, Anttila L. Hypothyroidism among infertile women in Finland. Gynecol Endocrinol. 2000;14:127–31.
25. Kachuei M, Jafari F, Kachuei A, Keshteli AH. Prevalence of autoimmune thyroiditis in patients with polycystic ovary syndrome. Arch Gynecol Obstet. 2012;285:853–6.
26. van den Boogaard E, Vissenberg R, Land JA, van Wely M, van der Post JA, Goddijn M, Bisschop PH. Significance of (sub)clinical thyroid dysfunction and thyroid autoimmunity before conception and in early pregnancy: a systematic review. Hum Reprod Update. 2011;17:605–19.
27. Haddow JE, Palomaki GE, Allan WC, Williams JR, Knight GJ, Gagnon J, O'Heir CE, Mitchell ML, Hermos RJ, Waisbren SE, Faix JD, Klein RZ. Maternal thyroid deficiency during pregnancy and subsequent neuropsychological development of the child. N Engl J Med. 1999;341:549–55.
28. Pedersen OM, Aardal NP, Larssen TB, Varhaug JE, Myking O, Vik-Mo H. The value of ultrasonography in predicting autoimmune thryroid disease. Thyroid. 2000;10(3):251–9.
29. Couto E, Cavichiolli F. Doenças da tireoide na gestação. São Paulo: Federação Brasileira das Associações de Ginecologia e Obstetrícia (FEBRASGO); 2018. (Protocolo FEBRASGO - Obstetrícia, no. 49/ Comissão Nacional Especializada em Gestação de Alto Risco).
30. Yassa L, Marqusee E, Fawcett R, Alexander EK. Thyroid hormone early adjustment in pregnancy (the THERAPY) trial. J Clin Endocrinol Metab. 2010;95:3234–41.
31. Cooper DS, Laurberg P. Hyperthyroidism in pregnancy. Lancet Diabetes Endocrinol. 2013;1:238–49.
32. Goodwin TM, Montoro M, Mestman JH. Transient hyperthyroidism and hyperemesis gravidarum: clinical aspects. Am J Obstet Gynecol. 1992;167:648–52.

33. Tan JY, Loh KC, Yeo GS, Chee YC. Transient hyperthyroidism of hyperemesis gravidarum. BJOG. 2002;109:683–8.
34. Hershman JM. Human chorionic gonadotropin and the thyroid: hyperemesis gravidarum and trophoblastic tumors. Thyroid. 1999;9:653–7.
35. Grun JP, Meuris S, De Nayer P, Glinoer D. The thyrotrophic role of human chorionic gonadotrophin (hCG) in the early stages of twin (versus single) pregnancies. Clin Endocrinol (Oxf). 1997;46:719–25.
36. Glinoer D, Spencer CA. Serum TSH determinations in pregnancy: how, when and why? Nat Rev Endocrinol. 2010;6:526–9.
37. Yoshihara A, Noh JY, Mukasa K, Suzuki M, Ohye H, Matsumoto M, Kunii Y, Watanabe N, Suzuki N, Kameda T, Sugino K, Ito K. Serum human chorionic gonadotropin levels and thyroid hormone levels in gestational transient thyrotoxicosis: is the serum hCG level useful for differentiating between active graves' disease and GTT? Endocr J. 2015;62:557–60.
38. Bouillon R, Naesens M, Van Assche FA, De Keyser L, De Moor P, Renaer M, De Vos P, De Roo M. Thyroid function in patients with hyperemesis gravidarum. Am J Obstet Gynecol. 1982;143:922–6.
39. Laurberg P, Bournaud C, Karmisholt J, Orgiazzi J. Management of Graves' hyperthyroidism in pregnancy: focus on both maternal and foetal thyroid function, and caution against surgical thyroidectomy in pregnancy. Eur J Endocrinol. 2009;160:1–8.
40. Davis LE, Lucas MJ, Hankins GD, Roark ML, Cunningham FG. Thyrotoxicosis complicating pregnancy. Am J Obstet Gynecol. 1989;160:63–70.
41. Millar LK, Wing DA, Leung AS, Koonings PP, Montoro MN, Mestman JH. Low birth weight and preeclampsia in pregnancies complicated by hyperthyroidism. Obstet Gynecol. 1994;84:946–9.
42. Andersen SL, Olsen J, Laurberg P. Foetal programming by maternal thyroid disease. Clin Endocrinol. 2015;83:751–8.
43. Momotani N, Noh JY, Ishikawa N, Ito K. Effects of propylthiouracil and methimazole on fetal thyroid status in mothers with graves' hyperthyroidism. J Clin Endocrinol Metab. 1997;82:3633–6.
44. Kempers MJ, van Tijn DA, van Trotsenburg AS, de Vijlder JJ, Wiedijk BM, Vulsma T. Central congenital hypothyroidism due to gestational hyperthyroidism: detection where prevention failed. J Clin Endocrinol Metab. 2003;88:5851–7.
45. Zwaveling-Soonawala N, van Trotsenburg P, Vulsma T. Central hypothyroidism in an infant born to an adequately treated mother with graves' disease: an effect of maternally derived thyrotrophin receptor antibodies? Thyroid. 2009;19:661–2.
46. Bliddal S, Rasmussen AK, Sundberg K, Brocks V, Feldt-Rasmussen U. Antithyroid drug-induced fetal goitrous hypothyroidism. Nat Rev Endocrinol. 2011;7:396–406.
47. Laurberg P, Bournaud C, Karmisholt J, Orgiazzi J. Management of Graves' hyperthyroidism in pregnancy: focus on both maternal and foetal thyroid function, and caution against surgical thyroidectomy in pregnancy. Eur J Endocrinol. 2009;160:1–8.
48. Luton D, Le Gac I, Vuillard E, Castanet M, Guibourdenche J, Noel M, Toubert ME, Leger J, Boissinot C, Schlageter MH, Garel C, Tebeka B, Oury JF, Czernichow P, Polak M. Management of graves' disease during pregnancy: the key role of fetal thyroid gland monitoring. J Clin Endocrinol Metab. 2005;90:6093–8.
49. McKenzie JM, Zakarija M. Fetal and neonatal hyperthyroidism and hypothyroidism due to maternal TSH receptor antibodies. Thyroid. 1992;2:155–9.
50. Mitsuda N, Tamaki H, Amino N, Hosono T, Miyai K, Tanizawa O. Risk factors for developmental disorders in infants born to women with graves disease. Obstet Gynecol. 1992;80:359–64.
51. Peleg D, Cada S, Peleg A, Ben-Ami M. The relationship between maternal serum thyroid-stimulating immunoglobulin and fetal and neonatal thyrotoxicosis. Obstet Gynecol. 2002;99:1040–3.
52. Zimmerman D. Fetal and neonatal hyperthyroidism. Thyroid. 1999;9:727–33.

53. Polak M, Le Gac I, Vuillard E, Guibourdenche J, Leger J, Toubert ME, Madec AM, Oury JF, Czernichow P, Luton D. Fetal and neonatal thyroid function in relation to maternal graves' disease. Best Pract Res Clin Endocrinol Metab. 2004;18:289–302.
54. Cohen O, Pinhas-Hamiel O, Sivan E, Dolitski M, Lipitz S, Achiron R. Serial in utero ultrasonographic measurements of the fetal thyroid: a new complementary tool in the management of maternal hyperthyroidism in pregnancy. Prenat Diagn. 2003;23:740–2.
55. Huel C, Guibourdenche J, Vuillard E, Ouahba J, Piketty M, Oury JF, Luton D. Use of ultrasound to distinguish between fetal hyperthyroidism and hypothyroidism on discovery of a goiter. Ultrasound Obstet Gynecol. 2009;33:412–20.
56. Tucker MA, Jones PH, Boice JD Jr, Robison LL, Stone BJ, Stovall M, Jenkin RD, Lubin JH, Baum ES, Siegel SE. Therapeutic radiation at a young age is linked to secondary thyroid cancer. The late effects study group. Cancer Res. 1991;51:2885–8.
57. Pacini F, Vorontsova T, Demidchik E, Molinaro E, Agate L, Romei C, Shavrova E, Cherstvoy ED, Ivashkevitch Y, Kuchinskaya E, Schlumberger M, Ronga G, Filesi M, Pinchera A. Post-Chernobyl thyroid carcinoma in Belarus children and adolescents: comparison with naturally occurring thyroid carcinoma in Italy and France. J Clin Endocrinol Metab. 1997;81:3563–9.
58. Bennedbaek FN, Perrild H, Hegedus L. Diagnosis and treatment of the solitary thyroid nodule. Results of a European survey Clin Endocrinol (Oxf). 1999;50:357–63.
59. Bennedbaek FN, Hegedus L. Management of the solitary thyroid nodule: results of a north American survey. J Clin Endocrinol Metab. 2000;85:2493–8.
60. Papini E, Guglielmi R, Bianchini A, Crescenzi A, Taccogna S, Nardi F, Panunzi C, Rinaldi R, Toscano V, Pacella CM. Risk of malignancy in nonpalpable thyroid nodules: predictive value of ultrasound and color-Doppler features. J Clin Endocrinol Metab. 2002;87:1941–6.
61. Belfiore A, La Rosa GL. Fine-needle aspiration biopsy of the thyroid. Endocrinol Metab Clin N Am. 2001;30:361–400.
62. Goellner JR, Gharib H, Grant CS, Johnson DA. Fine needle aspiration cytology of the thyroid, 1980 to 1986. Acta Cytol. 1987;31:587–90.
63. Atkinson BF. Fine needle aspiration of the thyroid. Monogr Pathol. 1993;35:166–99.
64. Solomon D. Fine needle aspiration of the thyroid: an update. Thyroid Today. 1993;16:1–9.
65. Oertel YC. Fine-needle aspiration and the diagnosis of thyroid cancer. Endocrinol Metab Clin N Am. 1996;25:69–91.
66. Singer PA. Evaluation and management of the solitary thyroid nodule. Otolaryngol Clin N Am. 1996;29:577–91.
67. Powers CN, Frable WJ. Fine needle aspiration biopsy of the head and neck. Boston, MA: Butterworth-Heinemann; 1996.
68. Choe W, McDougall IR. Thyroid cancer in pregnant women: diagnostic and therapeutic management. Thyroid. 1994;4:433–5.
69. Hamburger JI. Thyroid nodules in pregnancy. Thyroid. 1992;2:165–8.
70. Herzon FS, Morris DM, Segal MN, Rauch G, Parnell T. Coexistent thyroid cancer and pregnancy. Arch Otolaryngol Head Neck Surg. 1994;120:1191–3.
71. Moosa M, Mazzaferri EL. Outcome of differentiated thyroid cancer diagnosed in pregnant women. J Clin Endocrinol Metab. 1997;82:2862–6.
72. Yasmeen S, Cress R, Romano PS, Xing G, Berger-Chen S, Danielsen B, Smith LH. Thyroid cancer in pregnancy. Int J Gynaecol Obstet. 2005;91:15–20.
73. Amino N, Mori H, Iwatani Y, Tanizawa O, Kawashima M, Tsuge I, Ibaragi K, Kumahara Y, Miyai K. High prevalence of transient post-partum thyrotoxicosis and hypothyroidism. N Engl J Med. 1982;306:849–52.
74. Qaseem A, Snow V, Owens DK, Shekelle P. The development of clinical practice guidelines and guidance statements of the American College of Physicians: summary of methods. Ann Intern Med. 2010;153:194–9.
75. Patel J, Landers K, Li H, Mortimer RH, Richard K. Delivery of maternal thyroid hormones to the fetus. Trends Endocrinol Metab. 2011;22:164–70.

76. Mathieson L, Nielsen LK, Andersen JT, Grevys A, Sandlie I, Michaelsen TE, Hedegaard M, Knudsen LE, Dziegiel MH. Maternofetal transplacental transport of recombinant IgG antibodies lacking effector functions. Blood. 2013;122:1174–81.
77. Michalek K, Morshed SA, Latif R, Davies TF. TSH receptor autoantibodies. Autimmun Rev. 2009;9:113–6.
78. Brown RS, Bellisaro RL, Botero D, Fournier L, Abrams CA, Cowger ML, David R, Fort P, Richman RA. Incidence of transient congenital hypothyroidism due to maternal thyrotropin receptor-blocking antibodies in over one million babies. J Clin Endocrinol Metab. 1996;81:1147–51.
79. Derakhshan A, Peeters R, Taylor P, Bliddal S, Carty D, Meems M, Vaidya B, Chen L, Knight B, Ghafoor F, Popova PV, Mosso L, Oken E. Association of maternal thyroid function with birthweight: a systematic review and individual-participant data meta-analysis. Lancet Diabetes Endocrinol. 2020;8:501–10.
80. van Wassenaer AG, Stulp MR, Valianpour F, Tamminga P, Ris Stalpers C, de Randamie JS, van Beusekom C, de Vijlder JJ. The quantity of thyroid hormone in human milk is too low to influence plasma thyroid hormone levels in the very preterm infant. Clin Endocrinol. 2002;56:621–7.
81. Mandel SJ, Cooper DS. The use of antithyroid drugs in pregnancy and lactation. J Clin Endocrinol Metab. 2001;86:2354–9.
82. Howe DB, Beardsley M, Bakhsh S. 2008. Appendix U. model procedure for release of patients or human research subjects administered radioactive materials. In consolidated guidance about materials licenses. Program-specific guidance about medical use licenses. Final report. U.S. Nuclear Regulatory Commission Office of nuclear material safety and safeguards. NUREG-1556, vol. 9, rev. 2. Available at http://www.nrc.gov/reading-rm/doc-collections/nuregs/staff/sr1556/v9/r2/.

Chapter 28
Rheumatological Diseases

Nilson Ramires de Jesús, Marcela Ignacchiti Lacerda, Flavia Cunha dos Santos, Roger Abramino Levy, and Guilherme Ramires de Jesús

Several adaptations occur in a woman's immune system during pregnancy in order to maintain her defense capacity and at the same time to protect the fetus from immune rejection. This profound change can influence women who become pregnant with autoimmune diseases or are predisposed to the development of these diseases in different ways. The most worrisome is the worsening of a preexisting disease during pregnancy, while it is possible for one latent disease outbreak during this period.

Many autoimmune diseases are more frequent in women of childbearing age, so it is essential to assess the influence of the disease and its treatment on the pregnant woman and the fetus. Pregnancy is a delicate situation for women with systemic lupus erythematosus (SLE), rheumatoid arthritis (RA), or other systemic autoimmune disease and, when properly planned, it is possible to avoid several complications. There should be great interaction of obstetric and rheumatologic teams that are responsible for the patient and the decisions must be taken together.

Systemic Lupus Erythematosus

SLE is a chronic inflammatory autoimmune disease that can affect several organs and systems. It usually evolves with periods of flare and remission, and may have a relatively benign course, but patients have a shorter survival compared with general population. SLE predominantly affects women and its appearance is common during childbearing years, between the second and third decade of life, which justifies its study during pregnancy. Lupus is more common among blacks than whites, and

N. R. de Jesús (✉) · M. I. Lacerda · F. C. dos Santos · G. R. de Jesús
Department of Obstetrics, Universidade do Estado do Rio de Janeiro, Rio de Janeiro, Brazil

R. A. Levy
Immunology and Inflammation, GlaxoSmithKline (GSK), Upper Providence, PA, USA

© Springer Nature Switzerland AG 2022

R. A. Moreira de Sá, E. B. d. Fonseca (eds.), *Perinatology*,
https://doi.org/10.1007/978-3-030-83434-0_28

there is still an unclear trend toward an increase in the prevalence of SLE over the past few years. However, advances in treatment and follow-up have allowed many successful pregnancies, which has been prohibited in the past [1, 2].

Favorable gestational outcomes usually occur during the period of complete remission of SLE and when pregnancy is monitored by a multidisciplinary team, within a reference center with the necessary support for the mother and newborn. On the other hand, there are high rates of maternal morbidity and permanent damage to target organs when conception occurs during periods of severe disease activity [3], especially in patients with nephritis, impaired renal function, injury end-stage renal disease, pulmonary hypertension, restrictive lung disease, and cardiomyopathy [4, 5]. Maternal death can also occur, although today it is considered a rare event. The consequences for newborns are no less harmful, with high rates of prematurity, mortality [1, 6, 7] and malformations resulting from the use of teratogenic drugs used to treat active lupus. These are contraindicated in the gestational period, especially during the embryonic period [6, 8].

Several factors are identified as predisposing to the development of SLE: genetic predisposition, environmental factors, exposure to ultraviolet light the most well known, exposure to drugs, smoking, infections, and hormonal factors, which are of relevance for the study during the gestational period [9]. Some publications have linked pregnancy to disease flares, but this observation has not been confirmed in other studies [10–12].

Typical clinical manifestations of SLE include fatigue, fever, arthralgia, arthritis, malar rash, photosensitivity, pleuritic chest pain, Raynaud's phenomenon, glomerulonephritis, vasculitis, and hematological changes, such as thrombocytopenia, leukopenia, and autoimmune hemolytic anemia. Neurological manifestations, including seizures, psychosis, and chorea, can also occur, being considered a more severe form of the disease. Some symptoms may occur during pregnancy as the first manifestation of SLE or they may appear as disease activity during pregnancy. It is important to remember that many complaints and clinical manifestations related to SLE can be confused with physiological modifications resulting from adaptive changes in the body during pregnancy [3].

The classification criteria for SLE was recently updated by the American College of Rheumatology (ACR) and European League Against Rheumatism (EULAR) [13]. In this new criteria, which aims to include patients in studies and clinical trials, a positive antinuclear factor (ANA) (1/80) is mandatory at least once as an entry criterion. SLE's clinical manifestations were divided into seven clinical (constitutional, hematological, neuropsychiatric, mucocutaneous, serous, musculoskeletal, and renal) and three immunological groups (antiphospholipid antibodies, complement proteins, specific antibodies to SLE). Each domain can score between two and ten points, and at least 10 points are needed to classify the patient as having SLE (Table 28.1).

Lupus, especially if associated with antiphospholipid syndrome (APS), increases the risk of spontaneous abortion, intrauterine fetal death, preeclampsia, intrauterine growth restriction, and prematurity, and this last event may result from iatrogenic or from spontaneous delivery. When it occurs spontaneously, it is mainly due to the premature rupture of membranes (PROM) with great impact on pregnancy outcomes [8, 10, 14, 15].

Table 28.1 Classification criteria for systemic lupus erythematosus (ACR/EULAR 2019)

Entry criterion: Antinuclear antibodies (ANA) ≥1:80			
Clinical Domains	Points	Immunological domains	Points
Constitutional Fever	2	*Antiphospholipid antibodies* Anticardiolipin antibodies OR Anti-β2-glycoprotein I antibodies OR Lupus anticoagulant	2
Hematologic Leukopenia Thrombocytopenia Autoimmune hemolytic anemia	3 4 4	*Complement proteins* Low C3 OR low C4 Low C3 AND low C4	3 4
Neuropsychiatric Delirium Psychosis Seizure	2 3 5	*SLE specific antibodies* Anti-DNA antibody OR Anti-SM antibody	6
Mucocutaneous Non-scarring alopecia Oral ulcers Subacute cutaneous OR discoid lupus Acute cutaneous lupus	2 2 4 6		
Serosal Pleural or pericardial effusion Acute pericarditis	5 6		
Musculoskeletal Joint involvement	6		
Renal Proteinuria >0,5 g/24 h Renal biopsy class II or V lupus nephritis Renal biopsy class III or IV lupus nephritis	4 8 10		
Classify as systemic lupus erythematosus if score ≥10			

Obs. Only the highest score inside one domain should be considered
Adapted from Aringer et al. [13]

When only cutaneous manifestations are present, as in discoid lupus or chronic cutaneous lupus, there is no internal organ involvement. The use of certain medications can trigger drug-induced lupus syndrome. Hydralazine, hydantoin, lamotrigine and isoniazid are the most implicated in this situation. In general, these drugs stimulate the production of anti-histone antibodies, which have a nuclear homogeneous pattern in antinuclear antibodies (ANA) tests [16].

Fertility

In early stages of SLE development, as well as in other systemic autoimmune diseases, fertility can be considered normal. However, over the years, particularly in patients with SLE-associated nephritis, fertility can be reduced by the use of cyclophosphamide to induce remission of kidney or neurological disease. Premature ovarian failure occurs in 60% of women over 30 years of age submitted to the 6-month treatment protocol with cyclophosphamide, but the concomitant use of GnRH analogues may have a protective effect on ovarian function [17].

Treatment of nephritis with mycophenolate mofetil does not impose this risk on female fertility and may be an alternative of efficiency not inferior to cyclophosphamide, presenting a better safety profile. Nonhormonal anti-inflammatory drugs (NSAIDs) do not alter ovulation, but prevent the rupture of the follicle, as well as specific inhibitors of cycle oxygenase 2 (COX 2), which have a proven action in an animal model and affect the pre and post- implantation period [18].

Preconceptional Care

Patients with SLE should be reassured about the transmission of the disease to their children, making it clear that autoimmune diseases are multifactorial and depend on genetic, immunological, endocrine, and environmental factors. In any case, children born to women with SLE may have an increased risk of nonrheumatic autoimmune diseases versus controls [19]. This situation must be differentiated from neonatal lupus, which occurs due to the transference of anti-Ro/SS-A and/or anti-LaSS-B maternal autoantibodies to the fetus.

Pregnancy in SLE patients must be planned in advance, which means that the patient must use contraception until the disease is well controlled and used medication are appropriate for conception and pregnancy (Table 28.2). It is recommended that the patient should wait at least 6 months for clinical and laboratory remission before becoming pregnant, especially for kidney disease and disease of the central nervous system. In patients with previous kidney disease, conception is recommended after at least 6 months with proteinuria less than 500 mg/24 h, the same waiting time recommended after a thrombotic event. Pregnancy should be contraindicated in cases of advanced renal failure (creatinine >2.8 mg/dl), severe heart failure, pulmonary volume restriction syndrome (forced vital capacity <1 L), severe pulmonary arterial hypertension (systolic pulmonary artery pressure >50 mmHg) and myocarditis [1, 20].

Pregnancy should also be avoided in patients using cyclophosphamide, chlorambucil, mycophenolate mofetil, leflunomide, and methotrexate, as these drugs are related to fetal complications (Table 28.2). In these situations, the importance of contraception should be emphasized to the patient [3, 6, 22].

Corticosteroids should be used judiciously in patients who intend to become pregnant, in order to minimize adverse events. Azathioprine is a safe immunosuppressant for patients who need high doses of steroids, because it allows the reduction of the dose of prednisone and can be used for maintenance treatment of severe SLE manifestations in women of childbearing age who intend to become pregnant [23]. Blood pressure must be well controlled and the use of angiotensin-converting enzyme (ACE) inhibitors, angiotensin II receptor blockers and direct renin inhibitors should be suspended as soon as the pregnancy diagnosis is confirmed, being the

Table 28.2 Use of the main analgesics, immunosuppressants, and drugs that modify the biological response during pregnancy in patients with rheumatic diseases

Drug	Fetal risk	Clinical considerations	Data sources
Acetylsalicylic acid (low dose)	No	Prevention of preeclampsia in high-risk groups, recommended in antiphospholipid syndrome (APS)	Large prospective studies in humans
Paracetamol	No	Hepatotoxicity if high doses	Observational studies in humans
Nonsteroidal anti-inflammatory drug (NSAID) and COX-2 inhibitor	Closing of the ductus arteriosus in the third trimester, reduced fetal renal function	Platelet antiaggregant, reduced renal function	NSAID: Observational studies in humans COX-2 inhibitor: No studies
Hydroxychloroquine	No	Recommended in systemic lupus erythematosus (SLE), Sjögren's syndrome and anti-Ro/SSA (+). Maternal cutaneous hyperpigmentation	Small human case series, extensive clinical experience, systematic reviews
Corticosteroids (CE)	No. Transplacental passage is less than 10% of the maternal dose	Hypertension, gestational diabetes, osteopenia, immunosuppression, stretch marks, water retention, cataracts	Absence of fetal risk in prospective studies in humans
Azathioprine	No. the human fetal liver does not metabolize the drug	Used as a saver of CE in a well-monitored patient	Case series (1.000 cases) Clinical experience
Sulfasalazine	No. increased risk of kernicterus in your newborn 2 weeks before delivery	Myelotoxicity in patients with glucose-6-phosphate deficiency (G6 PD)	Prospective controlled study in humans
Cyclophosphamide	Yes. Abortamento, múltiplas malformações	Infertility Myelotoxicity Hemorrhagic cystitis	Case reports; animal studies
Methotrexate	Yes. Abortion, multiple malformations Yes. Abortion, abnormalities in the central nervous system, calvaria, limbs, growth restriction and mental retardation Dose-dependent	Myelotoxicity hepatotoxicity use 10 mg/day of folic acid during unintended pregnancy and monitor fetal health	Observational studies in humans, case reports, animal studies

(continued)

Table 28.2 (continued)

Drug	Fetal risk	Clinical considerations	Data sources
Leflunomide	Yes. Abortion, skeletal malformation, hydrocephalus	Myelotoxicity Hepatotoxicity Use cholestyramine in unintended pregnancy	Human reports
Mycophenolate mofetil	Yes. Mycophenolate embryopathy: microtia and atresia of the ear canal, orofacial clefts, micrognative, hypertelorism	Myelotoxicity Gastrointestinal changes	Animal data, human series. Report of cardiovascular, renal, CNS, and limb malformations
Anti-TNF	It is not teratogenic (certolizumab and etanercept have less placental transfer)	Used in inflammatory bowel diseases If used after 32 weeks, the baby can only be vaccinated for BCG after 6 months)	Case reports, extensive experience in inflammatory bowel disease, databases of rheumatoid arthritis (RA) and spondyloarthritis
Rituximab	It is not teratogenic, but can induce neonatal lymphopenia	Used in cases of clinical worsening of SLE, RA, APS and systemic sclerosis	Databases, case reports and series. Used in other indications besides RA and SLE: Lymphoma, multiple sclerosis, Castelman

Adapted from Schaefer et al. [21]

same recommended for statins [3]. The interruption of these medications can lead to increased proteinuria and possible uncontrolled blood pressure, which is undesirable, but inevitable. A patient on chronic use of thiazide diuretics can maintain it during pregnancy, but loop diuretics should be avoided [24].

Preconception Counseling and Contraception

When preconception counseling is provided for SLE patients, it is important to make it clear that the best strategy is to have a planned pregnancy and the contraceptive method to be used should be chosen based on the patient's risks and preference. It has long been questioned whether estrogens used in contraceptives are factors that worsen SLE activity, until the SELENA study (The Safety of Estrogen in Lupus Erythematosus: National Assessment) was designed to clarify this controversy. Women before menopause with quiescent SLE or with stable disease, without antiphospholipid antibodies, were randomized to receive oral contraceptives with low dose of estrogen or placebo for 1 year. There was no increase in SLE activity in the group exposed to estrogens, while the placebo group presented a higher number of renal disease activity [25]. Therefore, the current practice recommends avoiding estrogen-containing contraceptives only in women with SLE who are at high thrombotic risk (such as carriers of antiphospholipid antibodies), with kidney disease or history of thrombosis. It is worth mentioning that mycophenolate mofetil has an interaction with estrogen and progesterone, which may reduce their effectiveness [26].

A good contraceptive option for patients with SLE are methods containing only progesterone, especially in cases associated with APS and kidney disease in which the use of estrogens is contraindicated. The most used options are oral desogestrel and every 3-month injectable medroxyprogesterone [3]. The Food and Drug Administration (FDA) recommends that medroxyprogesterone should be used for a maximum period of 2 years due to the risk of osteoporosis with prolonged use. Apparently, there is no greater thrombotic risk in patients using methods containing only progesterone, despite controversial results with injectable progesterone [26].

There was a concern about an increased risk of intrauterine device (IUD) -associated infection in patients with chronic use of immunosuppressants; however, this risk has not been confirmed and its use is permitted. Despite few data in patients with rheumatological diseases, there also seems to be no restriction on the use of etonogestrel implant [26].

Effects of Pregnancy on the Activity of Systemic Lupus Erythematosus

There are some manifestations that occur during pregnancy which can simulate SLE manifestations, such as hemolytic anemia and thrombocytopenia found in HELLP syndrome, arterial hypertension and proteinuria in preeclampsia, convulsion associated with eclampsia, facial cutaneous lesion of the pregnant melasma and the characteristic alopecia of the puerperal period.

Studies remain controversial considering the influence of pregnancy on SLE activity, whether due to sample size, heterogeneity of studies, variations in disease activity assessment rates or population differences. Many publications have shown increased number of flares during pregnancy [11, 27] while others have not [12].

In most cases, SLE reactivation during pregnancy presents with mild predominantly mild cutaneous articular or hematological manifestations [2, 27] and there is a tendency to repeat the clinical manifestations presented before gestational period. Nevertheless, more serious reactivations can occur [28]. The main risk factors for reactivation during pregnancy are: SLE in activity up to 6 months preceding conception, multiple periods of activity before pregnancy, history of lupus nephritis, active lupus nephritis, and discontinuation of hydroxychloroquine or prednisone [12, 29, 30].

Nephropathy is the manifestation of SLE that is most often associated with worse maternal prognosis, which may lead to progressive decrease in creatinine clearance and chronic renal failure if not treated properly. Two studies carried out with 102 pregnancies of 75 patients who had a history of lupus nephritis, but who were in remission at the time of conception, showed activity rates with an increase in proteinuria between 45 and 50% and worsening of renal function between 17 and 21% of the cases [12].

A study developed in the cohort of pregnant women with SLE at the Hospital Universitário Pedro Ernesto – UERJ demonstrated that patients with proliferative nephritis (classes III and IV) had higher frequency of adverse maternal results, such as higher number of flares, greater need for hospitalization and a higher incidence of preeclampsia. On the other hand, patients with mesangial (class II) and membranous (class V) nephritis had similar pregnancy outcomes to patients with SLE but without nephritis [31].

Differentiation between SLE-related glomerulonephritis and preeclampsia based on clinical and laboratory data is necessary for better gestational results, because in the first case, treatment is performed with immunosuppressants, while in preeclampsia, delivery is recommended. However, this differentiation is still a challenge in clinical practice. Laboratory tests that suggest reactivation of SLE are positive anti-DNA, reduction of serum complement levels, urinary sediment with dysmorphic hematuria and/or hematic, pyocyte or granular cylinders. As for the clinical scenario, the following suggest SLE flare: fever, discoid lesion, subacute lupus lesions, cutaneous vasculitis, oral ulcers, polyserositis, lymphadenodegaly, myocarditis and pneumopathy. Other indicators of active nephritis are the appearance of urinary changes before mid-pregnancy and/or when there is no improvement after delivery. On the other hand, the lack of the clinical and laboratory findings described and the refractoriness of the condition to corticosteroids strengthen the diagnosis of preeclampsia [3].

It is important to note that these findings related to SLE activity may not always be present and the serum complement, normally reduced in glomerulonephritis, may be physiologically increased in pregnancy. A recent study demonstrated that patients with SLE and preeclampsia had the same angiogenic profile as patients without SLE, that is, elevation of sFlt-1 (Soluble fms-Like Tyrosine Kinase 1) and reduction of PIGF (Placental Growth Factor) and VEGF, (Vascular Endothelial Growth Factor) which indicates that these markers can be used to assist in the diagnosis differential with SLE nephritis [32].

Microangiopathic glomerulopathy with thrombotic background can also occur in patients with SLE-associated antiphospholipid syndrome (APS) and should be remembered as part of the differential diagnosis when the patient with SLE has proteinuria, hypertension and edema, which can also overlap with preeclampsia or SLE nephritis. HELLP syndrome is a complication related to preeclampsia that can be confused with SLE hematological activity and that can be differentiated by the presence of schizocytes in the peripheral blood smear, in addition to changes in liver enzymes and bilirubins that are not frequent in SLE [3].

Neurological manifestations of SLE, although potentially more severe, are less frequent than renal impairment and apparently there is no greater activity during pregnancy, with the adverse pregnancy outcome being directly related to the concomitant renal manifestation. It is worth mentioning that SLE convulsion is an important differential diagnosis with eclampsia, but in the first case, it has no association with hypertension and proteinuria [33].

Effects of Systemic Lupus Erythematosus on Obstetric Outcomes

There are several known risk factors for pregnancy complications in women with SLE. These include the presence of antiphospholipid antibodies or APS, lupus nephritis, hypocomplementenemia, hypertension, high doses of corticosteroids (above 20 mg/day) and active disease during conception [7, 34, 35]. SLE patients are considered to be at high gestational risk because they have higher abortion rates, fetal losses, intrauterine growth restriction and prematurity, in addition to maternal complications [36].

Preeclampsia is more prevalent in pregnant women with SLE and in those with active lupus nephritis than healthy pregnant women, and previous hypertension, APS and nephropathy are additional risk factors for this complication [6, 8, 37].

Several studies have reported that prematurity has been associated with SLE mainly in cases with disease flares during the gestational period [1, 2, 38]. A systematic review of 2751 pregnancies in 1842 SLE patients found a prematurity rate of 39.4% [8]. Premature deliveries can be performed as a way of protecting the health of the mother and/or the fetus, or occur spontaneously, most of them are related to premature rupture of membranes [39].

Chronic fetal distress caused by placental insufficiency that results in fetuses with low birth weight or small for gestational age newborns is quite common in patients with SLE and can occur between 6 and 35% of the cases [8, 36, 40].

Antiphospholipid antibodies significantly worsen the prognosis of pregnancy, which justifies their investigation in all pregnant women with SLE. It should be remembered that antiphospholipid antibodies in SLE patients without obstetric (recurrent miscarriage, fetal loss) or thrombotic events (deep vein thrombosis, arterial thrombosis) do not confer the diagnosis of APS or even indicate anticoagulation with heparin. Most authors recommend the use of low-dose acetylsalicylic acid (ASA) for these cases [3].

Active kidney disease at conception is often a predictor of adverse maternal and fetal outcomes in many cases [41, 42]. In the Johns Hopkins cohort, regardless of clinical activity, both low complement and positive anti-DNA in the second trimester were associated with fetal loss and preterm delivery. When combined with clinical activity, these parameters were even more predictors of adverse pregnancy outcomes [41].

A large multicenter, prospective study called PROMISSE (Predictors of Pregnancy Outcome: BioMarkers in Antiphospholipid Antibody Syndrome and Systemic Lupus Erythematosus) evaluated 385 pregnant women who presented for prenatal care in the first trimester using less than 20 mg/day of prednisone, less than 1 g/day of proteinuria, and/or less than 1.2 mg/dl of serum creatinine. SLE flares were classified by the SLEPDAI disease activity index (SLE Pregnancy Disease

Activity Index), which excludes physiological changes in pregnancy and incorporates components of the disease activity index as well as clinical changes, medication, and evaluation by the attending physician. Patients with severe disease activity were excluded from the study. Adverse gestational outcomes were reported in 19% of pregnant women and the predictive variables for these events were the presence of lupus anticoagulant, use of antihypertensive drugs, thrombocytopenia, and higher physician's global assessment (PGA) [43].

Although adverse pregnancy outcomes occur, a better understanding of the disease and, mainly, the improvement of treatment before and during pregnancy have resulted in a reduction in pregnancy losses in recent decades. Among one of the major advances considering SLE treatment is the use of hydroxychloroquine during pregnancy, which has been shown to be safe and effective to stabilize SLE and promote favorable pregnancy outcomes [44].

Neonatal Lupus Syndrome and Anti-Ro/SS-A and Anti-La/SS-B Antibodies

Neonatal lupus syndrome is defined by irreversible congenital atrioventricular block or photosensitive skin erythema in the newborn. The latter is self-limited and disappears around the sixth month of life, when maternal IgG is replaced by the child's own immunoglobulin. Other changes in the cardiac conduction system, as well as liver and hematological changes, are also related to neonatal lupus syndrome [45].

Positive ANA with nuclear speckled pattern is suggestive of antibodies against extractable nuclear antigens (ENA), which are polypeptides associated with small RNA particles. Ro/SS-A, La/SS-B, Sm, and RNP are part of the ENA, but anti-Ro/SS-A and anti-La/SS-B are usually described with a nuclear fine speckled ANA pattern. Anti-Ro/SS-A antibodies, whether or not accompanied by anti-La/SS-B antibodies, are found in some forms of SLE with cutaneous photosensitivity, subacute cutaneous lupus, primary or secondary Sjögren's syndrome, and neonatal lupus syndrome [16].

Most mothers of children with congenital atrioventricular block or neonatal lupus dermatitis, who invariably have anti-Ro/SS-A and/or anti-La/SS-B antibodies, have never had clinical manifestations of any of the diseases associated with these autoantibodies. However, almost half develop SLE or Sjögren's syndrome in the years following the birth of the child with the disease [46].

Apparently, there is a specific subtype of anti-Ro/SS-A antibody that is pathogenic, and even among patients who had children with congenital atrioventricular block, the probability of recurrence can vary between 12 and 17% [47]. In addition, there are reports in the literature about discordant congenital heart block in twins [47]. The pathogenic action of anti-Ro/SS-A antibodies is strongly suggested by the temporal relationship between the disappearance of dermatitis and the decrease in maternal IgG in the child's circulation. The direct action of the antibody is reinforced by the observation that the majority of anti-Ro/SS-A IgGs are from IgG1 subclass, which crosses the placental barrier. The induction of heart block in vitro is determined by antibodies against the 52 kDa Ro/SS-A protein, but probably some other factor participates as not all 52 kDa anti-Ro/ SS-A antibodies tested were able to induce the heart block [48].

When patients with positive anti-Ro/SS-A are considered, the frequency of neonatal lupus is low, affecting around 2% of the carriers of this autoantibody [49, 50]. On the other hand, neonatal lupus is responsible for 80 to 95% of atrioventricular blocks diagnosed in fetuses or newborns [47].

The most vulnerable period of occurrence of atrioventricular block for the fetus is between 18 and 24 weeks [47], and among the several techniques described for early detection of atrioventricular heart block, fetal Doppler echocardiography is more frequently used. Most authors recommend ultrasound evaluation of fetal heart for pregnant women with anti-Ro/SS-A and anti-La/SS-B antibodies weekly from the 16th to the 26th week, maintained thereafter every 2 weeks until 32 weeks of gestation.

In recent years, this weekly or biweekly fetal echocardiography during the follow-up of a pregnant woman with positive anti-Ro antibody has been questioned by some authors [51, 52]. It must be noticed that there seems to be a transition from incomplete atrioventricular block to third degree (total) atrioventricular block that can occur in a few hours or days. This means that weekly echocardiogram detection may be random or even unable to detect it [52, 53].

Another important point is that neonatal lupus phenotype with cardiac involvement is variable, ranging from silent first-degree atrioventricular block that remains stable even without treatment to third-degree atrioventricular block with cardiomyopathy that progresses to hydrops and fetal death in less than 1 week [48, 54].

Thus, the best surveillance strategy for patients who have positive anti-Ro/SS-A antibodies remains undefined, and further studies are to develop an appropriate protocol with good efficiency and low cost in monitoring a pathology with a low occurrence rate. Current proposal for follow-up with weekly echocardiography seems to be of little cost-effective considering the possibility of frequent surveillance of fetal heart rate on an outpatient basis, with referral only of abnormal cases for echocardiographic study, although this strategy is not being used by most of the centers [51].

Treatment of congenital atrioventricular block depends on the degree. In first degree atrioventricular blocks, the results reported in the literature are conflicting and there is no clear evidence that progression to total atrioventricular block occurs without treatment [48]. Therefore, treatment should be discussed with the family, considering mainly the possible side effects. Administration of fluorinated corticosteroids (betamethasone 3 mg/day or dexamethasone 4 mg/day) can be beneficial only in fetuses with second-degree heart block and should be started at the time of diagnosis, with maintenance until the end of pregnancy if there is a good response. Another situation in which the use of these steroids should be considered is in cardiomyopathy related to neonatal lupus. However, the effectiveness for these cases is still not well established [48].

Despite several proposed treatments, such as corticosteroid therapy and intravenous immunoglobulin, reversal of third-degree fetal atrioventricular block is not possible and most of these fetuses will need a pacemaker at birth. Many authors question intrauterine treatment at this advanced stage, given the lack of effectiveness and the large number of side effects [48].

Retrospective studies suggest that the use of hydroxychloroquine 400 mg/day throughout pregnancy appears to have a protective role in the development of the block [55]. In addition, a study found that hydroxychloroquine was able to reduce the recurrence of fetal atrioventricular block in 65% of the cases. The use of corticosteroids or intravenous immunoglobulin in a preventive manner, however, is not recommended due to the significant risks and ineffectiveness in preventing the heart block [56].

Prenatal Care

Facilities for pregnant women with SLE should have neonatal intensive care unit (ICU) and clinical assistance support, with intensive care resources for the pregnant woman. It also should have a multidisciplinary team, with an obstetrician trained in maternal–fetal medicine and a rheumatologist. Consultations should be done monthly until the 28th gestational week, biweekly until the 34th and weekly from that time until delivery. Interval between consultations can be reduced due to the presence or suspicion of disease activity or preeclampsia [3]. In the initial consultation, the following exams should be requested:

(a) Complete blood count, platelet count, prothrombin activation time, and partial thromboplastin time.
(b) Lupus anticoagulant, anticardiolipin antibody IgG and IgM, and anti-β2 glycoprotein I IgG and IgM (which must be repeated in 12 weeks if positive)
(c) Anti-Ro/SS-A, anti-La/SS- B, anti-Sm, and anti-RNP.
(d) Blood glucose, blood urea nitrogen (BUN), creatinine, uric acid, AST, and ALT.
(e) Anti-DNA, C3, C4, and CH50.
(f) Urinary sediment, 24-hour proteinuria or protein/creatinine ratio in a single urine sample, dysmorphic research erythrocyte in urine, creatinine clearance, and urine culture.

For quarterly consultations, the following exams are recommended:

(a) Complete blood count, platelet count.
(b) Anti-DNA, C3, C4, and CH50.
(c) Blood glucose, BUN, creatinine, uric acid, AST, and ALT.
(d) 24-hour proteinuria or protein/creatinine ratio in a single urine sample if preeclampsia or lupus nephritis is suspected, as well as research erythrocyte dysmorphism.

Ultrasound and Doppler velocimetry studies should be scheduled as follows:

(i) Monthly after 24 weeks: evaluation of fetal growth, amniotic fluid, and umbilical artery (fetal-placental flow)
(ii) Uterine artery evaluation at 24 weeks: screening tests for preeclampsia and intrauterine growth restriction.

Laboratory tests must be interpreted according to the knowledge of the changes imposed by pregnancy itself. Despite being used as a marker of inflammatory disease activity, the erythrocyte sedimentation rate (ESR) increases due to the pregnancy itself and, therefore, should not be used in pregnant women with SLE. Serum complement levels tend to increase in pregnancy and their fall should be assessed in relation to a baseline value. Incidental thrombocytopenia can occur in about 10% of pregnant women and it is difficult to differentiate it from that related to SLE activity [3].

Urinary proteins normally rise during pregnancy and a result up to 300 mg/24 h alone may have no clinical significance. In addition, pregnant women tend to have more urinary tract infections, and the use of immunosuppressants can inhibit leukocytosis and cell deviation [3]. Renal function should be assessed even in patients without a history of nephritis, as it may be asymptomatic or develop during pregnancy. A baseline evaluation at the beginning of pregnancy should be performed for further comparison in the case of renal injury during the course of pregnancy.

Hepatic involvement is uncommon in patients with SLE; however, the assessment of its function is necessary mainly in patients using azathioprine given its hepatotoxicity, with repetition of the tests at least every 3 months. Regarding the requested antibodies, antiphospholipid antibodies (LA, anticardiolipin and antib2glycoprotein I) are markers of adverse pregnancy outcomes and this investigation may help in the case of a thrombotic event during pregnancy. As described, anti-DNA and complement (C3, C4, CH50) are markers of disease activity and assist in clinical evaluation. ANA, anti-Ro/SS-A, anti-La/SS-B, anti-Sm, and anti-RNP do not change with the activity of the disease and, therefore, do not need to be repeated during follow-up [3].

Chronic fetal distress in pregnant patients with SLE follows the pattern of usual placental insufficiency and it is recommended to follow-up with ultrasound and monthly Doppler from 24 to 26 weeks to assess fetal growth, amniotic fluid and fetoplacental flow. Management of an altered Doppler study of umbilical artery is similar to woman without SLE, while a normal result of this exam has a high negative predictive value for fetal death [3].

Treatment

Some medications used to treat SLE that are contraindicated during pregnancy and should be replaced as soon as possible if pregnancy is not planned. In planned pregnancies, these medications have already been changed to safe ones to allow those patients to get pregnant. Drugs that should not be used during pregnancy are: cyclophosphamide, chlorambucil, mycophenolate mofetil, leflunomide and methotrexate [6, 8, 22].

Hydroxychloroquine is not only used to treat SLE but also to prevent reactivation of the disease. It is also recommended in pregnancies of women with some other autoimmune diseases, such as Sjögren's syndrome and rheumatoid arthritis. Current consensus is that its use is accepted and recommended for all pregnant women with SLE (Bertsias [5, 57]. It is safe for the fetus and should be continued or started in those pregnant women with SLE who are not yet using it. The use of hydroxychloroquine during pregnancy reduces the number of episodes of flares and hypertensive disorders. Levy and colleagues, in a double-blind randomized placebo study, reported a lower incidence of SLE activity and preeclampsia in the hydroxychloroquine group, in addition to not identifying complications in children exposed up to 3 years of age [44]. Despite being secreted in breast milk, there are no reports of adverse effects in breastfeeding infants whose mothers are using hydroxychloroquine [58].

Nonsteroidal anti-inflammatory drugs used to relieve arthralgia should, as far as possible, be replaced by common pain relievers. If there is still a benefit in their use, they should be used for the shortest possible time with the lowest possible dose and should be stopped completely at 32 weeks. After that time, there is a greater risk of maternal and fetal hemorrhage in addition to fetal renal dysfunction leading to oligohydramnios and premature closure of ductus arteriosus [59].

Azathioprine is a plausible therapeutic option for use in the case of SLE activation in pregnancy, being the immunosuppressant of choice in cases with severe disease or refractory to isolated use of corticosteroids. This medication, in addition to its immunosuppressive effect, is used as a steroid-sparing agent and is not associated with teratogenicity in humans, as the fetal liver is not able to metabolize azathioprine in the active form [23].

Corticosteroids are the medication group of choice as therapy in the case of SLE reactivation during pregnancy. Administration forms are preferably prednisone and prednisolone, which are inactivated in the placenta by 11-beta-dehydrogenase, reducing fetal exposure to less than 10% of the maternal dose [60]. For this reason, they cannot be chosen for use in fetal lung maturation, with this function being reserved to betamethasone and dexamethasone.

Whenever corticosteroids are used to treat SLE during pregnancy, the lowest dose necessary for treatment should be considered in order to minimize the adverse effects. Complications related to its use are the same as those that can occur in nonpregnant patients, especially in doses greater than 10 mg per day, such as avascular bone necrosis, osteopenia, immunosuppression, fluid retention, stretch marks, cataracts, dyslipidemia, and gestational complications such as maternal hyperglycemia and hypertension arterial, while doses greater than 40 mg per day supposedly predispose to premature rupture of membranes [61]. In cases of severe flare, it is possible to use venous methylprednisolone, as it has a faster action compared with prednisone. Prophylactic administration of corticosteroids during pregnancy has no proven benefits and is not recommended [20].

Calcium supplementation is necessary for those patients with long-term use of corticosteroids. For pregnant women who have used more than 5 mg/day of prednisone (or equivalent) for more than 3 weeks within the past year, doses of hydrocortisone are also recommended for emergency surgery, cesarean section and during labor to prevent adrenal insufficiency [17].

Delivery route in patients with SLE must have ordinary obstetric indications. In cases where well-being of the fetal maternal binomial is preserved, monitored spontaneous delivery is recommended. Suspension of low-dose aspirin to prevent bleeding is not necessary, as its action does not occur on fibrinolysis that regulates uterine bleeding. Management of childbirth and the complications inherent to the procedure must follow similar procedures to those indicated for pregnant women without SLE [3].

Lactation

Woman with SLE needs to be evaluated during immediate puerperium, since it is possible to reactivate the disease during this period and, therefore, new complementary exams must be performed to assess SLE activity. There is a higher rate of puerperal complications, including infections of the surgical wound and the urinary system, especially in those who use more than 10 mg/day of prednisone [6]. Excessive stress can also contribute to SLE flares and should be minimized through reassuring information.

During breastfeeding, some drugs are considered safe, such as acetaminophen, low-dose aspirin, prednisone less than 20 mg/day, azathioprine, warfarin, and heparins, in addition to antimalarials [3, 59]. Current recommendation is that hydroxychloroquine should be maintained, as well as azathioprine if necessary. Women who are breastfeeding and using doses greater than 20 mg of corticosteroids should wait 4 hours after administering the medication to breastfeed in order to decrease the concentration of the medication in the milk [59].

Cytotoxic substances are found in high concentrations in breast milk, and therefore, breastfeeding is contraindicated in women who are using cyclophosphamide, chlorambucil, mycophenolate mofetil, leflunomide, or methotrexate [62].

Rheumatoid Arthritis

Similar to SLE, rheumatoid arthritis (RA) tends to occur more in women than in men, especially in the reproductive period and affects up to 1% of the population. However, RA seems to hinder conception. Some studies report that disease activity and the use of certain medications for the treatment of RA can prolong the time for conception. In addition, it has also been established that RA patients can have earlier menopause than general population [63].

Between 50 and 70% of RA patients go into remission during pregnancy, with this improvement occurring in the first weeks and staying throughout pregnancy [64]. Some risk factors for flare during pregnancy are active disease and high C-reactive protein at the beginning of pregnancy, as well as suspension of anti-TNFs medications [65]. Apparently, patients with both negative rheumatoid factor (RF) and anti–cyclic citrullinated peptide (anti-CCP) are more likely to go into remission during pregnancy compared with patients who have one or both positive antibodies [66]. On the other hand, activation during the puerperium is very frequent and varies between 62 and 90%, usually in the first 3 months postpartum [63].

Part of these improvements reported during pregnancy is related to an improvement in the understanding of RA in recent decades with new therapeutic options and new clinical and radiological parameters for monitoring the disease. This allows patients to reach clinical remission more quickly and enter pregnancy in a low disease activity state [63].

There are several theories about the immunological and endocrinological changes in pregnancy that will affect RA activity. Immunological tolerance of the pregnant woman to the fetus, considered a semialogenic graft, results from the production of several anti-inflammatory enzymes such as interleukin-10 (IL-10). This fact, associated with the production of hormones, such as estrogen, progesterone and hCG, promotes the suppression of T-cell reactivity, which is essential for RA flares. During pregnancy, there is a predominance of monocytic activity over the activity of T lymphocytes, which also contributes to a lower RA activity, and the subsequent inversion of this pattern in the postpartum period may justify the high frequency of flares in this period. Other factors such as IgG galactosylation also appear to be involved in disease improvement during pregnancy [67].

Patients with RA in remission have gestational results comparable to the general population, however, those who become pregnant during disease activity may have a slightly worse gestational outcome than healthy women. A recent study showed a small increase in the incidence of abortion, which may be related to the use of medications such as methotrexate [63]. As for preeclampsia, the results are conflicting. A study looking at birth records in Sweden and Denmark showed a 5.0% risk of developing preeclampsia compared with the risk of 3.4% of women without the disease [68], but this difference was not found in other studies [66].

It has been reported that there is a greater probability that women with RA have newborns who are small for gestational age, showing a 10% risk compared with 3% of healthy women. In addition, the risk for intrauterine growth restriction is almost twice that of the patients without RA. Similar studies also showed an increased risk for premature birth and premature rupture of membranes, with prematurity being related to the severity of the disease and the use of corticosteroids [63, 69].

RA patients also have an increased risk of cesarean delivery, which is directly related to the disease activity. The incidence of congenital malformations and perinatal death, however, does not seem to be increased in these patients [63].

Currently available options for RA treatment have resulted in the improvement of disease control, which has been reflected in better pregnancy outcomes. Options include traditional therapeutic antirheumatic drugs (synthetic disease modifying antirheumatic drugs – s-DMARD) as initial treatment and biological drugs (Biologic disease modifying antirheumatic drugs - b-DMARD), which have anti-TNF agents as the best representatives and are usually reserved for those patients who do not respond to initial therapy. Not all therapeutic options provide definitive data about safety during pregnancy and lactation, so further studies are required in order to improve current knowledge. Medications for the treatment of RA will be discussed below.

Patients with RA should receive preconception counseling. It is important that the patient is instructed to become pregnant while the disease is in remission, which decreases the chance of flares during pregnancy. Thus, the use of medications to control RA should be optimized before conception, avoiding medications, such as methotrexate and leflunomide. It is also worth mentioning that the use of high-dose NSAIDs and corticosteroids can influence fertility [65].

Other Systemic Autoimmune Diseases

Undifferentiated Connective Tissue Disease (UCTD)

Undifferentiated connective tissue disease (UCTD), which usually affects women before the age of 40, is characterized by the presentation of clinical manifestations of one or more systemic autoimmune diseases, but does not meet the classification criteria for any specific one. UCTD can persist as an undifferentiated condition or migrate to a diagnosis defined as SLE, systemic sclerosis, Sjögren's syndrome, or RA. This definite diagnosis, when occurs, usually happens within the first 2 or 3 years of disease. Some studies have shown a disease activity rate between 24 and 32%, most of which are mucocutaneous and musculoskeletal. However, there are reports of severe forms of flares, such as hematological and glomerulonephritis [70].

Sjögren's Syndrome

It is an autoimmune inflammatory syndrome that, in addition to general and joint symptoms, is characterized by lymphocytic infiltration of exocrine glands. Clinically, it manifests with dryness of the oral and ocular mucous membranes, confirmed by objective tests. It can occur primarily or secondary to other diseases, mainly RA [70]. Little data are available on the activity of Sjögren's syndrome in pregnancy and obstetric complications, but it is noteworthy that the presence of anti-Ro/SSA antibodies (70–80%) is part of the diagnostic criterion and may even precede the clinical presentation. Thus, evaluation for congenital neonatal heart block is recommended in the same way as patients with SLE and positive anti-Ro/SSA [51].

Systemic Sclerosis

Systemic sclerosis is a rare and heterogeneous autoimmune disease, characterized by cutaneous fibrosis, vasculopathy, and visceral involvement, mainly pulmonary, gastrointestinal, and renal. Raynaud's phenomenon and digital ulcers usually improve because of the physiological changes in pregnancy, which result in increased cardiac output. Around 20% of patients may worsen the disease, usually with cutaneous involvement after delivery. Gastroesophageal reflux disease, which already occurs frequently in pregnant women without pathologies, generally worsens even more in patients with systemic sclerosis [70].

One of the most serious complication that occurs in pregnant women with systemic sclerosis is renal crisis. Abrupt onset of arterial hypertension and increased serum creatinine without proteinuria suggest this diagnosis, which is more common in patients with less than 3 years of disease with a diffuse cutaneous disease and positive antitopoisomerase antibodies (anti-Scl-70) [70].

Another serious complication is pulmonary hypertension, which has maternal mortality that can reach 50% of cases. Cardiologic evaluation should be performed before conception and its diagnosis during pregnancy can be an indication of therapeutic abortion. Despite these worrying conditions, pregnant women with systemic sclerosis generally have clinical outcome during the pregnant-puerperal period [70].

Considering obstetric results, a recent meta-analysis reported that patients with systemic sclerosis had a higher risk of miscarriage, restricted intrauterine growth, premature birth, gestational hypertension, and cesarean delivery [71].

Polymyositis and Dermatomyositis

Polymyositis (PM) is a systemic autoimmune disease characterized by the inflammation of proximal striated muscle. When this condition is associated with characteristic cutaneous manifestations, it is called dermatomyositis (DM). Myositis can start in childhood or more often in postmenopausal women, so data on pregnancy are from case reports and small retrospective series. Pregnant women with PM/DM had a higher risk of spontaneous abortion and premature birth, especially when the disease was active [72]. Apparently, there is no increased risk of disease flare during pregnancy, with some reports of clinical improvement in this period [70].

Mixed Connective Tissue Disease (DMTC)

DMTC is characterized by the superposition of clinical features of several systemic autoimmune diseases associated in patients with exclusively high titers of anti-RNP antibodies, which induce an ANA nuclear large/coarse speckled pattern. Prognosis of this disease tends to be better than that of SLE or systemic sclerosis and reports of worsening during pregnancy are very rare [70].

Systemic Vasculitis

Vasculitis often affects young women, especially Takayasu's arteritis and Behçet's disease. However, there are also reports of pregnancies in patients with antineutrophil cytoplasmic antibody (ANCA)–associated vasculitis, such as granulomatosis with polyangiitis (GPA), eosinophilic granulomatosis with polyangiitis (EGPA), and microscopic polyangiitis (MPA). Physiological changes in pregnancy can be both favorable and unfavorable in maternal disease, which ends up influencing the gestational outcome [73].

Behçet's Disease

Behçet's disease is characterized by a systemic inflammatory process, which results in genital and oral ulcerations, as well as ocular, gastrointestinal, thrombotic, and neurological manifestations. There is improvement of disease activity during pregnancy most of the time (60%), however, flares can occur in 30%. Gestational results are similar to those found in general population, with few reports of increased frequency of premature birth and pregnancy loss [73].

Takayasu's Arteritis

Takayasu's arteritis is a granulomatous vasculitis that preferably affects large vessels such as the aorta, its branches, and pulmonary arteries. Leukocyte infiltration of the intima of the artery and myofibroblastic proliferation result in vascular stenosis, but development of aneurysms is also possible in some cases. Frequent clinical manifestations are limb claudication, carotid involvement with vertigo and lipothymia, hypertension due to renal stenosis and aortic insufficiency. It typically affects women in the fertile period, so it is more common to be associated with pregnancy than with other systemic necrotizing vasculitis [74].

Pregnancy does not appear to have an influence on Takayasu's arteritis activity, but there are reports of serious complications, such as aortic dissection, renal failure, heart failure, and maternal death. The most frequent obstetric complications are hypertension and preeclampsia with a prevalence of approximately in 40% of cases, and intrauterine growth restriction, which affects up to 20% of the pregnant women. These complications are more frequent in patients with involvement of the abdominal aorta and renal artery [73, 74].

Granulomatosis with Polyangiitis (GPA), Formerly Wegener Granulomatosis

It is a necrotizing vasculitis of small vessels, with preference for the upper respiratory tract, lungs, and kidneys. It is more frequent in women between 40 and 50 years old, so pregnancy cases in patients with GPA are rare. Disease activity is common during pregnancy even in patients who were in remission, and almost all who were active at the time of conception present flares during pregnancy [70]. Associated obstetric complications are premature delivery, preeclampsia, spontaneous abortion, and antepartum hemorrhage, with worse gestational outcomes in patients with active disease [73].

Microscopic Polyangiitis (MPA)

It is an autoimmune necrotizing systemic vasculitis with a predilection for small vessels. Like polyangiitis with granulomatosis, it develops with the presence of ANCA, but in this case, the main detected antigen is not proteinase III but myeloperoxidase (MPO). Data about pregnancy in patients with MPA are very limited, but it seems to have a higher frequency of low birth weight and premature birth. There are reports of anti-MPO antibodies crossing the placenta and inducing a vasculitis in the neonate. As in other diseases, pregnancy that occurs when the disease is controlled usually have better outcomes than those who become pregnant with active disease or disease that develop during pregnancy [73].

Eosinophilic with Polyangiitis (EGPA), Formerly Churg-Strauss Syndrome

In EGPA, the systemic involvement of small vessels, mainly pulmonary, and the formation of extravascular necrotizing granulomas with asthma, allergic rhinitis, and hypereosinophilia is remarkable. As with other vasculitis, preterm delivery was highly frequent in this group, as well as fetal loss and intrauterine growth restriction. Around 24% of the patients in small published series presented flares, including reports of maternal death in pregnant women with heart and lung disease [70, 73].

Antirheumatics and their Use in Pregnancy and Lactation

Acetylsalicylic Acid and Paracetamol

Acetylsalicylic acid (ASA) is used only during pregnancy and puerperium in low doses (80–150 mg/day), as an antiplatelet agent in the prevention of fetal losses related to APS and for patients at high risk of preeclampsia. Paracetamol can be used throughout pregnancy and breastfeeding in the lowest possible dose, although there is recent work that associates its use with attention deficit hyperactivity disorder (ADHD) and autism. However, further investigation is needed.

Nonsteroidal Anti-Inflammatory Drugs and Cyclooxygenase 2 Inhibitors

When used in pregnancy, they should be used in the lowest possible dose and suspended around the 32nd week, due to the risks of fetal and maternal bleeding, in addition to reports of renal dysgenesis, oligodramnia, and premature closure of the ductus arteriosus. Anti-inflammatory drugs with shorter half-lives and inactive metabolites can be used more safely (e.g., ibuprofen, diclofenac) in the first two quarters. Some of them have been found safe by the American Academy of Pediatrics and can be used while breastfeeding, such as ibuprofen, indomethacin, and naproxen. Before the administration of these medications, the use of paracetamol for pain control should be considered. The COX 2 inhibitor celecoxib can influence renal formation and its use should be avoided in pregnancy.

Antimalarials

Antimalarials have been widely used in rheumatology for many decades. Although they are known to cross the placenta, fetal defects related to these substances have never been observed. Hydroxychloroquine is widely used in the treatment of SLE in pregnancy worldwide. Because it is a deposition substance, its suspension at the beginning of pregnancy does not prevent fetal exposure and, therefore, is not justified. In the Johns Hopkins cohort, there was no risk associated with the use of hydroxychloroquine in pregnancy [41]. There is no description of malformations, ocular involvement, or restriction in the growth of the fetus, despite the fact that there has been prolonged fetal exposure to hydroxychloroquine in numerous studies [75].

A systematic review that included randomized and observational clinical studies evaluated the safety of antimalarials in ocular function in the children of exposed women, with the GRADE system in the evaluation of the works. Twelve studies, with a total of 558 live births to mothers treated with chloroquine or hydroxychloroquine during pregnancy, met inclusion criteria. Five studies, with a total of 251 exposed fetuses, did not report any ocular abnormalities. In a controlled randomized clinical study, normally, visual acuity was reported in all cases. Therefore, current evidence suggests an absence of ocular toxicity from fetal exposure to antimalarials [76]. Although a small amount of hydroxychloroquine is detected in the milk of mothers who use the medication, it is considered compatible with breastfeeding and there are no reports of adverse effects on the infant [59].

Corticosteroids

The complications related to its use are the same as those that can occur in nonpregnant patients, including avascular bone necrosis, osteopenia, immunosuppression, water retention, hyperglycemia, stretch marks, and cataracts. They can also precipitate pregnancy complications, such as gestational diabetes, high blood pressure, and premature rupture of membranes [3, 39, 61]. It is recommended to use short-acting agents (prednisone, prednisolone) in the lowest possible dose, which are metabolized in the placenta by 11-beta-dehydrogenase, reducing fetal exposure to about 10% of the maternal dose [60]. Supplementation of calcium (up to 1200 mg of calcium carbonate) and vitamin D (up to 4000 U/day) is necessary for patients on long-term use of corticosteroids, as well as anticoagulants [17]. Patients using corticosteroids should receive hydrocortisone supplementation for emergency surgery, cesarean delivery, and prolonged labor. No teratogenic effect has been proven in long-term studies. Corticosteroids can be administered freely during lactation at doses less than 20 mg/day of prednisone or equivalent. When using higher doses, the mother must breastfeed 4 hours after taking the corticosteroid in order to reduce its concentration in breast milk [59].

Azathioprine

This corticosteroid-sparing and immunosuppressant is not associated with teratogenesis in humans. There are reports of teratogenesis in animals, but the human fetal liver is not able to metabolize azathioprine to its active form [59]. For this reason, several centers that treat high-risk pregnant women opt for azathioprine when safe and efficient immunosuppression is needed. Azathioprine (up to 200 mg/day) is the agent of choice in cases where the use of immunosuppressants is required for the treatment of difficult-to-control maternal disease or which requires a dose greater than 20 mg of corticosteroids for more than 1 month [77]. Azathioprine treatment is compatible with breastfeeding, without risks for the infant, since the concentration of the active metabolite in milk is very low [59].

Sulfasalazine

This medication can be maintained or started safely during pregnancy at doses of up to 2 g/day, being the first choice in patients with RA or spondyloarthropathies, including inflammatory bowel diseases, who intend to become pregnant or who have had the disease aggravated during pregnancy. An observational study of 300 women who used sulfasalazine during pregnancy did not reveal a higher risk of teratogenicity, but sulfasalazine is not recommended in the 2 weeks preceding delivery to avoid prolonged neonatal jaundice (Makol et al., 2011). Detectable levels of sulfasalazine can be found in the milk of mothers who use the medication while breastfeeding, and there was a case report of bloody diarrhea in an infant of a mother who was using the medication. Therefore, patients should use this medication with caution during this period [78].

Cyclophosphamide

This immunosuppressive agent is contraindicated for the treatment of rheumatic diseases in pregnancy and lactation, therefore, the fertile woman using cyclophosphamide must be well-oriented about the risks since its use can cause early menopause. Pregnancy testing is recommended before each venous cyclophosphamide pulse therapy and it should be suspended at least 3 months before the planned conception [79]. In extremely severe patients, its use has already been considered in the second and third trimesters, but most authors suggest termination of pregnancy for the proper treatment of the patient [80]. Cyclophosphamide should not be used during breastfeeding because in addition to being detected in breast milk, there are reports of hematological changes in the infant [78].

Methotrexate

Methotrexate is an antimetabolite agent that interferes with the synthesis of purines. It induces abortion and teratogenic effects, so it cannot be used in women who wish to become pregnant. Fertile women who will use methotrexate must be properly advised, as this medication is embryotoxic and must be discontinued at least 3 months before pregnancy [80]. In the case of accidental pregnancy using methotrexate, high doses of folic acid (10 mg/day) and detailed morphological ultrasound are recommended to assess neural tube closure defects [80]. The use of methotrexate during lactation is also contraindicated and, therefore, if there is an indication for treatment with methotrexate in the puerperium, breastfeeding should be suspended on days when methotrexate is used (which is used weekly) [80, 81]. Some recent publications suggest that the concentration of the drug excreted in milk is not so harmful, but more studies are needed to confirm this information [82].

Leflunomide

Leflunomide induces fetal effects similar to those of methotrexate, but with the possibility of having its effect reversed with the administration of cholestyramine (8 g VO, 3 times/day for 11 days). Then, two separate tests are performed to check whether the plasma levels of leflunomide are undetectable. If they remain elevated, more cholestyramine should be administered [83]. If there is no process for eliminating the substance, it should wait up to 3 months for conception. The experience reported by the OTIS database includes 63 pregnancies exposed to leflunomide compared with 108 unexposed patients and showed no difference in the frequency of microcephaly or other forms of embryopathy, although skeletal and craniofacial malformations have been observed in animal studies [83]. Its use is contraindicated during breastfeeding [81].

Mycophenolate Mofetil

Mycophenolate mofetil is a drug used to treat mainly lupus nephritis because it has a more favorable safety profile than cyclophosphamide. Studies in human pregnancies have proven the drug's teratogenicity, which causes a syndrome characterized by craniofacial malformations – affecting the oral cavity and ears and causing ocular anomalies. Changes in the limbs and cardiovascular, renal, and central nervous systems were also identified when the mothers were exposed in the first trimester [77, 84]. In the patient who plans to conceive, it must be withdrawn at least 6 weeks before conception and must not be administered during pregnancy, or during breastfeeding [81]. The switch from mycophenolate to azathioprine for patients who wish to become pregnant does not seem to be associated with greater SLE activity [3].

Biological Agents

So-called biological response modifiers or biological agents are monoclonal antibodies or receptor-blocking fusion proteins that interfere with the immune response. Targets can be cytokines, such as TNF, IL 1 and IL 6, cell presentation and survival flags, such as CTLA4 and BLyS, or cell flags, such as CD20. Most biological agents are IgG1 molecules and bind to the placental Fcγ receptor, being actively transported to the fetus during the second and third trimesters. This leads to concerns about a greater risk of opportunistic infections in the newborn and resulting from the use of live vaccines. On the other hand, due to their large complex structures, they are unlikely to cross the placenta during the first trimester and cause teratogenic effects.

Several new agents are under study and are expected to hit the market soon. These agents were introduced in the late twentieth century after many years of controlled and randomized clinical studies, which obviously did not include pregnant women.

The available data are from case reports, case series, and record banks. There are no reports of teratogenicity associated with these medications so far, but the precaution of use is justified by the lack of long-term effects. They are probably not excreted in breast milk, but there are little data on their use in lactation and should therefore be avoided during this period. It is important to remember that as these medications are actually proteins, they would be digested in the infant's stomach, without risk of absorption and adverse effects [77].

Anti-TNF

Anti-TNF drugs are the best studied biological agents during pregnancy and the safety data of these drugs are the most reassuring. Such agents have different structures and this is what will determine, besides the passage through the placenta, the level of detection in the fetal circulation through the analysis of cord blood.

The following drugs have the function of blocking tumor necrosis factor activity: infliximab (every 8 weeks, intravenous), adalimumab (every 2 weeks, subcutaneous), etanercept (weekly, subcutaneous), golimumab (monthly, subcutaneous), and certolizumab (biweekly, subcutaneous). None of them showed an increased risk of teratogenicity. Etanercept has a small placental passage, while certolizumab does not cross the placental barrier due to its different configuration compared with other medications. This makes this last medication the anti-TNF of choice for use during pregnancy according to some authors. Although evidence does not indicate the presence of malformations after exposure to golimumab, other medications should be considered as an alternative to replace it during pregnancy and lactation.

The use of anti-TNF medications during pregnancy should be carefully individualized, considering the absence of long-term data for most of these medications. Studies have not shown an increased risk of neonatal infection for newborns exposed to anti-TNFs in the third trimester, but vaccines for attenuated bacteria and viruses should be postponed for at least 6 months after birth.

Adalimumab, infliximab, and golimumab are whole monoclonal IgG1 antibodies. Etanercept has only part of the IgG Fcγ region and certolizumab does not have the Fc region. Active transport of anti-TNF across the placenta occurs as early as 18 weeks of gestation and increases throughout pregnancy, requiring the attachment of the Fcγ region to the placental Fcγ receptor. Certolizumab, as it does not have the Fc region, does not cross the placental barrier.

The EULAR task force recommends stopping adalimumab and infliximab at 20 weeks' gestation and etanercept at 30–32 weeks. The use of certolizumab is considered safe during pregnancy. The use of golimumab is not recommended due to the lack of greater safety information about its use during pregnancy.

When all data on anti-TNF were evaluated, there was no evidence of an increase in fetal malformations. A cohort of 30 women with RA exposed to adalimumab during pregnancy revealed live births in 90% of pregnancies, prematurity in 11% and two cases of congenital anomalies (microencephaly and absence of testicular migration), which was similar to a group control of RA patients without exposure to biological agents. The results from the infliximab database with an even greater number of patients did not demonstrate an increased risk.

Children of mothers who used anti-TNF agents during the second and third trimester of pregnancy should not be vaccinated with live attenuated virus vaccines until 6 months of age. Babies of mothers who have stopped taking medication until 22 weeks of gestational age can be vaccinated even with attenuated virus vaccines.

Breastfeeding is safe and released with the use of infliximab, adalilumabe, etanercept, and certolizumab [77].

Rituximab

Rituximab is a monoclonal antibody against CD20, expressed in an intermediate phase of B cell proliferation, and crosses the placenta. Due to lack of data on adverse effects with use before conception and in the first trimester, and as its use in the second and third trimesters seems to cause transient depletion in the B cells of the fetus, rituximab during pregnancy can be justified in cases of difficult-to-control RA, SLE nephritis, or ANCA-associated vasculitis, in addition to severe forms of APS, with thrombocytopenia, hemolytic anemia, and renal microangiopathy. Likewise, the EULAR task force confirms that as no evidence of an increased risk of malformations has been found, rituximab can be used in exceptional situations during the first trimester of pregnancy. On the other hand, the risk of cytopenias, infections, hypogammaglobulinemia and low vaccine response of babies contraindicate its use in the second and third trimesters. The British Society of Rheumatology recommends avoiding use during pregnancy and recommends the suspension of rituximab 6 months before the planned conception [77].

Belimumab

Belimumab is a monoclonal antibody that inhibits the B cell activation factor (BAFF/BLyS) and is an approved biological treatment for the treatment of SLE. The data on the use of belimumab during pregnancy are not sufficient to recommend it during pregnancy. When administered in supratherapeutic doses to monkeys, the only finding was neonatal transient lymphopenia, hence the recommendation to discontinue treatment at 32 weeks. Of the clinical studies, the 95 cases that occurred had results similar to the normal population. Clinical experience with the use of belimumab during pregnancy is still scarce. The task force of EULAR and the British society of rheumatology suggest that belimumab should be avoided during pregnancy [77].

References

1. Lateef A, Petri M. Managing lupus patients during pregnancy. Best Pract Res Clin Rheumatol. 2013;27(3):435–47.
2. Borella E, Lojacono A, Gatto M, Andreoli L, Taglietti M, Iaccarino L, et al. Predictors of maternal and fetal complications in SLE patients: a prospective study. Immunol Res. 2014;60(2–3):170–6.

3. de Jesus GR, Mendoza-Pinto C, de Jesus NR, Dos Santos FC, Klumb EM, Carrasco MG, et al. Understanding and managing pregnancy in patients with lupus. Autoimmune Dis. 2015;2015:943490.
4. Tincani A, Bazzani C, Zingarelli S, Lojacono A. Lupus and the antiphospholipid syndrome in pregnancy and obstetrics: clinical characteristics, diagnosis, pathogenesis, and treatment. Semin Thromb Hemost. 2008;34(3):267–73.
5. Bertsias GK, Tektonidou M, Amoura Z, Aringer M, Bajema I, Berden JH, et al. Joint European league against rheumatism and European renal association-European Dialysis and transplant association (EULAR/ERA-EDTA) recommendations for the management of adult and paediatric lupus nephritis. Ann Rheum Dis. 2012;71(11):1771–82.
6. Clowse ME, Jamison M, Myers E, James AH. A national study of the complications of lupus in pregnancy. Am J Obstet Gynecol. 2008;199(2):127.e1–6.
7. Moroni G, Doria A, Giglio E, Tani C, Zen M, Strigini F, et al. Fetal outcome and recommendations of pregnancies in lupus nephritis in the 21st century. A prospective multicenter study. J Autoimmun. 2016;74:6–12.
8. Smyth A, Oliveira GH, Lahr BD, Bailey KR, Norby SM, Garovic VD. A systematic review and meta-analysis of pregnancy outcomes in patients with systemic lupus erythematosus and lupus nephritis. Clin J Am Soc Nephrol. 2010;5(11):2060–8.
9. Costenbader KH, Kim DJ, Peerzada J, Lockman S, Nobles-Knight D, Petri M, et al. Cigarette smoking and the risk of systemic lupus erythematosus: a meta-analysis. Arthritis Rheum. 2004;50(3):849–57.
10. Clowse ME. Lupus activity in pregnancy. Rheum Dis Clin N Am. 2007;33(2):237–52, v.
11. Lockshin MD, Reinitz E, Druzin ML, Murrman M, Estes D. Lupus pregnancy. Case-control prospective study demonstrating absence of lupus exacerbation during or after pregnancy. Am J Med. 1984;77(5):893–8.
12. Tandon A, Ibañez D, Gladman DD, Urowitz MB. The effect of pregnancy on lupus nephritis. Arthritis Rheum. 2004;50(12):3941–6.
13. Aringer M, Costenbader K, Daikh D, Brinks R, Mosca M, Ramsey-Goldman R, et al. 2019 European league against rheumatism/American College of Rheumatology Classification Criteria for systemic lupus erythematosus. Arthritis Rheumatol. 2019;71(9):1400–12.
14. Clark CA, Spitzer KA, Laskin CA. Decrease in pregnancy loss rates in patients with systemic lupus erythematosus over a 40-year period. J Rheumatol. 2005;32(9):1709–12.
15. Vinet E, Clarke AE, Gordon C, Urowitz MB, Hanly JG, Pineau CA, et al. Decreased live births in women with systemic lupus erythematosus. Arthritis Care Res (Hoboken). 2011;63(7):1068–72.
16. Chan EK, Damoiseaux J, Carballo OG, Conrad K, de Melo Cruvinel W, Francescantonio PL, et al. Report of the first international consensus on standardized nomenclature of antinuclear antibody HEp-2 cell patterns 2014–2015. Front Immunol. 2015;6:412.
17. Andreoli L, Bertsias GK, Agmon-Levin N, Brown S, Cervera R, Costedoat-Chalumeau N, et al. EULAR recommendations for women's health and the management of family planning, assisted reproduction, pregnancy and menopause in patients with systemic lupus erythematosus and/or antiphospholipid syndrome. Ann Rheum Dis. 2017;76(3):476–85.
18. Micu MC, Micu R, Ostensen M. Luteinized unruptured follicle syndrome increased by inactive disease and selective cyclooxygenase 2 inhibitors in women with inflammatory arthropathies. Arthritis Care Res (Hoboken). 2011;63(9):1334–8.
19. Couture J, Bernatsky S, Scott S, Pineau CA, Vinet E. Brief report: risk of childhood rheumatic and nonrheumatic autoimmune diseases in children born to women with systemic lupus erythematosus. Arthritis Rheumatol. 2018;70(11):1796–800.
20. Ruiz-Irastorza G, Khamashta MA. Lupus and pregnancy: integrating clues from the bench and bedside. Eur J Clin Investig. 2011;41(6):672–8.
21. Schaefer C, Peters PWJ, Miller RK. Drugs during pregnancy and lactation : treatment options and risk assessment. 2nd ed. Amsterdam ; Boston: Elsevier Academic Press; 2007. p. xxv, 875.
22. Wallenius M, Salvesen K, Daltveit AK, Skomsvoll JF. Systemic lupus erythematosus and outcomes in first and subsequent births based on data from a national birth registry. Arthritis Care Res (Hoboken). 2014;66(11):1718–24.

23. Bitencourt N, Bermas BL. Pharmacological approach to managing childhood-onset systemic lupus erythematosus during conception. Pregnancy Breastfeeding Paediatr Drugs. 2018;20(6):511–21.
24. Umans JG, Lindheimer MD. Getting to safer and smarter medication use during pregnancy. Am J Obstet Gynecol. 2015;213(1):115–6.
25. Petri M, Kim MY, Kalunian KC, Grossman J, Hahn BH, Sammaritano LR, et al. Combined oral contraceptives in women with systemic lupus erythematosus. N Engl J Med. 2005;353(24):2550–8.
26. Sammaritano LR. Contraception and preconception counseling in women with autoimmune disease. Best Pract Res Clin Obstet Gynaecol. 2019.
27. Ruiz-Irastorza G, Lima F, Alves J, Khamashta MA, Simpson J, Hughes GR, et al. Increased rate of lupus flare during pregnancy and the puerperium: a prospective study of 78 pregnancies. Br J Rheumatol. 1996;35(2):133–8.
28. Petri M. The Hopkins lupus pregnancy center: ten key issues in management. Rheum Dis Clin N Am. 2007;33(2):227–35, v.
29. Clowse ME, Magder LS, Witter F, Petri M. The impact of increased lupus activity on obstetric outcomes. Arthritis Rheum. 2005;52(2):514–21.
30. Day CJ, Lipkin GW, Savage CO. Lupus nephritis and pregnancy in the 21st century. Nephrol Dial Transplant. 2009;24(2):344–7.
31. Rodrigues BC, Lacerda MI, Ramires De Jesús GR, Cunha Dos Santos F, Ramires De Jesús N, Levy RA, et al. The impact of different classes of lupus nephritis on maternal and fetal outcomes: a cohort study of 147 pregnancies. Lupus. 2019;28(4):492–500.
32. Mayer-Pickel K, Stern C, Eberhard K, Lang U, Obermayer-Pietsch B, Cervar-Zivkovic M. Angiogenic factors in pregnancies of women with antiphospholipid syndrome and systemic lupus erythematosus. J Reprod Immunol. 2018;127:19–23.
33. de Jesus GR, Rodrigues BC, Lacerda MI, Dos Santos FC, de Jesus NR, Klumb EM, et al. Gestational outcomes in patients with neuropsychiatric systemic lupus erythematosus. Lupus. 2017;26(5):537–42.
34. Ateka-Barrutia O, Khamashta MA. The challenge of pregnancy for patients with SLE. Lupus. 2013;22(12):1295–308.
35. Bramham K, Hunt BJ, Bewley S, Germain S, Calatayud I, Khamashta MA, et al. Pregnancy outcomes in systemic lupus erythematosus with and without previous nephritis. J Rheumatol. 2011;38(9):1906–13.
36. Peart E, Clowse ME. Systemic lupus erythematosus and pregnancy outcomes: an update and review of the literature. Curr Opin Rheumatol. 2014;26(2):118–23.
37. M KE, S BLM, L R, R JN, A LR, N AEM. Impacto da nefrite sobre os resultados gestacionais de mulheres com lúpus eritematoso sistêmico. Rev Bras Reumatol. 2005;45(3):107–13.
38. Pastore DEA, Costa ML, Surita FG. Systemic lupus erythematosus and pregnancy: the challenge of improving antenatal care and outcomes. Lupus. 2019;28(12):1417–26.
39. Clark CA, Spitzer KA, Nadler JN, Laskin CA. Preterm deliveries in women with systemic lupus erythematosus. J Rheumatol. 2003;30(10):2127–32.
40. Saavedra MA, Cruz-Reyes C, Vera-Lastra O, Romero GT, Cruz-Cruz P, Arias-Flores R, et al. Impact of previous lupus nephritis on maternal and fetal outcomes during pregnancy. Clin Rheumatol. 2012;31(5):813–9.
41. Clowse ME, Magder LS, Petri M. The clinical utility of measuring complement and anti-dsDNA antibodies during pregnancy in patients with systemic lupus erythematosus. J Rheumatol. 2011;38(6):1012–6.
42. Østensen M, Andreoli L, Brucato A, Cetin I, Chambers C, Clowse ME, et al. State of the art: reproduction and pregnancy in rheumatic diseases. Autoimmun Rev. 2015;14(5):376–86.
43. Buyon JP, Kim MY, Guerra MM, Laskin CA, Petri M, Lockshin MD, et al. Predictors of pregnancy outcomes in patients with lupus: a cohort study. Ann Intern Med. 2015;163(3):153–63.
44. Levy RA, Vilela VS, Cataldo MJ, Ramos RC, Duarte JL, Tura BR, et al. Hydroxychloroquine (HCQ) in lupus pregnancy: double-blind and placebo-controlled study. Lupus. 2001;10(6):401–4.

45. Lee LA. The clinical spectrum of neonatal lupus. Arch Dermatol Res. 2009;301(1):107–10.
46. Morel N, Lévesque K, Maltret A, Baron G, Hamidou M, Orquevaux P, et al. Incidence, risk factors, and mortality of neonatal and late-onset dilated cardiomyopathy associated with cardiac neonatal lupus. Int J Cardiol. 2017;248:263–9.
47. Brito-Zerón P, Izmirly PM, Ramos-Casals M, Buyon JP, Khamashta MA. The clinical spectrum of autoimmune congenital heart block. Nat Rev Rheumatol. 2015;11(5):301–12.
48. Friedman DM, Kim MY, Copel JA, Davis C, Phoon CK, Glickstein JS, et al. Utility of cardiac monitoring in fetuses at risk for congenital heart block: the PR interval and dexamethasone evaluation (PRIDE) prospective study. Circulation. 2008;117(4):485–93.
49. Costedoat-Chalumeau N, Amoura Z, Lupoglazoff JM, Huong DL, Denjoy I, Vauthier D, et al. Outcome of pregnancies in patients with anti-SSA/Ro antibodies: a study of 165 pregnancies, with special focus on electrocardiographic variations in the children and comparison with a control group. Arthritis Rheum. 2004;50(10):3187–94.
50. Izmirly PM, Saxena A, Kim MY, Wang D, Sahl SK, Llanos C, et al. Maternal and fetal factors associated with mortality and morbidity in a multi-racial/ethnic registry of anti-SSA/Ro-associated cardiac neonatal lupus. Circulation. 2011;124(18):1927–35.
51. Cuneo BF, Buyon JP. Keeping upbeat to prevent the heartbreak of anti-Ro/SSA pregnancy. Ultrasound Obstet Gynecol. 2019;54(1):7–9.
52. Cuneo BF, Sonesson SE, Levasseur S, Moon-Grady AJ, Krishnan A, Donofrio MT, et al. Home monitoring for fetal heart rhythm during anti-Ro pregnancies. J Am Coll Cardiol. 2018;72(16):1940–51.
53. Kan N, Silverman ED, Kingdom J, Dutil N, Laskin C, Jaeggi E. Serial echocardiography for immune-mediated heart disease in the fetus: results of a risk-based prospective surveillance strategy. Prenat Diagn. 2017;37(4):375–82.
54. Krishnan A, Arya B, Moak JP, Donofrio MT. Outcomes of fetal echocardiographic surveillance in anti-SSA exposed fetuses at a large fetal cardiology center. Prenat Diagn. 2014;34(12):1207–12.
55. Mekinian A, Lazzaroni MG, Kuzenko A, Alijotas-Reig J, Ruffatti A, Levy P, et al. The efficacy of hydroxychloroquine for obstetrical outcome in anti-phospholipid syndrome: data from a European multicenter retrospective study. Autoimmun Rev. 2015;14(6):498–502.
56. Gleicher N, Elkayam U. Preventing congenital neonatal heart block in offspring of mothers with anti-SSA/Ro and SSB/La antibodies: a review of published literature and registered clinical trials. Autoimmun Rev. 2013;12(11):1039–45.
57. Klumb EM, Silva CA, Lanna CC, Sato EI, Borba EF, Brenol JC, et al. Consensus of the Brazilian Society of Rheumatology for the diagnosis, management and treatment of lupus nephritis. Rev Bras Reumatol. 2015;55(1):1–21.
58. Noviani M, Wasserman S, Clowse ME. Breastfeeding in mothers with systemic lupus erythematosus. Lupus; 2016.
59. Makol A, Wright K, Amin S. Rheumatoid arthritis and pregnancy: safety considerations in pharmacological management. Drugs. 2011;71(15):1973–87.
60. Jain V, Gordon C. Managing pregnancy in inflammatory rheumatological diseases. Arthritis Res Ther. 2011;13(1):206.
61. Chakravarty EF, Colón I, Langen ES, Nix DA, El-Sayed YY, Genovese MC, et al. Factors that predict prematurity and preeclampsia in pregnancies that are complicated by systemic lupus erythematosus. Am J Obstet Gynecol. 2005;192(6):1897–904.
62. Hazes JM, Coulie PG, Geenen V, Vermeire S, Carbonnel F, Louis E, et al. Rheumatoid arthritis and pregnancy: evolution of disease activity and pathophysiological considerations for drug use. Rheumatology (Oxford). 2011;50(11):1955–68.
63. de Jong PH, Dolhain RJ. Fertility, pregnancy, and lactation in rheumatoid arthritis. Rheum Dis Clin N Am. 2017;43(2):227–37.
64. Jethwa H, Lam S, Smith C, Giles I. Does rheumatoid arthritis really improve during pregnancy? A systematic review and Metaanalysis. J Rheumatol. 2019;46(3):245–50.
65. Littlejohn EA. Pregnancy and rheumatoid arthritis. Best Pract Res Clin Obstet Gynaecol. 2019.

66. de Man YA, Bakker-Jonges LE, Goorbergh CM, Tillemans SP, Hooijkaas H, Hazes JM, et al. Women with rheumatoid arthritis negative for anti-cyclic citrullinated peptide and rheumatoid factor are more likely to improve during pregnancy, whereas in autoantibody-positive women autoantibody levels are not influenced by pregnancy. Ann Rheum Dis. 2010;69(2):420–3.
67. Förger F, Villiger PM. Immunological adaptations in pregnancy that modulate rheumatoid arthritis disease activity. Nat Rev Rheumatol. 2020;16(2):113–22.
68. Nørgaard M, Larsson H, Pedersen L, Granath F, Askling J, Kieler H, et al. Rheumatoid arthritis and birth outcomes: a Danish and Swedish nationwide prevalence study. J Intern Med. 2010;268(4):329–37.
69. de Man YA, Hazes JM, van der Heide H, Willemsen SP, de Groot CJ, Steegers EA, et al. Association of higher rheumatoid arthritis disease activity during pregnancy with lower birth weight: results of a national prospective study. Arthritis Rheum. 2009;60(11):3196–206.
70. Andreoli L, García-Fernández A, Chiara Gerardi M, Tincani A. The course of rheumatic diseases during pregnancy. Isr Med Assoc J. 2019;21(7):464–70.
71. Blagojevic J, AlOdhaibi KA, Aly AM, Bellando-Randone S, Lepri G, Bruni C, et al. Pregnancy in systemic sclerosis: results of a systematic review and Metaanalysis. J Rheumatol. 2019.
72. Zhong Z, Lin F, Yang J, Zhang F, Zeng X, You X. Pregnancy in polymyositis or dermatomyositis: retrospective results from a tertiary Centre in China. Rheumatology (Oxford). 2017;56(8):1272–5.
73. Machen L, Clowse ME. Vasculitis and pregnancy. Rheum Dis Clin N Am. 2017;43(2):239–47.
74. de Jesús GR, d'Oliveira IC, dos Santos FC, Rodrigues G, Klumb EM, de Jesús NR, et al. Pregnancy may aggravate arterial hypertension in women with Takayasu arteritis. Isr Med Assoc J. 2012;14(12):724–8.
75. Costedoat-Chalumeau N, Amoura Z, Huong DL, Lechat P, Piette JC. Safety of hydroxychloroquine in pregnant patients with connective tissue diseases. Rev Literat Autoimmun Rev. 2005;4(2):111–5.
76. Osadchy A, Ratnapalan T, Koren G. Ocular toxicity in children exposed in utero to antimalarial drugs: review of the literature. J Rheumatol. 2011;38(12):2504–8.
77. Balbi GGM, Domingues V, De Jesús GR, Levy RA. Use of synthetic and biologic DMARDs during pregnancy. Expert Rev Clin Immunol. 2019;15(1):27–39.
78. Drugs AAoPCo. Transfer of drugs and other chemicals into human milk. Pediatrics. 2001;108(3):776–89.
79. Harris EN. Antirheumatic drugs in pregnancy. Lupus. 2002;11(10):683–9.
80. Flint J, Panchal S, Hurrell A, van de Venne M, Gayed M, Schreiber K, et al. BSR and BHPR guideline on prescribing drugs in pregnancy and breastfeeding-part I: standard and biologic disease modifying anti-rheumatic drugs and corticosteroids. Rheumatology (Oxford). 2016.
81. Gotestam Skorpen C, Hoeltzenbein M, Tincani A, Fischer-Betz R, Elefant E, Chambers C, et al. The EULAR points to consider for use of antirheumatic drugs before pregnancy, and during pregnancy and lactation. Ann Rheum Dis. 2016.
82. Thorne JC, Nadarajah T, Moretti M, Ito S. Methotrexate use in a breastfeeding patient with rheumatoid arthritis. J Rheumatol. Canada2014;41:2332.
83. Brent RL. Teratogen update: reproductive risks of leflunomide (Arava); a pyrimidine synthesis inhibitor: counseling women taking leflunomide before or during pregnancy and men taking leflunomide who are contemplating fathering a child. Teratology. 2001;63(2):106–12.
84. Merlob P, Stahl B, Klinger G. Tetrada of the possible mycophenolate mofetil embryopathy: a review. Reprod Toxicol. 2009;28(1):105–8.

Chapter 29
Prophylaxis for Deep Venous Thrombosis During Pregnancy, Delivery, and Postpartum

Egle Couto and Renato Passini Junior

Pregnancy, the peripartum period and puerperium are high-risk periods for deep venous thrombosis (DVT) and pulmonary embolism (PE), collectively known as venous thromboembolism (VTE), which is an important cause of maternal morbidity and mortality.

Risk in pregnancy is increased due to venous stasis of the lower limbs, endothelial injury, and hypercoagulability, a triad described by Rudolf Virchow [1] in 1856.

All components of Virchow's Triad occur during pregnancy and the puerperium:

- Venous stasis, which is due to mechanical compression of the inferior vena cava and pelvic veins caused by an enlarged uterus, increased hormone-mediated venous capacitance and exaggerated compression of the left iliac vein by the right iliac vein
- Endothelial vascular injury, which occurs in preeclampsia and may also result from childbirth-related trauma
- Hypercoagulability, resulting from an increase in coagulation factors (VIII, IX, X, fibrinogen), reduction in natural anticoagulants (protein S, antithrombin) and fibrinolytic potential

Therefore, venous flow velocity in the lower limbs, from the beginning of the third trimester until 6 weeks postpartum, may be reduced by 50%. Approximately 90% of VTE in pregnancy occurs in the left side.

E. Couto (✉)
Department of Obstetrics and Gynecology, University of Campinas (UNICAMP), Campinas, SP, Brazil

Pontifical Catholic University of Campinas, Campinas, Brazil
e-mail: egle.couto@me.com

R. P. Junior
Department of Obstetrics and Gynecology, University of Campinas (UNICAMP), Campinas, SP, Brazil
e-mail: passini@caism.unicamp.br

© Springer Nature Switzerland AG 2022
R. A. Moreira de Sá, E. B. d. Fonseca (eds.), *Perinatology*,
https://doi.org/10.1007/978-3-030-83434-0_29

Table 29.1 Risk factors for VTE during pregnancy and postpartum period

Preexisting factors	Obstetric factors	Transient factors
Previous TEV	Preeclampsia	Surgery during pregnancy or postpartum
Known thrombophilia	Assisted reproduction	Hyperemesis
Comorbidities (cancer, renal failure, nephrotic syndrome, diabetes, connective tissue diseases, myeloproliferative diseases, sickle cell diseases)	Cesarean with hysterectomy or not	Ovarian hyperstimulation syndrome
Family history of unprovoked VTE	Multiple pregnancy	Systemic infection
Age > 35	Operative delivery	Prolonged immobilization
Obesity (BMI > 30 kg/m^2)	Labor >24 h	Dehydration
Parity ≥ 3	Postpartum hemorrhage and anemia	Hospital internment
Cigarette smoking	Premature delivery	
Extensive varicosities	Stillbirth	
Anatomic anomalies (May–Thurner syndrome)	Puerperal infection	

The state of hypercoagulation resulting from physiological alterations seems to be a protective evolutionary mechanism against hemorrhage during birth, although it creates a higher risk for VTE [2].

Complications during pregnancy or childbirth substantially increase the risk of VTE, such as those seen in Table 29.1.

The main risk for VTE in pregnancy is personal history [5]. From 15% to 25% of thromboembolic episodes associated with pregnancy are recurrent. This seems to be determined mainly by the clinical circumstances of the first episode: characteristics and age of the patient, and presence or absence of a triggering factor. Thrombophilia is the second most important risk factor. In about 20–50% of pregnancies complicated by thrombosis, at least one thrombophilia factor can be identified [16].

Thrombophilia, i.e., a higher tendency to develop thrombosis, may be due to acquired and/or inherited factors. The most common cause of acquired thrombophilia is antiphospholipid syndrome (APS). In inherited thrombophilia, factor V Leiden (FVL), G20210A mutation in the prothrombin gene, and deficiency of proteins C (PC), S (PS) and antithrombin (AT) have been associated with pregnancy complications in some studies [12, 17–28].

Acquired Thrombophilia—Antiphospholipid Syndrome

APS was described by Hughes [29] in 1983, and consisted in arterial and venous thrombosis, a positive direct Coombs test, thrombocytopenia, livedo reticularis and obstetric complications. More than 35 years after the original description, knowledge of the disease is still in development.

APS is a systemic autoimmune disease characterized by arterial or venous thrombosis and/or gestational loss in the persistent presence of antiphospholipid antibodies (aPL -lupus anticoagulant, anticardiolipin antibodies and anti-β2 glycoprotein 1).

In obstetric APS, recurrent abortion may be observed in up to 54% of women. Fetal death is considered to result from placental dysfunction induced by antibodies.

The origin of APS is still an enigma. However, it is probably due to loss of immune tolerance and disruption in the innate immune system, possibly triggered by infectious stimulation [30].

The first prothrombotic mechanism of action of aPL included the inhibition of natural anticoagulant activity, especially of the PC system. Antiphospholipid antibodies also inhibit heparin binding and antithrombin activation, as well as tissue factor inhibitor activity, and neutralize the ability of β2-glycoprotein 1 to stimulate tissue plasminogen activator, which inhibits fibrinolysis. Anti-β2-glycoprotein 1 antibodies also prevent the inhibition of platelet aggregation and complement activation [31–34].

In obstetric APS, the interaction of aPL leads to the production of proinflammatory cytokines, inhibition of migration and invasion of the trophoblast and a decrease in human chorionic gonadotropin production [35].

Although uteroplacental thrombosis with vascular insufficiency is a mechanism for adverse gestational outcomes, not all affected placentas demonstrate signs of thrombosis or infarction.

APL also interferes in complement activation, stimulating the release of tumor necrosis factor and antiangiogenic factors associated with impaired placentation. Anti-β2- glycoprotein 1 antibodies trigger the production of proinflammatory cytokines and chemokines [36].

Current clinical and laboratory criteria for diagnosis of APS may be seen in Box 29.1.

In addition to thrombosis, the clinical manifestations of APS may include cerebrovascular accident, thrombocytopenia, cardiac manifestations such as acute myocardial infarction and cardiomyopathy, pulmonary hypertension and infarction, livedo reticularis, renal disease and a very severe form of multisystemic thrombosis, known as catastrophic APS.

Obstetric APS may occur with recurrent abortions, fetal death, intrauterine growth restriction (IUGR), preeclampsia, eclampsia, preterm birth, and abruptio placentae.

The large amount of β2-glycoprotein 1 found in the fetomaternal interface may explain how low aPL titers are associated with gestational morbidity, while vascular events occur only in patients with medium or high titers [38].

Women with APS should receive counseling before pregnancy and vigilant monitoring of maternal thrombosis, renal manifestations, preeclampsia, and fetal growth during pregnancy.

Gestational morbidity may be a consequence of placental infarction due to aPL-mediated vascular thrombosis. Therefore, the standard of treatment for women with obstetric APS includes low-dose aspirin and low molecular weight heparin (LMWH) or unfractionated heparin (UFH), in prophylactic or intermediate doses.

Box 29.1 Clinical and laboratory criteria for diagnosis of APS [37]

Clinical criteria	Laboratory criteria
Vascular thrombosis One or more clinical episodes of arterial, venous or small vessel thrombosis	Lupus anticoagulant Presence in plasma, in more than 2 occasions at least 12 weeks apart, detected according to the *International Society on Thrombosis and Haemostasis* guidelines
Obstetric morbidity Unexplainable death of one or more morphologically normal fetuses, at 10 or more gestational weeks One or more premature morphologically normal newborn infants before 34 weeks of gestation, due to eclampsia or severe preeclampsia, or due to characteristics of placental insufficiency Three or more unexplainable consecutive spontaneous abortions until 10 weeks of gestation, excluding maternal anatomic or hormonal abnormalities, and paternal and maternal chromosomal disorders	Anticardiolipin antibody IgG or IgM, present in serum or plasma at medium or high titers (> 40 UI GPL or MPL, or >99th percentile), on more than two occasions, at least 12 weeks apart, measured by enzyme-linked immunosorbent assay (ELISA) Anti-β2 glycoprotein 1 antibody Present in the serum or plasma at titers above the 99th percentile, in more than two occasions, at least 12 weeks apart, measured by an ELISA
APS is diagnosed by the presence of at least one clinical and one laboratory criterion	

Women with a previous history of thrombosis require anticoagulation in intermediate or therapeutic dose to prevent new episodes.

Additional treatment in gestational loss has been proposed, despite conventional treatment with aspirin and heparin, to increase the rate of live births. The use of prednisolone [39], intravenous human immunoglobulin (IVIG) or plasmapheresis has not shown any conclusive results, as well as the use of statins.

Interest in the use of hydroxychloroquine as an immunomodulating drug for the treatment of APS has increased. This drug may be used in the primary prevention of thrombosis or as an adjuvant therapy. Retrospective studies have shown a reduction in abortion rates in the first trimester and improvement in the rate of live births, when hydroxychloroquine was associated with conventional treatment with low dose aspirin and LMWH. Thus, it has been used as therapy associated with heparin and aspirin in APS refractory to treatment [40–42].

Inherited Thrombophilia

Inherited thrombophilias are genetic conditions that increase the risk of thromboembolic disease during pregnancy and the postpartum period. Table 29.2 shows main inherited thrombophilias and their association with VTE during pregnancy.

A modest association between inherited thrombophilia and adverse gestational outcomes has been suggested, but controversy persists. It has been hypothesized that thrombophilia may increase the risk of thrombosis in the fetus–maternal

Table 29.2 Risk of venous thromboembolism with different inherited thrombophilias [3–15]

	VTE risk per pregnancy (no history) (%)	VTE risk per pregnancy (previous VTE) (%)	OR*
Factor V Leiden heterozygote	0.5–1.2	10	6.4
Factor V Leiden homozygote	4	17	35.8
Prothrombin gene heterozygote	<0.5	>10	5.1
Prothrombin gene homozygote	1–2	>17	21.1
Factor V Leiden/prothrombin both heterozygote	4–5	>20	21.2
Antithrombin deficiency	3–7	40	9.5
Protein C deficiency	0.1–0.8	4–17	9.3
Protein S deficiency	0.1	0–22	7.0

OR* Odds ratio for pregnancy- associated VTE, compared to with non-pregnant carriers

interface, resulting in placenta-mediated complications, such as gestational loss, preeclampsia, IUGR, and abruptio placentae.

Table 29.3 shows the association between pregnancy complications and thrombophilia. Despite that, causal relationship was not well established for most thrombophilias.

Clinically relevant inherited thrombophilias (total prevalence >10%) are deficiencies of coagulation-inhibiting proteins (antithrombin, proteins C and S), FVL and G20210A mutation in the prothrombin gene. Their effect on the coagulation cascade can be seen in Fig. 29.1.

Antithrombin is one of the most important inhibitors of thrombin and activated factor X (Xa). Type II AT deficiency results from decreased synthesis of biologically normal antithrombin. Type II AT deficiency is characterized by normal antithrombin levels, with reduced functional activity [44, 45].

AT deficiency is a rare disorder, occurring in about 1 in 5000 people. Affected individuals have approximately a 50% risk of thrombosis during their lifetime. It is the most thrombogenic of the inherited thrombophilias, and homozygotic mutation is lethal.

Owing to this risk, pregnant women with AT deficiency should receive heparin in therapeutic doses, irrespective of having a history of a prior thromboembolic event [46].

When discontinuation of anticoagulation is required, as during surgery or delivery, treatment with human recombinant antithrombin may prevent VTE [47].

Following AT deficiency, in decreasing order, the risks for VTE are homozygous FVL mutations, homozygous prothrombin, and both heterozygous present simultaneously.

Investigation of inherited thrombophilia in women with a history of obstetric complications and no history of thromboembolic disease is controversial. Association studies that were not very consistent, have suggested a modest absolute risk for the most frequent inherited thrombophilias. Nevertheless, obstetric complications give rise to indications for APS screening.

Some results may not be reliable during pregnancy, as can be seen in Table 29.4.

Table 29.3 Association between pregnancy complications and thrombophilia [12, 43]

Type of thrombophilia	Early loss	Recurrent first trimester loss	Non recurrent second trimester loss	Late loss	Preeclampsia	Placental abruption	Fetal growth restriction
Factor V de Leiden (homozygous)	2.71 (1.32–5.58)	–	–	1.98 (0.4–9.69)	1.87 (0.44–7.88)	8.43 (0.41–171.20)	4.64 (0.19–115.68)
Factor V de Leiden (heterozygous)	1.68 (1.09–2.58)	1.91 (1.01–3.61)	4.12 (1.91–8.81)	2.06 (1.10–3.86)	2.19 (1.46–3.27)	4.70 (1.13–19.59)	2.68 (0.59–12.13)
Prothrombin gene mutation (heterozygous)	2.49 (1.24–5.00)	2.70 (1.37–5.43)	8.60 (2.18–33.95)	2.66 (1.28–5.53)	2.54 (1.52–4.23)	7.71 (3.01–19.76)	2.92 (0.62–13.70)
MTHFR C677T (homozygous)	1.40 (0.77–2.55)	0.86 (0.44–1.69)	NA	1.31 (0.89–1.91)	1.37 (1.07–1.76)	1.47 (0.40–5.35)	1.24 (0.84–1.82)
Antithrombin deficiency	0.88 (0.17–4.48)	NA	NA	7.63 (0.30–196.36)	3.89 (0.16–97.19)	1.08 (0.06–18.12)	NA
Protein C deficiency	2.29 (0.20–26.43)	NA	NA	3.05 (0.24–38.51)	5.15 (0.26–102.22)	5.93 (0.23–151.58)	NA
Protein S deficiency	3.55 (0.35–35.72)	NA	NA	20.09 (3.70–109.15)	2.83 (0.76–10.57)	2.11 (0.47–9.34)	NA
Anticardiolipin antibodies	3.40 (1.33–8.68)	5.05 (1.82–14.01)	NA	3.30 (1.62–6.70)	2.73 (1.65–4.51)	1.42 (0.42–4.77)	6.91 (2.70–17.68)
Lupus anticoagulant	2.97 (1.03–9.76)	ND	14.28 (4.72–43.20)	2.38 (0.81–6.98)	1.45 (0.70–4.61)	NA	NA
Hyperhomocysteinemia	6.25 (1.37–28.42)	4.21 (1.28–13.87)	NA	0.98 (0.17–5.55)	3.49 (1.21–10.11)	2.40 (0.36–15.89)	NA

Data are presented as odds ratio (OR)

Bates et al. [12, 13

MTHFR methylene tetrahydrofolate reductase, *NA* not available

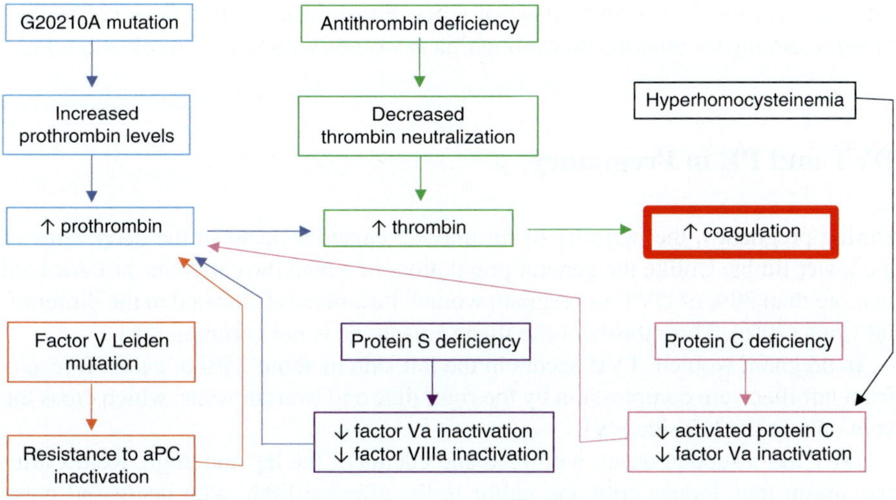

Fig. 29.1 Inherited thrombophilia and its effects on the coagulation cascade

Table 29.4 How to test for inherited thrombophilias [48]

Thrombophilia	Testing method	Is testing reliable during pregnancy?	Is testing reliable during acute thrombosis?	Is testing reliable with anticoagulation?
Factor V Leiden mutation	Activated protein C resistance assay (second generation)	Yes	Yes	No
	If abnormal: DNA analysis	Yes	Yes	Yes
Prothrombin G20210A mutation	DNA analysis	Yes	Yes	Yes
Protein C deficiency	Protein C activity (<65%)	Yes	No	No
Protein S deficiency	Functional assay (<55%)	No[a]	No	No
Antithrombin deficiency	Antithrombin activity (<60%)	Yes	No	No

[a]If screening in pregnancy is necessary, cutoff values for free protein S antigen levels in the second and third trimesters have been identified at less than 30% and less than 24%, respectively

The American College of Obstetricians and Gynecologists (ACOG) guidelines emphasize that women with recurrent fetal loss or abruptio placentae should not be investigated for inherited thrombophilia, due to insufficient clinical evidence that antepartum prophylaxis with heparin prevents recurrence [48]. Similarly, it is also recommended that women with IUGR or preeclampsia should not be investigated.

Furthermore, the American College of Chest Physicians (ACCP) does not recommend screening for inherited thrombophilia in women with prior complications [12].

DVT and PE in Pregnancy

During pregnancy, the majority of thrombotic episodes occur in the deep veins of the lower limbs. Unlike the general population, in which the calf veins are involved in more than 80% of DVT, in pregnant women thrombosis is located in the iliofemoral veins (70%). Thrombosis of the iliac veins alone is not common [16].

In pregnant women, TVE occurs in the left side in about 85% of cases. It results from left iliac vein compression by the right iliac and ovarian veins, which cross the vein only in the left side [49].

DVT has a sudden onset, with pain and edema of the leg and thigh. Reflex arterial spasm may induce cold and pallor in the affected limb, with decreased pulse pressure. The risk of sequelae after a DVT episode in pregnancy, such as chronic venous insufficiency or post-thrombotic syndrome, is higher in other periods of life.

Diagnostic imaging involves compression ultrasonography, which is the first-line imaging modality according to ACOG and ACCP guidelines, since it is a non-invasive technique [50].

Magnetic resonance imaging permits good anatomic details above the inguinal ligament and is useful for the diagnosis of iliofemoral and pelvic thrombosis [51].

D-dimer, a product of fibrin degradation, is generated during fibrinolysis and may be a useful marker in thrombosis. In pregnancy, however, D-dimer measurement is problematic. D-dimer serum levels may rise in advanced gestational age and are also affected by multifetal pregnancy, cesarean section, abruptio placentae, sickle cell disease and sepsis. Therefore, in pregnancy its measurement remains questionable [52].

Fig. 29.2 shows an algorithm for DVT during pregnancy.

About 30–60% of women with DVT in the lower limbs have asymptomatic PE. Pulmonary embolism accounts for around 10% of pregnancy-related deaths. Symptoms include dyspnea (82%), chest pain (49%), coughing (20%), syncope (14%), and hemoptysis (7%). Other clinical findings include tachypnea, tachycardia, and extreme apprehension.

Massive PE is defined as pulmonary embolism that causes hemodynamic instability. Acute mechanical obstruction of the pulmonary vasculature causes increased vascular resistance and pulmonary hypertension, followed by acute dilatation of the right ventricle. Circulatory collapse occurs after 75–80% of obstruction.

Investigation of PE should take into consideration the exposure of the mother and fetus to ionizing radiation. Intravascular pulmonary angiography is the gold standard for diagnosis of PE, but it requires catheterization of the right side of the heart and exposes the fetus to high doses of radiation. Computed tomography pulmonary angiography and ventilation/perfusion scintigraphy are options that generates less fetal radiation, but the results are still questionable in pregnant women [54–56].

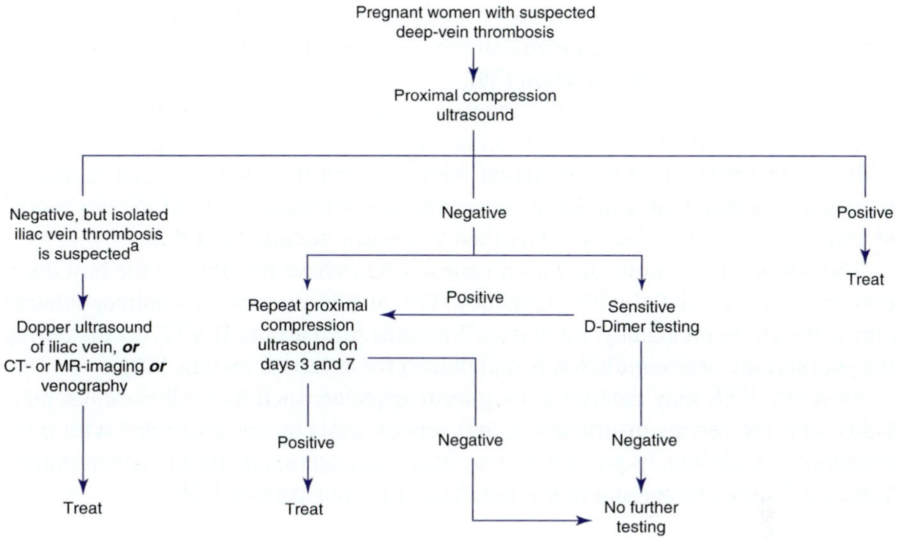

Fig. 29.2 Algorithm for evaluating TPV in pregnancy [53]

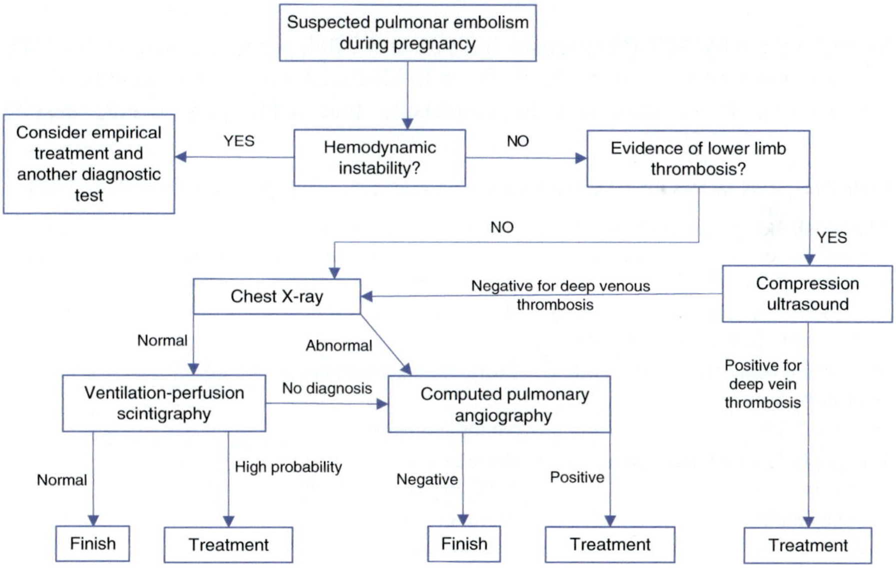

Fig. 29.3 Recommendations for suspected PTE in pregnancy, according to the American Thoracic Society and Society of Thoracic Radiology [56]

Figure 29.3 shows recommendations for suspected PE, from American Thoracic Society and Society of Thoracic Radiology [57].

Treatment of acute VTE during pregnancy requires full anticoagulation, usually performed with LMWH or UFH. The majority of studies suggest using LMWH, owing to greater safety and lower chance of side-effects [12].

Complementary procedures may be indicated, such as inferior vena cava filter, when the patient requires cesarean delivery, and the interruption of anticoagulation may result in another embolization [58].

There is little experience with thrombolysis and embolectomy in pregnancy, and case reports have described complication rates of up to 40% [59–61].

In the puerperium, anticoagulation with warfarin that does not contraindicate maternal breastfeeding is initiated concomitantly with heparin, until the target goal of anticoagulation is achieved. Only then is heparin discontinued [62].

The period of full anticoagulation varies. Studies have not defined the best duration for VTE associated with pregnancy. The ACCP recommends anticoagulation during the entire pregnancy, for at least 3 months postpartum. If VTE occurs during the puerperium, anticoagulation is maintained for at least 6 months [12].

Obstetric VTE may determine long-term sequelae, such as cardiovascular morbidity, chronic venous insufficiency, and venous stasis ulcers associated with post-thrombotic syndrome. Its prevention may decrease maternal morbidity and mortality. Table 29.5 shows major and minor risk factors for postpartum VTE.

Prophylaxis

As highlighted by ACCP consensus in 2001 and 2004, recommendations for VTE prevention during pregnancy should be individualized, taking into account all the risk factors. It is important to emphasize that VTE may occur, despite

Table 29.5 Risk factors for VTE resulting in a baseline risk of postpartum VTE > 3% [62–67]

Major risk factors: presence of at least one risk factor suggests a risk of postpartum VTE > 3%	Minor risk factors: presence of at least two risk factor or one risk factor in the setting of emergency cesarean section suggests a risk of postpartum VTE > 3%
Immobility (strict bed rest for 1 week or more in the antepartum period)	BMI > 30 kg/m^2
Postpartum hemorrhage >1000 mL with surgery	Postpartum hemorrhage >1000 mL
Previous VTE	Multiple pregnancy
Preeclampsia with fetal growth restrictions	Preeclampsia Fetal growth restriction
Thrombophilia Antithrombin deficiency Factor V Leiden Prothrombin G20210A	Thrombophilia Protein C deficiency Protein S deficiency
Medical conditions Systemic lupus erythematosus Heart disease Sickle cell disease	
Blood transfusion	
Postpartum infection	

antithrombotic prophylaxis. Galambosi et al. [68] evaluated 270 women in 369 pregnancies, who had a history of at least a prior PE. Recurrence was observed in 28 women (10.4%), 12 at the beginning of pregnancy, before the initiation of antithrombotic prophylaxis, and 16 during use of LMWH. Therefore, a selective screening strategy is required.

The ACOG recommends investigating thrombophilia when a personal history of VTE is associated with a nonrecurrent risk factor, such as fractures, surgeries and/or prolonged immobilization, or first-degree relatives with high-risk thrombophilia or VTE before the age of 50, in the absence of risk factors [48].

The first VTE episode may occur during pregnancy. A family history of VTE, especially in young individuals, suggests inherited thrombophilia, which may first manifest itself during pregnancy and the puerperium. In these cases, screening for thrombophilia is pertinent. There is a great disparity in recommendations for VTE prevention in pregnant women. Despite advances in prevention and treatment, over the past two decades maternal mortality resulting from VTE has remained constant.

Thromboprophylaxis requires evaluation in the antepartum, postpartum and at any time during pregnancy, in case hospital admission is required. It can be performed pharmacologically (anticoagulation) or mechanically (intermittent pneumatic compression or graduated compression stockings).

Pregnancy and puerperium are risk periods for the development of VTE. However, the majority of pregnant women do not require thromboprophylaxis, which is indicated for women considered at high risk for developing VTE during pregnancy. Indications for thromboprophylaxis are different in the antepartum and postpartum periods.

The majority of guidelines on thromboprophylaxis in pregnancy derive from consensus, but there is no general agreement as to which women should undergo treatment or be investigated for thrombophilias.

Tables 29.6 and 29.7 show the guidelines of the main medical associations regarding prophylaxis.

Bates et al. [70] reviewed the recommendations for VTE associated with pregnancy and showed that the majority derive from observational studies and extrapolated data obtained outside of the gestational period.

Similarly, a Cochrane review concluded that evidence is insufficient to definitively recommend thromboprophylaxis during pregnancy [71].

Nonpharmacological Thromboprophylaxis

The nonpharmacological measures recommended for thromboprophylaxis include adequate hydration, left lateral decubitus, early postpartum mobilization, use of elastic stockings, or pneumatic compression devices. The Royal College of Obstetrics and Gynaecology (RCOG) recommends the use of elastic stockings with graduated calf compression of 14–15 mmHg during pregnancy and the puerperal period [69].

Table 29.6 Royal College of Obstetricians and Gynaecologists recommendations for thromboprophylaxis in pregnant women with previous TEV and thrombophilia [68]

Risk	Thrombophilia	Recommendations
Very high	Previous VTE under anticoagulation Antithrombin deficiency	Enoxaparin 80 mg once daily antepartum and for 6 weeks postpartum
High	Previous TEV, except if associated with surgery Antiphospholipid syndrome with previous TEV	Enoxaparin 40 mg once daily antepartum and for 6 weeks postpartum
Intermediate	Factor V Leiden homozygous, Protein C or S deficiency without previous TEV	Consider LMWH prophylactic dose antepartum and postpartum
	Previous TEV associated with surgery	Consider LWMH prophylactic dose antepartum; antenatal prophylactic dose of LMWH from 28 weeks and 6 weeks postpartum is recommended
Low	Asymptomatic low risk thrombophilia	Postnatal prophylactic dose of LMWH for 10 days; consider postnatal prophylactic dose of LMWH if family history of VTE

VTE venous thromboembolism, *LMWH* low molecular weight heparin

In a study with 10 pregnant women, a Doppler ultrasound with venous blood flow study revealed that graduated compression stockings increased femoral venous flow velocity in late pregnancy [72]. It has been considered safe to use mechanical prophylaxis after cesarean section and in women hospitalized during pregnancy.

Pharmacological Thromboprophylaxis

The administration of pharmacological thromboprophylaxis before childbirth should consider the benefits of DVT prevention, risks of bleeding, and fetal complications.

There is no evidence to support the routine use of pharmacological thromboprophylaxis to all women hospitalized during pregnancy or postpartum period. Some women who do not fulfill the criteria for outpatient thromboprophylaxis may benefit from receiving this medication during hospital stay. The decision should be made on an individual basis.

Pharmacological prophylaxis may be considered for women with a history of a single idiopathic DVT, associated with pregnancy or the use of estrogen, and for women with a history of multiple VTE, irrespective of the cause. Furthermore, it should also be considered for women with known thrombophilia and for those with persistent risk factors for VTE.

Table 29.7 Recommendations for thromboprophylaxis during pregnancy and postpartum according to ACOG [48] and ACCP [12]

	Pregnancy		Postpartum	
Clinical setting	ACOG	ACCP	ACOG	ACCP
One previous TEV				
Risk factor no longer present	Surveillance	Surveillance	Postpartum anticoagulation	Prophylactic or intermediate dose of LMWH or warfarin with target INR between 2 and 3 for 6 weeks
Associated with pregnancy or use of estrogen or idiopathic, without long-term anticoagulation	Prophylactic or intermediate dose of LMWH or UFH	Prophylactic or intermediate dose of LMWH	Postpartum anticoagulation	Prophylactic or intermediate dose of LMWH or warfarin with target INR between 2 and 3 for 6 weeks
Using long term warfarin	Not specified	Adjusted dose of LMWH or 75% of therapeutic dose	Not specified	Resumption of long term warfarin
Associated with high-risk thrombophilia and without long-term anticoagulation, or with a history of VTE in a first-degree relative	Prophylactic, intermediate or adjusted dose of LMWH or UFH	Not specified	Postpartum anticoagulation or intermediate or adjusted dose of LMWH or UFH for 6 weeks	Prophylactic or intermediate dose of LMWH or UFH or warfarin with target INR between 2 and 3, for 6 weeks
Associated with low-risk thrombophilia without treatment	Prophylactic or intermediate dose of LMWH or UFH, or surveillance only	Not specified	Postpartum anticoagulation or intermediate dose of LMWH or UFH	Prophylactic or intermediate dose of LMWH or UFH or warfarin with target INR between 2 and 3, for 6 weeks
Two or more previous VTE, with or without thrombophilia				
No long-term treatment	Prophylactic or therapeutic dose of LMWH or UFH	Not specified	Postpartum anticoagulation or therapeutic dose of LMWH or UFH for 6 weeks	Prophylactic or intermediate dose of LMWH or warfarin with target INR between 2 and 3, for 6 weeks

(continued)

Table 29.7 (continued)

Clinical setting	Pregnancy		Postpartum	
	ACOG	ACCP	ACOG	ACCP
Receiving long-term anticoagulation	Therapeutic dose of LMWH or UFH	Adjusted dose of LMWH or 75% of therapeutic dose	Resume long-term anticoagulation	Resumption of long-term anticoagulation
Without previous VTE				
High-risk thrombophilia	Surveillance or prophylactic or intermediate dose of LMWH or UFH	Prophylactic or intermediate dose of LMWH or UFH	Postpartum anticoagulation	Intermediate dose of LMWH or warfarin with target INR between 2 and 3, for 6 weeks
Family history of VTE and homozygous FVL or homozygous prothrombin mutation	Not specified	Prophylactic or intermediate dose of LMWH or UFH	Not specified	Prophylactic or intermediate dose of LMWH or warfarin with target INR between 2 and 3, for 6 weeks
No family history and homozygous FVL or homozygous prothrombin mutation	Surveillance or prophylactic dose of LMWH or UFH	Surveillance	Postpartum anticoagulation	Prophylactic or intermediate dose of LMWH or warfarin with target INR between 2 and 3, for 6 weeks
Family history of VTE and low-risk thrombophilia	Surveillance	Surveillance	Postpartum anticoagulation or intermediate dose of LMWH or UFH	Prophylactic or intermediate dose of LMWH or, in women without CPD or DPS, warfarin with target INR between 2 and 3
Low-risk thrombophilia	Surveillance	Surveillance if no family history	Surveillance; postpartum anticoagulation if additional risk factors	Surveillance if no family history
Antiphospholipid antibodies				
History of previous VTE	Prophylactic dose of LMWH or UFH (plus low-dose aspirin)	Not specified	Prophylactic dose of LMWH or UFH	Not specified

Table 29.7 (continued)

	Pregnancy		Postpartum	
Clinical setting	ACOG	ACCP	ACOG	ACCP
No previous VTE	Surveillance or prophylactic dose of LMWH or UFH or prophylactic dose of LMWH or UFH plus low-dose aspirin if previous recurrent pregnancy loss or fetal death	Prophylactic or intermediate dose of LMWH or UFH or prophylactic dose of LMWH plus low-dose aspirin	Prophylactic dose of heparin plus low-dose aspirin for 6 weeks, if previous pregnancy loss or previous fetal death	Not specified

High-risk thrombophilia: antithrombin deficiency, homozygous factor V Leiden or homozygous prothrombin, factor V Leiden heterozygous compound with heterozygous prothrombin mutation; low-risk thrombophilia: heterozygous Leiden factor V, heterozygous prothrombin mutation, protein C or S deficiencies

LMWH low molecular weight heparin, *UFH* unfractionated heparin, *VTE* venous thromboembolism, *ACOG* American College of Obstetricians and Gynecologists, *ACCP* American College of Chest Physicians

Studies have reported a consistently higher incidence of VTE in women with variants of high-risk persistent thrombophilia, in those with a previous history of thromboembolism (Table 29.2).

When a transient risk factor can be identified, such as trauma, immobility or surgery, there is a low probability of VTE recurrence. In these cases, clinical vigilance is preferable to pharmacological thromboprophylaxis, except when more than one thromboembolic event occurs.

Women who are already receiving anticoagulant therapy outside of pregnancy require reassessment at the beginning of pregnancy. Should there be a need to maintain anticoagulation therapy, those using oral anticoagulants (direct thrombin inhibitors, activated factor X or warfarin) must switch to heparin.

During hospitalization, pregnant women considered at high risk for VTE are those admitted for clinical or surgical reasons, such as pneumonia, sepsis, orthopedic injuries, that require prolonged bed rest, or who have additional risks or multiple factors for VTE, including obesity, advanced age, severe disease, malignancies, ovarian hyperstimulation, and multiparity.

More than 200,000 pregnant women admitted to the hospital for reasons unrelated to labor had an 18-fold higher risk of VTE during hospitalization and a sixfold higher risk in the first 28 days after hospital discharge. The highest DVT rates were observed in women with a body mass index (BMI) above 30 kg/m^2, age over 35 years, admission in the third trimester and hospitalization for more than 3 days [73].

The choice of anticoagulant in pregnancy should take into account maternal and fetal safety in the peripartum period. In addition, labor is considered unpredictable and neuraxial analgesia is required for pain management.

Heparins are used in the majority of pregnant women. The reason is because these drugs do not cross the placenta and do not affect the fetus. LMWH is the anticoagulant of choice in pregnancy, due to its superior safety profile. It is effective at reducing the size of the thrombus, without increasing mortality rate or significant bleeding. UFH is chosen for women with severe renal insufficiency, since its metabolism is renal and hepatic. LMWH has an exclusively renal metabolism [74].

LMWH derives from UFH, with a molecular weight between 4000 and 5000 Da. Both exert anticoagulant activity by antithrombin activation. The primary difference is the relatively inhibitory action against activated factor X and thrombin: UFH has an equivalent activity against both, but LMWH has a higher activity against activated factor X than against thrombin. It also has a more predictable anticoagulant response with less bleeding complications than UFH, due to its better bioavailability, longer half-life and lower interference with platelets.

LMWH for use in pregnancy include enoxaparin, tinzaparin, and dalteparin. The pharmacokinetics of enoxaparin was studied in women with VTE during pregnancy or immediately postpartum [75], receiving 1 mg/kg twice a day. Anticoagulation was monitored by factor anti-Xa activity, with blood drawn 3 h after injection. The therapeutic goal of 0.4–1 U/mL was achieved by the majority of women evaluated. None developed recurrent VTE or hemorrhagic complications. After cesarean delivery, in women with a BMI of 35 kg/m^2 or more, a dose of 0.5 mg/kg was adjusted twice a day as recommended, to achieve the goal of 0.2–0.6 U/mL of anti-Xa [76].

UFH may be considered for the initial treatment of VTE and given close to the time of delivery or surgery, because it has a shorter half-life than LMWH, and its activity is more completely reversed. UFH may be used close to the time of delivery, when its reversibility and shorter half-life are desirable, enabling a more flexible administration of neuraxial anesthesia.

Heparins may be administered during pregnancy at different doses, depending on the risk of thromboembolism and degree of anticoagulation desired. Table 29.8 shows different anticoagulation regimens for LMWH and UFH.

When LMWH is administered for prophylaxis of VTE in patients without thrombophilia, prophylactic or intermediate doses are used. The therapeutic dose is provided when these doses are considered insufficient for prophylaxis in patients at high risk for thrombosis.

When indicated, pharmacological thromboprophylaxis should be maintained during the entire pregnancy. After delivery, the ACCP recommends continuing treatment for at least 6 weeks. Prophylaxis may be extended to 3 months, particularly in women with persistent risk factors for thrombosis [12].

Oral anticoagulants, such as antagonists of vitamin K and warfarin, are used for prolonged periods outside of pregnancy. These drugs cross the placenta and may cause hemorrhage and teratogenicity in the fetus. Embryopathy occurs in approximately 5% of the fetuses exposed between 6 and 12 weeks. They do not accumulate in human milk. When indicated, these drugs may be used safely during breastfeeding [77].

Table 29.8 Anticoagulation regimens definitions [48]

Anticoagulation regimens	Anticoagulation dosage
Prophylactic LMWH	Enoxaparin 40 mg SC once daily Dalteparin 5000 units SC once daily Tinzaparin 4500 units SC once daily Nadroparin 2850 units SC once daily
Intermediate-dose LMWH	Enoxaparin 40 mg SC every 12 h Dalteparin 5000 units SC every 12 h
Adjusted dose (therapeutic) LMWH	Enoxaparin 1 mg/kg every 12 h Dalteparin 200 units/kg once daily Tinzaparin 175 units/kg once daily Dalteparin 100 units/kg every 12 h Target an anti-Xa level in the therapeutic range of 0.6–1.0 U/mL 4 h after last injection for once-daily regimen; slightly higher doses may be needed for a once-daily regimen
Prophylactic UFH	UHF 5000–7500 units SC every 12 h in first trimester
	UHF 7500–10,000 units SC every 12 h in the second trimester
	UHF 10,000 units SC every 12 h in the third trimester, unless the aPTT is elevated
Adjusted dose (therapeutic) UFH	UFH 10,000 units or more SC every 12 h in doses adjusted to target aPTT in the therapeutic range (1.5–2.5 × control) 6 h after injection
Postpartum anticoagulation	Prophylactic, intermediate, or adjusted dose LMWH for 6–8 weeks as indicated. Oral anticoagulants may be considered postpartum based upon planned duration of therapy, lactation, and patient preference
Surveillance	Clinical vigilance and appropriate objective investigation of women with symptoms suspicious of deep vein thrombosis or pulmonary embolism. VTE risk assessment should be performed pre-pregnancy or early in pregnancy and repeated if complications develop, particularly those necessitating hospitalization or prolonged immobility

Abbreviations: *SC* subcutaneous, *LMWH* low molecular weight heparin, *UFH* unfractionated heparin, *VTE* venous thromboembolism, *aPTT* activated partial thromboplastin time

There is no evidence that the new anticoagulants, e.g., rivaroxaban, dabigatran, and apixaban are safe in pregnancy, and therefore these drugs should be avoided. Few studies have evaluated the new agents during pregnancy, and the reproductive risks to humans are unknown. Dabigatran crosses the human placenta, and the amount of drug excretion into human milk is unknown [78].

Complications of Anticoagulation

Three major complications associated with anticoagulation are hemorrhage, thrombocytopenia, and osteoporosis. The last two complications occur only with heparins and their risk may be reduced by the option for LMWH. The most serious complication is hemorrhage, more common in surgeries and lacerations. Bleeding may also occur in case of excessive heparin dose.

Heparin-Induced Thrombocytopenia

There are two types of thrombocytopenia. The most common is nonimmune and benign, developing in the first days of heparin use. It is reversed within 5 days of discontinuation of heparin. The second is the severe form of heparin-induced thrombocytopenia (HIT). It results from an immune reaction that involves IgG antibodies targeted against complexes composed of platelet factor 4 bound to platelet surface, and heparin. The diagnosis of HIT is based on a reduction in platelet numbers by more than 50% or thrombosis 5–10 days after the beginning of heparin treatment, associated with the emergence of platelet-activating antibodies. A decrease in platelet number occurs rapidly, within a period of 1–3 days, and typical values range from 40,000 to 80,000 platelets/μL. Table 29.9 shows the characteristics of these two types of thrombocytopenia.

The incidence of HIT is approximately 3–5% outside of pregnancy, in less than 0.1% of obstetric patients. The ACCP recommends monitoring platelets when the risk of HIT is lower than 1%. When it is above 1%, monitoring should be performed every 2–3 days, from the 4th to the 14th day of drug use.

When HIT is diagnosed, heparin should be switched to an anticoagulation alternative, to avoid platelet transfusions. The ACCP recommends the use of danaparoid, a heparinoid, as an option [12]. Nevertheless, Lindhoff-Last et al. [79] reported two maternal fatalities and three fetal deaths among 50 pregnant women using danaparoid. Magnani [80] reported two maternal deaths from hemorrhage among 83 pregnant women, and the drug was removed from the market in the United States.

Other alternative agents mentioned are fondaparinux and argatroban, and studies are mostly limited to case reports. Furthermore, danaparoid and fondaparinux have a prolonged half-life (24 h and 48 h, respectively).

Heparin-Induced Osteoporosis

Bone loss may develop with long-term heparin use, in general when administered for 6 months or more, with a higher prevalence in smokers. UFH may cause osteopenia, which occurs less frequently with LMWH. Women treated with any heparin

Table 29.9 Characteristics of the two types of heparin-induced thrombocytopenia [78]

	Type I	Type II
Frequency	10–20%	1–3%
Timing of onset	1–4 days	5–10 days after start of heparin
Nadir platelet count	100,000/μL	Usually >20,000/μL; median nadir 60,000/μL
Antibody mediated	No	Yes
Thromboembolic sequelae	None	30–80%
Hemorrhagic sequelae	None	Rare
Management	Observe	Cessation of heparin, alternative nonheparin anticoagulation to prevent thrombosis

should be encouraged to take a daily dose of 1500 mg of calcium supplementation [81].

Delivery Route and Anticoagulation

The delivery route in women undergoing anticoagulation is defined by obstetric conditions. When there is no maternal or fetal complication that precludes the vaginal route, delivery may occur. UFH or LMWH is usually discontinued at the beginning of labor. Less serious tissue injury and the possibility of early ambulation make vaginal delivery an excellent choice for women requiring anticoagulation during pregnancy.

In case of a cesarean indication, delivery may also occur, as long as rigorous hemostasis management is performed, similar to vaginal delivery. With the possibility of planned deliveries and discontinued use of heparin, some pregnant women opt for this route. The risk of DVT, particularly fatal VTE, is higher after cesarean delivery than after vaginal delivery. The lack of high-quality data generates considerable variation in the ACOG [48], RCOG [69], and ACCP [12] guidelines.

Cesarean delivery is associated with an increased risk of VTE, especially when performed in an urgent situation. Despite a higher relative risk, the absolute risk of VTE is low. Data suggest that the risk of clinically important events is similar to that seen in low-risk surgical patients. Thromboprophylaxis is not administered to these surgical patients, other than early ambulation.

When there is no indication for preterm delivery, it is recommended that the delivery (induction or cesarean section) should be scheduled for 39 weeks, to control the time when the patient is not taking antithrombotic drugs.

Pregnant women receiving a therapeutic dose of LMWH may switch to UFH between 36 and 37 weeks, due to its shorter half-life. Neuraxial anesthesia can be administered, minimizing bleeding in case of spontaneous delivery [48].

Anesthetic guidelines recommend at least a 24-h interval between the last therapeutic dose of LMWH and epidural catheter insertion, and at least 12 h for prophylactic UFH doses. The aim of switching LMWH to UFH at the end of the third trimester is mainly to prevent an epidural or spinal hematoma during the block, rather than to decrease the risk of maternal bleeding at the time of delivery.

Epidural hematoma is a rare complication of spinal anesthesia, with a reported incidence of 1: 200,000 to 250.000 deliveries [82]. It is more common during epidural anesthesia than spinal anesthesia, and usually occurs in situations of coagulation anomalies or anticoagulant administration. When neurologic deficits emerge due to a hematoma, decompression surgery is immediately recommended.

ACCP guidelines recommend that women with a planned delivery, receiving a therapeutic dose of LMWH or UFH twice a day, should discontinue heparin 24 h before the induction of labor or cesarean delivery [12]. ACOG guidelines recommend discontinuing the therapeutic dose 24 to 36 h before the procedure [48]. The American Society of Regional Anesthesia and Pain Medicine recommends avoiding neuraxial block, 10–12 h after a prophylactic dose of LMWH, and 24 h after a therapeutic dose. These approaches usually ensure that patients with prior thrombosis do not remain without anticoagulants for more than 48 h [83].

The effects of heparin on blood loss during delivery depend on the dose used, route and period of administration, number and depth of incisions and lacerations, intensity of postpartum myometrial contractions, and the presence of coagulation disorders.

Heparin effects rarely need to be reversed with protamine sulfate, and reversal is not indicated for prophylactic heparin doses. A slow intravenous administration of protamine sulfate generally reverses the effect of heparin rapidly and efficiently. Protamine should not be administered at higher doses than necessary to neutralize heparin, owing to its anticoagulant effect.

In women with APS, guidelines recommend low-dose aspirin combined with heparin for treatment. Interruption of aspirin seven to 10 days before delivery may prevent a slight increase in bleeding observed when the drug is continued.

References

1. Virchow RL. Gesammelte Abhandlungen zur wissenschaftlichen Medicin. Meidinger Sohn: Frankfurt; 1856.
2. Greer IA. Thrombophilia: implications for pregnancy outcome. Thromb Res. 2003;109:73–81.
3. Franco RF, Reitsma PH. Genetic risk factors of venous thrombosis. Hum Genet. 2001;109:369–84.
4. Gerhardt A, Scharf RE, Beckmann MW, Struve S, Bender HG, Pillny M, et al. Prothrombin and factor V mutations in women with a history of thrombosis during pregnancy and the puerperium. N Engl J Med. 2000;342:374–80.
5. Zotz RB, Gerhardt A, Scharf RE. Inherited thrombophilia and gestational venous thromboembolism. Best Pract Res Clin Haematol. 2003;16:243–59.
6. Haverkate F, Samama M. Familial dysfibrinogenemia and thrombophilia. Report on a study of the SSC Subcommittee on Fibrinogen. Thromb Haemost. 1995;73:151–61.
7. Friederich PW, Sanson BJ, Simioni P, Zanardi S, Huisman MV, Kindt I, et al. Frequency of pregnancy-related venous thromboembolism in anticoagulant factor-deficient women: implications for prophylaxis. Ann Intern Med. 1996;125:955–60.
8. Vossen CY, Preston FE, Conard J, Fontcuberta J, Makris M, van der Meer FJ, et al. Hereditary thrombophilia and fetal loss: a prospective follow-up study. J Thromb Haemost. 2004;2:592–6.
9. Paidas MJ, Ku DH, Lee MJ, Manish S, Thurston A, Lockwood CJ, et al. Protein Z, protein S levels are lower in patients with thrombophilia and subsequent pregnancy complications. J Thromb Haemost. 2005;3:497–501.
10. Dykes AC, Walker ID, McMahon AD, Islam SI, Tait RC. A study of protein S antigen levels in 3788 healthy volunteers: influence of age, sex and hormone use, and estimate for prevalence of deficiency state. Br J Haematol. 2001;113:636–41.
11. Goodwin AJ, Rosendaal FR, Kottke-Marchant K, Bovill EG. A review of the technical, diagnostic, and epidemiologic considerations for protein S assays. Arch Pathol Lab Med. 2002;126:1349–66.
12. Bates SM, Greer IA, Middeldorp S, Veenstra DL, Prabulos AM, Vandvik PO, American College of Chest Physicians. VTE, thrombophilia, antithrombotic therapy, and pregnancy: Antithrombotic Therapy and Prevention of Thrombosis, 9th ed: American College of Chest Physicians Evidence-Based Clinical Practice Guidelines. Chest. 2012;141(2 Suppl):e691S.

13. Robertson L, Greer I. Thromboembolism in pregnancy. Curr Opin Obstet Gynecol. 2005 Apr;17(2):113-6. https://doi.org/10.1097/01.gco.0000162177.30607.59. PMID: 15758600.
14. Gerhardt A, Scharf RE, Greer IA, Zotz RB. Hereditary risk factors for thrombophilia and probability of venous thromboem- bolism during pregnancy and the puerperium. Blood. 2016;128:2343–9.
15. Rheaume M, Weber F, Durand M, Mahone M. Pregnancy-related venous thromboembolism risk in asymptomatic women with antithrombin deficiency: a systematic review. Obstet Gynecol. 2016;127:649–56.
16. Marik PE, Plante LA. Venous thromboembolic disease and pregnancy. N Engl J Med. 2008;359(19):2025.
17. Christiansen SC, Cannegieter SC, Koster T, Vandenbroucke JP, Rosendaal FR. Thrombophilia, clinical factors, and recurrent venous thrombotic events. JAMA. 2005;293:2352.
18. Dalen JE. Should patients with venous thromboembolism be screened for thrombophilia? Am J Med. 2008;121:458.
19. Simone B, De Stefano V, Leoncini E, Zacho J, Martinelli I, Emmerich J, et al. Risk of venous thromboembolism associated with single and combined effects of factor V Leiden, prothrombin 20210A and methylenetethraydrofolate reductase C677T: a meta-analysis involving over 11,000 cases and 21,000 controls. Eur J Epidemiol. 2013;28:621.
20. Mahmoodi BK, Brouwer JL, Ten Kate MK, Lijfering WM, Veeger NJ, Mulder AB, et al. A prospective cohort study on the absolute risks of venous thromboembolism and predictive value of screening asymptomatic relatives of patients with hereditary deficiencies of protein S, protein C or antithrombin. J Thromb Haemost. 2010;8:1193.
21. Pernod G, Biron-Andreani C, Morange PE, Boehlen F, Constans J, Couturaud F, et al. Recommendations on testing for thrombophilia in venous thromboembolic disease: a French consensus guideline. J Mal Vasc. 2009;34:156.
22. Merriman L, Greaves M. Testing for thrombophilia: an evidence-based approach. Postgrad Med J. 2006;82:699.
23. Wu O, Robertson L, Twaddle S, Lowe G, Clark P, Walker I, et al. Screening for thrombophilia in high-risk situations: a meta-analysis and cost effectiveness analysis. Br J Haematol. 2005;131:80.
24. Lindhoff-Last E, Luxembourg B. Evidence-based indications for thrombophilia screening. Vasa. 2008;37:19.
25. Cohen W, Castelli C, Suchon P, Bouvet S, Aillaud MF, Brunet D, et al. Risk assessment of venous thrombosis in families with known hereditary thrombophilia: the MARseilles-NImes prediction model. J Thromb Haemost. 2014;12:138.
26. Davis SM, Branch DW. Thromboprophylaxis in pregnancy: who and how? Obstet Gynecol Clin North Am. 2010;37:333.
27. Culwell KR, Curtis KM, del Carmen Cravioto M. Safety of contraceptive method use among women with systemic lupus erythematosus: a systematic review. Obstet Gynecol. 2009;114:341.
28. Wu O, Robertson L, Langhorne P, Twaddle S, Lowe GD, Clark P, et al. Oral contraceptives, hormone replacement therapy, thrombophilias and risk of venous thromboembolism: a systematic review. The thrombosis: risk and Economic Assessment of Thrombophilia Screening (TREATS) Study. Thromb Haemost. 2005;94:17.
29. Hughes GR. Thrombosis, abortion, cerebral disease, and the lupus anticoagulant. Br Med J (Clin Res Ed). 1983;287(6399):1088–9.
30. Erkan D, Lockshin MD. What is antiphospholipid syndrome? Curr Rheumatol Rep. 2004;6(6):451.
31. Forastiero R, Martinuzzo M. Prothrombotic mechanisms based on the impairment of fibrinolysis in the antiphospholipid syndrome. Lupus. 2008;17(10):872.
32. Urbanus RT, Derksen RH, de Groot PG. Platelets and the antiphospholipid syndrome. Lupus. 2008;17(10):888.

33. Rand JH, Wu XX, Quinn AS, Taatjes DJ. Resistance to annexin A5 anticoagulant activity: a thrombogenic mechanism for the antiphospholipid syndrome. Lupus. 2008;17(10):922.
34. Bu C, Gao L, Xie W, Zhang J, He Y, Cai G, McCrae KR. beta2-glycoprotein I is a cofactor for tissue plasminogen activator-mediated plasminogen activation. Arthritis Rheum. 2009;60(2):559.
35. Abrahams VM, Chamley LW, Salmon JE. Emerging treatment models in rheumatology: antiphospholipid syndrome and pregnancy: pathogenesis to translation. Arthritis Rheumatol. 2017;69(9):1710.
36. Matrai CE, Rand JH, Baergen RN. Absence of distinct immunohistochemical distribution of annexin A5, C3b, C4d, and C5b-9 in placentas from patients with antiphospholipid antibodies, preeclampsia, and systemic lupus erythematosus. Pediatr Dev Pathol. 2019;22(5):431.
37. Miyakis S, Lockshin MD, Atsumi T, Branch DW, Brey RL, Cervera R, et al. International consensus statement on an update of the classification criteria for definite antiphospholipid syndrome (APS). J Thromb Haemost. 2006;4(2):295.
38. Di Simone N, Meroni PL, Del Papa N, Raschi E, Caliandro D, De Carolis S, et al. Antiphospholipid antibodies affect trophoblast gonadotropin secretion and invasiveness by binding directly and through adhered β2-glycoprotein I. Arthritis Rheum. 2000;43(1):140–50.
39. Branch DW, Silver RM, Blackwell JL, Reading JC, Scott JR. Outcome of treated pregnancies in women with antiphospholipid syndrome: an update of the Utah experience. Obstet Gynecol. 1992;80(4):614. Kutteh WH. Antiphospholipid antibody-associated recurrent pregnancy loss: treatment with heparin and low-dose aspirin is superior to low-dose aspirin alone. Am J Obstet Gynecol. 1996;174(5):1584.
40. Sciascia S, Hunt BJ, Talavera-Garcia E, Lliso G, Khamashta MA, Cuadrado MJ. The impact of hydroxychloroquine treatment on pregnancy outcome in women with antiphospholipid antibodies. Am J Obstet Gynecol. 2016;214(2):273.e1–8.
41. Bertolaccini ML, Contento G, Lennen R, Sanna G, Blower PJ, Ma MT, et al. Complement inhibition by hydroxychloroquine prevents placental and fetal brain abnormalities in antiphospholipid syndrome. J Autoimmun. 2016;75:30.
42. Ruffatti A, Tonello M, Hoxha A, Sciascia S, Cuadrado MJ, Latino JO, et al. Effect of additional treatments combined with conventional therapies in pregnant patients with high-risk antiphospholipid syndrome: a multicentre study. Thromb Haemost. 2018;118(4):639.
43. Robertson L, Wu O, Langhorne P, Twaddle S, Clark P, Lowe GD, et al. Thrombosis: risk and economic assessment of thrombophilia screening (TREATS) study. Thrombophilia in pregnancy: a systematic review. Br J Haematol. 2006;132(2):171–96.
44. Khor B, Van Cott EM. Laboratory tests for antithrombin deficiency. Am J Hematol. 2010;85(12):947.
45. Ambruso DR, Leonard BD, Bies RD, Jacobson L, Hathaway WE, Reeve EB. Antithrombin III deficiency: decreased synthesis of a biochemically normal molecule. Blood. 1982;60(1):78.
46. Lockwood CJ, Bauer KA. Inherited thrombophilias in pregnancy. In: Leung LLK, Berghella V, editors. UpToDate. Waltham: UpToDate Inc. https://www.uptodate.com. Accessed on 20 Jan 2020.
47. James AH, Konkle BA, Bauer KA. Prevention and treatment of venous thromboembolism in pregnancy in patients with hereditary antithrombin deficiency. Int J Womens Health. 2013;5:233–41.
48. ACOG Practice Bulletin No. 197: inherited thrombophilias in pregnancy. Obstet Gynecol. 2018;132(1):E18–E34.
49. Ginsberg JS, Brill-Edwards P, Burrows RF, Bona R, Prandoni P, Büller HR, et al. Venous thrombosis during pregnancy: leg and trimester of presentation. Thromb Haemost. 1992;67(5):519.
50. Polak JF, Wilkinson DL. Ultrasonographic diagnosis of symptomatic deep venous thrombosis in pregnancy. Am J Obstet Gynecol. 1991;165(3):625.
51. Torkzad MR, Bremme K, Hellgren M, Eriksson MJ, Hagman A, Jörgensen T, et al. Magnetic resonance imaging and ultrasonography in diagnosis of pelvic vein thrombosis during pregnancy. Thromb Res. 2010;126(2):107–12.

52. Chan WS, Lee A, Spencer FA, Chunilal S, Crowther M, Wu W, et al. D-dimer testing in pregnant patients: towards determining the next 'level' in the diagnosis of deep vein thrombosis. J Thromb Haemost. 2010;8(5):1004.
53. Huisman MV, Klok FA. Current challenges in diagnostic imaging of venous thromboembolism. Hematology Am Soc Hematol Educ Program. 2015;2015:202.
54. Cahill AG, Stout MJ, Macones GA, Bhalla S. Diagnosing pulmonary embolism in pregnancy using computed-tomographic angiography or ventilation-perfusion. Obstet Gynecol. 2009;114(1):124.
55. Revel MP, Cohen S, Sanchez O, Collignon MA, Thiam R, Redheuil A, et al. Pulmonary embolism during pregnancy: diagnosis with lung scintigraphy or CT angiography? Radiology. 2011;258(2):590.
56. Shahir K, Goodman LR, Tali A, Thorsen KM, Hellman RS. Pulmonary embolism in pregnancy: CT pulmonary angiography versus perfusion scanning. AJR Am J Roentgenol. 2010;195(3):W214.
57. Leung AN, Bull TM, Jaeschke R, Lockwood CJ, Boiselle PM, Hurwitz LM, et al. An official American Thoracic Society/Society of Thoracic Radiology clinical practice guideline: evaluation of suspected pulmonary embolism in pregnancy. Am J Respir Crit Care Med. 2011;184:1200. Official Journal of the American Thoracic Society.
58. Milford W, Chadha Y, Lust K. Use of a retrievable inferior vena cava filter in term pregnancy: case report and review of literature. Aust N Z J Obstet Gynaecol. 2009;49(3):331.
59. Turrentine MA, Braems G, Ramirez MM. Use of thrombolytics for the treatment of thromboembolic disease during pregnancy. Obstet Gynecol Surv. 1995;50(7):534.
60. Patterson DE, Raviola CA, D'Orazio EA, Buch C, Calligaro KD, Dougherty MJ, et al. Thrombolytic and endovascular treatment of peripartum iliac vein thrombosis: a case report. J Vasc Surg. 1996;24(6):1030.
61. Herrera S, Comerota AJ, Thakur S, Sunderji S, Disalle R, Kazanjian SN, et al. Managing iliofemoral deep venous thrombosis of pregnancy with a strategy of thrombus removal is safe and avoids post-thrombotic morbidity. J Vasc Surg. 2014;59(2):456–64.
62. Bates SM, Ginsberg JS. How we manage venous thromboembolism during pregnancy. Blood. 2002;100(10):3470.
63. Jacobsen AF, Skjeldestad FE, Sandset PM. Ante- and post- natal risk factors of venous thrombosis: a hospital-based case-control study. J Thromb Haemost. 2008;6(6):905–12.
64. Jacobsen AF, Drolsum A, Klow NE, Dahl GF, Qvigstad E, Sandset PM. Deep vein thrombosis after elective cesarean section. Thromb Res. 2004;113(5):283–8.
65. Lindqvist P, Dahlbäck B, Marŝál K. Thrombotic risk during pregnancy: a population study. Obstet Gynecol. 1999;94(4):595–9.
66. Simpson EL, Lawrenson RA, Nightingale AL, Farmer RD. Venous thromboembolism in pregnancy and the puerperium: incidence and additional risk factors from a London perinatal database. BJOG. 2001;108(1):56–60.
67. Knight M, UKOSS. Antenatal pulmonary embolism: risk factors, management and outcomes. BJOG. 2008;115(4):453–61.
68. Galambosi PJ, Ulander VM, Kaaja RJ. The incidence and risk factors of recurrent venous thromboembolism during pregnancy. Thromb Res. 2014;134(2):240–5.
69. Royal College of Obstetricians and Gynaecologists. Reducing the risk of venous thromboembolism during pregnancy and the puerperium – Green Top Guideline No 37a April 2015. https://www.rcog.org.uk/globalassets/documents/guidelines/gtg-37a.pdf. Accessed on 20 Jan 2020.
70. Bates SM, Middeldorp S, Rodger M, James AH, Greer I. Guidance for the treatment and prevention of obstetric-associated venous thromboembolism. J Thromb Thrombolysis. 2016;41(1):92–128.
71. Bain E, Wilson A, Tooher R, Gates S, Davis LJ, Middleton P. Prophylaxis for venous thromboembolic disease in pregnancy and the early postnatal period. Cochrane Database Syst Rev. 2014;(2):CD001689.

72. Norgren L, Austrell C, Nilsson L. The effect of graduated elastic compression stockings on femoral blood flow velocity during late pregnancy. Vasa. 1995;24(3):282.
73. Abdul Sultan A, West J, Tata LJ, Fleming KM, Nelson-Piercy C, Grainge MJ. Risk of first venous thromboembolism in pregnant women in hospital: population-based cohort study from England. BMJ. 2013;347:f6099.
74. Malhotra A, Weinberger SE. Deep vein thrombosis and pulmonary embolism in pregnancy: prevention. In: Leung LLK, Lockwood CJ, Mandel J, editors. UpToDate. Waltham: UpToDate Inc. https://www.uptodate.com. Accessed on 20 Jan 2020.
75. Rodie VA, Thomson AJ, Stewart FM, Quinn AJ, Walker ID, Greer IA. Low molecular weight heparin for the treatment of venous thromboembolism in pregnancy: a case series. BJOG. 2002;109(9):1020–4.
76. Overcash RT, Somers AT, LaCoursiere DY. Enoxaparin dosing after cesarean delivery in morbidly obese women. Obstet Gynecol. 2015;125(6):1371–6.
77. Basu S, Aggarwal P, Kakani N, Kumar A. Low-dose maternal warfarin intake resulting in fetal warfarin syndrome: in search for a safe anticoagulant regimen during pregnancy. Birth Defects Res A Clin Mol Teratol. 2016;106(2):142–7.
78. Cohen H, Arachchillage DR, Middeldorp S, Beyer-Westendorf J, Abdul-Kadir R. Management of direct oral anticoagulants in women of childbearing potential: guidance from the SSC of the ISTH. J Thromb Haemost. 2016;14(8):1673–6.
79. Lindhoff-Last E, Kreutzenbeck HJ, Magnani HN. Treatment of 51 pregnancies with danaparoid because of heparin intolerance. Thromb Haemost. 2005;93(1):63–9.
80. Magnani HN. An analysis of clinical outcomes of 91 pregnancies in 83 women treated with danaparoid(Orgaran). Thromb Res. 2010;125(4):297–302.
81. Pettilä V, Leinonen P, Markkola A, Hiilesmaa V, Kaaja R. Postpartum bone mineral density in women treated for thromboprophylaxis with unfractionated heparin or LMW heparin. Thromb Haemost. 2002;87(2):182.
82. Moen V, Dahlgren N, Irestedt L. Severe neurological complications after central neuraxial blockades in Sweden 1990–1999. Anesthesiology. 2004;101(4):950.
83. Horlocker TT, Vandermeuelen E, Kopp SL, Gogarten W, Leffert LR, Benzon HT. Regional anesthesia in the patient receiving antithrombotic or thrombolytic therapy: American Society of Regional Anesthesia and Pain Medicine Evidence-Based Guidelines (Fourth Edition). Reg Anesth Pain Med. 2018;43:263.

Chapter 30
Metabolomics Application in Fetal Medicine

G. Monni, F. Murgia, V. Corda, A. Iuculano, and L. Atzori

Introduction

In recent years, the holistic view has become the dominant perspective for the resolution of medical questions. High-throughput biologic technologies (−omics) such as metabolomics have begun to revolutionize many fields of biomedicine. The integrative analysis of an organism's response to a perturbation on the transcriptome, proteome, and metabolome levels will lead to a better understanding of the biochemical and biological mechanisms in complex systems. Metabolomics is a post-genomic research field based on methods of analysis for low molecular weight compounds in biological systems (the molecules include carbohydrates, amino acids, peptides, nucleic acids, organic acids, vitamins, lipids, and other biological species) [1] such as cells, organs, or organisms [2]. Metabolites are the by-product of biological processes that are influenced by external factors such as pathological status, therapies, life style, etc. Metabolomics is generally applied in the assessment of perturbations in biological systems, caused by diseases or treatments in comparison to unperturbed reference systems. The idea that various disease states can be reflected by changes in metabolite concentrations is in fact fundamental to metabolomics [3]. Although it is a relatively new field of research, the aims and expectations have been high from the beginning.

While several studies in the past have discussed the role of different metabolites in pregnancy, there has been limited use of metabolomics in obstetrics [4–6]. The

G. Monni (✉) · V. Corda · A. Iuculano
Department of Prenatal and Preimplantation Genetic Diagnosis and Fetal Therapy, Ospedale Pediatrico Microcitemico "A. Cao", Cagliari, Italy

F. Murgia · L. Atzori
Clinical Metabolomics Unit, Department of Biomedical Sciences, University of Cagliari, Cagliari, Italy
e-mail: federica.murgia@unica.it; latzori@unica.it

© Springer Nature Switzerland AG 2022

R. A. Moreira de Sá, E. B. d. Fonseca (eds.), *Perinatology*,
https://doi.org/10.1007/978-3-030-83434-0_30

aim of our review is to trace the application of metabolomics in several fields of prenatal medicine citing scientific articles which treated several pathological or physiological aspects of pregnancy.

Metabolomic Methods

The metabolome represents a wide variety of compound classes, including: amino acids, lipids, organic acids, nucleotides, etc. These compounds are extremely diverse in both their physical and chemical properties and occur in a wide concentration range. Their detection needs to be adequately addressed by a suitable analytic strategy. Metabolomics, the endpoint of the "omics cascade," is the closest to phenotype, and there is no single-instrument platform that currently can analyze all metabolites [7] in a single experiment. Moreover, two complementary approaches are used for metabolomic investigations: metabolic profiling and metabolic finger printing [8]. During the last 15 years, the development of robust, high-throughput analytical techniques, such as ^{1}H-nuclear magnetic resonance spectroscopy (^{1}H-NMR) and mass spectrometry (MS) has revolutionized the field. These modalities rapidly allow for the simultaneous measurement of large numbers of metabolites on a single biological sample [2]. NMR and MS are now the most commonly used techniques for measuring the metabolome. H-NMR is extremely valuable in detecting features of molecular structures, it has relatively limited sensitivity and measures only a small number of metabolites. Typically, only 100 or fewer high-abundance chemicals can be conveniently measured in biological samples using H-NMR. MS is usually combined with one of several separation techniques: liquid chromatography (LC), gas chromatography (GC), or capillary electrophoresis (CE) and allows for the measurement of hundreds to thousands of chemicals. MS has become a popular choice for performing metabolomics experiments [9].

A firm background in biostatistics and bioinformatics is necessary to interpret the biological data generated from the analytical platforms [10]. Metabolomics data are multivariate (many measurements per sample) and supervised learning multivariate analysis methods are needed [11]. In supervised learning, an algorithm is used to transform the multivariate data from metabolite profiles into something of biological interest (diseased vs. healthy or severity of disease). The goal of supervised learning is to find a "model" that will correctly associate the inputs with the targets. Partial least square discriminant analysis (PLS-DA) and projection to latent structures regression analysis (PLS) [12] are the most important approaches used with clinical data. Once key metabolite markers are identified, metabolic pathways (networks) analysis is performed. This will serve as a hypothesis starting point for a better understanding of the disease process [13].

Metabolomics in Fetal Medicine

Recently, omics sciences were introduced in obstetric clinical fields and in prenatal health. Metabolomic studies could improve the diagnostic power and clarify pathophysiological aspects in abnormal pregnancy. Pregnancy represents a complicated and insidious state, with various aspects to consider, including the well-being of the mother and child. During gestation, several types of biomaterials can be collected and investigated, including maternal blood (plasma or serum) [14], maternal urine, amniotic fluid (AF) [15, 16], cord blood [17], placenta [18], and cervicovaginal secretions. All of them enable the determination of the maternal and fetal state, but their biochemical interactions pose a number of challenges for the obstetric scientific world.

Based on literature, metabolomics has been employed for the study of physiological features occurring in normal pregnancy and pregnancy complications such as pre-eclampsia [19–21], chromosomal anomalies, preterm labor, stillbirth, etc. Metabolomics strategies have been increasingly exploited to understand the metabolic adaptations of the human organism to pregnancy and to characterize deviant behavior caused by prenatal complications. For these aims, the metabolomics studies in this field were focused on different trimesters of pregnancy.

Metabolomics and Normal Pregnancy

The human placenta differentiates in a physiologically low oxygen environment. Many changes in its development occur at the end of the first trimester when the maternal arterial circulation commences [22]. The oxygen tension within the intervillous space increases from 2.5% at 8 weeks to 8.5% at 12 weeks [23]. This rise is associated with a burst of oxidative stress in the placental tissues, along with a robust increase in antioxidant defences [24]. Moreover, the maternal metabolic profile changes from an anabolic to catabolic state to promote fetal growth, maturation, and development [25–27]. During this gestational period, metabolism seems to adapt itself to these conditions.

Jauniaux et al. [28] in line with our previously stated results [29], found an alteration related to the polyol pathways, which appears highly active in first trimester placental tissues. It has been hypothesized that polyols are the first source of carbohydrates for early life. This pathway could provide an important mechanism for the reoxidation of pyridine nucleotides under conditions of low oxygenation, enabling glycolysis to continue without an excessive rise in acidity.

Normal pregnancies are characterized also by changes in the levels of haematologically circulating free fatty acids, triglycerides, cholesterol and phospholipids and insulin resistance [30]. These adaptive metabolic changes are indispensable for the satisfying of the fetal energy demands necessary for rapid growth and to prepare the maternal body system for delivery and lactation [31]. Insulin resistance is a physiologic change during pregnancy that ensures an adequate fetal carbohydrate supply [32]. As pregnancy advances, insulin sensitivity gradually declines based on the effect of hormones [33] (estrogen and progesterone); however, intracellular mediators such as inositol and myo-inositol are also correlated with insulin sensitivity and could be implicated in glucose homeostasis [34–36].

Changes in maternal metabolic composition also reveal a linear positive correlation of myo-inositol and inositol levels with the Crown-Rump Lenght (CRL) [29], suggesting their biological role during pregnancy is closely linked to the glucose homeostasis as several studies have previously reported [30].

Metabolomics and Chromosomal Anomalies

Chromosomal defects, the most frequent fetal anomalies diagnosed in the first trimester of pregnancy, are characterized by a change in the number or structure of chromosomes. Routine screening for trisomies in pregnancy has been the standard of clinical care in developed countries [37]. The most common chromosomal aberration in newborns are certainly trisomies: 21 (T21, Down syndrome), 18 (T18, Edwards syndrome), and 13 (T13, Patau syndrome).

The identification of biomarkers that allow for the diagnosis and the clarification of the pathophysiologic features of these genetic disorders are a challenge in the metabolomics field [38]. Bahado-Singh et al. [39] planned a study with the purpose to determine whether metabolomic markers in maternal blood can distinguish T21 from normal pregnancies during the first trimester. After the analysis of 30 T21 serum samples and 60 controls serum samples with NMR technique, they found differences in 11 metabolites between the two classes. Among the potential biomarkers, the authors found two that were abnormal: 3-hydroxybutyrate (involved in brain growth and myelination) and 2-hydroxybutyrate (involved in the defence against oxidative stress).

The same group of Bahado-Singh studied chromosomal disorders in maternal serum with the following objectives: first to determine whether maternal first-trimester serum from T18 pregnancies had a qualitatively or quantitatively distinct metabolomic profile relative to normal pregnancies; second to evaluate the sensitivity and specificity of serum metabolite markers for the detection of T18; and finally to compare T18 with cases of Down syndrome to determine whether these two aneuploidies could be distinguished with the use of the first-trimester maternal serum metabolomic analysis [40]. In cases of T18, glycerol and 2-hydroxybutyrate were found as the most discriminating metabolites compared to euploid control specimens. In this study, the authors combined some discriminating metabolites with clinical and demographic parameters. When 2-hydroxybutrate was combined with Delta nuchal translucency (DNT), a sensitivity of 90.0% and a specificity of 100.0% were achieved.

Subsequently, threonine, trimethylamine, creatine, and methionine were found to be the most important molecules for distinguishing T18 from T21 cases. Similar metabolites were found significant when Troisi et al. [41] compared maternal serum samples of pregnancies complicated with different trisomies (treated as one group) with control pregnancies. Elaidic, stearic, linolenic, myristic, benzoic, citric and glyceric acid, mannose, 2-hydroxybutyrate, phenylalanine, proline, alanine, and 3-methylhistidine were selected as the most relevant metabolites in class separation suggesting a metabolic environment related to increased oxidative stress and a disturbance in the fetal central nervous system development [41]. Additionally, in the same study, the researchers investigated chromosomal disorders and specifically T21 with the focus on plasma lipid extracts. Chromosomal disorders cases were characterized by enhanced lipid β-oxidation (with increased ketone bodies) and underutilization of glucose, pyruvate and citrate. Moreover, lower circulating HDL levels were noted, together with changes in methanol and proline in the first trimester, and urea, creatinine, acetate and LDL + VLDL in the second trimester. T21 cases were indistinguishable from other chromosomal disorders in the first trimester, while in the second trimester increased methanol and albumin were found to be T21-specific.

Metabolomics and Preterm Delivery

Preterm delivery is an important and unexpected event in pregnancy. Every year approximately 10% of all neonates are born prematurely [42, 43] and this determines their exposure to a risk of short- and long-term pathological outcomes (including morbidity and mortality) [44]. The etiology of spontaneous preterm delivery (PTD) is still unknown. Only a few parameters which can individualize a risk group (e.g., uterine cervical length or comorbid diseases) are described [45].

Amniotic fluid (AF) represents a biomaterial which carries information about both the fetal and maternal state, and was the first choice for the study of preterm delivery metabolomics analyses [46–49].

Baraldi et al. [44] applied the metabolomics approach to define specific features in preterm delivery with and without bronchopulmonary dysplasia. While some signals were found to be significant, metabolites were only putatively identified. In another study, paired AF and maternal serum samples of preterm and no preterm delivery groups were compared. In AF, metabolites directly and indirectly involved in energy metabolism (pyruvic acid, glutamic acid, and glutamine) contributed to the classification of the two groups. In serum, increased levels of lipids and decreased levels of hypoxanthine, tryptophan, and pyroglutamic acid were observed in preterm delivery group [46]. The research group of Menon et al. evaluated differences in AF composition between early spontaneous preterm birth and term births in an African American population. They found metabolites significantly altered classified into steroids, bile acids, heme, xanthines, with the largest change (8-fold increase in preterm birth cases) observed for pantothenol [48].

Interestingly, metabolic profiling was performed to evaluate differences in AF composition between women with spontaneous preterm labor (PTL) at risk for preterm delivery, based on the presence or absence of intra-amniotic infection/inflammation (IAI). An increase in amino acids was a unique feature of PTL associated with IAI [47].

Graca et al. investigated specific metabolite characteristics in selected prenatal disorders, including preterm delivery. The authors found a decrease of citrate, myo-inositol, and amino acids and increase of allantoin and hexose that seems to be characteristic in the second trimester AF of PTD cases [50].

The metabolic analysis of blood samples obtained from pregnant women was used to identify metabolic changes in preterm delivery cases after spontaneous onset of labor. In the study by Lizewska et al. the increase of fatty acids in preterm birth cases seems to play a pivotal role in preterm delivery [51]. Tea et al. analyzed arterial and venous umbilical cord blood and maternal plasma obtained from full-term and preterm birth, focusing their attention on the very low birth weight (VLBW) cases. The metabolic signature of mothers delivering preterm reveals decreased levels of acetate and increased levels of lipids, glutamine, pyruvate, valine and threonine. On the other hand, decreased levels of lipoproteins, pyruvate, glucose, and increased levels of glutamine were observed in cord blood (both arterial and venous) of VLBW infants, together with decreased levels of several amino acids in arterial cord blood [52]. Small molecule biomarkers of preterm birth were also investigated in cervicovaginal secretions, but significant m/z–RT pairs were not even putatively identified [53].

Moreover, another study based on the NMR technique reveals high level of acetate in cervicovaginal fluids of women with symptoms of preterm labor. It appears predictive of preterm delivery, as well as delivery within 2 weeks of presentation [54].

Metabolomics and Preeclampsia

Preeclampsia (PE) according to the International Society for the Study of Hypertension in Pregnancy is defined as a multisystemic syndrome that develops during the second half of pregnancy. It is characterized by hypertension and proteinuria or in the absence of proteinuria, by hypertension associated with the finding of maternal organ dysfunction [55].

PE has a complex pathophysiology and is still not fully understood. PE develops in 2–5% of pregnancies and is a major cause of maternal and perinatal death throughout the world. The only treatment for PE is delivery [56, 57] and prevention before symptoms occur is critical.

More than 30 trials have investigated the benefit of low-dose aspirin for the prevention of preeclampsia. A meta-analysis of these studies showed that such therapy resulted in a 10% lower incidence of PE [58]. In recent years, the biggest prospective, randomized, placebo-controlled trial ever on the prophylactic use of aspirin in women at increased risk of preeclampsia (ASPRE STUDY) concludes that treatment with low-dose aspirin in women at high risk for preterm preeclampsia resulted in a lower incidence of this diagnosis than placebo [59].

Combined screening using maternal factors such as: mean arterial pressure (MAP), uterine Pulsatility Index (UTPI), and placental growth factor (PlGF) predicts about 90% of early PE (<34 weeks), 75% of preterm PE (<37 weeks) and 45% of term PE (≥37 weeks), at screen positive rate of 10%. Inclusion of PAPP-A and sFLT-1 does not improve the performance of screening.

Such detection rates are superior to the respective values of 49% (95% confidence interval, 43–55%) and 38% (34–41%) that were achieved by screening with maternal factors alone [60].

Further increase in this detection rate could be observed through the integration of new markers in this algorithm. While it is unlikely to find a single biomarker that could predict all cases of PE, metabolomics is increasingly being used to develop biomarkers for the detection, screening and monitoring of complex diseases.

Metabolomic analysis has the potential to allow for detailed phenotyping of the PE syndrome, however few metabolomics studies of women with active disease have thus far been undertaken.

Lipid metabolism and its related metabolites, inflammation and oxidative stress pathways, amino-acid metabolism, coagulation, and angiogenesis pathways were investigated and different samples, including plasma, serum, urine, placenta, and placental mitochondria have been used.

Metabolomic profiles from women with PE, normal pregnancies, and nonpregnant women were effectively discriminated by NMR metabolomics. Lipid metabolism results altered in PE patients in comparison with normal pregnancies: total, short and long-chain acylcarnitines, several polyunsaturated fatty acids, LDL and VLDL are increased in PE patients [19, 61–63].

The angiogenic imbalance characterized by increased maternal vascular inflammation and generalized endothelial dysfunction in PE patients results in increased levels of blood ketone bodies and decreased level of serum pyruvate, taurine and histidine-rich glycoprotein (HRG) [19, 64–67].

The levels of several amino acids such as arginine are reduced during PE, although further investigations are needed to understand if these alterations represent the cause or the effect of PE [68].

To date, comparison of the results from the different investigations present in literature is difficult because of the presence of technical and biological bias. In particular emerges the tendency in reporting and publishing only positive findings, as well as the lack of validation analysis for the identified metabolic biomarkers. This tendencies may cause misunderstanding in the biological interpretation of the results [69]. Therefore, further studies are necessary to recognize a combination of predictive and diagnostic biomarkers using "omic" technologies such as metabolomics and proteomics that can identify multiple markers simultaneously.

Metabolomics and Congenital Heart Disease

Congenital heart disease (CHD) has been defined as "a gross structural abnormality of the heart or intrathoracic great vessels that is actually or potentially of functional significance" by Mitchell et al. [70]. Normally, lesions such as hypertrophic or dilated cardiomyopathy are rarely detected during the foetal life but usually appear in childhood or adolescence.

The incidence of severe CHD is about 2.5 to 3/1000 live births while the moderately severe forms of CHD account for another 3 per 1000 live births [71]. Obviously, abortions after early diagnosis, misdiagnosis due to the intrinsic difficulties of the ultrasound analysis, developmental pathologies, are all factors that could influence epidemiological data.

Despite CHD being the most frequent and compromising fetal anomaly, evidence about maternal metabolomic profile in pregnancies carrying affected foetuses is very limited.

Differences in serum metabolomic profile of pregnancies with a chromosomally normal foetus compared with those affected with CHD have been determined. In particular, a significant disturbance in lipids homeostasis including phosphatidylcholine and various sphingolipids and choline metabolism were found in the pathological samples. These changes inevitably lead to an altered energetic process in both skeletal and myocardial muscles [72].

This study, despite its limitations, underlines the fact that metabolomics could play a pivotal role in developing biomarkers for the prediction of CHD.

Metabolomics and Mendelian Diseases

Another recent study proposed by Monni et al. exploited the metabolomics approach as a tool to investigate common and disabling genetic conditions such as thalassemia. In this study, the metabolome of chorionic villi was investigated to better understand the still unclear pathophysiological mechanisms of thalassemia. GC–MS analysis and multivariate statistics identified distinct metabolic profiles in the chorionic villi of foetuses affected by homozygous compared to heterozygous thalassemia and control fetuses. Glutamic acid, glycerol-1-phosphate, malic acid, arachidonic acid (ARA), glucose, and ribose were found to significantly increase in homozygous patients, while docosatetranoic acid and palmitoleic acid were found decreased. Penthose phosphate pathway, ARA metabolism, glutamine and glutamate metabolism, alanine, aspartate and glutamate metabolism, glycolysis, and gluconeogenesis were potentially altered in both the homozygous and heterozygous groups [73].

Conclusion

Based on recently published research it is clear that the field of prenatal metabolomics is moving in an exciting direction. We attempted to summarize the most important findings in this area hoping to create the contest to discuss the potential role of this emergent technique. The development of new approaches to find reliable biomarkers is crucial, not only to produce new knowledge, but also as a step to introduce new panels for the diagnosis and classification of different diseases.

References

1. Zhang A, Sun H, Wang P, et al. Modern analytic techniques in metabolomics analysis. Analyst. 2012;137:293–300.
2. Madsen R, Lundstedt T, Trygg J. Chemometrics in metabolomics—a review in human disease diagnosis. Anal Chim Acta. 2010;659:23–33.
3. Nicholson JK, Lindon JC. Nature. 2008;455:1054.
4. Haney RP, Skillman TG. Calcium metabolism in normal human pregnancy. J Clin Endocrinol Metabol. 1971;33:661–70.
5. Sheldon J, Bleicher MD, John B, et al. Carbohydrate metabolism in pregnancy — the interrelations of glucose, insulin and free fatty acids in late pregnancy and post partum. N Engl J Med. 1964;271:866–72.
6. Knopp RH, Warth MR, Charles D, et al. Lipoprotein metabolism in pregnancy, fat transport to the fetus, and the effects of diabetes. Biol Neonate. 1986;50:297–317.
7. Dettmer K, Aronov PA, Hammock BD. Mass spectrometry-based metabolomics. Mass Spectrom Rev. 2007;26:51–78.
8. Dettmer K, Hammock BD. Metabolomics—a new exciting field within the "omics" sciences. Environ Health Perspect. 2004;112:A396–7.
9. Moco S, Bino RJ, De Vos RCH, et al. Metabolomics technologies and metabolite identification. Trends Anal Chem. 2007;26(9):855–66.
10. Oresic M, Clish CB, Davidov EJ, et al. Phenotype characterisa-tion using integrated gene transcript, protein and meta-bolite profiling. Appl Bioinformatics. 2004;3:205–17.
11. Hastie T, Tibshirani R, Friedman J. The elements of statistical learning: data mining, inference and prediction. Berlin: Springer-Verlag; 2001. p. 50.
12. Manly BFJ. Multivariate statistical methods: a primer. London: Chapman & Hall; 1994. p. 215.
13. Hollywood K, Brison DR, Goodacre R. Metabolomics: current technologies and future trends. Proteomics. 2006;6:4716–23.
14. Luan H, Meng N, Liu P, et al. Pregnancyinduced metabolic phenotype variations in maternal plasma. J Proteome Res. 2014;13:1527–36.
15. Iuculano A, Murgia F, Peddes C, et al. Metabolic characterization of amniotic fluids of fetuses with enlarged nuchal translucency. J Perinat Med. 2019;47:311–8.
16. Diaz SO, Pinto J, Graça G, et al. Metabolic biomarkers of prenatal disorders: an exploratory NMR metabonomics study of second trimester maternal urine and blood plasma. J Proteome Res. 2011;10:3732–42.
17. Tea I, Le Gall G, Küster A, et al. ^{1}H-NMRbased metabolic profiling of maternal and umbilical cord blood indicates altered materno foetal nutrient exchange in preterm infants. PLoS One. 2012;7:e29947.
18. Horgan RP, Broadhurst DI, Dunn WB, et al. Changes in the metabolic footprint of placental explant-conditioned medium cultured in different oxygen tensions from placentas of small for gestational age and normal pregnancies. Placenta. 2010;31:893–901.
19. Kenny LC, Broadhurst DI, Dunn W, et al. Robust early pregnancy prediction of later preeclampsia using metabolomic biomarkers. Hypertension. 2010;56:741–9.
20. Dunn WB, Brown M, Worton SA, et al. The metabolome of human placental tissue: investigation of first trimester tissue and changes related to preeclampsia in late pregnancy. Metabolomics. 2011;8:579–97.
21. Bahado-Singh RO, Akolekar R, Mandal R, et al. First-trimester metabolomic detection of late-onset preeclampsia. Am J Obstet Gynecol. 2013;208:58.e1–7.

22. Burton GJ, Watson AL, Hempstock J, et al. Uterine glands provide histiotrophic nutrition for the human fetus during the first trimester of pregnancy. J Clin Endocrinol Metab. 2002;87:2954–9.
23. Jauniaux E, Watson AL, Hempstock J, et al. Onset of maternal arterial blood flow and placental oxidative stress; a possible factor in human early pregnancy failure. Am J Pathol. 2000;157:2111–22.
24. Burton GJ, Jauniaux E. Placental oxidative stress: from miscarriage to preeclampsia. J Soc Gynecol Investig. 2004;11:342–52.
25. Lain KY, et al. Metabolic changes in pregnancy. Clin Obstet Gynecol. 2007;50:938–48.
26. Herrera E, Ortega-Senovilla H. Lipid metabolism during pregnancy and its implications for fetal growth. Curr Pharm Biotechnol. 2014;15(1):24–31.
27. Zeng Z, Liu F, Li S. Metabolic adaptations in pregnancy: a review. Ann Nutr Metab. 2017;70:59–65.
28. Jauniaux E, Hempstock J, Teng C, et al. Polyol concentrations in the fluid compartments of the human conceptus during the first trimester of pregnancy: maintenance of redox potential in a low oxygen environment. J Clin Endocrinol Metab. 2005;90:1171–5.
29. Murgia F, Iuculano A, Peddes C, et al. Metabolic fingerprinting of chorionic villous samples in normal pregnancy and chromosomal disorders. Prenat Diagn. 2019;39:848–58.
30. Catalano P, Roman-Drago N, Amini S, et al. Longitudinal changes in body composition and energy balance in lean women with normal and abnormal glucose tolerance during pregnancy. Am J Obstet Gynecol. 1998;179:156–65.
31. Di Cianni G, Ghio A, Resi V, et al. Gestational diabetes mellitus: an opportunity to prevent type 2 diabetes and cardiovascular disease in young women. Womens Health. 2010;6:97–105.
32. McLachlan K, O'Neal D, Jenkins A, Alford F. Do adiponectin, TNFα, leptin and CRP relate to IR in pregnancy? Studies in women with and without gestational diabetes, during and after pregnancy. Diabetes Metab Res Rev. 2006;22:131–8.
33. Ryan EA, Enns L. Role of gestational hormones in the induction of IR. J Clin Endocrinol Metab. 1988;67:341–7.
34. Suzuki S, Kawasaki H, Satoh Y. Urinary chiro-inositol excretion is an index marker of insulin sensitivity in Japanese type II diabetes. Diabetes Care. 1994;17:1465–8.
35. Larner J, Brautigan DL, Thorner MO. d-Chiro-inositol glycans in insulin signaling and insulin resistance. Mol Med. 2010;16:543–51.
36. Corrado F, D'Anna R, Di Vieste G, et al. The effect of myoinositol supplementation on insulin resistance in patients with gestational diabetes. Diabet Med. 2011;28(8):972–5.
37. National Collaborating Centre for Women's and Children's Health. Antenatal care: routine care for the healthy pregnant woman. Clinical guideline. Commissioned by the National Institute for Clinical Excellence. London: Royal College of Obstetrics and Gynaecology Press; 2008. p. 218–27.
38. Troisi J, Sarno L, Martinelli P, et al. A metabolomics-based approach for non-invasive diagnosis of chromosomal anomalies; 2017.
39. Bahado-Singh O, Akolekar R, Mandal R, et al. Metabolomic analysis for first-trimester Down syndrome prediction. Am J Obstet Gynecol study with the cology. 2013;208:371.e1–371.e8.
40. Bahado-Singh RO, Akolekar R, Chelliah A, et al. Metabolomic analysis for first-trimester trisomy 18 detection. Am J Obstet Gynecol. 2013;209:65.e1–9.
41. Troisi J, Sarno L, Martinelli P, Di Carlo C, Landolfi A, Scala G, Rinaldi M, D'Alessandro P, Ciccone C, Guida M. A metabolomics-based approach for non-invasive diagnosis of chromosomal anomalies. Metabolomics. 2017;13:140.
42. Conde-Agudelo A, Romero R, Da Fonseca E, et al. Vaginal progesterone is as effective as cervical cerclage to prevent preterm birth in women with a singleton gestation, previous spontaneous preterm birth, and a short cervix: updated indirect comparison meta-analysis. Am J Obstet Gynecol. 2018;219:10–25.
43. Auray-Blais C, Raiche E, Gagnon R, et al. Metabolomics and preterm birth: what biomarkers in cervicovaginal secretions are predictive of high-risk pregnant women? Int J Mass Spectrom. 2011;307:33–8.

44. Baraldi E, Giordano G, Stocchero M, et al. Untargeted metabolomic analysis of amniotic fluid in the prediction of preterm delivery and bronchopulmonary dysplasia. PLoS One. 2016;11(10):e0164211.
45. Gervasi MT, Romero R, Bracalente G, et al. Midtrimester amniotic fluid concentrations of interleukin-6 and interferon-gamma-inducible protein-10: evidence for heterogeneity of intra-amniotic inflammation and associations with spontaneous early (<32 weeks) and late (>32 weeks) preterm delivery. J Perinat Med. 2012;40(4):329–43.
46. Virgiliou C, Gika HG, Witting M, et al. Amniotic fluid and maternal serum metabolic signatures in the second trimester associated with preterm delivery. J Proteome Res. 2017;16(2):898–910.
47. Romero R, Mazaki-Tovi S, Vaisbuch E, et al. Metabolomics in premature labor: a novel approach to identify patients at risk for preterm delivery. J Matern Fetal Neonatal Med. 2010;23(12):1344–59.
48. Menon R, Jones J, Gunst PR, et al. Amniotic fluid metabolomic analysis in spontaneous preterm birth. Reprod Sci. 2014;21(6):791–803.
49. Graca G, Duarte IF, Barros AS, et al. Impact of prenatal disorders on the metabolic profile of second trimester amniotic fluid: a nuclear magnetic resonance metabonomic study. J Proteome Res. 2010;9(11):6016–24.
50. Graca G, Goodfellow BJ, Barros AS, et al. UPLC-MS metabolic profiling of second trimester amniotic fluid and maternal urine and comparison with NMR spectral profiling for the identification of pregnancy disorder biomarkers. Mol Biosyst. 2012;8(4):1243–54.
51. Lizewska B, Teul J, Kuc P, et al. Maternal plasma metabolomic profiles in spontaneous preterm birth: preliminary results. Mediators Inflamm. 2018;2018:9362820.
52. Tea I, Le Gall G, Küster A, et al. 1H-NMR-based metabolic profiling of maternal and umbilical cord blood indicates altered materno-foetal nutrient exchange in preterm infants. PLoS One. 2012;7(1):e29947.
53. Auray-Blais C, Raiche E, Gagnon R, et al. Metabolomics and preterm birth: what biomarkers in cervicovaginal secretions are predictive of high-risk accepted manuscript pregnant women? Int J Mass Spectrom. 2011;307(1–3):33–8.
54. Amabebe E, Reynolds S, Stern VL, et al. Identifying metabolite markers for preterm birth in cervicovaginal fluid by magnetic resonance spectroscopy. Metabolomics. 2016;12:67.
55. Brown MA, Lindheimer MD, de Swiet M, et al. The classification and diagnosis of the hypertensive disorders of pregnancy: statement from the International Society for the Study of Hypertension in Pregnancy (ISSHP). Hypertens Pregnancy. 2001;20(1):IX–XIV.
56. Knight M, Kenyon S, Brocklehurst P, Neilson J, Shakespeare J, Kurinczuk JJ, editors. on behalf of MBRRACEUK. Saving lives, improving mothers' care - lessons learned to inform future maternity care from the UK and Ireland confidential enquiries into maternal deaths and morbidity 2009–12. Oxford: National Perinatal Epidemiology Unit, University of Oxford; 2014.
57. Donati S, Senatore S, Ronaconi A, the Regional Maternal Mortality Working Group. Maternal mortality in Italy: a record linkage study. BJOG. 2011;118:872–9.
58. Duley L, Henderson-Smart D, et al. Antiplatelet agents for preventing pre-eclampsia and its complications. Cochrane Database Syst Rev. 2007:CD004659.
59. Rolnik DL, Wright D, et al. Aspirin versus placebo in pregnancies at high risk for preterm preeclampsia. N Engl J Med. 2017;377:613–22.
60. O'Gorman N, Wright D, Syngelaki A, et al. Competing risks model in screening for preeclampsia by maternal factors and biomarkers at 11–13 weeks gestation. Am J Obstet Gynecol. 2016;214:103.e1–12.
61. Austdal M, Skråstad RB, Gundersen AS, et al. Metabolomic biomarkers in serum and urine in women with preeclampsia. PLoS One. 2014;9:e91923.
62. Thiele IG, Niezen-Koning KE, van Gennip AH, et al. Increased plasma carnitine concentrations in preeclampsia. Obstet Gynecol. 2004;103:876–80.
63. Zhou X, Han TL, Chen H, et al. Impaired mitochondrial fusion, autophagy, biogenesis and dysregulated lipid metabolism is associated with preeclampsia. Exp Cell Res. 2017;359:195–204.

64. Desforges M, Ditchfield A, Hirst CR, et al. Reduced placental taurine transporter (TauT) activity in pregnancies complicated by pre-eclampsia and maternal obesity. Taurine. 2013;8:81–91.
65. Bahado-Singh RO, Syngelaki A, Akolekar R, et al. Validation of metabolomic models for prediction of early-onset preeclampsia. Am J Obstet Gynecol. 2015;213:530.e531–530. E510.
66. Austdal M, Tangerås LH, Skråstad RB, et al. First trimester urine and serum metabolomics for prediction of preeclampsia and gestational hypertension: a prospective screening study. Int J Mol Sci. 2015;16:21520–38.
67. Bolin M, Åkerud P, Hansson A, et al. Histidinerich glycoprotein as an early biomarker of preeclampsia. Am J Hypertens. 2011;24:496–501.
68. Mukherjee R, Ray CD, Ray S, et al. Altered metabolic profile in early and late onset preeclampsia: an FTIR spectroscopic study. Pregnancy Hypertens. 2014;4:70–80.
69. Fatemeh B, Nobakht M. Gh application of metabolomics to preeclampsia diagnosis. Syst Biol Reprod Med. 2018;64:324–39.
70. Mitchell SC, Korones SB, Berendes HW. Congenital heart disease in 56,109 births. Incidence and natural history. Circulation. 1971;43:323–32.
71. Hoffman JJ, Kaplan S. The incidence of congenital heart disease. J Am Coll Cardiol. 2002;39:1890–900.
72. Bahado-Singh RO, Ertl R, Mandal R, et al. Metabolomic prediction of fetal congenital heart defect in the first trimester. Am J Obstet Gynecol. 2014;211:240.e1–14.
73. Monni G, Murgia F, Corda V, et al. Metabolomic investigation of β-thalassemia in chorionic villi samples. J Clin Med. 2019;8:798.

Part V
Pregnancy Complications: Prevention, Diagnosis and Management

Chapter 31
Prematurity: Relevant Aspects in Asymptomatic Patients

Rone Peterson Cerqueira Oliveira

Abbreviations

ACOG	American College of Obstetricians and Gynecologists
CI	Confidence interval
ENCIRCLE	Emergency Cerclage in Twin Pregnancies at Imminent Risk of Preterm Birth: an Open-Label Randomized Controlled Trial
EQUIPP	Evaluation of a Quantitative Instrument for the Prediction of Preterm Birth
fFN	Fetal fibronectin
LEEP	Loop electrosurgical excision procedure
NCIU	Neonatal intensive care unit
NNT	Numbers needed to treat
PECEP	The Pesario Cervical para Evitar Prematuridad
PD	Premature delivery
PROM	Premature rupture of membranes
QUIPP	Quantitative Instrument for the Prediction of Preterm Birth
RDS	Respiratory distress syndrome
RR	Relative risk

R. P. C. Oliveira (✉)
Department of Gynecology, Obstetrics and Human Reproduction, Federal University of Bahia, Salvador, Bahia, Brazil
e-mail: ronepeterson@bahiana.edu.br

© Springer Nature Switzerland AG 2022

R. A. Moreira de Sá, E. B. d. Fonseca (eds.), *Perinatology*,
https://doi.org/10.1007/978-3-030-83434-0_31

Introduction

There are roughly 15 million premature births (<37 weeks) every year [1]. Prematurity is the main cause of neonatal mortality and the second cause of mortality in children aged up to 5 years, decreasing the survivors' quality of life as a result of short- and long-term morbidities [2]. Premature births increase costs not only for the healthcare system but also for the families who also undergo considerable psychological difficulties [1]. Spontaneous premature births represent two-thirds of premature births and are often multifactorial in origin [3], making the use of prediction tools and prevention strategies difficult. Additionally, most women who undergo premature delivery are considered to be low risk [4], decreasing the effectiveness of strategies based on risk factors alone. As a consequence, prematurity predictors and preventive strategies evaluated in recent years have not reduced overall prematurity.

Being multifactorial, the prevalence of prematurity is affected by several characteristics in the studied population (e.g., single or multiple pregnancies), influencing the results of diagnostic tests and preventive measures. Thus, every prediction and prevention measure must be analyzed across several scenarios to effectively obtain external result validation.

The most commonly used prediction strategies involve recognizing risk factors for prematurity; biophysical measurements, such as ultrasound cervical length measurement; and biochemical methods, such as fetal fibronectin. The use of progesterone, cerclage, and pessary as preventive strategies has shown promising results, however, only in certain groups of patients.

This chapter reviews prediction and prevention strategy advances for a group of asymptomatic women, divided into single or multiple pregnancies to understand the progress of research and interpret research findings.

Prematurity Prediction in Asymptomatic Women

The multifactorial origin of prematurity allows for the influence of several risk factors in an isolated or associated manner. However, as most patients who suffer from prematurity show no identifiable risk factors, the presence of these factors does not increase the predictive value.

Some of the risk factors for prematurity are history of prematurity (which increases the risk two- to fivefold), multiple pregnancies (representing 15–20% of all premature births, 40–50% which occur spontaneously), short cervix, an interval between deliveries of <6 months, socioeconomic difficulties and low educational levels, lack of prenatal care, low body mass index, maternal infections, uterine malformations, cervical excisional procedures, second trimester maternal surgery, depression, smoking, drug use, black women, periodontal disease, and advanced age [3, 5].

The first models to combine clinical risk factors to create risk scores date from the early 1970s and were found to have low positive predictive values (38%) with high false-positive rates (17%) [6]. Also, a systematic review involving 67,390 women and 12 prediction systems concluded that the models were of low quality [7].

Despite these limitations, the recognition of risk factors during the care of asymptomatic women should be encouraged as it is easy and free of charge and gives rise to the possibility of using corrective measures directed to certain groups, leading to a possible reduction of the individual influence of each factor on the risk of prematurity. The various combinations of clinical characteristics allow for the stratification from population groups in which the validation of more advanced prediction and prevention strategies has been tested, such as prematurity history, twin pregnancies, and a short cervix.

Single Pregnancy Prediction

Biochemical Methods

Fetal fibronectin (fFN) is a glycoprotein produced in the extracellular matrix by cells located between the chorion and decidua. fFN is commonly present in the vaginal canal until 18 weeks of pregnancy; thereafter, levels begin to decrease before increasing again closer to delivery. However, in case of mechanical or inflammatory damage in this matrix, fFN levels rise and subsequently increase the risk of premature birth [8]. The main characteristic of the fFN level method is a high negative predictive value, while the positive predictive value is moderate [8]. A meta-analysis of 9 studies (1236 women) on fFN accuracy reported that in asymptomatic women without risk factors, this method presents with a sensitivity, specificity, positive, and negative probability ratio of 0.48 (95% CI 0.20–0.77), 0.96 (95% CI 0.86–0.99), 12.01 (95% CI 4.70–30.68), and 0.54 (95% CI 0.30–0.97), respectively [9]. The values in asymptomatic women with risk factors are conceptualized heterogeneously between the studies, with sensitivity, specificity, positive, and negative probability ratios of 0.34 (95% CI 0.24–0.43), 0.91 (95% CI 0.88–0.93), 3.47 (95% CI 2.84–4.24), and 0.75 (95% CI 0.68–0.82), respectively [9]. Despite the high capacity to predict outcomes in women without risk factors, it seems unlikely that the use of fFN alone as a screening tool is acceptable or feasible in this population. Furthermore, its use in asymptomatic women with risk factors has not altered clinical management thus far [9].

A more recent prospective study, the Evaluation of a Quantitative Instrument for the Prediction of Preterm Birth (EQUIPP), reported that fibronectin concentration in the vaginal canal is directly proportional to the risk of prematurity, offering a better prediction value than the qualitative test alone [8, 10]. This study demonstrated that values <10 ng/mL (present in 70% of asymptomatic women) represent a similar risk of premature birth to the general population of about 3.0%, with high sensitivity and negative predictive value. Values above 200 ng/mL represent a positive predictive value of only 38%, but higher than the value obtained with qualitative analysis [10]. Because of these characteristics, fFN can be associated with cervical length measurements to assist in the clinical management of women with short cervix [10].

Owing to the likely inflammatory origin of premature labor, several markers of inflammatory response, such as IL-6, IL-1α, IL-8, tumor necrosis factor alpha, and C-reactive protein, are collected from the blood, cervicovaginal fluids, or amniotic fluid [11]. However, these markers still need to be validated and better understood to determine their clinical usefulness [12].

A new line of research for the prediction premature births is that of genomic, transcriptomic, proteomic, and metabolomic technologies based on the study of genes and particles that are substrates of chemical reactions that may be associated with the onset of premature delivery [13]. Although promising, the results of their use, both isolated and associated with other prediction methods, are still conflicting, and there are no prevention measures related to these findings, limiting their use in clinical practice [11].

Biophysical Methods

Cervical length physiologically shortens with pregnancy; hence, the identification of a prematurely shortened cervix increases the chance of premature birth. Cervical length measurement is an operator-dependent examination that includes a series of criteria usually established by the Fetal Medicine Foundation. There is still discussion regarding the prediction capacity of this method, mainly due to its use in different populations and studies that use different cutoff points, preventing a broader meta-analysis and definitive conclusions.

The presence of a short cervix in low-risk women in the second trimester has been consistently associated with prematurity, resulting in a relative risk of 4 if <30 mm (P_{25}), 6 if <26 mm (P_{10}), 9 if <22 mm (P_5), and 14 if <13 mm ($P1_1$), with a positive predictive value of 6%–44% and a sensitivity of only 47% [14]. Thus, the identification of a short cervix, especially in advanced stages of pregnancy, is not related to premature birth. Additionally, cervical lengths <15 mm in low-risk populations are rare, present in only approximately 2% of the population [15, 16], making the use of cervical length measurements in these low-risk women questionable with regard to its cost-effectiveness. The clinical use of the examination in this group of women, however, seems to exist due to the use of progesterone, which can reduce prematurity by about 40% in low-risk women with short cervix [15, 17]. Considering these results, several studies have demonstrated that the use of cervical length measurement importantly reduces the costs related to prematurity through prevention measures, thus being cost-effective [17–20]. However, this is still not a formal recommendation in most guidelines [21].

There is a consensus on the use of transvaginal ultrasound for cervical length measurement in women at high risk for prematurity [21], which includes women with a history of prematurity, uterine anomalies, and cervical excisional treatments (loop electrosurgical excision procedure or cone biopsy) [14]. Serial cervical length measurements from 16 to 24 weeks of pregnancy seem to offer advantages over its isolated use in women with a history of prematurity <34 weeks [22]. The examination should be repeated every 2 weeks if cervical length remains >30 mm or weekly if it is between 25 and 29 mm [23]. This screening, associated with cerclage in cases with a cervix <25 mm, reduces births <24 weeks (RR 0.44, 95% CI 0.21–0.92), which in turn reduces perinatal death (RR 0.54, 95% CI 0.29–0.99), and when cervical length is <15 mm, the realization of cerclage to reduce birth <35 weeks (RR 0.23, 95% CI 0.08–0.66) [23–25].

Association of Methods: Prediction Models

The proposal of associating cervical length measurements and fibronectin dosage to improve the accuracy of these methods used individually in asymptomatic high-risk women was validated in 2016. This resulted in a prediction model that includes history of prematurity or premature rupture of membranes (PROM), cervical length measurement, and fibronectin dosage with an accuracy ranging from 77% to 99%. The model also has the ability to predict birth within 2–4 weeks, with a sensitivity of 75.0% (19.4–99.4%) and 63.6% (30.8–89.1%), specificity of 97.7% (96.2–98.8%) and 95.8% (93.9–97.2%), positive predictive value of 17.6% (3.8–43.4%) and 21.2% (9.0–38.9%), negative predictive value of 99.8% (99.1–100%) and 99.3% (98.3–99.8%), positive probability ratio of 33.3 (15.5–71.6) and 15.0 (8.4–27.0), and negative probability ratio of 0.3 (0.1–1.4) and 0.4 (0.2–0.8) for 2- and 4-week predictions, respectively [26]. The authors have also created an application called QUIPP to facilitate its use by physicians from all over the world [26]. However, initial research suggests that although the use of this application would double the use of preventive measures in the studied population, benefiting women who would progress to a premature delivery, it would also increase the inappropriate use of preventive measures in other subpopulations. Therefore, further research is necessary before its use in clinical practice [27].

Multiple Pregnancy Prediction

Biochemical Methods

The use of fFN in multiple pregnancies was evaluated in a meta-analysis of 15 studies including 1211 asymptomatic twin pregnancies, most of which (82%) underwent serial dosages between 22 and 34 weeks [28]. Most studies analyzed birth prediction before 34 weeks with a sensitivity of 35–45%, specificity of 81–94%, and positive and negative probability ratios of approximately 2.5 and 0.7, respectively, concluding that the accuracy of this test in this population is limited [28]. A more recent meta-analysis also stated that the accuracy of fFN in asymptomatic twin pregnancies is inconclusive [9].

Biophysical Methods

A short cervix (<25 m) at 22–24 weeks is more prevalent in women with twin pregnancies (18%) than in women with single pregnancies (9%), and the same cervical measurement seems to offer more risk of prematurity in twin than in single pregnancies [4]. The strong association between short cervix in asymptomatic women with twin pregnancies and the risk of prematurity was reported in a meta-analysis of 16 studies [29]. Findings indicated that cervical length measurement is a good predictor for prematurity, and the most accurate cutoff point for births <32 and <34 weeks is <20 mm between 20 and 24 weeks. The sensitivity, specificity, and positive and negative probability ratios for births <34 weeks were 39%, 96%, 10.1, and 0.64, respectively [29].

The use of cervical length measurements in asymptomatic women with twin pregnancies has helped to identify women at higher risk of prematurity and inspired studies to analyze the best prevention strategy. More recent publications have shown the possible benefits of prevention strategies in the subgroup of asymptomatic women with twin pregnancies and short cervix [30–32], encouraging the use of cervical length measurement in women with twin pregnancies between 19 and 24 weeks [21, 33]. However, further studies are still needed to conclusively prove the real benefits of prevention strategies and to show the cost-effectiveness of universal cervical screening to modify the current recommendations [4, 34]. Figure 31.1 summarizes the application of prediction methods in asymptomatic pregnant women according to the risk group.

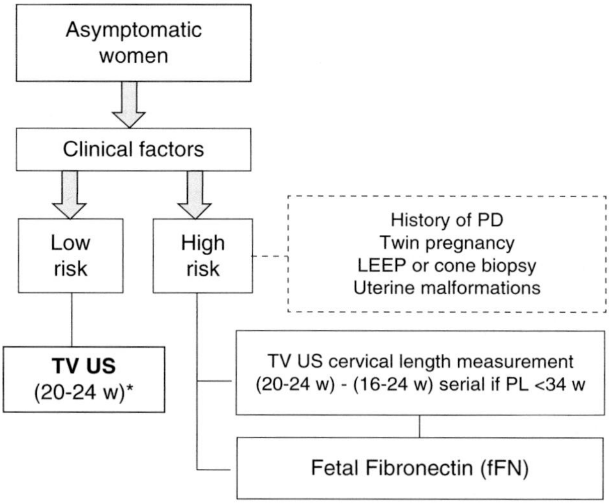

Fig. 31.1 Use of prematurity prediction methods in asymptomatic women. PD premature delivery, LEEP loop electrosurgical excision procedure, TV US transvaginal ultrasound, PL premature labor, * no consensus

Prevention Measures

Primary prevention measures are directed to all women [2], including recommendations to stop smoking, implantation of few embryos in in vitro fertilization, correction of maternal pathologies, treatment of infectious diseases, reduction of stress, and better socioeconomic conditions with access to health services.

Secondary prevention measures are directed to certain groups of women exposed to certain risk factors, including the use of cerclage, pessary, and progesterone, with different interpretations and outcomes in populations of asymptomatic women with single or twin pregnancies.

Prevention of Prematurity in Asymptomatic Single-Pregnancy Women

Cerclage

Cerclage consists of applying suture in the cervical region of the uterus to reinforce the structure of the cervix in women with cervical isthmus insufficiency. The suture is normally removed at 37 weeks of pregnancy. Cerclage can be performed transvaginally using the McDonald or Shirodkar's technique or abdominally by laparotomy or laparoscopy [35, 36]. Cerclage is generally indicated in the following three situations: based on history, ultrasound findings, or physical examination finding [35, 36].

Cerclage Indicated Due to History

History indication is based on reports of late second trimester losses or extreme premature deliveries and is considered a classic indication for cerclage. However, controversy exists as to the number of losses required as well as the effectiveness of this indication [37]. The Royal College of Obstetricians and Gynecologists recommends cerclage after 3 gestational losses [36], while the American College of Obstetricians and Gynecologists (ACOG) recommends prophylactic cerclage between 13 and 14 weeks for all women with a history of ≥1 second trimester losses, typically <24 weeks and without labor or placental detachment, or if there is a history of painless cervical dilatation cerclage in a previous pregnancy [35]. Neither of the guidelines recommend the use of resistance tests or radiographic examinations to diagnose cervical isthmus insufficiency [35, 36]. The Cochrane systematic review (2017) failed to demonstrate the effectiveness of cerclage indicated only due to history [38]. Approximately 40–70% of women with a history of second trimester loss or extreme premature births have a normal cervix up to 24 weeks of pregnancy, and of these, about 90% will have their deliveries after

34 weeks [36]. These data have supported the use of cerclage based on ultrasound findings, avoiding unnecessary procedures. Nevertheless, most pregnant women with a history of loss between 18 and 24 weeks usually undergo cerclage. Ultrasound screening for indication of cerclage is generally used on a more restricted group of women, in particular women with a history of prematurity between 24 and 34 weeks [35].

Cerclage Indicated Due to Ultrasound Findings

Cerclage indicated by ultrasonography is based on serial screening between 16 and 24 weeks to diagnose cervical shortening in women with a history of prematurity under 34 weeks [25, 37, 39]. If the cervix is shortened (<25 mm), cerclage should be performed to significantly reduce the risk of prematurity (RR 0.70, 95% CI 0.55–0.89) and perinatal morbidity and mortality (RR 0.64, 95% CI 0.45–0.91) [25]. However, cerclage should not be indicated if the cervix remains >25 mm or there is isolated presence of cervical funneling [36].

On the other hand, cerclage should not be indicated in the presence of a cervix <25 mm without a history of prematurity [35, 36, 40]. This recommendation was confirmed by a recent systematic review and meta-analysis published by Berghella et al. in 2017. The study included 419 women with single pregnancies and no history of prematurity and found no benefits for the use of cerclage [41]. However, these authors reported a reduction of births <35 weeks in women with a cervical length <10 mm (39.5% vs. 58.0%, RR 0.68, 95% CI 0.47–0.98), even without a history of prematurity. Further studies are required for a definitive conclusion because this study does not corroborate a previous randomized clinical trial (RCT) on 253 women to evaluate the efficacy of Shirodkar cerclage in women with cervix <15 mm in a population in which <20% of women had a history of prematurity between 16 and 32 weeks. The study concluded that it was not possible to demonstrate the benefits of cerclage [40].

Cerclage Indicated Due to Physical Examination

The presence of cervical dilatation during physical examination, without active labor or placental detachment, has also been as an indicator for emergency cerclage, if technically feasible, after ruling out the presence of uterine activity and intra-amniotic infection. However, there is limited data regarding this in the literature [35]. Counseling is recommended as it is a risky procedure with a higher prevalence of infection than cerclage indicated due to history or ultrasound (13–50% vs. 1–2%).

Ultrasound examination is recommended before any type of cerclage to evaluate fetal condition and confirm gestational age and fetal anatomy [42]. There is no evidence to suggest that the use of antibiotics and tocolytics associated with cerclage is beneficial [35]. Cerclage should preferably be performed under spinal anesthesia rather than general anesthesia [42], and there appears to be no advantage between

McDonald or Shirodkar cerclage sutures regarding prematurity prevention [43]. The McDonald's technique is preferred as it is easier to perform [42]. Mersilene™ or Ethibond™ sutures are commonly used and seem to provide similar results, although there are records detailing the successful use of absorbable rescue sutures. Meta-analysis results from six studies comparing the use of one or two sutures suggest that the use of two sutures reduces births <34 (OR 0.59, 95% CI 0.40–0.86) and <28 weeks (OR 0.43, 95% CI 0.26–0.73) without differences in neonatal morbidity and mortality [44]. Furthermore, patients were discharged on the day of the procedure or the following day if performed after 20 weeks [42].

Progesterone

Progesterone seems to act both on the myometrium, reducing the contractile response and frequency of contractions, and on the uterine cervix, reducing cervical remodeling. Remodeling occurs as a result of progesterone's local anti-inflammatory action, especially when administered vaginally, reducing inflammatory cytokines in circulation and the activity of inflammatory cells and enzymes at cervical level, which favor the cervical remodeling process [17, 45]. Due to its characteristics, progesterone has been tested in populations at high risk for prematurity, such as in women with cervix <25 mm, history of prematurity, and multiple pregnancies.

Some studies have used vaginal progesterone in asymptomatic women with single gestation and short cervix at doses of 90, 100, and 200 mg/day, the latter being the most studied [15, 16, 46]. Progesterone has a protective effect on risk of prematurity for this group of women regardless of the dose used [17]. A systematic review and meta-analysis published in 2012 showed that the use of vaginal progesterone in women with short cervix in the second trimester reduces the rate of birth before 28, 33, and 35 weeks. Furthermore, vaginal progesterone was also shown to reduce the number of neonatal intensive care unit (NICU) admissions by 52%, respiratory distress syndrome (RDS), and birth weight <1500 mg [17, 33]. These findings were reinforced by a systematic Cochrane review involving 36 RCTs (8523 women and 12,515 newborns) that included several risk profiles for prematurity and not only asymptomatic single pregnancies [47]. Of these, two studies reported the benefit of progesterone in relation to placebo in asymptomatic women with short cervix, reducing birth <28 (RR 0.59, 95% CI 0.37–0.93) and 34 weeks (RR 0.64, 95% CI 0.45–0.90) [47].

In 2016, the efficacy of progesterone in pregnant women with short cervix was questioned by a multicenter, double-blind, controlled RCT called OPPTIMUM. The study found no reduction in prematurity or improvement in neonatal outcomes in 1228 women with a history of prematurity or short cervix [48]. However, in 2018 a new meta-analysis was released with the largest number of individuals to date (974 women) and including data from the OPPTIMUM study. The meta-analysis included five studies on individual asymptomatic women with single pregnancies and cervix <25 mm, and analysis confirmed the efficacy of progesterone [17]. These authors demonstrated the important effect of vaginal progesterone on reducing births <33 weeks (14% vs. 22%, RR 0.62, 95% CI 0.47–0.81, $P = 0.0006$, I2 = 0%, numbers needed to treat [NNT] 12, 95% CI 8–23). The study also confirmed the reduction in births before 36, 35, 34, 32, 30, and 28 weeks regardless of prematurity history, thus being an alternative to cerclage in women with prematurity history and cervical shortening of <25 mm [17, 33]. The authors also demonstrated reduced RDS, neonatal composite morbidity, weight <1500 g, and <2500 g at NICU admission and a tendency to reduce mortality (RR 0.44, 95% CI 0.18–1.07, $P = 0.07$) [17]. Despite the tendency to reduce neonatal mortality by 40%–50%, intraventricular hemorrhage, and sepsis [17], these and other neonatal benefits still need to be better confirmed in women with this profile. Additionally, long-term follow-ups confirm that there is no evidence of malformations or development changes in children aged up to two years due to the use of progesterone [17, 48].

Consistent evidence regarding the benefits of progesterone for women with a history of prematurity and single pregnancies is shown in the systematic Cochrane review with reduced births <34 weeks (RR 0.31, 95% CI 0.14–0.69), <37 weeks, and a significant extension of pregnancy, in addition to several neonatal benefits such as reduced perinatal mortality (RR 0.50, 95% CI 0.33–0.75), birth <2500 g (RR 0.58, 95% CI 0.42–0.79), use of assisted ventilation, necrotizing enterocolitis, neonatal mortality, and NICU admission [47]. Although most RCTs demonstrate the advantage of using vaginal progesterone, the benefit of this therapy has been questioned by some studies, such as that by O'Brien et al. in 2007 and the PROGRESS study of 2017 [49]. The first study was a RCT with 611 women and analyzed the use of progesterone gel in women with a history of prematurity; their findings did not indicate reduced neonatal prematurity or morbidity [49]. The second study was also a multicenter RCT involving 39 centers and a progesterone dose of 100 mg in 787 women in which the primary finding was the occurrence of RDS. The study also reported no benefits with regard to the use of progesterone neither for this outcome nor for prematurity reduction. One of the questioning points in this study was the fact that about 2% of the sample was composed of twin pregnancies [46]. Divergent results lead to the need of meta-analysis with individual data to better understand the size of the vaginal progesterone effect in women with a history of prematurity [46]. Intramuscular progesterone (hydroxyprogesterone caproate) was initially used in women with a history of prematurity with good results. However, a recent RCT called PROLONG involving 1740 women in 9 countries could not demonstrate the benefits of this therapy [50]. After the publication of this study, the Food and Drug Administration recommended that hydroxyprogesterone caproate should not be used to prevent prematurity, although the ACOG still maintained the recommendation for use until further review of the data [51]. A recent systematic review and meta-analysis comparing two routes of progesterone administration in women with a history of prematurity reports better findings with vaginal use, which resulted in reduced incidence of prematurity, better neonatal results, and fewer side effects [52].

Pessary

A pessary is a flexible ring-shaped silicone device used to try to prevent premature birth. Most studies published to date used the Arabin pessary (CE0482, MED/CERT ISO 9003/EN 46003; Dr. Arabin GmbH and Co., KG) [53], but there are other alternatives, such as the pessary produced by Ingamed, which is the model used in an ongoing multicenter study in Brazil [54]. The most important advantages of a pessary are easy outpatient placement and removal that does not require anesthesia and not being invasive [55]. It acts by keeping the cervix closed and angulated, changing the direction of the cervical canal posteriorly, and focusing the weight on the anterior segment of the uterus [56, 57].

The use of a pessary in women with single pregnancies and short cervix has presented controversial results. The cervical pessary in pregnant women with a short cervix (PECEP) study was published by Goya et al. in 2012. It was one of the first RCT on the use of pessary for prematurity prevention and involved five Spanish hospitals [55]. A total of 380 women with single gestation and cervix <25 mm between 18 and 22 weeks were selected and randomly compared for pessary and placebo use, with an important reduction in births <34 weeks (6% vs. 27%, OR 0.18, 95% CI 0.08–0.37; $P < 0.0001$) in the pessary group [55].

In contrast, in a RCT by Hui et al. in 2013, analysis of 108 women indicated no advantages following the use of a pessary for birth prevention <34 weeks [58]. However, they did not reach the number of women intended for adequate power of the study (1120 women) due to interruptions early in the research process [58].

In 2016, a third multicenter RCT was published by Nicolaides et al. including women between 20 and 24 weeks +6 days with cervix <25 mm. Women with cervix <15 mm received vaginal progesterone. The authors did not identify differences in births <34 weeks and neonatal changes [59].

Some methodological differences between studies may explain the differences in results. A study by Goya et al. showed that 16% of the patients had their pessary repositioned, which did not occur in the other studies. Differences in the studied populations may also have occurred, with fewer women with a history of prematurity in the study by Goya et al. than in the study by Nicolaides et al. (10.8% vs. 16.8%, respectively) [55, 60]. The incidence of prematurity for the control group in the study by Goya et al. (26.8%) was much higher than that of other studies (5.5% in the study by Hui et al. and 10.8% in the study by Nicolaides et al.). Also, in the study by Goya et al. 20% of women were smokers, and 90% were Latin American, raising doubt about the fact that the women included in this study had difference characteristics from the women included in other studies. The study by Nicolaides et al. presented a high rate of pessary removal (24.5%), mainly due to the occurrence of premature membrane rupture or at the patient's request. After pessary removal most patients progressed to labor [59]. The pessary was also removed in cases of PROM in the study by Hui et al., in 14.5% of the women in the study group [58]. The study by Goya et al. maintained the device despite the occurrence of PROM and reported that the infection rate did not differ from the control group.

Unlike the other studies, the findings of Nicolaides et al. indicated that 45% of women (with cervix <15 mm) made concomitant use of vaginal progesterone in both groups, which may have reduced the effect of the pessary alone [59]. Likewise, the analysis of these RCTs does not allow definitive conclusions regarding the interpretations of the results by adequately stratifying the history of prematurity or cervical length ranges, which were divergent among the studies and must be considered for future studies [60].

Systematic reviews and meta-analyses published in 2017 by Saccone et al. [60] and Jin et al. [61] involving 3 RCTs and totaling 1420 women concluded that the use of the Arabin pessary in asymptomatic women with cervix <25 mm between 20 and 24 weeks +6 days does not reduce the rate of premature delivery or improve perinatal outcomes. However, it is worth noting that more than half of the meta-analysis sample came from the study by Nicolaides et al. (2016) and included women with and without a history of prematurity [60, 61].

Kabarsian et al. [62] tested the association of pessary use with the use of 400 mg vaginal progesterone in 144 women with single pregnancies and cervix <25 mm between 18 and 22 weeks. The pessary was removed in the presence of PROM and in women undergoing periodic cervical length measurements [62]. This study mixed women with and without a history of prematurity and 14.5% had PROM. The prematurity rate in the control group was 19.7% even with the use of progesterone and did not differ from the study group, thus showing no benefits from associating the pessary with the isolated use of progesterone [62].

To reduce population heterogeneity, Saccone et al. (2017) published a RCT on women with cervix <25 mm between 18 and 23 weeks +6 days and with no history of prematurity conducted in a single center and providing vaginal progesterone for women with cervix <20 mm in both groups [56]. In addition to training the team to place the pessary, it was maintained in case of PROM, and proper positioning was confirmed monthly through digital examination. Different from the meta-analysis published by the same author, this RCT showed a protective effect of the pessary for birth <34 weeks (7.3% vs. 15.3%, RR 0.48, 95% CI 0.24–0.95, $P = 0.04$) even with a mean cervical length lower than that in the study by Nicolaides et al. More than 80% of the sample was composed of cervix <20 mm and used progesterone. However, the authors recognized the limitation of external generalization of their results, since it was not a multicenter study, and also noted a high incidence of prematurity in the control group (32.7% <37 weeks and 15.3% <34 weeks).

A new meta-analysis published by Corrêa et al. in 2019 involving all five of the aforementioned RCTs concluded that although studies point to a lack of pessary efficacy, study heterogeneity allows no definitive conclusions, and better evaluation of its association with progesterone is still required [63].

Cruz-Melguizo et al. [64] published a RCT directly comparing the use of pessary and progesterone, which included 27 centers and 254 asymptomatic women with single pregnancies and cervix <25 mm between 19 and 22 weeks with a history of prematurity and ultrasound verification of pessary positioning; it did not consider PROM as a criterion for pessary removal [64]. The authors concluded that the use of a pessary is not inferior to progesterone even in cervical length or history of prematurity subgroups, but increases vaginal discharge and discomfort [64].

The population in which the use of the pessary shows its real effectiveness, or at least not inferior effectiveness to progesterone, has not yet been well established. New studies are needed to establish safety and advantages after PROM, to determine whether there are greater benefits in women with history of prematurity or with different cervical lengths (especially those <10 mm), where progesterone has reduced efficacy, and to confirm the efficacy of new pessary models [17, 33].

Comparison and Association of Prevention Strategies

Some studies, directly or indirectly, have tried to compare the abovementioned methods and the superiority of these strategies in relation to a placebo. An example of these studies was published by Alfiveric et al. [65] and compared the follow-up outcomes of women with a history of prematurity and short cervix assigned to different cohorts according to the prematurity prevention strategy used (progesterone, vaginal, or cerclage). The authors concluded that all strategies have similar effectiveness for this patient profile [65].

A meta-analysis published by Jarde et al. in 2018 with 40 RCTs (11,311 women) showed that progesterone (primarily when administered vaginally) is the best option to prevent prematurity and neonatal death in women with a history of prematurity or short cervix [66].

Strategies to Prevent Prematurity in Asymptomatic Women with Twin Pregnancy.

Cerclage

The use of cerclage in women with twin pregnancies is controversial as it is associated with increased gestational risks. Its placement is not routinely indicated as only some subgroups have been found to benefit from this method [24, 35, 36, 67].

Cerclage Indicated Due to Ultrasound Findings

A systematic Cochrane review published in 2014 and a meta-analysis published in 2015 by Saccone et al. [68] proved the risks of cerclage in women with twin pregnancies. However, they only included a few RCTs and therefore have a limited quality to allow for definitive conclusions. The negative points identified include a possibly increased incidence of births about 4 weeks earlier than in the control group and a higher number of newborns with a low birth weight and RDS [68, 69].

The number of women with a history of prematurity in the meta-analysis by Saccone et al. was extremely scarce and does not allow for conclusions. This point is important because cerclage indicated due to ultrasound only demonstrates benefits in women with single pregnancies and history of prematurity, especially prior to 34 weeks. Therefore, it is important that studies on twin pregnancies analyze the influence of short cervix, history of prematurity, and the phase in which prematurity occurred.

Although cerclage indicated due to ultrasound is not routinely recommended, a recent systematic review and meta-analysis published by Li et al. [70] including 16 studies and 1211 women suggested some positive points for cerclage in twin pregnancies [70]. Of the total studies included, 9 studies (3 RCT and 6 cohort studies) including 471 women were analyzed. Although the RCTs confirmed the lack of benefits, the cohort studies included in the meta-analysis showed that women with cervix <15 mm between 16 and 24 weeks had a significant pregnancy prolongation with reduced birth rates <37, <34, and <32 weeks when undergoing cerclage [70].

Cerclage Indicated Due to Physical Examination

Similar to that of single pregnancies, emergency cerclage seems to offer benefits when compared to expectant behavior, with scarce RCT literature on this topic. A meta-analysis of three cohort studies (244 women) evaluated the use of cerclage indicated due to cervical dilatation >10 mm at physical examination and reported a mean pregnancy prolongation of 6.8 weeks, reducing birth incidence <34, <28, <2, and improved perinatal outcomes [70]. A large RCT called Emergency Cerclage in Twin Pregnancies at Imminent Risk of Preterm Birth: An Open-Label Randomized Controlled Trial (ENCIRCLE) is in progress (ClinicalTrials.gov Identifier: NCT03818867) and intends to evaluate the real effect of emergency cerclage in twin pregnancies and the effect of cerclage in women with short cervix and twin-twin transfusion syndrome.

Cerclage Indicated Due to History

A case-control study with 82 women, of whom 41 underwent cerclage in the first trimester due to their history, demonstrated that the women who underwent cerclage presented with a higher gestational age at birth; lower birth rates <24, <28, 32, and 34 weeks; higher birth weight; and lower neonatal morbidity, NICU admission, RDS, intraventricular hemorrhage, necrotizing enterocolitis, and neonatal mortality compared with the control group [71]. However, the most recent meta-analysis on the subject states that it is not yet possible to demonstrate the real effectiveness of cerclage indicated only due to history as long as women present cervix >15 mm, and further studies are needed [70].

Progesterone

Progesterone has not demonstrated beneficial effects in unselected twin pregnancies either by intramuscular [72] or vaginal route, in either gel [66] or suppository form [15, 73, 74]. Increased doses of vaginal progesterone from 200 mg to 400 mg daily also showed no benefits [75], although they seem not to cause fetal or neurodevelopmental changes up to 4–5 years of life after being used during pregnancy [32, 73]. A recent Cochrane systematic review including 16 studies (4548 women) also concluded that the administration of vaginal or intramuscular progesterone does not seem to be associated with decreased prematurity or improved neonatal outcomes [76].

However, secondary meta-analysis data published in 2012 suggested that progesterone reduced perinatal composite morbidity and mortality (23.9% vs. 39.7%, RR 0.52, 95% CI 0.29–0.93) in the subgroup of women with twin pregnancies and short cervix [33]. Following this possibility, the study conducted by El-Rafaie et al. published the results of the largest RCT on the use of progesterone in women with twin pregnancies and short cervix (20–25 mm) screened between 20 and 24 weeks [30]. Although there are limitations regarding the risk of performance and detection bias due to the participants' lack of shielding and friction bias due to almost double follow-up losses in the control group [32], the authors reported that vaginal progesterone at a dose of 400 mg daily significantly reduced the incidence of births <34 weeks, <32 weeks, weight <1500 g at birth, RDS, need for mechanical ventilation, and early neonatal death [30]. The findings of this study had a strong impact on a new meta-analysis of individual data published in 2017 consisting of 6 RCTs and involving 303 women, showing a significant reduction of prematurity, neonatal and perinatal death, RDS, use of mechanical ventilation, and weight <1500 mg, with NNT of 6–12 women [32]. The study by El-Rafaie et al. represented 74% of this meta-analysis sample and its removal reduced result significance for birth prevention <33 weeks but maintained a reduction of about 39% in neonatal composite morbidity and mortality [32].

Current data considering the apparent absence of deleterious progesterone effects, the high risk of prematurity for women with twin pregnancies and cervix <25 mm between 20 and 24 weeks, and the apparent neonatal benefits show that the use of progesterone in this group of women seems acceptable. However, further studies on this population are required to clarify the real effectiveness of this prevention strategy, the appropriate dose, and the degree of benefit in different cervical length ranges.

Pessary

Since 2003, when Arabin published the results of his study showing reduced prematurity in women with short cervix in single or twin pregnancies, several studies tried to prove the effectiveness of this strategy. In 2013, Liem et al. published the results of a multicenter RCT called ProTWIN and showed a reduced risk of prematurity <28 and <32 weeks and poor perinatal outcomes in women with twin pregnancies and use of pessary when the cervical length <25th percentile, defined in the study as 38 mm [77]. Long-term evaluation did not show any neurodevelopment changes up to 3 years of age [78].

Furthermore, a large multicenter RCT published by Nicolaides et al. (2016) of 1180 women with unselected twin pregnancies concluded that the use of a pessary does not reduce the incidence of prematurity or perinatal morbidity and mortality in these women or even in the subgroup with cervical length <25 mm [79]. In this study, the authors recognized that adequate placement of the pessary could not be guaranteed, and it was removed in 22.3% of women before 34 weeks (8% secondary to PROM) [79]. However, in the same year, Goya et al. published the PECEP-TWIN study, a multicenter RCT on the use of pessary in 134 women with twin pregnancies and cervix <25 mm to be removed at 37 weeks, but maintaining the device in cases of PROM, which occurred in only 1.5% of women in the pessary group versus 9.1% of women in the control group [31]. The authors reported reduced birth <34 weeks (16.2% vs. 39.4%, RR 0.41, 95% CI 0.22–0.76), low birth weight, and neonatal composite morbidity. They reported no differences for births prior 28 weeks, which according to the authors could be due to the inefficacy of the pessary in a very short cervix [31].

A meta-analysis involving women with short cervix presented in the three RCTs described above showed no benefits for the use of a pessary to prevent prematurity or neonatal outcomes [80]. According to the data available so far, new RCTs directed at women with twin pregnancies and short cervix are needed, including adequate training and control for pessary positioning, standardizing cutoff points for short cervix definition, and stratifying results by history of prematurity. The real role and risks of pessary maintenance in women with PROM still need to be better clarified, and a focused study is required to achieve this.

Table 31.1 summarizes the application of prematurity prevention strategies for asymptomatic pregnant women according to the risk group.

Table 31.1 Use of secondary strategies to prevent prematurity in asymptomatic women

Pregnancy	Short cervix (<25 mm)	History of PD	Secondary prevention
Single	No	No	–
		Yes	Vaginal progesterone (200 mg/day)
	Yes	No	Vaginal progesterone (200 mg/day) and/or pessary[a]
		Yes	Cerclage and/or vaginal progesterone (200 mg/day)
Twin	No	No	–
		Yes	–
	Yes	No	Vaginal progesterone (200 to 400 mg/day) and/or pessary[a]
		Yes	Vaginal progesterone (200 to 400 mg/day) and/or pessary[a]

PD (spontaneous delivery <37 weeks)
[a]More studies are required

References

1. Chawanpaiboon S, Vogel JP, Moller AB, Lumbiganon P, Petzold M, Hogan D, et al. Global, regional, and national estimates of levels of preterm birth in 2014: a systematic review and modelling analysis. Lancet Glob Health. 2019;7(1):e37–46.
2. WHO recommendations on interventions to improve preterm birth outcomes. Available from: www.who.int/reproductivehealth.
3. Goldenberg RL, Culhane JF, Iams JD, Romero R. Epidemiology and causes of preterm birth. Lancet. 2008;371:75–84.
4. Son M, Miller ES. Predicting preterm birth: cervical length and fetal fibronectin. Semin Perinatol. 2017;41(8):445–51.
5. Vogel JP, Chawanpaiboon S, Moller AB, Watananirun K, Bonet M, Lumbiganon P. The global epidemiology of preterm birth. Best Pract Res Clin Obstet Gynaecol [Internet]. 2018;52:3–12. Available from: https://doi.org/10.1016/j.bpobgyn.2018.04.003.
6. Witkin SS, Moron AF, Ridenhour BJ, Minis E, Hatanaka A, Sarmento SGP, et al. Vaginal biomarkers that predict cervical length and dominant bacteria in the vaginal microbiomes of pregnant women. MBio. 2019;10(5):1–13.
7. Honest H, Bachmann LM, Sundaram R, Gupta JK, Kleijnen J, Khan KS. The accuracy of risk scores in predicting preterm birth - a systematic review. J Obstet Gynaecol (Lahore). 2004;24(4):343–59.
8. Hezelgrave NL, Shennan AH. Quantitative fetal fibronectin to predict spontaneous preterm birth: a review. Womens Health. 2016;12(1):121–8.
9. Dos Santos F, Daru J, Rogozińska E, Cooper NAM. Accuracy of fetal fibronectin for assessing preterm birth risk in asymptomatic pregnant women: a systematic review and meta-analysis. Acta Obstet Gynecol Scand. 2018;97(6):657–67.
10. Abbott DS, Hezelgrave NL, Seed PT, Norman JE, David AL, Bennett PR, et al. Quantitative fetal fibronectin to predict preterm birth in asymptomatic women at high risk. Obstet Gynecol. 2015;125(5):1168–76.
11. Souza RT, McKenzie EJ, Jones B, de Seymour JV, Thomas MM, Zarate E, et al. Trace biomarkers associated with spontaneous preterm birth from the maternal serum metabolome of asymptomatic nulliparous women – parallel case-control studies from the SCOPE cohort. Sci Rep. 2019;9(1):1–10.
12. Suff N, Story L, Shennan A. The prediction of preterm delivery: what is new? Semin Fetal Neonatal Med. 2019;24(1):27–32.
13. Cecatti JG, Souza RT, Sulek K, Costa ML, Kenny LC, McCowan LM, et al. Use of metabolomics for the identification and validation of clinical biomarkers for preterm birth: preterm SAMBA. BMC Pregnancy Childbirth [Internet]. 2016;16(1):1–9. Available from: https://doi.org/10.1186/s12884-016-1006-9.
14. Lim K, Butt K, Crane JM, Morin L, Bly S, Butt K, et al. Ultrasonographic cervical length assessment in predicting preterm birth in singleton pregnancies. J Obstet Gynaecol Canada [Internet] 2011;33(5):486–99. Available from: https://doi.org/10.1016/S1701-2163(16)34884-8.
15. da Fonseca EB, Celik E, Parra-Cordero M, Singh M, Nicolaides KH. Progesterone and the risk of preterm birth among women with a short cervix. N Engl J Med. 2007;357:462–9.
16. Hassan SS, Romero R, Vidyadhari D, Fusey S, Baxter J, Khandelwal M, et al. Vaginal progesterone reduces the rate of preterm birth in women with a sonographic short cervix: a multicenter, randomized, double-blinded, placebo-controlled trial. Ultrasound Obstet Gynecol. 2012;38(1):18–31.
17. Romero R, Conde-Agudelo A, Da Fonseca E, O'Brien JM, Cetingoz E. Vaginal progesterone for preventing preterm birth gestations with a short cervix : a meta-analysis of. Am J Obstet Gynecol. 2018;218(2):161–80.
18. Cahill AG, Odibo AO, Caughey AB, Stamilio DM, Hassan SS, Macones GA, et al. Universal cervical length screening and treatment with vaginal progesterone to prevent preterm birth: a

decision and economic analysis. Am J Obstet Gynecol [Internet]. 2010;202(6):548.e1–548.e8. Available from: https://doi.org/10.1016/j.ajog.2009.12.005.

19. Werner EF, Hamel MS, Orzechowski K, Berghella V, Thung SF. Cost-effectiveness of transvaginal ultrasound cervical length screening in singletons without a prior preterm birth: an update. Am J Obstet Gynecol [Internet]. 2015;213(4):554.e1–554.e6. Available from: https://doi.org/10.1016/j.ajog.2015.06.020.
20. Pizzi LT, Seligman NS, Baxter JK, Jutkowitz E, Berghella V. Cost and cost effectiveness of vaginal progesterone gel in reducing preterm birth: an economic analysis of the PREGNANT trial. Pharmacoeconomics. 2014;32(5):467–78.
21. Medley N, Poljak B, Mammarella S, Alfirevic Z. Clinical guidelines for prevention and management of preterm birth: a systematic review. BJOG. 2018;125:1361–9.
22. Owen J, Yost N, Berghella V, Thom E, Swain M, Dildy GA, et al. Mid-trimester endovaginal sonography in women at high risk for spontaneous preterm birth. JAMA. 2001;286(11):1340–8.
23. American College of Obstetricians and Gynecologists. Prediction and prevention of preterm birth. Pratice Bulletin No. 130. Obs Gynecol Gynecol. 2012;120(6):964–73.
24. Berghella V, Odibo AO, To MS, Rust OA, Althuisius SM. Cerclage for short cervix on ultrasonography: meta-analysis of trials using individual patient-level data. Obstet Gynecol. 2005;106(1):181–9.
25. Berghella V, Rafael TJ, Szychowski JM, Rust OA, Owen J. Cerclage for short cervix on ultrasonography in women with singleton gestations and previous preterm birth: a meta-analysis. Obstet Gynecol. 2011;117(3):663–71.
26. Kuhrt K, Smout E, Hezelgrave N, Seed PT, Carter J, Shennan AH. Development and validation of a tool incorporating cervical length and quantitative fetal fibronectin to predict spontaneous preterm birth in asymptomatic high-risk women. Ultrasound Obstet Gynecol. 2016;47(1):104–9.
27. Goodfellow L, Care A, Sharp A, Ivandic J, Poljak B, Roberts D, et al. Effect of QUiPP prediction algorithm on treatment decisions in women with a previous preterm birth: a prospective cohort study. BJOG. 2019;126(13):1569–75.
28. Conde-Agudelo A, Romero R. Cervicovaginal fetal fibronectin for the prediction of spontaneous preterm birth in multiple pregnancies: a systematic review and meta-analysis. J Matern Fetal Neonatal Med. 2010;23(12):1365–76.
29. Conde-Agudelo A, Romero R, Hassan SS, Yeo L. Transvaginal sonographic cervical length for the prediction of spontaneous preterm birth in twin pregnancies: a systematic review and meta-analysis. Am J Obstet Gynecol. 2010;203(2):128.e1–12.
30. El-refaie W, Abdelhafez MS, Badawy A. Vaginal progesterone for prevention of preterm labor in asymptomatic twin pregnancies with sonographic short cervix: a randomized clinical trial of efficacy and safety. Arch Gynecol Obstet. 2016;293(1):61–7.
31. Goya M, De La Calle M, Pratcorona L, Merced C, Rodó C, Muñoz B, et al. Cervical pessary to prevent preterm birth in women with twin gestation and sonographic short cervix: a multicenter randomized controlled trial (PECEP-Twins). Am J Obstet Gynecol. 2016;214(2):145–52.
32. Romero R, Conde-Agudelo A, El-Refaie W, Rode L, Brizot ML, Cetingoz E, et al. Vaginal progesterone decreases preterm birth and neonatal morbidity and mortality in women with a twin gestation and a short cervix: an updated meta-analysis of individual patient data. Ultrasound Obstet Gynecol. 2017;49(3):303–14.
33. Romero R, Nicolaides K, Conde-Agudelo A, Tabor A, O'Brien J, Elcin C, et al. Vaginal progesterone in women with an asymptomatic sonographic short cervix in the midtrimester decreases preterm delivery and neonatal morbity: a systematic review and meta-analysis of individual patient data Roberto. Am J Obstet Gynecol. 2012;206(2):124.e1–19.
34. McIntosh J, Feltovich H, Berghella V, Manuck T. The role of routine cervical length screening in selected high- and low-risk women for preterm birth prevention. Am J Obstet Gynecol [Internet] 2016;215(3):B2–7. Available from: https://doi.org/10.1016/j.ajog.2016.04.027.

35. Cerclage for the management of cervical insufficiency. Pratice Bulletin No. 142. American College of Obstetricians and Gylecologists. Obstet Gynecol. 2014;123(2):372–9.
36. Shennan A, To M. Green-top guideline no 60: cervical cerclage. RCOG 2011;
37. Goddijn M, Christiansen OB, Elson J et al. Recurrent pregnancy loss. Guideline of the European Society of Human Reproduction and Embryology. Eur Soc Hum Reprod Embryol. 2017;(November):0–153.
38. Alfirevic Z, Stampalija T, Medley N. Cochrane Database of Systematic Reviews Cervical stitch (cerclage) for preventing preterm birth in singleton pregnancy (Review) Cervical stitch (cerclage) for preventing preterm birth in singleton pregnancy (Review). 2017;(6). Available from: www.cochranelibrary.com.
39. Berghella V, Palacio M, Ness A, Alfirevic Z, Nicolaides KH, Saccone G. Cervical length screening for prevention of preterm birth in singleton pregnancy with threatened preterm labor: systematic review and meta-analysis of randomized controlled trials using individual patient-level data. Ultrasound Obstet Gynecol. 2017;49(3):322–9.
40. To MS, Alfirevic Z, Heath VCF, Cicero S, Cacho AM, Williamson PR, et al. Cervical cerclage for prevention of preterm delivery in women with short cervix: randomised controlled trial. Lancet. 2004;363(9424):1849–53.
41. Berghella V, Ciardulli A, Rust OA, To M, Otsuki K, Althuisius S, et al. Cerclage for sonographic short cervix in singleton gestations without prior spontaneous preterm birth: systematic review and meta-analysis of randomized controlled trials using individual patient-level data. Ultrasound Obstet Gynecol. 2017;50(5):569–77.
42. Berghella V, Ludmir J, Simonazzi G, Owen J. Transvaginal cervical cerclage: evidence for perioperative management strategies. Am J Obstet Gynecol. 2013;209(3):181–92.
43. Odibo A, Berghella V, To M, Rust O, Althuisius S, Nicolaides K. Shirodkar versus McDonald cerclage for the prevention of preterm birth in women with short cervical length. Am J Perinatol. 2007;24(1):55–60.
44. Pergialiotis V, Vlachos DG, Prodromidou A, Perrea D, Grioka E, Vlachos GD. Double versus single cervical cerclage for the prevention of preterm births. J Matern Fetal Med. 2015;28:379–85.
45. Furcron AE, Romero R, Plazyo O, Unkel R, Xu Y, Hassan SS, et al. Vaginal progesterone, but not 17α-hydroxyprogesterone caproate, has antiinflammatory effects at the murine maternal-fetal interface. Am J Obstet Gynecol [Internet]. 2015;213(6):846.e1–846.e19. Available from: https://doi.org/10.1016/j.ajog.2015.08.010.
46. Crowther CA, Ashwood P, McPhee AJ, Flenady V, Tran T, Dodd JM, et al. Vaginal progesterone pessaries for pregnant women with a previous preterm birth to prevent neonatal respiratory distress syndrome (the PROGRESS Study): a multicentre, randomised, placebo-controlled trial. PLoS Med. 2017;14(9):e1002390.
47. Dodd JM, Jones L, Flenady V, Crowther CA. Prenatal administration of progesterone for preventing preterm birth in women considered to be at risk of preterm birth. Cochrane Database Syst Rev. 2013;2013(7).
48. Norman JE, Marlow N, Messow CM, Shennan A, Bennett PR, Thornton S, et al. Vaginal progesterone prophylaxis for preterm birth (the OPPTIMUM study): a multicentre, randomised, double-blind trial. Lancet [Internet] 2016;387(10033):2106–16. Available from: https://doi.org/10.1016/S0140-6736(16)00350-0.
49. O'Brien JM, Adair CD, Lewis DF, Hall DR, DeFranco EA, Fusey S, et al. Progesterone vaginal gel for the reduction of recurrent preterm birth: primary results from a randomized, double-blind, placebo-controlled trial. Ultrasound Obstet Gynecol. 2007;30(5):687–96.
50. Blackwell SC, Gyamfi-Bannerman C, Biggio JR, Chauhan SP, Hughes BL, Louis JM, et al. 17-OHPC to prevent recurrent preterm birth in singleton gestations (PROLONG study): a multicenter, international, randomized double-blind trial. Am J Perinatol [Internet]. 2019;1(212). Available from: http://www.ncbi.nlm.nih.gov/pubmed/31652479.
51. American College of Obstetricians and Gynecologists' Committee on Practice Bulletins. Practice Advisory: Clinical guidance for integration of the findings of the PROLONG study: Progestin's

Role in Optimizing Neonatal Gestation [Internet]. 2019 [cited 2019 Dec 28]. Available from: https://www.acog.org/Clinical-Guidance-and-Publications/Practice-Advisories/Clinical-guidance-for-integration-of-the-findings-of-The-PROLONG-study-Progestins-Role-in-Optimizing?IsMobileSet=false.
52. Saccone G, Khalifeh A, Elimian A, Bahrami E, Chaman-Ara K, Bahrami MA, et al. Vaginal progesterone vs intramuscular 17α-hydroxyprogesterone caproate for prevention of recurrent spontaneous preterm birth in singleton gestations: systematic review and meta-analysis of randomized controlled trials. Ultrasound Obstet Gynecol. 2017;49:315–21.
53. ARABIN® Cerclage Pessary perforated [Internet]. [cited 2019 Dec 21]. Available from: https://dr-arabin.de/produkt/arabin-cerclage-pessary-perforated/?lang=en.
54. Pessário AM Ingamed® [Internet]. [cited 2019 Dec 21]. Available from: http://www.ingamed.com.br/produtos-detalhe/51/pessario-parto-prematuro.
55. Goya M, Pratcorona L, Merced C, Rodó C, Valle L, Romero A, et al. Cervical pessary in pregnant women with a short cervix (PECEP): an open-label randomised controlled trial. Lancet [Internet]. 2012;379(9828):1800–6. Available from: https://doi.org/10.1016/S0140-6736(12)60030-0.
56. Saccone G, Maruotti GM, Giudicepietro A, Martinelli P, Mazzarelli L, Visentin S, et al. Effect of cervical pessary on spontaneous preterm birth in women with singleton pregnancies and short cervical length a randomized clinical trial. JAMA J Am Med Assoc. 2017;318(23):2317–24.
57. Arabin B, Halbesma JR, Vork F, Hübener M, Van Eyck J. Is treatment with vaginal pessaries an option in patients with a sonographically detected short cervix? J Perinat Med. 2003;31(2):122–33.
58. Lao TT, Leung FRCOGTY. Hui S, Chor C, Lau T, Lao T, Leung T. Cerclage pessary for preventing preterm birth in women with a singleton pregnancy and a short cervix at 20 to 24 weeks: a randomized controlled trial. Am J Perinatol. 8 de agosto de 2012;30(04):283–8. 2013.
59. Nicolaides KH, Syngelaki A, Poon LC, Picciarelli G, Tul N, Zamprakou A, et al. A randomized trial of a cervical pessary to prevent preterm singleton birth. N Engl J Med. 2016;374(11):1044–52.
60. Saccone G, Ciardulli A, Xodo S, Dugoff L, Ludmir J, Pagani G, et al. Cervical pessary for preventing preterm birth in singleton pregnancies with short cervical length: a systematic review and meta-analysis. J Ultrasound Med. 2017;36(8):1535–43.
61. Jin XH, Li D, Huang LL. Cervical pessary for prevention of preterm birth: a meta-analysis. Sci Rep [Internet]. 2017;7(January):1–6. Available from: https://doi.org/10.1038/srep42560.
62. Karbasian N, Sheikh M, Pirjani R, Hazrati S, Tara F, Hantoushzadeh S. Combined treatment with cervical pessary and vaginal progesterone for the prevention of preterm birth: a randomized clinical trial. J Obstet Gynaecol Res. 2016;42(12):1673–9.
63. Corrêa TD, Amorim EG, Tomazelli JAG, Corrêa MD. Use of the pessary in the prevention of preterm delivery. Vol. 41, Revista Brasileira de Ginecologia e Obstetricia. Georg Thieme Verlag; 2019. p. 53–8.
64. Cruz-Melguizo S, San-Frutos L, Martínez-Payo C, Ruiz-Antorán B, Adiego-Burgos B, Campillos-Maza JM, et al. Cervical pessary compared with vaginal progesterone for preventing early preterm birth a randomized controlled trial. Obstet Gynecol. 2018;132(4):907–15.
65. Alfirevic Z, Owen J, Carreras Moratonas E, Sharp AN, Szychowski JM, Goya M. Vaginal progesterone, cerclage or cervical pessary for preventing preterm birth in asymptomatic singleton pregnant women with a history of preterm birth and a sonographic short cervix. Ultrasound Obstet Gynecol. 2013;41:146–51.
66. Jarde A, Lutsiv O, Beyene J, McDonald SD. Vaginal progesterone, oral progesterone, 17-OHPC, cerclage, and pessary for preventing preterm birth in at-risk singleton pregnancies: an updated systematic review and network meta-analysis. BJOG. 2019;126(5):556–67.
67. Huang X, Saravelos SH, Li TC, Huang R, Xu R, Zhou Q, et al. Cervical cerclage in twin pregnancy. Best Pract Res Clin Obstet Gynaecol [Internet]. 2019;59:89–97. Available from: https://doi.org/10.1016/j.bpobgyn.2019.06.001.

68. Saccone G, Rust O, Althuisius S, Roman A, Berghella V. Cerclage for short cervix in twin pregnancies: systematic review and meta-analysis of randomized trials using individual patient-level data. Acta Obstet Gynecol Scand. 2015;94(4):352–8.
69. Rafael TJ, Berghella V, Alfirevic Z. Cervical stitch (cerclage) for preventing preterm birth in multiple pregnancy. Cochrane Database Syst Rev. 2014;10(9).
70. Li C, Shen J, Hua K. Cerclage for women with twin pregnancies: a systematic review and metaanalysis. Am J Obstet Gynecol [Internet]. 2019;220(6):543–557.e1. Available from: https://doi.org/10.1016/j.ajog.2018.11.1105.
71. Rottenstreich A, Levin G, Kleinstern G, Zigron R, Rottenstreich M, Elchalal U, et al. History-indicated cervical cerclage in management of twin pregnancy. Ultrasound Obstet Gynecol. 2019;54(4):517–23.
72. Rouse D, Caritis S, Peaceman A, Sciscione A, Thom E, Spong C, et al. A trial of 17 alpha-hydroxyprogesterone caproate to prevent prematurity in twins. N Engl J Med. 2007;357:454–61.
73. Rode L, Klein K, Nicolaides KH, Krampl-Bettelheim E, Tabor A. Prevention of preterm delivery in twin gestations (PREDICT): a multicenter, randomized, placebo-controlled trial on the effect of vaginal micronized progesterone. Ultrasound Obstet Gynecol. 2011;38(3):272–80.
74. Brizot ML, Hernandez W, Liao AW, Bittar RE, Francisco RPV, Krebs VLJ, et al. Vaginal progesterone for the prevention of preterm birth in twin gestations: a randomized placebo-controlled double-blind study. Am J Obstet Gynecol [Internet]. 2015;213(1):82.e1–82.e9. Available from: https://doi.org/10.1016/j.ajog.2015.02.021.
75. Serra V, Perales A, Meseguer J, Parrilla JJ, Lara C, Bellver J, et al. Increased doses of vaginal progesterone for the prevention of preterm birth in twin pregnancies: a randomised controlled double-blind multicentre trial. BJOG. 2013;120(1):50–7.
76. Dodd JM, Grivell RM, OBrien CM, Dowswell T, Deussen AR. Prenatal administration of progestogens for preventing spontaneous preterm birth in women with a multiple pregnancy. Cochrane database Syst Rev. 2019;2019(11).
77. Liem S, Schuit E, Hegeman M, Bais J, De Boer K, Bloemenkamp K, et al. Cervical pessaries for prevention of preterm birth in women with a multiple pregnancy (ProTWIN): a multicentre, open-label randomised controlled trial. Lancet. 2013;382(9901):1341–9.
78. van't Hooft J, van der Lee JH, Opmeer BC, van Wassenaer-Leemhuis AG, van Baar AL, Bekedam DJ, et al. Pessary for prevention of preterm birth in twin pregnancy with short cervix: 3-year follow-up study. Ultrasound Obstet Gynecol. 2018;51(5):621–8.
79. Nicolaides KH, Syngelaki A, Poon LC, De Paco Matallana C, Plasencia W, Molina FS, et al. Cervical pessary placement for prevention of preterm birth in unselected twin pregnancies: A randomized controlled trial. Am J Obstet Gynecol [Internet]. 2016;214(1):3.e1–3.e9. Available from: https://doi.org/10.1016/j.ajog.2015.08.051.
80. Saccone G, Ciardulli A, Xodo S, Dugoff L, Ludmir J, D'Antonio F, et al. Cervical pessary for preventing preterm birth in twin pregnancies with short cervical length: a systematic review and meta-analysis. J Matern Neonatal Med [Internet] 2017;30(24):2918–25. Available from: https://doi.org/10.1080/14767058.2016.1268595.

Chapter 32
Prematurity: Relevant Aspects in the Symptomatic Patient

Renato Augusto Moreira de Sá and Eduardo Borges da Fonseca

Overview

Preterm is defined as babies born alive before 37 weeks of pregnancy are completed; however, the low-gestational age cutoff, or that used to distinguish preterm birth from spontaneous abortion, varies by location [1]. There are subcategories of preterm birth, based on gestational age [2] (Fig. 32.1):

- Extremely preterm (less than 28 weeks)
- Very preterm (28–32 weeks)
- Moderate to late preterm (32–37 weeks)

The incidence of prematurity varies from region to region, averaging around 10% of pregnancies. In almost all countries with reliable data, preterm birth rates are increasing, much of this increasing is explained by rising numbers of indicated preterm births [1]. The population characteristics may impact on incidence of preterm birth. For instance, nutritional status during pregnancy, described by indicators as body mass index (BMI), is associated with spontaneous preterm delivery. Low pre-pregnancy BMI is associated with a higher risk of spontaneous preterm birth. Obesity might be protective for spontaneous preterm labor, but increase the rate of medically indicated preterm birth [1, 3]. Contributing factors include the increasing frequency of births to women older than 35 years and the use of infertility treatments, with their significant enhancement of multiple birth rates [3].

R. A. Moreira de Sá (✉)
Fernandes Figueira Institut - FIOCRUZ, Rio de Janeiro, RJ, Brazil

E. B. d. Fonseca
Maternal Fetal Medicine Group - Nova Diagnóstico por Imagem, João Pessoa, PB, Brazil

Ob/Gyn Department, Federal University of Paraiba, João Pessoa, PB, Brazil

© Springer Nature Switzerland AG 2022

R. A. Moreira de Sá, E. B. d. Fonseca (eds.), *Perinatology*,
https://doi.org/10.1007/978-3-030-83434-0_32

DEFINITION	Preterm								Term						Postterm
SUB-CATEGORIES	Extremely Preterm				Very preterm		Moderate to late preterm		Early term		Full term		Late term		
VIABILITY	Periviable		Viable Preterm												
GA WEEKS	20 0/7	25 6/7	26 0/7	27 6/7	28 0/7	31 6/7	32 0/7	36 6/7	37 0/7	38 6/7	39 0/7	40 6/7	41 0/7	41 6/7	After 42 0/7

Gestational Age (weeks)

Fig. 32.1 Newborn classification by gestational age

An estimated 15 million babies are born prematurely every year. This is more than 1 in 10 babies. The morbidity and mortality in such group is high with serious illness or death during the neonatal period, especially for those born before 32 weeks. Without appropriate treatment, those who survive are at increased risk of lifelong disability and poor quality of life [1].

Preterm births account for 75% of perinatal mortality and more than half of the long-term morbidity. Approximately 1 million children die each year due to complications of preterm birth. Although most preterm babies survive, they are at increased risk of neurodevelopmental impairments and respiratory and gastrointestinal complications [1]. Many survivors face a lifetime of disability, including learning disabilities and visual and hearing problems. Globally, complications of prematurity are the single largest cause of neonatal death and the second leading cause of deaths among children under the age of 5 years [3]. The severity and incidence of adverse outcomes inversely correlate with gestational age, especially birth before 32 completed weeks of gestation. Beyond the enormous impact on affected families, the economic costs are staggering [3].

Inequalities in survival rates around the world are stark. In low-income settings, half of the babies born at or below 32 weeks (2 months early) die due to a lack of feasible, cost-effective care, such as warmth, breastfeeding support, and basic care for infections and breathing difficulties. In high-income countries, almost all of these babies survive. Suboptimal use of technology in middle-income settings is causing an increased burden of disability among preterm babies who survive the neonatal period [4].

The obstetric precursors leading to preterm birth are [4]:

1. Delivery for maternal or fetal indications, in which either labor is induced or the infant is delivered by prelabor cesarean section
2. Spontaneous preterm labor with intact membranes
3. Preterm premature rupture of the membranes (PPROM)

About 30–35% of preterm births are indicated, 40–45% follow spontaneous preterm labor, and 25–30% follow PPROM (Fig. 32.2); births that follow spontaneous labor and PPROM are together designated spontaneous preterm births, so considering both cause it is about 65–75% [4].

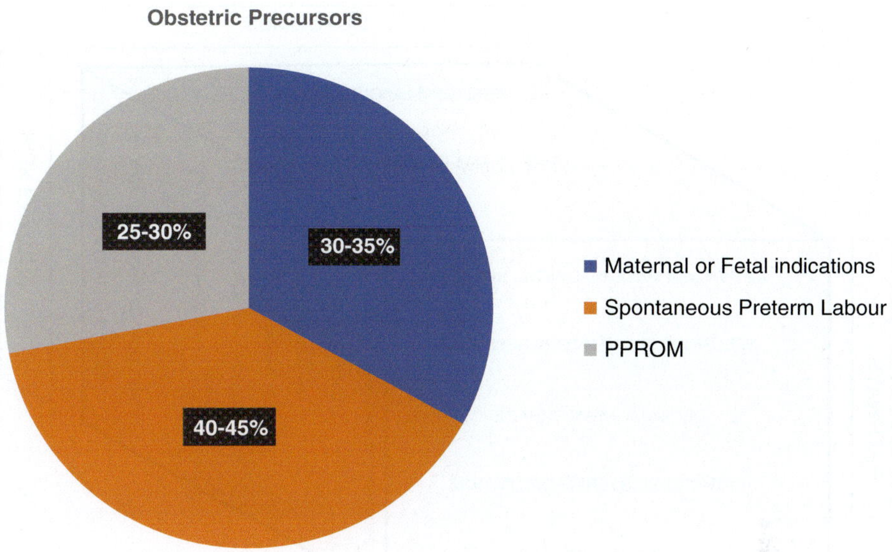

Fig. 32.2 Prevalence of preterm birth considering obstetric precursor cause

Pathogenesis of Spontaneous Preterm Birth

Compelling clinical and research evidence suggest that a number of pathogenic processes can lead to a final common pathway that results in spontaneous preterm labor [5]. In this context, at least five major pathophysiologic pathways have been described toward the shared outcome of preterm birth [4, 5]:

- Premature activation of the maternal or fetal hypothalamic-pituitary-adrenal (HPA) axis
- Exaggerated inflammatory response and/or infection
- Decidual hemorrhage
- Pathologic uterine distention
- Maternal genome

These pathophysiologic pathways may occur independently but more commonly are present in various degrees of combination [3]. Preterm labor is now thought to be a syndrome initiated by multiple mechanisms, including infection or inflammation, uteroplacental ischemia or hemorrhage, uterine overdistension, stress, and genome association. A precise mechanism cannot be established in most cases; therefore, factors associated with preterm birth, but not obviously in the causal pathway, have been sought to explain preterm labor. An increasing number of risk factors are thought to interact to cause a transition from uterine quiescence toward preterm labor or PPROM (Fig. 32.3) [4].

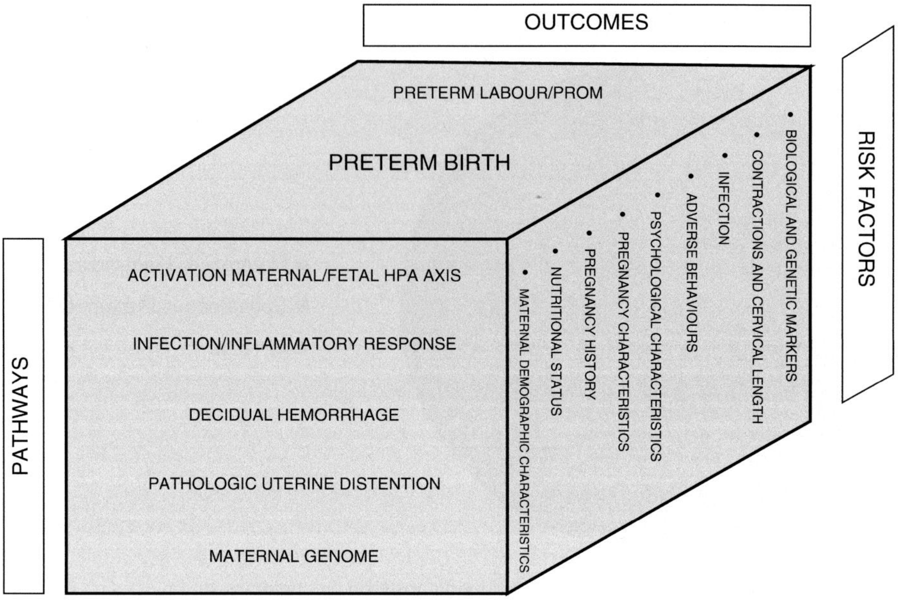

Fig. 32.3 Interactions of risk factors and pathways leading to preterm birth. (The elements shown here are selectively chosen, unweighted, and not intended to represent known quantifiable contributions or relationships). (Modified from Green et al. 2005). HPA hypothalamic-pituitary-adrenal

Premature Activation of the Maternal or Fetal HPA Axis

Stress is a common element activating a series of physiologic adaptive responses in the maternal and fetal compartments. From this perspective, premature activation of the hypothalamic-pituitary-adrenal (HPA) axis can initiate preterm birth. Two mechanisms underlie stress activation of HPA: high levels of psychological or social stress and uteroplacental ischemia [5].

Mothers experiencing high levels of psychological or social stress are at increased risk of preterm birth (generally <2–fold). Major maternal psychosocial stress can activate the maternal HPA axis and has been associated with a slightly higher rate of preterm birth [6]. The risk of preterm birth increases with increasing severity of depression, suggesting a "dose-response" effect. Furthermore, exposure to objectively stressful conditions, such as housing instability and severe material hardship, has also been associated with preterm birth. Although the mechanism underlying the association between psychological or social stress and increased risk of preterm birth is not completely known, a role for corticotropin-releasing hormone (CRH) has been proposed [3]. Women exposed to stressful conditions also have increased serum concentrations of inflammatory markers – such as C-reactive protein. Uteroplacental ischemia is a fetal stressor that can lead to premature fetal HPA activation and has a higher correlation with subsequent preterm than maternal psychosocial stress [3, 6].

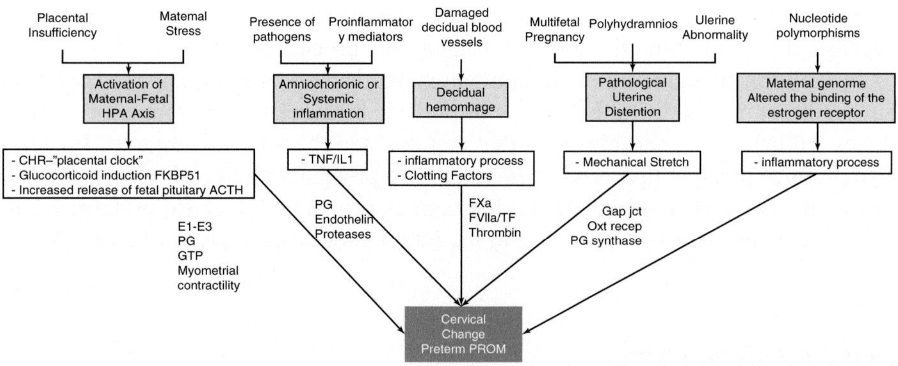

Fig. 32.4 Pathophysiologic pathways toward the shared outcome of preterm birth. (HPA hypothalamic-pituitary-adrenal, CHR corticotropin-releasing hormone, ACTH adrenocorticotropic hormone, E1-E3 estrone, estradiol, estriol, PG prostaglandin, GTP guanosine triphosphate, TNF-α tumor necrosis factor-alpha, IL-1 interleukin-1, F factor, TF tissue factor, Gap jct gap junction, Oxt recep oxytocin receptor)

These findings suggest that systemic inflammation might be a pathway by which stress could increase the risk of preterm birth. The mechanisms by which fetal HPA activation is thought to cause labor include (Fig. 32.4) [5]:

- Increased placental production and release of CRH, which appears to program a "placental clock"
- Glucocorticoid induction of the immunophilin cochaperone FK506-binding protein-51 (FKBP51), which binds to the ligand binding site on the progesterone receptor and glucocorticoid receptor to inhibit progesterone receptor and glucocorticoid receptor-mediated transcription in decidual cells [7]
- Increased release of fetal pituitary adrenocorticotropic hormone (ACTH) secretion, which stimulates production of placental estrogenic compounds and prostaglandins that may activate the myometrium and initiate labor [5]

Exaggerated Inflammatory Response and/or Infection

Intrauterine inflammatory process, associated or not to infection, is a frequent and important mechanism leading to preterm birth. The mechanisms by which they lead to preterm labor are related to proinflammatory mediators [8].

Noninfectious etiologies, such as placental hypoperfusion, also appear to increase production of proinflammatory mediators. Microorganisms are recognized by pattern-recognition receptors, which in turn elicit the release of inflammatory chemokines and cytokines – such as interleukin-8, interleukin-1β, and tumor necrosis factor (TNF)-α. Microbial endotoxins and proinflammatory cytokines stimulate the production of prostaglandins, other inflammatory mediators, and matrix-degrading enzymes. Prostaglandins stimulate uterine contractility. Accumulating evidence suggests that intra-amniotic infection is a chronic process [8, 9].

In addition to inducing an inflammatory response, some organisms may also have a direct role in the pathogenesis of preterm birth related to production of proteases, collagenases, and elastases that can degrade the fetal membranes. Bacteria also produce phospholipase A2 (which leads to prostaglandin synthesis) and endotoxin, substances that stimulate uterine contractions and can cause preterm labor. Degradation of extracellular matrix in the fetal membranes leads to PPROM [9].

Decidual Hemorrhage

Vaginal bleeding caused by placental abruption or placenta previa is associated with a very high risk of preterm delivery, but bleeding in the first and second trimesters that is not associated with either placental abruption or placenta previa is also associated with subsequent preterm birth [5]. Placental abruption (decidual hemorrhage) originates in damaged decidual blood vessels and presents clinically as vaginal bleeding or retroplacental hematoma formation [9, 10].

Decidual hemorrhage results in intense local thrombin generation. Hormonal factors such as progesterone play an important modulator role. Thrombin also induces synthesis of elements of the fibrinolytic system in decidual cells. However, the primary effect of thrombin is to inhibit fibrinolysis via generation of type-1 plasminogen inhibitor (PAI-1) to avoid hemorrhage in the setting of abruption, suggesting that abruption-associated decidual proteolysis and PPROM are mediated primarily by thrombin-enhanced matrix metalloproteinase expression [10, 11]. Decidual hemorrhage can be accompanied by an inflammatory process in the absence of infection. Proteases and free hemoglobin chains activate innate immunity and a feed-forward mechanism that reinforces the inflammatory process, leading to PPROM and preterm birth. In addition, thrombin is a potent inducer of IL-8 in decidual cells, accounting for the dense neutrophil infiltrate observed in abruption-associated PPROM in the absence of infection. The interactive effects of thrombin-enhanced metalloproteinases with neutrophil-derived proteases promote degradation of the fetal membrane extracellular matrix, which can result in PPROM [9, 10].

Pathologic Uterine Distention

Intra-amniotic pressure remains relatively constant throughout gestation despite the growth of the fetus and placenta. This has been attributed to progressive myometrial relaxation due to the effects of progesterone and endogenous myometrial relaxants such as nitric oxide [9, 11].

Multiple gestation, polyhydramnios, and other causes of excessive uterine distention are well-described risk factors for preterm labor. Uterine overdistension, resulting in contractions and PPROM, is believed to be the causative mechanism for the rate of increased spontaneous preterm births [9, 12]. Enhanced stretching of the myometrium induces formation of gap junctions, upregulation of oxytocin receptors, and production of inflammatory cytokines and prostaglandins, and myosin light chain kinase, which are critical events preceding uterine contractions and cervical dilation. Myometrial distention also increases expression of genes with important roles in collagenolysis and inflammation [9, 12].

Multiple gestations – accounting for only 2–3% of infants – carry a substantial risk of preterm delivery and result in 15–20% of all preterm births. Nearly 60% of twins are born preterm. Several lines of evidence indicate that women with twins and higher-order multiple pregnancies also represent a heterogeneous group. Some women suffer preterm labor associated with microbial invasion of the amniotic cavity. Others may have abnormalities of trophoblast invasion leading to vascular pathology with and without fetal growth disorders. These separate mechanisms of disease may operate in conjunction with uterine overdistension to activate the components of the common terminal pathway [9, 13].

Maternal Genome

Women who were themselves born prematurely have a higher risk of preterm birth, and this risk increases by 80 percent in women whose sisters had preterm birth [9].

Preterm birth demonstrates familial aggregation. A gene-environment interaction is said to be present when the risk of a disease (occurrence or severity) among individuals exposed (to both genotype and an environmental factor) is greater or lower than that which is predicted from the presence of either the genotype or the environmental exposure. A variety of single nucleotide polymorphisms, the majority associated with inflammation, have been linked to preterm birth. Gene-to-gene interactions may also play a role in modulating the inflammatory response and, therefore, may also play a role in preterm labor and delivery [5, 9].

Preventing Preterm Birth

Levels of prevention can be person oriented or oriented at the macro level of society. The main categories of prevention have been considered for physicians: primary, secondary, and tertiary.

Primary prevention – action taken to avoid or remove the cause of a health problem in an individual or a population before it arises

Secondary prevention – action taken to detect a health problem at an early stage in an individual or a population, thereby facilitating a cure or reducing or preventing its spread or long-term effects

Tertiary prevention – action taken to reduce the chronic effects of a health problem in an individual or a population [14]

Unfortunately physicians tend to overestimate the benefits and underestimate the harms of preventive and curative interventions. We need to be aware about the role of prevention and possible harm of medical activities implemented with preventive intention. The need to reduce these risks in the latter case was raised by Marc Jamoulle in 1986 with a new category of medical prevention: the quaternary prevention. It is defined as: "action taken to identify patient at risk of overmedicalization, to protect him from new medical invasion, and to suggest to him interventions, which are ethically acceptable" [14].

In this chapter we will address tertiary prevention interventions related to premature birth, observing the care to avoid overmedicalization.

Tertiary Interventions

Most obstetric interventions to reduce the morbidity and mortality of preterm birth are classified as tertiary. These measures are intended to reduce the burden of prematurity-related illness more than to reduce the rate of preterm birth. Tertiary interventions include early diagnosis of preterm labor although education programs directed at pregnant women to allow recognition of the earliest signs of preterm labor have not affected the rate of preterm births [15]. Treatment to arrest preterm labor without rupture of membranes often does not prolong pregnancy enough to allow additional intrauterine growth; however, it can defer preterm birth to allow for interventions that reduce neonatal morbidity and mortality: antenatal transfer to a neonatal intensive care unit, antibiotic treatment to prevent neonatal infection with group B streptococcus, and antenatal use of corticosteroids in the mother to promote fetal lung maturity [15].

Preterm premature rupture of membranes precedes 30% of preterm births. Management includes surveillance for labor, infection, and abruption; use of corticosteroids to promote fetal lung maturity; and use of antibiotics to treat infection. Continued suppression of contractions after acute tocolysis does not reduce the rate of preterm birth. Most evidence does not show that routine cesarean delivery of all preterm or very low-birth weight infants improves neonatal outcome [16].

Detection of conditions proximate to preterm birth offers another opportunity to improve outcome. The most common presenting complaints of preterm labor are uterine contractions, ruptured membranes, and vaginal spotting or bleeding. The last two are typically recognized, but detection of early preterm labor is a challenge because the symptoms and signs of preterm labor arise commonly in normal pregnancy [15].

We may consider as a tertiary interventions [15]:

1. Early diagnosis of preterm labor
2. Treatment of women with acute risk of preterm birth

    (a) Inhibition of acute preterm labor
    (b) Antibiotics

3. Antenatal administration of corticosteroids
4. Care after preterm premature rupture of the fetal membranes
5. Care after acute treatment for preterm labor
6. Delivery of preterm infants

Early Diagnosis of Preterm Labor

Programs to identify women at risk of preterm birth and to educate them to recognize the earliest signs and symptoms of labor did not affect the rate of preterm birth. Treatment to arrest preterm labor established by progressive cervical dilation and effacement or membrane rupture does not prolong pregnancy sufficiently to allow further intrauterine growth and maturation. Treatment can, however, defer preterm birth long enough to allow for interventions that reduce neonatal morbidity and mortality: antenatal transfer of the mother and fetus (especially those expected to be born before 32 weeks' gestation) to a hospital equipped to care for preterm infants in a regionalized system allowing training and development and maintenance of the necessary skilled personnel and facilities. This approach is associated with improved outcomes for preterm infants [15].

Preterm labor probably represents a syndrome rather than a diagnosis since the etiologies are varied. Identifying women with preterm labor who ultimately will give birth preterm is difficult. Approximately 30% of preterm labor spontaneously resolves, and 50% of patients hospitalized for preterm labor actually give birth at term [14].

Labor is defined as an increase in myometrial activity resulting in effacement and dilation of the uterine cervix and delivery of the products of conception. A definitive diagnosis of preterm labor is necessary before further treatment options are considered. Diagnosis requires the presence of both uterine contractions and cervical change (or, in nulliparous patients, an initial cervical exam >2 cm and/or >80% effacement in the setting of uterine contractions of increasing intensity and frequency). Uterine activity in the absence of cervical change should be regarded as preterm contractions and does not require further treatment [17].

The diagnosis of preterm labor is based upon clinical criteria of regular painful uterine contractions accompanied by cervical change (dilation and/or effacement). Vaginal bleeding and/or ruptured membranes in this setting increase diagnostic certainty [18].

The clinical findings of early labor are poorly predictive of the diagnosis; overdiagnosis is common until labor is well established. The following specific criteria are used for preterm labor diagnosis, and Table 32.1 summarizes the diagnostic components used on the labor unit or a labor triage unit [17].

- Uterine contractions (≥4 every 20 minutes or ≥8 in 60 minutes) plus:
  - Cervical dilation ≥3 cm or
  - Cervical length <20 mm on transvaginal ultrasound or
  - Cervical length 20 to <30 mm on transvaginal ultrasound and positive fetal fibronectin

Table 32.1 Clinical assessment of preterm labour

Diagnostic component	Consideration
History	Review history medical, surgical, obstetric, social considering risk factors associated with preterm birth
Maternal signs and symptoms	Pelvic pressure Lower abdominal cramping Lower back pain Vaginal loss – mucous, blood, fluid Regular uterine activity
Physical examination	Vital signs Abdominal palpation to assess: Uterine tone Contractions Fetal size Presentation Sterile speculum examination to: Confirm/exclude rupture of membranes Visualize cervix/membranes Assess amniotic fluid aspect Collect high vaginal swab for microscopy culture and sensitivity Perform test for the presence of fetal fibronectin (if not contraindicated) Collect combined low vaginal and anorectal swab for group B streptococcus [GBS] (insert swab 2 cm into vagina, and then insert same swab 1 cm into anus) Assess cervical dilatation by sterile digital vaginal examination unless contraindicated by ruptured membranes or suspected placenta previa
Fetal surveillance	Fetal heart rate Cardiotocography (take into account gestational age – interpret with caution if less than 28 weeks' gestation) Ultrasound examination
Laboratory investigations	High vaginal swabs Genital swab for GBS Midstream specimen of urine for bacteriology
Ultrasound examination	Fetal growth Fetal well-being Fetal number Presentation Amniotic fluid volume Placenta localization Fetal Doppler evaluation (for fetal well-being evaluation) Transvaginal cervical evaluation – measurement to women with identified or suspected preterm labor (where available) – consider therapeutic interventions when the cervix measures less than 25 mm
Fetal fibronectin testing	Symptomatic preterm labor patient: Between 22 + 0 and 36 + 0 weeks' gestation Intact membranes Cervical dilatation less than or equal to 3 cm

A definitive diagnosis of preterm labor is necessary before further treatment options are considered. Diagnosis requires the presence of both uterine contractions and cervical change [17]. The clinicians may use clinical judgment and appropriate consultation in assessing the need for admission. Consider the fetal fibronectin (fFN) result in the context of the overall clinical circumstances. Fetal fibronectin testing may improve assessment of overall risk, reduce unnecessary transfer, and ultimately reduce longer-term costs [18].

Fetal fibronectin is a glycoprotein thought to promote adhesion between the fetal chorion and maternal decidua. It is normally present in low concentrations in the cervicovaginal secretions between 18 and 34–36 weeks' gestation, rising as term approaches. Elevated levels off in cervicovaginal secretions after 22 weeks' gestation are associated with an increased risk of preterm labor. A negative fFN is associated with a 99.5% negative predictive value for preterm within 7 days and 99.2% in the next 14 days [18].

Uterine activity in the absence of cervical change should be regarded as preterm contractions and does not require further treatment [19].

Treatment of Women with Acute Risk of Preterm Birth

(a) Inhibition of acute preterm labor [1, 18] (Prevention of Preterm Labor: 2011 Update on Tocolysis, Drugs for the Treatment and Prevention of Preterm Labor, WHO, up to date)

Because the contracting uterus is the most frequently recognized antecedent of preterm birth, stopping contractions has been the focus of therapeutic approaches [20]. The inhibition of myometrial contractions is called tocolysis, and a drug administered to that end is referred to as a tocolytic agent. Tocolytics were initially characterized 60 years ago and are generally administered when a diagnosis of preterm labor is confirmed between 23 0/7 and 33 6/7 weeks' gestation. Although therapy that inhibits contractions does not prevent preterm birth, several goals may still be achieved [18, 20]:

- Delay delivery by at least 48 hours when it is safe to do so in order that antenatal corticosteroids (primary or rescue) given to the mother have time to achieve their maximum fetal/neonatal effects
- Provide time for safe transport of the mother, if indicated, to a facility that has an appropriate level of neonatal care if the patient delivers preterm
- Prolong pregnancy when it is safe to do so and when there are underlying, self-limited conditions that can cause labor, such as pyelonephritis or abdominal surgery, and are unlikely to cause recurrent preterm labor.

The mechanism of action of tocolytic agents involves the regulation of the myosin light chain kinase activity, specifically, calcium and cyclic AMP [20]. One of the two major pathways is used to abrogate myometrial contractility: by generation or alteration of intracellular messengers or by inhibiting the synthesis or blocking the action of a known myometrial stimulant agent (Fig. 32.5).

Maternal contraindications to tocolytics include:

- Severe preeclampsia
- Hemorrhage
- Significant cardiac disease as these medications create a greater risk for maternal hemodynamic compromise and collapse

Fetal contraindications to tocolysis include:

- Gestational age greater than or equal to 34 weeks
- Lethal fetal anomalies
- Intrauterine fetal demise
- Chorioamnionitis
- Fetal compromise that may necessitate immediate delivery

Selection of the appropriate tocolytic is determined by the efficacy, maternal and fetal risks, and the side effect profile of each medication. Administration of tocolytic drugs can reduce the strength and frequency of uterine contractions. Women in the early phases of acute preterm labor, when cervical dilation is not advanced, are optimum candidates for tocolytic therapy [18]. Tocolysis is indicated when the overall benefits of delaying delivery outweigh the risks. Based on the existing literature, the most common tocolytics drugs include oxytocin receptor antagonists, betamimetics, calcium channel blockers, magnesium sulfate, prostaglandin synthase (cyclooxygenase – COX) inhibitors, and nitric oxide (NO) donors [18–20]. Table 32.2 summarizes tocolytics use and effects. The National Institute for Health

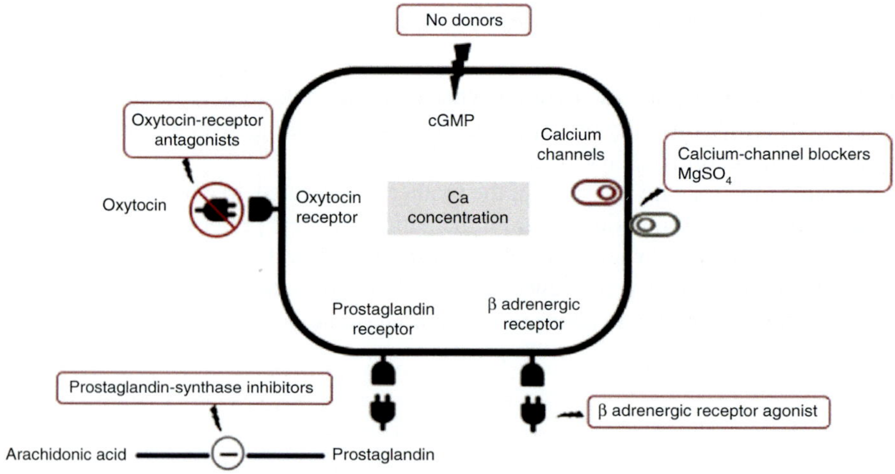

Fig. 32.5 Mechanisms of action of commonly used tocolytic drugs

and Care Excellence (NICE) guideline and the World Health Organization (WHO) recommend calcium channel blockers (nifedipine) as the first choice. However, in Europe, it is widely used in clinical practice because of its low side effects profile. Atosiban seems to be an adequate therapeutic choice for effective tocolysis with a low maternal and fetal adverse effects profile [16, 18].

Specific conditions are subject to discussion: in multiple pregnancies, expanded blood volume and anemia may predispose to pulmonary edema when tocolytic agents such as β-adrenergic receptor agonists, magnesium sulfate, and calcium channel blockers are prescribed [19]. In these pregnancies, atosiban, with its low side effects incidence, seems to be the safest choice [16].

(b) Antibiotics (Obstetric Clinical Algorithms, up to date)

Although subclinical genital tract infection clearly contributes to the pathogenesis of preterm birth, routine administration of prophylactic antibiotics to women in threatened preterm labor with intact membranes and without evidence of infection is not recommended [17]. If preterm labor ensues or there is imminent risk of preterm birth, give intrapartum antibiotic prophylaxis for prevention of early-onset group B streptococcal disease irrespective of GBS status or membrane status. Antibiotics for prolonging latency in preterm premature rupture of membranes and for treatment of clinical chorioamnionitis are discussed separately [19].

Intrapartum antibiotic prophylaxis can prevent early-onset GBS infection in GBS-positive women. The treatment of choice to prevent early-onset neonatal GBS infection is penicillin G (5 million units intravenously followed by 2.5 million units every 4 hours). A minimum of 4 hours of antibiotic is recommended, and it should be continued until delivery is complete [19].

Second-line antibiotics have been recommended for GBS prophylaxis in women who are allergic to penicillin, including clindamycin (900 mg IV every 8 hours), erythromycin (500 mg IV every 6 hours), and vancomycin (1 g every 12 hours). Approximately 20–30% of GBS isolates are resistant to erythromycin, and 10–20% are resistant to clindamycin [17]. If resistance to erythromycin or clindamycin is documented, vancomycin should be administered. An alternative approach is to perform penicillin skin testing in such woman, but this is rarely done [19].

(c) Antenatal administration of corticosteroids

Antenatal corticosteroids are associated with a significant reduction in rates of neonatal death, respiratory distress syndrome, and intraventricular hemorrhage. Routinely recommend corticosteroids to women with a viable fetus who are at increased risk of preterm birth from 24 + 0 to 34 + 6 weeks' gestation [18].

There is no evidence of long-term harm or benefit (in early childhood) from multiple courses of antenatal corticosteroids [19]. Corticosteroids use and management are discussed separately on Chap. 35.

(d) Care after preterm premature rupture of the fetal membranes

Premature rupture of the membranes (PROM) refers to rupture of the fetal membranes prior to the onset of labor. It can occur at term or preterm. Preterm PROM (pPROM) refers to PROM prior to 37 0/7 weeks of gestation. The management of pPROM is largely based on gestational age [9]. Contraindications to expectant management include intra-amniotic infection (chorioamnionitis), nonreassuring fetal

Table 32.2 Tocolytics use and effects

Agent or class	Side effects		Contraindications	Dose	Monitoring
	Maternal	Fetal			
Beta-agonists	Tachycardia and hypotension, tremor palpitations, shortness of breath, chest discomfort, pulmonary edema, hypokalemia, hyperglycemia	Tachycardia	Tachycardia-sensitive cardiac disease, women with poorly controlled hyperthyroidism or diabetes mellitus, risk for massive hemorrhage	Terbutaline is the most commonly used. The dose is variable, but generally, 0.25 mg is administered subcutaneously every 20–30 minutes, for up to four doses or until tocolysis has occurred. It can also be administered as a continuous intravenous infusion at a rate of 2.5–5 mg/min, increasing by 2.5–5 mg/min every 20–30 minutes to a maximum of 25 mg/min or until the contractions have quiesced	Cumulative fluid intake, urine output, and maternal symptoms, especially shortness of breath, chest pain, or tachycardia
COX inhibitors	Nausea, esophageal reflux, gastritis, and emesis; platelet dysfunction	In utero closure of ductus arteriosus, oligohydramnios	Platelet dysfunction or bleeding diathesis, hepatic dysfunction, gastrointestinal ulcerative disease, renal dysfunction, and asthma	Initial loading dose of 50–100 mg (orally or rectally), followed by 25 mg orally every 4–6 hours for 48 hours	Sonographic evaluation for oligohydramnios and narrowing of the fetal ductus arteriosus is warranted at least weekly
Ca channel blockers	Dizziness, flushing, hypotension	There are no data regarding fetal side effects with the oral doses commonly used for labor inhibition	Known hypersensitivity to the drugs, hypotension, or preload-dependent cardiac lesions and should be used with caution in women with heart failure with reduced ejection fraction	Initial loading dose of 20–30 mg orally, followed by an additional 10–20 mg orally every 4–8 hours for up to 48 hours, with a maximum dose of 180 mg/day	

Agent or class	Side effects		Contraindications	Dose	Monitoring
	Maternal	Fetal			
Oxytocin receptor antagonists	Hypersensitivity, injection-site reaction	There are no data regarding fetal side effects	There are no absolute contraindications to use of atosiban	Initial loading dose of a bolus of 6.75 mg intravenous, followed by a 300 mcg/min infusion for three hours, and then 100 mcg/min for up to 45 hours	
Magnesium sulfate	Flushing, diaphoresis, nausea, loss of deep-tendon reflexes, respiratory paralysis, cardiac arrest	There are no data regarding fetal side effects	Myasthenia gravis	Initial loading dose of 4 g intravenous over 20 minutes, followed by a continuous infusion of 1 or 2 g/hour	Signs and symptoms of magnesium toxicity can be assessed by history and physical examinations. Routine magnesium levels are not necessary
Nitric oxide donors	Dizziness, flushing, hypotension	There are no data regarding fetal side effects	Women with hypotension or with preload-dependent cardiac lesions, such as aortic insufficiency	10 mg glyceryl trinitrate patch applied to the skin of the abdomen. After one hour, if there is no reduction in contraction frequency or intensity, an additional patch is applied; no more than two patches are administered simultaneously. The patches can be left in place for 24 hours, after which they are removed and the patient reassessed	

Ca calcium, *COX* cCyclooxygenase

testing, clinically significant placental abruption, or active labor. The optimal gestational age for delivery is unclear and controversial [19]. Management of pPROM is discussed separately on Chap. 37.

(e) Magnesium sulfate for neuroprotection

The use of magnesium sulfate is recommended for women at risk of imminent preterm birth before 32 weeks of gestation for prevention of cerebral palsy. This recommendation applies to women carrying either singleton or multiple pregnancies [19].

Treatment should be started with a bolus of 4–6 g administered over 30 min, followed by a maintenance dose of 1–2 g for 12 h. Magnesium sulfate for neuroprotection is discussed separately on Chap. 36.

(f) Care after acute treatment for preterm labor

When preterm birth does not occur, the management of pregnancies after resolution of a suspected episode of acute idiopathic preterm labor needs to coordinate care and discharge planning with the family, relevant healthcare professionals, and the referring hospital [21]. However it lacks high-quality evidence on which to base the recommendations on Table 32.3.

(g) Delivery of preterm infants

Table 32.3 Management recommendations for pregnancies after resolution of a suspected episode of acute idiopathic preterm labor

Aspect	Considerations
Corticosteroids	The use of antenatal corticosteroids at various gestational ages and the indications for rescue/salvage/booster therapy in patients who have received a previous course of therapy are discussed in detail on Chap. 35 If corticosteroids are administered to women before the 29 + 0 week of gestation because of an imminent risk of preterm birth and steroids were administered more than 7 days previously, a further dose of steroids may be administered after the patient has been reassessed if the imminent risk of preterm birth is increasing
Progesterone	Continue the regimen of progesterone supplementation after resolution of an episode of suspected preterm labor if the pregnant woman received supplemental progesterone to reduce the risk of preterm birth because of a history of prior preterm birth or for a sonographic short cervix
Hospitalization	≥34 weeks' gestation after acute preterm labor resolves can be discharged as long as tests of fetal well-being are reassuring and there are no additional complications that warrant hospitalization <34 weeks' gestation: the duration of hospitalization is made on a case-by-case basis, depending on patient-specific factors including gestational age, cervical status, past obstetric history, distance between their residence and the hospital, and coexisting obstetric and medical problems
Cervical pessary	Consensus-based recommendation is to only utilize pessaries in the context of a clinical trial until a benefit in neonatal outcome is established, but there is some evidence from a prospective randomized study that placement of a cervical pessary in pregnant women previously treated for premature labor who have a shortened cervical length as measured by transvaginal ultrasound (<25 mm between and <20 mm between GW 24 + 0 and GW 29 + 6; <15 mm and <10 mm between GW 30 + 0 and GW33 + 6) may reduce the rate of preterm births for singletons and twins respectively. The decision whether or not to carry out cervical pessary must be made on a case-by-case basis, after acute treatment for preterm labor

Aspect	Considerations
Maintenance tocolysis	It is an unproven intervention. It does not prolong pregnancy, prevent preterm birth, or improve neonatal outcome. According to the information currently available, maintenance tocolysis (generally defined as tocolysis for more than 48 h) should not be used to reduce the rate of preterm births or neonatal morbidity and mortality rates
Discharge	Consider usual discharge criteria including: Maternal vital signs Signs of chorioamnionitis Membrane status Contractions infrequent/irregular Cervical change/TVCL (if measured) Normal CTG relevant to gestational age Provide the woman with information that: Aids her recognition of the signs and symptoms of preterm labor Identifies risk reduction measures appropriate to the circumstances Provides instruction about when to seek clinical advice Refer to Appendix B: Consumer advice after threatened preterm labor Determine follow-up and ongoing clinical surveillance requirements
Bed rest	There is a lack of evidence to advise bed rest for women with a recent episode of preterm labor of efficacy in order to prolong gestation or reduce preterm birth and the known significant risks of prolonged immobility. They may continue typical activities of daily living There is a general consensus that women at high risk for preterm birth should limit recreational exercise and avoid returning to work if their work involves working more than 40 hours per week, night shifts, prolonged standing, or heavy physical work

Fetal Monitoring

There is limited evidence about the usefulness of specific features to suggest hypoxia or acidosis in preterm babies. Fetal heart rate monitoring using either cardiotocography or external ultrasound may be offered to women in established preterm labor but with no other risk [22].

Mode of Birth

There is insufficient high-quality evidence about whether mode of birth affects neonatal morbidity and outcomes in established preterm labor [10]. Routine delivery by cesarean section for the purpose of improving preterm newborn outcomes is not recommended, regardless of cephalic or breech presentation. Preterm cesarean section is usually technically more difficult to perform and is not without risk to the baby as the lower segment is usually not well formed [22]. A vertical uterine incision may be required with risks to future pregnancies including scar dehiscence, uterine rupture, placental adherence, and maternal death [22].

Mode of delivery depends on fetal presentation and gestational age. Cesarean section for diagnosed or established preterm less than 25 + 0 weeks' gestation (vertex or breech) is not generally recommended for fetal indications alone [17]. The evidence regarding optimal mode of birth for preterm breech ≥26 + 0 weeks is conflicting and unclear due to a lack of high-quality studies; usually cesarean section is considered for women presenting established preterm labor between 26 + 0 and 36 + 6 weeks [17, 22].

Vaginal birth is recommended for cephalic presentation unless there are specific contraindications to vaginal birth or maternal conditions necessitating cesarean section if the fetus is aged ≥30 0/7 weeks of gestation. Delivery by cesarean section may be considered after carefully weighing up the risks/benefits in each individual case in cephalic presentation if the fetus is aged <30 0/7 weeks of gestation [22].

Timing of Cord Clamping for Preterm Babies

Clamp the cord as soon as possible if a preterm baby needs to be moved away from the mother for resuscitation or there is significant maternal bleeding. Wait at least 30 seconds, but no longer than 3 minutes, before clamping the cord of preterm babies if the mother and baby are stable [22]. Timing of cord clamping is discussed in detail on Chap. 54.

Preterm Labor Algorithms

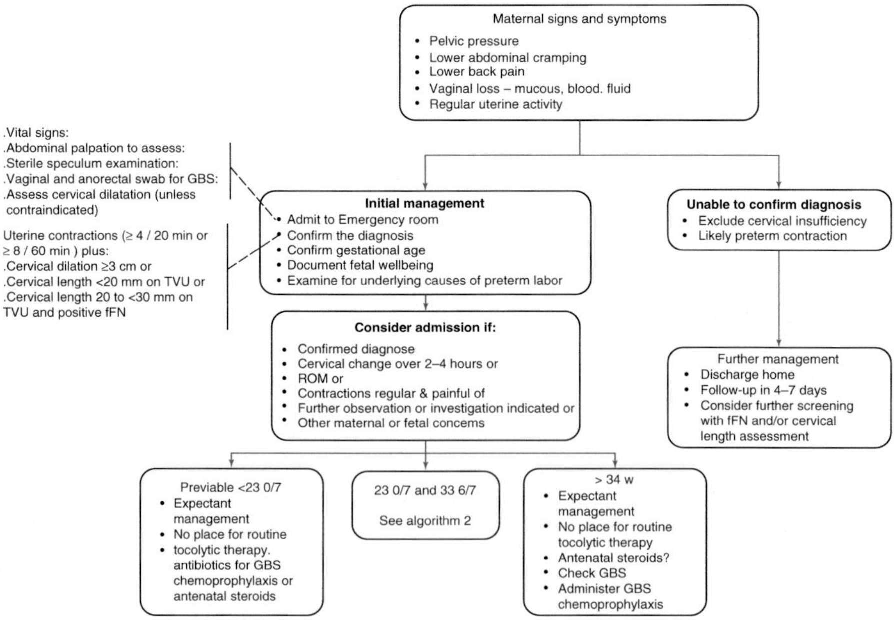

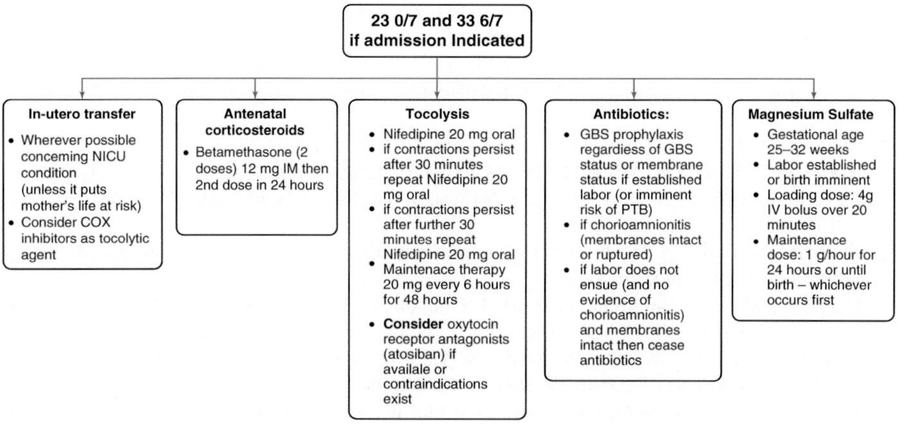

References

1. WHO. 2015. WHO recommendations on interventions to improve preterm birth outcomes. Geneva, Switzerland: World Health Organization. Retrieved from http://www.who.int/reproductivehealth/publications/maternal_perinatal_health/preterm-birth-guideline/en/.
2. ACOG Committee Opinion No. 579 (Reaffirmed 2019): definition of term pregnancy. Obstet Gynecol. 2013;122(5):1139–40.
3. Green NS, Damus K, Simpson JL, Iams J, Reece EA, Hobel CJ, Merkatz IR, Greene MF, Schwarz RH, March of Dimes Scientific Advisory Committee On Prematurity. Research agenda for preterm birth: recommendations from the March of Dimes. Am J Obstet Gynecol. 2005;193(3 Pt 1):626–35.
4. Goldenberg RL, Culhane JF, Iams JD, Romero R. Epidemiology and causes of preterm birth. Lancet. 2008;371(9606):75–84.
5. Lockwood CJ, Berghella V, Barss VA. Pathogenesis of spontaneous preterm birth. https://www.uptodate.com/contents/pathogenesis-of-spontaneous-...th/print?search=preterm%20labour&topicRef=6798&source=see_link.
6. Copper RL, Goldenberg RL, Das A, et al. The preterm prediction study: maternal stress is associated with spontaneous preterm birth at less than thirty-five weeks gestation. Am J Obstet Gynecol. 1996;175:1286–92.
7. Hähle A, Merz S, Meyners C, Hausch F. The many faces of FKBP51. Biomol Ther. 2019;9:35.
8. Bloomfield FH, Oliver MH, Hawkins P, Campbell M, Phillips DJ, Gluckman PD, et al. A periconceptional nutritional origin for noninfectious pre- term birth. Science. 2003;300:606.
9. Romero R, Espinoza J, Kusanovic J, Gotsch F, Hassan S, Erez O, Chaiworapongsa T, Mazor M. The preterm parturition syndrome. BJOG. 2006;113(Suppl. 3):17–42.
10. Romero R, Dey SK, Fisher SJ. Preterm labor: one syndrome, many causes. Science. 2014;345(6198):760–5.
11. Lockwood CJ, Kayisli UA, Stocco C, et al. Abruption-induced preterm delivery is associated with thrombin-mediated functional progesterone withdrawal in decidual cells. Am J Pathol. 2012;181:2138.
12. Phelan JP, Park YW, Ahn MO, Rutherford SE. Polyhydramnios and perinatal outcome. J Perinatol. 1990;10:347–50.
13. Besinger R, Carlson N. The physiology of preterm labor. In: Keith L, Papiernik E, Keith D, Luke B, editors. Multiple pregnancy: epidemiology, gestation and perinatal outcome. London: Parthenon Publishing; 1995. p. 415.

14. Martins C, Godycki-Cwirko M, Heleno B, Brodersen J. Quaternary prevention: reviewing the concept. Eur J Gen Pract. 2018;24(1):106–11.
15. Iams JD, Romero R, Culhane JF, Goldenberg RL. Preterm birth 2. Primary, secondary, and tertiary interventions to reduce the morbidity and mortality of preterm birth. Lancet. 2008;371:164–75.
16. Simhan HN, Caritis SN. Prevention of preterm delivery. N Engl J Med. 2007;357:477–87.
17. Norwitz ER, Saade GR, Miller H, Davidson CM. Preterm labor in obstetric clinical algorithms, 2nd edn. John Wiley & Sons, Ltd.; The Atrium, Southern Gate, Chichester, West Sussex 2017. p. 150–2.
18. Simhan HN, Caritis S. Inhibition of acute preterm labor. https://www.uptodate.com/contents/inhibition-of-acute-preterm-labor.
19. Berger R, Abele H, Bahlmann F, Bedei I, Doubek K, Felderhoff-Müser U, Fluhr H, Garnier Y, Grylka-Baeschlin S, Helmer H, Herting E, Hoopmann M, Hösli I, Hoyme U, Jendreizeck A, Krentel H, Kuon R, Lütje W, Mader S, Maul H, Mendling W, Mitschdörfer B, Nicin T, Nothacker M, Olbertz D, Rath W, Roll C, Schlembach D, Schleußner E, Schütz F, Seifert-Klauss V, Steppat S, Surbek D. Prevention and therapy of preterm birth. Guideline of the DGGG, OEGGG and SGGG (S2k Level, AWMF Registry Number 015/025, February 2019) - part 2 with recommendations on the tertiary prevention of preterm birth and the management of preterm premature rupture of membranes. Geburtshilfe Frauenheilkd. 2019;79(8):813–33.
20. Hubinont C, Debieve F. Prevention of preterm labour: 2011 update on tocolysis. J Pregnancy. 2011;2011:941057.
21. Simhan HN, Caritis S. Management of pregnant women after resolution of an episode of acute idiopathic preterm labor. https://www.uptodate.com/contents/management-of-pregnant-women-afterresolution-of-an-episode-of-acute-idiopathic-preterm-labor?-search=preterm%20labour&topicRef=6798&source=see_link.
22. National Institute for Health and Care Excellence (NICE). Preterm labour and birth. London: (UK); 2015 Nov. www.nice.org.uk/guidance/ng25.

Chapter 33
Prematurity: Evaluation of Fetal Well-Being and Delivery

Ana B. Bianchi and Miguel Ruoti

Preterm birth is defined by the World Health Organization (WHO) as a delivery before 37 completed weeks of gestation; extremely PTB is defined as occurring at less than 28 weeks, very preterm delivery as occurring between 28 and 32 weeks, and moderate to late PTB as occurring from 32 to 36 weeks [1, 2].

These distinctions are clinically important as there is a great increment in morbidity and mortality as the gestational age decreases among preterm births, and the obstetric management often differs at different stages of pregnancy. Prematurity has been the leading cause of neonatal mortality worldwide for at least a decade and has also become the leading cause of childhood mortality of children younger than 5 years of age.

Globally, each year, 15 million babies are born preterm, which is estimated to be about 11% of all deliveries. This 11% of babies born prematurely account for the 75% of all perinatal mortality and 50% of children with long-term neurologic impairment being responsible for most of the adulthood diseases of these children [3–5].

The leading cause of both neonatal and childhood morbimortality is a critical global problem in public health due to its implications for morbidity and mortality, as well as its socioeconomic liability.

Preterm birth is one of the great obstetric challenges. Despite the lack of strategies to predict and prevent infant morbimortality associated with preterm birth, it has decreased during the last years due to the management of neonatal intensive care of preterm infants which has improved the outcomes, for instance, maternal and fetal transportation to specialized health facilities in order to improve births with special neonatal units, the use of corticosteroids, progesterone administration to a mother at risk of preterm birth, etc. [6–8].

A. B. Bianchi (✉)
Perinatal Department, Pereira Rossell Hospital, Montevideo, Montevideo, Uruguay

M. Ruoti
University Asuncion, Asunción, Paraguay

© Springer Nature Switzerland AG 2022

R. A. Moreira de Sá, E. B. d. Fonseca (eds.), *Perinatology*,
https://doi.org/10.1007/978-3-030-83434-0_33

To determine that a PTB has occurred is a challenge in many settings in which ultrasound is not readily available for pregnancy dating. In many countries there is a great amount of difficulties to set up prenatal controls that allow physicians to determine the exact gestational age of the pregnancy. The gestational age distributions are derived from other dating methods such as last menstrual period (LMP).

The sequelae of PTB can be lifelong with poor long-term outcomes for premature infant survival including a high risk of cerebral palsy, learning disabilities, and visual disorders as well as the increase of chronic diseases in adulthood.

The incidence varies according to different continents. In Europe, for instance, the incidence is between the 5% and 7%. In the USA it is 11%. In Asia and Africa, it is 18%, especially in sub-Saharan Africa. In Latin America it is around 9–10% depending on the countries.

Preterm birth is a serious public health problem that involves several components of high impact. Primarily it exposes the newborn from the beginning to a series of complications that increase morbimortality. The impact for the mother, the family, and the environment constitutes a threat in respect to the concept of integral health. From a sanitary point of view, it is an indicator of the increment in health system costs.

Preterm birth may be classified into two general presentations: spontaneous and elective.

Between 70% and 80% of preterm births are spontaneous due to preterm labor (40–50%) or as a result of a premature rupture of ovular membranes (20–30%) [6–8]. The other 20 or 30% are indicated preterm births due to maternal or fetal problems in which the health of both the mother and the fetus is in danger and finish in interruption of pregnancy. Elderly age pregnant women would be carriers of great amounts of chronic diseases such as obesity, diabetes, and IUGR hypertension and are more likely to have high-risk pregnancies.

One of the measures which have shown to decrease incidence of elective preterm birth is to make protocols of specific maternal or ovular pathologies [9–12].

Prediction and Prevention of Preterm Birth

- Primary prevention – identification and treatment of risk factors
- Secondary prevention – early diagnosis of preterm labor
- Tertiary prevention – interventions to minimize complications of preterm birth

Most of the efforts are focused on the tertiary prevention.

Preterm birth represents a final common pathway for a number of pathogenic processes which are the real problems. It is a syndrome of multiple causes, it is difficult to predict and start an early and effective treatment that could reduce complications [13–16] (Table 33.1).

It is important to act upon risk factors for primary prevention in order to determine high-, medium-, or low-risk pregnancies knowing that around 2/3 of preterm

Table 33.1 Risk factors

Epidemiological
Low socioeconomic status
Inadequate nutrition
Physical and mental maternal stress
Family and gender violence
Lack of satisfaction at work due to long working hours
Consumption of toxic substances (cocaine was associated in 60% of preterm births)
Tobacco consumption
Climate and environmental factors
Maternal age (both extreme ages)
Short intergenesic period less than 12 months
Race (African American women have higher rates of preterm birth or PROM)
Previous obstetric records of preterm birth
Premature rupture of membranes
Cervical incompetence
Genital hemorrhage of trimesters 1 and 2
Multiple pregnancy
Hypertensive stages of pregnancy
Placental abruption/placenta pathologies
Placenta previa/polyhydramnios/oligohydramnios
Fetal malformations
Fetal growth restrictions
Assisted reproductive techniques (singleton or multiple pregnancy)
Infections/bacterial vaginosis
Diabetes
Maternal pathology
Gynecologic: Cervico-isthmic incompetence
Cervical surgery
Uterine myomatosis malformations
Surgical: Surgery during pregnancy
Infections
Maternal or fetal genetics/epigenetics

births do not have an associated factor. However, it is well known that a previous preterm birth history increases the recurrence of a second preterm birth in 30%, and in multiple pregnancy the risk is between 12% and 16% before 32/34 weeks of gestation [17–19].

Ideally the identification of modifiable and nonmodifiable risk factors for prematurity either in preconception or in the first weeks of gestation will lead to interventions which would help improve predictive capacity.

However, 2/3 of preterm births occur in women without known risk factors. The causality has been difficult to prove, and once preterm birth is triggered, the interventions are above all more focused on reducing the negative impact in the perinatal maternal health than avoiding a preterm birth [20, 21].

The most important risk independent factor is the reproductive history in which spontaneous preterm birth tends to be repeated.

Mother interventions must include preventive control and birth preparation in a third-degree neonatal maternal health facility [22, 23].

Maternal nutritional state, substance abuse, infections, social as well as working and economical stress, and climate changes worldwide are all highlighted to be risk factors.

Epigenetic factors would give information about the subjacent mechanisms to the changes of DNA methylation which can be indicators of a future health risk.

DNA methylation is an epigenetic change more widely studied. It is affected by the environment and is a modification characterized by the addition of a methyl group to the 5'position of a cytosine into a dinucleotide place of guanine-cytosine.

Understanding how the environmental risk factors affect DNA and the subsequent methylation of the genetic component will allow clinicians to evaluate the biomarkers suggested for prematurity [24–26] and help with prediction and prevention.

Maternal stress/gender violence during pregnancy is considered a predominant factor in preterm birth due to hypothalamic-pituitary-adrenal axis dysregulation that activates immune inflammatory pathways.

The activation of inflammatory and neuroendocrine pathways in response to stress or any other factor related to it results in the activation of a prostaglandin cytokine cascade in response to infection.

The risk of preterm birth was associated with the degree of maternal malnutrition, though this association could be mitigated by boosting the adequate weight during gestation.

The use of folic acid seems to have a positive impact in the fetus as it decreases premature rates (low weight at birth and small for gestational age). Even though nutritional requirements are improved, more randomized studies are needed in order to formalize them in an indication [27–30].

Risk Marker

Cervical Assessment by Ultrasonography

Cervical shortening as well as cervical opening can start weeks before birth labor. These modifications emerge from biochemical modifications of cervical tissue (these mechanisms are unknown). The transvaginal ultrasound is the most effective method for cervical assessment.

It is a reliable and reproducible method to assess cervical length.

Early asymptomatic dilation and effacement of the cervix (cervical *insufficiency*) is associated with an increase of preterm birth risk.

Transvaginal ultrasound must be performed during the morphologic ultrasound between 20 and 24 weeks. If a cervical shortening is found, it is determined as an independent risk factor of preterm birth and not as a predictive factor.

When cervical measure is lower than 20 mm between the cervical internal orifice and cervical external orifice (found in 5% of the population), it is considered a significant risk for pregnant women. There are authors who embrace 15 mm of length that is found in 1% of the population. Other authors embrace 25 mm which is found in 10% of the population.

Cervical length can be defined as:

- High-risk patients with a cervix below or equal to 15 mm
- Medium-risk patients with a cervix between 15 and 25 mm
- Low-risk patients with a cervix greater than 25 mm

Cervical shortening is associated with imminent preterm birth especially when cervical length is below 15 mm before 20 weeks of gestation. Vaginal ultrasound is accepted as the best tool to measure cervical length (Figs. 33.1 and 33.2).

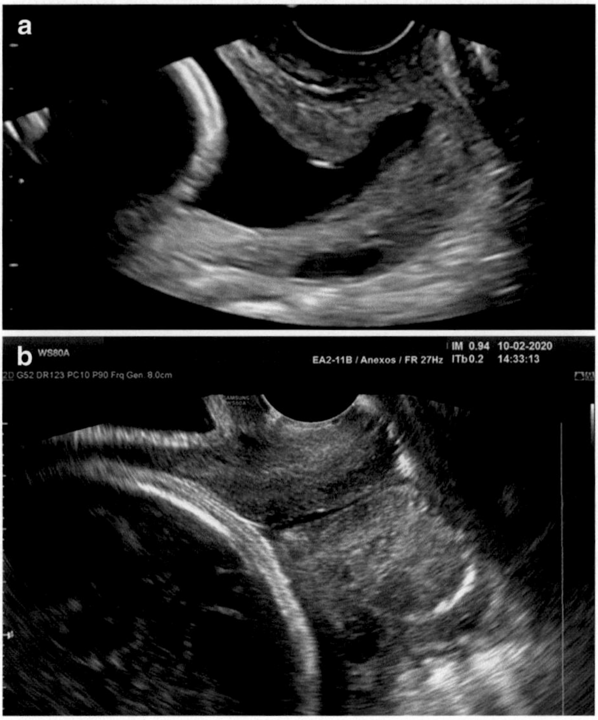

Figs. 33.1 and 33.2 Cervix assessed by transvaginal ultrasound (**a**) short cervix membrane protrusion. (**b**) measure of the cervix

Biochemical Markers

Fibronectin, a high molecular weight glycoprotein which is produced by the trophoblast, is the most used among the biochemical markers.

It is commonly present in the cervicovaginal content between 20 and 22 weeks of gestation. Then it disappears and later reappears at 36 weeks.

Its presence between 24 and 36 weeks increases the risk of preterm birth.

In risky population, fibronectin is a good predictor of preterm birth in contrast to other markers. It has also a great predictive negative value which is very useful to determine the risk of prematurity. Fibronectin and transvaginal cervical assessments together increase the predictive value as well as the risk assessment of a preterm birth. The fibronectin test, performed to symptomatic patients, enables to identify false positives and decreases unnecessary admissions.

Inflammation/Infection

There is clear evidence of the link between infection, inflammation, and prematurity, which is probably mediated by prostaglandins. Anatomo-pathological examinations of the placentas of a preterm group consistently revealed that between 20% and 75% of them had histological elements of chorioamnionitis and also in 30–60% membrane cultures were positive [31–33].

In the presence of a clinical or paraclinical diagnosis of bacterial vaginosis in symptomatic pregnant women, the treatment is fully indicated. Bacterial vaginosis is a common alteration of the vaginal flora and is associated with preterm birth and PROM.

However, in low-risk and asymptomatic patients, neither the treatment nor seeking of bacterial vaginosis is recommendable because it does not demonstrate a decrease in the occurrence of preterm birth.

Prevention and Management

It is a priority to try to determine the patients who have risk factors in order to perform the best interventions.

There are no uniformly effective interventions to prevent preterm labor. Prophylactic therapy including tocolytic drugs, bed rest, and hydration in asymptomatic women at high risk of preterm birth has not been shown to be effective.

Appropriate interventions should be offered to women based on either history or additional screening test by clinicians able to discuss the relevant risks and benefits according to up-to-date evidence and relevant guidance, for example, preterm clinical network guidance.

It is essential for the neonatal team to be well communicated with the family of the newborn in order to make appropriate decisions together. Moreover, it is necessary an adequate reference as well as a counter reference of the patient in order to attach discharge records or transferences and paraclinical and consents.

A suitable protocol for optimal cord clamping as well as implementing regionalization policies and an adequate and timely transfer optimizes perinatal outcomes [34, 35].

Transportation of preterm inside the womb decreases significantly the complications of transportation for preterm newborn and enables to maintain the binomial maternal-fetus-neonatal. This is the form of transportation that must be chosen if possible though risk-benefit assessment must be analyzed.

The pathway how to end a pregnancy in the gestation of a spontaneous preterm (vaginal delivery vs cesarean section) is a complex and controversial issue. This controversy not only lies in making the decision between vaginal delivery vs cesarean section but in the difficulty to implement what the scientific evidence defines and what is the reality of gestation.

If there is not a formal indication for C-section (double-layer closure, podalic, etc.), the birth must be vaginal. Elective cesarean section is associated with well-known risks for the mother, and there are no real proven benefits for preterm newborns with low weight and cephalic presentation [36–39].

The theoretical justification for a routine cesarean section for preterm with very low weight is based on the hypothesis that a C-section could prevent hypoxia and asphyxia as well as decrease the incidence of intraventricular hemorrhage. However, there is no solid evidence that supports this hypothesis. The evidence suggests that vaginal delivery is not a factor which affects the perinatal mortality or the post-neurodevelopment of these neonates.

Even if vaginal delivery for preterm is preferred, fetal intrapartum monitoring can become a complex challenge in early gestational ages, for it does not present the same aggravation diagnostic patterns of a full-term pregnancy.

Premature fetus produces patterns of fetal cardiac frequency which are normal for the gestational age, but slightly different from the typical patterns observed during full-term pregnancy due to the immature nervous system of the fetus.

Before 30 weeks, the cardiac frequency, amplitude, and duration of acceleration are reduced. Premature fetuses without aggravation may have little acceleration, and the peak can be of only 10 beatings/minute above the basal line and between 20 and 30 weeks may occasionally have a deceleration of fetal cardiac frequency which is not associated with uterine contractions.

On the other hand, the prophylactic use of episiotomy for premature deliveries is not associated with a better neonatal outcome.

In selected patients, the use of prenatal corticosteroids (PC) together with tocolysis, regionalization of policies, and transportation to neonatal care units have actually shown to reduce not the incidence but the premature morbimortality.

The use of magnesium sulfate reduces cerebral palsy in preterm. It is indicated between 24 weeks and 31 and 6 days of gestational age and in presence of an imminent birth within the next 24 hours. The effect would start, if birth occurs, after the first 4 hours of having administered the medication.

It is essential to set up clinical guidelines upon maternal and obstetric pathologies such as hypertensive stages of pregnancy, intrauterine growth restriction (IUGR), placenta previa, diabetes, and cardiopathies among others that contribute significantly to the preterm modality.

Multiple Pregnancy

The incidence of twin pregnancy has significantly increased worldwide in the recent years. One of the main associated problems is prematurity, which affects almost 50% of twin pregnancies and is the single most important cause of perinatal morbidity and mortality.

In multiple gestations, the results are less promising.

In patients with multiple pregnancy, progesterone treatment (intramuscular or vaginal) does not seem to either reduce the probability of a preterm delivery or improve the outcomes of neonates [40].

The use of cervical cerclage in women with multiple pregnancy has not improved the outcomes either for the mother or for the babies.

All trials which have recently been carried out have shown that pessary use has not been effective for multiple pregnancies.

Cervical Cerclage

Three types of cervical cerclage can be performed: prophylactic cerclage or based on clinical history which is indicated to patients with a regular history of cervical insufficiency. It is preferably to be performed between 12 and 14 weeks of GA.

The therapeutic cerclage or indicated through ultrasonography is very useful in single pregnancy and patients with a preterm birth history and cervical length ≤20 mm whose implantation is performed before 24 weeks of GA.

Finally, the emergency cerclage or through physical examination can be carried out in patients with cervical modifications and exposed fetal membranes, without uterine dynamics, and after ruling out intra-amniotic infection as a rescue measure to achieve fetal viability.

If endocervical culture is positive, the antibiotics will be administered before cerclage according to the antibiogram of the isolated germ.

An amniocentesis diagnostic of infection must be carried out before cerclage [41, 42].

Cerclage Contraindications

- Subclinical intra-amniotic infection or clinical chorioamnionitis suspicion.
- Relevant vaginal bleeding in the context of a placental pathology. Poor bleeding during cervical dilation process would not be a contraindication.
- Uterine dynamics.
- Premature rupture of membranes.
- Fetal death or legal interruption of gestation or severe fetal malformation not compatible with life.

Pessary

Pessary is a silicon device that is used vaginally, whose mechanism would be to change the angle of cervical canal to a more posterior position; thus, it would concentrate a greater weight towards the low anterior segment of the cervix helping it to collapse. Another theory suggests this device would act as an immunologic barrier between the amniochorionic space and the vaginal flora. The efficacy of Arabin pessary in preventing preterm birth is still controversial for unique pregnancy.

Current evidence does not support the use of cervical pessary to prevent preterm birth or improve perinatal outcomes in singleton with a short cervix. Further research is required before conclusive advice can be provided regarding the benefits of placing a cervical pessary in women at high risk.

Preterm Birth Treatment: Tocolytic

The uterine inhibitor agents are the keystone to manage preterm birth. The main objective is to delay birth for 2–7 days, enabling to administer a complete protocol of pulmonary maturity [43, 44] as well as to use magnesium sulfate for neuroprotection in order to decrease the incidence and severity of respiratory distress syndrome in the newborn as well as cerebral palsy and also the opportunity to transport the patient to a more complex health facility. The secondary objective is to decrease perinatal mortality and morbidity associated with prematurity.

If uterine dynamics is restarted, its reintroduction will be assessed. However, it does not have to be used for a long period of time due to the increment of maternal-fetal risk and because it does not offer a clear benefit [45]. Sixty years ago uterine dynamics were distinguished; now they are administered when there is a diagnosis of a preterm birth between 23 0/7 and 33 6/7 weeks of gestation [45].

However, in the presence of any contraindication (serious preeclampsia or hemorrhage and significantly cardiac disease), it's not appropriate to be used to prolong gestation because these drugs generate a greater risk of compromise as well as a maternal hemodynamic collapse. Fetal contraindications include gestational age greater or equal to 34 weeks, lethal fetal anomalies, intrauterine fetal death, chorioamnionitis, and fetal compromise symptoms which can require immediate preterm birth [46].

From Guyetvai and col. [47] in the 90s a meta-analysis has showed that the uterine inhibitors decrease preterm risk within the first 24 hours (OR 0.47 IC 95% 0.29–0.77), 48 hours (OR 0.57 IC 95% 0.38–0.83) and 7 days (OR 0.6 IC 95% 0.38–0.95), many studies reported [48, 49] endorsing the use of tocolytics in singleton gestations to delay premature birth.

Types of Tocolytics

Many tocolytic agents were reported as part of the therapeutic armamentarium, among them: beta-adrenergic, calcium channel blockers, prostaglandin synthesis inhibitors, nitrous oxide donors, oxytocin receptor antagonists, and magnesium sulfate.

Their election will be determined by maternal and fetal risks, collateral effects, and efficacy. Therefore each drug will be analyzed.

Calcium Channel Blockers

Nifedipine and nicardipine are the calcium channel blockers most commonly used for tocolysis. The first one belongs to hydropyridine family [50].

Mechanism of Action

These agents prevent the influx of calcium ions by literally blocking its transmembrane flux through the calcium channels located in the nonvascular smooth muscle of the myometrium. However, they are also found in other locations such as the bronchial smooth muscle and the gastrointestinal and urinary tracts, as well as the smooth muscle of arteries and veins. Their presence is also described in other tissues such as pancreas, pituitary adrenal glands, salivary glands, gastric mucosa, white cells, platelets, and tear tissue [51].

On the other hand, they inhibit the release of intracellular deposits of calcium from the sarcoplasmic reticulum, which leads to a reduction in the concentration of cytoplasmic calcium and an increase in the calcium flux of the cell. This interferes with actin-myosin interactions, inhibiting myometrial contractions and leading to myometrial relaxation [46].

Pharmacokinetics

Nifedipine, after its administration by oral route (OR), is almost completely absorbed (90%), and gastrointestinal absorption is rapid. Action starts, after dosing via OR, in 20 minutes with a maximum peak in 30–60 minutes, and its half-life is 2–3 hours. The 30–40% of the dose is excreted on its first pass through the liver, where it is metabolized to inactive substances which are then excreted in urine [52].

Sublingual absorption (SL) is very rapid being able to find the drug in the plasma in 3–5 minutes, and the action also starts in 3–5 minutes [53].

Although physiological changes of pregnancy can affect absorption, distribution, metabolism, and excretion, the pharmacokinetic parameters observed in the pregnant woman are similar to the parameters found in a non-pregnant woman. The half-life after sublingual administration is 81 minutes, and minimal blood levels are observed after 6 hours [52].

The drug crosses human placenta when the time interval between the last dose and the birth is equal or greater than 5 hours, and its levels in umbilical cord blood are very low, equal or lower than 6 ng/ml. As it is expected, when the interval is shorter, the concentrations are higher. 70% is excreted through urine and 30% through feces [53].

Dose and Administration

In order to avoid hypotension, a burden of 500 mL must be previously administered [54].

Optimum dose regimen was not yet determined; therefore, several alternatives are present:

- The current initial dose habitually used is 10–20 mg via OR, followed by 10 mg each 15 minutes. It is adjusted according to the clinical response of uterine contractions, with a maximum of 40 mg within the first hour, and then 20 mg each 6–8 hours during 48 hours [55].
- Initial dose of 30 mg OR and continuing with 10–20 mg each 4–6 hours with a maximum dose of 180 mg/day [45].
- In solution, initial dose of 2 ml OR followed by indication of 3 ml each 6–8 hours. If there is no response to initial treatment, 1.5 ml/15 minutes should be added within the first hour. If there is not a medical response, a change to the second line should be done, a maximum of 32 ml/day [56].

Efficacy

A Cochrane revision that included 38 randomly controlled trials of calcium channel blockers versus no treatment or placebo for preterm birth with a total of 3550 pregnant women concluded that the risk was reduced within 48 hours (RR 0.30 IC 95%

0.21–0.43). Premature (RR 0.89 IC 95% 0.80–0.98) and very premature (RR 0.78 IC 95% 0.66 a 0.93) decreased at birth as well as acute respiratory distress syndrome (RR 0.64 IC 95% 0.48–0.86); necrotizing enterocolitis (RR 0.21 IC 95% 0.05–0.96); intraventricular hemorrhage (RR 0.53 IC 95% 0.34–0.84); neonatal jaundice (RR 0.72 IC 95% 0.57–0.92); and neonatal intensive care unit admissions (NICN) (RR 0.74 IC 95% 0.63–0.87) [57].

However, there was not a statistically significant decrease in this outcome when calcium channel blockers were compared with other types of tocolytics (RR 0.86 IC 95% 0.67–1.10) [57].

In comparison with betamimetics, calcium channel blockers showed statistical benefits with respect to pregnancy prolongation (mean difference of 4.38 days; IC 95% 0.25–8.52), serious neonatal morbidity, and maternal adverse effects [57].

In general, calcium channel blockers have a more favorable profile of safety, maternal tolerance, and profile of secondary effects, and they are easier to administer compared with betamimetics for the treatment of premature birth labor [46].

Adverse Effects

In general, nifedipine is well tolerated by the mother, but as it specifically acts as a peripheral vasodilator, it can cause nauseas, blush, flushes, dizziness, and edema of the lower limbs [58]. Other adverse events not wished and more frequent are related to hypotension (especially supine) and headaches. The first one is generally mild and transitory; it is present 10 minutes after SL administration and 20 minutes after OR. Secondary adverse effects generally occur only with a higher dose of 60 mg/day [46].

Studies with animals showed a decrease of uterine blood flow and a late reduction in fetal saturation of oxygen with nifedipine use [52]. However, these findings could not be replicated in human studies assessing fetal maternal hemodynamics [59].

Contraindications

It is contraindicated in patients with impaired cardiac conduction as well as hepatic disease and hypotension (<90/50 mm Hg). It is not recommended to be used in combination with magnesium sulfate due to some cases that reported hypocalcemia, neuromuscular blocking, and cardiac toxicity including maternal death [60].

Agonists of Beta-adrenergic Receptors

Beta-adrenergic or beta-mimetic agonists used as uterine inhibitors include ritodrine and terbutaline among the most used in addition to isoxsuprine, hexoprenaline, fenoterol, orciprenaline, and salbutamol.

Action Mechanism

Beta-mimetics produce myometrial relaxation acting upon ß2 receptors, thus resulting in an increase of intracellular adenylyl cyclase. This action provokes protein kinase activation, which phosphorylates kinase proteins in the cytoplasm. Therefore, the global decrease of intracellular free calcium interrupts the activity of myosin light chain kinase which also alters the interaction between myosin and actin resulting in the decrease of myometrial contractility [46].

We must remember that there are three types of beta-adrenergic receptors: ß1 are located in the heart, small bowel, and adipose tissue and with a lipolysis activity, while ß2 are in the uterus, blood vessels, and bronchioles with a glycogenolysis activity. ß3 are in the gastrointestinal smooth muscle and urinary and respiratory tracts.

Tachyphylaxis is one of the characteristics of management with these uterine inhibitors, as pregnant women can develop tolerance to these drugs. Long time ago, it was demonstrated in animals of experimentation that, with a continued infusion, they are associated to a suppressed regulation of beta-adrenergic receptors and a decrease of adenylyl cyclase activity, which reduces the activity of uterine inhibitors [61].

Pharmacokinetics

Ritodrine with a steady intravenous (IV) administration reached 60–75% of the maximum levels in 20 minutes. At the end of perfusion, there was a rapid decrease of serum levels with an initial half-life of 6 minutes followed by a second stage with a half-life of 2.5 hours during the remaining elimination time with single variations which oscillated between 1 and 4 hours. The drug is conjugated in the liver under sulfate and glucuronide and is then excreted freely and conjugated through the kidney [62].

Terbutaline suffers an extensive first-step metabolism through the conjugation of sulfate (and some glucuronide) in the liver and intestinal wall. It is excreted partially in urine and feces as a conjugated inactive sulfate and partially as unaltered terbutaline. The proportion depends on the route the drug is administered through. It was reported that the half-life multiple doses is between 16 and 20 hours [63].

Dose and Administration

An infusion dose of 50 μg/min of ritodrine is administered intravenously and increased each 20 minutes. 350 μg/min is the maximum dose. Once preterm labor is inhibited, the infusion has to be maintained during 1 hour and to be decreased 50 μg/min later each 30 minutes until reaching the minimal effective dose (50 μg/min), which must be maintained for 12 hours. A dose of 5–10 mg 2–4 hours via intramuscular can be administered [54].

Terbutaline is administered through intravenous infusion in glucose (5%) preferably through a continuous infusion pump when the concentration is 100 μgr/ml. If it is not available, the concentration of infusion must be 10 μgr/ml. At the beginning, a 5 μgr/min of infusion speed is recommended and increased to 2.5 μgr/min through intervals of 20 minutes until contractions stop. Generally, until 10 μgr/min rate is considered enough. Infusion speed cannot be higher than 20 μgr/min, and if this maximum speed does not delay birth, then the infusion must be stopped. Once contractions have stopped, the infusion must be administered during 1 hour. Then the dose can be decreased to 2.5 μgr/min through intervals of 20 minutes until the lowest dose of maintenance produces a continuous suppression of contractions [63].

Maternal pulse must be controlled during the infusion in order to avoid a maternal cardiac frequency higher than 135 beatings/min. Also, a close monitoring of patient hydration must be done due to overburden of fluids which is considered a key risk factor for pulmonary edema [63].

Another alternative is to administer 0.25 mgr of terbutaline via subcutaneous route each 20–30 minutes, during a maximum of 4 doses or until tocolysis is produced [46]. In addition, the FDA recommends that terbutaline injection is not used in prolonged preterm labor (defined as 48–72 hours) due to possible severe secondary effects in the mother, specifically cardiac events and death [64].

Efficacy

The beta-mimetics have been studied in numerous randomized controlled trials, especially with ritodrine. Beta-mimetics were compared with placebo in a meta-analysis that included 12 studies with 1367 pregnant women. These studies showed a decrease in the number of pregnant women in premature preterm labor who gave birth within 48 hours (RR 0.68 IC 95% 0.53–0.88) [65].

There was a decrease in the number of births within 7 days (RR average 0.80 IC 95 0.65–0.98), but there was no evidence in the reduction of preterm premature labor (before 37 weeks of gestation) (RR 0.95 IC 95% 0.88–1.03). No benefit was shown either for perinatal death (RR 0.84 IC 95% 0.46–1.55) or neonatal death (RR 0.90 IC 95% 0.27–3.00). No significant effect was shown for infant respiratory distress syndrome (RR 0.87 IC 95% 0.71–1.08), probably because it delayed birth enough time to allow the administration cycle of prenatal corticosteroids [65].

Adverse Effects

They result from the stimulation of ß1 adrenergic receptors increasing maternal cardiac frequency, hence increasing cardiac output and thus increasing the oxygen demand which, on one hand, can produce myocardial ischemia and, on the other hand, stimulate ß2 adrenergic receptors causing peripheral vasodilation and bronchial relaxation as well as hypotension [46, 54, 58].

Multiple cases of pulmonary edema have been reported [66–69] as the most severe secondary effect when a prolonged and continued intravenous infusion of beta-mimetics is performed in preterm birth treatment either in singleton or multiple gestations [70].

Other mild secondary effects include nauseas and vomits, palpitations, tachycardia, cardiac arrhythmias, hypotension, tremor, hyperglycemia, hyperinsulinemia, hypokalemia, headaches, dyspnea, thyroid function alteration, and non-specific thoracic pain [47, 58]. A longer duration of tocolysis was significantly associated with an increase of maternal adverse effects [71].

Cross trough the placenta, they result in fetal secondary effects which are similar to the observed in the mother, more commonly: fetal tachycardia, hyperinsulinemia and hyperglycemia, neonatal hypoglycemia [72], hypokalemia, hyperbilirubinemia, intraventricular hemorrhage, hypotension, septal and myocardial hypertrophy, and myocardial and ileal ischemia [54]. However, this does not seem to affect negatively fetal acid base or the general neonatal result [73].

Contraindications

It is not possible to be used in women with cardiac disease and only with extreme precaution in pregnant women with a bad control of diabetes mellitus or thyroid pathologies. In women with controlled diabetes, serial glucose, potassium, and urine ketone tests must be required [54].

Inhibitors of Prostaglandin Synthesis

Cyclooxygenase inhibitors (COX) are nonsteroidal anti-inflammatory of which indomethacin is the most commonly used. Other less used agents of this family are ketorolac, ibuprofen, sulindac, and nimesulide.

Mechanism of Action

COX is an enzyme that converts arachidonic acid into prostaglandins, and by decreasing its production, it blocks the intracellular calcium flow, the interaction of the actin-myosin complex, and the stimulation of the formation of gap junctions that coordinate uterine muscle activity, therefore inhibiting myometrial contractions [54, 74].

There are two isoforms: COX-1 and COX-2. The first one constitutively expresses in most of the gestational tissues and the other in the decidua and myometrium which significantly increases during delivery.

Indomethacin, nonselective COX-1 and COX-2 inhibitor, is the most used tocolytic [46].

Selective COX-2 inhibition would be more effective than nonselective indomethacin, and moreover it helps in reducing fetal and maternal collateral effects [75]. Some of the agents which have been described are celecoxib and rofecoxib. There is not enough information upon which to base the decisions with respect to the role of COX-2 inhibition in women during premature preterm labor.

Pharmacokinetics

The drug can be administered through oral or rectal route. After the initial oral dose, the maximum blood levels are reached in 1–2 hours and more rapidly through rectal route [76]. The bioavailability of rectal suppositories in adults is comparable or slightly less than the bioavailability of oral dose pathways [77].

The drug joins with plasmatic proteins in 99%. The drug half-life in neonates (14.7 hours) is greater than the mother's (2.2 hours), possibly in relation with immature fetal liver. It crosses the human placenta, reaching similar fetal levels in blood to the levels observed in the mother. It is metabolized in the liver, and 10% is excreted without changes through urine [76, 77].

Dose and Administration

Indomethacin is started with 50–100 mg orally or 100–200 mg through rectal route. It continues with 25–50 mg each 4–6 hours during 48 hours [51]. In the protocol through the vagina a 100 mg suppository is administered in the posterior wall sac each 12 hours (two doses) [54].

Ketorolac is administered through intramuscular route with a starting dose of 60 mg, followed by 30 mg each 6 hours until the inhibition of uterine activity up to 48 hours [78], whereas 200 mg of sulindac is administered orally each 12 hours during 48 hours. Therapy with these agents is limited to a maximum of 48 hours and/or pregnancies below 32 weeks of gestation [54].

Efficacy

A systematic revision [79] done in the 1980s that included two randomized controlled trials of moderate to low methodological quality as well as a scarce number of pregnant women compared indomethacin with placebo. There were no differences in birth less than 48 hours after the admission to the study (RR average 0.20 IC 95% 0.03–1.28; 2 studies with 70 women). However, preterm birth was reduced (before completing the 37 weeks of gestation) in a small study (36 women) (RR 0.21 IC 95% 0.07–0.62; necessary number to treat [NNT] 2, IC 95% 2–4). Moreover, there were no differences among the groups with respect to neonatal adverse outcomes.

In comparative trials, indomethacin significantly decreased preterm birth in less than 37 weeks within the 48 hours after starting tocolytic treatment in comparison with any other beta-mimetic agent (RR 0.27 IC 95% 0.08–0.96) and seemed to be as effective as nifedipine (RR 1.08 IC 95% 0.58–2.01) [80]. However, no benefit was shown with respect to neonatal morbidity or mortality among these diverse tocolytic agents.

When it was compared with ritodrine [53, 81], the studies showed that both are equally effective to inhibit uterine contractions and delay delivery in patients in preterm premature labor and with intact membranes and whose gestational age is lower or equal to 34 weeks.

Another meta-analysis [82] reported that indomethacin and calcium channel blockers were tocolytics with the best possibility of classifying in the three main classes of medications due to the outcomes in delaying preterm birth, respiratory distress syndrome, neonatal mortality, and maternal secondary effects (all causes) within 48 hours.

Adverse Effects

COX inhibitors are associated with less maternal adverse outcomes in comparison with beta-mimetics, but there were no differences observed when COX inhibitors were compared with other tocolytics, as calcium channel blockers or magnesium sulfate [46].

The most common maternal secondary effects of indomethacin include platelet disease, nauseas, emesis, gastroesophageal reflux, and gastritis [83].

One of the most scary effects in the fetus is the premature closure of the ductus arteriosus [84–86] which is maintained dilated due to E series of prostaglandins that are produced in the placenta and the ductus as well. Ductus habitually closes in the first 24 hours after birth, as a result of the absence of placental prostaglandins and also the increase of pulmonary blood flow that generates concomitant pulmonary hypertension [76, 81]. However, in premature newborns the ductus can remain permeable as it is demonstrated in both the necessity of postnatal indomethacin therapy and the surgical ligature [77].

The risk of ductal constriction depends on the age of gestation. This fact is observed from week 27 of gestation and especially from week 32. It is more intense when the age of gestation is higher than 32–34 weeks [76].

On the other hand, evidence suggests that there is not a significant increase in risk of neonatal complications in the newborns who are exposed to indomethacin tocolysis in comparison with the control groups of infants who did not receive treatment or tocolysis with medications different from indomethacin [87, 88].

On the other hand, fetal diuresis decreases provoking oligohydramnios [81] since vasopressin action is intensified and the autoregulation of renal blood flow is modified. The effect is observed after a few hours of starting the treatment and rapidly disappears when drug administration is interrupted. If during the treatment the birth occurs, oliguria can affect the newborn in the first 2 or 3 days of life, disappearing spontaneously after these days [76].

In pregnant women with threat of preterm birth between 27 and 32 weeks [89], 100–150 mg/day administration was associated with a reduction of fetal urinary flow from a median value of 11.2 ml/hour to 2.2 ml/hour previous the start of the treatment at 5 hours of drug administration, settling in 1.8 ml/hour at 12 and 24 hours. At 24 hours of interrupting administration, the median urinary flow was 13.5 ml/hour. No correlation was observed among drug levels in maternal blood and fetal urinary flow.

Moreover, it has been demonstrated an increase of association with higher risk of intraventricular hemorrhage, periventricular leukomalacia and necrotizing enterocolitis [90], possible renal damage [91], or bronchopulmonary dysplasia [92, 93].

Contraindications

Maternal contraindications include hypersensitivity to nonsteroidal agents, alterations in coagulation as well as liver or renal function, and also gastrointestinal ulcerative disease and asthma in patients who are sensible to aspirin [54].

Use of indomethacin is not recommended in fetuses with cardiac malformations that affect the ductus arteriosus and fetal transfusion syndrome in twin pregnancy [76].

Antagonists of Oxytocin Receptors

These drugs are the only ones specifically designed for tocolysis. Atosiban is the commercially available drug. It is approved by the European Union agencies but not by the US Food and Drug Administration (FDA).

Action Mechanism

Atosiban is a nonapeptide that selectively blocks the oxytocin receptors of the myometrium and decidua, inhibiting the release of inositol triphosphate mediated by oxytocin from the cell membrane of the myometrium. Consequently, it reduces the intracellular release of stored calcium from the reticulum of the myometrial cells and the entry of calcium from the extracellular space [94, 95].

In addition, atosiban suppresses the release of prostaglandins E and F mediated by oxytocin via the decidua [96] (in both situations), therefore decreasing myometrial contractility.

Oxytocin receptors increase in the myometrium with gestational age and are relatively few at a lower gestational age of 28 weeks [97].

Pharmacokinetics

In pregnant women who are in preterm labor, atosiban reaches plasmatic concentrations at 60 minutes after the infusion starts and has a terminal half-life of 1.7 hours after suspending it [98]. Atosiban joins between the 46–48% with plasmatic proteins and crosses the placenta [51]. It is metabolized in an active metabolite, which is excreted through urine [98].

Dose and Administration

The protocol used for administration is carried out in three consecutive stages [60]: it is administered as an intravenous bolus of 6.75 mg/min, immediately followed by 18 mg/h (300 μg/min) through intravenous infusion for 3 hours, and finally 6 mg/h (100 μg/min) up to 45 hours. Full dose does not have to exceed 330 mg. Infusion will be continued at least for 6 hours after uterine contractions stop until a maximum of 12 hours.

Efficacy

A meta-analysis [99] that included 4 studies with 854 pregnant women compared the antagonists of oxytocin receptors (3 with atosiban and 1 with barusiban) with placebo as tocolytic agents in patients with premature preterm labor. The studies showed that with the use of these drugs, either the risk of preterm birth was reduced within 48 hours after treatment (RR 1.05 IC 95% 0.15–7.43), or the risk of preterm birth in less than 28 weeks of gestation (RR 3.11 IC 95% 1.02–9.51), or the risk of preterm birth less than 37 weeks of gestation (RR 1.17 IC 95% 0.99–1.37). In addition, neonatal morbidity and mortality outcomes were statistically similar in both groups.

The same systematical revision found that atosiban was as effective as the beta-mimetics in reducing preterm birth within 48 hours of treatment (RR 0.89 IC 95% 0.66–1.22). In addition, the use of atosiban was associated with a significantly lower risk of maternal secondary effects when compared with the beta-mimetics (RR 0.05 IC 95% 0.02–0.11).

A later trial (APOSTEL III) randomly assigned (1:1) women with premature preterm labor to oral nifedipine (254) versus intravenous atosiban (256) during 48 hours without considering a controlled group with placebo. The primary outcome occurred in 42 newborns (14%) in the nifedipine group and in 45 newborns (15%) in atosiban group (RR 0.91 IC 95% 0.61–1.37). 16 (5%) of them died in the first group and 7 (2%) in the second group (RR 2.20 IC 95% 0.91–5.33). However, it was considered unlikely that all deaths were related with the studied drug. Maternal adverse events were not different between both groups [100].

A similar result was obtained in a meta-analysis when the use of the drug to delay births in extreme premature (below 28 weeks) or to decrease mortality was analyzed [101].

At present APOSTEL VIII [102] is being held. It is an international, multicenter, randomized, double-blind, placebo-controlled clinical trial that estimates to recruit 757 pregnant women with preterm birth threat between 30 and 34 weeks of gestational ages. Treatment will be with atosiban or placebo during 48 hours. The primary outcome will be perinatal mortality and severe neonatal morbidity.

Adverse Effects

The most common maternal secondary effects associated with the use of atosiban are some reactions on the injection place as well as headaches, nausea, thoracic pain, and hypotension. The general frequency of secondary effects was significantly lower than any other uterine inhibitor [103].

A multicenter, double-blind [104] study that included 501 pregnant women who received intravenous atosiban ($n = 246$) or placebo ($n = 255$), followed by subcutaneous maintenance, revealed that atosiban was significantly better as a tocolytic at 24 hours, 48 hours, and 7 days after treatment (all $P <$ o = 0.008). However, a possible association between atosiban and fetal/neonatal deaths was shown. One of the cross-questions to this study was the association of these deaths to infection and extreme prematurity. Although a relation with atosiban could not been ruled out, it was observed that at randomization the gestational age had not been stratified. This provoked such an imbalance that most of very preterm gestations (below 26 weeks) were assigned to atosiban group (14 vs 5). Hence, the difference of mortality could be attributable to the lowest gestational age in this group and not to the drug [96].

A recent study [105] following APOSTEL III included a total of 117 neonates (of 102 women), 51 of which had been exposed to nifedipine and 66 to atosiban. This study showed that in children born before 32 weeks of gestation and after tocolytic use, the prevalence of brain injury was high. Brain injury was observed in 22 (43.1%) neonates of nifedipine group compared with 37 (56.1%) of atosiban group (OR 0.60 IC 95% 0.29–1.24). However, the sensitivity analysis, adjusted for maternal age and gestational age at randomization, showed no statistical differences between the groups for brain injury presence (OR 0.58 IC 95% 0.27–1.27).

Contraindications

This drug is absolutely not contraindicated for maternal use.

Nitric Oxide Donors

Nitric oxide (NO) is a vasodilator, neurotransmitter, and cytotoxic and cytostatic agent. They are more frequently used for uterine relaxation in pelvic presentation, uterine inversion, intrapartum version, and placenta retention.

Nitric oxide donors such as nitroglycerine or glyceryl trinitrate cause a rapid and reversible suppression of the uterine contraction.

Action Mechanism

NO synthetized in the endothelium, hepatocytes, macrophage, platelets, placenta, and umbilical vessels interacts with the guanylyl cyclase which leads to the increase of cyclic GMP which activates the protein kinase of the myosin light-chain kinase inside the smooth muscle producing the inhibition of calcium flow from extracellular space resulting in smooth muscle relaxation [106, 107].

Pharmacokinetics

The glyceryl trinitrate is rapidly absorbed from the oral mucosa, through the gastrointestinal tract and the skin. The bioavailability is lower at 100% when administered through any of these routes due to the presystemic clearance. The bioavailability is further reduced after oral use due to extensive first-pass metabolism in the liver.

The therapeutic effect is evident within 30–60 minutes of applying transdermal patches. These patches are designed to release a set quantity of medication during 24 hours [108].

Dose and Administration

Nitroglycerine is administered through transdermal patches or intravenous route. The optimal dose is unknown. Generally the dose and interval must be adjusted when contractions stop and while arterial pressure is properly maintained. Currently, a 10 mg of glyceryl trinitrate patch is applied transdermally on the abdomen. If contraction frequency/or intensity is not reduced within 1 hour, a second patch can be applied and left during 24 hours. An alternative method of administration is an intravenous infusion at a 20 mg/min speed until contractions stop [46], but this route is little used due to the high frequency of maternal failures and hypotension that compel to the suspension of this agent [54].

Efficacy

In a Cochrane revision [109], 12 studies were included with 1227 pregnant women at preterm birth risk. Three of them compared nitric oxide donors (glyceryl trinitrate) with placebo. Results showed that nitric oxide donors did not prolong the pregnancies for more than 48 hours (RR 1.19 IC 95% 0.74–1.90).

When nitric oxide donors were compared with other tocolytic drugs, there were no significant proof in which they obtain better outcomes than other tocolytics such as beta-mimetics, magnesium sulfate, and calcium channel blockers (or a combination of them) in terms of pregnancy prolongation. Neither were significant differences among the groups for the outcomes of infant morbidity or mortality.

Adverse Effects

As NO donors cause arterial smooth muscle dilation in all the body, they can produce headaches, dizziness, nauseas, vomits, flushing, palpitations, or maternal hypotension [46].

There is no clear evidence that indicate the neonates are affected. However, hypotension can be produced although there are no significant alterations in Apgar and umbilical cord gases [54].

Contraindications

The pregnant women with hypotension, myocardial insufficiency, augmented intracranial pressure, and hypersensitivity to these agents must be avoided.

Magnesium Sulfate

Action Mechanism

Although the accurate action mechanism is not fully understood until now and even after many years of research, it is affirmed that it depresses uterine contractility due to changes in uptake, binding, and distribution of calcium in smooth muscle cells. The increase of extracellular magnesium (Mg) concentration inhibits calcium uptake into smooth muscle cell (myometrial), without visibly altering calcium release from intracellular deposits. Therefore, the contractile process depending from extracellular calcium uptake would not be possible as it would be like a physiological antagonist of calcium [110].

Pharmacokinetics

With magnesium sulfate used as uterine inhibitor, efficient serum levels of magnesium are located between 5.5 and 7.5 mg/dl or 6 and 8 mEq/lit (1.2 mg/dl equivalent to 1 mEq/lit). However, it seems that the serum levels of the drug do not have correlation with the tocolytic effect, and they do not have to be used as a criterion to adjust doses [111].

Renal route is completely eliminated; therefore, the dose administered to patients with renal insufficiency must be adjusted. It freely crosses through the placenta, and fetal levels are similar or slightly lower than that of the mother's (70–100%). After birth, high levels of magnesium in blood of newborns can persist until 7 days, with a half-life of excretion of 43.2 hours [111].

Dose and Administration

A 4–6 gr intravenous bolus is administered during 20–30 minutes, followed by a continued 1–2 gr/h intravenous infusion [112]. Perfusion speed is determined according to the assessment of contraction frequency and maternal toxicity. The optimal regimen has not been determined [113].

Urine must be continuously monitored (keeping diuresis >30 ml/hour) as well as the presence of osteotendinous reflexes, pulse, respiratory frequency (keeping a respiratory frequency > 12/min), and a lung fields auscultation to search for pulmonary edema. The decrease of patellar reflex can be present with serum levels of 8 a 12 mg/dL and respiratory difficulty with higher serum levels of 15 mg/dL [111].

As it is excreted through the kidneys, in pregnant women with renal insufficiency, the dose must be adjusted. Pregnant women must receive a standard dose (because the distribution volume does not change) but with a decreased dose or even without maintenance. The clinical conditions of such patients must be controlled: a close control of the urine and the possibility to follow their concentration of magnesium serum each 6–8 hours to be considered.

In pregnant women with normal renal function, signs and symptoms of magnesium toxicity are assessed through clinical history and physical examination. The routine of serum magnesium levels is not indicated, but in the presence of life-threatening symptoms of toxicity due to magnesium, an intravenous dose of 1 gr calcium gluconate must be urgently administered during 5–10 minutes.

Efficacy

There is no evidence in literature that magnesium sulfate inhibits preterm premature labor or decreases fetal morbidity. A systematic Cochrane revision [114] compared magnesium sulfate with any placebo treatment, and results indicated that magnesium sulfate did not statistically decrease preterm birth ranges in less than 48 hours after treatment started (RR 0.56 IC 95% 0.27–1.14) nor improve neonatal and maternal outcomes, whereas the incidence of preterm births with less than 37 weeks of pregnancy at 48 hours after starting treatment was similar among the groups treated with magnesium as well as those who were not treated with it.

Adverse Effects

Among the maternal adverse effects are diaphoresis, hot flushes, nausea, vomit, headache, lethargy, nystagmus eye, blurry vision, diplopia, palpitations, and pulmonary edema [115, 116] especially related with rapid administration of the drug.

Fetal secondary effects include decrease of fetal breathing movements in fetal biophysical profile as well as a decrease in the frequency of fetal heart rate variability assessed through cardiotocography [78].

From a neonatal point of view, lethargy, respiratory difficulties, or alterations in bone mineralization detected by radiographies can be present in those who have been exposed to the drug for more than 7 days. In addition, statistically significant differences were observed at birth in the values of neonatal magnesium serum, phosphorus, calcium, and osteocalcin [117, 118].

However, these findings may be temporary [46]; more studies are needed to confirm or rule out long-term sequelae. Based on these findings, it is recommended that magnesium sulfate be used for no more than 48 hours and only in women who are between 24 and 34 weeks of gestation with a clinical diagnosis of preterm birth [119, 120].

Contraindications

It is contraindicated in women with a myasthenia gravis diagnosis and to those with myocardial compromise. It must be used with precaution in women with renal insufficiency because magnesium toxicity can be developed even with a standard dose [46].

Combination of Several Uterine Inhibitors

The possibility to use more than two uterine inhibitors is not recommended because its efficacy and safety have not been demonstrated. Therefore, more studies are needed to arrive to any specific conclusion upon the use of this combined tocolytic therapy for preterm birth [121]. In contrast, some studies have shown that they increase maternal morbidity [54].

Tocolysis Maintenance

It has been shown that treatment of maintenance with nifedipine [122, 123] or beta-adrenergics [124] when they are mainly used to prevent premature preterm labor recurrence after an initial cycle of successful treatment neither improves perinatal outcomes nor helps pregnancy prolongation effectively [125]. Therefore, eliminating or reducing this therapy routine of maintenance may substantially decrease costs and secondary effects associated with the management of preterm premature labor without compromising perinatal outcomes.

Twin Gestational Pregnancy

There is not enough evidence that tocolytic use in multiple gestations is useful or at least can improve neonatal outcomes. Also, there is a higher risk of maternal pulmonary edema. But due to proven benefits to delay birth at least 48 hours in singleton gestations, its use is as well recommended in complicated multiple gestations with a threat of preterm birth [45].

Prevention of Premature Preterm Labor

Progesterone

Progesterone was discovered in 1934, and its effect for uterine myometrial quiescence was not recognized until 1954. Fifty years after that, between 2003 and 2011, several randomized trials were published which evaluated progesterone effect in its diverse forms of preterm birth prevention despite the disparity of its outcomes (caproato 17-alpha hydroxyprogesterone caproate intramuscular [17P] versus vaginal progesterone versus oral progesterone) [126]. This specifically refers to progesterone supplementation in high-risk patients in the second trimester of pregnancy.

Although the accuracy of progesterone's mechanism of action to prevent preterm birth is not clear, it is estimated to have an anti-inflammatory effect that reduces the intrauterine inflammatory process which causes preterm birth or due to a mechanism that affects the isolated decrease of progesterone levels within myometrial tissues [126].

Use of Progesterone in Pregnant Women Without Previous History of Spontaneous Preterm Births

In women with singleton pregnancies, without history of previous preterm births and a short cervical length (lower or equal to 20 mm) assessed through transvaginal ultrasound in the weeks 18 0/7 and 23 6/7, vaginal progesterone administration was associated with a preterm birth reduction and perinatal morbimortality [126].

Da Fonseca and colleagues [127] in a randomized controlled double-blind study that included 142 singleton gestations of high-risk preterm birth (cervical length equal to or less than 15 mm) analyzed the use of 200 mg progesterone via vaginal vs placebo. There were statistically significant differences in the decrease of incidence of preterm birth lower than 34 weeks of gestation (18.6%–2.7%, respectively; p 0.05) and lower than 37 weeks of gestation (28.5% a 13.8%, respectively; $p < 0.05$).

Hassan and colleagues [128] used 90 mg of progesterone through vaginal gel compared with placebo in a randomized controlled study that included 458 singleton gestations with cervical length between 10 and 20 mm. The study showed that progesterone reduced preterm birth in the group with less than 33 weeks of gestation (15.3% a 7.6%, respectively; RR 0.50 IC 95% 0.27–0.90; $p < 0.02$). There were not statistically significant differences when a subgroup of pregnant women with previous spontaneous preterm births was analyzed (between 20 and 35 weeks) (15.8% vs 20.6%; RR 0.77; IC 95% 0.29–2.06; $p < 0.60$).

Although both studies support the use of vaginal progesterone, different doses and formulas were used.

In addition, the OPPTIMUM study [129], a randomized controlled, multicenter, double-blind study published years ago, which recruited 1228 pregnant women with previous history of preterm birth <34 weeks or cervical length <25 mm or positive fetal fibronectin, was randomized to use 200 mg vaginal progesterone or placebo. This study showed no differences in the groups in relation to births before 34 weeks (OR 0.86 IC 95% 0.61–1.22) as obstetric objective. With respect to neonatal follow-up, no differences were found either (OR 0.62 IC 95% 0.38–1.03).

In general, in women without preterm birth history, there is not enough evidence upon the advantages of progesterone preparation or the dose of vaginal progesterone as they were not compared face to face in a clinical trial. Therefore, the cost and preparation availability, as well as the patient preference and other factors, may influence progesterone's type and dose.

The Society for Maternal-Fetal Medicine [126] supports the use of vaginal progesterone to prevent preterm birth in women with shortened cervical length less than or equal to 20 mm in transvaginal ultrasound and without previous spontaneous preterm births. On the contrary, in a great number of studies, in women with previous spontaneous preterm births, vaginal progesterone has not shown to be useful in reducing preterm births; hence, it must not be recommended as a routine in this context.

tsc

A multicenter, double-blind, randomized, and controlled study [130], which involved pregnant women with singleton pregnancies and a previous spontaneous preterm birth, was randomized to 17P or placebo, showing a statistically significant decrease in the incidence of recurrent spontaneous preterm birth in less than 37 weeks in the 17P group (from 54.9% to 36.3%; RR 0.66 IC 95% 0.54–0.81), for the birth of less than 35 weeks of gestation (20.6%–30.7%; RR 0.67 IC 95% 0.48 a 0.93), and for the birth of less than 32 weeks of gestation (11.4% opposite to 19.6%; RR 0.58 IC 95% 0.37 a 0.91). In addition, the neonates of 17P group had significantly lower rates of necrotizing enterocolitis, intraventricular hemorrhage, and necessity of supplemental oxygen.

Therefore, in women with singleton pregnancies and a previous spontaneous preterm birth, a 17P supplementation is recommended. A 250 mg dose must be administered through intramuscular injection weekly from 16 to 20 weeks until

36 weeks of gestation. Moreover, vaginal progesterone must not be considered as a suitable substitute of 17P in these patients.

Follow-up studies of 4-year-old children who were exposed to 17P in the uterus to prevent recurrent preterm birth were done. None of them showed differences in the general physical examination, health condition, mental development, or skill performance (motor, problem-solving, interpersonal) compared with children exposed to placebo [131].

References

1. Blencowe H, Cousens S, Oestergaard MZ, Chou D, Moller AB, Narwal R, et al. National, regional and worldwide estimates of preterm birth rates in the year 2010 with time trends for selected countries since 1990: a systematic analysis and implications. Lancet. 2012;379:2162–72.
2. Nour N. Preterm delivery and the millennium development goal. Rev Obstet Gynecol. 2012;5:100–5.
3. World Health Organization. Newborn: reducing mortality. http://www.who.int/mediacentre/factsheets/fs333/en/. Accessed 10 Aug 2015.
4. Blencowe H, Cousens S, Chou D, Oestergaard M, Say L, Moller A-B, et al. Born too soon: the global epidemiology of 15 million preterm births. Reprod Health. 2013;10(Suppl 1):S2.
5. Shapiro-Mendoza CK, Barfield WD, Henderson Z, James A, Howse JL, et al. CDC grand rounds: public health strategies to prevent preterm birth. MMWR Morb Mortal Wkly Rep. 2016;65(32):826–30.
6. Yamashita M, Hayashi S, Endo M, Okuno K, Fukui O, Mimura K, et al. Incidence and risk factors for recurrent spontaneous preterm birth: a retrospective cohort study in Japan. J Obstet Gynaecol Res. 2015;41:1708–14.
7. Liu L, Johnson HL, Cousens S, et al. Global, regional, and national causes of child mortality: an updated systematic analysis for2010 with time trends since 2000. Lancet. 2012;379:2151–61.
8. Esplin MS, O'Brien E, Fraser A, et al. Estimating recurrence of spontaneous preterm delivery. Obstet Gynecol. 2008;112:516.
9. Bhattacharya S, Raja EA, Mirazo ER, et al. Inherited predisposition to spontaneous preterm delivery. Obstet Gynecol. 2010;115:1125.
10. Meenakshi, Srivastava R, Sharma NR, Kushwaha KP, Aditya V. Obstetric behavior and pregnancy outcome in overweight and obese women: maternal and fetal complications and risks in relation to maternal overweight and obesity. J Obstet Gynaecol India. 2012;62(3):276–80.
11. Behrman RE, Butler AS. Preterm birth: causes, consequences, and prevention. Washington, DC: The National Academies Press; 2007. p. 792.
12. Salihu HM, Mbah AK, Alio AP, Clayton HB, Lynch O. Low pre-pregnancy body mass index and risk of medically indicated versus spontaneous preterm singleton birth. Eur J Obstet Gynecol Reprod Biol. 2009;144:119–23.
13. Dunlop AL, Kramer MR, Hogue CJ, Menon R, Ramakrishan U. Racial disparities in preterm birth: Anoverview of the potential role of nutrient deficiencies. Acta Obstet Gynecol Scand. 2011;90:1332–41.
14. Vogel JP, Lee ACC, Souza JP. Maternal morbidity and preterm birth in 22 low and middle income countries: a secondary analysis of the World Health Organization Global Survey dataset. BMC Pregn Childbirth. 2014;14:1e14.
15. Marufu TC, Ahankari A, Coleman T, Lewis S. Maternal smoking and the risk of still birth: systematic review and meta-analysis. BMC Public Health. 2015;15:239.

16. Miller GE, Chen E, Zhou ES. If it goes up, must it come down? Chronic stress and the hypothalamicpituitary-adrenocortical axis in humans. Psychol Bull. 2007;133:25–45.
17. El Kady D, Gilbert WM, Xing G, Smith LH. Maternal and neonatal outcomes of assaults during pregnancy. Obstet Gynecol. 2005;105:357–63.
18. Di Mascio D, Magro-Malosso ER, Saccone G, et al. Exercise during pregnancy in normal-weight women and risk of preterm birth: a systematic review and meta-analysis of randomized controlled trials. Am J Obstet Gynecol. 2016;215:561.
19. Aune D, Schlesinger S, Henriksen T, et al. Physical activity and the risk of preterm birth: a systematic review and meta-analysis of epidemiological studies. BJOG. 2017;124(12):1816–26.
20. Han A, Stewart DE. Maternal and fetal outcomes of intimate partner violence associated with pregnancy in the Latin American and Caribbean region. Int J Gynaecol Obstet Off Organ Int Fed Gynaecol Obstet. 2014;124:6–11.
21. Shah PS, Shah J, Knowledge Synthesis Group on Determinants of Preterm/LBW Births. Maternal exposure to domestic violence and pregnancy and birth outcomes: a systematic review and meta-analyses. J Womens Health. 2010;19:2017–31.
22. Conde-Agudelo A, Rosas-Bermúdez A, Kafury-Goeta AC. Birth spacing and risk of adverse perinatal outcomes: a meta-analysis. JAMA. 2006;295:1809.
23. Wong LF, Wilkes J, Korgenski K, et al. Risk factors associated with preterm birth after a prior term delivery. BJOG. 2016;123:1772.
24. Parets SE, Bedient CE, Menon R, Smith AK. Preterm birth and its long-term effects: methylation to mechanisms. Biology. 2014;3:498–513.
25. Appleton AA, Armstrong DA, Lesseur C, Lee J, Padbury JF, Lester BM, Marsit CJ. Patterning in placental 11-b hydroxysteroid dehydrogenase methylation according to prenatal socioeconomic adversity. PLoS One. 2013;8:e74691.
26. Vidal AC, Benjamin Neelon SE, Liu Y, Tuli AM, Fuemmeler BF, Hoyo C, Murtha AP, Huang Z, Schildkraut J, Overcash F, et al. Maternal stress, preterm birth, and DNA methylation at imprint regulatory sequences in humans. Genet Epigenet. 2014;6:37–44.
27. Li Z, Ye R, Zhang L, Li H, Liu J, Ren A. Folic acid supplementation during early pregnancy and the risk of gestational hypertension and preeclampsia. Hypertension. 2013;61:873–9.
28. Chong MF, Wong JX, Colega M, Chen LW, van Dam RM, Tan CS, Lim AL, Cai S, Broekman BF, Lee YS, et al. Relationships of maternal folate and vitamin b12 status during pregnancy with perinatal depression: the gusto study. J Psychiatr Res. 2014;55:110–6.
29. Kim MW, Ahn KH, Ryu KJ, Hong SC, Lee JS, Nava-Ocampo AA, Oh MJ, Kim HJ. Preventive effects of folic acid supplementation on adverse maternal and fetal outcomes. PLoS One. 2014;9:e97273.
30. Siega-Riz AM, Savitz DA, Zeisel SH, Thorp JM, Herring A. Second trimester folate status and preterm birth. Am J Obstet Gynecol. 2004;191:1851–7.
31. Smaill F, Vazquez JC. Antibiotics for asymptomatic bacteriuria in pregnancy. Cochrane Database Syst Rev. 2007;(2):CD000490.
32. Sweeney EL, Kallapur SG, Gisslen T, et al. Placental infection with ureaplasma species is associated with histologic chorioamnionitis and adverse outcomes in moderately preterm and late-preterm infants. J Infect Dis. 2016;213:1340.
33. Valkenburg-van den Berg AW, Sprij AJ, Dekker FW, et al. Association between colonization with Group B Streptococcus and preterm delivery: a systematic review. Acta Obstet Gynecol Scand. 2009;88:958.
34. Lackritz EM, Wilson CB, Guttmacher AE, Howse JL, Engmann CM, Rubens CE, et al. A solution pathway for preterm birth: accelerating a priority research agenda. Lancet. 2013;1:e328e30.
35. Conde-Agudelo A, Romero R, Kusanovic JP. Nifedipine in the management of preterm labor: a systematic review and metaanalysis. Am J Obstet Gynecol. 2011;204(2):134–20.
36. Norman JE, Marlow N, Messow C-M, et al. Vaginal progesterone prophylaxis for preterm birth (the OPPTIMUM study): a multicentre, randomised, double-blind trial. Lancet (London, England). 2016;387(10033):2106–16.

37. American Academy of Pediatrics Committee on Fetus And Newborn. Levels of neonatal care. Pediatrics. 2012;130:587.
38. Anderson GD, Bada HS, Sibai BM, et al. The relationship between labor and route of delivery in the preterm infant. Am J Obstet Gynecol. 1988;158:1382.
39. Afors K, Chandraharan E. Use of continuous electronic fetal monitoring in a preterm fetus: clinical dilemmas and recommendations for practice. J Pregnancy. 2011;2011:848794.
40. Fogarty M, Osborn DA, Askie L, Seidler AL, Hunter K, Lui K, Tarnow-Mordi W. Delayed vs early umbilical cord clamping for preterm infants: a systematic review and meta-analysis. Am J Obstet Gynecol. 2018;218(1):1–18.
41. Berghella V, Alfirevic Z. Cervical stitch (cerclage) fo r preventing preterm birth in multiple pregnancy. Base de Datos Cochrane de Revisiones Sistemáticas. 2014;9:CD009166. https://doi.org/10.1002/14651858.CD009166.pub2.
42. Berghella V, Ludmir J, Simonazzi G, Owen J. Transvaginal cervical cerclage: evidence for perioperativemanagement strategies. Am J Obstet Gynecol. 2013;209(3):181–92.
43. Stoll BJ, Hansen NI, Bell EF, Walsh MC, Carlo WA, Shankaran S, et al. Trends in care practices, morbidity, and mortality of extremely preterm neonates, 1993-2012. JAMA. 2015;314(10):1039–51.
44. Wu F, Liu G, Feng Z, Tan X, Yang C, Ye X, et al. Short-term outcomes of extremely preterm infants at discharge: a multicenter study from Guangdong province during 2008-2017. BMC Pediatr. 2019;19(1):405.
45. Practice bulletin no. 171: management of preterm labor. Obstet Gynecol. 2016;128(4):e155–64.
46. Patel SS, Ludmir J. Drugs for the treatment and prevention of preterm labor. Clin Perinatol. 2019;46(2):159–72.
47. Gyetvai K, Hannah ME, Hodnett ED, Ohlsson A. Tocolytics for preterm labor: a systematic review. Obstet Gynecol. 1999;94(5 Pt 2):869–77.
48. Lam F, Gill P. Beta-agonist tocolytic therapy. Obstet Gynecol Clin North Am. 2005;32(3):457–84.
49. Haram K, Mortensen JH, Morrison JC. Tocolysis for acute preterm labor: does anything work. J Matern Fetal Neonatal Med. 2015;28(4):371–8.
50. Smith P, Anthony J, Johanson R. Nifedipine in pregnancy. BJOG. 2000;107(3):299–307.
51. Tsatsaris V, Cabrol D, Carbonne B. Pharmacokinetics of tocolytic agents. Clin Pharmacokinet. 2004;43(13):833–44.
52. Ruoti Cosp M. Nifedipina. En: Ruoti Cosp M, Calabrese E, Editores. Fármacos y embarazo, que medicamentos prescribir. AMOLCA. Caracas. 2015.p. 203–209.
53. Sweetman SC, Blake PS, McGlashan JM, et al., editors. Martindale: Guía completa de Consulta Farmacoterapeutica. 2da ed. Barcelona: Pharma Editores, SL; 2006. p. 1233.
54. Ortiz Ruiz ME, Labrador AM, Ayala YR. Uteroinhibidores actuales para el manejo de parto pretérmino. An Med (Mex). 2010;55(2):85–91.
55. Manual de recomendaciones en el embarazo y parto prematuro. Ministerio de Salud Pública Dirección General de la Salud Uruguay 2018.
56. Palacio M, Cobo T, Baños N, Migliorelli F. Amenaza de parto pretérmino En: Figueras F, Gratacós E, Puerto B. Actualización en Medicina Maternofetal. Barcelona. 2015. p. 247–260.
57. Flenady V, Wojcieszek AM, Papatsonis DN, Stock OM, Murray L, et al. Calcium channel blockers for inhibiting preterm labour and birth. Cochrane Database Syst Rev. 2014;(6):CD002255.
58. Di Renzo GC, Roura LC, European Association of Perinatal Medicine-Study Group on Preterm Birth. Guidelines for the management of spontaneous preterm labor. J Perinat Med. 2006;34(5):359–66.
59. Cornette J, Duvekot JJ, Roos-Hesselink JW, Hop WC, Steegers EA. Maternal and fetal haemodynamic effects of nifedipine in normotensive pregnant women. BJOG. 2011;118(4):510–40.
60. Di Renzo GC. Safety and efficacy of new drugs in preterm labor. Expert Rev Obstet Gynecol. 2007;2(1):19–24.

61. Caritis SN, Chiao JP, Kridgen P. Comparison of pulsatile and continuous ritodrine administration: effects on uterine contractility and beta-adrenergic receptors cascade. Am J Obstet Gynecol. 1991;139(4):1005–11.
62. Ruoti Cosp, M. Ritodrine. En: Ruoti Cosp M, Calabrese E, Editores. Fármacos y embarazo, que medicamentos prescribir. AMOLCA. Caracas. 2015. p. 1055–1059.
63. Sweetman SC, Pharm B, PharmS FR, editors. Terbutaline sulfate. Martindale: the complete drug reference. 36ª ed. China: Pharmaceutical Press; 2009. p. 1138–40.
64. US Food and Drug Administration. FDA drug safety communication: new warnings against use of terbutaline to treat preterm labor. Disponible en: http://www.fda.gov/Drugs/DrugSafety/ucm243539.htm#ds. Acceso Enero 17, 2019.
65. Neilson JP, West HM, Dowswell T. Betamimetics for inhibiting preterm labour. Cochrane Database Syst Rev. 2014;(2):CD004352.
66. Karaman S, Ozcan O, Akercan F, Terek MC, Yucebilgin MS, Firat V. Pulmonary edema after ritodrine therapy during pregnancy and subsequent cesarean section with epidural anesthesia. Clin Exp Obstet Gynecol. 2004;31(1):67–9.
67. Gezginç K, Gül M, Karatayli R, Cander B, Kanat F. Noncardiogenic pulmonary edema due to ritodrine usage in preterm labor. Taiwan J Obstet Gynecol. 2008;47(1):101–2.
68. Sweetman SC, Pharm B, PharmS FR, editors. Ritodrine hydrochloride. Martindale: the complete drug reference. 36ª ed. China: Pharmaceutical Press; 2009. p. 2017–8.
69. Pisani RJ, Rosenow EC 3rd. Pulmonary edema associated with tocolytic therapy. Ann Intern Med. 1989;110(9):714–8.
70. Shinohara S, Sunami R, Uchida Y, Hirata S, Suzuki K. Association between total dose of ritodrine hydrochloride and pulmonary oedema in twin pregnancy: a retrospective cohort study in Japan. BMJ Open. 2017;7(12):e018118.
71. Shigemi D, Aso S, Yasunaga H. Inappropriate use of ritodrine hydrochloride for threatened preterm birth in Japan: a retrospective cohort study using a national inpatient database. BMC Pregnancy Childbirth. 2019;19(1):204.
72. Shimokawa S, Sakata A, Suga Y, Isoda K, Itai S, Nagase K, et al. Incidence and risk factors of neonatal hypoglycemia after ritodrine therapy in premature labor: a retrospective cohort study. J Pharm Health Care Sci. 2019;5:7.
73. Golichowski AM, Hathaway DR, Fineberg N, Peleg D. Tocolytic and hemodynamic effects of nifedipine in the ewe. Am J Obstet Gynecol. 1985;151(8):1134–40.
74. Sawdy RJ, Sullivan MH, Bennett PR. The effects of non-steroidal anti-inflammatory compounds on human myometrial contractility. Eur J Obstet Gynecol Reprod Biol. 2003;109(1):33–40.
75. Conde-Agudelo A, Romero R. Transdermal nitroglycerin for the treatment of preterm labor: a systematic review and metaanalysis. Am J Obstet Gynecol. 2013;209(6):551.e1–551.e18.
76. Ruoti Cosp, M. Indometacina. En: Ruoti Cosp M, Calabrese E, Editores. Fármacos y embarazo, que medicamentos prescribir. AMOLCA. Caracas. 2015.p.944–949.
77. Sweetman SC, Pharm B, PharmS FR, editors. Indometacin. Martindale: the complete drug reference. 36ª ed. China: Pharmaceutical Press; 2009. p. 66–9.
78. Hearne A, Nagey D. Therapeutic agents in preterm labor: Tocolytic agents. Clin Obstet Gynecol. 2000;43(4):787–801.
79. Reinebrant HE, Pileggi-Castro C, Romero CL, Dos Santos RA, Kumar S, et al. Cyclooxygenase (COX) inhibitors for treating preterm labour. Cochrane Database Syst Rev. 2015;(6):CD001992.
80. Zuckerman H, Shalev E, Gilad G, Katzuni E. Further study of the inhibition of premature labor by indomethacin. Part II double-blind study. J Perinat Med. 1984;12(1):25–9.
81. Besinger RE, Niebyl JR, Keyes WG, Johnson TR. Randomized comparative trial of indomethacin and ritodrine for the long-term treatment of preterm labor. Am J Obstet Gynecol. 1991;164(4):981–6.
82. Haas DM, Caldwell DM, Kirkpatrick P, McIntosh JJ, Welton NJ. Tocolytic therapy for preterm delivery: systematic review and network meta-analysis. BMJ. 2012;345:e6226.

83. Rundell K, Panchal B. Preterm labor: prevention and management. Am Fam Physician. 2017;95(6):366–72.
84. Vermillion ST, Scardo JA, Lashus AG, Wiles HB. The effect of indomethacin tocolysis on fetal ductus arteriosus constriction with advancing gestational age. Am J Obstet Gynecol. 1997;177(2):256–9.
85. Dathe K, Hultzsch S, Pritchard LW, Schaefer C. Risk estimation of fetal adverse effects after short-term second trimester exposure to non-steroidal anti-inflammatory drugs: a literature review. Eur J Clin Pharmacol. 2019;75(10):1347–53.
86. Beaute JI, Friedman KG. Indomethacin induced ductus arteriosus closure in midgestation fetus. Clin Case Rep. 2018;6(3):506–8.
87. Loe SM, Sanchez-Ramos L, Kaunitz AM. Assessing the neonatal safety of indomethacin tocolysis: a systematic review with meta-analysis. Obstet Gynecol. 2005;106(1):173–9.
88. Vermillion ST, Newman RB. Recent indomethacin tocolysis is not associated with neonatal complications in preterm infants. Am J Obstet Gynecol. 1999;181(5 Pt 1):1083–6.
89. Kirshon B, Moise KJ Jr, Wasserstrum N, Ou CN, Huhta JC. Influence of short-term indomethacin therapy on fetal urine output. Obstet Gynecol. 1988;72(1):51–3.
90. Hammers AL, Sanchez-Ramos L, Kaunitz AM. Antenatal exposure to indomethacin increases the risk of severe intraventricular hemorrhage, necrotizing enterocolitis, and periventricular leukomalacia: a systematic review with metaanalysis. Am J Obstet Gynecol. 2015;212(4):505.e1–13.
91. van der Heijden BJ, Carlus C, Narcy F, Bavoux F, Delezoide AL, Gubler MC. Persistent anuria, neonatal death, and renal microcystic lesions after prenatal exposure to indomethacin. Am J Obstet Gynecol. 1994;171(3):617–23.
92. Eronen M, Pesonen E, Kurki T, Teramo K, Ylikorkala O, Hallman M. Increased incidence of bronchopulmonary dysplasia after antenatal administration of indomethacin to prevent preterm labor. J Pediatr. 1994;124(5 Pt 1):782–8.
93. Jensen EA, Dysart KC, Gantz MG, Carper B, Higgins RD, Keszler M, et al. Association between use of prophylactic indomethacin and the risk for bronchopulmonary dysplasia in extremely preterm infants. J Pediatr. 2017;186:34–40.e2.
94. López Gómez L, Marín Gabriel MA, Encinas B, de la Cruz Troca JJ, Rodríguez MB. Oxytocin receptor antagonist (Atosiban) in the threat of preterm birth: does it have any effect on breastfeeding in the term newborn? Breastfeed Med. 2018;13(2):123–8.
95. Phaneuf S, Asbóth G, MacKenzie IZ, Melin P, López BA. Effect of oxytocin antagonists on the activation of human myometrium in vitro: atosiban prevents oxytocin-induced desensitization. Am J Obstet Gynecol. 1994;171(6):1627–34.
96. Aguarón G, Aguarón A, Melchor JC. Manejo de la Amenaza de Parto Pretérmino: ¿Atosiban o Nifedipino? En: Gallo Vallejo Editores. Embarazo y Parto Pretérmino. Editorial AMOLCA.
97. Arrowsmith S, Wray S. Oxytocin: its mechanism of action and receptor signalling in the myometrium. J Neuroendocrinol. 2014;26(6):356–69.
98. Sweetman SC, Pharm B, PharmS FR editors. Atosiban. Martindale: the complete drug reference. 36ª ed. China: Pharmaceutical Press; 2009. p. 2005–6.
99. Flenady V, Reinebrant HE, Liley HG, Tambimuttu EG, Papatsonis DN. Oxytocin receptor antagonists for inhibiting preterm labour. Cochrane Database Syst Rev. 2014;(6):CD004452.
100. van Vliet EOG, Nijman TAJ, Schuit E, Heida KY, Opmeer BC, Kok M, et al. Nifedipine versus atosiban for threatened preterm birth (APOSTEL III): a multicentre, randomised controlled trial. Lancet. 2016;387(10033):2117–24.
101. Miyazaki C, Garcia RM, Ota E, Swa T, Oladapo OT, Mori R. Tocolysis for inhibiting preterm birth in extremely preterm birth, multiple gestations and in growth-restricted fetuses: a systematic review and meta-analysis. Reprod Health. 2016;13:4.
102. Klumper J, Breebaart W, Roos C, Naaktgeboren CA, van der Post J, Bosmans J, et al. Study protocol for a randomised trial for atosiban versus placebo in threatened preterm birth: the APOSTEL 8 study. BMJ Open. 2019;9(11):e029101.

103. de Heus R, Mol BW, Erwich JJ, van Geijn HP, Gyselaers WJ, Hanssens M, et al. Adverse drug reactions to tocolytic treatment for preterm labour: prospective cohort study. BMJ. 2009;338:b744.
104. Romero R, Sibai BM, Sanchez-Ramos L, Valenzuela GJ, Veille JC, Tabor B, et al. An oxytocin receptor antagonist (atosiban) in the treatment of preterm labor: a randomized, double-blind, placebo-controlled trial with tocolytic rescue. Am J Obstet Gynecol. 2000;182(5):1173–83.
105. Nijman TAJ, Goedhart MM, Naaktgeboren CN, de Haan TR, Vijlbrief DC, Mol BW, et al. Effect of nifedipine and atosiban on perinatal brain injury: secondary analysis of the APOSTEL-III trial. Ultrasound Obstet Gynecol. 2018;51(6):806–12.
106. Shaikh S, Shaikh AH, Akhter S, Isran B. Efficacy of transdermal nitroglycerine in idiopathic pre-term labour. J Pak Med Assoc. 2012;62(1):47–50.
107. Yallampalli C, Dong YL, Gangula PR, Fang L. Role and regulation of nitric oxide in the uterus during pregnancy and parturition. J Soc Gynecol Investig. 1998;5(2):58–67.
108. Sweetman SC, Pharm B, PharmS FR, editors. Glyceryl Trinitrate. Martindale: the complete drug reference. 36ª ed. China: Pharmaceutical Press; 2009. p. 1298–9.
109. Duckitt K, Thornton S, O'Donovan OP, Dowswell T. Nitric oxide donors for treating preterm labour. Cochrane Database Syst Rev. 2014;(5):CD002860.
110. Lemancewicz A, Laudańska H, Laudański T, Karpiuk A, Batra S. Permeability of fetal membranes to calcium and magnesium: possible role in preterm labour. Hum Reprod. 2000;15(9):2018–22.
111. Ruoti Cosp M. Magnesio, Sulfato de En: Ruoti Cosp M, Calabrese E, Editores. Fármacos y embarazo, que medicamentos prescribir. AMOLCA. Caracas. 2015.p. 1038–1040.
112. Elliott JP, Lewis DF, Morrison JC, Garite TJ. In defense of magnesium sulfate. Obstet Gynecol. 2009;113(6):1341–8.
113. McNamara HC, Crowther CA, Brown J. Different treatment regimens of magnesium sulphate for tocolysis in women in preterm labour. Cochrane Database Syst Rev. 2015;(12):CD011200.
114. Crowther CA, Brown J, McKinlay CJ, Middleton P. Magnesium sulphate for preventing preterm birth in threatened preterm labour. Cochrane Database Syst Rev. 2014;(8):CD001060.
115. Kim MK, Lee SM, Oh JW, Kim SY, Jeong HG, Kim SM, et al. Efficacy and side effect of ritodrine and magnesium sulfate in threatened preterm labor. Obstet Gynecol Sci. 2018;61(1):63–70.
116. Shepherd E, Salam RA, Manhas D, Synnes A, Middleton P, et al. Antenatal magnesium sulphate and adverse neonatal outcomes: a systematic review and meta-analysis. PLoS Med. 2019;16(12):e1002988.
117. Holcomb WL Jr, Shackelford GD, Petrie RH. Magnesium tocolysis and neonatal bone abnormalities: a controlled study. Obstet Gynecol. 1991;78(4):611–4.
118. Schanler RJ, Smith LG Jr, Burns PA. Effects of long-term maternal intravenous magnesium sulfate therapy on neonatal calcium metabolism and bone mineral content. Gynecol Obstet Invest. 1997;43(4):236–41.
119. American College of Obstetricians and Gynecologists Committee on Obstetric Practice Society for Maternal-Fetal Medicine. Committee Opinion No. 573: magnesium sulfate use in obstetrics. Obstet Gynecol. 2013;122(3):727–8.
120. Elliott JP, Morrison JC, Bofill JA. Risks and benefits of magnesium sulfate tocolysis in preterm labor (PTL). AIMS Public Health. 2016;3(2):348–56.
121. Vogel JP, Nardin JM, Dowswell T, West HM, Oladapo OT. Combination of tocolytic agents for inhibiting preterm labour. Cochrane Database Syst Rev. 2014;(7):CD006169.
122. van Vliet E, Dijkema GH, Schuit E, Heida KY, et al. Nifedipine maintenance tocolysis and perinatal outcome: an individual participant data meta-analysis. BJOG. 2016;123(11):1753–60.
123. Parry E, Roos C, Stone P, Hayward L, Mol BW, McCowan L. The NIFTY study: a multicenterrandomised double-blind placebo-controlled trial of nifedipine maintenance tocolysis in fetal fibronectin-positive women in threatened preterm labour. Aust N Z J Obstet Gynaecol. 2014;54(3):231–6.

124. Younger JD, Reitman E, Gallos G. Tocolysis: present and future treatment options. Semin Perinatol. 2017;41(8):493–504.
125. Sanchez-Ramos L, Huddleston JF. The therapeutic value of maintenance tocolysis: an overview of the evidence. Clin Perinatol. 2003;30(4):841–54.
126. Society for Maternal-Fetal Medicine Publications Committee, with assistance of Vincenzo Berghella. Progesterone and preterm birth prevention: translating clinical trials data into clinical practice. Am J Obstet Gynecol. 2012;206(5):376–86.
127. da Fonseca EB, Bittar RE, Carvalho MH, Zugaib M. Prophylactic administration of progesterone by vaginal suppository to reduce the incidence of spontaneous preterm birth in women at increased risk: a randomized placebo-controlled double-blind study. Am J Obstet Gynecol. 2003;188(2):419–24.
128. Hassan SS, Romero R, Vidyadhari D, Fusey S, Baxter JK, et al. Vaginal progesterone reduces the rate of preterm birth in women with a sonographic short cervix: a multicenter, randomized, double-blind, placebo-controlled trial. Ultrasound Obstet Gynecol. 2011;38(1):18–31.
129. Norman JE, Marlow N, Messow CM, Shennan A, Bennett PR, Thornton S, et al. Vaginal progesterone prophylaxis for preterm birth (the OPPTIMUM study): a multicentre, randomised, double-blind trial. Lancet. 2016;387(10033):2106–16.
130. Meis PJ, Klebanoff M, Thom E, Dombrowski MP, Sibai B, Moawad AH. Prevention of recurrent preterm delivery by 17 alpha-hydroxyprogesterone caproate. N Engl J Med. 2003;348(24):2379–85.
131. Northen AT, Norman GS, Anderson K, Moseley L, Divito M, Cotroneo M, et al. Follow-up of children exposed in utero to 17 alpha-hydroxyprogesterone caproate compared with placebo. Obstet Gynecol. 2007;110(4):865–72.

Chapter 34
Antenatal Corticosteroid

Viviane P. Monteiro, Luciana C. Cima, and Mariane T. Tauile

Introduction

Respiratory distress syndrome (RDS) is the main cause of death among the preterm newborn and is a consequence of surfactant deficiency in the pulmonary alveoli. Other factors, such as immaturity of the lung parenchyma, are also involved in the pathophysiology of this condition.

The benefits of administering corticosteroid therapy before preterm delivery include reduction of perinatal mortality and incidence of complications, such as respiratory distress syndrome, intraventricular hemorrhage, need for ventilatory support, admission to the neonatal intensive care unit (NICU), and neonatal systemic infections in the first 48 hours after birth [1].

The only corticosteroids capable of crossing the placental barrier, in an equally effective manner, are betamethasone and dexamethasone. Therefore, other corticosteroids are not *recommended* to reduce neonatal risks related to prematurity.

Recommended Dosage

Currently, regimens of 2 doses of intramuscular 12 mg betamethasone taken every 24 hours (total of 2 doses) and dexamethasone 6 mg intramuscularly every 12 hours (total of 4 doses) are the currently recommended regimens (as recommended by the National Institutes of Health) [2].

V. P. Monteiro (✉)
Instituto Fernandes Figueira / Fiocruz, Rio de Janeiro, RJ, Brazil

L. C. Cima · M. T. Tauile
Perinatal/Rede D'or, Rio de Janeiro, RJ, Brazil

© Springer Nature Switzerland AG 2022

R. A. Moreira de Sá, E. B. d. Fonseca (eds.), *Perinatology*,
https://doi.org/10.1007/978-3-030-83434-0_34

The most effective period of action occurs between 24 hours and 7 days after the administration of the last dose of corticosteroids [3].

Multiple courses of corticosteroids are not recommended due to the risk of maternal and fetal damage [4]. Some studies suggest deleterious effects on cerebral myelination, lung growth, and function of the hypothalamic-pituitary-adrenal axis [5].

Corticotherapy Recommendations

The recommendation for antenatal administration of corticosteroid includes all pregnant women between 24 and 34 weeks at risk of premature delivery within 7 days [6].

Previable Gestation

In pregnancies of less than 24 weeks, with risk of premature birth, the use of corticosteroids should be considered if it has been decided with the family to resuscitate the newborn [7].

Local limits of fetal viability are a relevant predictor when determining the lowest gestational age for administration of corticosteroids for lung maturation. It should be noted that even in high-resource settings, the level of "intact survival" (survival without morbidity) is low [8].

Late Preterm

Pregnant women between 34 and 36 weeks +6 days of gestation (late preterm) at risk of delivery within 7 days, and who have not previously undergone corticosteroid therapy, can undergo a single course of corticosteroids, as it has been shown that it lowers neonatal morbidity in this group. However, there are no long-term studies that ensure the safety of the use of the drug in this [8, 9].

Term Gestation

When there is a need for elective termination of pregnancy and in the absence of labor between 37 and 38 weeks +6 days, a single course of corticosteroids should be considered as a strategy for reducing the risk of RDS in patients who have not undergone previous corticosteroid therapy [10].

The risk of adverse respiratory outcome is also greater in cesarean deliveries when compared to vaginal delivery, especially when cesarean delivery takes place before labor begins [11].

The American College of Obstetricians and Gynecologists (ACOG) recommends that elective cesarean sections should not take place before 39 weeks' gestation, since the timing of the delivery relates to infant outcomes, and have an important impact on public health issues [12].

Multi-fetal Gestation

For twin pregnancies, in the absence of contraindications, the same corticosteroid regimen is recommended for all patients between 24 and 34 weeks at risk of childbirth within 7 days, as it is for singleton gestations [7].

Preexisting or Gestational Diabetes

The use of corticosteroids for fetal lung maturation is not contraindicated in diabetic women. Insulin-dependent diabetic patients must be strictly monitored for the risk of glycemic control and must have their insulin dose adjusted according to established protocols [13].

Fetal Growth Restriction

Although evidence shows a significant reduction in the risk of RDS, intraventricular hemorrhage, and intrauterine death, data on the administration of corticosteroids in fetuses with growth restriction are still conflicting, requiring the individualization of each case [14].

Rescue Dosage

According to the WHO, a new corticosteroid cycle can be considered if premature birth does not occur within 7 days after the first course and a new risk of childbirth is identified after that period [8]. The American College of Obstetricians and Gynecologists (ACOG) recommends that a new course can be taken after 14 days of the first cycle in pregnant women under 34 weeks of age with a new risk of premature delivery within 1 week [12].

The use of antenatal corticosteroids has proven to be a very clinically efficient and cost-effective way of preventing neonatal respiratory complications. Pregnant women with clinical symptoms of premature labor should be carefully evaluated, and measurements of uterine cervix and fibronectin should be considered. Corticosteroids should only be administered if there is strong clinical suspicion of preterm delivery in the following 2–7 days [15].

References

1. Crowley P, Chalmers I, Keise MJ. The effects of corticosteroid administration before preterm delivery: an overview of the evidence from controlled trials. Br J Obstet Gynaecol. 1990;97:11–25.
2. Gilstrap LC, Christensen R, Clewell WH, et al. Effect of corticosteroids for letal maturation on prenatal outcomes. NIH Consensus Development Panel on the effect of corticosteroids for fetal maturation on perinatal outcomes. JAMA. 1995;273:413–8.
3. Di Renzo GC, FIGO. Good clinical practice advice: antenatal corticosteroids for fetal lung-maturation. Int J Gynaecol Obstet. 2019;144(3):352–5.
4. American College of Obstetricians and Gynecologists' Committee on Practice Bulletins-Obstetrics. Practice bulletin N0. 171: management of preterm labor. Obstet Gynecol. 2016;128:e155–64.
5. National Institutes of Health Consensus Development Panel. Antenatal corticosteroids revisited: repeat courses – National Institutes of Health Consensus Development Conference Statement, August 17–18, 2000. Obstet Gynecol. 2001;98:144–50.
6. Roberts D, Dalziel SR. Antenatal corticosteroids for accelerating fetal lung maturation for women at risk for preterm birth. Cochrane Database Syst Rev. 2006;(19):CD004454.
7. Committee on Obstetric Practice. Committee Opinion No. 713: antenatal corticosteroid therapy for fetal maturation. Obstet Gynecol. 2017;130:e102–9.
8. World Health Organization. WHO recommendations on interventions to improve preterm birth outcomes. Geneva: WHO; 2015.
9. Gyamfi-Bannerman C, Thom EA, Blackwell SC, et al.; NICHD Maternal-Fetal Medicine Units Network. Antenatal betamethasone for women at risk for late preterm delivery. N Engl J Med. 2016;374:1311–20.
10. Saccone G, Berghella V. Antenatal corticosteroids for maturity of term or near term fetuses: systematic review and meta-analysis of randomized controlled trials. BMJ. 2016;355:i5044.
11. Tita AT, Landon MB, Spong CY, et al.; Eunice Kennedy Shriver NICHD Maternal-Fetal Medicine Units Network. Timing of elective repeat cesarean delivery at term and neonatal outcomes. N Engl J Med. 2009;360:111–20.
12. American College of Obstetricians and Gynecologists' Committee on Obstetric Practice; Society for Maternal-Fetal Medicine. Committee Opinion No. 677: antenatal corticosteroids therapy for fetal maturation. Obstet Gynecol. 2016;128:e187–e194.
13. National Institute for Health and Care Excellence. Diabetes in pregnancy; management from preconception to the postnatal period (NG3). London: NICE; 2015.
14. Magann EF, Haram K, Ounpraseuth S, Mortensen JH, Spencer HJ, Morrison JC. Use of antenatal corticosteroids in special circumstances: a comprehensive review. Acta Obstet Gynecol Scand. 2017;96:395–409.
15. Di Renzo GC, Cabero Roura L, Facchinetti F, et al. Preterm labor and birth management: recommendations from the European Association of Perinatal Medicine. J Matern Fetal Neonatal Med. 2017;30:2011–30.

Chapter 35
Magnesium Sulfate in Prevention of Cerebral Palsy

Ingrid Schwach Werneck Britto
and Mario Henrique Burlacchini de Carvalho

Cerebral palsy is the most prevalent chronic childhood motor disability. Cerebral palsy is defined by the International Committee on Cerebral Palsy Classification as a group of developmental disorders of movement and posture causing limitations that can be attributed to nonprogressive disturbances occurring in the developing fetal or infant brain [1]. There are two patterns of frequent changes in the nervous system related to prematurity: intraventricular hemorrhage and white matter injury.

The severe degrees of ventricular hemorrhage (3 and 4) are associated with motor changes and cognitive impairment and occur more frequently in babies born at or before 28 weeks' gestation. Others adverse clinical findings related to prematurity are deafness, blindness, development delay, motor disabilities, and learning difficulties [2]. Cerebral palsy is a symptom complex of nonprogressive motor impairment syndrome secondary to brain injury with an estimated cost nearly $ 1 million per person. Spasticity, movement disorders, ataxia, and muscle weakness are signs of cerebral palsy [2]. Deliveries before 32 weeks are associated with one third of new cases of cerebral palsy [1]. Others risk factors are multiple gestation, intrauterine growth restriction, intracranial hemorrhage, infection, genetic syndromes, birth asphyxia, and trauma.

Magnesium sulfate causes cerebral vasodilation, reduction of oxygen free radicals and inflammatory cytokines, and nuclear factor kappa-B (NF-KB) activation and inhibits the entry of calcium into cells [3, 4]. Magnesium also affects the brain endothelium by relaxing the smooth muscle of the vessels and causes N-methyl-D-aspartate (NMDA) inhibition which reduces ischemia associated with brain damage [5]. Neuroprotection is related to decreased NMDA receptor excitotoxicity and reduced proinflammatory cytokine levels and oxidative stress [5]. In a

I. S. W. Britto · M. H. B. de Carvalho (✉)
Department of Obstetrics and Gynecology, Faculty of Medical Sciences of Santa Casa of São Paulo, São Paulo, São Paulo, Brazil
e-mail: mario.burlacchini@hc.fm.usp.br

© Springer Nature Switzerland AG 2022

R. A. Moreira de Sá, E. B. d. Fonseca (eds.), *Perinatology*,
https://doi.org/10.1007/978-3-030-83434-0_35

recent study, the half-life of magnesium was 2.7 hours in nonpreeclamptic women and 3.9 hours in preeclamptic women [6]. This study showed that magnesium sulfate maternal level can be affected by maternal weight. However, gestational age and maternal creatinine did not influence maternal magnesium level.

Historically, magnesium sulfate has been used as a tocolysis agent and to treat eclampsia. In 2002, a Cochrane review concluded that magnesium sulfate is not effective in preventing premature birth [7]. Observational studies reported that women treated for preeclampsia with magnesium sulfate showed a reduction in the occurrence of neonatal cerebral palsy compared to newborns of mothers without preeclampsia and without exposure to magnesium sulfate.

From 2002 to 2008, multiple randomized trials were carried out and concluded that magnesium sulfate exposure significantly decreases the risk of cerebral palsy [8–19].

The Beneficial Effects of Antenatal Magnesium Sulfate (BEAM) trial showed a decrease in moderate cerebral palsy in patients treated with $MgSO_4$, from 3.5% to 1.9%, respectively [10]. The number of cases studied was 2336, and the average gestational age of delivery was 28 weeks. In the PREterm brain protection by MAGnesium sulfate (PREMAG) trial, children treated for neuroprotection at 2 years of age showed a reduction from 30.8% to 25.6% in the combined rate of death and motor dysfunction [9]. The number of cases studied was 573, and median gestational age of delivery was 30 weeks.

The American College of Obstetricians and Gynecologists (ACOG) conclude that there is level A evidence suggesting that fetal neuroprotection with $MgSO_4$ reduces severity and risk of cerebral palsy when delivery is anticipated before 32 weeks gestation [13]. The three main trials that recommend the use of magnesium sulfate used different treatment doses [8–10]. For this reason, ACOG advise hospitals to develop uniform, specific guidelines addressing inclusion criteria, treatment, tocolysis, and monitoring in accordance with one of the larger clinical trials.

Different protocols were used in each of the tree main trials (BEAM, PREMAG, and ACTOMgSO4). BEAM trial recommends a loading dosage of 6 grams over 20–30 minutes and a maintenance dose of 2 g/h until birth or for 12 hours [10]. PREMAG trial recommends a loading dosage of 4 grams over 30 minutes and no maintenance dose [9]. ACTOMgSO4 trial recommends a loading dosage of 4 grams over 20 minutes and a maintenance dose of 1 g /h until birth or for 24 hours [8]. Retreatment was recommended only in the BEAM trial.

A Cochrane meta-analysis showed reduced risk of cerebral palsy (relative risk, 0.68; 95% confidence interval, 0.51–0.91) associated with maintenance dosing of $MgSO_4$ [12]. A 6 grams loading dose and a higher maintenance dose were associated with reduced risk of cerebral palsy (relative risk, 0.59; 95% confidence interval, 0.40–0.85) Despite this, a recent meta-analysis found no difference in neonatal prognosis related to dose [17].

Therefore, the absence of a clear consensus on the magnesium sulfate dose for neuroprotection remains a challenge, and there are no data in the literature to date indicating a universal standard treatment for all cases [5].

Most authors recommend an attack dose and maintenance dose of magnesium sulfate when there is risk of imminent delivery and gestational age is below 32 weeks. Pharmacological model suggests that the optimal level of $MgSO_4$ for neuroprotection occurs in 5.5–18 hours of continuous treatment [5].

Magnesium sulfate for fetal neuroprotection was not associated with an increase in infant death [19]. Randomized controlled trials demonstrated no other differences in neonatal morbidity such as necrotizing enterocolitis, respiratory distress syndrome, and seizures [19]. Exposure to magnesium sulfate for less than 48 hours is usually not related to complications to neonates; however, complications such as hypotonia, lethargy, and respiratory depression may occur, especially in prolonged regimens.

To prevent 1 case of cerebral palsy, 46 women must be treated with magnesium sulfate when at risk for preterm delivery [5].

Contraindications for the use of magnesium sulfate are hypersensitivity to the drug, hepatic coma, myasthenia gravis, and fetus with lethal malformations or chromosomal abnormalities. Women with renal impartment should be monitored.

The most common side effects of using magnesium sulfate are flushing, sweating, nausea, vomiting, maternal hypotension, tachycardia, respiratory depression, discomfort, mouth dryness, blurred vision, and problems at the injection site. Maternal side effects are dose-related. Some women have discontinued use due to side effects; however, no case of death or cardiac arrest was described in the trials [19]. Side effects may be reduced by lower-dose regimens.

Antenatal magnesium sulfate administration should be considered for fetal neuroprotection when women present at <31 + 6 weeks with imminent preterm birth. Magnesium sulfate should be discontinued if delivery is no longer imminent or a maximum of 24 hours of therapy has been administrated.

Magnesium sulfate should be started within 4 hours before birth. If necessary emergency delivery for fetal or maternal indications, delivery should not be delayed in order to administer antenatal magnesium sulfate for fetal neuroprotection.

Women receiving magnesium sulfate for fetal neuroprotection should be monitored by care providers using preeclampsia/eclampsia protocols until the standardization of the treatment regimen is established.

References

1. Bax M, Goldstein M, Rosenbaum P, et al. Proposed definition and classification of cerebral palsy. April 2005. Dev Med Child Neurol. 2005;47(8):571–6.
2. Magee L, Sawchuck D, Synnes A, von Dadelszen P. Magnesium sulphate for fetal neuroprotection. SOGC Clinical Practice Guideline. J Obstet Gynaecol Can. 2011;33(5):516–29.
3. Suzuki-Kakisaka H, Sugimoto J, Tetarbe M, et al. Magnesium sulfate increases intracellular magnesium reducing inflammatory cytokine release in neonates. Am J Reprod Immunol. 2013;70(3):213–20.

4. Sugimoto J, Romani AM, Valentin-Torres AM, et al. Magnesium decreases inflammatory cytokine production: a novel innate immunomodulatory mechanism. J Immunol. 2012;188(12):6338–46.
5. Jameson RA, Bernstein HB. Magnesium sulfate and novel therapies to promote neuroprotection. Clin Perinatol. 2019;46:187–201.
6. Brookfield KF, Elkomy M, Su F, et al. Optimization of maternal magnesium sulfate administration for fetal neuroprotection: application of a prospectively constructed pharmacokinetic model to the BEAM cohort. J Clin Pharmacol. 2017;57(11):1419–24.
7. Crowther CA, Brown J, McKinlay CJD, et al. Magnesium sulphate for preventing preterm birth in threatened preterm labour. Cochrane Database Syst Rev. 2014;(8):CD001060. https://doi.org/10.1002/14651858.CD001060.pub2.
8. Crowther CA, Hiller JE, Doyle LW, et al. Effect of magnesium sulfate given for neuroprotection before preterm birth: a randomized controlled trial. JAMA. 2003;290:2669–76.
9. Marret S, Marpeau L, Zupan-Simunek V, et al. Magnesium sulphate given before very-preterm birth to protect infant brain: the randomised controlled PREMAG trial. BJOG. 2007;114(3):310–8.
10. Rouse DJ, Hirtz DG, Thom E, et al. A randomized, controlled trial of magnesium sulfate for the prevention of cerebral palsy. N Engl J Med. 2008;359(9):895–905.
11. Costantine MM, Weiner SJ. Effects of antenatal exposure to magnesium sulfate on neuroprotection and mortality in preterm infants: a meta-analysis. Obstet Gynecol. 2009;114:354–64.
12. Doyle LW, Crowther CA, Middleton P, et al. Magnesium sulphate for women at risk of preterm birth for neuroprotection of the fetus. Cochrane Database Syst Rev. 2009;(1):CD004661.
13. American College of Obstetricians and Gynecologists Committee on Obstetric. Practice, Society for Maternal-Fetal Medicine. Committee opinion no. 455: magnesium sulfate before anticipated preterm birth for neuroprotection. Obstet Gynecol. 2010;115(3):669–71.
14. Reeves SA, Gibbs RS, Clark SL. Magnesium for fetal neuroprotection. Am J Obstet Gynecol. 2011;204(3):202.e1–4.
15. Bain E, Middleton P, Crowther CA. Different magnesium sulphate regimens for neuroprotection of the fetus for women at risk of preterm birth. Cochrane Database Syst Rev. 2012;(2):CD009302.
16. Zeng X, Xue Y, Tian Q, et al. Effects and safety of magnesium sulfate on neuroprotection: a meta-analysis based on PRISMA guidelines. Medicine (Baltimore). 2016;95(1):e2451.
17. Crowther CA, Middleton PF, Voysey M, et al. Assessing the neuroprotective benefits for babies of antenatal magnesium sulphate: an individual participant data meta-analysis. PLoS Med. 2017;14(10):e1002398.
18. Shepherd E, Salam RA, Middleton P, et al. Antenatal and intrapartum interventions for preventing cerebral palsy: an overview of Cochrane systematic reviews. Cochrane Database Syst Rev. 2017;(8):CD012077.
19. Conde-Agudelo A, Romero R. Antenatal magnesium sulfate for the prevention of cerebral palsy in preterm infants less than 34 weeks' gestation: a systematic review and metaanalysis. Am J Obstet Gynecol. 2009;200(6):595–609.

Chapter 36
Premature Rupture of Membranes

Juliana Silva Esteves

Introduction

Prelabor rupture of membranes (PROM) complicates 7–8% of pregnancies and is defined as rupture of membranes before the onset of labor. Preterm prelabor rupture of membranes (PPROM) before 37 weeks is the leading identifiable cause of preterm birth and accounts for 30–40% of cases [1–3].

Management of PROM is influenced by gestational age and the presence of complicating factors such as maternal infection, abnormal fetal testing, labor, or abruptio placentae.

Preterm birth involves a heterogeneous group with a wide range of characteristics, management, and outcomes. Considering that, the executive summary of proceedings from a joint workshop sponsored by the Society for Maternal-Fetal Medicine and the Eunice Kennedy Shriver National Institute of Child and Human Development (NICHD), in association with other entities, defined previable birth as delivery occurring from 20^{+0} weeks to 25^{+6} weeks of gestation. Approximately 0.5% of all births occur at this time of pregnancy, and these very early deliveries result in the majority of neonatal and infant deaths [5].

An accurate assessment of gestational age and knowledge of the maternal, fetal, and neonatal risks are essential to appropriate evaluation and care of these patients. Management and counseling of PPROM have been a clinical dilemma in the last decades, as strong predictors of neonatal and maternal outcomes remain unclear [4, 6, 7].

J. S. Esteves (✉)
Hospital Federal dos Servidores do Estado - Ministry of Health, Rio de Janeiro, RJ, Brazil

© Springer Nature Switzerland AG 2022

R. A. Moreira de Sá, E. B. d. Fonseca (eds.), *Perinatology*,
https://doi.org/10.1007/978-3-030-83434-0_36

Etiology

During the first weeks of gestation, the amnion is contained within the gestational sac separated from the chorion by chorionic fluid and in turn encloses the fetus and amniotic fluid in a separate space within a sac. This fusion of the chorionic space normally occurs around the 14th week of gestation, although fusion could be delayed in some pregnancies up to the 15th week. This persistence of separation in the second trimester is termed chorioamniotic separation and can be detected on high-resolution ultrasound [8]. These connected membranes can always be easily mechanically separated from each other, and are never truly fused, cellularly speaking, and after the delivery the chorioamniotic membranes can be manually separated from each other. The situation with the defect of only one membrane frequently occurs and is related to inexistent obliteration between fetal membranes (Pre-PPROM).

Membrane rupture may occur for a variety of reasons. Although membrane rupture at term can result from a normal physiologic weakening of the membranes combined with shearing forces created by uterine contractions, preterm PROM can result from a wide array of pathologic mechanisms that act individually or in concert.

The most prevalent site of rupture of amniotic membranes is the supracervical area, where membrane overlying the ostium of cervical area. At this site, the amniotic membrane is structurally altered and easily disrupted. However, clinical experience has shown that not all cases of PPROM follow this classic pattern of rupture, which can explain cases where patients with positive PPROM test maintain a normal amniotic fluid on ultrasound examination.

Altered membrane morphology including marked swelling and disruption of the collagen network which is seen with PPROM can be triggered by bacterial products or/and pro-inflammatory cytokines. Activation of matrix metalloproteinases (MMP) has been implicated in the mechanism of PPROM. Inflammatory mediators likely play a causative role in both disruption of fetal membrane integrity and activation of uterine contraction [9, 10].

Intra-amniotic infection has been shown to be commonly associated with preterm PROM, especially at earlier gestational ages. The propagation of bacteria is an important contributing factor not only in PPROM but also in adverse neonatal and maternal outcomes after PPROM. A history of preterm PROM is a major risk factor for preterm PROM or preterm labor in a subsequent pregnancy [11, 12]. Additional risk factors associated with preterm PROM are similar to those associated with spontaneous preterm birth and include short cervical length, second-trimester and third-trimester bleeding, low body mass index, low socioeconomic status, cigarette smoking, and illicit drug use [13]. Although each of these risk factors is associated with preterm PROM, the condition often occurs in the absence of recognized risk factors or an obvious cause.

Diagnosis

Most cases of PROM can be diagnosed on the basis of the patient's history and physical examination. A report of watery leakage from the vagina, confirmed by sterile speculum examination and by the observation of either fluid accumulation in the posterior vaginal fornix or direct leakage from the cervical canal with pressure from uterine fundus, is evidence of rupture.

Examination should be performed in a manner that minimizes the risk of introducing infection. Digital cervical examinations should be avoided because of its association with an increased risk of chorioamnionitis by ascending infection and reduction of the latency period by 9 days on average. Sterile speculum examination provides an opportunity to inspect for cervicitis and prolapse of the umbilical cord or fetal parts, assess cervical dilatation and effacement, and obtain cultures as appropriate [14].

Additional testings, such as nitrazine or the ferning tests, may be applied, if the diagnosis is uncertain; however, contaminating substances could produce a false-positive result in the presence of blood, semen after coitus, alkaline-based antiseptics, or bacterial vaginosis. Normal vaginal pH varies between 4.4 and 6.0, whereas pH of amniotic fluid is 8.0.

Based on clinical evaluation, the diagnosis of PROM can be equivocal in 10–20% of cases. According to the National Institute for Health and Care Excellence (NICE), when a pool of amniotic fluid is not clearly observed, consideration should be given to testing for insulin-like growth factor binding protein 1 (IGFBP-1) or placental alpha-microglobulin 1 (PAMG-1) if these tests are available. NICE emphasizes that the test results for IGFBP-1 or PAMG-1 should not be used alone to decide what care to offer the woman and that clinical condition, medical and pregnancy history, and gestational age should be taken in to account [15].

Several commercially available tests for amniotic proteins are currently on the market, with reported high sensitivity for PROM [8].

No studies were identified specifically addressing ultrasound to determine amniotic fluid volumes in women presenting with suspected PPROM. Ultrasound examination demonstrating oligohydramnios may be useful to support the clinical diagnosis of PPROM [16].

Term Prelabor Rupture of Membranes

At term, PROM complicates approximately 8% of pregnancies and generally is followed by the prompt onset of spontaneous labor and delivery [17].

In 1996, the TERMPROM Study Group showed that one half of women with term PROM who were managed expectantly had an interval of membrane rupture to delivery of 33 hours, and 95% gave birth within 94–107 hours of membrane rupture with the use of oxytocin or prostaglandin when, during expectant management, induction was indicated or an endpoint of 4 days of expectant management was reached [18].

Once the diagnostic of term PROM was done, gestational age and fetal position should be confirmed, and fetal heart rate monitoring should be used, to assess fetal status. Group B streptococcal prophylaxis should be given based on prior culture results or intrapartum risk factors if cultures have not been performed previously for women who are GBS positive, administration of antibiotics for GBS prophylaxis should not be delayed while awaiting labor, and immediate induction rather than expectant management may be recommended [7, 16].

A meta-analysis of 23 randomized controlled trials (8615 women) found that induction of labor reduced the time from rupture of membrane to birth and the rates of chorioamnionitis or endometritis, or both, and also reduced admission to the neonatal intensive care unit without increasing the rates of cesarean birth or operative vaginal delivery. Induction of labor with vaginal prostaglandins has been shown to be equally effective for labor induction compared with oxytocin but was associated with higher rates of chorioamnionitis (Cochrane 2017). However, the authors concluded that there was low-quality evidence to suggest that planned early birth (with induction methods such as oxytocin or prostaglandins) reduces the risk of maternal infectious morbidity compared with expectant management for PROM at 37 weeks' gestation or later, without an apparent increased risk of cesarean section. Evidence was mainly downgraded due to the majority of studies contributing data having some serious design limitations, and for most outcomes estimates were imprecise.

In your last guideline, the ACOG defends the idea that in women with PROM at 37 0/7 weeks of gestation or more, if spontaneous labor does not occur near the time of presentation in those who do not have contraindication to labor, labor induction should be recommended, although the choice of expectant management for a short period of time may be appropriately offered. In the cases in which expectant management is chosen, given that nearly 80% and 95% of patients start labor spontaneously within 12 hours and 24 hours respectively, a period of 12–24 hours of expectant management is reasonable as long as the clinical and fetal conditions are reassuring, and the patient is adequately counseled regarding the risks of prolonged PROM and the limitations of available data [7].

Preterm Premature of Membranes

Preterm prelabor rupture of membranes (PPROM) before 37 weeks is the leading identifiable cause of preterm birth and accounts for one third of cases [4]. Regardless of obstetric management or clinical presentation, birth within 1 week of membrane rupture occurs in at least one half of patients with preterm PROM. Latency after membrane rupture is inversely correlated with the gestational age at membrane rupture.

Among women with preterm PROM, clinically evident intra-amniotic infection occurs in 15–35% of cases, and postpartum infection occurs in approximately 15–25% of cases. The incidence of infection is higher at earlier gestational ages, and abruptio placentae complicates 2–5% of pregnancies with preterm PROM [19, 20].

The most significant risks to the fetus after preterm PROM are complications of prematurity. Preterm PROM has been associated with an increased risk of neurodevelopmental impairment, and respiratory distress has been reported to be the most common complication of preterm birth. Sepsis, intraventricular hemorrhage, and necrotizing enterocolitis also are associated with prematurity but are less common near term. However, there are no data that suggest immediate delivery after presentation with PROM will avert these risks. A large cohort study suggests that prolonged latency duration, when adjusted for gestational age, does not worsen neonatal prognosis with respect to survival, survival without morbidity, and early-onset sepsis [21, 22].

Antibiotics

A Cochrane review investigating the role of antibiotics for women with confirmed PPROM found that the use of antibiotics is associated with a statistically significant reduction in chorioamnionitis (RR 0.66, 95% CI 0.46–0.96). There was a significant reduction in the numbers of babies born within 48 hours (RR 0.71, 95% CI 0.58–0.87) and 7 days (RR 0.79, 95% CI 0.71–0.89). Neonatal infection, use of surfactant, oxygen therapy, and abnormal cerebral ultrasound prior to discharge from hospital were also reduced. There was no significant reduction in perinatal mortality or on the health of the children at 7 years of age [23, 24].

The optimal antibiotic regimen is unclear because multiple regimens have demonstrated benefit. Based on available information, to reduce maternal and neonatal infections and gestational-age-dependent morbidity, a 7-day course of therapy of latency antibiotics with a combination of intravenous ampicillin and erythromycin followed by oral amoxicillin and erythromycin is recommended during expectant management of women with preterm PROM who are at less than 34 0/7 weeks of gestation ([24]; Cochrane 2013).

The regimen used in the Eunice Kennedy Shriver National Institute of Child Health and Human Development Maternal Fetal Medicine Units Network trial was intravenous ampicillin (2 g every 6 hours) and erythromycin (250 mg every 6 hours) for 48 hours followed by oral amoxicillin (250 mg every 8 hours) and erythromycin base (333 mg every 8 hours) [7]. Some centers have replaced the use of erythromycin with azithromycin (such as a single oral dose of azithromycin 1 g) in situations in which erythromycin is not available or not tolerated, and this substitution is a suitable alternative; there is no difference in latency or secondary outcomes such as neonatal survival, sepsis, or respiratory distress between the two medications [25, 26]. The use of amoxicillin-clavulanic acid should be avoided as it is associated with an increased risk of neonatal necrotizing enterocolitis [24]. Antibiotics should not be given unless the diagnosis of PPROM is confirmed [16].

Antenatal Infection

One of the risks associated with PPROM is ascending infection leading to chorioamnionitis and subsequent fetal and neonatal infection. The National Institute for Health and Care Excellence (NICE) recommends that a combination of clinical assessment (pulse, blood pressure, temperature, and symptoms like abdominal or fundal tenderness), maternal blood tests (C-reactive protein and white blood cell count), and fetal heart rate should be employed to diagnose clinical infection. The results should not be considered alone, so if they are not in agreement to the clinical assessment or if any of the tests are not consistent with each other, it is recommended that the woman should continue to be observed and consideration should be given to repeating the tests [15]. Unfortunately, there is no consensus on the optimal frequency of assessment.

A study investigating several maternal serum markers for predicting histological chorioamnionitis after PPROM concluded that a raised C-reactive protein was most informative. However, a systematic review and meta-analysis of 13 observational studies found that C-reactive protein has a sensitivity of only 68.7% and specificity of 77.1% in diagnosing histological chorioamnionitis [27, 28].

So, when cared for as an inpatient, women with PPROM should have their vital signs, including pulse, blood pressure, respiratory rate, and temperature, recorded on an obstetric early warning chart. They should also be observed for clinical symptoms and signs of infection. It's important to remember that white blood cell count will rise 24 hours following administration of corticosteroids and should return to baseline 3 days following administration [16].

Management

After clinical assessment, a management strategy should be developed to define whether to prolong the pregnancy or delivery because of signs of chorioamnionitis and/or fetal distress. Once the option was conservative management, a vaginal-rectal swab for GBS culture should be obtained at the time of initial presentation and GBS prophylaxis.

The short-term benefits of conservative management of PPROM with antenatal corticoids and maternal systemic antibiotic treatment are well established.

Corticosteroids administration for the lung maturation between 24/0 and 34/0 weeks' gestation is the gold standard. The exact moment for antenatal corticosteroids is still unknown. Most of the guidelines indicate at the moment of PPROM diagnostic.

According to the ACOG, a single course of corticosteroids is recommended for pregnant women between 34 0/7 weeks of gestation and 36 6/7 weeks of gestation at risk of preterm birth within 7 days and who have not received a previous course of antenatal corticosteroids if proceeding with induction or delivery in no less than 24 hours and no more than 7 days [7].

To reduce maternal and neonatal infections and gestational-age-dependent morbidity, a 7-day course of therapy of latency antibiotics with a combination of intravenous ampicillin and erythromycin followed by oral amoxicillin and erythromycin (or azithromycin) is recommended during expectant management of women with preterm PROM who are at less than 34 0/7 weeks of gestation, as discussed above. Women with preterm PROM and a viable fetus who are candidates for intrapartum GBS prophylaxis should receive intrapartum GBS prophylaxis to prevent vertical transmission regardless of earlier antibiotic treatments.

Neuroprotection with magnesium sulfate should be considered for women with preterm PROM before 32 0/7 weeks of gestation who are thought to be at risk of imminent.

Abnormal results from fetal testing, clinical intra-amniotic infection, and significant abruptio placentae are clear indications for delivery. Otherwise, gestational age is a primary factor when considering delivery versus expectant management, and 34 weeks of gestation is used to be the threshold.

Recently a Cochrane review of 3617 women explored the effect of planned early delivery versus expectant management for women with PROM before 37 weeks. The authors conclude that in women with PPROM with no contraindications to continuing the pregnancy, expectant management with careful monitoring is associated with better outcomes for the mother and baby. The review found no differences between early birth and expectant management in neonatal sepsis or infection. Early delivery increased the incidence of respiratory distress syndrome and increased the rate of cesarean section. There were no differences in overall perinatal mortality or intrauterine deaths when comparing early delivery with expectant management. Early birth was associated with a higher rate of neonatal death and need for ventilation [29].

The PPROMPT trial randomized 1839 women that evaluated immediate delivery (shortly after diagnosis and preferably within 24 hours) versus expectant management in patients with PROM between 34 0/7 weeks of gestation and 36 6/7 weeks of gestation suggests benefits to expectant management. There was no significant difference in neonatal sepsis (primary outcome) or in neonatal morbidity (secondary outcome) between the two groups. Infants in the immediate delivery group had higher rates of respiratory distress and mechanical ventilation and spent more days in intensive care (4 days versus 2 days). However, maternal adverse outcomes, such as hemorrhage and infection, were approximately twofold higher with expectant management, although the rate of cesarean birth was lower [30].

According to the authors, the findings suggest that if expectant management until 37 weeks is chosen, it should include careful monitoring of symptoms and signs of maternal infection, chorioamnionitis, and antepartum hemorrhage.

Midtrimester Premature Rupture of Membranes

Midtrimester premature rupture of membrane is an uncommon complication, occurring in less than 1% of pregnancies. Despite this low incidence, midtrimester PPROM is a major perinatal complication that involves maternal-fetal morbidity and mortality. Pregnancies complicated by PPROM usually involve high risks of miscarriage, stillbirth, and neonatal death. The survival rate is low and in most cases associated with neonatal morbidity, such as intraventricular hemorrhage (IVH), retinopathy of prematurity (ROP), bronchopulmonary dysplasia (BPD), and need for home care. Besides that, women with PPROM are also exposed to the risk of chorioamnionitis and sepsis as a consequence of the expectant management necessary for better neonatal outcomes [6, 31, 32].

Management and counseling of PPROM have been a clinical dilemma in the last decades, as strong predictors of neonatal and maternal outcomes remain unclear. On the other hand, advances in neonatal care have enhanced survival, also increasing a wide variety of morbidities.

In a review involving pregnancies with PROM between 14 weeks of gestation and 24 weeks of gestation, perinatal deaths were more or less equally divided in stillbirths and neonatal deaths. Neonatal survival rates in patients expectantly managed were much higher following membrane rupture after 22 weeks of gestation compared with membrane rupture before 22 weeks of gestation (57.7% versus 14.4%, respectively) [33].

A second retrospective study of patients between 20 weeks of gestation and 24 weeks of gestation with periviable PROM who elected expectant management showed similar results, with neonatal survival rate of 22% for newborns of patients with membrane rupture before 22 weeks of gestation and 58% for those with membrane rupture at 22 and 23 weeks of gestation [34].

Latency periods appear to be prolonged with midtrimester preterm PROM compared with PROM during later gestational ages. However, 40–50% of this patients will give birth within the first week, and approximately 70–80% will give birth within 2–5 weeks after membrane rupture [35, 36].

As consequences, most of births still occurring under 28 weeks of gestation, with all complications that involve prematurity. So, the RCOG and ACOG suggest that women with midtrimester PPROM and their partners should be offered access to additional emotional support, both during pregnancy and postnatally [7, 16].

Maternal and Neonatal Outcomes

Taylor et al. first described in 1984 a live birth rate of 34% and 25% of neonate survival after PROM below 26 weeks. In 2009, a meta-analysis revealed a live birth rate of 68%, similar to the live birth rate found in 2006, but better perinatal survival rate (44% versus 21%) [33].

Despite advances in neonatal care and apparent improvement in neonatal outcomes, longer-term neonatal outcomes of children delivered following early midtrimester PPROM are largely unknown.

Maternal infections such as chorioamnionitis and sepsis impact on neonatal outcomes, according to other studies.

It has been reported that midtrimester deliveries, especially with less than 23 weeks, had more association with retained placentae. It can also be added that 67% of all pregnancies with midtrimester PROM before 22 weeks had stillbirth/ miscarriage [31]. A recent systematic review showed an overall frequency of clinical chorioamnionitis of 47% and that complications such as retained placentae and curettage were found to be more common in midtrimester PROM before 20 weeks [6].

In a published report of 53 neonatal ICUs, the presence of maternal clinical chorioamnionitis was associated with significantly increased respiratory distress syndrome (RDS) (69% vs. 60.2%), early-onset neonatal sepsis (10.2% vs. 2.8%, OR 3.1), necrotizing enterocolitis (NEC) (11.2% vs. 7.7%, OR 1.3), severe intraventricular hemorrhage (IVH) (14.5% vs. 8.4%), periventricular leukomalacia (PVL) (8.4% vs. 5.7%), and retinopathy of prematurity (ROP, stage >2) (5.3% vs. 3.2%) in live-born infants ≤1500 g. Half of the neonates from mothers with chorioamnionitis required oxygen at 28 days (46% vs. 30%), and they had a higher rate of BPD (23.2% vs. 14.9%) as well. Chorioamnionitis was associated with increased infant mortality (14.2% vs. 22.6%) and reduced survival without major morbidity, including IVH, PVL, BPD, NEC, or ROP >2 from 57.1% to 42.0% [37].

Severe oligohydramnios during midtrimester pregnancies inhibits a crucial phase of fetal pulmonary development and has been associated with lower perinatal survival rate [38]. Recently, Sim et al. and Cobo et al. proposed that the average post-rupture amniotic fluid index (AFI) was higher for survivors compared to non-survivors and that anhydramnios at any time during the latency period was significantly associated with poor survival outcome [32, 39].

Van Teeffelen et al. tried to estimate the ability of imaging parameters in the prediction of lethal pulmonary hypoplasia secondary to midtrimester prelabor rupture of fetal membranes. The authors concluded that the estimated ROC curves for the chest circumference/abdominal circumference ratio and other parameters showed limited accuracy in the prediction of pulmonary hypoplasia [40].

Birth weight and gestational age at birth were recently described as predictor factors for survival rate [41]. So, in the absence of any symptoms of chorioamnionitis, all of the efforts should be focused on prolonging the latency period (e.g., hospitalization and use of antibiotic prophylaxis) and increasing the birth weight and gestational age. However, it should be noted that the fetal birth weight only influences the neonatal mortality and not morbidity, which remains a concern for these neonates.

References

1. Goldenberg RL, Culhane JF, Iams JD, Romero R. Epidemiology and causes of preterm birth. Lancet. 2008;371:75–84.
2. Raju TN, Mercer BM, Burchfield DJ, Joseph GF Jr. Periviable birth: executive summary of a joint workshop by the *Eunice Kennedy Shriver* National Institute of Child Health and Human Development, Society for Maternal-Fetal Medicine, American Academy of Pediatrics, and American College of Obstetricians and Gynecologists. Obstet Gynecol. 2014;123:1083–96.
3. Middleton P, Shepherd E, Flenady V, McBain RD, Crowther CA. Planned early birth versus expectant management (waiting) for prelabour rupture of membranes at term (37 weeks or more). Cochrane Database Syst Rev. 2017;(1):CD005302.
4. Manuk TA, Varner MW. Neonatal and early childhood outcomes following early vs later preterm premature rupture of membranes. Am J Obstet Gynecol. 2014;211(3):308.
5. Kaimal A, Mercer BM, Blackwell SC, de Regnier RA, Farrell RM, Grobman WA, Resnik JL, Sciscione AC. Periviabel birth: American College of Obstetricians and Gynecologists and the Society for Maternal-Fetal Medicine care consensus. Am J Obstet Gynecol. 2015;213(5):604–14.
6. Sim WH, Araujo Junior E, Da Silva CF, Sheehan PM. Maternal and neonatal outcomes following expectant management of preterm rupture of membranes before viability. J Perinat Med. 2017;45(1):29–44.
7. ACOG Committee on Practice Bulletins. Clinical management guidelines for Obstetrician and Gynecologists number 217: premature rupture of membranes. Obstet Gynecol. 2020;135(3):e80–97.
8. Tchirikov M, Schlabritz-Loutsevitch N, Maher J, Buchmann J, Naberezhnev Y, Winarni AS, et al. Mid-trimester preterm premature of membranes (PPROM): etiology, diagnosis, classification, international recommendations of treatment options and outcome. J Perinat Med. 2018;46(5):465–88.
9. DiGiulio DB, Romero R, Kusanovic JP, Gomez R, Kim CJ, Seok KS, et al. Prevalence and diversity of microbes in the amniotic fluid, the fetal inflammatory response, and pregnancy outcome in women with preterm pre-labor rupture of membranes. Am J Reprod Immunol. 2010;64:38–57.
10. Romero R, Miranda J, Chaemsaithong P, Chaiworapongsa T, Kusanovic JP, Dong Z, et al. Sterile and microbial-associated intra-amniotic inflammation in preterm prelabor rupture of membranes. J Matern Fetal Neonatal Med. 2015;28:1394–409.
11. Lee T, Carpenter MW, Heber WW, Silver HM. Preterm premature rupture of membranes: risks of recurrent complications in the next pregnancy among a population- based sample of gravid women. Am J Obstet Gynecol. 2003;188:209–13.
12. Mercer BM, Goldenberg RL, Meis PJ, Moawad AH, Shellhaas C, Das A, et al. The Preterm Prediction Study: prediction of preterm premature rupture of membranes through clinical findings and ancillary testing. The National Institute of Child Health and Human Development Maternal Fetal Medicine Units Network. Am J Obstet Gynecol. 2000;183:738–45.
13. Harger JH, Hsing AW, Tuomala RE, Gibbs RS, Mead PB, Eschenbach DA, et al. Risk factors for preterm premature rupture of fetal membranes: a multicenter case-control study. Am J Obstet Gynecol. 1990;163:130–7.
14. Chauleur C, Rochigneux S, Seffert P, Chene G, Billiemaz K, Collet F. Neonatal outcomes and four-year follow-up after spontaneous or iatrogenic preterm prelabor rupture of membranes before 24 weeks. Acta Obstet Gynecol Scand. 2009;88:801–6.

15. National Institute for Health and Care Excellence. Preterm labour and birth. NICE guideline 25. London: NICE; 2015.
16. Thomson AJ, on behalf of the Royal College of Obstetricians and Gynaecologists. Care of women presenting with suspected preterm prelabour rupture of membranes from 24^{+0} weeks of gestation. BJOG. 2019;126:e152–66.
17. Mercer BM. Preterm premature rupture of the membranes. Obstet Gynecol. 2003;101:178–93.
18. Hannah ME, Ohlsson A, Farine D, Hewson SA, Hodnett ED, Myhr TL, et al. Induction of labor compared with expectant management for prelabor rupture of the mem- branes at term. TERMPROM Study Group. N Engl J Med. 1996;334:1005–10.
19. Ramsey PS, Lieman JM, Brumfield CG, Carlo W. Chorioamnionitis increases neonatal morbidity in pregnancies complicated by preterm premature rupture of membranes. Am J Obstet Gynecol. 2005;192:1162–6.
20. Ananth CV, Oyelese Y, Srinivas N, Yeo L, Vintzileos AM. Preterm premature rupture of membranes, intrauter- ine infection, and oligohydramnios: risk factors for placental abruption. Obstet Gynecol. 2004;104:71–7.
21. Drassinower D, Friedman AM, Obican SG, Levin H, Gyamfi-Bannerman C. Prolonged latency of preterm prelabour rupture of membranes and neurodevelopmental outcomes: a secondary analysis. BJOG. 2016;123:1629–35.
22. Lorthe E, Ancel PY, Torchin H, Kaminski M, Langer B, Subtil D, et al. Impact of latency duration on the prognosis of preterm infants after preterm premature rupture of membranes at 24 to 32 weeks' gestation: a national population-based cohort study. J Pediatr. 2017;182:47–52.e2.
23. Kenyon S, Boulvain M, Neilson JP. Antibiotics for preterm rupture of membranes. Cochrane Database Syst Rev. 2013;(2):CD001058.
24. Kenyon S, Pike K, Jones DR, Brocklehurst P, Marlow N, Salt A, et al. Childhood outcomes after prescription of antibiotics to pregnant women with preterm rupture of the membranes: 7-year follow-up of the ORACLE I trial. Lancet. 2008;372:1310–8.
25. Navathe R, Schoen CN, Heidari P, Bachilova S, Ward A, Tepper J, et al. Azithromycin vs erythromycin for the management of preterm premature rupture of membranes. Am J Obstet Gynecol. 2019;221:144.e1–8.
26. Pierson RC, Gordon SS, Haas DM. A retrospective comparison of antibiotic regimens for preterm premature rupture of membranes. Obstet Gynecol. 2014;124:515–9.
27. Caloone J, Rabilloud M, Boutitie F, Traverse-Glehen A, Allias-Montmayeur F, Denis L, et al. Accuracy of several maternal seric markers for predicting histological chorioamnionitis after preterm premature rupture of membranes: a prospective and multicentric study. Eur J Obstet Gynecol Reprod Biol. 2016;205:133–40.
28. Sabogal CP, Fonseca J, Garcia-Perdomo HA. Validation of diagnostic tests for histologic chorioamnionitis: systematic review and meta-analysis. Eur J Obstet Gynecol Reprod Biol. 2018;228:13–26.
29. Bond DM, Middleton P, Levett KM, van der Ham DP, Crowther CA, Buchanan SL, et al. Planned early birth versus expectant management for women with preterm prelabour rupture of membranes prior to 37weeks' gestation for improving pregnancy outcome. Cochrane Database Syst Rev. 2017;3(3):CD004735.
30. Morris JM, Roberts CL, Bowen JPJ, Bond DM, Algert CS, Thornton JG, Crowther CA. Immediate delivery compared with expectant management after preterm pre-labour rupture of the membranes close to term (PPROMT trial): a randomised controlled trial. Lancet. 2016;387:444–52.
31. Dotters-Katz SK, Panzer A, Grace MR, Smid MC, Keku JA, Vladutiu CJ, Boggess KA, Manuck TA. Maternal morbidity after Previable prelabor rupture of membranes. Obstet Gynecol. 2017;129(1):101–6.
32. Sim WH, Araujo Júnior E, Da Silva CF, Sheehan PM. Maternal and neonatal outcomes following expectant management of preterm prelabour rupture of membranes before viability. J Perinat Med. 2017;45(1):29–44.
33. Waters TP, Mercer BM. The management of preterm pre- mature rupture of the membranes near the limit of fetal viability. Am J Obstet Gynecol. 2009;201:230–40.

34. Kibel M, Asztalos E, Barrett J, Dunn MS, Tward C, Pittini A, et al. Outcomes of pregnancies complicated by preterm premature rupture of membranes between 20 and 24 weeks of gestation. Obstet Gynecol. 2016;128:313–20.
35. Muris C, Girard B, Creveuil C, Durin L, Herlicoviez M, Dreyfus M. Management of premature rupture of membranes before 25 weeks. Eur J Obstet Gynecol Reprod Biol. 2007;131:163–8.
36. Taylor J, Garite TJ. Premature rupture of membranes before fetal viability. Obstet Gynecol 1984;64:615–20.
37. Garcia-Munoz Rodrigo F, Galan Henriquez G, Figueras Aloy J, Garcia-Alix PA. Outcomes of very-low-birth-weight infants exposed to maternal clinical chorioamnionitis: a multicentre study. Neonatology. 2014;106:229–34.
38. Linehan LA, Walsh J, Morris A, Kenny L, O'Donoghue K, Dempsey E, et al. Neonatal and maternal outcomes following midtrimester preterm premature rupture of the membranes: a retrospective cohort study. BMC Pregnancy Childbirth. 2016;16:25.
39. Cobo T, Munros J, Rios J, Ferreri J, Migliorelli F, Banos N, et al. Contribution of amniotic fluid along gestation to the prediction of perinatal mortality in women with early preterm premature rupture of membranes. Fetal Diagn Ther. 2018;43(2):105–12.
40. van Teeffelen ASP, van der Heijden J, Oei SG, Porath MM, Willekes C, Opmeer B, et al. Accuracy of imaging parameters in the prediction of lethal pulmonary hypoplasia secondary to mid-trimester prelabor rupture of fetal membranes: a systematic review and meta-analysis. Ultrasound Obstet Gynecol. 2012;39:495–9.
41. Esteves JS, De Sá RA, Carvalho PR, Coca Velarde GC. Neonatal outcome in women with preterm premature rupture of membranes (PPROM) beween 18 and 26 weeks. J Matern Fetal Neonatal Med. 2016;29(7):1108–12.

Chapter 37
Fetal Growth Restriction

Eva Meler, Leticia Benítez, Judith Martínez, and Francesc Figueras

Identification of Small-for-Gestational Age (SGA)

Antenatal detection of babies with defective growth often falls short, missing up to 75% of babies at risk of SGA before delivery [1]. In low-risk pregnancies, the detection rate is worse (~15%) [2]. Such poor performance takes a toll, as most instances of avoidable stillbirth are linked to failures in antenatal SGA detection [3].

Current third-trimester strategies to monitor growth involve symphysis-fundal height measurement, an easy and affordable system. However, it can just be used in 75% of pregnancies because of maternal and gestational characteristics [4], and only 16% of SGA infants are detected in low-risk populations when using this system [5]. In order to minimize its heterogeneity and to improve its detection capacity, Morse K et al. [4] presented a standardized protocol of measurement by tape and plotting on customized charts.

Third-trimester ultrasound (US) monitoring of fetal growth is done routinely in some countries, boosting detection rates up to 40–80% [6, 7]. In a designed prospective cohort study comparing universal vs. selective (based on risk factors), third-trimester screening provides evidence that universal screening triples (57% vs. 20%) the detection rate of SGA [8]. However, another observational study [9] found that a contingent strategy based on selecting for third-trimester growth assessment of the 50% of the population at highest risk as accrued by the first- and second-trimester screening yields similar performance than universal screening.

However, the impact of third-trimester ultrasound on perinatal outcomes remains unclear. A meta-analysis of randomized trials fails to demonstrate any real benefit from routine third-trimester scanning [10, 11]. However, it may be argued that the older pooled data holds limited contemporary validity. The most recent study [12]

E. Meler · L. Benítez · J. Martínez · F. Figueras (✉)
BCNatal - Barcelona Center for Maternal-Fetal and Neonatal Medicine (Hospital Clínic and Hospital Sant Joan de Deu), University of Barcelona, Barcelona, Spain
e-mail: ffiguera@clinic.cat

© Springer Nature Switzerland AG 2022

R. A. Moreira de Sá, E. B. d. Fonseca (eds.), *Perinatology*,
https://doi.org/10.1007/978-3-030-83434-0_37

(included in the meta-analysis mentioned above) claimed a 30% reduction in FGR when third-trimester US was performed. Furthermore, many of the studies involved no change in management if a diagnosis of FGR was made, which does not reflect current modes of practice. And finally, just three of the included trials [12–14] (contributing only 12% of subjects overall) routinely performed US studies after 34 weeks, which is when FGR due to placental insufficiency is more likely to be phenotypically apparent and thus more readily detected by ultrasound. In fact, a randomized study [15] comparing routine 32- vs. 36-week scan found that the latter strategy doubles the detection rate of SGA and severe SGA, with similar false-positive rate. Some recent studies [16–18] corroborated that the detection performance for SGA neonate of routine third-trimester scan is better when it is carried out at 36 weeks than at 32 weeks.

Akolekar R et al. [19] recently presented a two-stage approach for improving the screening of SGA neonate by routine ultrasound examination at 35–37 weeks. Pregnancies with and increased risk (EFW < 40th percentile) were stratified into management groups based on findings of EFW and Doppler indices (pulsatility index in the uterine arteries, umbilical artery and fetal middle cerebral artery). They achieved detection rates up to 89% and 88% of birth weight <3rd and <10th centiles, respectively. The predictive performance for adverse perinatal outcome of EFW <10th percentile was also improved by the new approach proposed, predicting up to 31% of adverse perinatal outcomes when the scan is done within 2 weeks before the delivery.

A recent systematic review and meta-analysis found that abdominal circumference is comparable to EFW in finding out SGA [20]. However, the largest prospective study included [21] confirms EFW as superior method over individual biometric measures. Also in a more recent study carried out by Cianobau et al. [16], fetal abdominal circumference did not show superiority to EFW as a screening method.

The most recent researches have focused on growth velocity as a possible tool to improve the SGA neonate detection rates. However, estimated growth velocity does not add benefit when it is calculated neither from 32 to 36 weeks' gestation nor from 20 to 36 weeks [17, 18]. Fetal abdominal growth velocity in the lowest centile could identify a subset of SGA fetuses with increased risk of neonatal morbidity [8], but it is not known whether this prediction capacity remains when usual Doppler parameters are used for the same purpose.

Delter RL et al. [35] suggested the *Individualized Growth Assessment* as a method to estimate the fetal growth potential using each individual as its own control. Sonographic fetal size parameters calculated in two times in the second trimester with an interval of at least 2–3 weeks are used to calculate the growth velocity and predict the third-trimester measurements that can be compared with the real ones. The Individualized Growth Assessment Program is a free software developed to interpret the data. Currently, Individualized Growth Assessment is a research approach, and there are not available studies about the clinical use of this tool to characterize abnormal growth and its relationship to physiologic changes, perinatal complications, and long-term disabilities.

An early detection of SGA has several potential benefits. First, the suspicion of an impaired growth will prompt further investigations, such as the umbilical artery Doppler study, which has been shown to reduce stillbirth and increase preterm delivery without increasing neonatal mortality [22]. Secondly, an early diagnosis will lead the clinician and the mother to deliberate the optimal timing of delivery. A population-based study in the USA reported a significantly increased risk of stillbirth in pregnancies complicated by SGA when delivered after the 37th week [23]. Third, the fact of identifying the problem has also shown to reduce adverse outcomes [24]: in the UK 92,218, where normally formed singletons (including 389 stillbirths) were analyzed, a reduced stillbirth rate (per 1000 births) of 9.7 was found with antenatal FGR detection, compared to 19.8 when undetected. The impact of timely recognition and delivery of SGA babies is also underscored by the fact that in this study, gestational age in instances of detected vs. non-detected SGA differed by only 10 days (270 vs. 280 days) but resulted in a 50% lower incidence of stillbirths. Similarly, another large single-center retrospective study by Lindqvist et al. [6] found that fetuses with severe FGR (i.e., weight deviation $\leq -22\%$ or approximately <3rd percentile) that went undetected before delivery showed a fourfold increase in risk of adverse fetal outcome. More recently, another large population-based study has shown that SGA detection was followed by a 52% reduction of stillbirth [25].

The detection of SGA is therefore key for an optimal management and improvement of outcomes of this entity. Nevertheless, as the detection rate is far from being excellent, the identification of those patients at risk of SGA early in the pregnancy may improve the detection. Several strategies have been proposed.

The cross-sectional assessment of first- and second-trimester uterine Doppler velocimetry has clinical utility for the detection of pregnancies at high risk of delivering a SGA neonate, especially when preeclampsia is concomitant [26]. In the second trimester, pulsatility index increased is the best predictor for intrauterine growth restriction in low-risk patients, and resistance index increased is the best for high-risk patients [27]. Also maternal circulating angiogenic markers can be useful showing the declining levels of placental function in the first half of gestation [26]. Uterine Doppler velocimetry and angiogenic factors (PlGF and sFlt-1) were combined with maternal characteristics in a screening model achieving an overall early-onset growth restriction detection rate of 86.4% (94.7% for growth restriction with preeclampsia) [28]. For late-onset growth restriction, the model achieved a detection rate of 65.8% (70.2% linked with preeclampsia) for a 10% false-positive rate in both cases [28]. These results improve the detection rates found in previous studies [29, 30].

During the third trimester, maternal characteristics, biochemical markers (PlGF, lipocalin-2, and estriol), and uterine Doppler velocimetry could be useful too; combined with EFW, it may improve the performance of EFW alone [31]. A combined screening model including these variables increased the prediction rates of SGA and late-onset growth restriction compared with EFW alone from 52% to 61% for SGA and from 64% to 77% for late-onset growth restriction, keeping a 10% false-positive rate [31].

In the first- and second-trimester, a simpler combined model was evaluated in a recent retrospective study; combining maternal factors, PAPP-A levels, and uterine Doppler velocimetry in the first trimester, the prediction of overall late-onset growth restriction was 36.7%, and adding the second-trimester biometrics and uterine Doppler velocimetry, the prediction rate reached 59.6%, with 10% false-positive rate in both cases [32]. At the second trimester, using fetal biometry, estimated fetal weight <10th centile, and abnormal uterine Doppler velocimetry or cerebroplacental ratio detected 20.1% of late SGA for 25% false-positive rate [33].

Although the studies carried out in the last years show optimistic results and promising lines of research, nowadays early screening for late-onset growth restriction is of limited value. Growth restriction in late pregnancy is still largely overlooked [29, 32] while accounting for the largest fraction of adverse perinatal outcomes and stillbirths [34, 35]. Within this subset, the chief correlate in stillbirth, perinatal complications, and abnormal neurodevelopment is severe growth restriction (generally birth weight <3rd percentile).

Definition Issues

Distinction Between "Fetal Growth Restriction (FGR)" and SGA

SGA represent a heterogeneous population that comprises several phenotypes: (i) Those with congenital malformations (including chromosomopathies) or infections are a small proportion; in severe and early-onset cases (especially when other markers and/malformations are present), a genetic causation should be suspected. Some studies [36, 37] found that a genetic array (based either on CGH or SNPs) has a 3–10% of incremental yield over conventional karyotyping; in those severe cases with early onset or with other markers of infection, ruling out a cytomegalovirus infection seems appropriate. In setting where malaria is endemic, this agent should be also considered. Other TORCH screening is not required in the absence of other markers of infection. (ii) Some of the SGA fetuses do not achieved their endowed growth potential mainly due to placental insufficiency. Thus, they could be considered true cases of fetal growth restriction. (iii) Finally, a large fraction of the small babies are only constitutionally small (i.e., they have a low growth potential). By convention, these last two groups are normally referred to as FGR versus SGA.

From a clinical point of view, the distinction between late-onset FGR versus SGA is relevant because of the correlation with perinatal outcome. Whereas FGR represents a pathological condition associated with adverse perinatal outcome, SGA merely are the end of the spectrum of healthy babies. While conceptually FGR and SGA are clearly distinct conditions, from a clinical point of view their differentiation is rather challenging.

Placental Insufficiency that Appears Early in the Pregnancy

There is a good evidence that umbilical artery Doppler captures well the placental insufficiency that appears early in the pregnancy. Indeed, a survey on 45 experts in the field found a good agreement that before 32 weeks a severely abnormal umbilical artery Doppler (defined as an absent/reversed end-diastolic flow) as a standalone could be considered a criterion for FGR [38]. Alternatively, there was also substantial agreement that a pulsatile waveform (above the 95th centile) plus a defective fetal growth also qualifies for FGR [38]. There is a good evidence that the use of umbilical Doppler in high-risk pregnancies improves a number of adverse outcomes, among them a 30% reduction in perinatal mortality [39]. The inclusion of other Doppler parameters in the distinction between early FGR and SGA is more debatable. Among the candidates, the uterine Doppler has the advantage that reflects placental insufficiency from the maternal side and that captures the placental insufficiency secondary to other pathophysiologic mechanisms other than early defective trophoblastic invasion [40]. The agreement to include this parameter into the definition of early FGR is also substantial [38].

Placental Insufficiency that Appears Late in the Pregnancy

On the other hand, there is a sizable body of evidence showing that the umbilical artery does not reliably reflect placental insufficiency and does not predict adverse outcome in late-onset FGR [41, 42]. It is intriguing that while most cases of late-onset SGA present signs of placental underperfusion [43], this is not reflected in the umbilical artery Doppler. One could speculate that the degree of the extension is what accounts for this finding. Indeed, animal [44] and mathematical [45] experimental models of placental vessel obliteration have suggested that umbilical artery Doppler becomes abnormal only if an extensive part of the placenta is involved.

The use of middle cerebral artery (MCA) Doppler in this setting is supported by recent studies that have demonstrated that 15–20% of term SGA fetuses with normal UA Doppler have reduced impedance in MCA blood flow and that this sign is associated with poorer perinatal outcome [46, 47] and neurobehavior, both at birth [48] and at two years of age [49]. Furthermore, the cerebroplacental ratio (CPR), which combines the pulsatility index of the middle cerebral and umbilical arteries, has demonstrated to be more sensitive to hypoxia than its individual components [50] and it correlates better with adverse outcome [51, 52]. In addition to these brain Doppler parameters, abnormal uterine artery (UtA) Doppler has been associated with an increased risk of intrapartum fetal distress, emergency cesarean delivery, and admission to intensive care unit [46, 53, 54]. Finally, evidence also exists that very low estimated fetal weight (EFW) centile by itself predicts a higher risk of adverse perinatal outcome in term SGA fetuses without Doppler signs of brain redistribution and normal umbilical and uterine artery Doppler [54, 55].

The clinical relevance of using a combined model is the significant improvement in prediction over using a single predictor (a detection rate for adverse outcome of 83% for a 48% of false positives) [56] without excessive technical sophistication; the estimation of the fetal weight is an integrated part of the third-trimester echography and Doppler interrogation of the UA, MCA, and UtA and is easily accomplished in the great majority of cases. Such algorithm allows profiling of the general population of late SGA fetuses in two risk-differing groups. While SGA fetuses with moderate growth restriction (>3rd centile) and normal placental function on both the fetal (normal CPR) and maternal (normal uterine Doppler) sides could be considered low risk and managed as constitutionally small babies, those with either severe growth restriction or evidence of placental dysfunction should be considered high risk. In our series, constitutional smallness accounted for 40% of the population, in which only 17% of adverse outcomes occurred, whereas late-onset FGR represented the remaining 60% of the population, which concentrated 83% of instances of adverse outcome.

Some evidence coming from observational studies suggests that growth velocity is a good predictor of adverse outcome in SGA [8, 42], outperforming some of the Doppler parameters that are discussed below. However, when the use of Doppler parameters is in place to differentiate between constitutional SGA and growth restriction, the added value of growth velocity remains unclear [57].

It is likely that in the future years, maternal blood biomarkers are incorporated as a diagnostic criterion of FGR in composite algorithms, as a marker of placental involvement [58]. Indeed, it has been shown in late-onset FGR that the angiogenic factors correlate with placental findings secondary to underperfusion [59, 60].

A recent consensus [38] reached by 45 experts in the field established that there is also substantial agreement to define late-onset FGR when at least two of the following are met: (i) estimated fetal weight or abdominal circumference below the 10th centile; (ii) a declining fetal growth (defined as when the growth trajectory crosses two quartile); or (iii) an abnormal cerebroplacental ratio (<5th centile).

Distinction Between Early and Late-Onset FGR

Over the last decade, two different patterns of clinical presentation, determined primarily by the gestational age of disease onset and the pattern of umbilical artery Doppler, have been more clearly characterized [41, 61, 62].

Fetal growth restriction has a different phenotypic expression, evolution, and outcome when it starts early in gestation. The typical pattern of deterioration progresses from escalating abnormalities in UA and venous Doppler parameters to abnormal biophysical parameters. The rate of deterioration of Doppler parameters determines the overall speed of deterioration in early-onset FGR, often necessitating preterm delivery. In addition, there is a high association with preeclampsia and perinatal mortality [29, 61, 62].

Table 37.1 Summary of the main differences between early- and late-onset forms of FGR

Early-onset FGR	Late-onset FGR
Challenge: management Prevalence: ~1%	Challenge: diagnosis Prevalence: 3–5%
Severe placental disease: UA Doppler abnormal, high association with PE, angiogenic profile	Mild placental disease: UA Doppler normal, low association with PE, angiogenic profile
Severe hypoxia ++: systemic CV adaptation	Mild hypoxia: central CV adaptation
High mortality and morbidity	Lower mortality (but common cause of late stillbirth)
Low maternal cardiac output and high vascular peripheral resistance	Normal or increased maternal cardiac output

Abbreviations: *PE* preeclampsia, *CV* cardiovascular

In contrast, late-onset FGR is normally associated with less severe placental disease, so that normal or minimally elevated UA Doppler indices are usually observed. Overt cardiovascular adaptation does not extend beyond the cerebral circulation, manifesting as decreased cerebroplacental ratio (CPR). The association between late-onset FGR with preeclampsia (PE) is minimal in comparison with early-onset forms [30].

A study [65] aimed at setting the optimal cutoff to differentiate early and late forms has shown that a cutoff of 32 weeks at diagnosis or 34 weeks at delivery maximizes differences between early- and late-onset FGR, but resulted in substantial overlapping of cases with similar characteristics. Umbilical artery Doppler discriminated better than gestational age in two groups with different timing, natural history, and rate of adverse outcome. A survey on 45 experts in the field of FGR found good agreement (89%) that early FGR is that diagnosed before 32 weeks [38] (Table 37.1).

Clinical Management

There is evidence form one randomized trial [66] that when compared with monitoring every 2 weeks, twice-a-week monitoring results in more inductions without any improvement in the perinatal outcomes. Thus, the standard of care for those low-risk SGA would be this latter regime. However, in late-onset FGR, such definition of “low-risk SGA” could not be reliably trusted on the umbilical Doppler, and, therefore, some other markers are needed.

Amniotic Fluid

In a large study on late SGA [67], it was found that about one third of the pregnancies had oligohydramnios, as defined by an amniotic fluid index below 5. However, it could be argued that such a substantial proportion of cases does not represent fetuses at higher risk of progression but an overdiagnosis. In fact, evidence [68] shows that compared with the single deepest vertical pocket, the amniotic fluid index results in more inductions and cesarean sections without any improvement in the perinatal outcomes.

A meta-analysis [69] of 18 randomized studies demonstrated that a reduced amniotic fluid index is associated with abnormal 5-minute Apgar score, but failed to demonstrate an association with acidosis or perinatal death in those with cases associated with SGA (RR 1.6 [95% CI 0.9–2.6]).

Because there is limited evidence on the role of oligohydramnios to predict perinatal complications in SGA fetuses already managed with umbilical artery Doppler, its inclusion in management protocols is doubtful.

Doppler Parameters

Umbilical Artery (UA) Doppler

There is compelling evidence that using UA Doppler in high-risk pregnancies improves perinatal outcomes, with a 29% reduction in perinatal deaths [70]. Absent or reversed end-diastolic velocities, the end of the spectrum of the abnormalities of the umbilical artery Doppler, have been reported to be present on average 1 week before the acute deterioration [71]. There is an association between reversed end-diastolic flow in the umbilical artery and adverse perinatal outcome (with a sensitivity and specificity of about 60%), which seems to be independent of prematurity [72]. After 30 weeks the risk of stillbirth of a fetus with isolated reversed end-diastolic velocities in the umbilical artery Doppler overcomes the risks of prematurity [73–75], and therefore delivery seems justified.

Middle Cerebral Artery (MCA) Doppler/Cerebral-Placental Ratio (CPR)

MCA informs about the existence of brain vasodilation, a surrogate marker of hypoxia. There is an association between abnormal MCA-PI and adverse perinatal and neurological outcome, but it is unclear whether delivering before term could add any benefit. MCA is particularly valuable for the identification of [41] and prediction of adverse outcome among [47, 76] late-onset FGR, independently of the UA Doppler, which is often normal in these fetuses. Fetuses with abnormal MCA-PI had a sixfold risk of emergency cesarean section for fetal distress when compared with SGA fetuses with normal MCA-PI [77], which is particularly relevant because labor induction at term is the current standard of care of late-onset FGR [65, 77]. Late-onset FGR with abnormal MCA-PI have poorer neurobehavioral competence at birth and at 2 years of age [76, 79]. MCA is considered a rather late manifestation, with acceptable specificity but low sensitivity, which is improved by the use of CPR.

The CPR improves remarkably the sensitivity of UA and MCA alone. Thus, the CPR is already decreased when its individual components suffer mild changes but are still within normal ranges [50, 51]. In late-SGA fetuses, abnormal CPR is present before delivery in 20–25% of the cases [80], and it is associated with a higher risk of adverse outcome at induction, although to a lesser degree than MCA [77].

Ductus Venosus (DV) Doppler

DV is the strongest single Doppler parameter to predict the short-term risk of fetal death in early-onset FGR. Longitudinal studies have demonstrated that DV flow waveforms become abnormal only in advanced stages of fetal compromise [61, 71, 72, 81]. Absent-reversed velocities during atrial contraction are associated with perinatal mortality independently of the gestational age at delivery [82] with a risk ranging from 40% to 100% in early-onset FGR [73, 83]. Thus, this sign is normally considered sufficient to recommend delivery at any gestational age, after completion of steroids. In about 50% of cases, abnormal DV precedes the loss of short-term variability in cCTG [61], and in about 90% of cases, it is abnormal 48–72 hours before the BPP [81]. Hence, it is considered to provide a better window of opportunity for delivering fetuses in critical conditions at very early gestational ages.

Aortic Isthmus (AoI) Doppler

This vessel reflects the balance between the impedance of the brain and systemic vascular systems [84, 85]. Reverse AoI flow is a sign of advanced deterioration and a further step in the sequence starting with the UA and MCA Doppler. AoI has an association with both adverse perinatal [86] and neurological outcome [87]. However, longitudinal studies show that the AoI precedes DV abnormalities by 1 week [88, 89], and consequently it is not as good to predict the short-term risk of stillbirth [73]. In contrast, AoI seems to improve the prediction of neurological morbidity [87]. Among early-onset FGR with positive DV atrial velocities, a reverse AoI indicated an increased risk of late neonatal neurological injury (57% vs. 9.7%) [73].

Fetal Heart Rate (FHR) Analysis by Conventional and Computerized Cardiotocography (CTG and cCTG)

Early studies on high-risk pregnancies showed that, though highly sensitive, cardiotocography has a 50% rate of false positives for the prediction of adverse outcome [90]. In addition, a meta-analysis [91] on high-risk pregnancies failed to demonstrate any beneficial effect in reducing perinatal mortality. Hence, there is no evidence to support the use of traditional FHR monitoring or "non-stress tests" in FGR fetuses. A main limitation of CTG is the subjective interpretation of the FHR, which is extremely challenging in very preterm fetuses with a physiologically reduced variability.

cCGT has represented a step forward and has provided new insights into the pathophysiology and management of FGR. cCGT evaluates short-term variability of the FHR, an aspect that subjective evaluation cannot assess. Current evidence suggests that cCGT is sensitive to detect advanced fetal deterioration, and it provides a value similar to DV reverse atrial flow for the short-term prediction of fetal death. Short-term variability becomes abnormal, coinciding with the ductus venosus, whereas in about half of cases, abnormal ductus venosus precedes the loss of short-term FHR variability; the latter is the first to become abnormal in the other cases [61].

Biophysical Profile

Early observational studies reported a very low risk of false positives for acidosis and perinatal death, but more recent studies on early-onset very preterm FGR fetuses raise concerns over the false-positive rate, with up to 23% of instances of IUFD in fetuses with BPP >6 and 11% in those with BPP >8 [92]. A meta-analysis [93] showed no significant benefit of biophysical profile in high-risk pregnancies. Consequently, whenever Doppler expertise and/or cCTG are available, the incorporation of BPP in management protocols of FGR is questionable.

Prevention and Treatment: Evidence on Timing of Delivery

Prevention

Several trials have evaluated the effect of heparin for the prevention and treatment of SGA and FGR. The two best conducted trials were the EPPI trial (AAS + Calcium vs. AAS + Calcium + Heparin) and the HEPEPE trial (AAS vs. AAS + Heparin). The EPPI trial included high-risk women (defined as a recent pregnancy complicated with preterm preeclampsia, preterm SGA <10th centile, or SGA <3rd centile). They were randomly assigned to standard high-risk care (including daily low-dose aspirin) or high-risk care plus enoxaparin 40 mg daily, not seeing any improvement in the prevention of preeclampsia or SGA. Similarly, the HEPEPE trial demonstrated that enoxaparin added to low-dose aspirin versus aspirin alone had no impact in the reduction in maternal death, perinatal death, preeclampsia, SGA, or placental abruption, in women with previous severe preeclampsia [94].

Groom et al. [95] also published that the addition of heparin to standard high-risk care does not reduce the risk of recurrence of preeclampsia and SGA in patients with a previous history of placental dysfunction.

Prevention of SGA neonates using aspirin was evaluated in the ASPREE trial [96]. The use of aspirin reduced the overall incidence of SGA defined as <10th centile by about 40% in babies born below 37 weeks and by 70% in babies born below 32 weeks. No significant effect was shown in neonates at term. Nevertheless, this decrease was mainly due to the prevention of pre-eclampsia, as the coexistence of these two conditions is well known, especially in preterm cases. Therefore, no evidence exists about the prevention of this entity with AAS.

Therefore, at the moment, no evidence has been published about an effective prevention of SGA/FGR.

Treatment

Finding an effective treatment for placental insufficiency has always been a main field of interest in fetal growth restriction, showing no benefit in terms of birth weight nor delaying delivery [97–101]. Recently, some promising studies have been published.

A recent meta-analysis based on two studies about the use of heparin as a therapy showed a significantly higher birth weight and significant increase of gestational age at birth in women treated with heparin [102]. This limited evidence requires further research on this field, and RCT has been initiated among early severe FGR fetuses [103].

On the other hand, the STRIDER trials [104] are a series of international randomized controlled studies with the goal of assessing the ability of sildenafil to improve pregnancy outcomes in severe early-onset FGR. Five studies were initially planned (in the UK, New Zealand and Australia, the Netherlands, Ireland, and Canada), each with slightly different eligibility criteria and protocols. They did not prove any benefit in terms of prolonging pregnancy nor improving pregnancy outcome. The Dutch trial was stopped after 183 patients because a higher than expected neonatal mortality (19/71 [27%] with sildenafil vs. 9/63 [14%] with placebo) and high rates of persistent pulmonary hypertension of the neonate (PPHN) in the sildenafil group (17/64 [27%] sildenafil vs. 3/58 [5%] placebo).

Finally, the EVERREST trial [105] has been designed to demonstrate the efficacy and safety of maternal vascular endothelial growth factor (VEGF) gene therapy in severe early-onset FGR defined as EFW <3rd centile between 20+0 and 26+6 weeks of gestation. Preclinical studies have shown that VEGF gene therapy, delivered via an adenoviral vector into the maternal uterine arteries, increases uterine artery volume blood flow and vasodilates the uterine arteries in pregnant sheep through increased expression of endothelial nitric oxide synthase and perivascular adventitial angiogenesis. In animal models of FGR, it has also been shown to safely increase fetal growth velocity. However, as it would be the first clinical trial using gene therapy during pregnancy and it is an invasive therapy, it raises important ethical questions [106].

Statins have also received considerable attention. In vitro and animal models suggest a beneficial effect on improving the angiogenic profile. However, in clinical terms the evidence is still scarce, as a treatment for placental insufficiency. Costantine et al. [107, 108] have reported a small safety and pharmacokinetic trial of pravastatin for the treatment of preeclampsia (10 women receiving pravastatin, 10 receiving placebo) and found no adverse effects on the mother or baby. Although this was a secondary outcome, preeclampsia was reported in four of the women receiving placebo but none in those receiving pravastatin; birth weight was similar in the two groups, but placental weight was not reported. The STAMP study [109] was an RCT that recruited 62 women with early-onset preeclampsia and failed to find any effect of pravastatin in improving the angiogenic profile.

Thus, so far, assessment of fetal well-being and timely delivery remain as the main management strategy.

Timing of Delivery

The gestational age and the severity of the disease will be the two main pillars for decision making in the management of FGR fetuses. In early FGR fetuses, DV and cCTG will be crucial in the management of those, as they will precede deterioration of biophysical variables and stillbirth. In late-onset FGR, those fetuses at higher risk of adverse outcomes will be identified, as mentioned before, by severe growth restriction (EFW <3rd centile), by impaired fetal Doppler in the umbilical, middle cerebral artery or CPR or impaired uterine Doppler.

The Growth Restriction Intervention Trial (GRIT) study [74] was a multicenter randomized controlled trial that aimed to compare the effect of delivering early with delaying birth for as long as possible when the diagnosis of FGR was made. The study observed similar stillbirth rate and perinatal outcomes between both groups. However, when evaluating those neonates at 2 years of age, there was a trend towards more disability in the immediate delivery group [75].

A standard management of FGR and SGA, timing the best moment for delivery has proved to improve outcome and prevent stillbirth [110].

Between 24 and 26 weeks, FGR fetuses should be considered as periviable. Neonatal survival is below 50%, and the rate of major complications is around 80% [110]. The increase in neonatal survival per day gained in utero is 2%. Therefore, as the neonatal prognosis is poor, delivery will be indicated for maternal indications. Planned delivery for fetal indication should only be considered after a full assessment to the parents from a multidisciplinary approach.

Between 26 and 28 weeks of gestation, the increase in survival per day gained in utero ranges 2% per day (range 1.0–2.1%) [63]. Above 28 weeks, the daily gain in survival decreases to 0.7% per day because the intact survival is significantly improved at that time.

Regarding early-onset FGR, a randomized study [111] compared three strategies to determine delivery in early-onset FGR (<32 weeks): short-term variation below

3.5–4 msec (depending on the gestational age) at the computerized CTG (cCTG); early changes in the DV (pulsatility index above the 95th centile); and late changes in the DV (absent/reversed atrial flow). While there were no differences in the rate of survival without neurological impairment, neurodevelopmental impairment was less likely in survivors of the DV groups compared to those in the cCTG group. However, it should be stressed that all pregnancies had a cCTG evaluation (as a safety net) and a substantial fraction of babies in the DV groups were in fact delivered by an abnormal cCTG. On the contrary a DV evaluation was not performed in those babies allocated to the cCTG groups. One important finding of this trial was that, overall, better perinatal and neonatal outcomes than expected were observed (70% of survival without severe neonatal morbidity at discharge), compared with the previous series on the same population [64]. It suggests that when a protocol is set up, there is a secondary improvement in care. The second important conclusion of this study is that cCTG and DV should be combined in the management of early FGR fetuses.

Regarding late-onset FGR, one randomized equivalence trial exists comparing the effect of induction of labor or expectant monitoring in women after 37 weeks of gestation with suspected SGA [67]. They found negligible differences in perinatal and neonatal outcomes between induction of labor and expectant monitoring [67, 78]. At 2 years of age, no differences between both strategies were found [112]. While it is seemingly reasonable to offer delivery after 37 weeks in SGA, it should also be acknowledged that further studies differentiating true FGR from other causes of SGA not associated with poor perinatal outcome are required. It seems also reasonable to deliver at term those fetuses at high risk of adverse outcomes according to EFW or Doppler findings.

A Stage-Based Protocol for Managing FGR/SGA

While strong evidence is lacking to support firm recommendation on the timing of delivery, a protocol that integrates the best available evidence can help reducing clinical practice variation. One approach is to group in stages those indices or signs that are associated with similar fetal risks, since they should indicate similar follow-up intervals and timing of delivery. Thus, we suggest to profile several stages, or prognostic groups, which define different management strategies.

The timing of delivery and the mode of delivery are defined by the finalization when the prematurity risk overcomes the stillbirth risk, as shown in the TRUFFLE study [63].

It is very important to differentiate late-onset FGR versus SGA because their risks of intrauterine fetal demise and perinatal adverse outcomes are not comparable as we mentioned before. Classifying only by umbilical artery is not enough to identify the proportion of perinatal adverse outcomes. When we use UtA, CPR, and EFW below the 3rd centile, fetuses meeting any of these criteria show a 40% of risk of poor outcome, compared to only an 11% of risk in fetuses with a normal value of these three parameters and an 8% risk in control fetuses [55].

SGA Defined as EFW in the 3rd centile or above and under the 10th centile, with normal Doppler. Fortnightly Doppler and growth assessment is safe [66] and constitutes standard practice. Labor induction should be recommended at 40 weeks.

***Stage I FGR* [severe smallness or mild placental insufficiency]** Defined as EFW below the 3rd centile or between the 3rd and the 10th centile with at least one of the following: UtA >95th centile or CPR <5th centile or PI MCA <5th centile. Available evidence suggests a low risk of fetal deterioration before term. Labor induction beyond 37 weeks is acceptable, but the risk of intrapartum fetal distress is increased [77]. If PI MCA <5th centile, emergency cesarean section rate is 50%. Regarding the method of labor induction in FGR cases, the use of mechanical methods has showed to increase vaginal delivery rate and to avoid hypersystolia and CTG abnormalities [113].

***Stage II FGR* [severe placental insufficiency]** This stage is defined by UA AEDV. Delivery should be recommended after 34 weeks. The risk of emergent caesarean section at labor induction exceeds 50%, and, therefore, elective caesarean section is a reasonable option. Monitoring twice a week is recommended.

***Stage III FGR* [advanced fetal deterioration, low-suspicion signs of fetal acidosis]** The stage is defined by reverse diastolic flow in the UA (REDV) or DV-PI>95th centile. There is an association with a higher risk of stillbirth and poorer neurological outcome. However, since signs suggesting a very high risk of stillbirth within days are not present yet, it seems reasonable to delay elective delivery to reduce as possible the effects of severe prematurity. We suggest delivery should be recommended by cesarean section after 30 weeks [114]. Monitoring every 24–48 hours is recommended.

***Stage IV FGR* [high suspicion of fetal acidosis and high risk of fetal death]** There are spontaneous FHR decelerations, reduced short-term variability (<3 ms) in the cCTG, or reverse atrial flow in the DV Doppler. Delivery is after 26 weeks by cesarean section at a tertiary care center under steroid treatment for lung maturation (and prophylaxis of cerebral palsy with magnesium sulfate). Intact survival exceeds 50% only after 26–28 weeks, and before this threshold parents should be counseled by multidisciplinary teams. Monitoring every 12–24 hours until is recommended.

References

1. Hepburn M, Rosenberg K. An audit of the detection and management of small-for-gestational age babies. BJOG. 1986;93(3):212–6.
2. Backe B, Consultant JN. Effectiveness of antenatal care: a population based study. BJOG. 1993;100(8):727–32.

3. Richardus JH, Graafmans WC, Verloove-Vanhorick SP, Mackenbach JP, Masuy-Stroobant G, Alderdice F, et al. Differences in perinatal mortality and suboptimal care between 10 European regions: results of an international audit. BJOG. 2003;110(2):97–105.
4. Morse K, Williams A, Gardosi J. Fetal growth screening by fundal height measurement. In: Best practice and research: clinical obstetrics and gynaecology, vol. 23; 2009. p. 809–18.
5. Kean LH, Liu DTY. Antenatal care as a screening tool for the detection of small for gestational age babies in the low risk population. J Obstet Gynaecol (Lahore). 1996;16(2):77–82.
6. Lindqvist PG, Molin J. Does antenatal identification of small-for-gestational age fetuses significantly improve their outcome? Ultrasound Obstet Gynecol. 2005;25(3):258–64.
7. Souka AP, Papastefanou I, Pilalis A, Michalitsi V, Kassanos D. Performance of third-trimester ultrasound for prediction of small-for-gestational-age neonates and evaluation of contingency screening policies. Ultrasound Obstet Gynecol [Internet]. 2011/08/23. 2012;39(5):535–42. Available from: http://www.ncbi.nlm.nih.gov/entrez/query.fcgi?cmd=Retrieve&db=PubMed&dopt=Citation&list_uids=21858886.
8. Sovio U, White IR, Dacey A, Pasupathy D, Smith GCS. Screening for fetal growth restriction with universal third trimester ultrasonography in nulliparous women in the Pregnancy Outcome Prediction (POP) study: a prospective cohort study. Lancet (London, England). 2015;386(10008):2089–97.
9. Triunfo S, Crovetto F, Scazzocchio E, Parra-Saavedra M, Gratacos E, Figueras F. Contingent versus routine third-trimester screening for late fetal growth restriction. Ultrasound Obstet Gynecol [Internet]. 2015/09/15. 2016;47(1):81–8. Available from: http://www.ncbi.nlm.nih.gov/entrez/query.fcgi?cmd=Retrieve&db=PubMed&dopt=Citation&list_uids=26365218.
10. Bricker L, Neilson JP, Dowswell T. Routine ultrasound in late pregnancy (after 24 weeks' gestation). Cochrane Database Syst Rev [Internet]. 2008 Oct 8 [cited 2019 May 30];(4):CD001451. Available from: http://www.ncbi.nlm.nih.gov/pubmed/18843617.
11. Skråstad RB, Eik-Nes SH, Sviggum O, Johansen OJ, Salvesen KÅ, Romundstad PR, et al. A randomized controlled trial of third-trimester routine ultrasound in a non-selected population. Acta Obstet Gynecol Scand. 2013;92(12):1353–60.
12. McKenna D, Tharmaratnam S, Mahsud S, Bailie C, Harper A, Dornan J. A randomized trial using ultrasound to identify the high-risk fetus in a low-risk population. Obstet Gynecol. 2003;101(4):626–32.
13. Duff GB. A randomized controlled trial in a hospital population of ultrasound measurement screening for the small for dates baby. Aust N Z J Obstet Gynaecol. 1993;33(4):374–8.
14. Neilson JP, Munjanja SP, Whitfield CR. Screening for small for dates fetuses: a controlled trial. Br Med J. 1984;289(6453):1179–82.
15. Roma E, Arnau A, Berdala R, Bergos C, Montesinos J, Figueras F. Ultrasound screening for fetal growth restriction at 36 *vs* 32 weeks' gestation: a randomized trial (ROUTE). Ultrasound Obstet Gynecol [Internet]. 2015 Oct [cited 2018 Jul 13];46(4):391–7. Available from: http://www.ncbi.nlm.nih.gov/pubmed/26031399.
16. Ciobanu A, Khan N, Syngelaki A, Akolekar R, Nicolaides KH. Routine ultrasound at 32 *vs* 36 weeks' gestation: prediction of small-for-gestational-age neonates. Ultrasound Obstet Gynecol. 2019;uog.20258.
17. Ciobanu A, Formuso C, Syngelaki A, Akolekar R, Nicolaides KH. Prediction of small-for-gestational-age neonates at 35–37 weeks' gestation: contribution of maternal factors and growth velocity between 20 and 36 weeks. Ultrasound Obstet Gynecol. 2019;53(4):488–95.
18. Ciobanu A, Anthoulakis C, Syngelaki A, Akolekar R, Nicolaides KH. Prediction of small-for-gestational-age neonates at 35–37 weeks' gestation: contribution of maternal factors and growth velocity between 32 and 36 weeks. Ultrasound Obstet Gynecol. 2019;53(5):630–7.
19. Akolekar R, Panaitescu AM, Ciobanu A, Syngelaki A, Nicolaides KH. Two-stage approach for prediction of small-for-gestational-age neonate and adverse perinatal outcome by routine ultrasound examination at 35–37 weeks' gestation. Ultrasound Obstet Gynecol. 2019;54(4):484–91.

20. Blue N, Yordan J, Holbrook B, Nirgudkar P, Mozurkewich E. Abdominal circumference alone versus estimated fetal weight after 24 weeks to predict small or large for gestational age at birth: a meta-analysis. Am J Perinatol [Internet]. 2017 Sep 3 [cited 2018 May 14];34(11):1115–24. Available from: http://www.ncbi.nlm.nih.gov/pubmed/28672412.
21. Fadigas C, Saiid Y, Gonzalez R, Poon LC, Nicolaides KH. Prediction of small-for-gestational-age neonates: screening by fetal biometry at 35–37 weeks. Ultrasound Obstet Gynecol [Internet]. 2015/03/03. 2015;45(5):559–65. Available from: http://www.ncbi.nlm.nih.gov/entrez/query.fcgi?cmd=Retrieve&db=PubMed&dopt=Citation&list_uids=25728139.
22. Alfirevic Z, Neilson JP. Doppler ultrasonography in high-risk pregnancies: systematic review with meta-analysis. Am J Obstet Gynecol. 1995;172(5):1379–87.
23. Trudell AS, Cahill AG, Tuuli MG, Macones GA, Odibo AO. Risk of stillbirth after 37 weeks in pregnancies complicated by small-for-gestational-age fetuses. Am J Obstet Gynecol [Internet]. 2013 May [cited 2018 Jul 12];208(5):376.e1–376.e7. Available from: http://www.ncbi.nlm.nih.gov/pubmed/23523099.
24. Gardosi J, Madurasinghe V, Williams M, Malik A, Francis A. Maternal and fetal risk factors for stillbirth: population based study. BMJ [Internet]. 2013 Jan 24 [cited 2018 Jul 12];346:f108. Available from: http://www.ncbi.nlm.nih.gov/pubmed/23349424.
25. Nohuz E, Rivière O, Coste K, Vendittelli F. Is prenatal identification of small-for-gestational-age fetuses useful? Ultrasound Obstet Gynecol [Internet]. 2019 Apr 4 [cited 2019 Jul 22];uog.20282. Available from: https://onlinelibrary.wiley.com/doi/abs/10.1002/uog.20282.
26. Triunfo S, Crovetto F, Rodriguez-Sureda V, Scazzocchio E, Crispi F, Dominguez C, et al. Changes in uterine artery Doppler velocimetry and circulating angiogenic factors in the first half of pregnancies delivering a small-for-gestational-age neonate. Ultrasound Obstet Gynecol [Internet]. 2017 Mar [cited 2017 Aug 26];49(3):357–63. Available from: http://doi.wiley.com/10.1002/uog.15978.
27. Cnossen JS, Morris RK, ter Riet G, Mol BWJ, van der Post JAM, Coomarasamy A, et al. Use of uterine artery Doppler ultrasonography to predict pre-eclampsia and intrauterine growth restriction: a systematic review and bivariable meta-analysis. CMAJ. 2008;178(6):701–11.
28. Crovetto F, Triunfo S, Crispi F, Rodriguez-Sureda V, Roma E, Dominguez C, et al. First-trimester screening with specific algorithms for early- and late-onset fetal growth restriction. Ultrasound Obstet Gynecol [Internet]. 2016 Sep [cited 2018 Jul 12];48(3):340–8. Available from: http://www.ncbi.nlm.nih.gov/pubmed/26846589.
29. Poon LCY, Syngelaki A, Akolekar R, Lai J, Nicolaides KH. Combined screening for preeclampsia and small for gestational age at 11-13 weeks. Fetal Diagn Ther. 2013;33(1):16–27.
30. Crovetto F, Crispi F, Scazzocchio E, Mercade I, Meler E, Figueras F, et al. First-trimester screening for early and late small-for-gestational-age neonates using maternal serum biochemistry, blood pressure and uterine artery Doppler. Ultrasound Obstet Gynecol [Internet]. 2014 Jan [cited 2017 Aug 26];43(1):34–40. Available from: http://doi.wiley.com/10.1002/uog.12537.
31. Miranda J, Rodriguez-Lopez M, Triunfo S, Sairanen M, Kouru H, Parra-Saavedra M, et al. Prediction of fetal growth restriction using estimated fetal weight *vs* a combined screening model in the third trimester. Ultrasound Obstet Gynecol. 2017;50(5):603–11.
32. Sotiriadis A, Figueras F, Eleftheriades M, Papaioannou GK, Chorozoglou G, Dinas K, et al. First-trimester and combined first- and second-trimester prediction of small-for-gestational age and late fetal growth restriction. Ultrasound Obstet Gynecol. 2019;53(1):55–61.
33. Hernandez-Andrade E, Maymon E, Erez O, Saker H, Luewan S, Garcia M, et al. A low cerebroplacental ratio at 20-24 weeks of gestation can predict reduced fetal size later in pregnancy or at birth. Fetal Diagn Ther. 2018;44(2):112–23.
34. Clausson B, Cnattingius S, Axelsson O. Preterm and term births of small for gestational age infants: a population-based study of risk factors among nulliparous women. BJOG. 1998;105(9):1011–7.

35. Clausson B, Gardosi J, Francis A, Cnattingius S. Perinatal outcome in SGA births defined by customised versus population-based birthweight standards. Br J Obstet Gynaecol. 2001;108(8):830–4.
36. de Wit MC, Srebniak MI, Joosten M, Govaerts LCP, Kornelisse RF, Papatsonis DNM, et al. Prenatal and postnatal findings in small-for-gestational-age fetuses without structural ultrasound anomalies at 18–24 weeks. Ultrasound Obstet Gynecol. 2017;49(3):342–8.
37. Shaffer LG, Rosenfeld JA, Dabell MP, Coppinger J, Bandholz AM, Ellison JW, et al. Detection rates of clinically significant genomic alterations by microarray analysis for specific anomalies detected by ultrasound. Prenat Diagn. 2012;32(10):986–95.
38. Gordijn SJ, Beune IM, Thilaganathan B, Papageorghiou A, Baschat AA, Baker PN, et al. Consensus definition of fetal growth restriction: a Delphi procedure. Ultrasound Obstet Gynecol. 2016;48(3):333–9.
39. Westergaard HB, Langhoff-Roos J, Lingman G, Marsál K, Kreiner S. A critical appraisal of the use of umbilical artery Doppler ultrasound in high-risk pregnancies: use of meta-analyses in evidence-based obstetrics. Ultrasound Obstet Gynecol. 2001;17(6):466–76.
40. Llurba E, Turan O, Kasdaglis T, Harman CR, Baschat AA. Emergence of late-onset placental dysfunction: relationship to the change in uterine artery blood flow resistance between the first and third trimesters. Am J Perinatol. 2013;30(6):505–11.
41. Oros D, Figueras F, Cruz-Martinez R, Meler E, Munmany M, Gratacos E. Longitudinal changes in uterine, umbilical and fetal cerebral Doppler indices in late-onset small-for-gestational age fetuses. Ultrasound Obstet Gynecol. 2011;37(2):191–5.
42. Chang TC, Robson SC, Spencer JAD, Gallivan S. Prediction of perinatal morbidity at term in small fetuses: comparison of fetal growth and Doppler ultrasound. BJOG. 1994;101(5):422–7.
43. Parra-Saavedra M, Crovetto F, Triunfo S, Savchev S, Parra G, Sanz M, et al. Added value of umbilical vein flow as a predictor of perinatal outcome in term small-for-gestational-age fetuses. Ultrasound Obstet Gynecol [Internet]. 2013 Aug [cited 2017 Aug 26];42(2):189–95. Available from: http://doi.wiley.com/10.1002/uog.12380.
44. Morrow RJ, Adamson SL, Bull SB, Ritchie JWK. Effect of placental embolization on the umbilical arterial velocity waveform in fetal sheep. Am J Obstet Gynecol. 1989;161(4):1055–60.
45. Thompson RS, Stevens RJ. Mathematical model for interpretation of Doppler velocity waveform indices. Med Biol Eng Comput. 1989;27(3):269–76.
46. Severi FM, Bocchi C, Visentin A, Falco P, Cobellis L, Florio P, et al. Uterine and fetal cerebral Doppler predict the outcome of third-trimester small-for-gestational age fetuses with normal umbilical artery Doppler. Ultrasound Obstet Gynecol. 2002;19(3):225–8.
47. Hershkovitz R, Kingdom JC, Geary M, Rodeck CH. Fetal cerebral blood flow redistribution in late gestation: identification of compromise in small fetuses with normal umbilical artery Doppler. Ultrasound Obstet Gynecol. 2000;15(3):209–12.
48. Cruz-Martinez R, Figueras F, Oros D, Padilla N, Meler E, Hernandez-Andrade E, et al. Cerebral blood perfusion and neurobehavioral performance in full-term small-for-gestational-age fetuses. Am J Obstet Gynecol. 2009;201(5):474.e1–7.
49. Eixarch E, Batalle D, Illa M, Muñoz-Moreno E, Arbat-Plana A, Amat-Roldan I, et al. Neonatal neurobehavior and diffusion MRI changes in brain reorganization due to intrauterine growth restriction in a rabbit model. Baud O, editor. PLoS One [Internet]. 2012 Feb 8 [cited 2017 Aug 26];7(2):e31497. Available from: http://dx.plos.org/10.1371/journal.pone.0031497.
50. Arbeille P, Maulik D, Fignon A, Stale H, Berson M, Bodard S, et al. Assessment of the fetal PO2 changes by cerebral and umbilical Doppler on lamb fetuses during acute hypoxia. Ultrasound Med Biol. 1995;21(7):861–70.
51. Gramellini D, Folli MC, Raboni S, Vadora E, Merialdi A. Cerebral-umbilical Doppler ratio as a predictor of adverse perinatal outcome. Obstet Gynecol. 1992;79(3):416–20.
52. Bahado-Singh RO, Kovanci E, Jeffres A, Oz U, Deren O, Copel J, et al. The Doppler cerebroplacental ratio and perinatal outcome in intrauterine growth restriction. Am J Obstet Gynecol. 1999;180(3 Pt 1):750–6.

53. Ghosh GS, Gudmundsson S. Uterine and umbilical artery Doppler are comparable in predicting perinatal outcome of growth-restricted fetuses. BJOG. 2009;116(3):424–30.
54. Vergani P, Roncaglia N, Andreotti C, Arreghini A, Teruzzi M, Pezzullo JC, et al. Prognostic value of uterine artery Doppler velocimetry in growth-restricted fetuses delivered near term. Am J Obstet Gynecol. 2002;187(4):932–6.
55. Savchev S, Figueras F, Cruz-Martinez R, Illa M, Botet F, Gratacos E. Estimated weight centile as a predictor of perinatal outcome in small-for-gestational-age pregnancies with normal fetal and maternal Doppler indices. Ultrasound Obstet Gynecol [Internet]. 2011/11/22. 2011;39(3):299–303. Available from: http://www.ncbi.nlm.nih.gov/entrez/query.fcgi?cmd=Retrieve&db=PubMed&dopt=Citation&list_uids=22102177.
56. Figueras F, Savchev S, Triunfo S, Crovetto F, Gratacos E. An integrated model with classification criteria to predict small-for-gestational-age fetuses at risk of adverse perinatal outcome. Ultrasound Obstet Gynecol [Internet]. 2015 Mar [cited 2017 Aug 26];45(3):279–85. Available from: http://doi.wiley.com/10.1002/uog.14714.
57. Caradeux J, Eixarch E, Mazarico E, Basuki TR, Gratacos E, Figueras F. Longitudinal growth assessment for the prediction of adverse perinatal outcome in SGA-suspected fetuses. Ultrasound Obstet Gynecol [Internet]. 2017.; Available from: http://www.ncbi.nlm.nih.gov/entrez/query.fcgi?cmd=Retrieve&db=PubMed&dopt=Citation&list_uids=28782171.
58. Aviram R, Biron Shental T, Kidron D. Placental aetiologies of foetal growth restriction: clinical and pathological differences. Early Hum Dev. 2010;86(1):59–63.
59. Benton SJ, Hu Y, Xie F, Kupfer K, Lee S-W, Magee LA, et al. Angiogenic factors as diagnostic tests for preeclampsia: a performance comparison between two commercial immunoassays. Am J Obstet Gynecol. 2011;205(5):469.e1–8.
60. Triunfo S, Lobmaier S, Parra-Saavedra M, Crovetto F, Peguero A, Nadal A, et al. Angiogenic factors at diagnosis of late-onset small-for-gestational age and histological placental underperfusion. Placenta [Internet]. 2014 Jun [cited 2017 Aug 26];35(6):398–403. Available from: http://linkinghub.elsevier.com/retrieve/pii/S0143400414001301.
61. Hecher K, Bilardo CM, Stigter RH, Ville Y, Hackelöer BJ, Kok HJ, et al. Monitoring of fetuses with intrauterine growth restriction: a longitudinal study. Ultrasound Obstet Gynecol [Internet]. 2001 Dec [cited 2019 May 19];18(6):564–70. Available from: http://www.ncbi.nlm.nih.gov/pubmed/11844190.
62. Turan OM, Turan S, Gungor S, Berg C, Moyano D, Gembruch U, et al. Progression of Doppler abnormalities in intrauterine growth restriction. Ultrasound Obstet Gynecol [Internet]. 2008;32(2):160–7. Available from: http://doi.wiley.com/10.1002/uog.5386.
63. Lees C, Marlow N, Arabin B, Bilardo CM, Brezinka C, Derks JB, et al. Perinatal morbidity and mortality in early-onset fetal growth restriction: cohort outcomes of the trial of randomized umbilical and fetal flow in Europe (TRUFFLE). Ultrasound Obstet Gynecol [Internet]. 2013/10/01. 2013;42(4):400–8. Available from: http://www.ncbi.nlm.nih.gov/entrez/query.fcgi?cmd=Retrieve&db=PubMed&dopt=Citation&list_uids=24078432.
64. Baschat AA, Cosmi E, Bilardo CM, Wolf H, Berg C, Rigano S, et al. Predictors of neonatal outcome in early-onset placental dysfunction. Obstet Gynecol. 2007;109(2 Part 1):253–61.
65. Savchev S, Figueras F, Sanz-Cortes M, Cruz-Lemini M, Triunfo S, Botet F, et al. Evaluation of an optimal gestational age cut-off for the definition of early- and late-onset fetal growth restriction. Fetal Diagn Ther [Internet]. 2014 [cited 2017 Aug 26];36(2):99–105. Available from: https://www.karger.com/?doi=10.1159/000355525.
66. McCowan LME, Harding JE, Roberts AB, Barker SE, Ford C, Stewart AW. A pilot randomized controlled trial of two regimens of fetal surveillance for small-for-gestational-age fetuses with normal results of umbilical artery Doppler velocimetry. Am J Obstet Gynecol. 2000;182(1 I):81–6.
67. Boers KE, Vijgen SM, Bijlenga D, van der Post JA, Bekedam DJ, Kwee A, et al. Induction versus expectant monitoring for intrauterine growth restriction at term: randomised equivalence trial (DIGITAT). BMJ [Internet]. 2010;341:c7087. Available from: http://www.ncbi.nlm.nih.gov/entrez/query.fcgi?cmd=Retrieve&db=PubMed&dopt=Citation&list_uids=21177352.

68. Nabhan AF, Abdelmoula YA. Amniotic fluid index versus single deepest vertical pocket as a screening test for preventing adverse pregnancy outcome. Cochrane Database Syst Rev. 2008;(3):CD006593.
69. Chauhan SP, Sanderson M, Hendrix NW, Magann EF, Devoe LD. Perinatal outcome and amniotic fluid index in the antepartum and intrapartum periods: a meta-analysis. Am J Obstet Gynecol. 1999;181(6):1473–8.
70. Alfirevic Z, Stampalija T, Dowswell T. Fetal and umbilical Doppler ultrasound in high-risk pregnancies, vol. 2017, Cochrane Database of Systematic Reviews. Wiley; 2017.
71. Ferrazzi E, Bozzo M, Rigano S, Bellotti M, Morabito A, Pardi G, et al. Temporal sequence of abnormal Doppler changes in the peripheral and central circulatory systems of the severely growth-restricted fetus. Ultrasound Obstet Gynecol [Internet]. 2002 Feb [cited 2019 May 19];19(2):140–6. Available from: http://www.ncbi.nlm.nih.gov/pubmed/11876805.
72. Cosmi E, Ambrosini G, D'Antona D, Saccardi C, Mari G. Doppler, cardiotocography, and biophysical profile changes in growth-restricted fetuses. Obstet Gynecol [Internet]. 2005;106(6):1240–5. Available from: http://content.wkhealth.com/linkback/openurl?sid=WKPTLP:landingpage%7B&%7Dan=00006250-200512000-00006.
73. Cruz-Lemini M, Crispi F, Van Mieghem T, Pedraza D, Cruz-Martínez R, Acosta-Rojas R, et al. Risk of perinatal death in early-onset intrauterine growth restriction according to gestational age and cardiovascular Doppler indices: a multicenter study. Fetal Diagn Ther [Internet]. 2012 [cited 2017 Aug 26];32(1–2):116–22. Available from: http://www.karger.com/doi/10.1159/000333001.
74. GRIT Study Group. A randomized trial of timed delivery for the compromised preterm Fetus: short-term outcomes and Bayesian interpretation. Obstet Gynecol Surv. 2003;58(7):449–50.
75. Thornton JG, Hornbuckle J, Vail A, Spiegelhalter DJ, Levene M, GRIT study group. Infant wellbeing at 2 years of age in the Growth Restriction Intervention Trial (GRIT): multicentred randomised controlled trial. Lancet (London, England). 2004;364(9433):513–20.
76. Eixarch E, Meler E, Iraola A, Illa M, Crispi F, Hernandez-Andrade E, et al. Neurodevelopmental outcome in 2-year-old infants who were small-for-gestational age term fetuses with cerebral blood flow redistribution. Ultrasound Obstet Gynecol. 2008;32(7):894–9.
77. Cruz-Martínez R, Figueras F, Hernandez-Andrade E, Oros D, Gratacos E. Fetal brain Doppler to predict cesarean delivery for nonreassuring fetal status in term small-for-gestational-age fetuses. Obstet Gynecol. 2011;117(3):618–26.
78. Boers KE, van Wyk L, van der Post JAMM, Kwee A, van Pampus MG, Spaanderdam MEAA, et al. Neonatal morbidity after induction vs expectant monitoring in intrauterine growth restriction at term: a subanalysis of the DIGITAT RCT. Am J Obstet Gynecol [Internet]. 2012;206(4):344.e1–7. Available from: http://linkinghub.elsevier.com/retrieve/pii/S0002937812000270.
79. Oros D, Figueras F, Cruz-Martinez R, Padilla N, Meler E, Hernandez-Andrade E, et al. Middle versus anterior cerebral artery Doppler for the prediction of perinatal outcome and neonatal neurobehavior in term small-for-gestational-age fetuses with normal umbilical artery Doppler. Ultrasound Obstet Gynecol. 2010;35(4):456–61.
80. Cruz-Martinez R, Figueras F, Hernandez-Andrade E, Puerto B, Gratacós E. Longitudinal brain perfusion changes in near-term small-for-gestational-age fetuses as measured by spectral Doppler indices or by fractional moving blood volume. Am J Obstet Gynecol. 2010;203(1):42.e1–6.
81. Baschat AA, Gembruch U, Harman CR. The sequence of changes in Doppler and biophysical parameters as severe fetal growth restriction worsens. Ultrasound Obstet Gynecol [Internet]. 2001 Dec [cited 2019 May 19];18(6):571–7. Available from: http://www.ncbi.nlm.nih.gov/pubmed/11844191.
82. Schwarze A, Gembruch U, Krapp M, Katalinic A, Germer U, Axt-Fliedner R. Qualitative venous Doppler flow waveform analysis in preterm intrauterine growth-restricted fetuses with ARED flow in the umbilical artery - correlation with short-term outcome. Ultrasound

Obstet Gynecol [Internet]. 2005;25(6):573–9. Available from: http://doi.wiley.com/10.1002/uog.1914.
83. Baschat AA, Gembruch U, Weiner CP, Harman CR. Qualitative venous Doppler waveform analysis improves prediction of critical perinatal outcomes in premature growth-restricted fetuses. Ultrasound Obstet Gynecol [Internet]. 2003;22(3):240–5. Available from: http://doi.wiley.com/10.1002/uog.149.
84. Mäkikallio K, Jouppila P, Räsänen J. Retrograde aortic isthmus net blood flow and human fetal cardiac function in placental insufficiency. Ultrasound Obstet Gynecol. 2003;22(4):351–7.
85. Fouron JC, Skoll A, Sonesson SE, Pfizenmaier M, Jaeggi E, Lessard M. Relationship between flow through the fetal aortic isthmus and cerebral oxygenation during acute placental circulatory insufficiency in ovine fetuses. In: American Journal of Obstetrics and Gynecology. Mosby Inc.; 1999. p. 1102–7.
86. Del Río M, Martínez JM, Figueras F, Bennasar M, Olivella a, Palacio M, et al. Doppler assessment of the aortic isthmus and perinatal outcome in preterm fetuses with severe intrauterine growth restriction. Ultrasound Obstet {&} Gynecol Off J Int Soc Ultrasound Obstet Gynecol [Internet]. 2008;31(1):41–7. Available from: http://www.ncbi.nlm.nih.gov/pubmed/18157796.
87. Fouron J-C, Gosselin J, Raboisson M-J, Lamoureux J, Tison C-A, Fouron C, et al. The relationship between an aortic isthmus blood flow velocity index and the postnatal neurodevelopmental status of fetuses with placental circulatory insufficiency. Am J Obstet Gynecol. 2005;192(2):497–503.
88. Figueras F, Benavides A, Del Rio M, Crispi F, Eixarch E, Martinez JM, et al. Monitoring of fetuses with intrauterine growth restriction: longitudinal changes in ductus venosus and aortic isthmus flow. Ultrasound Obstet Gynecol [Internet]. 2009;33(1):39–43. Available from: http://www.ncbi.nlm.nih.gov/pubmed/19115231.
89. Cruz-Martinez R, Figueras F, Hernandez-Andrade E, Oros D, Gratacos E. Changes in myocardial performance index and aortic isthmus and ductus venosus Doppler in term, small-for-gestational age fetuses with normal umbilical artery pulsatility index. Ultrasound Obstet Gynecol. 2011;38(4):400–5.
90. Evertson LR, Gauthier RJ, Schifrin BS, Paul RH. Antepartum fetal heart rate testing. I. Evolution of the nonstress test. Am J Obstet Gynecol. 1979;133(1):29–33.
91. Pattison N, McCowan L. Cardiotocography for antepartum fetal assessment. Cochrane Database Syst Rev. 2000;(2):CD001068.
92. Kaur S, Picconi JL, Chadha R, Kruger M, Mari G. Biophysical profile in the treatment of intrauterine growth-restricted fetuses who weigh <1000 g. Am J Obstet Gynecol. 2008;199(3):264.e1–4.
93. Alfirevic Z, Neilson JP. Biophysical profile for fetal assessment in high risk pregnancies. Cochrane Database Syst Rev. 2000;(2):CD000038.
94. Haddad B, Winer N, Chitrit Y, Houfflin-Debarge V, Chauleur C, Bages K, et al. Enoxaparin and aspirin compared with aspirin alone to prevent placenta-mediated pregnancy complications. Obstet Gynecol. 2016;128(5):1053–63.
95. Groom KM, McCowan LM, Mackay LK, Lee AC, Said JM, Kane SC, et al. Enoxaparin for the prevention of preeclampsia and intrauterine growth restriction in women with a history: a randomized trial. In: American Journal of Obstetrics and Gynecology. Mosby Inc.; 2017. p. 296.e1–296.e14.
96. Tan MY, Poon LC, Rolnik DL, Syngelaki A, de Paco Matallana C, Akolekar R, et al. Prediction and prevention of small-for-gestational-age neonates: evidence from SPREE and ASPRE. Ultrasound Obstet Gynecol. 2018;52(1):52–9.
97. Say L, Gülmezoglu AM, Hofmeyr GJ. Plasma volume expansion for suspected impaired fetal growth. Cochrane Database Syst Rev. 1996;(2):CD000167.
98. Gülmezoglu AM, Hofmeyr GJ. Betamimetics for suspected impaired fetal growth. Cochrane Database Syst Rev. 2001;(4):CD000036.

99. Laurin J, Persson PH. The effect of bedrest in hospital on fetal outcome in pregnancies complicated by intra-uterine growth retardation. Acta Obstet Gynecol Scand. 1987;66(5):407–11.
100. Say L, Gülmezoglu AM, Hofmeyr GJ. Maternal nutrient supplementation for suspected impaired fetal growth. Cochrane Database Syst Rev. 2003;(1):CD000148.
101. Say L, Gülmezoglu AM, Hofmeyr GJ. Maternal oxygen administration for suspected impaired fetal growth. Cochrane Database of Systematic Reviews. John Wiley and Sons Ltd; 2009.
102. Mazarico E, Molinet-Coll C, Martinez-Portilla RJ, Figueras F. Heparin therapy in placental insufficiency: Systematic review and meta-analysis. Acta Obstet Gynecol Scand. 2019;aogs.13730.
103. Mazarico E, Peguero A, Camprubí M, Rovira C, Gomez Roig MD, Oros D, et al. Study protocol for a randomised controlled trial: treatment of early intrauterine growth restriction with low molecular weight heparin (TRACIP). BMJ Open. 2018;8(10):e020501.
104. Sharp A, Cornforth C, Jackson R, Harrold J, Turner MA, Kenny LC, et al. Maternal sildenafil for severe fetal growth restriction (STRIDER): a multicentre, randomised, placebo-controlled, double-blind trial. Lancet Child Adolesc Health. 2018;2(2):93–102.
105. Spencer R, Ambler G, Brodszki J, Diemert A, Figueras F, Gratacós E, et al. EVERREST prospective study: a 6-year prospective study to define the clinical and biological characteristics of pregnancies affected by severe early onset fetal growth restriction. BMC Pregnancy Childbirth [Internet]. 2017 Jan 23 [cited 2017 Aug 26];17(1):43. Available from: http://bmcpregnancychildbirth.biomedcentral.com/articles/10.1186/s12884-017-1226-7.
106. Sheppard M, Spencer RN, Ashcroft R, David AL, EVERREST Consortium. Ethics and social acceptability of a proposed clinical trial using maternal gene therapy to treat severe early-onset fetal growth restriction. Ultrasound Obstet Gynecol. 2016;47(4):484–91.
107. Costantine MM, Cleary K, Hebert MF, Ahmed MS, Brown LM, Ren Z, et al. Safety and pharmacokinetics of pravastatin used for the prevention of preeclampsia in high-risk pregnant women: a pilot randomized controlled trial. Am J Obstet Gynecol. 2016;214(6):720.e1–720.e17.
108. Sisó C, Goncé A, Bosch J, Salvia MD, Hernández S, Figueras F. Listeriosis in pregnancy: a secular trend in a tertiary referral hospital in Barcelona. Eur J Clin Microbiol Infect Dis [Internet]. 2012 Sep 13 [cited 2019 Feb 15];31(9):2125–32. Available from: http://link.springer.com/10.1007/s10096-012-1545-6.
109. Ahmed A, Williams D, Cheed V, Middleton L, Ahmad S, Wang K, et al. Pravastatin for early-onset pre-eclampsia: a randomised, blinded, placebo-controlled trial. BJOG [Internet]. 2019 Dec 14 [cited 2019 Dec 24];1471-0528.16013. Available from: https://onlinelibrary.wiley.com/doi/abs/10.1111/1471-0528.16013.
110. Baschat AA. Planning management and delivery of the growth-restricted fetus. Best Pract Res Clin Obstet Gynaecol. 2018;49:53–65.
111. Lees CC, Marlow N, van Wassenaer-Leemhuis A, Arabin B, Bilardo CM, Brezinka C, et al. 2 year neurodevelopmental and intermediate perinatal outcomes in infants with very preterm fetal growth restriction (TRUFFLE): a randomised trial. Lancet (London, England). 2015;385(9983):2162–72.
112. van Wyk L, Boers KE, van der Post JAM, van Pampus MG, van Wassenaer AG, van Baar AL, et al. Effects on (neuro)developmental and behavioral outcome at 2 years of age of induced labor compared with expectant management in intrauterine growth-restricted infants: long-term outcomes of the DIGITAT trial. Am J Obstet Gynecol. 2012;206(5):406.e1–7.
113. Villalain C, Herraiz I, Quezada MS, Gómez Arriaga P, Simón E, Gómez-Montes E, et al. Labor induction in late-onset fetal growth restriction: Foley balloon versus vaginal dinoprostone. Fetal Diagn Ther. 2019;46(1):67–74.
114. Caradeux J, Martinez-Portilla RJ, Basuki TR, Kiserud T, Figueras F. Risk of fetal death in growth-restricted fetuses with umbilical and/or ductus venosus absent or reversed end-diastolic velocities before 34 weeks of gestation: a systematic review and meta-analysis. 2018 [cited 2019 Dec 24]; Available from: https://doi.org/10.1016/j.ajog.2017.11.566.

Chapter 38
Perinatal Hemolytic Disease

Mário Dias Corrêa Júnior, Gabriel Martins Cruz Campos, and Priscila Chaves Pita

Introduction

The main cause of Perinatal Hemolytic disease's main cause is Rh alloimmunization, which is caused by the exposure of Rh(D)-negative pregnant women to Rh(D)-positive red blood cells, leading to the development of antibodies that cross the placental barrier and cause fetal red blood cell destruction. The consequence of this process is the emergence of intrauterine anemia and, later, hyperbilirubinemia in the newborn, a condition known as perinatal hemolytic disease, associated with high rates of morbidity and mortality. The advances in medicine made possible to know the causes of the disease, the appropriate treatment, and a way of prevention, as shown in Fig. 38.1.

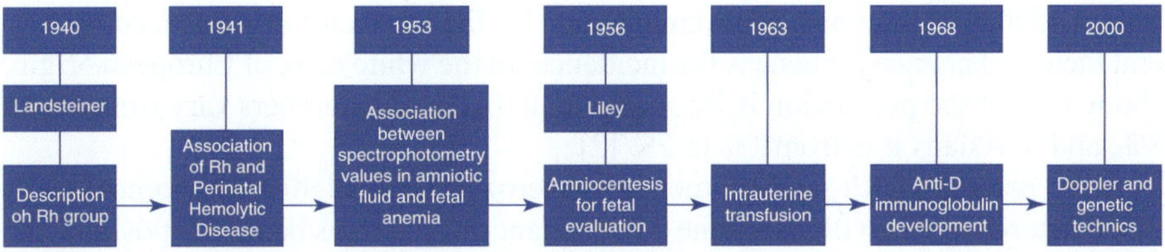

Fig. 38.1 Evolution of perinatal hemolytic disease management

M. Dias Corrêa Júnior (✉)
Obstetrics and Gynecology Department – Faculdade de Medicina da UFMG, Belo Horizonte, Brazil

G. M. C. Campos
Fetal Medicine Residence – Hospital das Clínicas da UFMG, Belo Horizonte, Brazil

P. C. Pita
Ultrasonography Residence – Hospital das Clínicas da UFMG, Belo Horizonte, Brazil

© Springer Nature Switzerland AG 2022

R. A. Moreira de Sá, E. B. d. Fonseca (eds.), *Perinatology*,
https://doi.org/10.1007/978-3-030-83434-0_38

Alloimmunization evolves in a different, peculiar way; it does not show signs or symptoms in the pregnant woman. However, normal fetuses undergo progressive morbid changes that can be mild and disappear completely after birth or that can lead to serious impairments, which can determine fetal or neonatal death. The emergence of fetal anemia, fetal hydrops, or hemolytic disease in the newborn is strongly associated with fetal morbidity and mortality. With the advent of ultrasound and Doppler velocimetry, it was possible to diagnose fetal anemia, without the need for invasive procedures, improving the neonatal prognosis. In addition, intrauterine transfusions significantly changed the neonatal prognosis with a survival rate of 90% and a survival rate of 80% even in hydropic fetuses.

When alloimmunization is identified in the prenatal period, the degree of fetal anemia should be assessed. Previously, this was done by amniocentesis with measurement of the optical density of the amniotic fluid to detect bilirubin levels. Currently, with easy access to ultrasound, amniocentesis has been replaced by Doppler velocimetry, with the assessment of the peak systolic velocity of the middle cerebral artery (MCA PSV).

The reduction of Rh hemolytic disease has become possible since the advent of Rh(D) immunoglobulin [1].

Rh disease is technically preventable, and that should be the goal. To achieve this goal, it is necessary to recognize patients at risk and adopt the recommended measures. In practice, however, immunization by the Rh factor still occurs due to failures in obstetric care or immunization by other antibodies.

Epidemiology and Relevance

The incidence of maternal alloimmunization by the Rh factor is influenced by several factors. The race influences the incidence: in the white race, of European origin, about 15% of the population is Rh-negative; in black, the numbers vary from 5% to 8%, and in Asians it is from 1% to 2% [2].

Sixty percent of Rh-positive men are heterozygous, and 40% are homozygous. Since heterozygotes will determine a 50% chance of the fetus being Rh-positive, the overall chance of the fetus being Rh-positive is approximately 70% [2]. Genetic predisposition also influences the incidence. Up to 30% of Rh-negative individuals do not respond immunologically and do not become sensitive, even when stimulated with large volumes of Rh-positive blood [3].

The incompatibility in the ABO system provides partial protection against Rh sensitization. In the first pregnancy with incompatibility in the ABO system and Rh-positive fetus, the incidence of immunization is only 1–2%. It seems that the incompatible red blood cells in the ABO system are quickly eliminated from the maternal circulation, before sensitization by the Rh factor can be established [4].

Fetal-maternal transplacental hemorrhage plays an important role in the incidence of immunization. Approximately 50% of normal deliveries have transplacental hemorrhage before or during delivery [5].

If the amount of blood is less than 0.1 ml, the incidence of immunization up to six months after delivery is only 3%. If more than 0.1 ml enters the maternal circulation, the incidence is approximately 14%. For Rh-negative women regardless of transplacental hemorrhage, in the first pregnancy with Rh-positive fetus and compatible in the ABO system, the risk is 7–8%. In the second pregnancy, the risk is 15–16% [5].

The routine use of Rh(D) immunoglobulin is responsible for reducing the rate of erythrocyte alloimmunization in economically developed countries. First introduced in the 1970s, postpartum Rh(D) immunoglobulin administration reduced the rate of alloimmunization in high-risk pregnancies from approximately 13–16% to approximately 0.5–1.8% [6].

Pathophysiology

Maternal alloimmunization by the Rh factor results from the formation of anti-Rh antibodies in the circulation. Antibodies are produced when fetal red blood cells with the positive Rh factor (in general, the D antigen) enter the maternal circulation, through transplacental hemorrhages, stimulating their immune system.

The Rhesus (Rh) system has five major antigens, named by the Fisher-Race nomenclature as "C," "c," "D," "E," and "e," and many other variant antigens. An antigen "d" was never found, and the use of the letter "d" indicates the absence of an evident allelic product. Rh alloimmunization, in most cases, is the result of incompatibility with antigen D, causing severe hemolytic disease in the fetus and the newborn [6].

Transplacental hemorrhages occur in about 75% of pregnant women [7]. The primary response is slow, usually takes several weeks to develop, is weak, and predominantly produces IgM, which does not cross the placenta. In a second exposure to Rh-positive red blood cells, the secondary immune response is rapid (days) and very strong and produces IgG, which crosses the placenta. The second dose may be minimal (fraction of ml) [7]. When IgG crosses the placenta, it opsonizes the Rh-positive fetal red blood cell and produces extravascular hemolysis, primarily in the spleen through macrophage phagocytosis. As hemolysis increases, the fetus responds increasing the production of red blood cells, primarily in the liver and spleen. The titer (quantity) and constant binding (avidity for anti-D) of the maternal antigen determine the degree of hemolysis and, therefore, the severity of the hemolytic disease. In 50% of cases, the disease is so mild that the newborn survives without treatment. In 25%, fetuses are in good condition at the end of pregnancy, but after birth, they either die of kernicterus or survive with severe mental disorders. The remaining 25% have higher degrees of hemolysis and develop hydropsy [7].

The initiation of the primary response depends on both the frequency and the quantity of Rh-positive red blood cells from the fetus that enter the maternal bloodstream. Doses of 0.1 ml of Rh-positive red blood cells are enough to trigger the primary response. The secondary response requires doses smaller than 0.01 ml [8].

Etiology

Rh alloimmunization etiology is due to maternal exposure to fetal antigens after transplacental hemorrhage [2]. There are several factors involved in generating primary immune response in addition to blood volume. Fetal red blood cell immunogenicity and an appropriate maternal immune response are required [9]. Interestingly, AIDS patients may be unable to generate antibodies to the anti-D antigen [10]. The Rh group D antigen is primarily responsible for intrauterine hemolysis; however, more than 50 other antigens present on the surfaces of red blood cells have already been linked to the appearance of perinatal hemolytic disease (Table 38.1).

Maternal alloimmunization by the Rh factor occurs when red blood cells (RBC), with D antigen on their surface, enter the bloodstream of a Rh-negative woman, stimulating her immune system to produce antibodies against that antigen. This is possible in the following situations:

- In incompatible blood transfusion. Although very rare, it still happens: human failures in the classification of donor and recipient blood or, exceptionally, in emergencies where urgent transfusion is required and there is no compatible blood in the Rh system [11].

Table 38.1 Antigens causing fetal hemolytic disease requiring treatment

Common
Rhesus family: D, C, E, c, e
Kell
Uncommon
JK^a (Kidd)
Fy^a (Duffy)
$Kp^{a \text{ or } b}$
k
S
Rare
Do^a
$Di^{a \text{ or } b}$
Fy^b
Hutch
Jk^b
Lu^a
M
N
s
U
yt
Never
$Le^{a \text{ or } b}$
p

- During pregnancy. When fetal-maternal hemorrhages occur, fetal Rh(D)-positive red blood cells enter the maternal circulation whose red blood cells are Rh-negative. This immunization occurs in 1.3% of pregnancies and almost always in the third trimester [12]. The frequency and volume of maternal-fetal transfusions increase proportionally to the gestational age.
- At delivery. This is the moment when there is a greater possibility of immunization, about 92% of the cases [12]. The risk increases in cesarean sections with manual extraction of the placenta; in intrapartum hemorrhages – placental abruption and placenta previa; and in twin pregnancy.
- Before birth, intrauterine. There is a theoretical risk when Rh-negative fetuses receive Rh-positive blood from their mother, through maternal-fetal transplacental transfusion, or twin pregnancy with fetuses with and without the Rh factor. Intrauterine sensitization is very rare. The fetus immune system is immature and is generally unable to recognize maternal antigens or produce antibodies. Rh-negative newborns, children of Rh-positive mothers, had anti Rh(D) antibody titers detected by special techniques [13].

A study carried out at the Fetal Medicine Center of Hospital das Clínicas, UFMG, in 2005 evaluated the causes of maternal alloimmunization, showing that the majority of cases is related to the absence of postpartum prophylaxis (72.3% of cases) [14], followed by incompatible transfusion, which represented 13.3% of the sample.

The Rh factor was discovered in 1940 by Landsteiner and Wiener [15]. In 1991, Cherif-Zahar and colleagues located the locus of the Rh group on the short arm of chromosome 1 [16]. Two genes were identified – RhD and RhCE. There are several variations of the D antigen, called weak D or partial D, depending on the type of expression. The best known type of weak D is the Du variant. This variant can be falsely typed as Rh-negative. This is of clinical importance since Du-positive erythrocytes can stimulate the production of anti Rh(D) antibodies in Rh-negative individuals which can lead to failures in prevention with Rh(D) immunoglobulin. Rh(D)-negative, but Du-positive, individuals must be followed as Rh(D)-positive [17].

In addition to the antigens of the Rh and ABO systems, our red blood cells have more than 50 antigens on their surface, many of which are less important, because they are less common or because they have less antigenicity (ability to stimulate the production of antibodies). With the greater application of anti-Rh(D) prophylaxis in recent years, alloimmunization by other antigens has gained greater importance (Table 38.1).

Diagnosis

The first step in diagnosis is to request the pregnant woman's blood typing. The next step is to check whether or not the pregnant woman has anti-Rh antibodies in her bloodstream. This is achieved through the qualitative determination of anti-Rh antibodies – indirect qualitative Coombs test. The negative test means that the pregnant woman is not immunized; the reverse – positive Coombs test – means the pregnant woman is already immunized. The test should be repeated between 16 and 18 weeks and then monthly until the end of pregnancy in non-immunized pregnant women.

The indirect Coombs test is based on patient blood sample being exposed to red blood cells known to be D-positive. Anti-D antibodies adhere to these red blood cells and after washing and suspension in another ligand immunoglobulin (Coombs reagent), the red blood cells are agglutinated.

Care of Unimmunized Pregnant Women

Prenatal Care

In addition to standard prenatal care, non-immunized Rh-negative pregnant women should be investigated about previous history of blood transfusion, previous surgeries, previous pregnancies, use of anti-Rh immunoglobulin, and finally the history of newborns – hydropic, stillborn, or newborn babies with severe jaundice. We can also determine fetal Rh(D) in maternal blood by analyzing fetal DNA circulating in the maternal bloodstream. If the fetus is Rh(D)-negative, no special monitoring is necessary.

Because of the risk of immunization during pregnancy, the administration of Rh immunoglobulin is recommended in Rh-negative pregnant women who are not immunized in the 28th week of pregnancy, and the dose should be repeated in the postpartum period when the newborn is Rh-positive [18]. The half-life of the antibodies is approximately 12 weeks.

A study that evaluated the dose of 300 mcg given at the 28th week of gestation and after delivery showed that the sensitization rate in the group that received both doses was 0.32% against 1.8% in the group that received only postpartum prophylaxis – a reduction of 82% [19]. Antenatal prophylaxis programs have led to a significant reduction in anti-D alloimmunization.

The immunoglobulin administered during pregnancy usually produces anti-D titers of 1:1 or 1:2. With these titers, newborns are not compromised with hemolysis or anemia.

Labor and Delivery Care

When conducting labor in unimmunized Rh-negative pregnant women, there is no indication of immediate umbilical cord clamping. It is recommended to collect blood from the umbilical cord to perform some tests: blood group, Rh factor, and anti-Rh(D) antibodies screening – direct Coombs test. During the delivery, whenever possible, manual extraction of the placenta should be avoided. This maneuver could increase fetal-maternal bleeding.

Postpartum Care

After delivery, the next step, of fundamental importance, is the administration of human anti-Rh(D) immunoglobulin, aiming at the prevention of maternal isoimmunization by the Rh factor, under the dose of 250–300 mcg, applied to the muscle up to 72 hours after delivery. Prevention is ensured by the destruction of fetal red blood cells linked to exogenous antibodies, before endogenous antibodies are produced. The red cells linked to the antibodies are directed to the red pulp of the spleen, where they are quickly removed from the circulation and destroyed before the sensitization process takes place. Red blood cells not linked to exogenous antibodies circulate until they undergo apoptosis, releasing fragments that may reach the white pulp of the spleen, where the process of antigen recognition occurs. About 90% of immunizations happen at the time of delivery. The conditions for administering immunoglobulin to the parturient are:

- Rh-negative mother
- Indirect Coombs test – negative during the whole pregnancy
- Rh-positive newborn
- Direct Coombs test in umbilical cord blood – negative for Rh factor

If the indirect Coombs test is positive, we must request a panel of red blood cells that identifies which antibodies are present. If anti-Rh(D) is present, sensitization has already occurred, and immunoglobulin should not be applied as it will not bring any benefit.

If for some reason prophylaxis is not performed within 72 hours, it is still suggested to administer immunoglobulin until the 28th day after delivery [20] as long as the indirect Coombs remains negative.

The usual doses of immunoglobulin administered in the postpartum period are able to prevent immunization in about 85–90% of cases [21]. Large transplacental hemorrhages require larger doses of immunoglobulin. There is evidence that the 300 mcg dose of immunoglobulin prevents immunization if fetal-maternal hemorrhage is up to 25 ml Rh-positive blood or 12 ml fetal red blood cells [18].

With the diagnosis of massive transplacental hemorrhage (through the Kleihauer test), 300 mcg should be administered in hemorrhages below 25 ml, 600 mcg when between 25 and 49 ml, and 900 mcg between 50 and 74 ml [18].

Bowman [12] recommends that these tests are performed when major transplacental hemorrhages are suspected: cesarean section with manual extraction of the placenta and pre- and intrapartum hemorrhages (placenta previa, placental abruption).

Figure 38.2 summarizes prenatal and postpartum care for non-immunized pregnant women.

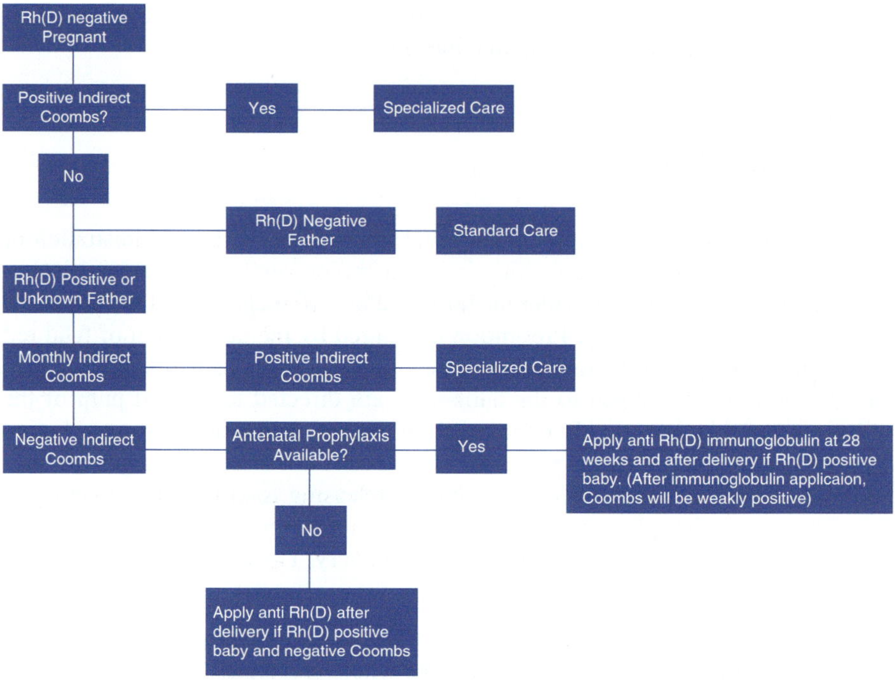

Fig. 38.2 Monitoring of Rh(D)-negative pregnant women by the traditional method and by the method using genetic determination tests

Care of Immunized Pregnant Women

Prenatal Care

The presence of anti-Rh antibodies in the blood of a Rh-negative pregnant woman means that she is already immunized. Her prenatal care has to be special, differentiated, in order to avoid serious problems in the fetus and/or the newborn. In the anamnesis, it is necessary to ask about the transfusion history, especially in nulliparous women. Complementary exams can assess fetal conditions and their degree of impairment, and non-invasive and invasive methods can be used.

In addition to tests to assess fetal anemia, a panel of red blood cells should be performed to identify which antibodies are responsible for alloimmunization and schedule follow-up according to the likelihood of that antibody causing hemolysis.

The blood typing of fetal red blood cells can be done through analysis of maternal blood in search of Fetal DNA, after 10 weeks of gestation.

Due to the risks of invasive procedures, since the 1960s, a way to safely diagnose fetal anemia through non-invasive methods has been sought. Several methods have been studied, and more recently, Doppler velocimetry has received the greatest attention from researchers.

The non-invasive methods also aim to detect fetal anemia before the development of hydrops, since the edematous fetus responds worse to treatment than the non-edematous fetus. The non-invasive diagnosis of fetal anemia is based on the pathophysiological changes that the anemic fetus undergoes. These changes are metabolic, hematopoietic, and hemodynamic.

Nicolaides et al. [22] established through cordocentesis studies that fetal hemoglobin is, on average, 12 g/dL at 20 weeks and 16 g/dL at 40 weeks, and therefore, to classify the fetus as anemic, we should not use a fixed value of hemoglobin. Therefore, the concept of hemoglobin deficit was also created where the definition of anemia would be based on the difference between the mean hemoglobin value and the hemoglobin found in the fetus. The 2.5th percentile corresponds to a deficit of 2 g regardless of gestational age, and moderate and severe anemia would be observed with a deficit of 5 and 7 g, respectively.

The adaptations that the fetus undergoes to compensate for anemia are installed according to the degree of hemolysis and anemia.

Starting from the normal hemoglobin value and reaching a deficit of 2 g/dL, the fetus begins to present hemodynamic changes to compensate for anemia such as increased cardiac output. The decrease in blood viscosity caused by the decrease in hematocrit associated with increased cardiac output leads to the hyperdynamic state of the fetus that can be detected on Doppler. The study of blood speed in fetal vessels allows the diagnosis of the degree of anemia [15].

With a hemoglobin deficit greater than 5 g/dL, the fetus begins to undergo hematological changes such as the extramedullary production of red blood cells in the liver and spleen and the release into the blood of immature forms or erythroblasts, which are part of the classic syndrome of perinatal hemolytic disease, also called fetal erythroblastosis. Ultrasonography detects enlargement of the liver and spleen caused by extramedullary hematopoiesis [2].

With a deficit greater than 7 g/dL or severe anemia, the fetus begins to present hypoalbuminemia and increased pressure in the portal vein due to the obstruction of the hepatic sinuses by the extramedullary production of red blood cells and can then begin to lose fluid to the extravascular space accumulating liquid in several cavities such as abdominal, pleural, and pericardial, a condition known as hydrops – the most severe form of the disease. Ultrasonography diagnoses hydrops by visualizing fetal effusions, such as subcutaneous edema, ascites, pericardial effusion, and pleural effusion. It can also show increased cardiac area. Venous Doppler can show overload and heart failure, and cardiotocography shows myocardial hypoxia [15].

Generally, fetuses with a hemoglobin deficit greater than 10 g/dL are not found because those values are associated with intrauterine death [2].

The most widely used non-invasive method today is the Doppler of the middle cerebral artery (Fig. 38.3). This exam has several characteristics that bring it closer to the ideal. It is a method of easy execution, widely available, and capable of detecting fetal anemia in its initial stages, allowing the installation of early treatment using the criteria shown in Table 38.2. In addition, the position of the middle cerebral artery allows its evaluation in angle close to zero – fundamental for the evaluation of blood velocity.

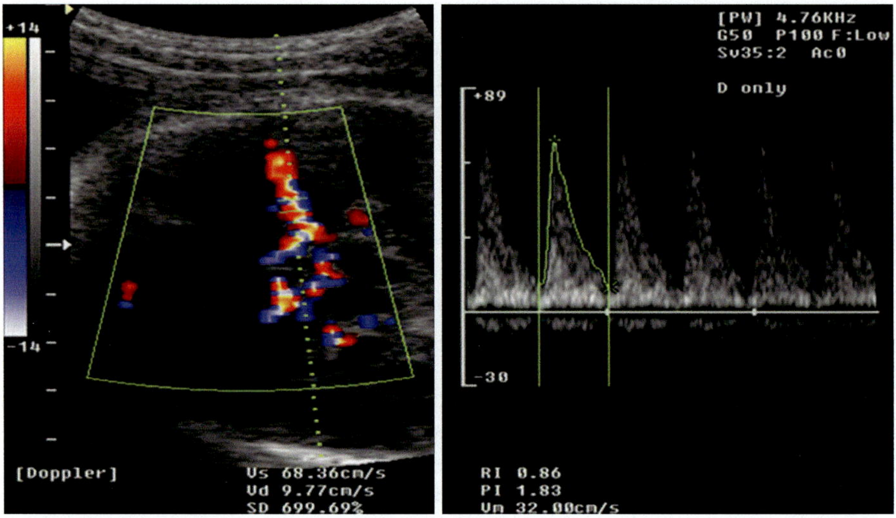

Fig. 38.3 Middle cerebral artery Doppler

Table 38.2 Criteria for assessing fetal anemia by means of Doppler of the middle cerebral artery

Fetus at rest and apnea
Enlarging the image enough to view the entire path of the vessel
Insonation with an angle as close to zero as possible and always below 30° (for angles between 0 and 30°, use the angle corrector)
Insonate the vase close to its origin in the Willis polygon
Delimit peak systolic speed manually
Make 3 measurements and use the largest

Mari et al. [21] demonstrated that when the peak systolic velocity (PSV) in the middle cerebral artery was greater than 1.5 multiples of the median for gestational age, the positive predictive value in the prediction of moderate and severe fetal anemia was 100%, with a false-positive rate only 12%. If the anemia is moderate or severe, intrauterine transfusion or anticipation of delivery depending on the gestational age is indicated. Table 38.3 shows the reference values for MCA PSV.

Subsequent studies confirmed that the measurement of PSV in MCA was a superior method, when compared to invasive methods in the diagnosis of fetal anemia, with the advantage of being less aggressive [23].

However, the prediction of fetal anemia using MCA Doppler has some problems. In pregnancies over 34 weeks, the evaluation becomes less reliable due to changes in fetal hemodynamics. Another problem is the assessment of anemia after intrauterine transfusion, since the introduction of adult red blood cells into the fetal circulation changes the rheological properties of the blood (viscosity, density, etc.), changing the Doppler interpretation [24].

Table 38.3 Peak systolic velocity × degree of fetal anemia

Middle cerebral artery PSV (cm/s)				
Degree of anemia		Mild	Moderate	Severe
Weeks	Mean	1,29 MoM	1,5 MoM	1,55 MoM
14	19,3	24,9	28,9	29,9
15	20,2	26,1	30,3	31,3
16	21,1	27,2	31,7	32,7
17	22,1	28,5	33,2	34,3
18	23,2	29,9	34,8	36,0
19	24,3	31,3	36,5	37,7
20	25,5	32,9	38,2	39,5
21	26,7	34,4	40,0	41,4
22	27,9	36,0	41,9	43,2
23	29,3	37,8	43,9	45,4
24	30,7	39,6	46,0	47,6
25	32,1	41,4	48,2	49,8
26	33,6	43,3	50,4	52,1
27	35,2	45,4	52,8	54,6
28	36,9	47,6	55,4	57,2
29	38,7	49,9	58,0	60,0
30	40,5	52,2	60,7	62,8
31	42,4	54,7	63,6	65,7
32	44,4	57,3	66,6	68,8
33	46,5	60,0	69,8	72,1
34	48,7	62,8	73,1	75,5
35	51,1	65,9	76,6	79,2
36	53,5	69,0	80,2	82,9
37	56,0	72,2	84,0	86,8
38	58,7	75,7	88,0	91,0
39	61,5	79,3	92,2	95,3
40	64,4	83,1	96,6	99,8

MoM multiples of median

In order to solve these problems, the UFMG group has been working with the association of non-invasive markers. The association of non-invasive parameters allows the evaluation other aspects of the pathophysiology of fetal anemia and increases the diagnostic accuracy.

The evaluation of the cardiac area, by measuring the external biventricular diameter (LVBD) of the fetus' heart, proved to be a good parameter to assess fetal anemia, even after intrauterine transfusions [25, 26].

A study published in 2010 showed that the measurement of the cardio femoral index (CFI), which corresponds to the direct ratio between LVDB and the length of the femur, has a sensitivity of 91.7% for severe anemia. However, MCA PSV was more specific for the detection of mild anemia [27].

We currently use an association of non-invasive methods: PSV from MCA and CFI. Alloimmunized pregnant women from 28 weeks onwards undergo weekly ultrasounds to assess the likelihood of severe anemia through the combination of non-invasive methods. If both MCA PSV and the CFI are altered or the fetus shows signs of hydrops, cordocentesis is proposed, once the risk of severe fetal anemia is high.

Labor and Delivery Care

The decision as to when to deliver or to treat the fetus depends on the intensity of the fetal anemia and the gestational age. There are three management strategies in immunized Rh-negative pregnant women:

- Assistance to spontaneous delivery at term
- Premature anticipation of pregnancy
- Intrauterine treatment

In Rh-negative fetuses (heterozygous father), identified by intrauterine typing, or in Rh-positive fetuses with mild disease – proven by any of the propaedeutic resources used, with antibody titers below the critical levels and non-invasive follow-up showing low probability of anemia – pregnancy can progress to term.

In pregnancies over 34 weeks, hydrops fetalis or non-invasive tests showing a high probability of severe anemia, anticipation is indicated after corticosteroid therapy.

In pregnancies below 34 weeks with non-invasive follow-up showing a high probability of fetal anemia, invasive propaedeutic is indicated to determine anemia and possible transfusion.

Intrauterine Treatment

In compromised fetuses in pregnancies below 34 weeks, intrauterine treatment is mandatory. Fetal blood transfusion to decrease anemia should be performed, until enough maturity is reached and delivery is possible. This treatment, idealized and performed by Liley in 1963, has been used, with increasingly better results. Initially, blood was injected into the abdominal cavity of the fetus (intraperitoneal transfusion). From the 1980s, whenever conditions permit and using ultrasound to guide the procedure, blood is introduced directly into the umbilical cord vessels (intravascular transfusion).

The overall survival rates described range from 76% to 94%. Perinatal survival of non-hydropic fetuses exceeds 90%, and approximately 75% of hydropic survives after treatment [2].

Intrauterine blood transfusion is an extreme resource for treating severely compromised fetuses. It should only be performed in referral centers, by qualified and experienced medical staff.

Transfusion is indicated if the fetal hematocrit is less than 30% or the hemoglobin deficit is greater than 5 mg/dL for gestational age. The most used type of transfusion is intravascular. By this technique, the umbilical vein is punctured with a 20 g needle guided by ultrasound. The best sites for puncture are placental insertion of the cord and the insertion into the abdomen of the fetus. Whenever possible, transplacental puncture should be avoided as it has a higher rate of complications. The purpose of intravascular transfusion is to increase the hematocrit to 50–55%.

The blood used is O Rh(D)-negative, also negative for other antigens, if the sensitization is by irregular antigens, and negative for infections. The blood is phenotyped in addition to being concentrated to reach a hematocrit of 70–80%, which allows a smaller volume to be infused into the fetus, reducing the risks of post-transfusion cardiac decompensation due to hypervolemia. In addition, leukocytes are removed (delucotization), and the blood is irradiated to prevent a graft-versus-host reaction.

The volume of blood to be transfused can be calculated with the following formula [28]:

- Transfusion volume = 18.2 + 13.4 × pre-IUT hemoglobin +6 × GA (weeks).

In non-hydropic fetuses, two transfusions are usually performed every 15 days to ensure the correction of anemia. Thereafter, new transfusions are performed every 3–4 weeks until the 34th week when delivery occur [29].

The rate of drop in hematocrit is approximately 2% per day after transfusions. After a few transfusions, most of the blood circulating in the fetus comes from the donor and not from himself; this reduces the rate of hemolysis, reduces the need for new transfusions, but can also lead to a block in the production of new red blood cells. In neonatal follow-up, periodic transfusions are usually performed until the bone marrow has recovered.

Fetuses with hydrops may present cardiac decompensation after transfusion, so it is recommended that the final hematocrit in the first transfusion does not exceed 25% or a 4× increase in pre-transfusion values. Thus, the objective of the first transfusion is to increase the hematocrit to 25%. A second transfusion is performed in 48 hours to raise the hematocrit to 35% and a third in a week to reach 50%, if the hydrops has disappeared [29].

Phenobarbital to Accelerate Liver Maturity

After birth, the main problem of the newborn, son of an alloimmunized mother, becomes hyperbilirubinemia, because while he is still inside the uterus, bilirubin passes through the placenta and is eliminated by the mother. In newborns, whose liver is often immature, the accumulation of bilirubin can lead to the development of kernicterus resulting in permanent sequelae for that individual. The treatment of hyperbilirubinemia is the exchange of blood with low hematocrit and high bilirubin for transfused blood – exsanguinotransfusion.

Some research has shown that the administration of phenobarbital to the mother can reduce the need for exanguineotransfusion due to hyperbilirubinemia in the newborn. Phenobarbital stimulates the enzyme glucuronyl transferase in the newborn's liver, increasing the ability to conjugate and eliminate bilirubin. In a study with 71 alloimmunized pregnant women, 1 group received phenobarbital, 30 mg, 3 times a day, for 7–10 days before delivery, and another did not receive any medication. In the treated group, 9% of newborns required blood transfusion, while in the untreated group, the procedure was performed in 52% of cases – a 75% reduction [12].

Figure 38.4, synthetizes the care of a sensitized mother.

Other Situations

Abortion and Threatened Abortion

There is a risk of immunization in abortions and even in the threat of miscarriage, when pregnancy continues its evolution. Fetal circulation is established by the fourth week of pregnancy and the Rh antigen has already been demonstrated in the fetal red blood cell, 38 days after conception [29].

The risk of immunization in patients with spontaneous or induced abortions is 3%–6%, increasing with advancing gestational age [30].

All non-sensitized Rh-negative women should receive 50 mcg of Rh immunoglobulin within 72 hours after induced or spontaneous abortion, which occurs in the first trimester. In the second trimester, with 13 weeks or more, the total dose of 250–300 mcg should be routinely administered [2].

The threat of abortion in the first trimester appears to increase the risk of immunization. A case of sensitization after threatened abortion in the first trimester has been described [2].

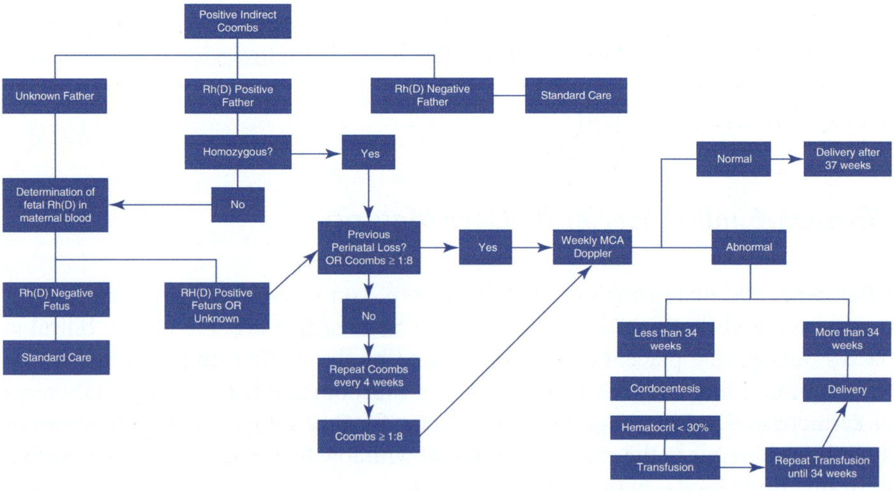

Fig. 38.4 Management of Rh(D)-negative sensitized pregnant women

In the absence of a 50 mcg dose, a 250–300 mcg dose is used in abortion regardless of gestational age. In case of miscarriage, it is recommended to administer a dose of 250 or 300 mcg. If the pregnancy continues, the dose is repeated every 12 weeks until the end of the pregnancy.

Other Types of Antepartum Hemorrhages

In all types of gestational hemorrhage, immunoglobulin administration is recommended. All non-immunized Rh-negative pregnant women, with hemorrhage before delivery without loss of conceptus, are at risk of transplacental hemorrhage and, therefore, of immunization. A full dose of Rh immunoglobulin should be administered and repeated every 12 weeks until delivery [18].

In the previous placenta with bleeding and in invasive therapeutic procedures – amniocentesis, cordocentesis, and villous chorion biopsy – in non-immunized Rh-negative pregnant women, it is recommended to administer Rh immunoglobulin.

All non-immunized Rh-negative pregnant women submitted to amniocentesis should receive 300 mcg of immunoglobulin unless they are known to be Rh-negative as well. The dose should be repeated 12 weeks later, if there is no delivery, or in 6 weeks, if another amniocentesis is performed [31].

In the placenta previa, the regimen is also 300 mcg, and if delivery does not happen within 12 weeks, the dose is repeated.

Ectopic Pregnancy

Once the Rh(D) antigen has been present in fetal red blood cells since the sixth week of conception, there is a potential risk of sensitization in ectopic pregnancy, and at least one case has been reported [32].

In 9 of the 38 (24%) women with ectopic pregnancy, between 6 and 10 weeks of gestation, a significant number of fetal red blood cells were found in the maternal circulation [30].

It is recommended that all Rh-negative pregnant women not immunized with ectopic pregnancy be treated with Rh immunoglobulin [33].

Gestational Trophoblastic Disease

Using special techniques, by immunofluorescence, Goto [34] demonstrated the presence of Rh antigen in the chorial villi of the human placenta of gestation between 12 and 14 weeks. The red cell antigenicity increases with fetal maturity.

In the embryonic hydatidiform mole, the administration of immunoglobulin is recommended; when there is no embryo, its use is questioned. Rh immunoglobulin is not believed to be necessary in the hydatidiform mole; however, its use is not harmful [35].

Tubal Ligation

Rh-negative women not yet immunized at reproductive age and submitted to postpartum tubal ligation should receive Rh(D) immunoglobulin. There is a risk of failure, or, later, the woman may undergo recanalization of the tubes and become pregnant again.

Table 38.4 lists the indications and doses of anti-Rh(D) immunoglobulin.

Table 38.4 Indications and doses of anti-Rh(D) immunoglobulin

Indication	Dose
Postpartum	100–300 mcg
Rh(D)-negative pregnant woman	(with the 100 mcg dose, it is mandatory to check the volume of maternal fetus hemorrhage)
Rh(D)-positive newborn	
Negative indirect Coombs	
Positive indirect Coombs if received immunoglobulin during pregnancy or if the RBC panel shows sensitization by an antigen other than Rh(D)	
Even if tubal ligation is performed	
During pregnancy	300 mcg (single dose at the 28th week)
Rh(D)-negative pregnant woman	
Rh(D)-positive or unknown fetus	100 mcg (one dose at the 28th and another at the 34th week)
Negative indirect Coombs	
Prophylactic at 28th week (or 28th and 34th weeks)	
Post-bleeding during pregnancy	
Abortion	Below 13 weeks the dose can be 50 mcg
Ectopic pregnancy	
Molar pregnancy	
Threat of abortion	If the risk factor persists, the dose should be repeated every 12 weeks
Previous placenta	
Post-procedures during pregnancy	
Amniocentesis	
Chorial villus biopsy	
Cordocentesis	
Fetal surgery	
Post-incompatible transfusion	10 mcg of immunoglobulin for each ml of incompatible blood transfused
Rh(D)-negative woman	
Negative indirect Coombs	

References

1. Moise KJ Jr. Hemolytic disease of the fetus and newborn. In: Creasy RK, Resnik R, Iams JD, editors. Maternal-fetal medicine: principles and practice, vol. 26. 6th ed. Philadelphia: Saunders; 2009. p. 477–503.
2. Jackson M, Branch DW. Isoimunização na Gravidez. In: Gabbe SG, Niebyl JR, Simpson JL, editors. Obstetrícia – Gestações Normais e Patológicas. 3rd ed. Rio de Janeiro: Guanabara-Koogan; 1999. p. 657–80.
3. Rote NS. Pathophysiology of Rh immunization. Clin Obstet Gynecol. 1982;25:243–53.
4. Nevanlina HR, Vainio T. The influence of mother-child ABO incompatibility on Rh immunization. Vox Sang. 1956;1:26–32.
5. Bowman JM. The management of Rh-immunization. Obstet Gynecol. 1978;52:1–8.
6. ACOG Practice Bulletin No. 192: management of alloimmunization during pregnancy - prevention of Rh D alloimmunization.
7. Bowman JM. Antenatal supression of Rh alloimmunization. Clin Obstet Gynecol. 1991;34:296–303.
8. Gorman JC. Analysis of failures with Rh immuneglobulin. Clin Obstet Gynecol. 1971;14:635–46.
9. Kumpel BM. On the imunnologic basis of Rh imune globulin (anti-D) Prophylaxis.
10. Boctor FM, et al. Absence of D-alloimunization in AIDS patients receiving D-mismatched RBCs. Transfusion. 2003;43:173–6.
11. Queenan S. Rhesus incompatibility, example of progressive perinatal medicine. In: Carrera JM, Cabero L, Baraibar R, editors. The perinatal medicine of the new millennium. Bologna: Monduzzi Editore; 2001. p. 416–23.
12. Bowman J. The prevention of Rh immunization. Transfus Med Rev. 1988;2:129–50.
13. Acott JR, Beer AE, Guy LR, Ligsh M, Elbert G. Pathogenesis of Rh immunization in primigravida – feto maternal versus materno-fetal bleedings. Obstet Gynecol. 1977;49:9–12.
14. Cabral ACV, Melo IG, Osanan GC, Dantas JBPD, Taveira MR, Leite HV. Estudo das causas da isoimunização materna por antígenos eritrocitários entre gestantes acompanhadas no serviço de medicina fetal do HC-UFMG. Rev Med Minas Gerais. 2005;15(1):10–2.
15. Corrêa Jr MD. Avaliação da Anemia Fetal Pela Dopplervelocimetria da Artéria Esplênica. 2006. 135p. Tese (Doutorado em Ginecologia e Obstetrícia) - Faculdade de Medicina da Universidade Federal de Minas Gerais.
16. Cherif-Zahar B, Mattei MG, Le Van Kim C, Bailly P, Cartron JP, Colin Y. Localization of the human Rh blood group gene structure to chromosome region 1p34.3-1p36.1 by in situ hybridization. Hum Genet. 1991;86:398–400.
17. Van Kim C, Cartron JP. Rh proteins: key structural and functional components of the red cell membrane. Blood Rev. 2006;20:93–110.
18. Bowman JM. Controversies in Rh prophylaxis. Who needs Rh immnuneglobulin and when should, it, be given? Am J Obstet Gynecol. 1985;151:289–94.
19. Bowman JM, Pollock JM. Failures of intravenous Rh immunoglobulin prophylaxis: an analyses of the reasons for such failures. Transfus Med Rev. 1987;1:101–12.
20. Bowman J. Rh-immunoglobulin: Rh prophylaxis. Best Pract Res Clin Haematol. 2006;19:27–34.
21. Mari G, Deter RL, Carpenter RL, Rahman F, Zimmerman R, Moise KJ Jr, et al. Noninvasive diagnosis by Doppler ultrasonography of fetal anemia due to maternal red-cell alloimmunization. Collaborative Group for Doppler Assessment of the Blood Velocity in Anemic Fetuses. N Engl J Med. 2000;342:9–14.
22. Nicolaides KH, Soothill PW, Clewell WH, Rodeck CH, Mibashan RS, Campbell S. Fetal haemoglobin measurement in the assessment of red cell isoimmunisation. Lancet. 1988;1(8594):1073–5.
23. Oepkes D, Seaward G, Vandenbussche FPHA, Windrim R, Kingdon J, Beyene J, et al. Doppler ultrasonography versus amniocentesis to predict fetal anemia. N Engl J Med. 2006;355:156–64.

24. Mari G. Middle cerebral artery peak systolic velocity for the diagnosis of fetal anemia: the untold story. Ultrasound Obstet Gynecol. 2005;25:323–30.
25. Cabral AC, Reis ZS, Leite HV, Lage EM, Ferreira AL, Melo IG. Cardiofemoral index as an ultrasound marker of fetal anemia in isoimmunized pregnancy. Int J Gynaecol Obstet. 2008;100(1):60–4.
26. Van Dongen H, Klumper FJ, Sikkel E, Vandenbussche FP, Oepkes D. Non-invasive tests to predict fetal anemia in Kell-alloimmunized pregnancies. Ultrasound Obstet Gynecol. 2005;25:341–5.
27. Cabral AC, Reis ZS, Apocalypse IG, Osanan GC, Lage EM, Leite HV. Combined use of the cardio femoral index and middle cerebral artery Doppler velocimetry for the prediction of fetal anemia. Int J Gynaecol Obstet. 2010;111(3):205–8.
28. Santiago MD, Rezende CA, Cabral AC, Leite HV, Vitral ZN, Apocalypse IM. Cálculo do volume de sangue necessário para a correção de anemia fetal em gestantes isoimunizadas. Rev Bras Ginecol Obstet. 2008;30:196–200.
29. Schumacher B, Moise KJ Jr. Fetal transfusion for red blood cell alloimmunization.
30. Katz J, Marcus RG. Incidence of Rh immunization following abortion. Possible detection of lymphocyte priming to Rh antigen. Am J Obstet Gynecol. 1973;117:261–7.
31. Bowman JM. Suppression of the Rh immunization. Obstet Gynecol. 1978;52:385–8.
32. Aborjaily NA. Rh sensitization after tubal pregnancy. N Engl J Med. 1969;28:1076–80.
33. ROCG Green top guideline. Use of Anti-D Immunoglobulin for Rh Prophylaxis. Disponível em: http://www.rcog.org.uk/womens-health/clinical-guidance/use-anti-d-immunoglobulin-rhprophylaxis-greentop-22. Consulta em julho de 2009.
34. Goto J, Mishi H, Tomada Y. Blood group Rh-D factor in human throphoblast determines by immunoflorescent method. Am J Obstet Gynecol. 1980;137:707–12.
35. Moise K Jr. Management of rhesus alloimmunization in pregnancy. Obstet Gynecol. 2008;112:164–76.

Chapter 39
Disorders of Amniotic Fluid Volume: Oligoamnios and Polyhydramnios

Mario S. F. Palermo, Ana Espinosa, and Mónica Trasmonte

Amniotic fluid (LA) is a complex of necessary and essential substances for the complete development of intrauterine life; it occupies the amniotic cavity from the early stages of gestation creating a physical space around the embryo and subsequently the fetus. It contains nutrients and growth factors.

The production and absorption processes of amniotic fluid are due to multiple factors, being a reason for increasing research in recent decades.

The volume of amniotic fluid is determined by the fluid that flows into and out of the amniotic cavity.

Alterations in amniotic fluid volume may reflect a problem in fluid production or circulation, such as occurs in the presence of a fetal abnormality or maternal factors. Both its marked decrease (oligoamnios) and the exaggerated increase (polyhydramnios) are accompanied by an increased risk of an adverse perinatal outcome.

Function and Production of Amniotic Fluid

The amniotic cavity appears on the eighth day of gestation. In the early stages of pregnancy, the amniotic cavity fills up with a liquid of a composition similar to that of extracellular fluid, with a crystalline appearance partly produced by amniotic cells but mainly originated from maternal blood [1].

M. S. F. Palermo (✉)
Diagnomed Affiliated Institution Faculty of Medicine of Buenos Aires, Teaching and Research, Buenos Aires, Argentina

A. Espinosa
Institution Matersur, Teaching and Research, Bahía Blanca, Buenos Aires, Argentina

M. Trasmonte
Hospital Nacional Prof. Dr. A. Posadas, MATERNAL CHILD, Buenos Aires, Argentina

© Springer Nature Switzerland AG 2022
R. A. Moreira de Sá, E. B. d. Fonseca (eds.), *Perinatology*,
https://doi.org/10.1007/978-3-030-83434-0_39

During the first half of pregnancy, there is transfer of water and other small molecules through the amnion (transmembrane flow), through the fetal vessels on the placental surface (intramembrane flow), and through the fetal skin. Fetal diuresis begins between 11 and 12 weeks at which time renal function is complete, but does not become a substantial component of amniotic fluid until the second trimester. This last observation explains why fetuses with lethal renal abnormalities do not manifest severe oligoamnios until after 18 weeks. Water transport through fetal skin continues until keratinization occurs between 22 and 25 weeks. This is why extremely premature infants can lose significant amounts of fluid through the skin (Fig. 39.1).

The amount of amniotic fluid varies from 30 ml at 10 weeks, going from 450 ml at 20 weeks to 800 ml- 1 liter at the end at 37 weeks. The maximum peak is at 34 weeks (Fig. 39.2) [1–3].

During the initial stages of gestation and up to 22 weeks, before the development of fetal urination and swallowing, amniotic fluid is a result of osmotic gradients; there is a transudation through the fetal skin and the placental surface. In later stages, when the skin is keratinized, most of the fluid is produced from fetal urine, where the fetal kidney produces 800–1200 ml/day, and the secretion of pulmonary fluid is 340 ml/day. A part of this fluid is reabsorbed and another part is dumped into the amniotic cavity. Swallowing absorbs between 500 ml at 1 l/day (Fig. 39.3).

Now, the amount of amniotic fluid is not justified with the simple balance of diuresis and swallowing. In recent decades, research has been carried out on the intramembrane route. Intramembrane absorption is mainly unidirectional, vesicular; it is a process of bulk transport mediated through the activation of vascular endothelial growth factor (VEGF) of transcytotic transport through caveolae actively and passively by transcellular transfer of water that is supplied by the aquaporin water channels located in the cell membrane of the amnion [2]. This route regulates up to 500 ml/day. A very small amount of fluid 10 ml/day is regulated by the transmembrane route (Fig. 39.4).

In the third trimester, the membranes are pressed against the uterine wall, and by constant osmotic difference of the amniotic fluid in relation to the plasma of 30 mOsm/kg, the net flow of the exchanges is an exit of the liquid from the amniotic cavity toward the mother 0.3–0.7 ml/h (transmembrane route). Controlled prolactin plays a predominant role in the regulation of these passages [4].

The inconveniences that appear in the circulation of the amniotic fluid, such as an obstruction in the fetal digestive system or a defect in the central nervous system- which makes swallowing difficult for the fetus-, would give rise in the amount of amniotic fluid, called polyhydramnios.

A severe renal malformation or obstruction of the urinary tract, on the contrary, would cause a decrease in the fluid, giving rise to oligoamnios.

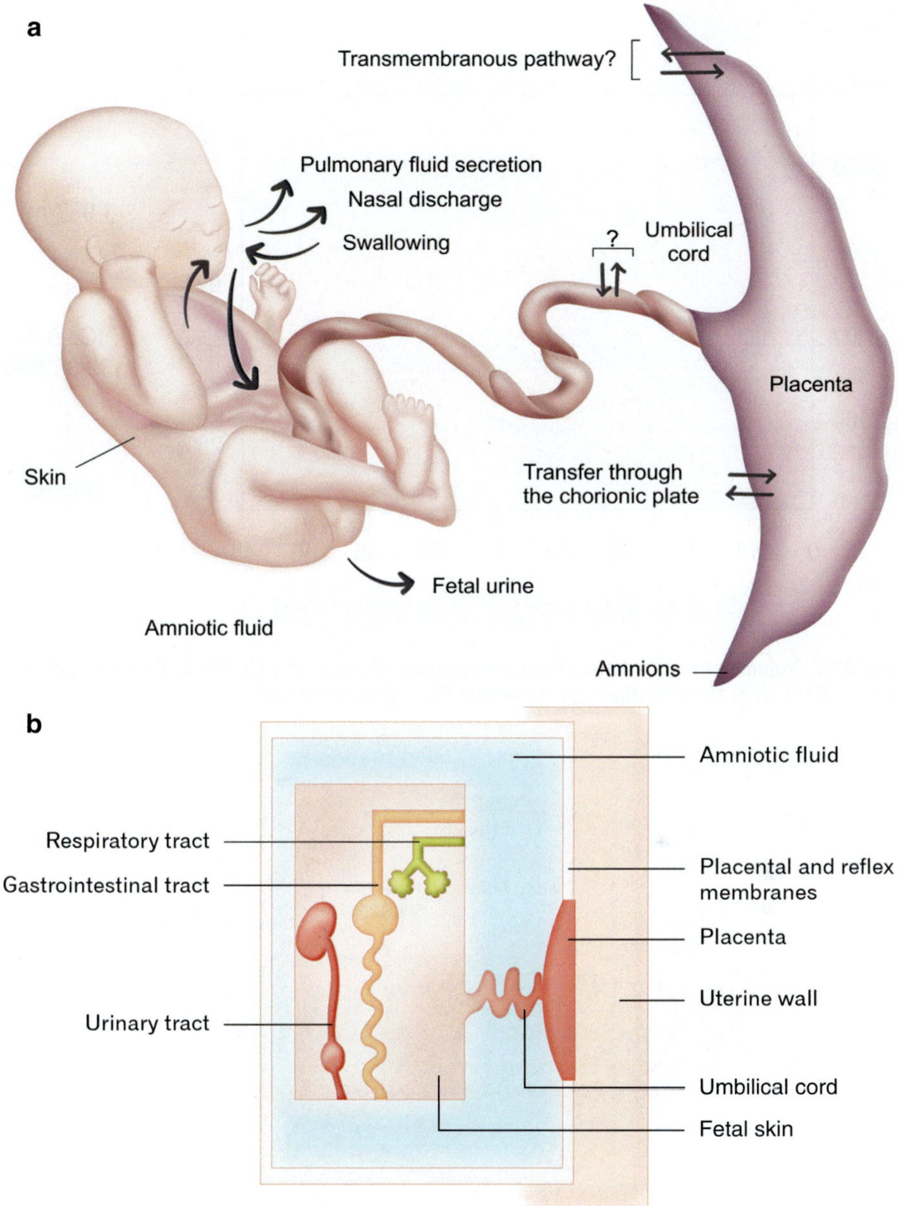

Fig. 39.1 Formation of amniotic fluid in the second half of gestation (**a**); Scheme of the umbilical cord function (**b**). Illustrated by Dr. Mario Palermo and Miss Karina Barbieri as Graphic illustrator. (Adapted from Callen [3] and Madar [4])

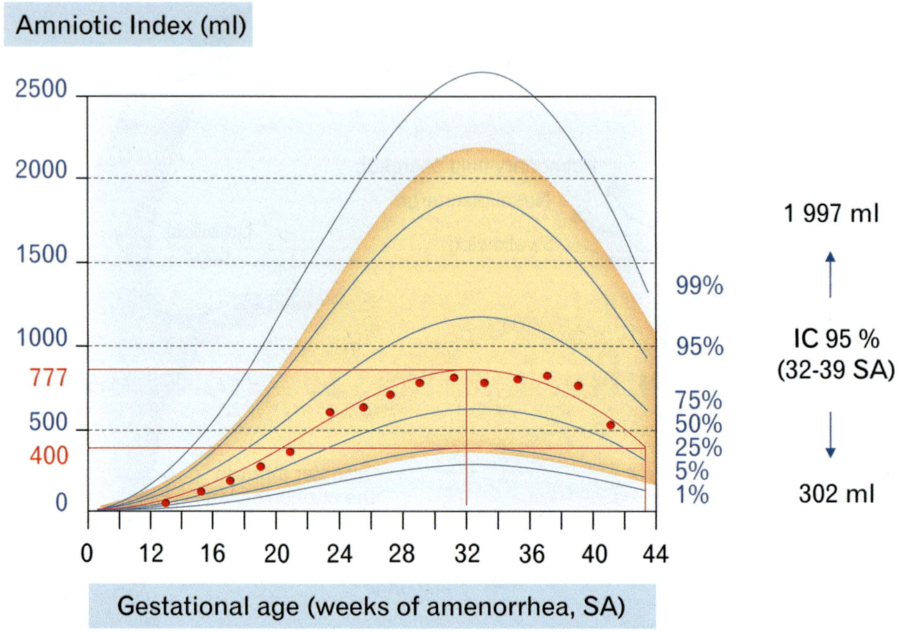

Fig. 39.2 Volume of amniotic fluid during pregnancy. Illustrated by Dr. Mario Palermo and Miss Karina Barbieri as Graphic illustrator. (Adapted from Madar et al. [4])

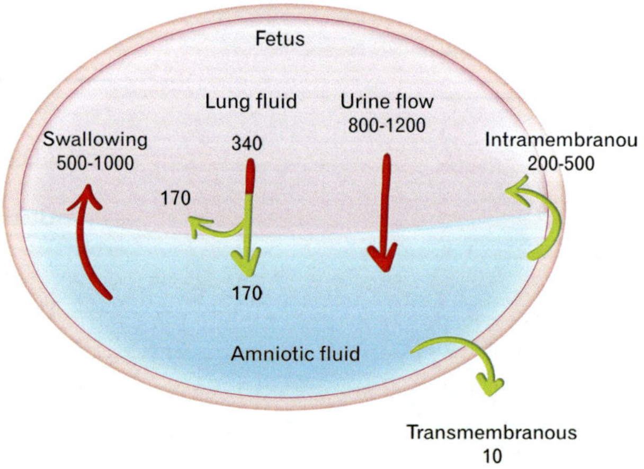

Fig. 39.3 Production and absorption routes of amniotic fluid. The numbers express ml/day. (Illustrated by Dr. Mario Palermo and Miss Karina Barbieri as Graphic illustrator. Adapted from Gilbert [5])

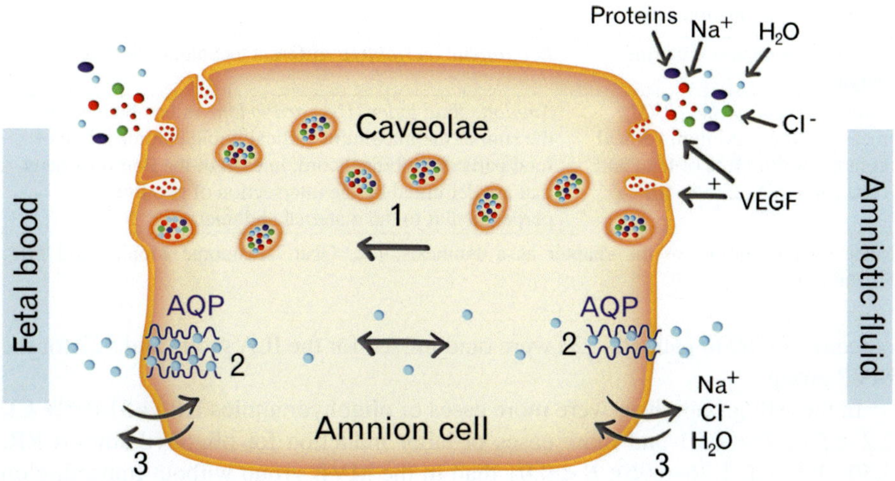

Fig. 39.4 Schematic representation of the transport of amniotic fluid through amniocytes. (1) VEGF unidirectional caveolar activated transcytosis (2). Water transport facilitated by aquaporin channels (3). Bidirectional diffusion of water and solutes. Illustrated by Dr. Mario Palermo and Miss Karina Barbieri as Graphic illustrator. (Adapted from Brace and C.Y. Cheung [12])

Echographic Evaluation of the Amniotic Fluid Volume

Examination of amniotic fluid volume has become an integral part of routine and diagnostic ultrasound in maternal fetal medicine.

It can be easily and inexpensively evaluated through ultrasonography, where the fluid surrounding the fetus, the umbilical cord, and the chorial surface of the placenta are seen. Ultrasonography is the only method to examine the volume of amniotic fluid during pregnancy.

The absolute volume of amniotic fluid by EG [6] is calculated and estimated by dilution and mathematical calculations.

In ultrasound there are subjective or qualitative and semiquantitative methods to assess the amount of amniotic fluid. This point has been one of the great challenges of ultrasound for more than 40 years.

The limitation of ultrasound in the assessment of AF is the three-dimensionality of its distribution, where the experience of the operator is essential. Therefore, various methods for estimating quantity measurement have been discussed. The objective of these methods is to track pregnancy in the timeline, mainly, regardless of the experience of the operators.

Subjective assessment of LA volume is excellent when the sonographer is adept.

The most widely used semiquantitative methods are the amniotic fluid index (ILA or Phelan index or four quadrants) [7] and the measurement of the maximum vertical amniotic fluid pocket (MVP) (Table 39.1).

The S.A.F.E study is a randomized open multicenter controlled trial on the comparison of MVP vs ILA as an evaluation test to predict the adverse pregnancy

Table 39.1 Evaluation

Clinic (presumptive): uterine height	*Ecographic (certainty):* different techniques are used
Major vertical pocket (BVM): measures the maximum vertical column of fluid free of fetal and cord parts (VN: 2 to 8–10)	*Amniotic fluid index (ILA) or Phelan:* value obtained from the sum of the maximum vertical liquid columns, free of fetal parts or umbilical cord, in each of the four quadrants that are delimited by the intersection of two lines perpendicular to the maternal abdomen (VN: 5–25)

Made by the authors of the chapter as a synthesis. Lic. Obst. Trasmonte Mónica and Prof. Dr. Palermo

outcome. Of 6930 patients, 525 were randomized for the ILA group and 527 for the MVP group.

In the AFI group, there were more cases of oligohydramnios RR, 4.51 (95% CI, 2.2–8.57); $P < 0.01$ and more cases of labor induction for oligohydramnios RR, 3.50 (95% CI, 1.76–6.96); $P < 0.01$ than in the MVB group without impacting on better perinatal results [8].

There are two meta-analyses comparing both ILA and MBV methods. The first was carried out by Cochrane on 3226 patients [9] and the second by Sekhon et al. with 4228 patients [10]. The results were the MVP as the best method for the diagnosis of oligoamnios when it is less than 2 cm versus less than 5 cm from the ILA, without statistically significant differences in other parameters such as the presence of meconium, admission to a neonatal UTI, etc. In the first, the ILA vs MVP, the RR was 2.39 (95% CI 1.73, 3.28), and in the second, the MVP vs ILA, the RR was 0.38 (95% CI 0.27–0.53).

Taking into account that MVP is the best method for evaluating amniotic fluid, we will make the definitions:

Oligoamnios: the MVP does not exceed 2 cm in pregnancy.

Polyhydramnios: greater vertical pocket is equal to or greater than 8 cm before 20 weeks and greater than 10 cm thereafter.

Measurement method: consists of measuring the depth (vertical diameter) of the maximum pocket of amniotic fluid perpendicularly, without interposition of the umbilical cord or small parts, preferably after 5–10 minutes from the start of the ultrasound.

Alterations of the Amniotic Fluid (AF)

Oligoamnios

Oligoamnios refers to the volume of amniotic fluid that is less than expected for gestational age. It is usually diagnosed by ultrasound examination and can be described qualitatively or with the description of MVP less than 2 cm.

Fetal urine is the most important source of AF in pregnancy, and any condition that disrupts urine formation or leakage or diuresis into the amniotic sac results in oligoamnios.

The Potter sequence, characterized by pulmonary hypoplasia and skeletal deformities secondary to prolonged and severe oligoamnios, anhydramnios, in the second trimester is the most serious manifestation of this condition. In the facies, low implantation of the ears, epicanthic folds of the eyes, flat nose, micrognathia, and severe postural defects in the limbs are observed. It is incompatible with extrauterine life.

Incidence

Oligoamnios complicates 0.5–8% of pregnancies. Although the reported rates of oligoamnios are influenced by variations in the diagnostic criteria, the study population (low or high risk, detection, or indicated ultrasound examination), the threshold used, and the gestational age at the time of the ultrasound examination (preterm, term, or post-term).

The most likely etiologies of oligoamnios vary depending on the severity and the quarter in which they are diagnosed. Table 39.2 summarizes the main causes of each trimester.

First Trimester

The presence of oligoamnios is a sign of a poor prognosis.

Second Trimester

Prognosis and management depend on the underlying etiology and extent of amniotic fluid reduction Fig 39.5. Compression of the cord can cause suffocation and stillbirth.

Serial ultrasound examinations every one to two weeks are helpful in following the natural history of the process, which may stabilize, resolve, or progress toward the development of oligoamnios or concomitant fetal growth restriction (IUGR).

Table 39.2 Main causes of oligoamnios. Made by the authors of the chapter as a synthesis. Lic. Obst. Trasmonte and Prof. Dr. Palermo Mario [28]

First trimester	*Second trimester*	*Third trimester*
Unknown	Kidney malformations	Rupture of the fetal membranes
Chromosomopathies	Urinary malformations	Uteroplacental insufficiency
	Maternal factors	Fetal growth restriction
	Placental factors	Drugs and medications
	Rupture of the fetal membranes	Fetal malformations with pulmonary hypoplasia
	Chromosomal disorders	Idiopathic post-term [28]

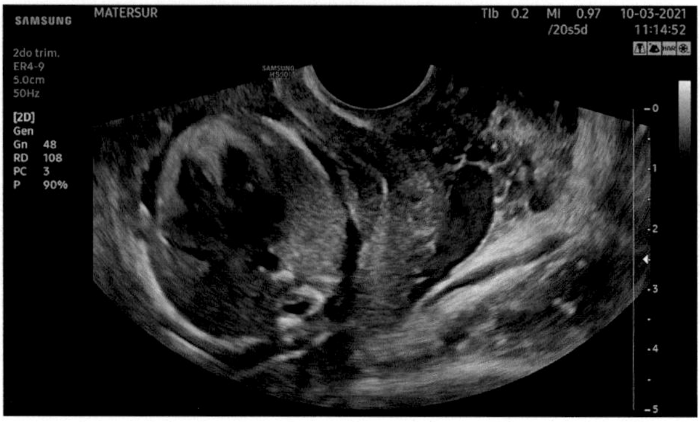

Fig. 39.5 Oligoamnios

If there are anhydramnios, the risk of pulmonary hypoplasia and fetal deformities increases dramatically.

Third Trimester

There appears to be an inverse relationship between the volume of amniotic fluid in the third trimester and the incidence of adverse perinatal outcomes.

Adverse outcomes are related to umbilical cord compression, uteroplacental insufficiency, and meconium aspiration. In particular, uteroplacental insufficiency and cord compression are associated with fetal heart rate abnormalities resulting in cesarean delivery and low Apgar scores.

The Duration of Oligoamnios Is Also a Prognostic Factor

Patients who present with idiopathic oligoamnios at an earlier gestational age have a higher risk of adverse perinatal outcomes compared to those who present later in gestation. Still undetermined and possibly of clinical importance is the infrequent documentation of a full fetal bladder in the presence of oligoamnios [11].

The presence of an oligoamnios with intact membranes warrants detailed evaluation to detect possible fetal and placental abnormalities, IUGR, or aneuploidy.

Idiopathic oligoamnios may be associated with alterations in cell organization and immune function as well as increased activity of the vesicular transport pathways through the amnion [12].

In a meta-analysis carried out by Rabie et al. [13], the results showed an increase in the adverse effects with oligoamnios in low-risk pregnancies (admission to the NICU, cesarean delivery due to fetal distress, and meconium aspiration), but did not provide enough data to determine the optimal moment of delivery in such cases.

First trimester: The etiology of first trimester oligohydramnios is often unclear.

Reduction of amniotic fluid before 10 weeks' gestation is rare because fluid from the gestational sac is derived primarily from the fetal surface of the placenta, trans-amniotic flow from the maternal compartment, and secretions from the surface of the embryo's body.

At the beginning of the *second trimester*, fetal urine begins to enter the amniotic sac, and the fetus begins to swallow amniotic fluid. Therefore, disorders related to the fetal urinary/renal system begin to play a prominent role in the etiology of oligohydramnios. These abnormalities include intrinsic kidney disorders (cystic kidney disease) and obstructive lesions of the lower urinary tract (posterior urethral valves, urethral atresia, prune belly syndrome). Maternal and placental factors, as well as ruptured fetal membranes, are also common causes of oligohydramnios in the second trimester [28].

Third trimester: Oligohydramnios first diagnosed in the third trimester is often associated with PPROM or uteroplacental insufficiency due to conditions such as preeclampsia or other maternal vascular diseases. Oligohydramnios frequently accompany fetal growth restriction related to uteroplacental insufficiency.

Fetal abnormalities and placental abruption also play a role in this gestational age.

The volume of amniotic fluid normally decreases after delivery, so oligohydramnios can develop in these pregnancies.

Also, many cases of third trimester oligohydramnios are idiopathic.

If the diagnosis of isolated oligoamnios is given at the pregnancy term, it may be an indication to terminate the gestation. A meta-analysis carried out by Shrem et al. found that patients had significantly higher rates of labor induction (OR 7.56, IC 4.58–12.48) and cesarean sections (OR 2.07, IC 1.78–2.42). The newborn had Apgar score rates below 7, both at 1 minute and at 5 minutes (OR1.53, IC 1.03–2.26 and OR 2.01, IC 1.3–3.09, respectively); also had more chances of being in neonatal intensive care unit (OR 1.47, IC 1.17–1.84) [14].

Prenatal Care

The pregnancy-specific complications associated with oligoamnios are managed as appropriate for the condition.

In a systematic review and meta-analysis carried out by Morris et al. [15], they showed an association of oligoamnios and neonatal (total OR 8.72, 95% CI 2.43–31.26) and perinatal mortality in high-risk pregnancies (total OR 11.54, 95% CI 4.05–32.90).

Considerations in the Oligoamnios for the Calculation of Fetal Weight

With the evidence that we have at the moment, oligoamnios does not seem to impact the calculation of fetal weight in fetuses of gestational age at the limit of viability [16].

Strategies to Increase the Volume of Amniotic Fluid

Maternal hydration (MH) In cases of isolated oligoamnios (OA) in which delivery is not indicated, oral hydration with one or two liters of water may temporarily increase the volume of amniotic fluid and may have some benefit, especially in dehydration patients. This approach is easier and safer than intravenous fluid administration.

Hydration with water appears to reduce maternal plasma osmolarity and sodium concentration, resulting in osmotically driven maternal-fetal water flow.

In a meta-analysis carried out by Gizzo et al. [17], they conclude that while other studies should be conducted to reach more robust conclusions, the available data suggests that MH may be a safe, well-tolerated, and useful strategy for improving LA volume, especially in cases of OA. Oral hydration is preferred as it appears to be more effective and potentially more feasible, avoiding invasion and the need for hospitalization of parenteral hydration and potentially increasing adherence to treatment. Hypotonic solutions should be preferred to isotonic solutions and administered in low doses (around 1500 ml per day) for long periods (ideally for 2 weeks).

Sildenafil Its use in isolated oligoamnios seems promising. Maher et al. conducted a randomized controlled study of sildenafil and hydration vs parenteral hydration alone. Follow-up was completed in 166 patients (90%): 82 in the sildenafil group and 84 in the hydration group. LA volume was higher in the sildenafil group in the final evaluation (11.5 compared to 5.4 cm, $P = 0.02$). Deliveries in the sildenafil group were at higher EG (38.3 compared to 36.0 weeks gestation, $P = 0.001$) and had a lower cesarean section rate (28% compared to 73%), and neonates were less likely to be admitted to the neonatal intensive care unit (11% compared to 41%, $P = 0.001$) [18].

Ins-3 polyunsaturated fatty acids There is a line of research with very promising results in a randomized controlled study with improvements at the fourth week [19].

Amnioinfusion

Transcervical route in chorioamnionitis. Although there were no major maternal complications, the studies are still small to obtain sufficient evidence for clinical use outside of research protocols [20].

Premature rupture of membranes. In a Cochrane review [21] using either of the two types of amnioinfusion, both abdominal and transcervical versus control, favorable results were observed in the reduction of fetal distress, death, and neonatal morbidity without unfavorable impact on maternal health. RR 0.30 (95% CI 0.14–0.66), there was a 70 percent reduction with respect to neonatal death.

Recommendations

- Maternal history and physical examination and a comprehensive ultrasound evaluation for all pregnancies with oligohydramnios.
- The use of additional tests (e.g., karyotype, dye instillation, evidence of an infection-related etiology) depends on individual clinical circumstances.
- There is no effective long-term treatment for oligohydramnios.
- In idiopathic oligohydramnios, maternal treatment such as oral hydration or amnioinfusion may lead to short-term improvement. These procedures can be useful under certain circumstances, such as facilitating diagnostic ultrasound evaluation, when the fetal anatomical study is suboptimal.
- The reduction of amniotic fluid in the first trimester seems to be a sinister finding. We advise these patients regarding poor prognosis, discuss the signs of miscarriage, and follow the pregnancy with serial ultrasound examinations to determine its course.
- The prognosis and management of second trimester oligohydramnios depend on the underlying etiology and severity of oligohydramnios.

Also known as hydramnios, it is defined as the excessive volume of amniotic fluid, or 8 or 10 cm MBV, in advanced pregnancies. It complicates approximately 0.5–1% of all pregnancies.

The prognosis depends on the cause. When the diagnosis is made, careful evaluation of the fetal anatomy is required.

Polyhydramnios

Any condition that results in a relative increase in daily fetal urine output or a decrease in fetal swallowing can result in a marked increase in amniotic fluid volume Fig. 39.6.

At the end of pregnancy, the main sources of amniotic fluid production are fetal urination and pulmonary fluid secretion.

The most frequent cause is idiopathic.

Among the fetal causes we can find:

1. Pathologies of the central nervous system (26%, swallowing would be altered by central disorder)
2. Gastrointestinal (39%)
3. Heart failure (22%)
4. Some respiratory malformations such as cystic adenomatous malformation or laryngeal atresia (CHAOS)
5. Twin-to-twin transfusion syndrome (TTTS)

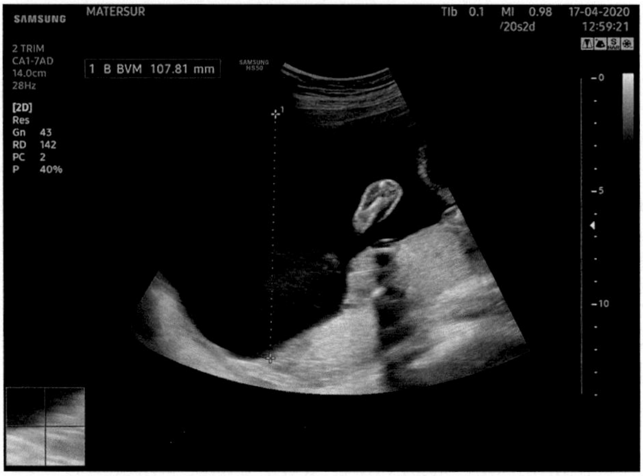

Fig. 39.6 Polyhydramnios

6. Fetal structural anomaly/anomalies
7. Fetal chromosomal abnormality (e.g., trisomy 18)
8. A high state of fetal cardiac output (e.g., any condition that causes anemia)
9. Fetal infection (e.g., parvovirus)
10. Fetal Bartter syndrome

Maternal Causes

Drug abuse (due to depression of the central nervous system with decreased swallowing of the amniotic fluid and alteration of the production-reabsorption cycle)

1. Metabolic diseases (DBT the most frequent)
2. Abundant intake of xanthines (coffee, tea, etc.)
3. Polydipsia
4. Maternal infections (TORCH)

In a series of 272 singleton pregnancies with polyhydramnios, approximately one third found a congenital abnormality, and a quarter was associated with maternal diabetes; the remaining 40 percent were considered idiopathic. After birth, an abnormality is diagnosed in up to 25 percent of prenatally idiopathic cases [22].

Fetal anemia, Bartter syndrome, infection, and neuromuscular disorders represent some cases considered prenatally idiopathic and should be considered in the differential diagnosis if structural abnormality and maternal diabetes are excluded, although Bartter syndrome and neuromuscular diseases are quite rare and infection (TORCH, parvovirus) is rarely associated with isolated polyhydramnios.

Abnormalities of the central nervous system, gastrointestinal tract, and skeletal muscle system should always be ruled out, mainly in the context of severe polyhydramnios.

Mild idiopathic polyhydramnios usually presents with a good perinatal result, but there is an association with macrosomia and cesarean section.

The combination of intrauterine growth restriction and polyhydramnios suggests trisomy 18. Generally more echographic markers appear in this trisomy.

Other aneuploidies have also been associated with polyhydramnios, most commonly trisomy 21, toward later gestational ages in the second trimester. Anatomical detail will be very important for the search for other markers.

Offer karyotype analysis in cases of severe polyhydramnios or if there are associated anatomic abnormalities; knowledge of the karyotype will be very important for management.

There is an increase in urine output in states of high fetal cardiac output (e.g., fetal anemia due to alloimmunization, parvovirus infection, fetomaternal hemorrhage, alpha-thalassemia, hemolysis secondary to glucose-6-phosphate dehydrogenase deficiency) or, rarely, from entities such as the Bartter syndrome fetus.

The most common prenatal type of Bartter syndrome is a rare autosomal recessive tubular disorder associated with intrauterine presentation of renal tubular hypokalemic alkalosis. As a result, the fetus develops subsequent polyuria and polyhydramnios between 24 and 30 weeks of gestation.

Infants exhibit postnatal polyuria and persistent loss of kidney salt, requiring lifelong treatment. A severe but transient form of prenatal Bartter syndrome has been attributed to mutations in MAGED2, which maps to the X chromosome and appears to be essential for reabsorption of fetal kidney salt and maintenance of normal homeostasis of amniotic fluid. This X-linked disorder has a very early onset of severe polyhydramnios (median 19–20 weeks' gestation), often resulting in premature birth (median gestational age 22–34 weeks), but the signs and symptoms of renal dysfunction resolve spontaneously after delivery [23].

The mechanism of polyhydramnios in pregnancies complicated by maternal diabetes is unclear. Fetal hyperglycemia leading to polyuria is a likely etiology and is supported by observation that is often associated with high levels of maternal glycated hemoglobin (A1C) and fetal macrosomia.

Decreased fetal swallowing and an imbalance in the movement of water between the maternal and fetal compartments in diabetic pregnancies are other possible mechanisms.

A retrospective study that included 1545 patients with polyhydramnios found that only 8.5 percent of the cases could be attributed to diabetes and those patients had mild polyhydramnios [24].

Polyhydramnios is associated with an increased risk of various adverse pregnancy outcomes, including premature delivery, placental abruption, and macrosomia.

Clinical Importance

Many idiopathic cases resolve spontaneously, especially if they are mild. However, polyhydramnios has been associated with an increased risk of various adverse outcomes in addition to poor outcomes related to associated morphological abnormalities.

- Maternal respiratory compromise
- Preterm labor, antepartum membrane rupture (PROM), preterm labor
- Fetal malposition
- Macrosomia (which can lead to shoulder dystocia)
- Prolapse of the umbilical cord
- Detachment due to rupture of membranes
- Second longest stage of labor
- Postpartum uterine atony

These complications increase the risk of cesarean delivery and admission to neonatal intensive care.

Although preterm labor and PROM can lead to spontaneous preterm delivery, preterm delivery in affected pregnancies is also caused by an iatrogenic intervention for the management of pregnancy complications.

The risk of stillbirth in non-abnormal pregnancies affected by polyhydramnios increases five and a half times more, compared to pregnancies with normal amniotic fluid at each gestational age, with the highest increase at term (adjusted odds ratio 5.5, 95% CI 4.1–7.6) [25].

The combination of a small fetus for gestational age and polyhydramnios has a particularly poor prognosis (including perinatal death) due to the high prevalence of fetal chromosome and structural abnormalities in this setting. In a study by Gezer et al., they found that the myocardial performance index appeared to be significantly higher in polyhydramnion fetuses compared to controls and was an early indicator of adverse perinatal outcomes in pregnancies complicated by idiopathic polyhydramnios [26].

Management options in the polyhydramnios patient depend on the underlying cause. Faced with severe polyhydramnios or symptoms of preterm delivery with a fetus that does not present a fetal abnormality incompatible with life, performing an amniodrainage (amnioreduction) reduces maternal discomfort and decreases the frequency of preterm delivery.

Ballantyne syndrome (mirror syndrome). It is characterized by the association of fetal hydrops, placental edema, and maternal edema. It is a rare condition that can appear in a polyhydramnios accompanying the hydrops. The maternal compartment reacts in a "mirror" to the hydrops of the fetus, causing severe edema, hypertension, anemia, sudden weight gain, dyspnea, and, in more severe conditions, headaches and platelets.

Management of Pregnancy with Polyhydramnios

Management of idiopathic polyhydramnios depends on gestational age, severity, presence of symptoms, and cause.

Antepartum fetal monitoring: No randomized trial has evaluated whether pregnancies complicated by idiopathic polyhydramnios benefit from any method of prenatal surveillance.

In mild to moderate polyhydramnios, we performed a stress-free test (NST) at diagnosis and then every 1–2 weeks until 37 weeks and then weekly from 37 weeks to delivery.

Procedures to reduce the volume of amniotic fluid:

Amnioreduction

There is no consensus on how much fluid to remove, how quickly to remove it, on the use of tocolytic medications, or the use of antibiotics during amnioreduction.

A common technique is to clean the site with a surgical scrub and then administer local anesthesia to the skin and subcuticular tissues.

Under continuous ultrasound guidance to minimize fetal contact, an 18 gauge needle is inserted with the tip pointed into the fluid. A hard-walled arterial line tube is attached to the needle with a three-way stopcock and connected to a vacuum suction bottle. Liquid can be sucked directly into the container or alternatively withdrawn with a 50 ml syringe under controlled suction, but this can be tedious when there is a lot of liquid. A reasonable guideline is to flush no more than 2–2.5 liters at a time and flush fluid no faster than 1000 ml for 20 minutes, although rates of 100–125 ml/min have been reported.

The procedure ends when the MBV is less than 8 cm or when the intra-amniotic pressure is less than 20 mmHg. Sometimes the procedure will need to be ended prematurely due to patient discomfort, a blocked needle, or separation of the membrane. We do not use antibiotic prophylaxis, and we initiate tocolytic drugs only if greater contractions occur.

Indometacina

Los metaanálisis de la terapia de indometacina para el parto prematuro están asociados con un riesgo mayor de morbilidades neonatales, hemorragia intraventricular incluida, leucomalacia periventricular y enterocolitis necrotizante. Por las complicaciones neonatales reportadas, y en ausencia de datos sobre mejores resultados maternos o neonatales, se recomienda el uso de la indometacina con el único propósito de disminuir el líquido amniótico en el contexto de un polihidramnios [27].

Delivery Management

During labor, we check the fetal position frequently to confirm maintenance of vertex presentation due to the possibility of conversion to breech presentation or transverse situation.

Spontaneous rupture of the membranes can cause sudden severe uterine decompression with risk of prolapse or cord shedding.

Controlled amniotomy is performed using a small-gauge needle to pierce the fetal membranes at one or more locations in an operating room with continuous FCF monitoring.

Figure 39.5 provides a summary of recommendations and the degree of evidence from the Society for Maternal-Fetal Medicine.

Recommendation	Grade
The polyhydramnios in singleton pregnancies be defined as either a DUP of >= 8 cm or an amniotic fluid index of >= 24cm.	2C Week Recommendation Low quality evidence
The amnioreduction be considered only for the induction of severe maternal dosconfort dysnea, or both in the setting of severe polyhydramnios.	1C Strong Recommendation Low quality evidence
Indometacin shoud not be used for the sole purpose of decresing amniotic fluid in the setting of polyhydramnios.	1B Strong Recommendation Moderate quality evidence.
Antenatal fetal surveillance is not required for the sole indication of mild idiopathic polyhydramnios.	2C Weak Recommendation Low quality evidence
Labor should be allowed to occur spontaneously at term for women with mild idiopathic polyhydramnios, that induction if planned should not occur at < 39 weeks of gestation in the absence of other indications, and that mode of delivery should be determined based on usual obstetric indications.	1C Stron recommendations Low qua lity evidence.
The women severe polyhydramnios deliver at a tertiary center due to the significant possibility that fetal anomalies may be present.	1C Stron Recommendation Low quality evidence

Fig. 39.7 Summary of recommendations. Made by the authors of the chapter. Adapted from SMMF 27

Summary and Recommendations

- If there is a subjective impression of polyhydramnios, we suggest that an objective measurement be made, such as an amniotic fluid index. We use a single bag deeper than ≥8 cm.
- Objective indices are standardized and provide a measurement that can be followed in serial examinations, despite sensitivity and positive predictive value (PPV) being suboptimal.
- Comprehensive ultrasound evaluation to determine if there are fetal abnormalities or hydrops fetalis.
- The outcome of pregnancies complicated by polyhydramnios varies depending on the severity and underlying etiology of excess fluid accumulation. Possible complications include maternal respiratory compromise, premature delivery, premature rupture of the membranes (PROM), fetal malposition, and prolapse of the umbilical cord and/or postpartum uterine atony.
- Offer karyotype analysis in cases of severe polyhydramnios or if there are associated anatomic abnormalities, if knowledge of the karyotype will affect management.

Biochemical analyses of amniotic fluid can aid in the diagnosis of esophageal atresia and Bartter syndrome.

- Treatment of polyhydramnios in single pregnancies only if there is premature delivery or significant maternal discomfort (Grade 2C). The therapeutic option is determined by gestational age and the degree of discomfort [28].

Conclusions

Amniotic fluid gives us important maternal-fetal information due to the factors involved in its production and in maintaining its balance.

Ultrasonography allows us to evaluate it easily, to achieve adequate perinatal management, thus avoiding adverse perinatal results.

Bibliography

1. Sadler TW. Langman's medical embryology. 13th ed. Philadelphia: Wolters Kluwer Health; 2015.
2. Zhang L, Ducsay CA, editors. Advances in fetal and neonatal physiology. In: Advances in experimental medicine and biology, Vol. 814. New York: Springer Science+Business Media; 2014. p. 49. https://doi.org/10.1007/978-1-4939-1031-1_5.
3. Callen P. Ultrasonography in Obstetrics and Ginecology, 4th edition. 2000 W. B. Saunders Company. Trad. Ed. Medica Panamericana.

4. H. Madar, S. Brun, F. Coatleven, P. Chabanier, H. Gomer, A. Nithart, M.A. Coustel, B. Merlot, J. Horovitz, D. Dallay. Mahieu-Caputo† D, Sentilhes L. Fisiología y regulación del Líquido Amniótico. EMC-Ginecología-Obstetricia. 2016;52(4):1–10. https://doi.org/10.1016/S1283-081X(16)80903-0.
5. Gilbert WM, et al. Amniotic fluid dynamics. Fetal Med Rev. 1991;3:89.
6. Sandlin AT, Ounpraseuth ST, Spencer HJ, Sick CL, Lang PM, Magann EF. Amniotic fluid volume in normal singleton pregnancies: modeling with quantile regression. Arch Gynecol Obstet. 2014;289(5):967–72. https://doi.org/10.1007/s00404-013-3087-2.
7. Phelan JP, Ahn MO, Smith CV, Rutherford SE, Anderson E. Amniotic fluid index measurements during pregnancy. J Reprod Med. 1987;32(8):601–4.
8. Kehl S, Schelkle A, Thomas A, et al. Single deepest vertical pocket or amniotic fluid index as evaluation test for predicting adverse pregnancy outcome (SAFE trial): a multicenter, open-label, randomized controlled trial. Ultrasound Obstet Gynecol. 2016;47(6):674–9. https://doi.org/10.1002/uog.14924.
9. Nabhan AF, Abdelmoula YA. Amniotic fluid index versus single deepest vertical pocket as a screening test for preventing adverse pregnancy outcome. Cochrane Database Syst Rev. 2008;(3). Art. No.: CD006593. https://doi.org/10.1002/14651858.CD006593.pub2.
10. Sekhon S, Rosenbloom JI, Doering M, et al. Diagnostic utility of maximum vertical pocket versus amniotic fluid index in assessing amniotic fluid volume for the prediction of adverse maternal and fetal outcomes: a systematic review and meta-analysis [published online ahead of print, 2019]. J Matern Fetal Neonatal Med. 2019:1–10. https://doi.org/10.1080/14767058.2019.1691988.
11. Sherer DM. A review of amniotic fluid dynamics and the enigma of isolated oligohydramnios. Am J Perinatol. 2002;19(5):253–66. https://doi.org/10.1055/s-2002-33084.
12. Cheung CY, Brace RA. Altered proteomics profile in the amnion of patients with oligohydramnios. Physiol Rep. 2020;8(4):e14381. https://doi.org/10.14814/phy2.14381.
13. Rabie N, Magann E, Steelman S, Ounpraseuth S. Oligohydramnios in complicated and uncomplicated pregnancy: a systematic review and meta-analysis. Ultrasound Obstet Gynecol. 2017;49(4):442–9. https://doi.org/10.1002/uog.15929.
14. Shrem G, Nagawkar SS, Hallak M, Walfisch A. Isolated oligohydramnios at term as an indication for labor induction: a systematic review and Meta-analysis. Fetal Diagn Ther. 2016;40(3):161–73. https://doi.org/10.1159/000445948.
15. Morris RK, Meller CH, Tamblyn J, Malin GM, Riley RD, Kilby MD, Robson SC, Khan KS. Association and prediction of amniotic fluid measurements for adverse pregnancy outcome: systematic review and meta-analysis. BJOG. 2014;121:686–99.
16. Huber C, Zdanowicz JA, Mueller M, Surbek D. Factors influencing the accuracy of fetal weight estimation with a focus on preterm birth at the limit of viability: a systematic literature review. Fetal Diagn Ther. 2014;36(1):1–8. https://doi.org/10.1159/000358518.
17. Gizzo S, Noventa M, Vitagliano A, et al. An update on maternal hydration strategies for amniotic fluid improvement in isolated oligohydramnios and normohydramnios: evidence from a systematic review of literature and meta-analysis. PLoS One. 2015;10(12):e0144334. Published 2015 Dec 11. https://doi.org/10.1371/journal.pone.0144334.
18. Maher MA, Sayyed TM, Elkhouly N. Sildenafil citrate therapy for oligohydramnios: a randomized controlled trial. Obstet Gynecol. 2017;129(4):615–20. https://doi.org/10.1097/AOG.0000000000001928.
19. Ismail AM, Ramadan MF, Ali MK, Abbas AM, El Saman AM, Makarem MH. A randomized controlled study of the efficacy of 4 weeks of supplementation with ω-3 polyunsaturated fatty acids in cases of unexplained oligohydramnios. J Perinatol. 2016;36(11):944–7. https://doi.org/10.1038/jp.2016.134.
20. Hofmeyr GJ, Kiiza JAK. Amnioinfusion for chorioamnionitis. Cochrane Database Syst Rev. 2016;(8). Art. No.:CD011622. https://doi.org/10.1002/14651858.CD011622.pub2.

21. Hofmeyr GJ, Eke AC, Lawrie TA. Amnioinfusion for third trimester preterm premature rupture of membranes. Cochrane Database Syst Rev. 2014;(3). Art. No.: CD000942. https://doi.org/10.1002/14651858.CD000942.pub3.
22. Abele H, Starz S, Hoopmann M, et al. Idiopathic polyhydramnios and postnatal abnormalities. Fetal Diagn Ther. 2012;32:251.
23. Laghmani K, Beck BB, Yang SS, et al. Polyhydramnios, transient antenatal Bartter's syndrome, and MAGED2 mutations. N Engl J Med. 2016;374:1853.
24. Moore LE. Amount of polyhydramnios attributable to diabetes may be less than previously reported. World J Diabetes. 2017;8:7.
25. Pilliod RA, Page JM, Burwick RM, et al. The risk of fetal death in nonanomalous pregnancies affected by polyhydramnios. Am J Obstet Gynecol. 2015;213:410.e1.
26. Gezer C, Ekin A, Ozeren M, et al. Can the myocardial performance index be used as a new predictive factor for a poor prognosis in fetuses with idiopathic polyhydramnios? J Ultrasound Med. 2016;35:2649.
27. Society for Maternal-Fetal Medicine (SMFM). Electronic address: pubs@smfm.org, Dashe JS, Pressman EK, Hibbard JU. SMFM consult series #46: evaluation and management of polyhydramnios. Am J Obstet Gynecol. 2018;219(4):B2–B8. https://doi.org/10.1016/j.ajog.2018.07.016.
28. Ron Beloosesky, MD y col This topic last updated: Mar 20, 2019.

Chapter 40
Preeclampsia

Liliana Susana Voto and Moises Gabriel Zeitune

Physiopathology

Various genetic, angiogenic, structural, and metabolic pathways have been implicated in the pathogenesis of preeclampsia, including spiral artery remodeling, placental oxygenation, redox and immune tolerance at the maternal-fetal interface, and the balance of angiogenic and antiangiogenic factors.

The pathophysiological alterations characteristic of preeclampsia are manifested both at a local level (defective placentation and reduced placental perfusion) and at a systemic level (angiogenic imbalance and vascular endothelium dysfunction). These changes raise endothelial sensitivity to vasopressor substances, platelet activity, and thrombogenesis.

Reduced placental perfusion enhances oxidative stress, and anomalous fetal and maternal vascular endothelium leads to vasodilator prostacyclin deficiency. The increase of oxidative stress and prostacyclin and nitric oxide deficit results in vascular endothelium dysfunction, impairing other organs such as the placenta, kidneys, liver, pancreas, lung, brain, and the hematopoietic system. Thus, the different clinical signs of preeclampsia stem from the dysfunction of all these organs, and hypertension would, therefore, be the homeostatic response of the fetoplacental unit to these alterations and should then be considered a consequence rather than a cause of the disease.

L. S. Voto (✉) · M. G. Zeitune
Maternal and Childbirth Department, Hospital General de Agudos Dr. Juan A. Fernández, School of Medicine, University of Buenos Aires, Buenos Aires, Argentina
e-mail: lvoto@intramed.net

© Springer Nature Switzerland AG 2022

R. A. Moreira de Sá, E. B. d. Fonseca (eds.), *Perinatology*,
https://doi.org/10.1007/978-3-030-83434-0_40

Defective Placentation and Reduced Placental Perfusion

Preeclampsia is thought to originate in the placenta, and two facts support the hypothesis of a central involvement of placenta in the pathogenesis of preeclampsia: (1) the only definitive cure for preeclampsia is delivery of the placenta, and (2) women who experience a hydatidiform molar pregnancy – in which a placenta develops without a fetus – frequently develop severe preeclampsia [1].

Another unique characteristic of the disease is that preeclampsia is a human disease and is not present in other species. The reason for this selectivity is thought to be the unique ratio of the brain and bodyweight of the human fetus, which requires 60% of nutritional exchange from the mother in the third trimester in comparison with only 20% of nutritional exchange in other animals. Thus, normal placentation is the result of the structural and functional adaptations of the maternal vessels to accommodate the requisite blood flow to the developing fetus [1–3].

The radial arteries of the uterus divide into two or more branches, which either terminate in the myometrium or decidua (basal arteries) or open into the intervillous space (spiral arteries). In normal pregnant women, vasodilation of the spiral arteries can be up to four times their usual gauge, which reduces their peripheral resistance and favors intervillous space perfusion [2–4]. This is due to the trophoblastic invasion of the spiral arteries in early pregnancy and ends at 20–21 weeks' gestation, destroying the vascular musculoelastic layer and the continuity of the endothelial lining, thus preventing the action of vasopressor agents. Transformation of the spiral arteries from small muscular arteries to large tortuous vessels is hypothesized to be required to accommodate the enormous blood flow requirements of the placenta and to override the vasomotor control of the maternal arteries [2–4].

In contrast, in preeclampsia, *the second trophoblastic migration does not take place*; therefore, the musculoelastic layer remains intact, reducing the gauge of blood vessels and giving rise to atheromatous plaques due to decreased blood flow. The superficial invasion of the decidua results in narrow and undilated proximal segments of the spiral arteries, which ultimately leads to uterine hypoperfusion and higher-than-normal velocity of blood flow to the intervillous space [1–4].

Endothelial Dysfunction

As stated early in the 1970s by Gant [5], preeclamptic pregnant women develop vascular sensitivity to angiotensin II. His studies demonstrated that in these patients, the balance between prostacyclin (vasodilator) and thromboxane A2 (TXA2) (vasoconstrictor) is lost in favor of TXA2. As a result, blood pressure increases, and the coagulation chain is activated [5, 6]. This responsiveness may be augmented by circulating sFLT1 [7, 8]. Increased responsiveness to vasopressors has now been shown to continue postpartum, with women with a history of hypertensive pregnancy showing increased blood pressure, aldosterone levels, and sFLT1 levels in response to these agents [1, 6].

Preeclampsia is a truly endothelial disorder, and among the multiple functions of the endothelium, secretion of prostaglandins, endothelins, nitric oxide, and protein C is one of the most important. When a noxa causes endothelial damage, anticoagulant and vasodilator substance production decreases. Alterations in intercellular unions and in the water and protein transport expel these elements outside the cells. Endothelin 1 levels – a vasoactive peptide released from the vascular endothelium that serves as a regulator of blood pressure and vascular tone by promoting vasoconstriction – have been shown to be more elevated in preeclamptic than in normal pregnant women, whereas prostacyclin and nitric oxide, the most important vasodilating and anti-aggregating factors, are markedly reduced [1, 7, 8]. We might then conclude that there is an inadequate expansion in plasma volume, an increased sensitivity to angiotensin II, a ruptured prostacyclin/thromboxane balance, and an untimely activation of the coagulation mechanism, leading to a decreased multiorgan perfusion.

As described above, the paths to hypertension in pregnancy lead to endothelial dysfunction. The alterations found in the plasminogen activator and in the equilibrium between the plasminogen activator and the inhibiting function of the prostacyclin/ thromboxane balance lead to an increase in the platelet aggregation and vasoconstriction. These morphological and functional changes in endothelial cells would be responsible for triggering a clinical syndrome characterized by arterial vasospasm, increased platelet aggregation, and capillary permeability, expressed clinically as hypertension, edema, proteinuria, and, sometimes, thrombocytopenia and organic hypoperfusion [1, 6–8].

It has been suggested that abnormal endothelial function – as evidenced by reduced vasodilation, decreased circulating NO, and increased cholesterol levels – may precede pregnancy in women who later develop preeclampsia. This hypothesis is supported by the fact that such endothelial dysfunction is also present in women with recurrent miscarriage, who have an increased risk of future cardiovascular disease despite an absence of hypertension and end-organ damage that is seen in preeclampsia [1, 7, 8]. Thus, endothelial dysfunction before pregnancy may be a common link between conditions with defective placentation and cardiovascular disease.

Therefore, pregnancy-induced hypertension is likely to be caused by an abnormal trophoblastic invasion which leads to decreased uteroplacental blood flow, placental ischemia, placental release of cytokines, endothelial dysfunction due to an increase in endothelin 1 and thromboxane A2 (two potent vasoconstrictors), a reduction in prostacyclin and NO levels (two powerful vasodilators), and a rise in vascular sensitivity to angiotensin II.

Immunological Maladaptation of the Fetal Graft

There exists a consensus that the immunological maladaptation – lack of immunological tolerance that is required at the maternal-placental interface – of the fetal graft plays a major role in the defective placentation that gives rise to placental ischemia. This ischemia can be caused by several factors, the most important of which are (a) immunological maladaptation, (b) genetic predisposition, and (c) vascular mediators.

Epidemiologic findings seem to confirm the presence of a maladaptation syndrome [1]:

- Preeclampsia is more frequent in primigravidas, but less frequent in subsequent gestations if pregnant by the same husband.
- Women with a history of abortion and blood transfusions are at a lower risk of preeclampsia.
- There is an inverse relationship between the length of cohabitation and the incidence of preeclampsia.
- Women who use barrier contraceptive methods are twice as likely to develop preeclampsia compared with those who do not.
- The incidence of preeclampsia is higher in women who have conceived with donor semen.

Normal fetal trophoblast cells express HLA-C molecules, which interact with killer Ig-like receptors (KIRs) expressed on maternal uterine natural killer cells. HLA-C is inherited from both the mother and the father, and certain groups of HLA-C molecules, as well as certain haplotypes of KIRs, seem to be more frequently expressed in preeclamptic pregnancies than in normal pregnancies [9]. Normal placentation requires allorecognition by maternal KIRs of paternal HLA-C63, and the maladaptation syndrome could be related to reduced paternal antigen exposure [10].

Normal placentation is also characterized by a characteristic profile of T cells and their respective cytokines. Preeclampsia is characterized by an imbalance in the T cell profile, with a predominance of T helper 1 cells and their associated cytokines such as IFNγ and TNF67. This imbalance likely contributes to poor placentation and the ensuing maternal inflammation and endothelial dysfunction [10, 11].

Complement activation has been implicated in pathological pregnancies such as preeclampsia and intrauterine fetal growth restriction [1, 11, 12]. Women with Bb complement activation fragment levels in the top decile were four times more likely to develop preeclampsia than those with lower levels, whereas complement dysregulation also occurs in atypical hemolytic uremic syndrome, thrombotic microangiopathy (TMA) with histological similarities to severe preeclampsia, and HELLP syndrome [11, 12].

In normal pregnancies, 40% of all decidual lymphocytes are CD56+ uterine natural killer cells, 60% are CD3+ T-lymphocytes, and about 30% are CD8+ T cells. In contrast, in preeclamptic pregnancies plus intrauterine growth retardation (IUGR), there is a higher proportion of CD56+ uterine natural killer cells and CD8+ T lymphocytes in the decidua (70% of all CD3+ cells). In pregnancies without IUGR, no increase in CD56+ uterine natural killer cells has been observed, while CD8+ T lymphocytes have been found to be significantly elevated compared with the normal level (50% of all CD3+ cells) [11, 12].

Placental ischemia and the activation of polynuclear neutrophils appear to be the last and most severe consequences of the altered maternal immune response, which in turn activates a chain of events ending up in endothelial damage and dysfunction and in typical preeclamptic symptomatology.

Genetic Predisposition

Some families have a strong history of preeclampsia, and having a family history of preeclampsia significantly increases an individual woman's risk of preeclampsia by between 24% and 163% [1, 13]. Population studies of families reveal clear transmission of preeclampsia across generations; however, the exact inheritance pattern is unknown [13, 14]. The tendency to develop preeclampsia can be affected by genetic variations carried by the parents and genetic variations carried by the unborn child. Immune maladaptation, inadequate placentation, oxidative stress, and thrombosis are all influenced by genetic factors.

To date, numerous genetic studies, using both the candidate gene and genome-wide approach, have been undertaken to tease out the genetic basis of preeclampsia, to find potential markers of the disease and understand its origins. Such studies have identified some promising candidate genes as markers of early detection: the untargeted cellular mRNA signature was consistently increased in early preeclampsia after 22 weeks of gestation, and individual mRNAs of this signature were significantly increased as early as 11–17 weeks of gestation. Several single-cell placental signatures predicted future development of the disease at 11–17 weeks and were also increased in women already diagnosed at 32–34 weeks of gestation [15]. It has been also proposed that gene-specific hypomethylation may be a common phenomenon in early-onset preeclampsia placentas and that TIMP3 promoter could serve as a potential prenatal diagnostic marker for early-onset preeclampsia [16].

Although the exact cause is still unknown, epigenetic features are implicated in the pathogenesis of preeclampsia. Mutations in STOX1 were identified in some unique familial cases of preeclampsia with apparent maternal-only transmission of susceptibility. Epigenetic alterations of non-imprinted genes have also been suggested to be involved. For example, the SERPINA3 promoter was found to be hypomethylated in preeclampsia-associated placenta, suggesting that the epigenetic alteration of this gene may be associated with reduced trophoblastic invasion and implicating this change as a potential biomarker for preeclampsia. A recent systematic review describing the differences between normal and preeclampsia placental gene expression by using mRNA microarrays identified a subset of genes that are downregulated in preeclampsia placenta only and further identified the expression of another 88 genes that were highly associated with preeclampsia [17].

Researchers are studying whether variations in genes involved in fluid balance, the functioning of the vascular endothelium, or placental development affect the risk of developing preeclampsia or its severity. Additional genes with no known function in pregnancy have also been associated with preeclampsia risk [18]. Nevertheless, research faces challenges of replicating these genetic associations in different populations and performing the functional validation of identified genetic variants to determine their causality in preeclampsia.

Vasopressor Substances

Normal pregnancy is associated with a rise in plasma renin activity and concentration, renin substrate, and angiotensin II, and in normal gestations, angiotensin stimulates prostacyclin production through the walls of the uterine and systemic arterial blood vessels. In contrast, preeclampsia is responsible for the suppression of the renin-angiotensin system. Preeclampsia would, therefore, suggest a defective production of angiotensin II: Ito et al. [19] demonstrated that angiotensin-converting enzyme (ACE) is present mainly in venous endothelial cells of placental villous stem cells and that ACE activity, ACE protein expression, and ACE mRNA expression are higher in preeclamptic placentas than in normal pregnancy. Furthermore, they also found that, in vitro, hypoxia promotes the expression of ACE mRNA and its activity in endothelial vein cells. Consequently, venous endothelial cells in the placenta and the umbilical vein would play a major role in the regulation of the fetoplacental renin-angiotensin system, and, in hypoxic conditions such as preeclampsia, the fetus can induce placental ACE activity. Thus, the hypertension that occurs in preeclampsia does not seem to be mediated through the renin-angiotensin-aldosterone system (RAAS) as the levels of renin, aldosterone, and angiotensin II are reduced in affected pregnancies compared with their physiological increases in normal pregnancy [19]. Rather, this hypertension might be mediated via antiangiogenic factors and agonistic autoantibodies that bind to the angiotensin II type 1 receptor (AT1-AAs). The administration of these autoantibodies into pregnant mice induces hypertension, proteinuria, and glomerular endotheliosis. Levels of AT1-AAs do not fully regress postpartum and may contribute to the increased cardiovascular risk that is seen in women with a history of preeclampsia [20–22].

Another important mediator of endothelial dysfunction in preeclampsia is the potent vasodilator and antioxidant NO, which has been shown to mediate the effects of PlGF and VEGF. Circulating levels of NO are reduced in women with preeclampsia. Polymorphisms and changes in the expression of eNOS have also been implicated in preeclamptic pregnancies [23, 24].

Endothelin 1 (ET1) is a potent vasoconstrictor, and ET1 levels are elevated in women with preeclampsia, whereas ET1 production has been shown to mediate the hypertension that is caused by sFLT1 and AT1-AAs [25].

The hydrogen sulfide (H2S) system is another key mechanistic pathway in vasodilation and angiogenesis. Decreased circulating levels of H2S have been demonstrated in women with preeclampsia, as has reduced placental expression of cystathionine γ-lyase, the enzyme that is responsible for H2S production [26]. The effects of H2S in pregnancy may be mediated through VEGF, as administration of the H2S donor sodium hydrosulfide (NaHS) to sFLT1-overexpressing rats attenuated hypertension, proteinuria, and glomerular endotheliosis [27].

Hypoxia

Despite relative hypoxia, energy demands throughout gestation are uncompromised, and low oxygen tension triggers cytotrophoblast proliferation via mechanisms involving the transcription factor hypoxia-inducible factor 1α (HIF1α). HIF1α and HIF2α are the products of a common oxygen-sensing pathway. They regulate the expression of hypoxia-induced genes including erythropoietin, vascular endothelial growth factor (VEGF), and nitric oxide (NO) synthase [28]. Expression of HIF1α in human placentae is increased in the first trimester and decreases at around 9 weeks when circulation and thus oxygenation to the fetus increase [29]. Persistently elevated HIF1α levels may indicate placental stress and precedes the development of preeclampsia. Indeed, preeclamptic placentae have been shown to overexpress HIF1α and HIF2α and fail to downregulate their expression upon oxygenation [29]. Furthermore, overexpression of HIF1α is associated with elevated levels of antiangiogenic factors such as soluble FLT1 (sFLT1; also known as sVEGFR1) and soluble endoglin (sENG)43. Hypoxia-induced increases in the level of sFLT1 were demonstrated in both in vitro and in vivo models of placental hypoxia, including in placentae from early-first-trimester pregnancies in women living at high altitude and from women with preeclampsia [29, 30]. Thus, HIF1α seems to be a pathogenic mediator in preeclamptic pregnancies.

Oxidative Stress

Oxidative stress also occurs at the maternal-fetal interface and is thought to have a key role in normal and defective placental development. Normal regression of the peripheral villi (where placental blood flow begins) early in gestation is postulated to occur via a mechanism involving oxidative stress and apoptosis [31]. In preeclampsia, an imbalance seems to exist between antioxidant and pro-oxidant mechanisms. This imbalance may be due to the defective spiral artery remodeling that is seen in affected pregnancies, which is thought to lead to repetitive ischemia-reperfusion injuries owing to the retention of contractile segments of the spiral arteries in the myometrium [32]. The heme oxygenase (HO) pathway is an important mediator of oxidative stress. HO exists as an inducible isoform (HO1), a constitutive isoform (HO2), and an isoform with unknown function (HO3) [33]. HO1 and HO2 oxidize heme to produce biliverdin and carbon monoxide (CO). Biliverdin is converted to bilirubin, which has antioxidant effects including inhibition of LDL lipid oxidation, whereas CO is a signaling molecule with pleiotropic effects, including vasorelaxation and cardioprotection [33]. The level of HO1 protein is substantially reduced in preeclamptic placentae compared with the placentae of normotensive controls [32], and overexpression of HO1 in endothelial cells inhibited placental release of antiangiogenic factors, whereas induction of HO1 in an animal model of preeclampsia attenuated hypertension induced by placental ischemia, suggesting a role of HO1 in the downstream effects of such ischemia on the maternal endothelium [34]. Taken together, these findings support the role of the HO system as an important mediator of oxidative stress in normal pregnancy as well as a key factor in the pathogenesis of abnormal placentation in preeclampsia.

Imbalance of Angiogenic Factors

There is a consensus in considering a pathological role for an imbalance in circulating angiogenic factors in the etiology of preeclampsia. Elevated levels of the antiangiogenic factor sFLT1, which is produced in the placenta and released into the maternal circulation, induce maternal endothelial dysfunction leading to preeclamptic signs and symptoms. sFLT1 is a soluble splice variant of the membrane-bound receptor VEGFR1 that binds to the proangiogenic proteins VEGF and placental growth factor (PlGF); therefore, sFLT1 acts as a ligand trap and antagonizes ligand-mediated angiogenic signaling via the cell surface receptors. Higher maternal levels of sFLT1 are associated with more severe forms of the disease, and high plasma sFLT1/PlGF ratios are also strong predictors of disease severity and adverse clinical outcomes [35]. Together, these findings indicate that high levels of circulating sFLT1 and low levels of circulating proangiogenic factors (VEGF and PlGF) produce an antiangiogenic state that contributes to the clinical manifestations of preeclampsia [35, 36].

The antiangiogenic protein sENG, which inhibits transforming growth factor-β (TGFβ) signaling, is expressed at high levels in preeclampsia and in eclampsia. Elevated levels of both sENG and sFLT1 are also associated with more severe forms of preeclampsia. Overexpression of sFLT1 and sENG interfered with endothelial cell stability and led to the development of periventricular edema that resembled the cerebral edema that is seen in patients with eclampsia [36–38]. In addition, sENG may downregulate a TGFβ signaling pathway and further attenuate endothelial NO synthase (eNOS) activity, resulting in decreased NO availability and increased vascular permeability [38].

Pathological Anatomy of the Placenta in Preeclampsia

Pregnancy is associated with a tenfold increase in uterine blood flow, 90% of which goes to the intervillous space. Towards the end of gestation, blood flow may reach 750 ml/min. The number of spiral arteries can be predicted early in pregnancy (about 120). During the first trimester, in their adaptation to the increased blood flow, the decidual segment of spiral arteries undergoes degeneration of the internal elastic medial wall, as well as the disappearance of the smooth muscle and of elastin in the inner and outer medial tunic. A change is observed in the structure of vascular walls due to hyaline and fibrin. During the second trimester, the second adaptation phase takes place, which is characterized by intense trophoblastic invasion limited to the internal part of the medial tunic of spiral arteries. Whereas blood pressure in the radial arteries is 70–80 mmHg, in the villous spaces it is about 10 mmHg, which shows a gradient that clearly benefits the fetus. Normal morphological changes in the placental bed prevent maternal spiral vessels from responding to vasopressor agents by reducing the number of smooth muscle cells capable of responding to them.

Placentas from preeclamptic patients with acute atherosclerosis show discontinuity of endothelial cells, focal interruption of the basal membrane, platelet deposits, mural thrombosis, and fibrinoid necrosis. There are also disorderly proliferative changes in the vascular intima cells, resulting in hyperplasia of the myointimal and medial tunic smooth muscle cells, which could be caused by the mitogenic effects of platelet growth factors. The marked reduction in fetal villous cell subendothelial fibronectin is a clear indicator of extensive endothelial damage in preeclampsia. An important characteristic of acute atherosis is the extensive lipoid necrosis of smooth muscle and myointimal cells, resulting from chronic hypoxia and/or from cytotoxic action. Acute atherosis is found not only in preeclamptic primigravidas but also in the preeclamptic placentas of women with either chronic hypertension, diabetes, renal failure, or lupus, and it can lead to reduced intervillous blood flow, increased intrinsic vascular resistance, and an elevated response to vasopressor substances [1–4].

The extravillous trophoblast encompasses all the trophoblastic cells which are not in contact with the basal membrane of chorionic villi. It has two components: the interstitial trophoblast and the endovascular trophoblast. The giant multinuclear cells of the interstitial trophoblast infiltrate into the placental bed. Early in 1967 Brosens described the trophoblastic permeation of decidual and myometrial spiral arteries by extravillous trophoblast, which penetrates the spiral arteries migrating through the distal end of decidual vessels at 9 weeks' gestation and reaching myometrial vessels at 14–15 weeks' gestation [39]. Trophoblastic invasion leads to the destruction of the muscular elastic tissue and of the nervous tissue, turning the uteroplacental vasculature into a low resistance, low pressure, and high blood flow system without maternal vasomotor control. Five years later, Brosens demonstrated the absence of a physiological transformation of uteroplacental arteries in preeclampsia.

In addition, vascular lesions such as atherosis and vascular endothelial infiltration by macrophages were also early described [1–4]. In addition to atherosis, there is fibrinoid necrosis: over 60% of preeclamptic placentas show vascular atherosis mainly in decidual necrosis and infarcted areas. The endothelium is disrupted in 80% of the patients with preeclampsia, probably resulting from increased oxidative stress and production of vasoactive substances as well as from alterations in cytokine production [1–4]. The vascular bed in preeclamptic patients is characterized by a higher number of basal and spiral arteries with greater tortuosity and by a reduction in their luminal diameter. More frequently than atherosis, medial disorganization and hyperplasia in myometrial arteries are also displayed.

Clinical Aspects

Maternal Syndrome and Fetal Syndrome

In the clinical setting, we face three different situations: (a) women who have chronic hypertension and become pregnant; (b) pregnant women who present with pure gestational hypertension, without clinical or fetal impact; and (c) pregnant women with preeclampsia, *which is always a severe stage*, because it simultaneously impacts the mother and the fetus by putting both at risk. Therefore the most important challenge is to keep in mind that we have to handle two different syndromes – a maternal syndrome and a fetal syndrome – and these two syndromes often do not progress simultaneously: sometimes we can reasonably manage the disease in the mother, but we are not able to control the fetal syndrome; in other situations the fetal impact is not so severe, but the mother goes into emergency due to hypertension or, in a more complicated scenario, both the mother and the fetus being in serious trouble and we not being able to control the disease.

Another way to differentiate if preeclampsia will affect the mother's health more than that of the fetus is to identify those cases of early-onset preeclampsia (EOPE) and differentiate them from those of late-onset PE (LOPE) or late clinical manifestations. EOPE is associated with the highest rate of maternal complications both in the short and long term and with an increased risk of perinatal morbidity and mortality. Although LOPE is associated with a lower incidence of severe morbidity, its higher incidence and the fact that in a larger proportion it affects women with previous conditions, it makes their prediction no less important.

If we take into account each of these aspects, we could also say that when we face pure chronic hypertension or pure gestational hypertension with little impact on the fetus, the most important point is to manage arterial hypertension; in these cases we must manage the antihypertensive medication, and of course, we will always be monitoring the fetal health.

Preeclampsia is a disease with an endothelial impact, therefore affecting systemically both the mother and the fetus, presenting two well-differentiated syndromes: maternal syndrome which presents a raise in the arterial blood pressure levels and liver and neurological damage and the presence of HELLP syndrome, that is, a very severe endothelial impact.

On the other hand, fetal syndrome is expressed by a growth disorder and changes in fetal hemodynamics, evidenced by a restriction of intrauterine growth (IUGR), oligohydramnios, and fetal hypoxia, which could have a high impact on neonatal fetal survival.

There are several lines of ongoing research studying the causes of preeclampsia and IUGR, all of which help us to prevent or identify cases earlier. A hypothesis of why in some cases there would be more fetal involvement proposed that the degree of endothelial involvement and the presence or absence of metabolic syndrome before pregnancy would be the responsibility of the greatest maternal or fetal involvement. Also, the presence of a greater maternal involvement and the previous existence of some degree of metabolic syndrome – a composite of adiposity, insulin resistance, hyperglycemia, hyperlipidemia, and coagulopathy – would lead to a greater degree of maternal involvement during pregnancy and even later, with increased cardiovascular risk in the postpartum and after during the entire life [40]. On the contrary, the IUGR develops in the absence of prenatal metabolic syndrome, and the mother would not develop a clinically apparent disease [41].

In other series of studies, which account for a maternal pro-inflammatory profile in both patients with preeclampsia and associated IUGR, cytokines like TNF-alpha, IL-6, and IL-8 are elevated in both preeclampsia and IUGR cases [42, 43]. This pro-inflammatory profile can also be seen in psychophysical stress, in metabolic syndrome, and in systemic hypertension, making even more complex to separate risk factors. In another recently published study which evaluates the degree of systemic inflammation by assessing free fetal DNA in maternal blood, it was shown that the levels found were higher in those patients with preeclampsia compared with those who developed IUGR. The authors suggested that it is evidence that the low maternal systemic inflammation would be used to differentiate one syndrome from the other [44].

It remains to be elucidated what factors in combination lead to this maternal pro-inflammatory state: whether it is a psychological stress (affecting the hypothalamus adrenal pituitary axis, the autonomous nervous system, and the immune system), or there are associated nutritional factors that induce alterations in the maternal microbiota, which in combination with an increased intestinal permeability, would induce a low degree of intestinal and systemic inflammation. Another alternative considers that these nutritional factors, by generating obesity and increased insulinemia (pro-inflammatory conditions), would be the basis to develop preeclampsia. The importance of the uterine microbiota has been increasingly stressed and how the endometrial microbiome in periconceptional stages could be a generator of local pro-inflammatory states: the results of several studies suggest that the immune responses triggered by a pathogenic endometrial microbiota would have a direct impact on implantation, placentation, and, ultimately, on maternal and neonatal outcomes, including preeclampsia [45].

Clinical Evaluation

The peculiarity of the existence of these two syndromes that may not appear in parallel is that we could face different clinical situations: (a) a severe maternal morbidity with a medium fetal impact, (b) a very impacted fetus with a manageable maternal syndrome, (c) both the mother and the fetus in relatively good condition, or (d) both the mother and the fetus in very bad conditions.

Thus, it will be neccesary to permanently assess the risk to both the mother and the fetus, choosing between intensive or expectant behaviors, depending on the mother's risk, or when a Doppler study marks an alteration of fetus hemodynamics of 28 weeks or more of gestation with a significant risk and an imminent intrauterine death, to think to induce the elective termination of pregnancy and get a better survival within the neonatology setting. When the high risk is equal for both the mother and the fetus, elective termination of pregnancy is imposed, taking preventive measures of fetal lung maturation.

Early and Late Preeclampsia

Since the late 1970s, two different forms of presentation and evolution of the disease have been described. At present, and following the latest updated worldwide classifications, preeclampsia can be differentiated according to its onset and its pathophysiology in two different entities: early-onset preeclampsia (EOPE) – the one that develops before 34 weeks of gestation – and late-onset preeclampsia (LOPE), which develops after 34 weeks of gestation [46].

Although the presentation characteristics could overlap, EOPE and LOPE are associated with different maternal and perinatal outcomes, biochemical markers, genetics, and clinical characteristics. In the following paragraphs, we will review these differences and similarities that led us to determine what clinical conduct will be more appropriate in each case, to make a timely diagnosis, to obtain favorable perinatal results, and to implement prevention measures.

Epidemiology and Risk Factors

Worldwide, the incidence of preeclampsia ranges between 2% and 10% of pregnancies. However, the incidence varies greatly geographically: the WHO estimates the incidence of preeclampsia to be seven times higher in developing countries (2.8% of live births) than in developed countries (0.4%) [47, 48]. The incidence of eclampsia in the developed countries of North America and Europe is similar and estimated to be about 5–7 cases per 10,000 deliveries. On the other hand, the incidence of eclampsia in developing nations varies widely, ranging from 1 case per 100 pregnancies to 1 case per 1700 pregnancies [49].

Both epidemiology and risk factors differ in EOPE and LOPE: prevalence of EOPE was estimated 0.3% and LOPE was 0.6–1.5%. These figures were similar to those reported by other authors, in which both the incidence and risk factors were evaluated: prevalence was 0.38% for EOPE and 2.72% for LOPE, and the rate of presentation of EOPE was also substantially lower than that of LOPE (the different series estimated 5–20% of EOPE vs 75–80% of LOPE). Besides, gestational age also relates to the incidence, the curve of the appearance of PE rises until the end of pregnancy, with a more abrupt trend from week 34 [50].

Among the risk factors found in patients with EOPE, we can mention the history of preeclampsia, primigesta, African American race, chronic hypertension, and congenital anomalies. On the other hand, patients with diabetes, family history of preeclampsia, maternal age under 20 or over 40 years, multiparity, obesity, gestational diabetes, maternal anemia, smoking, excessive weight gain during pregnancy, and metabolic syndrome have an increased risk of LOPE [51]. Smoking was strikingly cited as a protective factor as well as some dietary factors [50, 52].

Although some previous suggestions of an increase in its prevalence, preeclampsia did not appear to be influenced by maternal age > 45 years: there was no significant difference in prevalence between women aged >45 years and <45 years (OR 1.86; 95% 0.9–3.6; $p = 0.052$) [53] nor conception by assisted reproductive technology; after stratification by plurality, the difference in gestational hypertension/preeclampsia rates between ART and non-ART mothers was not statistically significant, with a OR 1.05 (95% CI, 0.98–1.12) for mothers of singletons [54].

Pathogenesis

In EOPE, the intricate neuro-immuno-endocrine network makes us question whether the alteration at the level of oxidative stress and the pro-inflammatory state in maternal tissues are the causes or the consequences of previous factors acting before the gestation (see section "Physiopathology").

On the other hand in LOPE patients, where previous concomitant maternal conditions associated with overweight, obesity, and even morbid obesity, the psycho-neuro-immuno-endocrine networks would work differently: either by the release of a pro-inflammatory substance from the maternal adipose tissue or due to the pro-inflammatory effect of insulin and associated hyperlipidemia [55–57]. Alternatively, a pro-inflammatory and obesogenic effect of an altered microbiome by the underlying pathologies induces endothelial dysfunction [45]. In this case, it is clear that low-grade inflammation is prior to pregnancy.

Due to the mechanism described, a relative placental insufficiency would then be generated, where the placenta is unable to meet the increased fetal requirements. On the other hand, the fetus, seeking a new balance to counteract the placental deficiency, produces proangiogenic molecules that generate an improvement on placental perfusion. Adenosine produced by the fetus has been proposed as the molecule that would improve placental perfusion, increase maternal cardiac output, and raise blood pressure in cases of LOPE [55–57]. This strategy of the fetus to increase the contributions of nutrients would also generate an unfavorable fetal programming, which would lead him in adult life to suffer from chronic noncommunicable diseases [58–61], bringing the epigenetic basis of an intrauterine fetal programming of adult disease.

As pointed out in previous sections of this chapter, it should be addressed that the evaluation of biomarkers involved in the pathophysiology of endothelial disease still offer very different results among the published reports.

Clinical Aspects

As we pointed out previously, in EOPE fetal syndrome predominates over maternal syndrome, presenting placental hypoflux, intrauterine growth restriction, low birth weight, iatrogenic premature delivery, and perinatal death. In the ultrasonography, in addition to the characteristics of intrauterine growth restriction and oligohydramnios, we will find signs of redistribution of flow in the fetal Doppler and alteration of the pulsatility of the uterine arteries. At the level of the pathological placental anatomy, the findings include decreased placental volume, thrombosis, and vascular atherosis, among others.

L0PE, however, is more associated with an underlying maternal constitutional disorder, where obesity, metabolic syndrome, hyperlipidemia, insulin resistance, and gestational diabetes are imposed, and often with normal placenta, without clear evidence of atherosis or signs of hypoperfusion, normal or greater placental volume than expected and normal fetal growth, normal uterine and umbilical arteries under Doppler evaluation, adequate or slightly elevated newborn weight at birth, and more favorable maternal and neonatal outcomes.

Although the termination of pregnancy is the way in which preeclampsia begins its stage of involution or reversal of symptoms, nowadays expectant management in cases of EOPE with severe maternal and fetal involvement was promising and has been set over the early active behavior.

The aim is to reduce the neonatal complications derived from iatrogenic prematurity – respiratory distress syndrome, bronchopulmonary dysplasia, intraventricular hemorrhage, and increased neonatal mortality – a strategy that implies the induction of the delivery before the end, and in turn to prevent in the pregnant woman the onset of HELLP syndrome, the detachment of placenta normoinserta, pulmonary edema, disseminated intravascular coagulation, and renal insufficiency.

The decision to move from the expectant behavior to the induction of labor depends on the continuous monitoring and evaluation in real time of the physical exam, laboratory, and Doppler results from both the mother and the fetus. Expectant behavior includes magnesium sulfate, antihypertensive treatment, glucocorticosteroids for maturation, continuous AP monitoring, routine laboratory screening, and frequent fetal Doppler. Maternal indications for induction of labor during expectant management included major maternal complications and fetal death, eclampsia, placental abruption, persistent or severe headache, increased proteinuria, upper abdominal pain or visual changes two hours after controlling eclampsia, diagnosis of HELLP syndrome, disseminated intravascular coagulation, heart failure, massive ascites and pleural effusion, pulmonary edema, and acute renal failure. In addition, patients with severe uncontrolled hypertension should be taken into account. For this group, the measurement of plasma albumin and the identification of hydrothorax instead of the 24-hour urine protein levels or the serum creatinine levels were used to determine the termination of pregnancy. Fetal indications for termination of pregnancy may include non-reactive fetal monitoring decelerations or decreased variability, severe intrauterine restriction, color Doppler ultrasound resulting from the absence of end-diastolic velocity of the fetal umbilical artery, and severe oligohydramnios or when there was a lack of fetal growth for two weeks [1, 61].

The expectant strategy reported a mean of prolongation of labor in an average of around 19 days and resulted in 80% of live newborns with an average gestational age at birth of around 27/28 weeks and with an average birth weight of 1582 g. Neonatal mortality of live newborns was 14.5% which was associated with gestational age and birth weight: fetal deaths occurred around 26/27 weeks with an average birth weight of 850 g. The maternal and perinatal results obtained considering immediate delivery or expectant management seem also to depend on both the gestational age range (<34 weeks and between 34 and 37 weeks) and the election of the time of delivery before 34 weeks of pregnancy, the maternal results were similar, but the perinatal results were significantly worse when immediate delivery occurred. However, between 34 and 37 weeks of gestation, the progression to severe maternal disease was slightly higher among women who underwent expectant management, achieving better perinatal outcomes [62].

Perinatal and maternal morbidity and mortality could be different in patients diagnosed with E0PE or LOPE: in EOPE patients fetal syndrome is more frequent and more severe and presents severe placental lesions in the first weeks of pregnancy and more adverse perinatal results. Around 3% of the decision to terminate the pregnancy in EPE was due to fetal causes, 34% when evidencing alterations in Doppler velocimetry; cesarean section rate was 88.9%, postpartum hospitalization time was significantly longer in the EOPE, and the perinatal outcome was significantly worse than in L0PE patients: 89.66% of newborns entered intensive care units, 32.76% of infants presented low birth weight, and 100% of newborns of preterm and neonatal mortality amounted to 8.62%. LOPE on the other hand, which is characterized by maternal alterations in the third trimester, has a secondary impact on fetal health, but less frequent and less severe: 91% terminated pregnancies due to maternal causes, (uncontrolled proteinuria 45% and 28% due to uncontrolled hypertension) and the cesarean section rate was 63%. Whereas 19.05% of infants entered the intensive care unit, there were only 6.61% of newborns with low birth weight, 17.14% prematurity in this group, with no perinatal deaths [62].

According to ACOG recommendations [63], delivery is recommended instead of expectant behavior in women with gestational hypertension or preeclampsia without severity, with 37 0/7 weeks gestation, (Level A), or in women with gestational hypertension or severe preeclampsia diagnosed at 34 weeks or more after the clinical stabilization of the mother, or in patients with labor or premature rupture of membranes. It is not necessary to perform MPF in these cases if the spontaneous evolution of labor is allowed and act accordingly (Level B).

ACOG guidelines of expectant management of severe preeclampsia before 34 weeks of gestation recommend taking this behavior based on strict criteria for selection of maternal and fetal health, with appropriate resources for maternal and neonatal care. Because expectant management is intended to provide a neonatal benefit at the expense of maternal risk, expectant management is not advised when the feto-neonatal prognosis is ominous. During expectant management, termination of pregnancy is recommended at any time when there is evidence of deterioration in maternal or fetal health (Level B) [63].

Finally, we would like to highlight at least three controversial points that arise in LPE patients and the decision of termination of pregnancy and the responsibility of each treating team: (1) There is no certainty if planned immediate delivery or expectant management has better maternal and neonatal outcomes if preeclampsia develops between 34 and 37 weeks of pregnancy. (2) Labor should be induced between 34 and 37 weeks of pregnancy if a woman develops severe refractory hypertension and presents altered hematological or biochemical indices and evidence of fetal compromise or other indicators of severe preeclampsia. (3) An important advice important for our daily practice: precise information to women and their families with preeclampsia should be always provided so they can be alert for new symptoms of maternal worsening and fetal movements that may decrease or be absent in cases of severity.

To sum up: to improve perinatal outcomes, when no evidence of severe maternal involvement or parameters that indicate a fetal compromise exist – especially before 34 weeks – pregnancy should be carefully monitored and delivery postponed. Between 34 and 37 weeks, the decision about the time to delivery should be shared with the pregnant woman and her family, after providing clear information about the risks and adverse outcomes associated with preeclampsia and prematurity. EOPE is associated with the highest rate of maternal complications – both in the short and long term – and with an increased risk of perinatal morbidity and mortality. Although LOPE is associated with a lower incidence of severe morbidity, its higher incidence and the fact that it affects women with previous comorbidities make their prediction also very important. Differences between EPE and LPE are summarized in Table 40.1.

Early Prediction

Prediction of preeclampsia has proven to be difficult due to the complex nature of the disease. Early diagnosis has major implications for the long-term health of the mother and the newborn since preeclampsia is associated with an elevated risk to develop cardiovascular diseases later in life.

Ideally, a marker to predict preeclampsia must be sensitive and specific and should detect the anomaly, while prevention of the clinical development of the

Table 40.1 Summary of the main differences between early preeclampsia (EOPE) and late preeclampsia (LOPE)

	EOPE	LOPE
Incidence	0.38%	2.72%
Prevalence	5–20%	75–80%
Risk factors	Extreme maternal ages Single Afro-American Nullipara Fetal and neonatal death Tobacco	Chronic hypertension Diabetes Fertility treatment Male fetus Tobacco
Biomarkers[i]		
PIGF	↓	↓
SFit-1	↑↑	↑
Endoglin	↑	↑
Tie-2	↓	↓
VEGFR	↑↑	↑
PP13	↓↓	↓
Endostatin	↑	ND
sFLT1	↑	ND
sENG	↑	ND
Prediction	Decreased PIGF from second trimester sFit-1/PIGF ratio between 26 and 28 weeks	Elevated serum sFit-1 in first trimester
Morbidity	High	Low
Mother	Multiorgan dysfunction Adverse maternal evolution	Good evolution, associated to previous conditions
Fetus	IUGR, low birth weight, perinatal death	Normal weight and growth or elevated weight, macrosomia
Placenta	Reduction of placental volume	Normal placentation, elevated or normal placental volume
Uterine arteries	Increased resistance	Normal resistance or slightly elevated
Recurrence	High	Low

disease is still possible. The tool should be safe, simple, inexpensive, and appropriate for the patient. Unfortunately, in preeclampsia, none of the tools available leads to accurate diagnosis either in low- or high-risk patients; they do not comply with the criteria mentioned above. Given the multiple factors leading to preeclampsia, it is difficult to develop a sole test that is at the same time predictive, sensitive, and specific. As a consequence, the decision to implement prophylactic measures in certain patients – i.e., calcium or aspirin – should be based on the presence of risk factors stemming from preexisting diseases, from their obstetric history, or from their current gestation associated with an increased risk for pregnancy-induced hypertension.

Until the last few years, the core criteria of preeclampsia have been considered to be a new-onset hypertension after the 20th gestational week combined with proteinuria ≥300 mg per day. However, due to the heterogeneity of the disorder, new diagnostic criteria have recently been introduced. According to the new guidelines, the diagnosis of preeclampsia no longer requires the detection of high levels of protein in the urine (proteinuria). Evidence shows organ problems with the kidneys and livers can occur without signs of protein in urine and that the amount of protein in the urine does not predict how severely the disease will progress. Prior to this time, most healthcare providers traditionally adhered to a rigid diagnosis of preeclampsia based on blood pressure and proteinuria. However, preeclampsia is now to be diagnosed by persistent high blood pressure that develops during pregnancy or during the postpartum period that is associated with a lot of protein in the urine or the new development of decreased blood platelets, trouble with the kidney or liver, fluid in the lungs, or signs of brain trouble such as seizures and/or visual disturbances. Thus, proteinuria has been questioned as an exclusive criterion for diagnosis, and according to the two new diagnostic criteria by the American College of Obstetricians and Gynecologists (ACOG) [63] and the International Society for the Study of Hypertension in Pregnancy (ISSHP) [64], new-onset hypertension *in the absence of proteinuria* but combined with hematological complications, renal insufficiency, impaired liver function, neurological symptoms, or uteroplacental dysfunction also fulfills diagnostic criteria for preeclampsia. This is to provide a more broad definition of preeclampsia for clinical practice, and a more sensitive recognition is beneficial considering the potential severity of the disorder.

Currently, preeclampsia is diagnosed based on clinical characteristics, but biomarkers and genetic variants are expected to provide more specific criteria in the future: according to current guidelines, there is no test or set of tests that can early predict the development of all cases of preeclampsia; however, a combination of maternal risk factors, BP, placental growth factor (PlGF) levels, and uterine artery Doppler can select women who may benefit from 150 mg/d of aspirin to prevent preterm (before 37 weeks' gestation) but not term preeclampsia [63, 64]. These current guidelines also discourage the routine clinical use of rule-in or rule-out tests (specifically PlGF or sFlt-1 [soluble fms-like tyrosine kinase-1]/PlGF ratio) for preeclampsia, which should continue to be evaluated within the context of clinical trials [63, 64]. However, the NICE 2016 diagnostics guidance [66] recommended that the Elecsys immunoassay for the sFlt-1/PlGF ratio, or the Triage PlGF test, be used with a standard clinical assessment to help rule out proteinuric preeclampsia or preeclampsia requiring delivery within the next 7 (for the sFlt-1/PlGF ratio) or 14 days (for Triage PlGF) in women with suspected preeclampsia between 20 and 34 + 6 weeks' gestation. This recommendation was based primarily on two multicenter studies of women with a broad definition of suspected preeclampsia at <34 + 6 weeks' gestation: the PROGNOSIS study (Prediction of Short-Term Outcome in Pregnant Women With Suspected Preeclampsia Study) and the PELICAN study (Plasma Placental Growth Factor [PlGF] in the Diagnosis of Women With Pre-eclampsia Requiring Delivery Within 14 Days) [66]. ISSHP guidelines recommend the PIERS model (Preeclampsia Integrated Estimate of RiSk) as a useful adjunct in the initial assessment of women with preeclampsia which is aimed to predict the likelihood of a composite severe adverse maternal outcome using variables gathered from 0 to 48 hours after admission with preeclampsia [64]. Similarly, the PREP Collaborative Network (Prediction of Complications in Early-Onset Preeclampsia) published prognostic models that assist in predicting the overall risk of women with established preeclampsia to experience a complication using logistic regression (PREP-L) and in predicting the time to adverse maternal outcome using a survival model (PREP-S) [67].

Prevention of Preeclampsia

The efforts made to prevent a disease depend on its prevalence and on the consequences it has in both the individual and the community. Prevention will be successful if it allows us to determine the cause of the disease, to detect the early and latent stage of the pathology, and to establish effective and safe intervention measures. Preeclampsia occurs in 2–8% of pregnancies, and eclampsia is observed in 5–8 out of 10,000 gestations. The main risk entailed by pregnancy-induced hypertension is conversion into preeclampsia and therefore results in potentially severe complications in both the mother and the fetus/neonate.

Preeclampsia affects different systems of the body and is characterized by vasoconstriction, blood flow disorders, endothelial cell dysfunction, and hemostatic system alterations. Maternal morbidity and mortality may occur either due to renal failure, liver dysfunction, heart and lung failure, seizures (eclampsia), cerebral hemorrhage, and death. Perinatal morbidity and mortality, on the other hand, may occur due to abruptio placentae, intrauterine fetal growth retardation, acute and chronic fetal distress, and elective preterm delivery. These disorders are found to be more serious in low-income countries with health budget restrictions where prenatal care is not easily accessible.

Early Recognition of Risk Factors

Prevention of preeclampsia can be obtained also by early recognition of the known risk factors for gestational hypertensive disorders. Thus, a maternal history of nulliparity or previous preeclampsia/eclampsia or for multiparas short intervals between gestations may alert. Partners also account for the risk of preeclampsia, as a partner with whom the patient has had a preeclamptic pregnancy or a new smoker partner, as well as women older than 40 years or younger than 20 years, is more prone to develop preeclampsia. A close family relative with preeclampsia precedents, like a mother or sister with a history of preeclampsia/ eclampsia, could also increase the risk. Several previous medical conditions like chronic hypertension or renal disease, obesity, insulin resistance/diabetes mellitus (gestational or type 1), factor V Leiden and protein S deficiency, antiphospholipid antibodies, lupus anticoagulant, and hyperhomocysteinemia are recognized as risk factors. Fetal factors can also account for the risk as multiple gestation, hydatidiform mole, and chromosomal abnormalities (trisomy 13, triploidy) [1].

Biomarkers

Early recognition of biomarkers for preeclampsia may have also a potential preventive value. These markers must be sensitive and specific and should detect the anomaly, while prevention of the clinical development of the disease is still possible. The test should be safe, simple, inexpensive, and appropriate for the patient. Unfortunately, in preeclampsia, none of the tests available leads to accurate diagnosis either in low- or high-risk patients; they do not comply with all criteria mentioned above. However, and based in the finding that women with preeclampsia have abnormal blood flow in their uterine arteries and reduced maternal serum levels of placental products, placental growth factor (PlGF) is the most discriminating biomarker for preeclampsia – and for early-onset preeclampsia in particular – that researchers have found to date [68]. PlGF levels are significantly lower in pregnant women who go on to develop preeclampsia, and researchers have used PlGF combined with other factors to achieve a 93% detection rate for the risk of developing preeclampsia in the first trimester, with a false-positive ratio of 5% [64–68]. The other factors included the abovementioned risk factors of maternal history, prior and family history of preeclampsia, maternal blood pressure, uterine artery pulsatility index, and pregnancy-associated plasma protein-A (PAPP-A). The antiangiogenic factor soluble fms-like tyrosine kinase 1 (sFlt1) and the sFlt-1/PlGF ratio have also shown promise in clinical research as biomarkers for predicting and diagnosing preeclampsia in the second and third trimesters [69].

Specific Preventive Approaches

The term prevention refers not only to primary prevention (stopping the disease from developing) but also to the act of reversing or slowing the process of the disease before it becomes clinically manifest (secondary prevention). Primary prevention is achieved only if the cause of the disease is recognized and then prevented or manipulated; therefore, such an approach is not feasible for gestational hypertension since its etiology is unknown. We are still unable to determine if it is a defective bound between the trophoblast and maternal tissue leading to disorders in uteroplacental adaptation and trophoblastic invasion and also to an exaggerated inflammatory response with endothelial damage in the mother leading to preeclampsia. Secondary prevention, on the other hand, is possible in preeclampsia and can be summarized as follows:

- Lifestyle intervention
- Reduced physical activity and stress
- Diet interventions: low-sodium diet, energizers, protein, magnesium, zinc, calcium, vitamin, linoleic acid, and fish oil supplementation
- Pharmacological interventions: diuretics, antihypertensive drugs, anticoagulants and nitric oxide donors, acetylsalicylic acid, and pravastatin

Lifestyle Intervention

There is no evidence that changes in lifestyle have a preventive effect on the development of pregnancy-induced hypertension. However, the risk of developing gestational hypertension in primigravid and multiparous women is inversely proportional to the length of sexual cohabitation [70].

Diet Interventions and Supplements

Diet observational studies indicate that a balanced diet with an adequate daily calorie intake benefits both the pregnant mother and the baby [71]. Although there is no clinical evidence that sodium restriction in the patients' diets have the prophylactic effect, clinical experimental studies indicate that strict sodium restriction in pregnancy may not be completely harmless as it interferes with the physiological increase in cardiac one-minute volume and the expansion of plasma volume, which are already markedly reduced in preeclamptic patients [72]. While there seems to be no reason to prescribe a low-sodium diet in healthy pregnant women, it should be recommended in patients sensitive to salt who suffer from chronic hypertension and are already on a sodium-restricted diet [72].

Although some studies show that a high-energy intake is associated with an increased risk for preeclampsia, in controlled studies there is no clear evidence that weight loss or reduced weight gain might lead to a decrease in the incidence of pregnancy-induced hypertension [73]. It is important to note that a severe limitation in weight gain reduces birth weight and, therefore, might be dangerous for the fetus.

Recent controlled clinical trials have demonstrated the efficacy of magnesium sulfate in the prevention of eclampsia in preeclamptic women and the management of eclampsia. However, the prevention of hypertensive disorders of pregnancy with the use of magnesium supplements has so far been unsuccessful: the systematic review of 7 controlled clinical trials involving 2689 women did not show any beneficial effect of the daily oral intake of a magnesium supplement during pregnancy [74].

Zinc is an essential oligo-element in many metabolic pathways. In a recent cohort study, no association was found between maternal plasma concentrations of zinc and any pregnancy outcome parameters in almost 3500 women from a low socioeconomic class [75].

Calcium supplementation in pregnancy is supposed to reduce parathyroid hormone secretion (xxx) which in turn would decrease the levels of free ionized calcium in the smooth muscle and lead to a reduced response of vasopressor agents and vasodilation. A meta-analysis of 14 controlled but heterogeneous clinical studies involving a total of 1218 pregnant women who received a daily 1.5–2 g calcium supplementation or placebo showed a reduction in both systolic and diastolic arterial blood pressure, with an odds ratio for preeclampsia of 0.38 (95% CI: 0.22–0.65), as compared with the control group. The same analysis also demonstrated that there is a tendency towards a lower incidence of preterm deliveries, IUGR, and perinatal death [76]. Almost all these studies included populations with a low-calcium diet, which would explain why a similar randomized controlled study of the use of a daily 2 g calcium supplement in healthy nulliparous pregnant women from week 21 to delivery carried out in the United States did not differ from the use of placebo [77]. To sum up, currently available data seem to indicate that calcium supplements in pregnancy reduces the risk of preeclampsia in communities with low incomes and hence calcium intake. No beneficial effects on perinatal outcomes have been demonstrated so far.

Controlled clinical studies carried out to assess their possible beneficial effects in gestational hypertension have demonstrated that the use of fish oil supplements helps to prolong the length of gestation [78]. However, fish oil has not been found to prevent the development of either preeclampsia or its complications [79]. The same conclusions apply to vegetable oils.

Oxidative stress is known to be a major pathophysiological mechanism leading to endothelial damage and malfunctioning in preeclampsia. Vitamins C and E are powerful inhibitors of reactive oxygen and lipid peroxidation. The levels of both these vitamins are rather low in preeclamptic patients. However, results were disappointing, and in large randomized clinical trials, compared with a placebo group, no difference was found in the incidence of pregnancy-induced hypertension in both groups [80].

Pharmacological Interventions

Diuretics: Diuretics are known to reduce blood pressure and edema, which does not necessarily imply they have a beneficial effect on the pathophysiology of preeclampsia. Furthermore, meta-analyses of controlled studies agree that there is not enough evidence to support a probable preventive effect of diuretics on the development of preeclampsia and its complications [81]. On the other hand, no deleterious effects on the fetus or gestation have been found with the use of diuretics. Therefore, treatment with diuretics may be continued in pregnant women who require it due to a preexisting pathology.

Antihypertensives: Given the high risk for such serious complications as abruptio placentae, cerebral hemorrhage, and hepatic and renal failure, antihypertensive drug medication must be prescribed immediately if blood pressure rises over 160/110 mmHg. Although the administration of antihypertensive drugs in patients with mild or moderate hypertension can prevent the development of severe hypertension, there is no evidence available in the literature that the use of antihypertensive treatment in women with mild or moderate hypertension, whether chronic or gestational, might prevent the development of preeclampsia and eclampsia [82].

Angiotensin-converting enzyme inhibitors and, therefore, angiotensin II receptor antagonists seem to be the only contraindicated antihypertensive drugs during gestation as they are associated with fetal skull ossification defects, fetal growth restriction, oligohydramnios, and neonatal renal failure [83].

Aspirin: Acetylsalicylic acid (aspirin) produces irreversible and non-selective inhibition of cyclooxygenases (COX) – the key enzyme in the arachidonic acid cascade – and prevents prostanoid synthesis like thromboxanes (TXA2) in platelets where it decreases the TXA2/PGI2 ratio and induces an antithrombotic effect. The inhibition of prostanoid synthesis depends on aspirin dose: at low daily doses (0.5–1.5 mg/kg body weight) aspirin produce a dose-dependent inhibition in platelet TxA2 synthesis, reaching almost complete inhibition at 1.5 mg/kg [84]. As platelets lack a cellular nucleus, they are unable to resynthesize TxA2; consequently, recovery of TxA2 depends on new platelet production by the bone marrow. In contrast, this low concentration of aspirin does not affect endothelial cell production of PGI2, even when aspirin is no longer present in the patient's circulation. 100–300 mg/day inhibits TXA2 and to a lesser extent PGI2 [84]. In 1994, CLASP carried out a multicenter controlled clinical trial of a daily dose of 60 mg of aspirin among 8021 women with mixed parity and at low to moderate risk for hypertensive disorders of pregnancy and/or fetal growth restriction. It is important to note that the reduction in the incidence of proteinuric preeclampsia (12%), fetal growth restriction (11%), and perinatal death (20%) observed in the group treated with aspirin, when compared with the placebo group, was not statistically significant. However, low-dose aspirin was found to reduce significantly the rate of preterm delivery (20%). Post hoc analysis of the data in the CLASP trial showed that the earlier the onset of treatment, the greater the reduction in the development of preeclampsia. The results of this trial showed that aspirin had no therapeutic effect in 1343 women with pregnancy-induced hypertension or IUGR. The differences observed were not statistically significant in women with either moderate or low risk among a population of 28,000 women [85].

Through meta-analysis, it can be concluded that the results of the randomized controlled studies conducted in over 30,000 pregnant women at low, moderate, or high risk of developing preeclampsia indicate that prophylactic use of low-dose aspirin from the 12th week of gestation will prevent the development of preeclampsia in about 15% of high-risk women [86]. It will also lead to a similar reduction in the rate of low birth weight for gestational age and preterm deliveries. A lower but not statistically significant decrease in perinatal mortality has been also observed. In Table 40.2, the number needed to treat (NNT) for aspirin for three levels of risk for preeclampsia, IUGR, and preterm birth is presented. It should be noted that neither in the CLASP trial nor any other report has the prophylactic use of low-dose aspirin been associated with any deleterious effect on gestation, delivery, or the newborn. Furthermore, follow-up of those babies from delivery to date has not revealed any aspirin-related complication [85, 86].

Table 40.2 Number needed to treat for three levels of risk for preeclampsia, IUGR, and preterm birth

Outcome	Risk of outcome	RR	Absolute change in risk	Risk after change	NNT benefit (95% CI)	NNT harm (95% CI)
Preeclampsia	0.10	0.76	−0.02	0.08	42 (26, 200)	NA
	0.18	0.76	−0.04	0.14	23 (15, 111)	NA
	0.23	0.76	−0.06	0.17	18 (11, 87)	NA
IUGR	0.07	0.80	−0.01	0.06	71 (41, 1429)	NA
	0.13	0.80	−0.03	0.10	38 (22, 769)	NA
	0.24	0.80	−0.05	0.19	21 (12, 417)	NA
Preterm birth	0.11	0.86	−0.02	0.09	65 (38, 455)	NA
	0.19	0.86	−0.03	0.16	38 (22, 263)	NA
	0.31	0.86	−0.04	0.27	23 (13, 161)	NA
Abruption (in women at increased risk)	0.015	1.12	0.002	0.017	NA	556(145 harm to ∞ to 476 benefit)
	0.020	1.12	0.002	0.022	NA	417(109 harm to ∞ to 357 benefit)
Abruption (across all risk levels)	0.015	1.17	0.0026	0.018	NA	392(139 harm to ∞ to 952 benefit)
	0.020	1.17	0.0034	0.023	NA	294(104 harm to ∞ to 714 benefit)

Abbreviations: IUGR intrauterine growth restriction, *NNT* number needed to treat, *RR* relative risk. Taken from: Low-Dose Aspirin for the Prevention of Morbidity and Mortality From Preeclampsia: A Systematic Evidence Review for the U.S. Preventive Services Task Force [Internet].Evidence Syntheses, No. 112.Henderson JT, Whitlock EP, O'Conner E, et al.Rockville (MD): Agency for Healthcare Research and Quality (US); 2014 Apr.

Discrepancies Among Clinical Studies of Aspirin

The decision to publish articles in the literature is usually biased towards those which report positive results even though the populations involved may be small. It is also a fact that in the large populations analyzed in multicenter studies, high-risk patients may be overlooked, and others may be wrongly classified as preeclamptic, thus underestimating the preventive effect of low-dose aspirin. Sources of discrepancy among reported results include:

(a) Gestational age at the time of inclusion in the trial (before or after 20 weeks' gestation).
(b) Chronotherapy: The time of the day when aspirin is administered. Several controlled studies have demonstrated a more marked effect on blood pressure when aspirin is taken 8 h after waking up; even better results have been obtained if aspirin is taken at bedtime perhaps because of the reduced renin-angiotensin system activity; thus, a 100 mg dose administered at bedtime to pregnant woman reduced systolic blood pressure to 12.4 mmHg and diastolic blood pressure to 8.1 mmHg [87].
(c) Dose: Early trials conducted in small populations reported the use of daily doses of 100–150 mg, while later large multicenter studies have used much lower doses (50–75 mg daily). This dose will inhibit platelet thromboxane but may not be enough to affect placental thromboxane [84]. We still do not know if a higher dose of aspirin might have other benefits without increasing side effects.
(d) Aspirin resistance: Clinical resistance to aspirin occurs when an adverse cardiological event occurs despite taking aspirin in the recommended doses [88]. Factors that could be associated with aspirin resistance include insufficient inhibition of platelet TXA2, less enteral absorption (due to the enteric coat film of the tablets), genetic polymorphism, smoking, erythrocyte-induced platelet activation, COX2 mRNA overexpression, low expression of COX-1, and increased norepinephrine activity [88]. Doses of aspirin <100 mg presented an increase of the prevalence of biochemical resistance compared with 150–300 mg doses [89], and 30% of pregnancies showed aspirin resistance at doses below 100 mg. The dose recommended for aspirin-resistant patients ranges between 75 and 150 mg/day.
(e) Treatment compliance: It is well known that there is a variable compliance – 20–80% – in obstetric drug treatments, and compliance to aspirin treatment use is below 20–45% [90]. Thus, before determining if a given patient is resistant to aspirin, we must check the compliance to treatment. Usually, it is difficult to corroborate treatment compliance and protocol adherence in large multicenter studies. On the other hand, small randomized clinical studies enable better control over eligibility criteria, objectives, time of treatment administration, and protocol adherence by both researchers and patients [91].

Statins: Although statins are currently contraindicated in the current medical practice in both pregnancy and lactation, statins are taken during pregnancy, in particular lipophilic statins which have been linked with major congenital malformations [92]. Early promising results obtained from experimental and pilot clinical studies encouraged several investigators to scale the research to more ambitious designs in human clinical research. Thus, statins reduced sFlt-1 secretion from endothelial and trophoblast cells in vitro [93]; the administration of pravastatin in vivo to animals prevented the preeclampsia-like syndrome and overexpression of sFlt-1 [94] and in the clinical setting. Pravastatin 10 mg in a pilot prevention trial in high-risk pregnancies demonstrated improved pregnancy outcomes and a favorable angiogenic profile [95]. However, the randomized controlled trials designed recently as treatment or prevention protocol studies did not confirm the expectations of the first-mentioned studies. Thus, although limited by the lack of statistical power, the study StAmP which randomized women with preeclampsia between 24 and 31 weeks to either pravastatin (40 mg; $n = 30$) or placebo ($n = 32$) did not show any significant reductions in sFlt1 or improvement in clinical outcomes [96]. Despite the study couldn't reach the primary outcome – mean concentration of soluble FMS-like tyrosine kinase (sFlt1) during the first 3 days after randomization – safety results confirm the support of pravastatin use in high-risk pregnancies. There were no major adverse neonatal outcomes related with the use of the drug and – as previously reported in the aforementioned pravastatin prevention trial – there was a limited transplacental transfer of pravastatin that shows that the drug is not being concentrated in the fetus [95, 96]. As pointed out by Constatine [95], however, the lack of efficacy in the StAmP trial should not impact the prevention trials because a medication may still be effective as a prevention strategy when it is not as effective as a treatment (e.g., aspirin for preeclampsia and progesterone for preterm birth). In a more recent preventive protocol study, however, the addition of pravastatin 20 mg to aspirin 80 mg did not seem to be synergic since the two groups did not differ from each other in preventing preeclampsia nor in the maternal outcomes and in decreasing angiogenic marker (endothelin 1) levels. Similarly to the StAmP trial, no differences were found in fetal outcomes such as preterm birth and fetal growth retardation between the two groups [97].

Conclusions

Preventive measures require the accurate identification of potential high-risk patients – about 2–8% of healthy nulliparous pregnant women. So far this selection can only be based on their obstetric and clinical histories and on the presence of known maternal and fetal risks. Unfortunately, no reliable biophysical or biochemical markers are available to acutely predict the development of a hypertensive disorder during pregnancy.

At the present time, the main medical society guidelines on the use of aspirin for preeclampsia prevention differ in the dose of aspirin recommended – 81 mg ACOG [63], 75 mg NICE and WHO [65], and 75–162 mg SOGC [98] – but all the recommendations coincide in that treatments should be initiated early between 12 and 28 weeks' gestation. Perhaps the main finding of ASPRE trial [99] is that aspirin started between 11 and 14 weeks' gestation of high risk for preterm preeclampsia has the maximum effect on the reduction of incidence for preeclampsia with no effect on neonatal outcome or adverse events of aspirin. Current evidence supports the recommendation of low-dose aspirin (75–150 mg/day, according to the different guidelines) prophylaxis in women at high risk of preeclampsia and should be initiated optimally before 16 weeks and continued daily until delivery. Low-dose aspirin prophylaxis should also be considered for women with more than one of several moderate risk factors for preeclampsia. In the absence of high-risk factors for preeclampsia, current evidence does not support the use of prophylactic low-dose aspirin for the prevention of early pregnancy loss, fetal growth restriction, stillbirth, or preterm birth. A daily low dose of aspirin before week 16 to delivery seems to be safe and effective when used in a definite group of high-risk patients to either prevent preeclampsia or delay its development and reduce its severity and complications. In addition, when using aspirin to prevent preeclampsia, it will be necessary to consider in detail the mechanism of action of aspirin, the optimal dosage, the appropriate time to start the treatment, the chronotherapy, and the factors that can induce resistance and lack of adherence to treatment.

Calcium supplement appears to be effective only in high-risk pregnant women with a low dietary calcium intake. The recommended treatment protocol can be summarized as follows: (1) Daily administration of 81 mg of aspirin from week 12 to delivery in pregnant women with (a) a history of severe preeclampsia or eclampsia before 32 weeks' gestation; (b) a history of severe fetal growth restriction, with or without preeclampsia, due to reduced uteroplacental blood flow; (c) a close family history of preeclampsia/eclampsia (mother or sister); and (d) severe chronic hypertension and/or renal disease. (2) Daily administration of 1.5–2 g elemental calcium supplement in high-risk women –selected as described above – and with a low dietary calcium intake, assessed according to their consumption of milk and other dairy products.

Clinical evidence seems to confirm the maternal and fetal/neonatal safety profile when statins are administered in high-risk pregnant women; however, up to now, treatment and preventive randomized controlled studies failed to confirm early assumptions of benefits to prevent or to treat preeclampsia.

Antihypertensive Treatments

Treatment of Chronic Hypertension

Despite the difficulties in accurately determining the benefit/risk balance for the mother and the fetus/neonate of the different interventions available for the treatment of chronic hypertension of pregnancy, the short- and long-term risks of complications have displaced the conservative trend of non-intervention towards the application of pharmacological and non-pharmacological tools for the treatment of chronic mild to moderate hypertension.

There is some level of consensus that antihypertensive treatment in chronic hypertension of pregnancy should be started or reestablished only when systolic blood pressure >150 mm Hg and/or diastolic pressure >100 mm Hg are detected. However, if evidence of target organ damage exists (e.g., kidney disease, proteinuria, left ventricular hypertrophy, retinopathy), it would be reasonable to start treatment with diastolic blood pressure values of >90 mm Hg [63–65].

Other authors [100], however, suggested not starting treatment for blood pressure values below or less than 170/110 mmHg, since women are unlikely to experience any complications, in the short or long term, during their pregnancy.

The lack of information obtained from adequately controlled clinical trials monitored by safety and data monitoring committees prevents us from adopting an appropriate therapeutic measure and from evaluating the real impact of antihypertensive treatment on mild to moderate chronic hypertension on maternal and perinatal outcomes. However, the results of the CHIPS study [101] clearly indicate that patients with moderate hypertension who were not treated with strict control of blood pressure had an increased risk of severe hypertension (adjusted odds ratio: 1.8) when blood pressure was not strictly controlled. Thus, some evidence from RCTs seems to indicate that antihypertensive medication in mild and moderate clinical forms halves the risks of progression to more severe forms of the disease;hence this could have a benefit in preventing brain vascular damage of the mother. There is also consensus that antihypertensive medication is useful in treating hypertensive emergency to decrease the risk of stroke and death of the mother (*see 6.2 treatment of gestacional hypertensive emergency*).

Despite the epidemiological data indicating an increased risk of severe complications for the mother, fetus, and newborn, it is necessary to note that there are currently difficulties in determining whether the proposed pharmacological treatments have an adequate risk-benefit balance, since the aim of the treatment is to reduce the risk of maternal complications without affecting the well-being of the fetus/neonate due to intrauterine exposure to antihypertensive medication and extreme measures to control the mother's blood pressure.

Therefore, regarding the benefits, it is important to point out that according to the available evidence, it is not clear whether a particular treatment used in gestational chronic hypertension – although successful in terms of lowering blood pressure – prevents superimposed preeclampsia or maternal proteinuria or decreases perinatal mortality, prenatal hospitalization, neonatal respiratory distress syndrome, or intrauterine growth restriction [82]. Likewise, regarding the risks, it cannot be specified whether the pharmacological treatments available (antihypertensive drugs, aspirin) are safe for the mother and the fetus/neonate, since the potential adverse effects have not been quantified in detail or were only reported in case reports – with significant methodological biases – or from drug surveillance reports and almost none from RCTs [82].

With these safety and efficacy concerns and precautions in mind, initial antihypertensive therapy should be monotherapy with first-line medications: oral labetalol, oral methyldopa, long-acting oral nifedipine, or other oral beta-blockers if labetalol is not available (acebutolol, metoprolol, pindolol, and propranolol, although these drugs have been associated with low birth weight, especially when administered during the first trimester of pregnancy). Other antihypertensive medications may be considered second-line medications, such as clonidine, hydralazine, and thiazide diuretics. Angiotensin-converting enzyme inhibitors (ACEIs) and angiotensin receptor blockers should not be used during pregnancy due to their teratogenicity, but during the postpartum period they are a valid alternative for the management of hypertension [102]. Other drugs may be used as third-line agents and should be reserved for the treatment of special situations: α1-adrenergic antagonists such as prazosin or doxazosin and oral hydralazine. Nitroprusside and diazoxide are used only in some cases of emergencies.

Most of the non-pharmacological interventions, as well as expectant of non-intervention and non-evidence-based strategies used in the management of complications of chronic hypertension, have not been sufficiently exposed to experimental contrast in RCTs, so their utility in the management of hypertensive pregnant patient remains unknown.

Table 40.3 summarizes the recommendations for the use of the first-line pharmacological interventions in the control of gestational chronic hypertension.

Treatment of Gestational Hypertensive Emergency

Hypertensive emergencies are the most severe clinical conditions of the gestational hypertension syndrome. Appropriate diagnosis and timely therapeutic measures can help to prevent the worst outcome – maternal death – as a result of bleeding and cerebral infarction that occurs primarily from increased systolic blood pressure.

A hypertensive emergency is a condition in which sudden rise in blood pressure levels equal to or greater than 160/110 mmHg that persists for more than 15 minutes is accompanied by clinical symptoms such as intense headaches, scotomas, blurred vision, photopsia, tinnitus, increased osteotendinous reflexes, and epigastralgia [1]. Hypertensive emergency is a condition associated with severe preeclampsia, HELP, or in the exacerbation of a preexisting chronic hypertension, whether or not it has superimposed preeclampsia [1]. In its management, initially, it would not be necessary to look for cardiological support, but in the absence of a good response, a therapist, cardiologist, or anesthetist should be called immediately according to the patient's condition.

The objective of the emergency treatment is to reach blood pressure levels in the range of 140–150 mmHg systolic and 90–100 mm Hg diastolic to restabilize brain self-regulation and prevent stroke. It can be treated with various drugs, but in all cases, a sudden decrease in blood pressure – as the one indicated by nifedipine – should be avoided as it can have a deleterious effect on the fetus. Thus, strict control of fetal hemodynamics must be maintained throughout the treatment.

Antihypertensive treatment must begin immediately in the prenatal, prepartum, and immediate postpartum periods to avoid severe injuries in the pregnant woman. In addition to antihypertensive medication and especially in the crisis that accompanies preeclampsia, the administration of magnesium sulfate should be added to prevent seizures, but not as an antihypertensive drug.

The ACOG Committee Opinion [103] recommended labetalol, in the first place, and hydralazine as drugs of choice for the treatment of hypertensive emergency. Nifedipine would be indicated in case of not having accessible routes but taking into account that the route of choice for the administration of antihypertensive

Table 40.3 Guide for the use of antihypertensive medication in chronic hypertension

Drug	*Methyldopa*
Properties and use	Central action antihypertensive. First-line choice for the management of hypertension generated during pregnancy; however, more recent work would indicate that labetalol would be superior No adverse effects on cognitive development up to the age of 7.5 years of children exposed in utero
Adult dose	250 mg PO, bid/tid; increase q2d prn; maximum dose: 3 g/d
Pediatric dose	10 mg/kg/d PO, divided bid/qid; increase q2d prn maximum dose: 65 mg/kg/d
Pregnancy category	Category B. Usually safe, but benefits should overcome risks
Precautions	Adverse effects include drowsiness and dry mouth; 15% of women do not tolerate therapeutic doses and may induce hemolytic anemia and liver disease. Reduce dose in kidney disease
Contraindications	Documented hypersensibility to the drug or acute liver disease
Interactions with other drugs	The co-administration of barbiturates and ADTs can decrease the hypotensive effect, while that of iron supplements, MAOIs, sympathomimetics, phenothiazine, and beta-blocker drugs can produce elevation of blood pressure
Drug	*Labetalol*
Properties and uses	Also considered a first-line drug in the treatment of hypertension during pregnancy. It has mixed alpha-beta adrenergic blocker properties. Unlike other beta-blockers, labetalol has not been associated with restrictions to fetal growth. Oral and IV forms are used as an alternative to hydralazine in severe eclampsia and preeclampsia emergencies
Adult dose	100 mg IV bid; not exceed 2400 mg/d For BP values >170/110 mmHg: 20 mg IV bolus; subsequently, administer 40 mg doses, followed by 80 mg IV. It can be administered at 10–20 min intervals to control BP. It can also be administered as a continuous infusion at 1 mg/kg/h
Pediatric dose	Not available
Pregnancy	Category C – safety has not been established
Precautions	Treatment should be interrupted if signs of hepatic dysfunction appear
Contraindications	Known hypersensitivity, cardiogenic shock, lung edema, bradycardia, AV block, CHF; untreated asthma, severe COPD
Interactions with other drugs	Decreases the effects of diuretics. Increases the toxicity of methotrexate, lithium, and salicylates. Decreases reflex tachycardia induced by nitroglycerin without affecting its hypotensive effect. Cimetidine can increase plasma levels of labetalol. Glutethimide may decrease the effects of labetalol by microsomal enzyme induction
Drug	*Nifedipine*
Properties and uses	It produces vasodilation by blocking the flow of calcium into the vascular and visceral smooth muscle cell. Due to this effect, it is also used to treat preterm uterine contractions
Adult dose	Capsules: 10–30 mg PO tid. Maximum dose: 120–180 mg/d. Tablets: 30–60 mg PO qd. Maximum dose: 90–120 mg/d. PA >170/110 mmHg: start with 10 mg PO; repeat dose every 30 min prn
Pediatric dose	0.25–0.5 mg/kg, PO tid/qid prn

Table 40.3 (continued)

Pregnancy	Category C – safety has not been established
Precautions	Can induce leg edema and allergic hepatitis (very rare)
Contraindications	Known hypersensitivity
Interactions with other drugs	Co-administration of any other hypotensive agent (including opioids) can potentiate nifedipine hypotensive effects. Cimetidine can increase toxicity. Do not use together with magnesium salts as it can cause deep hypotension (antidote: IV calcium gluconate)

Abbreviations: *bid* twice a day, *tid* three times a day, *qid* 4 times a day, *prn* as demand, *q2d* every other day, *q4-6h* every 4–6 hours, *IV* intravenous, *PO* orally, *PA* blood pressure, *COPD* chronic obstructive pulmonary disease, *CHF* congestive heart failure

drugs in the crisis is the IV. If the intravenous line is not accessible and nifedipine immediate release is not available, 200 mg of labetalol may be used by mouth, which can be repeated after 30 minutes if necessary. If the treatment of the three drugs given in succesive appropriate doses, fail to relieve the acute-onset of the severe hypertension and no response is obtained, i.e., resistant hypertension, emergent consultation with an anesthesiologist, maternal-fetal medicine subspecialist, or critical care subspecialist to discuss second-line intervention and the use of the second alternative like nicardipine and labetalol by infusion pump is recommended [103].

If it is decided to terminate the pregnancy by cesarean section, the emergency must be controlled, and the pregnant woman must be transferred to the surgery room with antihypertensive medication since anesthesia intubation is a procedure that could increase blood pressure and could trigger the hypertensive crisis.

Systematic reviews of the clinical trials with the first-line drugs used in the gestational hypertensive emergency denotes, however, that there is a need for studies designed to compare head to head the efficacy of drugs for the treatment of severe hypertension in pregnancy [104]. Also, several limitations were found in the studies analyzed as lack of a precise and common definition of preeclampsia, different pretreatment blood pressure values, lack of analysis of potential differences between the response of primigravids and multigravida, lack of fetal outcomes as distress, congenital anomalies, and IUGR [104].

Protocol for the Treatment of Hypertensive Emergencies

The management of the hypertensive emergency exceeds the mere reduction of the blood pressure under the threshold level and includes different clinical situations from seizure control and cardiovascular/renal decompensation to pregnancy interruption. Thus multidisciplinary interventions are needed to avoid the worst maternal outcome.

Induction of Labor

Assessment of fetal growth and vitality: The fetus will be affected by the disease and will show alterations in both growth and vitality. Ultrasound scans should be used to follow fetal growth and to study amniotic fluid volume and any changes that might occur in it. Any reduction in amniotic fluid volume will be an indication of compromised vitality and a sign of an adverse outcome. Fetal vitality can be evaluated before the third trimester through the study of blood flow velocity waves: an increase in systolic peak and a reduction in end-diastolic flow will be an indication of a higher resistance in the uteroplacental and umbilical beds and, therefore, of imminent compromise in fetal vitality. During the third trimester, evaluation of fetal vitality using antepartum non-stress tests is recommended since its effectiveness is not affected by the use of hypotensive drugs (xx). After these maneuvers are completed, criteria for pregnancy interruption will include patients with moderate hypertension with a mature fetus (over 37 weeks' gestation) or with severe hypertension with a fetus over 34 weeks gestational age or severe hypertension with an immature fetus in the presence of damaged maternal health and/or treatment failure or eclampsia.

Route of Delivery

The route of delivery will depend on the hypertensive condition and the degree of fetal distress and/or IUGR. In the presence of mild or moderate hypertension there is no contraindication to vaginal delivery unless there exists an obstetric indication for surgical delivery. In cases with severe hypertension, the route of delivery will depend on the degree of fetal distress and of IUGR: if the fetus is highly compromised, surgical delivery through the abdominal wall is recommended. If the vaginal route is attempted, intrapartum fetal monitoring is mandatory. However, any complication in the progress of labor and/or any sign of intrapartum fetal distress must be taken as an indication for a cesarean section.

Anesthesia: general anesthesia is preferred in cases of severe hypertension and eclampsia. In mild or moderate hypertension, however, an epidural can be used if a sudden hypotension is avoided and if the dose is fractioned and administered through a catheter.

General measures for the treatment of eclampsia: measures to prevent tongue biting and pharynx suction; oxygen administration; routine urine and blood test; Foley catheter to measure urine output.

Magnesium sulfate (MgSO4) administration: (a) If the patient presents seizures, start with a slow intravenous bolus (7–14 drops per minute) of 4–6 g of MgSO4, diluted in 10 cm^3 of 5% dextrose solution. If seizures recur within 2 h, the same diluted bolus can be repeated. (b) In the absence of seizures but with prodromic signs, a MgSO4 infusion is recommended instead of the bolus administration. Magnesium sulfate is not recommended as an antihypertensive agent, but magnesium sulfate remains the drug of choice for seizure prophylaxis for women with acute-onset severe hypertension during pregnancy and the postpartum period. Starting magnesium should not be delayed in the setting of acute severe hypertension; it is recommended regardless of whether the patient has gestational hypertension with severe features, preeclampsia with severe features, or eclampsia. If the patient presents signs and/or symptoms of MgSO4 toxicity (xx), MgSO4 administration should be interrupted immediately, maintaining adequate oxygenation, performing an ECG (arrhythmias are likely), and administering diuretics and IV calcium gluconate as an adequate antidote of the MgSO4. Treatment with MgSO4 should be administered for at least 24 h after achieving its therapeutic effect or until the cause of its indication has ceased. Other medications different from MgSO4 for the treatment of seizures include sodium thiopental (slow 250 mg IV diluted bolus) or diazepam (100 mg/ 500 cm^3 of 5% dextrose solution, 5–7 drops per minute, or a slow IV bolus of 40 mg is also possible). Caution is recommended since diazepam is a fetal and maternal respiratory depressant. If the patient presents high blood pressure and seizures, a simultaneous parenteral administration of a hypotensive medication is recommended.

Despite these measures, the patient's prognosis, however, can be complicated by several clinical conditions like pulmonary edema, weak and fast pulse, pulmonary stertor, blood pressure reduction, prolonged coma, cerebral hemorrhage, renal failure, and reduced urinary output.

Antihypertensive Treatment of the Emergency

According to ACOG recommendation [103], intravenous (IV) labetalol and hydralazine have long been considered first-line medications for the management of acute-onset, severe hypertension in pregnant women and women in the postpartum period. Immediate-release oral nifedipine also may be considered as a first-line therapy, particularly when IV access is not available. The use of any of the three drugs does not require cardiac monitoring.

Labetalol IV, hydralazine IV, and oral immediate-release nifedipine were the drugs most studied in hypertensive emergency clinical settings. Although labetalol seemed to be the preferred choice, systematic reviews and meta-analysis failed to found major differences between the drugs in both maternal and fetal-neonatal outcomes [104]. Although all three medications are appropriately used for the treatment of hypertensive emergencies in pregnancy, each agent can be associated with specific adverse effects and eventually contraindications (*see* Table 40.4).

When urgent treatment is needed before the establishment of intravenous access or in low-resource environments where venous access and careful fetal monitoring might not be feasible, all three oral drugs – methyldopa, nifedipine, and labetalol – showed to be viable initial options for treating severe hypertension in low-resource settings [105]. In this scenario, it is recommended that the oral nifedipine algorithm can be initiated as intravenous access is being obtained, or a 200-mg dose of

Table 40.4 Drugs of choice used in the hypertensive emergency

Drug	Mechanism of action	Precautions/adverse events/ contraindications	Dosing scheme
Labetalol	Alpha 1 and beta adrenergic antagonist	IV labetalol should be avoided in women with asthma, heart disease, or congestive heart failure Neonatal bradycardia	Initial dose: 2 min IV 20 mg bolus Followed by 20–40 mg IV to a maximum single dose of 80 mg according to response Interval between each dose: 10–20 min Maintenance dose: 1–2 mg/min, IV infusion Maximum total cumulative dose: 300 mg
Nifedipine	Calcium channel blocker	Maternal tachycardia Marked hypotension Should be avoided in cardiovascular shock, prepartum hemorrhage, and placenta previa	Initial dose: 10 mg, orally Continues: 10 mg every 20 min Maximum dose: 50 mg *Sublingual route is contraindicated*
Hydralazine	Direct vasodilator	Increased risk for maternal hypotension with parenteral hydralazine	Initial dose: 5 mg IV bolus in 2 minutes Continued: repeated doses of 5 mg IV every 20 min Maximum dose: 20 mg IV Maintenance dose: 2 mg/hour IV

labetalol can be administered orally. Labetalol can be repeated in 30 minutes if the appropriate improvement is not observed [105].

Labetalol: There are several reports of the effectiveness of the use of labetalol, which seems to have become the "drug of choice" in the treatment of hypertensive emergencies – the initial dosing scheme is 20 mg. If blood pressure still exceeds the threshold, it is reasonable to consider increasing the dose every 10 minutes in increments of 20–40 mg to a maximum single dose of 80 mg. A maximum total cumulative dose of 300 mg is still recommended in this scenario.

Hydralazine: This drug used to be the most widely used all over the world in hypertensive emergencies in preeclampsia pregnant women; however, it is less effective in patients with preexisting hypertension. Initial dose: slow 5 mg IV bolus (dilute the 20 mg ampoule in 10 cm^3 of dextrose solution). After 15–20 min, if blood pressure still exceeds the threshold, repeat 5–10 mg at 20-min intervals until a total cumulative 40 mg dose is given. Maintenance dose should be the same as the initial dose which resulted in a favorable response.

Nifedipine: Immediate-release oral nifedipine also may be considered as a first-line therapy, particularly when IV access is not available. Initial dose: 10 mg orally immediate release, continue with 10 mg every 20 min. Maximum dose: 50 mg, *sublingual route is contraindicated.*

Other drugs studied include:

Clonidine: initial dose, slow 0.25 mg IV bolus; maintenance dose, 0.75 mg/500 cm^3 of dextrose solution at a rate of 7 drops/min.

Vasodilators like sodium nitroprusside and diazoxide but are no longer used at present or used as a second alternative when the first-choice drugs fail.

Converting enzyme inhibitors such as intravenous enalapril are not recommended as they can result in acute fetal renal failure and even intrauterine fetal death. However, enalapril has been described as effective and safe in cases of acute ventricular failure, as well as in the treatment of a hypertensive emergency during puerperium [102].

References

1. Voto LS, Ortí J. Hypertension in pregnancy. In: Kurjak A, Chervenak FA, editors. Textbook of perinatal medicine, vol. 1. 2nd ed. London: Informa UK Ltd; 2006. p. 2051–65.
2. Brossens I, Robertson WB, Dixon HG. The role of the spiral arteries in the pathogenesis of pre-eclampsia. Obstet Gynecol Annu. 1972;1:177–91.
3. Ridder A, Giorgione V, Khalil A, Thilaganathan B. Preeclampsia: the relationship between uterine artery blood flow and trophoblast function. Int J Mol Sci. 2019;20:3263.
4. Ditisheim A, Sibai B, Tatevian N. Placental findings in postpartum preeclampsia: A comparative retrospective study. Am J Perinatol. 2019. https://doi.org/10.1055/s-0039-1692716.
5. Gant NF, Chand S, Whalley PJ, et al. The nature of pressor responsiveness to angiotensin II in human pregnancy. Obstet Gynecol. 1974;43:854–60.
6. Gant NF, Richard JW, Royice BE, Macdonald PC. Control of vascular responsiveness during human pregnancy. Kidney Int. 1980;18:253–8.
7. Tomimatsu T, Mimura K, Matsuzaki S, et al. Preeclampsia: maternal systemic vascular disorder caused by generalized endothelial dysfunction due to placental antiangiogenic factors. Int J Mol Sci. 2019;20:4246. https://doi.org/10.3390/ijms20174246.
8. Boeldt DS, BirdI M. Vascular adaptation in pregnancy and endothelial dysfunction in preeclampsia. J Endocrinol. 2017;232:R27–44.
9. Bouças AP, de Souza BM, Bauer AC, Crispim D. Role of innate immunity in preeclampsia: a systematic review. Reprod Sci. 2017;10:1362–70.
10. Matthiesena L, Berga G, Ernerudhb J, et al. Immunology of preeclampsia. In: Markert UR, editor. Immunology of pregnancy. Chem Immunol Allergy, vol. 89. Basel: Karger; 2005. p. 49–61.
11. Hui-Qing L, Rong H. The role of immunity in the pathogenesis and development of preeclampsia. Scand J Immunol. 2019;90:e12756.
12. Kobayashi H, Ichikawa M, Akasaka J, et al. Immune-related pathophysiological causes relevant to a subset of patients with preeclampsia (Review). World Acad Sci J. 2019;1:59–66.
13. Williams PJ, Pipkin FB. The genetics of pre-eclampsia and other hypertensive disorders of pregnancy. Best Pract Res Clin Obstet Gynaecol. 2011;25(4–4):405–17.
14. Ehret G. Genes for preeclampsia: an opportunity for blood pressure genomics. Hypertension. 2018;72(2):285–6.
15. Brew O, Sullivan MHF, Woodman A. Comparison of normal and pre eclamptic placental gene expression: a systematic review with meta analysis. PLoS One. 2016;11(8):e0161504. https://doi.org/10.1371/journal.pone.0161504.
16. Yuen RKC, Aherrera MSP, von Dadelszen P, et al. DNA methylation profiling of human placentas reveals promoter hypomethylation of multiple genes in early-onset preeclampsia. Eur J Hum Genet. 2010;18:1006–12.

17. Apicella C, Camino SM, Ruano Méhats C, et al. The role of epigenetics in placental development and the etiology of preeclampsia. Int J Mol Sci. 2019;20:2837.
18. Laissue P, Vaiman D. Exploring the molecular aetiology of preeclampsia by massive parallel sequencing of DNA. Curr Hypertens Rep. 2020;22:31. https://doi.org/10.1007/s11906-020-01039-z.
19. Ito M, Itakura A, Ohno Y, et al. Possible activation of the renin-angiotensin system in the feto-placental unit in preeclampsia. J Clin Endocrinol Metab. 2002;87(4):1871–8.
20. Xia Y, Kellems RE. Angiotensin receptor agonistic autoantibodies and hypertension: preeclampsia and beyond. Circ Res. 2013;113(1):78–87.
21. Campbell N, LaMarca B, Cunningham MW. The role of agonistic autoantibodies to the angiotensin II type 1 receptor (AT1-AA) in pathophysiology of preeclampsia. Curr Pharm Biotechnol. 2018;19(10):781–5.
22. Cunningham MW Jr, Williams JM, Amaral L, et al. Agonistic autoantibodies to the angiotensin II type 1 receptor enhance angiotensin II–induced renal vascular sensitivity and reduce renal function during pregnancy. Hypertension. 2016;68(5):1308–13.
23. Dymara-Konopka W, Laskowska M. The role of nitric oxide, ADMA, and homocysteine in the etiopathogenesis of preeclampsia—review. Int J Mol Sci. 2019;20:2757. https://doi.org/10.3390/ijms20112757.
24. Sutton EF, Gemmel M, Powers RW. Nitric oxide signaling in pregnancy and preeclampsia. Nitric Oxide. 2020;95:55–62.
25. Granger JP, Spradley FT, Bakrania BA. The endothelin system: a critical player in the pathophysiology of preeclampsia. Curr Hypertens Rep. 2018;20(4):32. https://doi.org/10.1007/s11906-018-0828-4.
26. Wang K, Ahmad S, Cai M, et al. Dysregulation of hydrogen sulfide producing enzyme cystathionine γ-lyase contributes to maternal hypertension and placental abnormalities in preeclampsia. Circulation. 2013;127(25):2514–22.
27. Katsouda A, Bibli SI, Pyriochou A, et al. Regulation and role of endogenously produced hydrogen sulfide in angiogenesis. Pharmacol Res. 2016;113(Pt A):175–85.
28. Tirpe AA, Gulei D, Ciortea SM, et al. Hypoxia: overview on hypoxia-mediated mechanisms with a focus on the role of HIF genes. Int J Mol Sci. 2019;20(24):6140. https://doi.org/10.3390/ijms2024614013.
29. Tal R. The role of hypoxia and hypoxia-inducible factor-1alpha in preeclampsia pathogenesis. Biol Reprod. 2012;87(6):134. https://doi.org/10.1095/biolreprod.112.102723.
30. Sriyanti R, Mose JC, Masrul M, Suharti N. The difference in maternal serum hypoxia-inducible factors-1α levels between early onset and late-onset preeclampsia. J Med Sci. 2019;7(13):2133–7.
31. Mendes S, Timóteo-Ferreira F, Almeida H, Silva E. New insights into the process of placentation and the role of oxidative uterine microenvironment. Oxid Med Cell Longev. 2019;2019:9174521. https://doi.org/10.1155/2019/9174521.
32. Ahmada IM,. Zimmermanb MC and Moorec TA (2019). Oxidative stress in early pregnancy and the risk of preeclampsia. Pregnancy Hypertens 18: 99–10.
33. George EM, Granger JP. Heme oxygenase in pregnancy and preeclampsia. Curr Opin Nephrol Hypertens. 2013;22(2). https://doi.org/10.1097/MNH.0b013e32835d19f7.
34. Mannaerts D, Faes E, Gielis J, et al. Oxidative stress and endothelial function in normal pregnancy versus pre-eclampsia, a combined longitudinal and case control study. BMC Pregnancy Childbirth. 2018;18:60. https://doi.org/10.1186/s12884-018-1685-5.
35. Herraiz I, Llurba E, Verlohren S, Galindo A. Update on the diagnosis and prognosis of preeclampsia with the aid of the sFlt-1/PlGF ratio in singleton pregnancies. Fetal Diagn Ther. 2018;43(2):81–9.
36. Lopes Perdigao J, Chinthala S, Mueller A. Angiogenic factor estimation as a warning sign of preeclampsia-related peripartum morbidity among hospitalized patients. Hypertension. 2019;73(4):868–77.

37. Agarwal I, Karumanchi SA. Preeclampsia and the anti-angiogenic state. Pregnancy Hypertens. 2011;1(1):17–21.
38. Umapathy A, Chamley LW, James JL. Reconciling the distinct roles of angiogenic/anti-angiogenic factors in the placenta and maternal circulation of normal and pathological pregnancies. Angiogenesis. 2020;23(2):105–17.
39. Brosens I, Robertson WB, Dixon HG. The physiological response of the vessels of the placental bed to normal pregnancy. J Pathol Bacteriol. 1967;93(2):569–79.
40. Mazar RM, Srinivas SK, Sammel MD, et al. Metabolic score as a novel approach to assessing preeclampsia risk. Am J Obstet Gynecol. 2007;197(4):411.e1–5.
41. Ness RB, Sibai BM. Shared and disparate components of the pathophysiologies of fetal growth restriction and preeclampsia. Am J Obstet Gynecol. 2006;195(1):40–9.
42. Raghupathy R, Al-Azemi M, Azizieh F. Intrauterine growth restriction: cytokine profiles of trophoblast antigen-stimulated maternal lymphocytes. Clin Dev Immunol. 2012;2012:734865. https://doi.org/10.1155/2012/734865.
43. Raghupathy R. Cytokines as key players in the pathophysiology of preeclampsia. Med Princ Pract. 2013;22(Suppl 1):8–19.
44. Rafaeli-Yehudai T, Imterat M, Douvdevani A, et al. Maternal total cell-free DNA in preeclampsia and fetal growth restriction: evidence of differences in maternal response to abnormal implantation. PLoS One. 2018;13(7):e0200360. https://doi.org/10.1371/journal.pone.0200360.
45. Bardos J, Fiorentino D, Longman RE, Paidas M. Immunological role of the maternal uterine microbiome in pregnancy: pregnancies pathologies and alterated microbiota. Front Immunol. 2020;10:2823. https://doi.org/10.3389/fimmu.2019.02823.
46. Duley L. The global impact of pre-eclampsia and eclampsia. Semin Perinatol. 2009;33(3):130–7.
47. Vousden N, Lawley E, Seed PT, et al. Incidence of eclampsia and related complications across 10 low- and middle-resource geographical regions: secondary analysis of a cluster randomised controlled trial. PLoS Med. 2019;16(3):e1002775. https://doi.org/10.1371/journal.pmed.1002775.
48. Osungbade KO, Ige OK. Public health perspectives of preeclampsia in developing countries: implication for health system strengthening. J Pregnancy. 2011. https://doi.org/10.1155/2011/481095.
49. Robillard PY, Dekker G, Scioscia M, Bonsante F, Iacobelli S, Boukerrou M, Hulsey TC. Validation of the 34-week gestation as definition of late onset preeclampsia: testing different cutoffs from 30 to 37 weeks on a population-based cohort of 1700 preeclamptics. Acta Obstet Gynecol Scand. 2020. https://doi.org/10.1111/aogs.13846.
50. Lisonkova S, Joseph KS. Incidence of preeclampsia: risk factors and outcomes associated with early- versus late-onset disease. Am J Obstet Gynecol. 2013;209(6):544.e1–544.e12.
51. Aksornphusitaphong A, Phupong V. Risk factors of early and late onset pre-eclampsia. J Obstet Gynaecol Res. 2013;39(3):627–31.
52. Grum T, Hintsa S, Hagos G. Dietary factors associated with preeclampsia or eclampsia among women in delivery care services in Addis Ababa, Ethiopia: a case control study. BMC Res Notes. 2018;11:683. https://doi.org/10.1186/s13104-018-3793-8.
53. Carolan MC, Davey MA, Biro M, et al. Very advanced maternal age and morbidity in Victoria, Australia: a population based study. BMC Pregnancy Childbirth. 2013;13:80.
54. Wang YA, Chughtai AA, Farquhar CM, et al. Increased incidence of gestational hypertension and preeclampsia after assisted reproductive technology treatment. Fertil Steril. 2016;105(4):920–26 e2.
55. Redman CW. Early and late onset preeclampsia: two sides of the same coin. Pregnancy Hypertens. 2017;7:58.
56. Raymond D, Peterson E. A critical review of early-onset and late-onset preeclampsia. Obstet Gynecol Surv. 2011;66(8):497–506.

57. Valensise H, Vasapollo B, Gagliardi G, Novelli GP. Early and late preeclampsia two different maternal hemodynamic states in the latent phase of the disease. Hypertension. 2008;52:873–80.
58. Bernardes TP, Mol BW, Ravelli ACJ, van den Berg P, Boezen HM, Groen H. Early and late onset pre-eclampsia and small for gestational age risk in subsequent pregnancies. PLoS One. 2020;15(3):e0230483.
59. Amaral LM, Cunningham MW Jr, Cornelius DC, LaMarca B. Preeclampsia: long-term consequences for vascular health. Vasc Health Risk Manag. 2015;11:403–15.
60. Herzoga EM, Egginka AJ, Reijnierse A, et al. Impact of early- and late-onset preeclampsia on features of placental and newborn vascular health. Placenta. 2017;49:72–9.
61. Bassily E, Bell C, Verma S, Patel N, Patel A. Significance of obstetrical history with future cardiovascular disease risk. Am J Med. 2019;132(5):567–71. WHO recommendations: policy of interventionist versus expectant management of severe pre-eclampsia before term. Geneva: World Health Organization; 2018. Licence: CC BY-NC-SA 3.0 IGO.
62. Churchill D, Duley L, Thornton JG, Moussa M, Ali HSM, Walker KF. Interventionist versus expectant care for severe pre-eclampsia between 24 and 34 weeks' gestation. Cochrane Database Syst Rev. 2018;(10). Art. No.: CD003106. https://doi.org/10.1002/14651858.CD003106.pub3.
63. ACOG Practice Bulletin No. 202: Gestational hypertension and preeclampsia.Obstet Gynecol. 2019;133(1):e1–e25.
64. Brown MA, Magee LA, Kenny LC, et al. Hypertensive disorders of pregnancy ISSHP classification, diagnosis, and management recommendations for international practice. Hypertension. 2018;72:24–43.
65. Hypertension in pregnancy: diagnosis and management NICE guideline. 2019. Published: 25 June www.nice.org.uk/guidance/ng133.
66. PlGF-based testing to help diagnose suspected pre-eclampsia (Triage PlGF test, Elecsys immunoassay sFlt-1/PlGF ratio, DELFIA Xpress PlGF 1-2-3 test, and BRAHMS sFlt-1 Kryptor/BRAHMS PlGF plus Kryptor PE ratio). Diagnostics guidance [DG23] Published date:11 May 2016. https://www.nice.org.uk/guidance/dg23.
67. Thangaratinam S, Allotey J, Marlin N, et al. Prediction of complications in early-onset pre-eclampsia (PREP): development and external multinational validation of prognostic models. BMC Med. 2017;15:68. https://doi.org/10.1186/s12916-017-0827-3.
68. Duhig KE, Myers J, Seed PT, et al. Placental growth factor testing to assess women with suspected pre-eclampsia: a multicentre, pragmatic, stepped-wedge cluster-randomised controlled trial. Lancet. 2019;393:1807–18.
69. Nikuei P, Rajaei M, Roozbeh N, et al. Diagnostic accuracy of sFlt1/PlGF ratio as a marker for preeclampsia. BMC Pregnancy Childbirth. 2020;20:80. https://doi.org/10.1186/s12884-020-2744-2.
70. Allen R, Rogozinska E, Sivarajasingam P, Khan KS, Thangaratinam S. Effect of diet- and lifestyle-based metabolic risk-modifying interventions on preeclampsia: a meta-analysis. Acta Obstet Gynecol Scand. 2014;93(10):973–85.
71. Achamrah N, Ditisheim A. Nutritional approach to preeclampsia prevention. Curr Opin Clin Nutr Metab Care. 2018;21(3):168–73.
72. Duley L, Henderson-Smart DJ, Meher S. Altered dietary salt for preventing pre-eclampsia, and its complications. Cochrane Database Syst Rev. 2005;(4). Art. No.: CD005548. https://doi.org/10.1002/14651858.CD005548.
73. Furber CM, McGowan L, Bower P, et al. Antenatal interventions for reducing weight in obese women for improving pregnancy outcome. Cochrane Database Syst Rev. 2013;(1). Art. No.: CD009334. https://doi.org/10.1002/14651858.CD009334.pub2.
74. Makrides M, Crosby DD, Shepherd E, Crowther CA. Magnesium supplementation in pregnancy. Cochrane Database Syst Rev. 2014;(4). Art. No.: CD000937. https://doi.org/10.1002/14651858.CD000937.pub2.

75. Ota E, Mori R, Middleton P, et al. Zinc supplementation for improving pregnancy and infant outcome. Cochrane Database Syst Rev. 2015;(2). Art. No.: CD000230. https://doi.org/10.1002/14651858.CD000230.pub5.
76. Hofmeyr GJ, Manyame S, Medley N, Williams MJ. Calcium supplementation commencing before or early in pregnancy, for preventing hypertensive disorders of pregnancy. Cochrane Database Syst Rev. 2019;(9). Art. No.: CD011192. https://doi.org/10.1002/14651858.CD011192.pub3.
77. Hofmeyr GJ, Betrán AP, Singata-Madlik M, et al. Prepregnancy and early pregnancy calcium supplementation among women at high risk of pre-eclampsia: a multicentre, double-blind, randomised, placebo-controlled trial. Lancet. 2019;393:330–9.
78. Middleton P, Gomersall JC, Gould JF, et al. Omega-3 fatty acid addition during pregnancy. Cochrane Database Syst Rev. 2018;(11):Art. No.: CD003402. https://doi.org/10.1002/14651858.CD003402.pub3.
79. Chen B, Ji X, Zhang L, et al. Fish oil supplementation does not reduce risks of gestational diabetes mellitus, pregnancy-induced hypertension, or pre-eclampsia: a meta-analysis of randomized controlled trials. Med Sci Monit. 2015;21:2322–30.
80. Shennan AH, Duckworth S. Use of vitamin C and E to prevent preeclampsia obstetric. Medicine. 2010;3:121–2.
81. Churchill D, Beevers GDG, Meher S, Rhodes C. Diuretics for preventing pre-eclampsia. Cochrane Database Syst Rev. 2007;(1). Art. No.: CD004451. https://doi.org/10.1002/14651858.CD004451.pub2.
82. Abalos E, Duley L, Steyn DW, Gialdini C. Antihypertensive drug therapy for mild to moderate hypertension during pregnancy. Cochrane Database of Syst Rev. 2018;10:CD002252. https://doi.org/10.1002/14651858.CD002252.pub4.
83. Cooper WO, Hernandez-Diaz S, Arbogast PG, et al. Major congenital malformations after first-trimester exposure to ACE inhibitors. N Engl J Med. 2006;354(23):2443–51.
84. Cadavid AP. Aspirin: the mechanism of action revisited in the context of pregnancy complications. Front Immunol. 2017;8:261. https://doi.org/10.3389/fimmu.2017.00261.
85. CLASP: a randomised trial of low-dose aspirin for the prevention and treatment of pre-eclampsia among 9364 pregnant women. CLASP (Collaborative Low-dose Aspirin Study in Pregnancy) Collaborative Group. Lancet. 1994;343(8898):619–29.
86. Duley L, Henderson-Smart DJ, Knight M, King JF. Antiplatelet agents for preventing pre-eclampsia and its complications. Cochrane Database Syst Rev. 2003;(4). Art. No.: CD004659. https://doi.org/10.1002/14651858.CD004659.
87. Hermida RC, Ayala DE, Iglesias M, et al. Time-dependent effects of low-dose aspirin administration on blood pressure in pregnant women. Hypertension. 1997;30(3 Pt 2):589–95.
88. Macchi L, Sorel N, Christiaens L. Aspirin resistance: definitions, mechanisms, prevalence, and clinical significance. Curr Pharm Des. 2006;12(2):251–8.
89. Navaratnam K, Alfirevic A, Alfirevica Z. Low dose aspirin and pregnancy: how important is aspirin resistance? BJOG. 2016;123(9):1481–7.
90. Shanmugalingam R, Mengesha Z, Notaras S, et al. Factors that influence adherence to aspirin therapy in the prevention of preeclampsia amongst high-risk pregnant women: a mixed method analysis. PLoS One. 2020;15(2):e0229622. https://doi.org/10.1371/journal.pone.0229622.
91. Institute of Medicine. Small clinical trials: issues and challenges. Washington, DC: The National Academies Press; 2001. https://doi.org/10.17226/10078.
92. Karalis DG, Hill AN, Clifton S, Wild RA. The risks of statin use in pregnancy: a systematic review. J Clin Lipidol. 2016. https://doi.org/10.1016/j.jacl.2016.07.002.
93. Brownfoot FC, Tong S, Hannan NJ, et al. Effects of pravastatin on human placenta, endothelium and women with severe preeclampsia. Hypertension. 2015;66:687–97.
94. Kumasawa K, Ikawa M, Kidoya H, et al. Pravastatin induces placental growth factor (PGF) and ameliorates preeclampsia in a mouse model. PNAS. 2011;108:1451–5.

95. Costantine MM. Pravastatin to prevent obstetrical complications in women with antiphospholipid syndrome. J Clin Invest. 2016;126(8):2792–4.
96. Ahmed A, Williams DJ, Cheed V, et al. Pravastatin for early-onset pre-eclampsia: a randomised, blinded, placebo-controlled trial. BJOG. 2020;127(4):478–88.
97. Riu DS, Sunarno I, Lukas E, Wewengkang ET, Amalia R. The effect of pravastatin on endothelin-1 levels and pregnancy outcomes in women who have a high risk for preeclampsia: a randomized control trial. Enferm Clin. 2020;30 Suppl 2:499–505.
98. Diagnosis, evaluation, and management of the hypertensive disorders of pregnancy. Society of Obstetricians and Gynaecologists of Canada (SOGC) Clinical Practice guideline. J Obstet Gynaecol Can. 2008;30(7):S. http://www.sogc.org/guidelines/documents/gui206CPG0803_001.pdf.
99. Rolnik D, Wright D, Poon LC, et al. Aspirin versus placebo in pregnancies at high risk for preterm preeclampsia. N Engl J Med. 2017;377:613–22.
100. Homuth V, Dechend R, Luft FC. When should pregnant women with an elevated blood pressure be treated? Nephrol Dial Transplant. 2003;18(8):1456–7.
101. Magee LA, von Dadelszen P, Singer J, et al. The CHIPS randomized controlled trial (Control of Hypertension in Pregnancy Study) is severe hypertension just an elevated blood pressure? Hypertension. 2016;68:1153–9.
102. James R, Nelson-Piercy C. Management of hypertension before, during, and after pregnancy. Heart. 2004;90:1499–504.
103. ACOG Committee Opinion No. 767: Emergent Therapy for Acute-Onset, Severe Hypertension During Pregnancy and the Postpartum Period. Obstet Gynecol. 2019;133(2):e174–e180.
104. Duley L, Meher S, Jones L. Drugs for treatment of very high blood pressure during pregnancy. Cochrane Database Syst Rev. 2013;(7). Art. No.: CD001449. https://doi.org/10.1002/14651858.CD001449.pub3.
105. Easterling T, Mundle S, Bracken H. Oral antihypertensive regimens (nifedipine retard, labetalol, and methyldopa) for management of severe hypertension in pregnancy: an open-label, randomised controlled trial. Lancet. 2019;394:1011–21.

Chapter 41
Gestational Diabetes

Renato Augusto Moreira de Sá and Eduardo Borges da Fonseca

Introduction

The prevalence of diabetes in pregnancy has been increasing. The majority is gestational diabetes mellitus (GDM) with the remainder primarily preexisting type 1 diabetes and type 2 diabetes. We may concern that the rise in GDM and type 2 diabetes occurs in parallel with obesity worldwide. Type 1 diabetes and type 2 diabetes in pregnancy confer significantly greater maternal and fetal risk than GDM, with some differences according to type of diabetes [1].

In general, specific risks of uncontrolled diabetes in pregnancy include spontaneous abortion, fetal anomalies, preeclampsia, fetal demise, macrosomia, neonatal hypoglycemia, and neonatal hyperbilirubinemia, among others. In addition, diabetes in pregnancy may increase the risk of obesity and type 2 diabetes in offspring later in life [2].

Gestational Diabetes

GDM develops during pregnancy in women whose pancreatic function is insufficient to overcome the insulin resistance associated with the pregnant state. It is characterized by increased risk of macrosomia and birth complications and an increased risk of maternal type 2 diabetes after pregnancy. Macrosomia and birth complications risks increase with progressive hyperglycemia [3].

R. A. Moreira de Sá (✉)
Fernandes Figueira Institut - FIOCRUZ, Rio de Janeiro, RJ, Brazil

E. B. d. Fonseca
Maternal Fetal Medicine Group - Nova Diagnóstico por Imagem, João Pessoa, PB, Brazil

Ob/Gyn Department, Federal University of Paraiba, João Pessoa, PB, Brazil

© Springer Nature Switzerland AG 2022

R. A. Moreira de Sá, E. B. d. Fonseca (eds.), *Perinatology*,
https://doi.org/10.1007/978-3-030-83434-0_41

The term "gestational diabetes" has been defined as any degree of glucose intolerance with the onset or first recognition during pregnancy. Women with probable preexisting diabetes that is first recognized during early pregnancy may be distinguish from those whose disease is a transient manifestation of pregnancy-related insulin resistance and diagnosed in the late second or the third trimester [4]. GDM is defined when diabetes is diagnosed in the second or third trimester of pregnancy and was not clearly overt diabetes prior to gestation [5].

The prevalence varies worldwide and among racial and ethnic groups, generally in parallel with the prevalence of type 2 diabetes [6].

Risk factors for GDM defined by the American Diabetes Association (ADA) and American College of Obstetricians and Gynecologists (ACOG) include a prior history of GDM, glycated hemoglobin ≥5.7 percent (impaired glucose tolerance or impaired fasting glucose on previous testing), a family history (first degree relative) of diabetes, a prior macrosomic or large-for-gestational age infant, sustained glycosuria, a prior unexplained late intrauterine fetal demise, hypertension, polycystic ovary syndrome, or obesity [body mass index (BMI) ≥25 kg/m^2]. Such patients should have early testing for GDM at 16–20 weeks. If the early testing is negative, this should be repeated at 24–28 weeks [5, 6].

GDM diagnosis is based on the results of the fasting 75 g oral glucose tolerance test (OGTT) performed during pregnancy at 24–28 weeks of gestation (IADPSG: International Association of the Diabetes and Pregnancy Study Groups; ADA: American Diabetes Association), for women who have not been previously diagnosed with diabetes. Although it is also universally used to diagnose diabetes outside of pregnancy, this is an imprecise test with poor reproducibility, and there is no consensus regarding the optimum thresholds for a positive test. One or more elevated level is sufficient for a diagnosis of GDM (Table 41.1). If a fasting glucose test has been performed for other reasons and shows an elevated value, this may be accepted as diagnostic of GDM [5].

Table 41.1 International Association of the Diabetes and Pregnancy Study Groups and American Diabetes Association criteria for a positive 2-hour 75 gram oral glucose tolerance test for the diagnosis of gestational diabetes

Diagnosis	Time	Plasma glucose level (one or more)
GDM	Fasting	≥92 mg/dL to 125 (5.1–6.9 mmol/L)
	1 hour	≥180 mg/dL (10.0 mmol/L)
	2 hours	≥153 mg/dL (8.5 mmol/L)

Management of Gestational Diabetes Mellitus

The risk of GDM may be reduced by diet, exercise, and lifestyle counseling, particularly when interventions are started during the first or early in the second trimester. Table 41.2 summarizes the management of gestational diabetes. Glucose monitoring aims for the following targets [1]:

- Fasting glucose <95 mg/dL (5.3 mmol/L)
- One-hour postprandial glucose <140 mg/dL (7.8 mmol/L)
- Two-hour postprandial glucose <120 mg/dL (6.7 mmol/L)

Table 41.2 Management of gestational diabetes for mother control

Aspect	Considerations
Models of care	A multidisciplinary team approach is ideal Women without other risk factors and with well-managed diet-treated GDM may be suitable for low risk models of care although closer surveillance/more frequent antenatal contact is still required
Lifestyle management	After diagnosis, treatment starts with medical nutrition therapy, physical activity, and weight management depending on pregestational weight Glucose monitoring aims for the targets recommended above
Nutrition therapy	The food plan should provide adequate calorie intake to promote fetal/neonatal and maternal health, achieve glycemic goals, and promote adequate weight gain The food plan should be based on a nutrition assessment with guidance from the Dietary Reference Intakes (DRI). The DRI for all pregnant women recommends a minimum of 175 g of carbohydrate, a minimum of 71 g of protein, and 28 g of fiber. The diet should not be high in saturated fat
Pharmacologic therapy	Insulin: both multiple daily insulin injections and continuous subcutaneous insulin infusion are reasonable delivery strategies, and neither has been shown to be superior to the other during pregnancy. Treatment of GDM with lifestyle and insulin has been demonstrated to improve perinatal outcomes Sulfonylureas are known to cross the placenta and have been associated with increased neonatal hypoglycemia. Concentrations of glyburide in umbilical cord plasma are approximately 50–70% of maternal levels. Glyburide was associated with a higher rate of neonatal hypoglycemia and macrosomia than insulin or metformin Metformin was associated with a lower risk of neonatal hypoglycemia and less maternal weight gain than insulin in systematic reviews. However, metformin readily crosses the placenta, resulting in umbilical cord blood levels of metformin as high or higher than simultaneous maternal levels. Metformin exposure may be associated to smaller neonates with acceleration of postnatal growth resulting in higher BMI in childhood. Due to the potential for growth restriction or acidosis in the setting of placental insufficiency, metformin should not be used in women with hypertension or preeclampsia or at risk for intrauterine growth restriction

The dose of insulin varies in different individuals because of varied rates of obesity, ethnic characteristics, degree of hyperglycemia, and other demographic criteria, but the majority of studies have reported a total insulin dose ranging from 0.7 to 2 units per kg (present pregnant weight) to achieve glucose control. For women with gestational diabetes mellitus, common practice is to initiate insulin therapy when target glucose levels are exceeded despite nutritional therapy. The dose and type of insulin used is calculated based upon the specific abnormality of blood glucose noted during monitoring. One principle we have found useful is to start with the simplest regimen and increase the complexity as needed to address the particular situation [7].

The insulin can be divided 50 percent as intermediate-acting insulin, such as neutral protamine hagedorn (NPH) (given in two equal doses before breakfast and before bedtime), and 50 percent as three preprandial rapid-acting insulin injections; however, it may be possible to omit the lunchtime dose in some patients [7].

For patients whose glucose levels are not well controlled, an alternative approach to insulin therapy is described below:

- If insulin is required because the fasting blood glucose concentration is high, an intermediate-acting insulin, such as NPH insulin, is given before bedtime; an initial dose of 0.2 unit/kg body weight is utilized [7].
- If postprandial blood glucose concentrations are high, rapid-acting insulin analogs such as insulin aspart or insulin lispro are given before meals at a dose calculated to be 1.5 units per 10 g carbohydrate in the breakfast meal and 1 unit per 10 g carbohydrate in the lunch and dinner meals [7].
- If both preprandial and postprandial blood glucose concentrations are high or if the woman's postprandial glucose levels can only be blunted if starvation ketosis occurs, then a six injection per day regimen is utilized. The total starting dose is 0.7 units/kg up to week 12, 0.8 units/kg for weeks 13–26, 0.9 units/kg for weeks 26–36, and 1.0 unit/kg for weeks 36 to term. In obese women with higher body mass indexes (BMIs), the initial doses of insulin may need to be increased to 1.5–2.0 units/kg to overcome the combined insulin resistance of pregnancy and obesity [7].

Preexisting Diabetes (Type 1 and Type 2) in Pregnancy

The term "preexisting diabetes in pregnancy" refers to diabetes diagnosed before pregnancy. The prevalence of preexisting diabetes has increased in the past decade primarily as a result of the increase in type 2 diabetes. Women with preexisting diabetes show higher rates of complications compared to the general population, including perinatal mortality, congenital malformations, hypertension, preterm delivery, large-for-gestational-age (LGA) infants, cesarean delivery, and other neonatal morbidities. There is an increase in insulin requirements in the first trimester, followed by a decrease. In the second trimester, there is a rapidly increasing insulin resistance, requiring weekly increases in insulin dose of about 5% per week to achieve glycemic targets. There is roughly a doubling of insulin requirements by the late third trimester [8].

Women with type 1 diabetes have an increased risk of hypoglycemia in the first trimester and, like all women, have altered counterregulatory response in pregnancy that may decrease hypoglycemia awareness. Despite of this, pregnancy is a ketogenic state, and women with type 1 diabetes, and to a lesser extent those with type 2 diabetes, are at risk for diabetic ketoacidosis at lower blood glucose levels than in the nonpregnant state [5, 8].

Type 2 diabetes is often associated with obesity. Glycemic control is often easier to achieve in women with type 2 diabetes than in those with type 1 diabetes but can require much higher doses of insulin, sometimes necessitating concentrated insulin formulations [8].

Insulin is the preferred agent for the management of both type 1 diabetes and type 2 diabetes in pregnancy because it does not cross the placenta and because oral agents are generally insufficient to overcome the insulin resistance in type 2 diabetes and are ineffective in type 1 diabetes [5, 8].

Frequent self-monitoring of blood glucose in pregnant women with type 1 diabetes is essential during pregnancy in order to achieve the glycemic control associated with better outcomes. Preprandial testing is used to guide mealtime insulin dose adjustment and postprandial testing to meet postprandial targets. Due to the increased risk of nocturnal hypoglycemia with any intensive insulin therapy, self-monitoring of blood glucose during the night is often necessary in pregnant women with diabetes receiving insulin [8].

Self-monitoring of blood glucose four to seven times per day is also recommended for pregnant women with type 2 diabetes (i.e., fasting, preprandial, and 1 or 2 hours' postprandially) to achieve good glycemic control, which is associated with less macrosomia and reduced preeclampsia. An important first step in achieving optimal glycemic control is to set target blood glucose levels. However, optimal targets for fasting, preprandial, and postprandial blood glucose levels in women with preexisting diabetes vary in clinical practice [8].

In women suspected of preterm delivery, two doses of betamethasone is often given to aid in the maturation of the fetal lungs. Table 41.3 shows a management of

Table 41.3 Management of pregnant women with diabetes on insulin receiving betamethasone

Day (Following the first dose of betamethasone)	Adjustment
01	Increase the night insulin dose by 25%
02	Following the first dose of betamethasone
03	
04	Increase all insulin doses by 20%
05	Increase all insulin doses by 10–20%
06	Gradually taper insulin doses to pre-betamethasone doses
07	

pregnant women with diabetes on insulin receiving betamethasone to prevent severe hyperglycemia and severe hypoglycemia [9].

Fetal Environment

Pathophysiological Aspects

The fetal hemodynamic repercussions on diabetes during pregnancy are still not completely understood. Fetal injuries or even death can result from hyperglycemia with hyperinsulinemia [3]. In diabetes, maternal predisposition and placental factors result in progressively decreased glucose tolerance with secondary fetal repercussions that normally appear in the third trimester. The underlying concept is related to a subclinical pathology that progresses to clinical manifestation that also results in fetal involvement and that has a placental component as part of its etiology [10].

The degree of preexisting vulnerability to metabolic deterioration determines the time of onset, the severity of the clinical disease, and the potential for placental and fetal complications. However, the relationship between the degree of glycemic control and placental changes remains unclear. Figure 41.1 shows the short-term fetal and neonatal complications of intrauterine exposure to maternal hyperglycemia

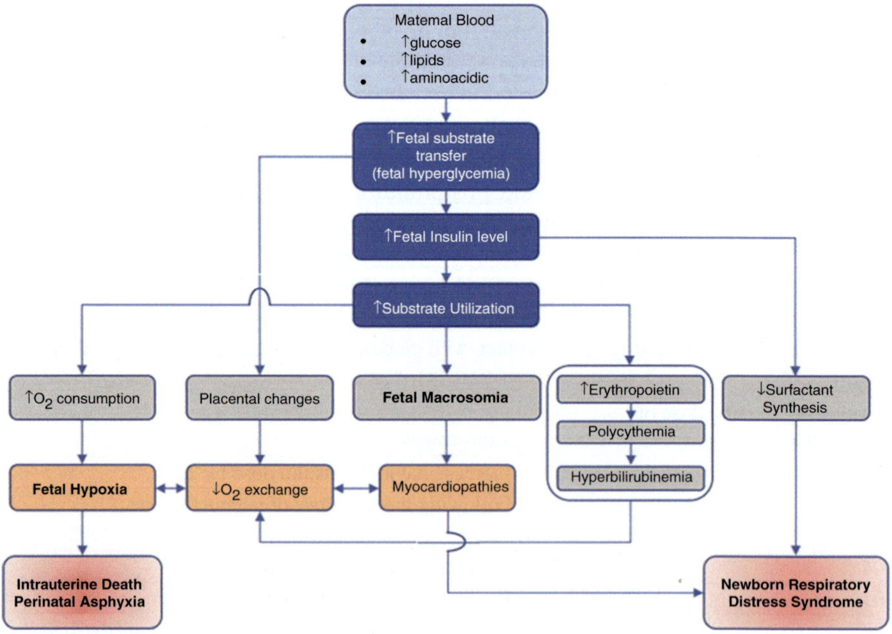

Fig. 41.1 Sequence of changes related to fetal complications in diabetes

[11]. While some studies support the concept that the degree of damage is proportional to the degree of hyperglycemia, others have shown that even under strict glycemic control regimen, there are still histological differences in the placentas of diabetic pregnant women compared to nondiabetic ones [12, 13].

Macroscopically, the diabetic placenta is characterized by an increase in size and weight, resulting in an increase in the relationship between the weight of the placenta and the fetus. These changes are proportional to the degree of hyperglycemia and suggest that, in the diabetic environment, the placenta grows first and then contributes to fetal growth accelerated by the increase in glucose, as well as the transfer of other nutrients [10].

Microscopically and independently of the maternal glycemic state, various degrees of changes in the syncytiotrophoblast, cytotrophoblast, trophoblastic basement membrane, and fetal vessels are observed in all ranges of diabetic severity; the lesions found in the placentas of diabetic women are [10]:

1. Villous fibrinoid necrosis: a condition in which the villous stroma is replaced by fibrinoid material and villous immaturity is observed with a decrease in the formation of terminal villi. These changes can affect the maternal-fetal distribution of nutrients and gas exchange and, consequently, can be precursors of unexpected fetal complications, such as stillbirth.
2. Chorioangiosis and vascular hyperplasia of the chorionic villi or, if so, a proliferation of capillaries in the terminal villi in the placenta, which translates into an attempt to supply a possible fetal hypoxia, may be the result of increased vascular recruitment that occurs with placental overgrowth.
3. Placental infarction and evidence of ischemia or Tenney-Parker alterations: Tenney-Parker alterations are representative of syncytiotrophoblast hypertrophy and are characterized by the formation of prominent syncytial nodes and numerous clusters of nuclei in the veins, which signal the premature aging of the placenta, resulting in increased maturation of branched villi, as well as an increase in the number of fetal nucleated red blood cells as a marker of chronic fetal hypoxemia.

In general, the placenta of the diabetic pregnant woman is subjected to opposite stimuli, on the one hand the acceleration of growth mediated by glucose and on the other hand the decrease in vascular development. Thus, the increase in the size of the placenta and the increase in the distance of interventional diffusion in immature villi predispose the fetus to sudden changes in the exchange of gases and nutrients due to inadequate perfusion [10].

The glucose metabolism, in the fetus and placenta, is characterized by an adequate balance between exogenous glucose (from the mother and the placenta) and its use by the fetus (directly or by lactate production). The utilization and oxidation of glucose by the fetus is mediated by the maternal concentration of glucose and insulin which, acting synergistically, substitute the oxidation of glucose for that of other energy substrates and direct the metabolization of glucose to glycogen, fat, and protein [14].

Relative fetal hypoxia, secondary to high insulin-induced glucose uptake and metabolic rate, causes increased erythropoietin secretion and, as a consequence, increased fetal red blood cell production. The incidence and severity of polycythemia are associated with poor maternal glycemic control [11].

Fetal hyperinsulinemia increases the supply of glucose to the placenta, its use by the fetus, and the consumption of oxygen and, as a consequence, decreases the amount of arterial oxygen. Hyperglycemia, in turn, is responsible for gross changes in oxygen transport and fetal metabolism, causing a plasma decrease in pH, an increase in pCO_2, lactate concentration, and erythropoietin. The main hypothesis for the onset of fetal distress in these cases is the occurrence of edema of the chorial villi induced by osmolarity, hindering placental gas exchange [15].

In addition, clinical complications of diabetes can increase the supply of acid radiocarbons to the fetus, such as ketoacidosis. Another relevant factor is the proportionality between the rate of use of O_2 and the body mass of the fetus. Normal O_2 levels for AGA fetuses may be insufficient for macrosomic fetuses, with increased metabolism as a result of hyperglycemia and hyperinsulinemia. Fetal death occurs when your metabolic O_2 needs are greater than your placental transport capacity. An inverse correlation is observed between maternal glycemia in uncontrolled diabetic pregnant women and the newborn's pH, that is, the higher the mother's glycemic levels, the lower the newborn's pH [15]. Both hyperinsulinemia and hyperglycemia by independent mechanisms negatively influence fetal development, resulting in fetal macrosomia and hypoxia. High glucose levels are accompanied by oxidative stress with changes in the activities of antioxidant enzymes, impaired glutathione metabolism, and decreased levels of ascorbic acid. Free radicals oxidize components of the lipid membrane and produce changes in the lipid bilayer of cell membranes, changing their adaptability to capillary circulation, promoting platelet hyperaggregation, and shortening the half-life mainly in erythrocytes. These circumstances also contribute to fetal hypoperfusion [16].

Another relevant factor in the fetal response is the propensity to develop hypertrophic myocardiopathy (most of the time asymptomatic) due to exposure to maternal hyperglycemia and hyperinsulinism. Cardiomyopathy mainly affects the interventricular septum, but it can extend to the myocardium and sometimes lead to severe morbidity and mortality, according to the severity of the aortic obstruction and the extent of cardiac hypertrophy [11].

Evaluation of the Fetal Response

All procedures available to assess fetal well-being in gestational diabetes and also preexisting diabetes lack precision. They are not liable to identify true fetal distress, with false positive rates ranging from 25% to 50%. So far, the evidence indicates that the normalization of maternal glycemia is the main factor to improve perinatal results. Perinatal mortality in the controlled diabetic population, if corrected by congenital malformations, is similar to that of nondiabetic pregnant women [15].

Fetal Management

The main objective of antenatal management in diabetic pregnant women should be the prevention of congenital anomalies, fetal macrosomia, hypertrophic cardiomyopathy, respiratory distress syndrome in the newborn, and fetal/neonatal death. The strongest evidence suggests that the best way to guarantee fetal well-being is to maintain normal, or close to normal, maternal glycemic levels at all stages of pregnancy [17].

The use of biophysical tests, on the other hand, is no less confusing. There is not enough data in the literature to ensure the best tests and the interval at which they should be repeated. Doppler velocimetry does not show the same efficiency in monitoring fetuses compromised by diabetes as when used in the evaluation of fetuses suffering from placental insufficiency [18].

The protocol proposed in Fig. 41.2 is what seems, at the moment, the most appropriate for the diagnosis of the health of the child born to a diabetic mother [19, 20]. Furthermore, it should be noted that:

- ***Childbirth*** should be scheduled according to the severity of the diabetes and cesarean section should be indicated whenever fetal vitality is compromised at gestational age compatible with a viable concept.
- Strict control of maternal blood glucose is imperative, a conduct that most contributes to reducing perinatal mortality and morbidity.

Intrapartum Management

Changes in glucose and insulin requirements during labor mandate monitoring blood glucose concentration in women who have been treated with insulin or oral antihyperglycemic drugs during pregnancy. The frequency of monitoring depends on the phase of labor, diet, and whether exogenous insulin is being administered. Capillary blood glucose measurements are convenient and reasonably accurate over the normal range of blood glucose concentrations. Overt hypoglycemia (<50 mg/dL [2.8 mmol/L]) or hyperglycemia (>180 mg/dL [10 mmol/L]) detected in capillary blood should be treated promptly [21].

The optimum frequency of glucose monitoring required to maintain target glucose levels has not been established. Glycemic control depends on endogenous insulin secretion and insulin resistance; thus, closer monitoring is required in women with type 1 diabetes than in many women with type 2 or gestational diabetes. Table 41.4 summarizes glucose control during labor phases [21].

Postpartum

After delivery of the placenta, the insulin-resistant state that characterizes pregnancy rapidly dissipates and insulin requirements drop precipitously. Glucose targets can be relaxed to avoid hypoglycemia from overtreatment. All diabetes

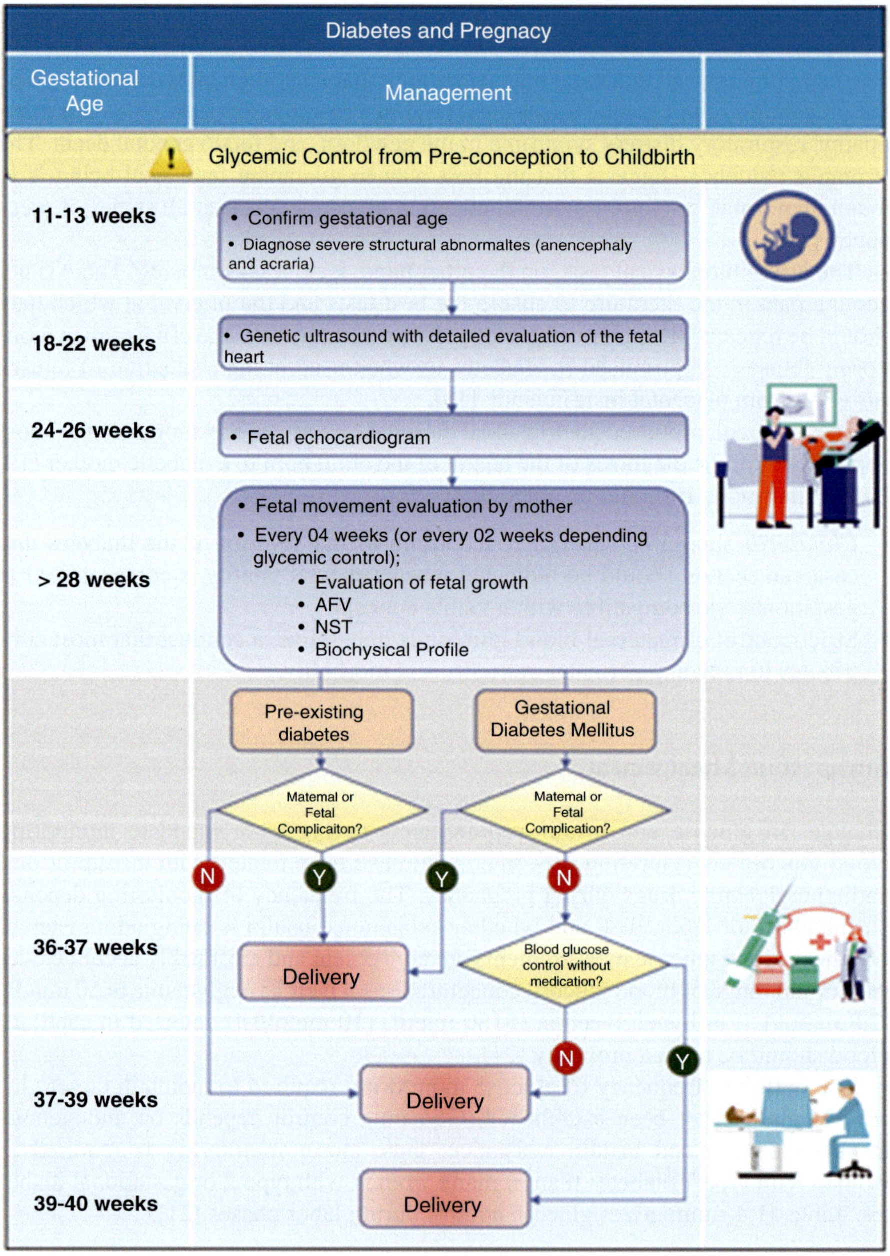

Fig. 41.2 Flowchart for fetal monitoring and guidance on the time of delivery in pregnancy complicated by diabetes. AFV amniotic fluid volume, NST nonstress test

Table 41.4 Blood glucose control during labor phases

Classification	Management
Pregestational diabetes	Latent phase: measure glucose levels every 2–4 hours in women with reduced oral intake and type 1 or type 2 diabetes or diabetes diagnosed in early pregnancy (as these women are likely to have undiagnosed type 2 diabetes). If the woman is eating, monitor capillary glucose levels before and after meals Active phase: measure glucose levels every hour in women receiving insulin supplementation either by infusion or subcutaneous injection
Gestational diabetes	Women with gestational diabetes who have maintained euglycemia antenatally on diet, lifestyle, and/or medical therapy rarely develop intrapartum hyperglycemia A blood glucose level is measured on admission Latent phase: monitor capillary glucose levels before and after meals in women who are eating. In the absence of significant oral intake, check glucose levels no more frequently than every 4–6 hours, which is as efficacious as hourly assessment when the goal is to avoid neonatal hypoglycemia. Monitoring frequency can be decreased in women with glucose values consistently within the target range. Women with glucose levels below or above target ranges should receive appropriate therapy and more frequent monitoring Active phase: similar to latent phase

medications should be stopped after delivery for women with GDM. Women with type 1 diabetes have markedly reduced insulin requirements for the first 24 to 48 hours after delivery and need frequent monitoring of glucose levels to avoid hypoglycemia. Postoperative patients should receive a 5 percent dextrose (0.45 normal saline) solution with no more than half of their basal insulin until adequate oral intake is resumed. Glucose levels should be checked every 4–6 hours and hyperglycemia treated with insulin prescribed using sliding scales. Similarly, patients on insulin pumps should have basal rates reduced by at least one-half and can administer correction doses via their pump using the prescribed sliding scale [21].

After approximately 24–48 hours, standard diabetes management can be resumed with calculated total daily dose of insulin at 0.6 units/kg postpartum weight or approximately 50 percent of the insulin dose prior to delivery. Women delivering vaginally generally resume normal oral intake after delivery. They can be restarted on their multiple daily dosing regimen but require one-third to one-half of their predelivery long-acting or intermediate-acting insulin dose to meet postpartum basal needs and one-third to one-half of their predelivery short- or rapid-acting insulin premeal doses [21].

Glucose levels tend to be normal or modestly elevated in postpartum women with type 2 diabetes. Fasting, preprandial, and postprandial glucose levels should be measured. Hyperglycemia is treated with insulin prescribed using a sliding scale [21].

Women with GDM should be encouraged to breastfeed immediately after delivery and for at least 4 months postpartum, as this may contribute to the reduction of neonatal hypoglycemia and offspring obesity and prevent the development of metabolic syndrome and type 2 diabetes in the mother [20].

Longer duration and more intense breastfeeding are associated with less diabetes in the mother. Furthermore, offspring that are breastfed for at least 4 months have lower incidence of obesity and diabetes longer term. However, GDM is associated with either similar or poor initiation rates compared to those without diabetes, as well as poor continuation rates. Factors associated with cessation of breastfeeding before 3 months include breastfeeding challenges at home, return to work, inadequate support, cesarean section, and lower socioeconomic status [20].

Women with preexisting diabetes tend to have delayed milk production. There is a greater delay in lactation onset in mothers with type 1 diabetes who had poor glycemic control. Women with type 1 diabetes also discontinue breastfeeding at a higher rate during the first week postpartum. Overall, women with any form of diabetes during pregnancy have more nursing difficulties with lower milk supply than women without diabetes. However, once established, lactation persists and duration is similar in mothers with and without diabetes [20].

In conclusion, women with GDM and preexisting diabetes should be encouraged to breastfeed as long as possible as intensity and duration of nursing have both infant and maternal benefits, but more support is needed as this group is at risk for early cessation.

Newborn Care

Risk of neonatal hypoglycemia correlates with quality of glycemic management more than type of diabetes and is increased if insulin is required during labor. Newborn must be kept warm (36.5–37.2 °C), and early skin-to-skin contact and drying the newborn after birth are important [22].

Initiate early feeds within 30–60 minutes of birth and encourage feeding at least 3 hourly or more frequently [21].

Perform blood glucose control prior to second feed or within 3 hours of birth if baby has fed effectively, at 2 hours of age if the baby has not fed effectively, and every 4–6 hours pre-feeds until monitoring ceases. If feeding is unsuccessful, recheck blood glucose and observe for signs of neonatal hypoglycemia, and initiate additional blood glucose control monitoring if hypoglycemia is detected [21].

Final Considerations

Diabetes in pregnancy is associated with risks to the woman and to the developing fetus. Miscarriage, preeclampsia, and preterm labor are more common in women with preexisting diabetes. In addition, diabetic retinopathy can worsen rapidly during pregnancy. Stillbirth, congenital malformations, macrosomia, birth injury, perinatal mortality, and postnatal adaptation problems (such as hypoglycemia) are more common in babies born to women with preexisting diabetes.

Figure 41.3 summarizes recommendations for managing diabetes in pregnancy. We must pay attention on areas where additional or different care should be offered to women with diabetes and their newborn babies.

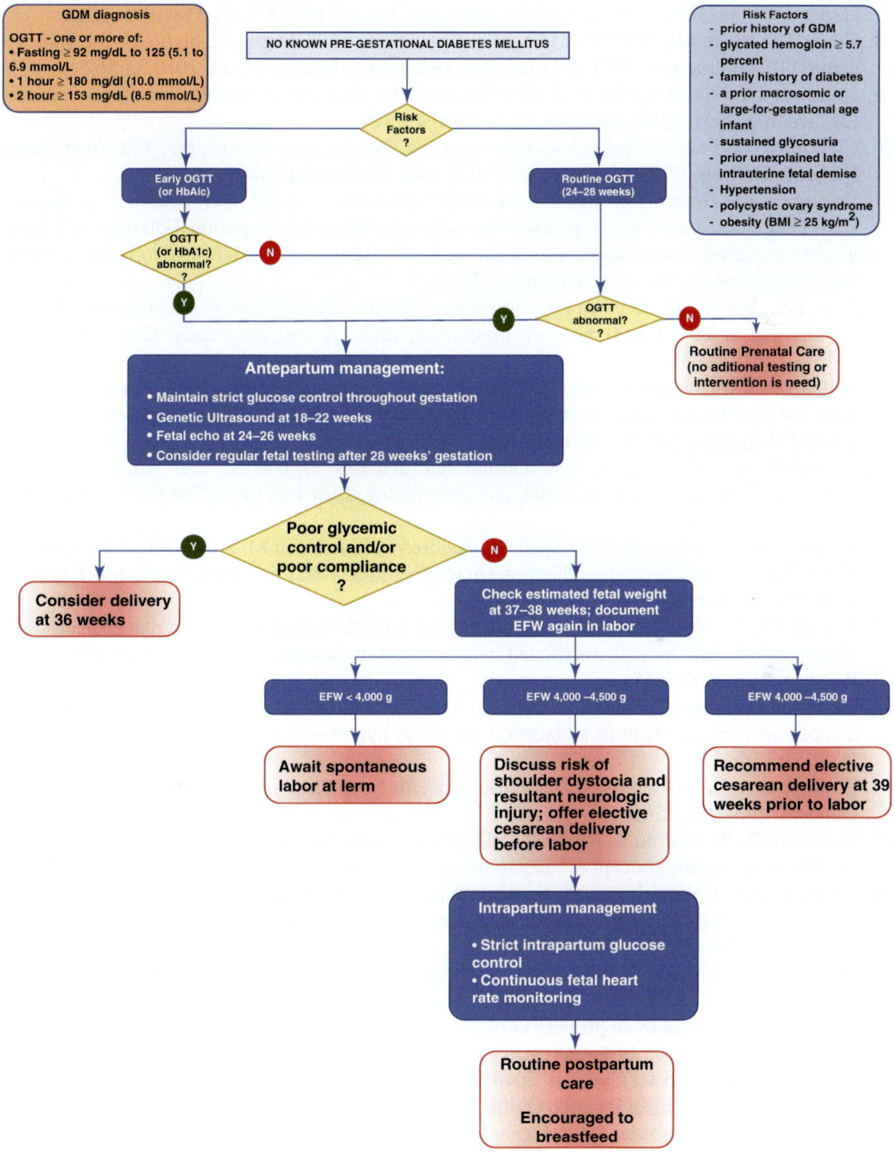

Fig. 41.3 Flowchart of managing diabetes in pregnancy. GDM gestational diabetes mellitus, OGTT oral glucose tolerance test, EFW estimated fetal weight

References

1. American Diabetes Association. 14. Management of diabetes in pregnancy: standards of medical care in diabetes-2020. Diabetes Care. 2020;43(Suppl 1):S183–92.
2. Dabelea D, Hanson RL, Lindsay RS, et al. Intrauterine exposure to diabetes conveys risks for type 2 diabetes and obesity: a study of discordant sibships. Diabetes. 2000;49:2208–11.
3. Metzger BE, Lowe LP, Dyer AR, HAPO Study Cooperative Research Group, et al. Hyperglycemia and adverse pregnancy outcomes. N Engl J Med. 2008;358:1991–2002.
4. Cowie CC, Rust KF, Byrd-Holt DD, et al. Prevalence of diabetes and high risk for diabetes using A1C criteria in the U.S. population in 1988–2006. Diabetes Care. 2010;33:562.
5. American Diabetes Association. 2. Classification and diagnosis of diabetes: standards of medical care in diabetes-2020. Diabetes Care. 2020;43:S14.
6. Committee on Practice Bulletins—Obstetrics. ACOG Practice Bulletin No. 190: Gestational Diabetes Mellitus. Obstet Gynecol. 2018;131:e49. Reaffirmed 2019.
7. Durnwald C. Gestational diabetes mellitus: glycemic control and maternal prognosis. UpToDate. Available in: https://www.uptodate.com/contents/gestational-diabetes-mellitus-glycemic-control-and-maternal-prognosis?search=gestational%20diabetes&topicRef=6797&source=see_link. Assessed at September 2020.
8. Feig DS, Berger H, Donovan L, Diabetes Canada Clinical Practice Guidelines Expert Committee, et al. Clinical practice guidelines. diabetes and pregnancy. Can J Diabetes. 2018;42(2018):S255–82.
9. Mathiesen ER, Christensen AB, Hellmuth E, et al. Insulin dose during gluco- corticoid treatment for fetal lung maturation in diabetic pregnancy: test of an algorithm [correction of analgoritm]. Acta Obstet Gynecol Scand. 2002;81:835–9.
10. Gabbay-Benziv R, Baschat AA. Gestational diabetes as one of the "great obstetrical syndromes"--the maternal, placental, and fetal dialog. Best Pract Res Clin Obstet Gynaecol. 2015;29(2):150–5.
11. Mitanchez D, Yzydorczyk C, Siddeek B, Boubred F, Benahmed M, Simeoni U. The offspring of the diabetic mother-short- and long-term implications. Best Pract Res Clin Obstet Gynaecol. 2015;29(2):256–69.
12. Laurini RN, Visser GHA, van Ballegooie E, et al. Morphological findings in placentas of insulin-dependent diabetic patients treated with continuous subcutaneous insulin infusion (CSII). Placenta. 1987;8:153e65.
13. Desoye G, Korgun ET, Ghaffari-Tabrizi N, et al. Is fetal macrosomia inadequately controlled diabetic women the result of a placental defect? A hypothesis. J Matern Fetal Neonatal Med. 2002;11:258e61.
14. Kontopoulos E, Vintzileos A. Condition-specific antepartum fetal testing. Am J Obstet Gynecol. 2004;191:1546–51.
15. Yessoufou A, Moutairou K. Maternal diabetes in pregnancy: early and long-term outcomes on the offspring and the concept of "metabolic memory". Exp Diabetes Res. 2011;2011:218598.
16. Torres-Cuevas I, Parra-Llorca A, Sánchez-Illana A, Nuñez-Ramiro A, Kuligowski J, Cháfer-Pericás C, Cernada M, Escobar J, Vento M. Oxygen and oxidative stress in the perinatal period. Redox Biol. 2017;12:674–81.
17. Nurain MN, Marmuji LZ, Mastura I, Michael FH, Barakatun-Nisak MY, Yusof M, Rohana AG, Norasyikin AW, Nazatul SI, Adam NL, Mustafa N, Balchin I, Dhalliwal R. Management of diabetes in pregnancy in primary care. Malays Fam Physician. 2019;14(3):55–9.
18. Committee on Practice Bulletins—Obstetrics: ACOG Practice Bulletin No. 190: gestational diabetes mellitus. Obstet Gynecol. 2018;131(2): e49–e64.
19. Diabetes Canada Clinical Practice Guidelines Expert C, Feig DS, Berger H, et al. Diabetes and pregnancy. Can J Diabetes. 2018;42 Suppl 1:S255–S82.
20. Hod M, Kapur A, Sacks DA, et al. The International Federation of Gynecology and Obstetrics (FIGO) initiative on gestational diabetes mellitus: a pragmatic guide for diagnosis, management, and care. Int J Gynaecol Obstet. 2015;131 Suppl 3:S173–211.

21. Kjos S. Pregestational (preexisting) and gestational diabetes: intrapartum and postpartum glycemic control. UpToDate. Available in: https://www.uptodate.com/contents/pregestational-preexisting-and-gestational-diabetes-intrapartum-and-postpartumglycemic-control?search=gestational%20 diabetes&topicRef=6790&source=see_link. Assessed at September 2020.
22. Queensland Clinical Guidelines. Neonatal hypoglycaemia. Guideline No. MN13.8-V4-R18. Queensland Health. 2013. Available from: http://www.health.qld.gov.au/qcg/.

Chapter 42
Complications of Monochorionic Twin Pregnancy: Double Trouble?

Alexandra Matias and Miguel Pereira-Macedo

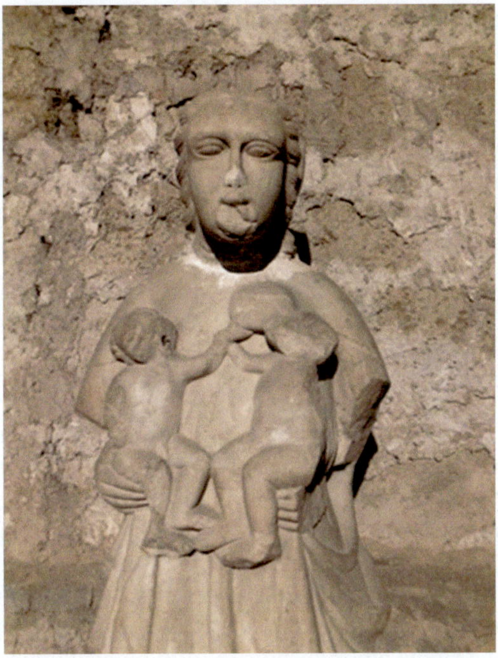

Somewhere in Naples…

A. Matias (✉)
Department of Obstetrics, Gynecology and Pediatrics, Faculty of Medicine University of Porto, Centro Hospitalar Universitário Hospital of S. João, Porto, Portugal

M. Pereira-Macedo
Centro Hospitalar Universitário Lisboa Central, Lisbon, Portugal

© Springer Nature Switzerland AG 2022
R. A. Moreira de Sá, E. B. d. Fonseca (eds.), *Perinatology*,
https://doi.org/10.1007/978-3-030-83434-0_42

Monochorionicity: What We Know

Multiple pregnancy has boomed since the 1980s up until the early 2000s, especially in the United States. According to the National Center for Health Statistics, the number of twin pregnancies soared more than 75% in the last 30 years, and, in 2018, in the United States, there were about 33 twins born per 1000 births. An "epidemic" of multiple pregnancies was observed in the world in the last 30 years, as a consequence of the increase in the reproductive age of pregnant women [116] and the widespread use of ovulation induction and assisted reproduction techniques (ART) [6, 9, 12, 29]. However, 2019 data revealed that, for the first time in almost 40 years, the US twin birth rate dropped by 4% from 2014 to 2018, after decades of constant growth.

The growing concern with multiple pregnancies is mainly related to the higher mortality and greater incidence of adverse perinatal outcomes when compared to singleton pregnancies [16, 32, 42, 94, 105]. Though multiple pregnancies represent 1–2% of the population, they heavily contribute to 12.6% of perinatal mortality. Perinatal loss still remains six times higher than in singleton pregnancies. Even more striking, the perinatal mortality of monochorionic twins (260 per 1000) remains three- to fivefold higher than in dichorionic pregnancies (90 per 1000): the rate of perinatal loss before 24 weeks in monochorionic compared with dichorionic pregnancies is 12.2% versus 1.8% [94]. This should prompt a more differentiated and specialized surveillance [16, 43].

Monozygosity: A Reproductive Anomaly

The human female was programmed to ovulate once in every menstrual cycle, leading to mono-fetal pregnancies and to the nurturing of one infant at a time. Therefore, in about 99% of spontaneous pregnancies, a unique fetus will derive from a single zygote. As a consequence of a *reproductive disorder,* which occurs in about 0.8% of spontaneous conceptions, more than an oocyte is released and fertilized in each cycle, resulting in a polyzygotic multiple pregnancy. In another 0.4% of spontaneous pregnancies, as a result of a *reproductive anomaly*, a single ovum normally destined to produce a single embryo splits to form monozygotic multiples.

The prevalence of MZ twinning is fairly constant worldwide suggesting strongly that MZ twinning stems from an intrinsic "anomalous" property of human zygotes. In spontaneous conceptions, the rate of MZ twins represents about a third of all twin pregnancies, that is, about 4:1000 births, and about two thirds of MZ twin pregnancies will develop a monochorionic placentation, that is, 2–3:1000 births.

With regard to iatrogenic pregnancies, it was noticed that the early embryonic/fetal loss was slightly superior in the pregnancies resulting from ART than in spontaneous pregnancies. But whenever the end result of ART was a twin pregnancy, this early loss rate appeared importantly reduced. Thus, multiple pregnancy may be looked as a marker of reproductive advantage [70, 71]. It may well be that the higher levels of placental hormones produced by a larger placental mass in twin gestations would improve the implantation capacity of the egg. Several studies support this evidence [51, 53, 70, 71, 80, 117, 125], showing loss rates of 24% for singleton pregnancies versus 3–11% in twin pregnancies, that is, the early fetal loss rate associated with ART is two to five times higher in singleton pregnancies.

In certain cases, a familial tendency to MZ twinning was described, probably due to molecular mechanisms that cause post-zygotic cells to disaggregate more easily than usual, forming two or more internal masses.

Why does the division of a single zygote occur? Presently, four theories are available to explain the mechanism of zygotic splitting, but all of them still remain speculative: the so-called *repulsion hypothesis* [44] in which cells in the developing zygote express genetic differences that cause repulsive forces and lead to the splitting of the zygote; the existence of codominant axes [2] in which the continuous *presence of a codominant axis* will cause the zygote to split; *depressed calcium levels* in the early embryo [107]; and the *blastomere herniation* hypothesis in which the integrity of the zona pellucida is breached during embryonic development, thereby losing its sequestering and protective role and permitting herniation of pluripotent cells through a gap in the zona pellucida [45, [9]. All these theories are, however, not convincingly clear to explain the origin of monozygotic triplets and quadruplets and do not clarify the higher rate of MZ twins related to ART techniques. This particular difficulty is due to the inexistence of animal models of monozygosity, in which, with the exception of the human race and the nine-banded armadillo (*D. novemcinctus*), in no other mammals is this process expected to occur. More recently another hypothesis has been put forward (*zona pellucida-assisted binary fission theory*): human fertilized oocytes more prone to splitting are able to undergo one or two successive binary fissions or various combinations offered by subsequent secondary fissions, just as the case for the nine-banded armadillo [13]. This latter theory would be able to explain monozygotic triplets and quadruplets [109] as well as some midline asymmetries in MZ twins [17].

Time Matters in Zygotic Splitting: Sharing Levels and a Model of Placentation

The timing of MZ twinning events can be inferred from the type of membranes and placentation, according to Corner's hypothesis which was never proven, since no evidence of such a split exists in observations from in vitro fertilization.

Dizygotic twins (fraternal or nonidentical) result from the fertilization of two ova by different spermatozoids, showing a different genetic content. The type of placenta resulting from this process of fertilization, in which the trophoblast formation precedes the egg implantation, has two chorions and two amniotic sacs, defining a dichorionic diamniotic pregnancy.

Monozygotic twins are uniovular twins that result from the early division of a single egg (originating from the fertilization of an oocyte and a single spermatozoid) in two cell masses that are more or less identical since theoretically they contain the same genotype. This cleavage will occur between the fertilization and the gastrulation period. However, the placentation inherent to these twins is more complex, depending on the moment in which the separation occurs.

Dichorionic diamniotic (DC-DA) MZ twins (about 25%) have separate membranes and placentas and result from abnormal splitting at the two cells to morula stages (day 0 to 3). Consequently, each twin receives trophoblastic and somatic stem cells into their cell masses. Therefore, twinning must have happened before the differentiation and physical separation of somatic and trophoblastic cells into the outer and inner cell masses, respectively, in the cavitated blastocyst at about 3 days postconception. Dichorionic diamniotic placentas are derived from the splitting of about eight blastomeres.

Splitting at any time thereafter results in a single MC placenta that continues as such even in the face of subsequent MZ twinning of the inner cell mass. *Monochorionic diamniotic* (MC-DA) twins (~75%) separate at the inner cell mass level, after the chorion has formed (day 4 to 7). Consequently two fetuses will develop with a single placenta and two amniotic cavities, considering the fact that the amniotic cavity will be formed after the eighth day after conception. The sharing of a single placenta is in itself an anomaly, creating unequal vascular territories for each twin and a more common eccentric location of the umbilical cords [25]. Eventually 5–15% will develop a twin-to-twin transfusion syndrome, and a late discrepancy in fetal growth can be quite a frequent finding [28].

If the division occurs between the 9th and 12th day, at the late blastocyst stage, a single placenta and a unique amniotic cavity will be formed, resulting in a *monochorionic-monoamniotic* (MC-MA) twin pregnancy (~1%).

The highest level of structure sharing occurs when the division happens circa the 13th day, resulting in the incomplete division of the embryonic disc, originating *conjoined twins* (estimated prevalence of 1 in 100,000). After that time, the undivided egg will maintain its expected course to produce a singleton pregnancy.

In fact perinatal mortality and morbidity are related directly with the level of sharing, that is, the greater the level of sharing, the greater the risk of pregnancy adverse outcomes. Whereas MZ with dichorionic placentation and dizygotic twins present pregnancies with similar risks, those with monochorionic placentation have an important increase in adverse outcomes, mainly if the shared circulation is unbalanced or if we are dealing with monoamniotic or conjoined twins [94].

How Identical Are MZ Twins? The Combination of Genetic, Epigenetic, and Environmental Factors

Contrary to what might first be deduced, it is incorrect to consider MZ twins as "genetically identical." Although an equal number of founder cells are exposed to the same internal milieu, different genetic, post-zygotic, epigenetic, and environmental factors of prenatal occurrence can determine differing genetic and phenotypic properties [75, 101].

MZ twins may even be of a different chromosomal composition (heterokaryotypic twins) either due to a mitotic error occurring before the twinning event (the mosaic will be present in both fetuses with different distribution between the twins) or due to a mitotic error occurring after the twinning event (the mosaic will be present in only one twin) [91].

Various post-zygotic events determine a discordant phenotype for MZ twins, which are not so identical as would be expected, such as:

- Concordant or reciprocal X chromosome inactivation
- Chromosomal mosaicism
- Genomic imprinting
- Trinucleotide repeat sequence discordance
- Phenotypic discordance for a single gene mutation
- Epigenetics
- Unequal placental territoriality

Discordance for Major Malformations

MC twins show an increased rate of structural abnormalities compared to both DC twins and to singletons [77, 94]. In MC twins, the incidence of congenital anomalies is reported to be up to 10%, compared to a 3–4% rate in DC twins and a 2–3% in singletons [20, 55].

Congenital abnormalities in MC twins are discordant in most of the cases (approximately 85%), and this phenomenon implies a careful and complex clinical management [40, 55, 89]. This discordance can be attributed to the following:

1. Variable gene expression (post-zygotic mutation, asymmetrical X inactivation)
2. Asymmetric splitting of the cellular mass
3. Splitting after laterality gradients have been established (midline defects and cardiac)
4. Hemodynamic factors in monochorionic gestations with twin-to-twin transfusion syndrome (TTTS)

MZ are usually discordant for malformations such as cardiac and urinary tract defects, omphalocele, and neural tube defects. Recently Gijtenbeek et al. [36] demonstrated that MC twins were 6.3 times more likely to be born with a congenital heart disease (CHD) (59.3 per 1000 live-born twins; relative risk (RR) 6.3; 95% confidence interval (CI): 4.4–9.1) and TTTS twins had a 12-fold increased risk of having a CHD at birth (87.3 per 1000 live births; RR 12.4, 95% CI: 8.6–17.8) [36]. On the contrary, MZ are usually concordant for malformations such as cloacal dysgenesis and omphalocele-exstrophy-imperforate anus-spinal defect syndrome.

Disruptions in MZ twins including limb reduction defects, hemifacial microsomia, and amyoplasia may be the result of shared placental circulation leading to secondary disruptions and sometimes to single intrauterine fetal death.

Finally, clubfeet, dislocated hips, and craniosynostosis are deformations associated with spatial constraint and intrauterine crowding, which are apparently related to limited space in utero consequence of two fetuses in a pregnancy.

In about 25% of MZ twins, the development of normal lateralization may be impaired by the twinning process itself in such a way that for some of the asymmetrical features, the resulting twins would not be duplicated, but mirror images.

The Limits of Zygosity Testing: Postnatal Importance

The estimation of MZ twins is frequently based on the number of monochorionic twins observed in obstetric ultrasound. All monochorionic placentas correspond to MZ twins, and all twin pairs of different sex are DZ. However in the majority of like-sexed twins with dichorionic placentation, we are blind to their zygosity. The "gold standard" for the determination of zygosity should be based on several genetic markers (including "DNA fingerprinting") in buccal swabs or blood sampling. This may be, however, a somewhat misleading approach as all MZ twins share vascular placental connections and might have exchanged DNA (chimerism).

In reality, the final diagnosis of zygosity cannot be accomplished in about 43% of cases without DNA evaluation [31]. In daily practice, the estimation of MZ twins is based roughly on chorionicity and fetal sex, leaving about one-third of MZ twins undetected. Presently therefore whatever method is employed will underestimate the real incidence of MZ twins.

Chorionicity: A (Re)definition of Perinatal Prognosis

Clearly, it is chorionicity rather than zygosity that determines several aspects of antenatal management and perinatal outcomes. Thus, the routine assignment of chorionicity and the earliest possible diagnosis of monochorionic twinning are highly desirable [68, 73].

Zygosity refers to the type of conception whereas chorionicity reflects the type of placentation.

Caution should be taken when using the number of chorionic sacs and the number of yolk sacs alone to determine the number of embryos. Shortly after the sixth postmenstrual week, embryonic heartbeats are visible, and one can confidently count the number of embryos by the number of beating hearts. To determine the number of amnions in a monochorionic twin pregnancy, in which two embryos are seen within the chorionic sac, it is wise to wait until the eighth postmenstrual week to ascertain amnionicity. The amniotic membrane is so thin that it may remain inconspicuous until 8–9 weeks, leading to the incorrect consideration of a monochorionic-monoamniotic gestation.

After that gestational age, it becomes clear that no amniotic membrane is present between the embryos and only one yolk sac is visualized. When two embryos or fetuses assume a parallel, head-to-head position, conjoined twins should be suspected. A jerk with the probe should be inflicted to induce movement between the two fetuses, away from each other or close together when conjoined twins are in question. From then on, it is important to look for sonographic signs of cord entanglement, potentially depicted as early as 12 weeks, with the help of color Doppler.

At 10–14 weeks, the gold standard "window" for chorionicity definition, the chorion frondosum is sufficiently thick to be identified between the two layers of amnion in a dichorionic twin pregnancy (not an obligatorily dizygotic twin pregnancy), yielding the fully diagnostic "twin peak" or "lambda" or "delta" sign [98, 124, 106] (Fig. 42.1a). However, the number of "twin-peak" signs is no secure indication of how many chorionic sacs exist within a given pregnancy. If two fused layers of amnion, without any chorion interposed, are found in the scan creating a T-shape (T sign), showing a very thin membrane with strictly two layers, a monochorionic twin pregnancy can be diagnosed with a 100% certainty [32] (Fig. 42.1b).

After 16 weeks, the chorion frondosum physiologically regresses and chorionicity becomes a more uncertain issue (in the second trimester, a false characterization of chorionicity will occur in about 10% cases) [88, 124]. The delta sign disappears [4, 99] and, if sexes are alike, monochorionicity can be wrongly inferred. Therefore, an adequate first-trimester scan of a multifetal pregnancy makes the subsequent second- and third-trimester evaluation simpler, faster, and much more meaningful.

Later in pregnancy, identifying a single placenta with a paper-thin, reflective hairlike septum less than 2 mm without chorion between the two amnions and like-sex twins indicates monochorionicity. In contrast, if one finds two separate placentas of different location or two fetuses of a different sex or a thick interfetal membrane >2 mm with more than two layers, dichorionicity is strongly suspected. Note that a membrane placed parallel to the ultrasonic beam will appear thinner and

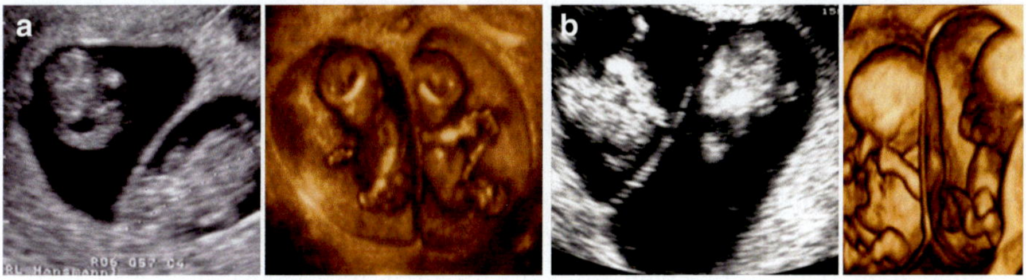

Lambda sign: dichorionic placentation T sign: monochorionic placentation

Fig. 42.1 Diagnosis of chorionicity: lambda sign (dichorionic placentation) and T sign (monochorionic placentation) in the first trimester of pregnancy. (**a**) Lambda sign: dichorionic placentation. (**b**) T sign: monochorionic placentation

poorly imaged, rendering it impossible to be sure about the number of layers of the intertwin membrane.

When chorionicity is established, stratification of risk is possible, anticipating the complications characteristic of each type of placenta. Recently an update on the management of twin pregnancies was published in two papers, discussing the peculiarities of MC twin clinical orientation [50, 114].

Prenatal Screening and Diagnosis of Aneuploidies: Does Chorionicity Matter?

Having correctly established chorionicity, specific aspects of prenatal screening and diagnosis can be adequately programmed in multiple pregnancies, since chromosomal abnormalities in twin pregnancies arise different clinical, ethical, and moral problems that need to be addressed [70].

The overall probability that a multiple gestation contains an aneuploid fetus is directly related to its zygosity. In *dizygotic* pregnancies, each fetus has an independent risk of aneuploidy; thus, the maternal age-related risk for chromosomal abnormalities for each twin may be the same as in singleton pregnancies, but the chance that at least one fetus will be affected by a chromosomal defect is twice as high as in singleton pregnancies [70] (Fig. 42.2). This means that for dizygotic twin pregnancies, the pregnancy-specific risk is calculated by *adding* the individual risk estimates for each fetus. The 10% of dichorionic twin pregnancies that are monozygotic will incorrectly have their risks calculated by the summing rather than the averaging method. However, the ultimate effect on overall screening performance and clinical meaning will be a negligible one.

In *monozygotic* twins, the risk of an affected fetus is similar to the maternal age risk of a singleton pregnancy, and, in the vast majority of cases, the risk for one fetus is the same as the risk for the other [67]. The most reliable and reproducible method of screening is nuchal translucency (NT), and it is therefore appropriate to take the average of the two NT measurements, so that a single risk estimate can be calculated (averaging method).

This ignores the small possibility of heterokaryotypic monozygotic twins resulting from a mitotic nondisjunction after the zygote splits.

If the pregnancy is dichorionic, then the parents should be counseled that the risk of discordance for a chromosomal abnormality is about twice that of a singleton pregnancy, whereas the risk that both fetuses would be affected is a much rarer event, corresponding to the singleton risk squared. However, with higher risk conditions, such as autosomal recessive disorders, this could be as high as 1 in 16. For example, a 40-year-old pregnant woman with a risk for trisomy of about 1 in 100 based on maternal age would in a dizygotic twin pregnancy have a risk that one fetus is affected of 1 in 50 (1 in 100 plus 1 in 100), whereas the risk that both fetuses would be affected is 1 in 10,000 (1 in 100 × 1 in 100). This is, however, an oversimplification since, unlike all monochorionic pregnancies that are always monozygotic, only about 90% of dichorionic pregnancies are dizygotic.

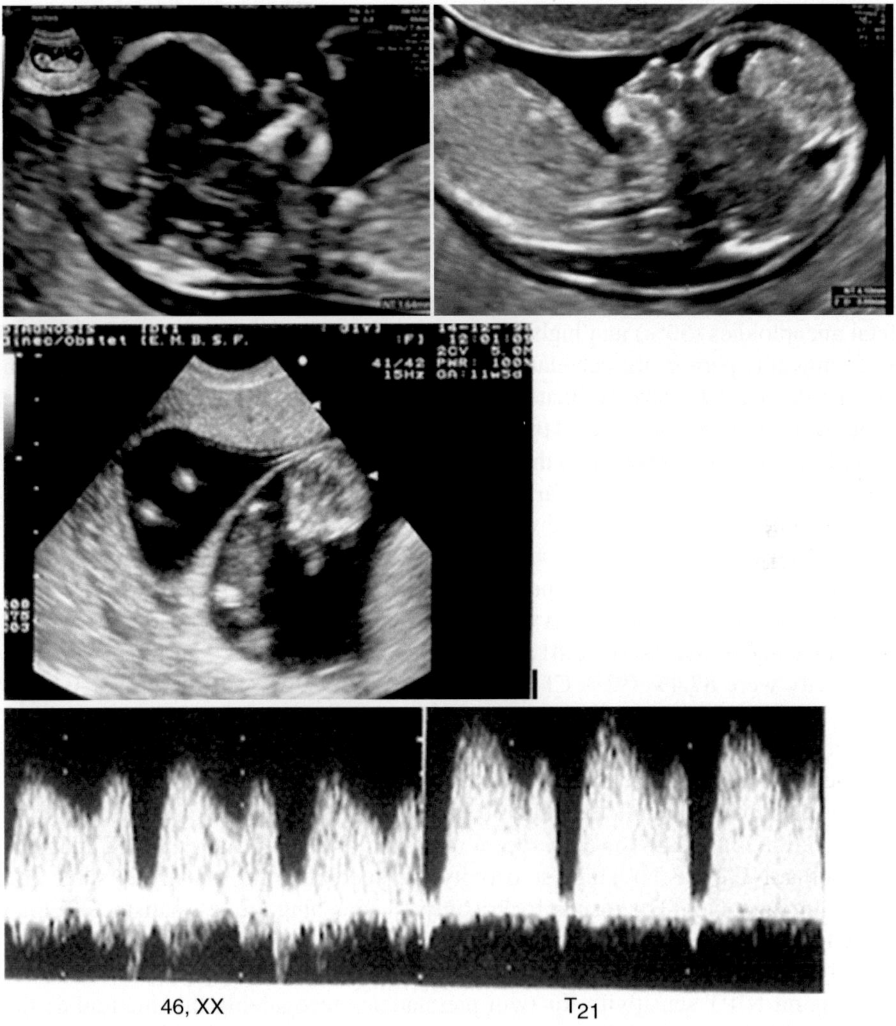

Fig. 42.2 Screening for trisomy 21 in dichorionic twins (summing method): the lambda sign is evident at 10–14 weeks. We can observe discrepant nuchal translucencies (NT = 1.1 and 4.1 mm). Ductus venosus Doppler blood flow is abnormal in the fetus with increased NT that eventually revealed to be a fetus affected by trisomy 21

When calculating the risk of higher-order multiples, estimates can be made by multiplying the singleton risk by the number of fetuses [76]. This method assumes unique chorionicity for each fetus, though monozygosity can occur more frequently than previously thought due to higher rates in ART multiple gestations [14, 15].

The possibility of deriving a risk for trisomy 21 from NT assessment in the first trimester of pregnancy shifted the focus from a pregnancy-specific risk to a fetus-specific risk [93]. This assumption was based on the observation that the distribution of NT measurements in twin fetuses with trisomy 21 was similar to that in singletons [81,

93]. The higher rate of false positives for NT among MC twins (8.4%) should be ascribed to the possibility of early hemodynamic imbalance (the risk of developing TTTS if NT is increased is augmented three- to fivefold) [21, 48, 100, 102].

Assessing nasal bones in multiple pregnancies can be more demanding; however, they can be combined with NT and biochemical screening for first-trimester risk calculation [37]. With the addition of nasal bone evaluation, sensitivity for trisomy 21 screening increased from 79% to 89%, for the same false positive rate of 5% [24, 100].

In contrast, although biochemical screening was the first alternative to age-derived risk in twins, it can still be a source of confusion and has a lower detection rate for fetal aneuploidies (50%) and higher rates of false positives [103, 104]. This kind of screening only permits the calculation of a pregnancy and not a fetus-specific risk. In twin pregnancies, the levels of maternal serum markers are, on average, expected to be about twice as high in unaffected twin pregnancies as in unaffected singleton pregnancies [27], that is, proportional to the number of fetoplacental units. Therefore, as biochemical screening in twins is far less powerful than in singletons, it should not be recommended in general practice without extensive counseling [63, 78].

However the systematic review from Prats et al. [87] brought a different light to the cumulative evidence on the performance of the combined test in twin pregnancies. The performance of the test was good (summary receiver operating characteristic area under the curve: 0.817). In monochorionic twins, the sensitivity and specificity were 87.4% (95% CI 0.526–0.977) and 95.4% (95% CI 0.943–0.963), respectively. Therefore, nowadays, it still is the best first-trimester screening test available for twin pregnancies [87].

The more recent application of noninvasive prenatal test (NIPT) in twin pregnancies is much more complicated than its use in singleton pregnancies. Normally the fetal fraction in twins is lower. A recent meta-analysis from Liao et al. [57] demonstrated that NIPT has both high sensitivity and specificity for trisomy 21 screening in twin pregnancies. The results for trisomy 18 screening are less satisfactory than those for trisomy 21. The performance for trisomy 13 screening could not be determined as only three cases were identified [57]. In 2021 our group published a meta-analysis on NIPT sensitivity for twin pregnancies recognizing this method as the most sensitive for aneuploidiy screening [19].

Twin-to-Twin Transfusion Syndrome (TTTS): A Disease for Two

An example of a complication unique almost to monozygotic twinning is twin-to-twin transfusion syndrome (TTTS). A MC twin placenta is designed and built for a singleton fetus; hence, attempts to cater for the needs of two fetuses can often be suboptimal. Twin fetal circulations are seldom separate, and several intertwin vascular communications may be present. Quite often there is an unequal sharing of placental parenchyma. Thus, interfetal transfusion is a normal event in monochorionic twin pregnancies. By way of an imbalance in these intertwin vascular connections, blood is transfused in excess from the *donor*, who becomes growth-restricted and develops high-output cardiac insufficiency and oligohydramnios (depleted-donor twin), to the recipient, who develops circulatory overload with congestive heart failure and polyhydramnios (volume and an overfilled recipient twin). Therefore TTTS reflects primarily a circulatory imbalance that develops chronically between hemodynamically connected monochorionic twin fetuses.

Twin-to-twin transfusion syndrome (TTTS) affects about 5–15% of monochorionic twin pregnancies (1:400 pregnancies) and thus occurs in 1 in 1600 deliveries. This syndrome accounts for 17% of perinatal mortality, nearly 12% of neonatal deaths, and 8.4% of infant deaths in twins. This is three to ten times higher than that attributed to singletons.

Though clinically identifiable, this condition is still far from being effectively anticipated and treated. TTTS presents unique characteristics and greatest therapeutic challenges in perinatal medicine:

- It affects *two* fetuses, not one.
- It affects *structurally normal* fetuses.
- Its basis resides in the *placenta*, not in the fetuses.
- It is associated with important *perinatal morbidity* and *mortality*.
- It is amenable to *curative* therapy.

More than a century ago, Schatz [90] suggested that TTTS is due to discordant hemodynamics, secondary to transfusional imbalance. Later Bajoria et al. [1] related TTTS with unbalanced intertwin transfusion mediated by one or more arteriovenous (AV) anastomoses in association with absent bidirectional superficial anastomoses: those affected by TTTS had fewer arterio-arterial (AA) anastomoses present in 24% versus 84% of monochorionic twins without TTTS [30]. Seventy-eight percent of monochorionic pregnancies in this series with one or more AV anastomoses and no AA anastomoses developed TTTS [30]. When an AA anastomosis is found, the risk of developing TTTS is reduced ninefold.

The progressive nature of TTTS in utero is thought to be due to one twin (the donor) slowly pumping blood to the other (the recipient) through these anastomoses. Net result of transfusion between twins depends on the following:

1. *Vascular anastomoses*: in some cases, the normal transfusion from the donor's arterial to the recipient's venous circulation is not adequately compensated by the opposite flow by other deep or superficial anastomoses [1, 108].
2. *Placental sharing*: unequal placental sharing, both by discrepant size of placental territory and/or by velamentous insertion of umbilical cord, may further impair growth in TTTS fetuses [54].
3. *Asymmetry* in the progressive reduction of an initially large number of bidirectional AV connections.

4. *Unbalanced renin-angiotensin system* (RAS): upregulation of RAS (donor) and downregulation of RAS (recipient) with transfer of angiotensin II may cause or contribute to the development of TTTS [64].
5. *Incomplete remodeling* and defective trophoblastic invasion of maternal spiral arteries.

The pathophysiology of TTTS is poorly understood, and, although transfusion has been confirmed in vivo, TTTS includes more than shunting of blood from donor to recipient. A vicious cycle of hypervolemia-polyuria-hyperosmolality is established, leading in about one-third of the cases to the development of acute polyhydramnios/oligohydramnios sequence in the second trimester of pregnancy.

Diagnosis of TTTS

In the past, diagnosis of the syndrome was made only after delivery of the affected twin pair and careful examination of the placenta. The standard neonatal criteria comprised of the following:

- A difference in *cord hemoglobin* concentrations of 5 g/dl or more
- A difference in *birth weights* of 20% or more (this criterion is not necessarily present in the acute form of fetofetal transfusion syndrome that occurs in labor)

Considering the many pitfalls of neonatal findings in TTTS and the more consistent sonographic antenatal criteria, Wittmann et al. [123] proposed as discriminating findings in TTTS the discrepancy in the sizes of twins and the polyhydramnios surrounding the larger twin. Brennan et al. [18] added to the former criteria disparity in size of the vessels in the umbilical cords, same sex, single placenta showing different echogenicity of the cotyledons supplying the two cords, and evidence of hydrops in either twin or congestive heart failure in the recipient.

More recently, more useful sonographic criteria were adopted:

Discordance in Amniotic Fluid Volume *(Oligohydramnios Sequence)*

In 1988 Chescheir and Seeds [22] noted that fetuses affected by TTTS had concurrent polyhydramnios and oligohydramnios: the congestive heart failure in the recipient will overperfuse the kidneys with consequent polyuria and excess of amniotic fluid; hypovolemia in the donor causes inadequate perfusion of the kidneys with decrease in urinary output and oligohydramnios (Fig. 42.3).

Quantitative criteria for amniotic fluid volume assessment have been proposed for a more accurate definition: oligohydramnios if the deepest vertical pool in the donor sac was <2 cm and polyhydramnios, if the deepest vertical pool would be

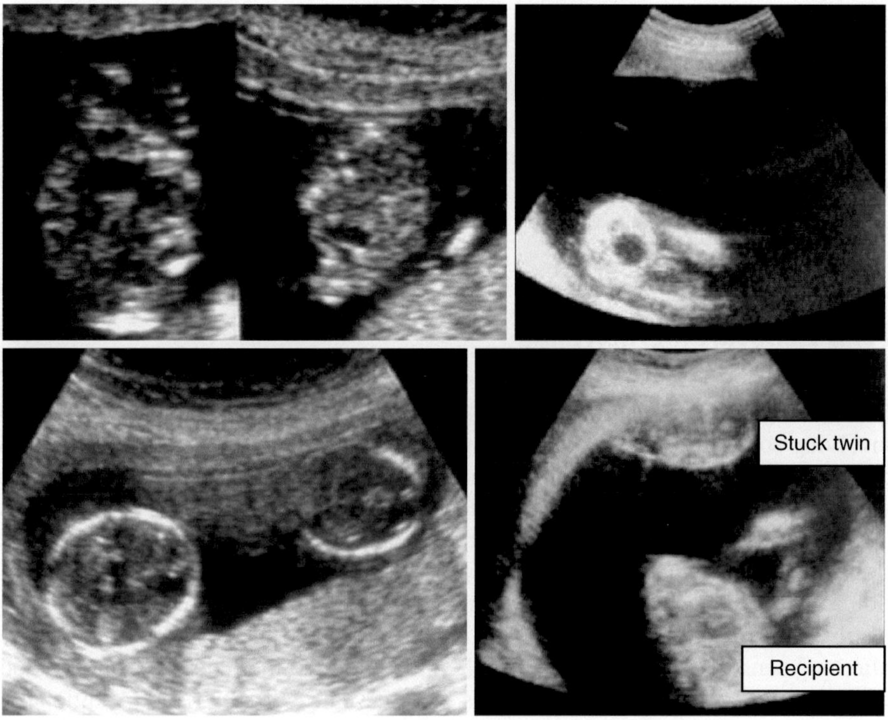

Fig. 42.3 Discrepancy in growth and amniotic fluid between a pair of monochorionic diamniotic twins in a case of twin-to-twin transfusion syndrome. Note the polyhydramnios of the recipient and the stuck twin

>8 cm in the recipient's sac. Not infrequently, anhydramnios in the donor sac results in it becoming "stuck," shrouded by the intertwin membrane, while the recipient's sac becomes severely polyhydramniotic.

Other related confirmatory features include a small or non-visible bladder due to hypovolemia and renal hypoperfusion in the donor, along with a distended urinary bladder with resulting excessive micturition in the recipient.

Discordance in Fetal Size

Discordant growth is a common complication of twin pregnancies. Abdominal circumference rather than head measurements of twins was proposed as the most reproducible and meaningful one. Besides, considering that fetal weight estimations based on singleton growth charts may be inadequate for twins, the abdominal circumference criterion should be definitely used for the sonographic diagnosis of divergent twin growth. A cutoff value of 20 mm for the difference in abdominal circumference between twins indicated growth discordance of more than 20%.

Abnormal Doppler Findings

Alterations in cardiac hemodynamics are indirectly represented by alterations in venous blood flow waveforms. The receptor presents with pulsatility in the umbilical vein and absent or reverse flow in the ductus venosus [47] as signs of congestive heart failure due to hypervolemia and increased preload from placental vascular anastomotic transfusion.

Fetal Echocardiography

Considering the hemodynamic imbalance between the circulations of the twins involving some excess of blood flowing from the donor to the recipient fetus, cardiac involvement is expected [66]. Echocardiography is a well-established tool for antenatal assessment of structural and functional heart disease.

Zosmer et al. [126] showed that some surviving twins of TTTS had a persistent right ventricular hypertrophic cardiomyopathy and proposed that cardiac dysfunction could be induced in utero by sustained strain upon the heart by TTTS, predominantly affecting the right ventricle. The right ventricle is stiffer and more afterload-sensitive than the left ventricle, mostly due to the redistribution of blood in the cerebral arteries which decreases the left ventricular afterload. Additionally recipients remain at increased risk of pulmonary artery stenosis and maintain a slightly reduced early diastolic ventricular filling as compared to donors (diastolic dysfunction) [121].

In contrast, the significant reduction of blood flow velocity in the umbilical artery recorded in the “donor” is consistent with hypovolemia and increased placental resistance, increasing cardiac afterload and decreasing umbilical venous return. This is in good agreement with some studies which show that the donor twin has a trend toward a lower Tei index than in the normal population. Finally, there have been speculations about an increased incidence of aortic coarctation in donors due to a lower venous return from the placenta and hence a decreased loading of the left ventricular outflow tract [120, 121].

After birth about half of the recipients showed biventricular hypertrophy, with prevalent left ventricular hypertrophic cardiomyopathy [33, 34, 126]. A smaller subgroup will develop right ventricular tract obstruction (functional pulmonary stenosis) and pulmonary hypertension in the neonatal period, which may be aggravated by systolic right ventricular dysfunction.

Since there is an increased incidence of CHDs in MC twins due mainly to the risk of right ventricular outflow tract obstruction (35/1000 TTTS twin live births vs. 0.5/1000 singleton live births), an expert fetal echocardiogram in all MC twins, follow-up scans in the event of TTTS, and a postnatal cardiac evaluation in all TTTS survivors should be warranted [36].

Abnormalities of vascular distensibility were described in survivors of TTTS in infancy [34]. The donor fetus showed evidence of chronic hypovolemia resulting in activation of the renin-angiotensin system. This upregulation initially attempts to correct volume depletion, and transfusion of increased concentrations of angiotensin II will probably cause increased vascular stiffness in the surviving donor in childhood.

Signs of Hydrops in the Recipient Twin

In advanced stages of TTTS, the recipient twin affected by congestive heart failure may present signs of serosa effusions, such as ascites, pleural effusion, and subcutaneous edema.

Other Ultrasonographic Findings

- Identification of cord insertion: velamentous insertion of the cord is a frequent finding (Fig. 42.4).
- Difference in color of the placentas: due to blood transfusion from one twin to the other, the placenta of the donor twin tends to be whitish ("pale") and the placenta of the recipient of a denser color (excess of blood).

Treatment of TTTS

Fetoscopic laser coagulation of intertwin vascular anastomoses (Solomon technique) in monochorionic placentas is the preferred treatment for twin-to-twin transfusion syndrome [3]). Several postoperative complications can occur when intertwin vascular anastomoses remain patent including twin anemia polycythemia sequence or recurrent twin-to-twin transfusion syndrome, but they are less prevalent using the Solomon technique [102]. No differences in survival or neurodevelopmental impairment between both techniques were found [119].

Lopriore et al. [59] presented important data concerning the psychomotor development of survivors from TTTS evaluated until school entry. From a total of 29 children affected in utero by TTTS and evaluated during 8 years, 41% presented cerebral anomalies disclosed by ultrasound and about 21% had cerebral palsy [59]. This figure rose to 50% in the cases of TTTS complicated by intrauterine fetal demise of the co-twin, whereas rates of 14% of cerebral palsy were found in the cases in which both twins survived. Bamberg and Hecher [3] in a recent review reported that a long-term neurodevelopmental impairment occurs in about 10% of

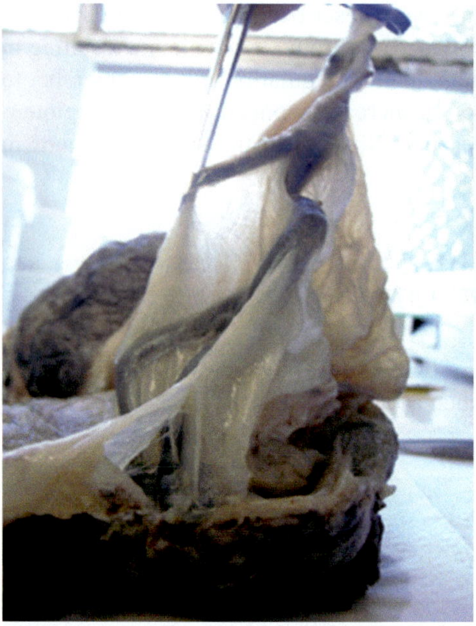
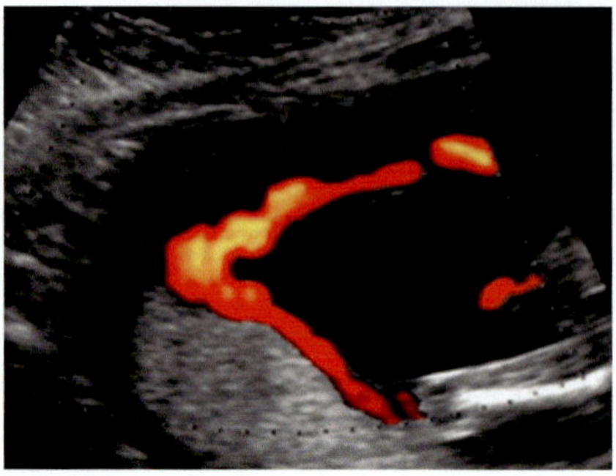

Fig. 42.4 Pathological specimen illustrating a velamentous insertion that was already diagnosed in a second-trimester ultrasound (see vessel highlighted with power Doppler)

children after laser surgery in good accordance with Schou [92] that demonstrated in a retrospective study that children after TTTS treated with laser appeared to have a higher risk of severe neurodevelopmental impairment and scored significantly lower on psychological questionnaires compared to monochorionic twins from uncomplicated pregnancies [92].

Prediction of TTTS

Targeted surveillance of monochorionic twins at earlier stages of gestation could anticipate and provide timely management of the pregnancies at risk of one of the most devastating type-specific complications: twin-to-twin transfusion syndrome (TTTS).

Both increased nuchal translucency [95, 96], and abnormal flow in the ductus venosus in monochorionic twins may be early manifestations of hemodynamic imbalance between donor and recipient. In these pregnancies, in addition to NT measurement at 11–14 weeks, the Doppler assessment of DV blood flow increases relevantly the performance of screening for those at risk of developing twin-to-twin transfusion syndrome [68, 69, 72] (Fig. 42.5). Recently, Stagnati et al. [106] published a systematic review and a meta-analysis to evaluate the performance of each ultrasonographic early marker (intertwin NT discrepancy, NT > 95th percentile,

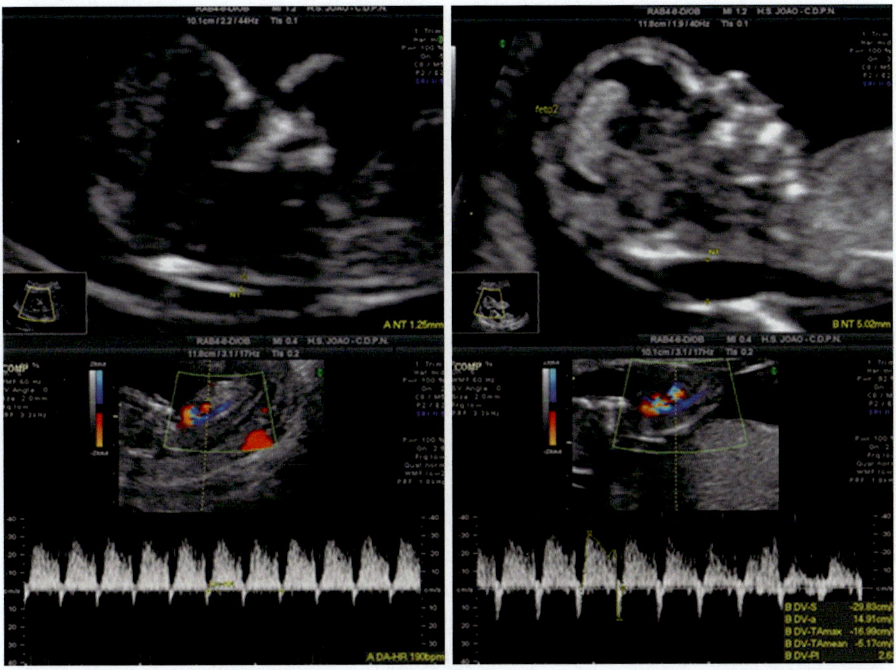

Fig. 42.5 Screening for trisomy 21 in monochorionic twins (averaging method). We can observe discrepant nuchal translucencies (NT = 1.25 and 5.02 mm). Ductus venosus Doppler blood flow is abnormal in the fetus with increased NT. This pair of twins was chromosomally normal and developed a twin-to-twin transfusion syndrome at 16 weeks

intertwin CRL discrepancy >10%, or abnormal DV flow) in the prediction of TTTS in the first trimester of pregnancy. An increased risk of TTTS was associated with intertwin NT discrepancy (positive likelihood ratio (LR+), 1.92 (95% CI, 1.25–2.96); negative likelihood ratio (LR-), 0.65 (95% CI, 0.50–0.84)); NT > 95th percentile (LR+, 2.63 (95% CI, 1.51–4.58); LR-, 0.85 (95% CI, 0.75–0.96)); CRL discrepancy >10% (LR+, 1.80 (95% CI, 1.05–3.07); LR-, 0.92 (95% CI, 0.81–1.05)); and abnormal DV flow (LR+, 4.77 (95% CI, 1.33–17.04); LR-, 0.49 (95% CI, 0.17–1.41)). The highest sensitivities were observed for intertwin NT discrepancy (52.8% (95% CI, 43.8–61.7%)) and abnormal DV flow (50.0% (95% CI, 33.4–66.6%)) [106].

Twin Anemia-Polycythemia Sequence (TAPS)

TAPS is another hemodynamic disorder unique to monochorionic placentation, first reported in 2007. It is another form of chronic intertwin transfusion. The pathogenesis is based on tiny AV anastomoses causing unbalanced slow intertwin transfusion. TAPS is associated with a high risk of perinatal mortality and morbidity and long-term sequelae, warranting increased surveillance in the antenatal period as well as postnatally [60, 111, 112].

In contrast with chronic TTTS, TAPS twins have normal pockets of amniotic fluid and do not show oligo-polyhydramnios sequence [60, 122]. TAPS may be diagnosed antenatally in the presence of abnormalities on Doppler ultrasound: the donor has signs of fetal anemia (increased middle cerebral artery peak systolic velocity: MCA-PSV >1.5 multiples of the median (MoM)), while the recipient has signs of polycythemia (decreased MCA-PSV <1.0 MoM) [97]. Most recently, Tollennar et al. [113] proposed the delta MCA-PSV >0.5 MoM as having a greater diagnostic accuracy for predicting TAPS compared to the current MCA-PSV cutoff criteria [112].

TAPS may be missed antenatally and only become clearly apparent at birth in the presence of a pale and a plethoric twin pair. In addition, color difference of the maternal side of the placenta could help to differentiate between TAPS and acute peripartum TTTS. In TAPS twins, the donor's placenta share is pale while the recipient's placenta share is reddish.

Another hematological complication which can occur in TAPS twins is thrombocytopenia (platelet count <150 × 10^9/L). Within TAPS twins, recipients have more often thrombocytopenia compared to donor twins caused by impaired platelet production secondary due to hypoxia. An explanation for thrombocytopenia in donors is impaired platelet production due to repression of megakaryocytes associated with increased erythropoiesis.

Twin Reversed Arterial Perfusion (TRAP)

Twin reversed arterial perfusion (TRAP) sequence is a unique and rare complication of monozygotic pregnancies with monochorionic placentation in which the surviving twin keeps its deceased co-twin alive through retrograde perfusion [118]. Its prevalence is estimated in about 1 in 10,000 pregnancies. In the first-trimester scan, one usually finds one structurally normal and one grossly abnormal twin with massive cystic edema and reversed flow in the umbilical artery toward rather than away from the abnormal twin.

If one of a monochorionic pair dies very early in the embryonic period, the surviving twin (pump twin) may continue to perfuse its deceased co-twin's body through a large arterio-arterial anastomosis. The deceased twin therefore continues to grow and becomes a true parasite without any functional cardiac activity of its own. Through the arterio-arterial anastomosis, deoxygenated blood will flow from the pump towards the acardiac twin in the opposite direction [56].

This reversed perfusion may cause high-output cardiac failure in the pump twin as evidenced by cardiomegaly, tricuspid regurgitation, polyhydramnios, and hydrops (Fig. 42.6). Severely deoxygenated blood usually flows back to the pump twin through a direct veno-venous anastomosis, bypassing the placenta.

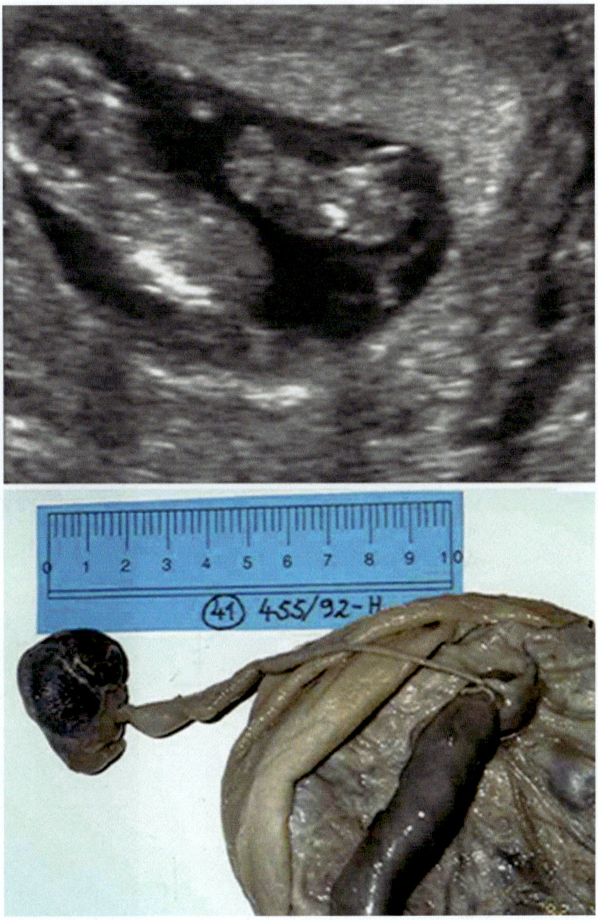

Fig. 42.6 Example of a TRAP in the first trimester with a normal fetus and a grossly abnormal fetus in a monochorionic-monoamniotic twin pregnancy. Pathological specimen showing the umbilical cord of the acardiac twin entangling the cord of the pump twin

Conjoined Twins

Conjoined twins always have a monochorionic-monoamniotic placentation and show fusion of any portion of their bodies as a result of an incomplete division of the embryonic disk, after the 13th day of conception. The term conjoined is actually a misnomer because this kind of twins seems to result from a failure of complete separation rather than from a fusion of the twins [110].

This is a rare condition and the reported frequency varies from 0.1 to 0.35 per 10,000 births. If stillborns are excluded, the estimate is 0.05 per 10,000 births. Females are more commonly affected, with a male-to-female ratio of 1.6–3 to 1. No association with maternal age, race, parity, or heredity has been observed. The recurrence risk is negligible.

Several sonographic signs can be observed in this condition at the time of the first-trimester ultrasound scan [35, 73] (Fig. 42.7):

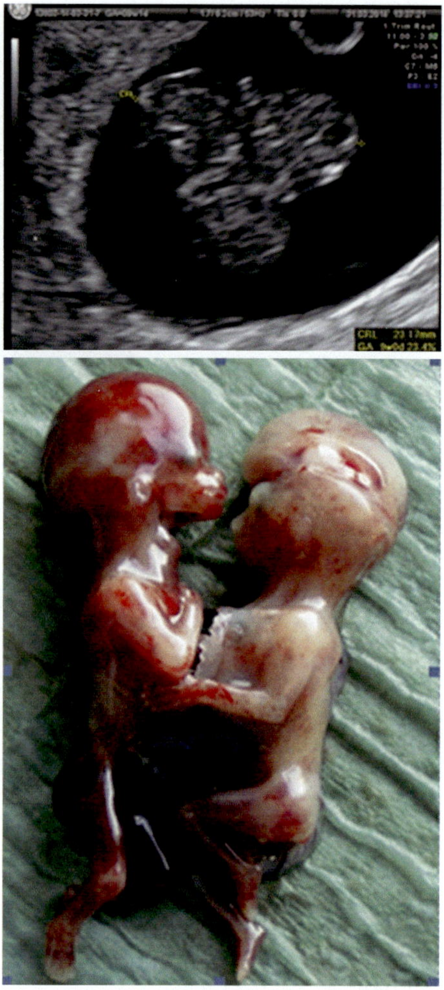

Fig. 42.7 Ultrasound image showing conjoined twins at 10 weeks' gestation. Necropsic specimen after termination of pregnancy of the abovementioned twins at 12 weeks (omphalopagus)

- Absence of an amniotic membrane between the twins.
- Inability to separate fetal bodies.
- Fixed position of the fetuses relative to one another, even after external stimulation or maternal movement.
- Bifid appearance of the first-trimester fetal pole (V- or Y-shaped twin pregnancy) and continuous skin contours at the same anatomic level.
- The heads and bodies of both twins are seen at the same level (Fig. 42.7).
- Unusual extension of the spines.
- Unusual proximity of the extremities.
- Presence of a single heart.
- Abnormal number of vessels (more than three) in the umbilical cord.

Although the diagnosis of conjoined twins is easier during the first trimester, the type and severity of the condition is better accomplished during the second trimester, when a more precise evaluation of the shared organs can be performed. Termination of pregnancy can be offered to couples.

Conjoined twins are classified according to the area of the bodies where the fusion takes place. The symmetrical and equal forms, in which the twins have equal or nearly equal duplication of structures, are called duplicata completa. Whenever there is an unequal duplication of structures, the twins are called duplicata incompleta, and this category includes the most severe types of conjoined twins in which just a few organ systems are duplicated. The most frequent varieties of conjoined twins are thoracopagus (40–74%), omphalopagus (10–33%), pygopagus (18%), ischiopagus (6%), and craniopagus (1–6%).

Discordance of Fetal Growth: Adaptation, Promotion, and Growth Restriction in Multiples

The restriction of intrauterine fetal growth is more frequently found in multiple pregnancies: about 52% of twins and 92% of triplets present low birth weight (<2500 g) compared to 6% of singletons, whereas 10% of twins and 32% of triplets are born with very low birth weight (<1000 g), when compared to 1% of singletons [10].

The common growth curves show that deviations from singleton standards only occur after 28 weeks [5]. The uterine milieu, comprising uteroplacental, maternal, and fetal components, limits physiologically the growth potential of the individual fetus in a multiple pregnancy. This concept implies that most multiples delivered after 28 weeks are growth restricted compared to singletons, as a result of an adaptive process. The total twin and total triplet birth weights exceed that of the 90th birth weight centile for singletons as early as 25 weeks' gestation (data derived from 3.6 million singletons from Matria database). The uterine potential adaptation to a multiple pregnancy is also appreciated by realizing that the average singleton birth weight at 40 weeks is reached as early as 32 weeks in twins and as early as 29 weeks in triplets.

Consequently, the individual multiple is relatively *growth restricted* compared to singletons, whereas the entire pregnancy is *growth promoted* [7]. This physiological restriction (reduction in fetal size) is a way to promote a more advanced gestation as long as possible, to overcome the tremendous increase in volume, the uterine overdistension, and the higher frequency of preterm delivery in multiples [5]. The variables that most strongly influence uterine adaptation are parity (less in nulliparas), maternal age, maternal height, and weight gain.

Discordant growth is another potential way to reduce uterine volume in order to promote an advanced gestational age at birth. The problem is to distinguish between natural variation and pathological growth restriction. Differences as large as 15% may be normal, whereas 15–25% discordance may denote adaptation and differences of more than 25% reveal the inability to maintain growth [10]. This latter group presents the best correlation with adverse outcome, namely, neonatal mortality and morbidity and intensive care admission [8, 11].

The risk of a fetal growth restriction in a multiple pregnancy is ten times greater than in a singleton pregnancy [62], being even greater in a monochorionic (34%) compared to a dichorionic pregnancy (23%) [94]. More recently, our group showed that in uncomplicated MC twin pregnancies, abnormal DV flow in at least one of the fetuses seems to be associated, later in pregnancy, with a higher discordance in birth weight than in those with normal flow in both fetuses [74]. In fact, in pregnancies with abnormal DV flow in at least one of the fetuses, the median discordance in birth weight was higher than in those with normal DV flow in both twins (13.2% vs. 7.8%, $p = 0.006$).

Currently used criteria for FGR in twins are EFW less than the 10th centile of one of the twins, abdominal circumference (AC) of one twin less than the 10th centile, EFW discordance of 25% or more, and umbilical artery (UA) pulsatility index (PI) of the smaller twin above the 95th centile. According to the published International Society of Ultrasound in Obstetrics and Gynecology (ISUOG) twin pregnancy guideline, sFGR is diagnosed when the EFW of one of the twins is less than the 10th centile and the EFW discordance is 25% or more [50]. In the case of selective FGR, three types are considered (I, II, and III) according to the Doppler finding of the end-diastolic flow in the umbilical artery of the small fetus. It is normal in type I, absent or reversed (AREDF) in type II, or intermittent AREDF in type III [39]. Pregnancies complicated by type II or III sFGR treated with fetoscopic laser ablation have a higher rate of mortality but lower rate of morbidity compared with those managed expectantly, supporting the use of fetal therapy at gestations remote from neonatal viability [115].

In what concerns early growth discordance, Grande et al. [38] demonstrated that early discordant twin pregnancies were at a significantly higher risk of chromosomal (OR 11.42; 95%CI: 2.78–46.94) and structural anomalies (OR 5.91; 95%CI: 2.25–15.54), spontaneous fetal loss (OR 4.23; 95%CI: 1.79–10.01), birth weight discordance (OR 2.8; 95%CI: 1.48–5.65), and small-for-gestational age (OR 3.48; 95%CI 1.78–6.79). In fact crown-rump length (CRL) discordance (≥ 10%) presented with higher rates of structural anomalies, stillbirth, birth weight discordance, and small newborns. Fetal anomalies and growth restriction increased in severe CRL discordance (≥ 16%) [38]. More recently Curado et al. [28] showed that compared to late-onset sFGR in monochorionic twin pregnancies, early-onset sFGR is slightly more common and associated with a worse perinatal outcome. The incidence of type II and III is more common in early sFGR [28].

A recent study from Litwinska et al. [58] demonstrated that a large discordance in CRL is associated with a high risk for fetal loss. In DC twins, CRL discordance of ≥15% is associated with increased risk of fetal loss before 20 weeks' gestation, and in MCDA twins CRL discordance of ≥10%, and more so if discordance is above 15% and 20%, is associated with a very high risk of fetal loss or endoscopic laser surgery at <20 weeks.

The meaning of fetal growth discordance in multiples depends on chorionicity. The abdominal circumference is the most reliable sonographic criterion for the establishment of growth discrepancy. A difference of 20 mm translates in a birth weight discrepancy of 20% or more. In a dichorionic twin pregnancy (dizygotic in 90%) may be ascribed to a different genetic constitution of the twins or to an unequal placental function. In a monochorionic pregnancy, as the genetic content is the same, growth discordance may be due to an unequal division of the cellular mass (unequal sharing of the placenta), velamentous insertion (VCI) of the cord, vasa previa, or the unbalanced transfusion of blood through the vascular anastomoses. Our group recently demonstrated that VCI is not associated with the development of TTTS but increases the risk of adverse outcomes. Both VCI and TTTS independently increased the prevalence of intrauterine fetal death and lower gestational age at birth in a similar way, showing that VCI is an important indicator of adverse perinatal outcome in monochorionic twins [25, 26].

Importantly this growth restriction among twins, mainly the monochorionic subgroup, has well-known ominous consequences for fetal neurodevelopment [59, 83–86, 99]. The prognosis is even worse if adding to the growth restriction, the discordance in growth between twins is over 25% [8]. What's new is that this issue has a negative impact on all three areas of development: cognition, language, and motor skills [46]. In a recent systematic review, it was demonstrated that MC twins with birth weight discordance (BWD) had a sixfold higher risk of cerebral palsy compared to DC twins, but even so, the authors concluded that the evidence for such dismal prognosis was moderate [41]. MC twins with sFGR/BWD are in fact at increased risk of long-term neurodevelopment impairment as compared to BWD DC or concordant MC twins, with a within-pair disadvantage for the smaller twin [41].

Death of a Co-twin

In MC twin pregnancies, the risk of single or double fetal death is higher than in DC twins, and in both MC and DC twin pregnancies, the rate of early preterm birth is higher in those with one fetal death than in those with two live fetuses. In both MC and DC twins with one fetal death, the interval to delivery is inversely related to the gestational age at fetal death [23, 49]. In fact the demise of the co-twin in utero in a monozygotic pregnancy can compromise significantly the surviving twin outcome.

The sudden hypotension with the "drain back" of blood from the surviving twin to the low resistance territory of the dead fetus will cause acute exsanguination of the surviving twin into the circulation of the dead twin through vascular anastomoses. Such abrupt hypotension may cause irreversible brain damage in about 50% of the surviving co-twin and death in 38% of the cases [79]. In the central nervous system (CNS), ventriculomegaly, porencephaly, cerebral atrophy, cystic encephalomalacia, or microcephaly can occur in about half of the cases. Extracranial abnormalities include small bowel atresia, gastroschisis, limb amputation, hydrothorax, aplasia cutis, and renal cortical necrosis.

Cordocentesis performed in the survivor showed anemia within 24 hours after death. The results of coagulation screening tests on the surviving newborn twin at delivery are almost always normal.

Conclusion

In clinical terms, the assignment of chorionicity is more relevant than zygosity determination in twin pregnancies. Chorionicity, established according to the type of placentation, is the feature that will most dramatically influence perinatal morbidity and mortality. In fact, about 30% of MC twin pregnancies are complicated by TTTS, isolated discordant growth, twin anemia-polycythemia sequence, congenital defects, or intrauterine demise of the co-twin. About 15% will be eligible for invasive fetal therapy. Combining several sonographic markers, ultrasound examination in the first and early second trimester can differentiate monochorionic twins at high risk for adverse outcome from those likely to follow an uneventful development. This is of utmost importance in patient counseling and planning of care [52, 61]. The stratification of fetus-specific risks by early prenatal screening, the possibility of discordant congenital anomalies, and asymmetrical fetal growth by unique hemodynamic designs make twin pregnancies much more than just a double trouble.

References

1. Bajoria R, Wigglesworth J, Fish NM. Angioarchitecture of monochorionic placentas in relation to twin-to-twin transfusion syndrome. Am J Obstet Gynecol. 1995;172:856–63.
2. Baldwin VJ. Anomalous development of twins. In: Baldwin VJ, editor. Pathology of multiple pregnancy. New York: Springer; 1994. p. 169–97.
3. Bamberg C, Hecher K. Update on twin-to-twin transfusion syndrome. Best Pract Res Clin Obstet Gynaecol. 2019;58:55–65.
4. Blickstein I. The twin-twin transfusion syndrome. Obstet Gynecol. 1990;76:714–22.
5. Blickstein I. Normal and abnormal growth of multiples. Semin Neonatol. 2002;7:177–85.
6. Blickstein I. The worldwide impact of iatrogenic pregnancy. Int J Gynecol Obstet. 2003;82:307–17.
7. Blickstein I. Is it normal for multiples to be smaller than singletons? Best Pract Res Clin Obstet Gynecol. 2004;18:613–23.
8. Blickstein I. Do multiple gestations raise the risk of cerebral palsy? Clin Perinatol. 2004;31:395–408.
9. Blickstein I. Estimation of iatrogenic monozygotic twinning rate following assisted reproduction: pitfalls and caveats. Am J Obstet Gynecol. 2005;192:365–8.
10. Blickstein I. Growth aberration in multiple pregnancy. Obstet Gynecol. 2005;32:39–54.

11. Blickstein I, Keith LG. Neonatal mortality rates among growth-discordant twins, classified according to the birth weight of the smaller twin. Am J Obstet Gynecol. 2004;190:170–4.
12. Blickstein I, Keith LG. The decreased rates of triplet births: temporal trends and biologic speculations. Am J Obstet Gynecol. 2005;193:327–31.
13. Blickstein I, Keith LG. On the possible cause of monozygotic twinning: lessons from the 9-banded armadillo and from assisted reproduction. Twin Res Hum Genet. 2007;10(2):394–9.
14. Blickstein I, Verhoeven HC, Keith LG. Zygotic splitting following assisted reproduction. N Engl J Med. 1999;340:738–9.
15. Blickstein I, Jones C, Keith LG. Zygotic splitting rates following single embryo transfers in in-vitro fertilization: a population-based study. N Engl J Med. 2003;348:2366–7.
16. Blickstein I, Arabin B, Lewi L, Matias A, Kavak ZN, Basgul A, Kalish R, Vladareanu R, Ville Y. A template for defining the perinatal care of monochorionic twins: the Istanbul international ad hoc committee. J Perinat Med. 2010;38(2):107–10.
17. Blokage CE. Embryogenesis of chimeras, twins and anterior midlines asymmetries. Hum Reprod. 2006;21:579–91.
18. Brennan JN, Diwan RV, Rosen MG, Bellon EM. Fetofetal transfusion syndrome: prenatal ultrasonographic diagnosis. Radiology. 1982;143:535–6.
19. Caroto T, Santos V, Matias A. Accuracy of non-invasive prenatal test (NIPT) for detection of trisomy 21, 18 and 13 in twin pregnancies: a systematic review. Obstet Gynecol 2021 (in press).
20. Casati D, Faiola S, Lanna M. Major discordant anomalies in MZ twins: management and outcome. In: Matias A, Blickstein I, editors. Developmental and fetal origins of differences in monozygotic twins: from genetics to environmental factors. Elsevier Inc; 2020. (in press).
21. Cheng PJ, Huang SY, Shaw SW, Hsiao CH, Kao CC, Chueh HY, Hsieh TT. Difference in nuchal translucency between monozygotic and dizygotic spontaneously conceived twins. Prenat Diagn. 2010;30(3):247–50.
22. Chescheir NC, Seeds JW. Polyhydramnios and olygohydramnios in twin gestations. Obstet Gynecol. 1988;71:882–4.
23. Cimpoca B, Syngelaki A, Chi Mu A, Savvoulidou E, Nicolaides KH. Twin pregnancies with two live fetuses at 11-13 weeks: effect of one fetal death on pregnancy outcome. Ultrasound Obstet Gynecol. 2019. https://doi.org/10.1002/uog.21925.
24. Cleary-Goldman J, Rebarber A, Krantz D, Hallahan T, Saltzman D. First-trimester screening with nasal bone in twins. Am J Obstet Gynecol. 2008;199(3):283.e1–3.
25. Costa-Castro T, De Villiers S, Montenegro N, Severo M, Oepkes D, Matias A, Lopriore E. Velamentous cord insertion in twin-to-twin transfusion syndrome: does it matter? Placenta. 2013;34(11):1053–8.
26. Costa-Castro T, Zhao DP, Lipa M, Haak M, Oepkes D, Severo M, Montenegro N, Matias A, Lopriore E. Velamentous cord insertion in dichorionic and monochorionic twin pregnancies – does it make a difference? Placenta. 2016;42:87–92. https://doi.org/10.1016/j.placenta.2016.04.007. Epub 2016 Apr.
27. Cuckle H. Down's syndrome screening in twins. J Med Screen. 1998;5(1):3–4.
28. Curado J, Sileo F, Bhide A, Thilaganathan B, Khalil A. Early and late selective fetal growth restriction in monochorionic diamniotic twin pregnancies: natural history and diagnostic criteria. Ultrasound Obstet Gynecol. 2019; https://doi.org/10.1002/uog.20849.
29. de Mouzon J, Goossens V, Bhattacharya S, Castilla JA, Ferraretti AP, Korsak V, Kupka M, Nygren KG, Nyboe Andersen A, European IVF-monitoring (EIM) Consortium, for the European Society of Human Reproduction and Embryology (ESHRE). Assisted reproductive technology in Europe, 2006: results generated from European registers by ESHRE. Hum Reprod. 2010;25(8):1851–62.
30. Denbow ML, Cox P, Taylor M, Hammal DM, Fisk NM. Placental angioarchitecture in monochorionic twin pregnancies: relationship to fetal growth, fetofetal transfusion syndrome, and pregnancy outcome. Am J Obstet Gynecol. 2000;182(2):417–26.

31. Derom C, Derom R. The east flanders prospective twin survey. In: Blicktein I, Keith LG, editors. Multiple pregnancy. 2nd ed. London, UK: Taylor & Francis; 2005. p. 39–47.
32. Dudenhausen JW, Maier RF. Perinatal problems in multiple births. Deutsch Arztebl Int. 2010;107(38):663–8.
33. Fesslova V, Villa L, Nava S, Mosca F, Nicolini U. Fetal and neonatal echocardiographic findings in twin-twin transfusion syndrome. Am J Obstet Gynecol. 1998;179:1056–62.
34. Gardiner HM, Taylor MJ, Karatza A, Vanderheyden T, Huber A, Greenwald SE, Fisk NM, Hecher K. Twin-twin transfusion syndrome: the influence of intrauterine laser photocoagulation on arterial distensibility in childhood. Circulation. 2003;107:1–6.
35. Gica N, Gana N, Mat C, Panaitescu AM, Peltecu G, Vayna AM. Conjoined twins - early prenatal diagnosis. J Obstet Gynaecol. 2019;12:1–2. https://doi.org/10.1080/01443615.2019.1650012.
36. Gijtenbeek M, Shirzada MR, Ten Harkel ADJ, Oepkes D, Haak M. Congenital heart defects in monochorionic twins: a systematic review and meta-analysis. J Clin Med. 2019;8:902.
37. Goncé A, Borrell A, Fortuny A, Casals E, Martínez MA, Mercadé I, Cararach V, Vanrell JA. First-trimester screening for trisomy 21 in twin pregnancy: does the addition of biochemistry make an improvement? Prenat Diagn. 2005;25(12):1156–61.
38. Grande M, Goncé A, Stergiotou I, Bennasar M, Borrell A. Intertwin Crown Rump Length discordance in the prediction of fetal anomalies, fetal loss and adverse perinatal outcome. J Matern Fetal Neonatal Med. 2015;15:1–20.
39. Gratacós E, Lewi L, Muñoz B, Acosta-Rojas R, Hernandez-Andrade E, Martinez JM, Carreras E, Deprest J. A classification system for selective intrauterine growth restriction in monochorionic pregnancies according to umbilical artery Doppler flow in the smaller twin. Ultrasound Obstet Gynecol. 2007;30(1):28–34.
40. Gratacós E, Ortiz JU, Martinez JM. A systematic approach to the differential diagnosis and management of the complications of monochorionic twin pregnancies. Fetal Diagn Ther. 2012;32(3):145–55. https://doi.org/10.1159/000342751. Epub 2012 Sep 24.
41. Groene SG, Tollenaar LSA, Oepkes D, Lopriore E, van Klink JMM. The impact of selective fetal growth restriction or birth weight discordance on long-term neurodevelopment in monochorionic twins: a systematic literature review. J Clin Med. 2019;8(7):944. https://doi:10.3390/jcm8070944.
42. Hack KE, Derks JB, Elias SG, Franx A, Roos EJ, Voerman SK, Bode CL, Koopman-Esseboom C, Visser GH. Increased perinatal mortality and morbidity in monochorionic versus dichorionic twin pregnancies: clinical implications of a large Dutch cohort study. BJOG. 2008;115(1):58–67.
43. Hack KE, Vereycken MEMS, Torrance HL, Koopman-Esseboom C, Derks JB. Perinatal outcome of monochorionic and dichorionic twins after spontaneous and assisted conception: a retrospective cohort study. Acta Obstet Gynecol Scand. 2018;97(6):717–26. https://doi.org/10.1111/aogs.13323. Epub 2018 Mar 23.
44. Hall JG. Twinning: mechanisms and genetic implications. Curr Opin Genet Dev. 1996;6(3):343–7.
45. Hall JG. Twinning.Lancet. 2003 Aug 30;362(9385):735–43. https://doi.org/10.1016/S0140-6736(03)14237-7.
46. Halling C, Malone FD, Breathnach FM, Stewart MC, McAuliffe FM, Morrison JJ, Dicker P, Manning F, Corcoran JD, Perinatal Ireland Research Consortium. Neuro-developmental outcome of a large cohort of growth discordant twins. Eur J Pediatr. 2015. [Epub ahead of print].
47. Hecher K, Ville Y, Snijders R, Nicolaides KH. Doppler studies of the fetal circulation in twin-to-twin transfusion syndrome. Ultrasound Obstet Gynecol. 1995;5:318–24.
48. Kagan O, Gazzoni A, Sepulveda-Gonzalez G, Sotiriades A, Nicolaides K. Discordance in nuchal translucency thickness in the prediction of severe twin-to-twin transfusion syndrome. Ultrsound Obstet Gynecol. 2007;29(5):527–32.
49. Karageyim Karsidag AY, Kars B, Dansuk R, Api O, Unal O, Turan MC, Goynumer G. Brain damage to the survivor within 30 min of co-twin demise in monochorionic twins. Fetal Diagn Ther. 2005;20(2):91–5.

50. Khalil A, Rodgers M, Baschat A, Bhide A, Gratacos E, Hecher K, Kilby MD, Lewi L, Nicolaides KH, Oepkes D, Raine-Fenning N, Reed K, Salomon LJ, Sotiriadis A, Thilaganathan B, Ville Y. ISUOG Practice Guidelines: role of ultrasound in twin pregnancy. Ultrasound Obstet Gynecol. 2016;47(2):247–63. https://doi.org/10.1002/uog.15821.
51. La Sala GB, Nicoli A, Villani MT, Gallinelli A, Nucera G, Blickstein I. Spontaneous embryonic loss rates in twin and singleton pregnancies after transfer of top- versus intermediate-quality embryos. Fertil Steril. 2005;84:1602–5.
52. Lam JR, Liu B, Bhate R, Fenwick N, Reed K, Duffy JMN, Khalil A, Global Twins and Multiples Priority Setting Partnership Collaborators. Research priorities for the future health of multiples and their families: the Global Twins and Multiples Priority Setting Partnership. Ultrasound Obstet Gynecol. 2019;54(6):715–21. https://doi.org/10.1002/uog.20858.
53. Lambers MJ, Mager E, Goutbeek J, McDonnell J, Homburg R, Schats R, Hompes PG, Lambalk CB. Factors determining early pregnancy loss in singleton and multiple implantations. Hum Reprod. 2006;22(1):275–9.
54. Lewi L, Cannie M, Blickstein I, Jani J, Huber A, Hecher K, Dymarkowski S, Gratacós E, Lewi P, Deprest J. Placental sharing, birthweight discordance, and vascular anastomoses in monochorionic diamniotic twin placentas. Am J Obstet Gynecol. 2007;197(6):587e.1–8.
55. Lewi L, Lewi P, Diemert A, Jani J, Gucciardo L, Van Mieghem T, Doné E, Gratacós E, Huber A, Hecher K, Deprest J. The role of ultrasound examination in the first trimester and at 16 weeks' gestation to predict fetal complications in monochorionic diamniotic twin pregnancies. Am J Obstet Gynecol. 2008;199(5):493.e1–7.
56. Lewi L, Couck I, Deprest J. Twin reversed arterial perfusion sequence: different identical twins. In: Matias A, Blickstein I, editors. Developmental and fetal origins of differences in monozygotic twins: from Genetics to Environmental factors. Elsevier Inc.; 2020. (in press).
57. Liao H, Liu S, Wang H. Performance of non-invasive prenatal screening for fetal aneuploidy in twin pregnancies: a meta-analysis. Prenat Diagn. 2017;37(9):874–88.
58. Litwinska E, Syngelaki A, Cimpoca B, Sapantzoglou I, Nicolaides KH. Intertwin discordance in fetal size at 11-13 weeks' gestation and pregnancy outcome. Ultrasound Obstet Gynecol. 2020 Feb;55(2):189–197. https://doi.org/10.1002/uog.21923.
59. Lopriore E, Nagel HT, Vandenbussche FP, Walther FJ. Longterm neurodevelopmental outcome in twin-to-twin transfusion syndrome. Am J Obstet Gynecol. 2003;189:1313–8.
60. Lopriore E, Middeldorp JM, Oepkes D, Kanhai HH, Walther FJ, Vandenbussche FP. Twin anemia-polycythemia sequence in two monochorionic twin pairs without oligo-polyhydramnios sequence. Placenta. 2007;28:47–51.
61. Lopriore E, Lewi L, Khalil A. Monochorionic twins: a delicate balance. J Clin Med. 2019;8(10). pii: E1711.
62. Luke B, Keith LG. The contribution of singletons, twins and triplets to low birth weight, infant mortality and handicap in the United States. J Reprod Med. 1992;37:661–6.
63. Madsen H, Ball S, Wright D, Tørring N, Petersen O, Nicolaides K, Spencer K. A re-assessment of biochemical marker distributions in T21 affected and unaffected twin pregnancies in the first trimester. Ultrasound Obstet Gynecol. 2010;37(1):38–47.
64. Mahieu-Caputo D, Muller F, Joly D, Gubler MC, Lebidois J, Fermont L, Dumez Y, Dommergues M. Pathogenesis of twin-twin transfusion syndrome: the renin-angiotensin system hypothesis. Fetal Diagn Ther. 2001;16(4):241–4.
65. Malone FD. Monochorionic pregnancy – where have we been? Where are we going? Am J Obstet Gynecol. 2003;189:1308–9.
66. Martins Y, Silva S, Matias A, Blickstein I. Cardiac morbidity in twin-twin transfusion syndrome? J Perinat Med. 2012;40(2):107–14.
67. Matias A, Montenegro N. Down's syndrome screening in multiple pregnancies. Obst Gynecol Clin North Am. 2005;32(1):81–96.
68. Matias A, Montenegro N, Areias JC. Anticipating twin-twin transfusion syndrome in monochorionic twin pregnancy. Is there a role for nuchal translucency and ductus venosus blood flow evaluation at 11-14 weeks? Twin Res. 2000;3(2):65–70.

69. Matias A, Ramalho C, Montenegro N. Search for hemodynamic compromise at 11-14 weeks in monochorionic twin pregnancy: is abnormal flow in the ductus venosus predictive of twin-twin transfusion syndrome? J Matern Fetal Neonatal Med. 2005;18(2):79–86.
70. Matias A, Oliveira C, da Silva JT, Silva J, Barros A, Blickstein I. The effect of ICSI, maternal age, and embryonic stage on early clinical loss rate of twin versus singleton pregnancies. Eur J Obstet Gynecol Reprod Biol. 2006;130:212–5.
71. Matias A, La Sala G, Blickstein I. Early loss rates of the entire pregnancy are lower in singleton pregnancies following assisted reproduction. Fertil Steril. 2007;88:1452–4.
72. Matias A, Montenegro N, Loureiro T, Cunha M, Duarte S, Freitas D, Severo M. Screening for twin-twin transfusion syndrome at 11-14 weeks of pregnancy: the key role of ductus venosus blood flow assessment. Ultrasound Obstet Gynecol. 2010;35(2):142–8.
73. Matias A, Jeanty P, Toy E. Sonography in multiple gestation. In: Fleischer AC, Toy EC, Lee W, Manning FA, Romero RJ, editors. Sonography in obstetrics and gynecology. 7th ed. Mc Graw Hill; 2011. p. 337–74.
74. Matias A, Maiz N, Montenegro N, Nicolaides KH. Ductus venosus flow at 11-13 weeks in the prediction of birthweight discordance in monochorionic twins. J Perinat Med. 2011;39(4):467–70.
75. Matias A, Silva S, Blickstein I. Mechanisms of discordance in MZ twins: why and when? In: Matias A, Blickstein I, editors. Developmental and fetal origins of differences in monozygotic twins: from Genetics to Environmental factors. Elsevier Inc; 2020. (in press).
76. Maymon R, Jauniaux E. Down's syndrome screening in pregnancies after assisted reproductive techniques: an update. Reprod Biomed Online. 2002;4(3):285–93.
77. McNamara HC, Kane SC, Craig JM, Short RV, Umstad MP. A review of the mechanisms and evidence for typical and atypical twinning. Am J Obstet Gynecol. 2016;14(2):172–91.
78. Nicolaides KH, Spencer K, Avgidou K, Faiola S, Falcon O. Multicenter study of first-trimester screening for trisomy 21 in 75 821 pregnancies: results and estimation of the potential impact of individual risk-orientated two-stage first-trimester screening. Ultrasound Obstet Gynecol. 2005;25(3):221–6.
79. Odibo AO. Single intrauterine fetal death in twin pregnancies is associated with increased risk of preterm birth and abnormal antenatal brain imaging in the surviving co-twin. BJOG. 2019;126(5):579. https://doi.org/10.1111/1471-0528.15599.
80. Oliviennes F. Avoiding multiple pregnancies in ART double trouble: yes a twin pregnancy is an adverse outcome. Hum Reprod. 2000;15:1663–5.
81. Pandya PP, Snijders RJ, Johnson SP, De Lourdes BM, Nicolaides KH. Screening for fetal trisomies by maternal age and fetal nuchal translucency thickness at 10 to 14 weeks of gestation. Br J Obstet Gynaecol. 1995;102(12):957–62.
82. Park YH, Kim YN, Im DH, Kim DH, Byun JM, Jeong DH, Lee KB, Sung MS. Neonatal outcomes between discordant monochorionic and dichorionic twins. J Matern Fetal Neonatal Med. 2021;34(13):2080–88. https://doi.org/10.1080/14767058.2019.1657085. Epub 2019 Aug 28.
83. Pharoah P. Neurological outcome in twins. Semin Neonatol. 2002;7:223–30.
84. Pharoah P. Risk of cerebral palsy in multiple pregnancies. Clin Perinatol. 2006;33(2):301–13.
85. Pharoah P. Twins and locomotor disorder in children. J Bone Joint Surg Br. 2006;88(3):295–7.
86. Pharoah PO, Cooke RW. A hypothesis for the aetiology of spastic cerebral palsy - the vanishing twin. Dev Med Child Neurol. 1997;39:292–6.
87. Prats P, Rodríguez I, Comas C, Puerto B. Systematic review of screening for trisomy 21 in twin pregnancies in first trimester combining nuchal translucency and biochemical markers: a meta-analysis. Prenat Diagn. 2014;34(11):1077–83. https://doi.org/10.1002/pd.4431.
88. Pretorious D, Budorick N, Sciosia A, Krabble JK, Ko S, Myhre CM. Twin pregnancies in the second trimester in an α-fetoprotein screening program: sonographic evaluation and outcome. Am J Roentgenol. 1993;161:1007–13.
89. Rustico MA, Lanna M, Faiola S, Casati D, Spaccini L, Righini A, Parazzini C, Napolitano M, Scelsa B, Lista G, Corti C, Riccipetitoni G, Cetin I. Major discordant structural anomalies in monochorionic twins: spectrum and outcomes. Twin Res Hum Genet. 2018;21(6):546–55.
90. Schatz F. Clinical for the physiology of the fetus. Berlin: Hirschwald; 1890.

91. Schmid O, Trautmann U, Ashour H, Ulmer R, Pfeiffer RA, Beinder E. Prenatal diagnosis of heterokaryotypic mosaic twins discordant for fetal sex. Prenat Diagn. 2000;20(12):999–1003.
92. Schou KV, Lando AV, Ekelund CK, Jensen LN, Jørgensen C, Nørgaard LN, Rode L, Søgaard K, Tabor A, Sundberg K. Long-term neurodevelopmental outcome of monochorionic twins after laser therapy or umbilical cord occlusion for twin-twin transfusion syndrome. Fetal Diagn Ther. 2019;46(1):20–7.
93. Sebire NJ, Snidjers RJM, Hughes K, Sepulveda W, Nicolaides KH. Screening for trisomy 21 in twin pregnancies by maternal age and fetal nuchal translucency thickness at 10-14 weeks of gestation. Br J Obstet Gynecol. 1996;103:999–1003.
94. Sebire NJ, Snijders RJM, Hughes K, Sepulveda W, Nicolaides KH. The hidden mortality of monochorionic twin pregnancies. Br J Obstet Gynecol. 1997;104:1203–7.
95. Sebire NJ, D' Ercole C, Hughes K, Carvalho M, Nicolaides KH. Increased nuchal translucency thickness at 10-14 weeks of gestation as predictor of severe twin-to-twin transfusion syndrome. Ultrasound Obstet Gynecol. 1997;10:86–9.
96. Sebire NJ, Souka A, Skentou H, Geerts L, Nicolaides KH. Early prediction of severe twin-to-twin transfusion syndrome. Hum Reprod. 2000;15:2008–10.
97. Senat MV, Loizeau S, Cooudere S, Bernard JP, Ville Y. The value of middle cerebral artery peak systolic velocity in the diagnosis of fetal anemia after intrauterine death of one monochorionic twin. Am J Obstet Gynecol. 2003;189:1319–23.
98. Sepulveda W, Sebire N, Hughes K, Odibo A, Nicolaides KH. The lambda sign at 10-14 weeks of gestation as a predictor of chorionicity in twin pregnancies. Ultrasound Obstet Gynecol. 1996;7:421–3.
99. Sepulveda W, Sebire N, Hughes K, Kalogeropoulos A, Nicolaides KH. Evolution of the lambda or twin-chorionic peak sign in dichorionic twin pregnancies. Obstet Gynecol. 1997;89:439–41.
100. Sepulveda W, Wong AE, Casasbuenas A. Nuchal translucency and nasal bone in first-trimester ultrasound screening for aneuploidy in multiple pregnancies. Ultrasound Obstet Gynecol. 2009;33(2):152–6.
101. Silva S, Martins Y, Matias A, Blickstein I. Why are monozygotic twins different? J Perinat Med. 2011;39(2):195–202.
102. Slaghekke F, Lopriore E, Lewi L, Middeldorp JM, van Zwet EW, Weingertner AS, Klumper FJ, DeKoninck P, Devlieger R, Kilby MD, et al. Fetoscopic laser coagulation of the vascular equator versus selective coagulation for twin-to-twin transfusion syndrome: an open-label randomised controlled trial. Lancet. 2014;383:2144–51.
103. Spencer K, Salonen R, Muller F. Down's syndrome screening in multiple pregnancies using alpha-fetoprotein and free beta hCG. Prenat Diagn. 1994;14:537–42.
104. Spencer K, Kagan KO, Nicolaides KH. Screening for trisomy 21 in twin pregnancies in the first trimester: an update of the impact of chorionicity on maternal serum markers. Prenat Diagn. 2008;28(1):49–52.
105. Sperling L, Kiil C, Larsen LU, Qvist I, Schwartz M, Jorgensen C, Skajaa K, Bang J, Tabor A. Naturally conceived twins with monochorionic placentation have the highest risk of fetal loss. Ultrasound Obstet Gynecol. 2006;28:644–52.
106. Stagnati V, Zanardini C, Fichera A, Pagani G, Quintero RA, Bellocco R, Prefumo F. Early prediction of twin-to-twin transfusion syndrome: systematic review and meta-analysis. Ultrasound Obstet Gynecol. 2017;49(5):573–82.
107. Steinman G, Valderrama E. Mechanisms of twinning. III. Placentation, calcium reduction and modified compaction. J Reprod Med. 2001;46(11):995–1002.
108. Taylor MJ, Denbow ML, Tanawattanacharoen S, Gannon C, Cox PM, Fisk NM. Doppler detection of arterio-arterial anastomoses in monochorionic twins: feasibility and clinical application. Hum Reprod. 2000;15:1632–6.
109. Teplica D, Peekna K. The mirror phenomenon in monozygotc twins. In: Blickstein I, Keith LG, editors. Multiple pregnancy. 2nd ed. London, UK; 2005. p. 277–88.
110. The International Clearinghouse for Birth Defects Monitoring Systems. Conjoined twins- an epidemiological study based on 312 cases. Acta Genet Med Gemellol. 1991;40:325–35.

111. Tollenaar LSA, Slaghekke F, van Klink JMM, Groene SG, Middeldorp JM, Haak MC, Klumper FJCM, Oepkes D, Lopriore E. Twin-twin transfusion syndrome with anemia-polycythemia: prevalence, characteristics, and outcome. J Clin Med. 2019;8(8). pii: E1129.
112. Tollenaar LSA, Lopriore E, Middeldorp JM, Haak MC, Klumper FJ, Oepkes D, Slaghekke F. Improved prediction of twin anemia-polycythemia sequence by delta middle cerebral artery peak systolic velocity: new antenatal classification system. Ultrasound Obstet Gynecol. 2019;53(6):788–93.
113. Tollenaar LSA, Lopriore E, Slaghekke F, Oepkes D, Middeldorp JM, Haak MC, Klumper FJC, Tan RNG, Rijken M, van Klink JMM. High risk of long-term impairment in donor twins with spontaneous twin anemia polycythemia sequence. Ultrasound Obstet Gynecol.2020 Jan;55(1):39–46. https://doi.org/10.1002/uog.20846.
114. Townsend R, Khalil A. Ultrasound surveillance in twin pregnancy: an update for practitioners. Ultrasound. 2018;26(4):193–205.
115. Townsend R, D'Antonio F, Sileo FG, Kumbay H, Thilaganathan B, Khalil A. Perinatal outcome of monochorionic twin pregnancy complicated by selective fetal growth restriction according to management: systematic review and meta-analysis. Ultrasound Obstet Gynecol. 2019;53(1):36–46. https://doi.org/10.1002/uog.20114.
116. Tromp M, Ravelli AC, Reitsma JB, Bonsel GJ, Mol BW. Increasing maternal age at first pregnancy planning: health outcomes and associated costs. J Epidemiol Community Health. 2010;65(12):1083–90.
117. Tummers P, De Sutter P, Dhont M. Risk of spontaneous abortion in singleton and twin pregnancies after IVF/ICSI. Hum Reprod. 2003;18:1720–3.
118. van Gemert MJ, van den Wijngaard JP, Vandenbussche FP. Twin reversed arterial perfusion sequence is more common than generally accepted. Birth Defects Res A Clin Mol Teratol. 2015;103:641–3.
119. van Klink JM, Slaghekke F, Balestriero MA, Scelsa B, Introvini P, Rustico M, Faiola S, Rijken M, Koopman HM, Middeldorp JM, Oepkes D, Lopriore E. Neurodevelopmental outcome at 2 years in twin-twin transfusion syndrome survivors randomized for the Solomon trial. Am J Obstet Gynecol. 2016;214(1):113.e1–7.
120. Van Mieghem T, Lewi L, Gucciardo L, Dekoninck P, Van Schoubroeck D, Devlieger R, Deprest J. The fetal heart in twinto-twin transfusion syndrome. Int J Pediatr. 2010;2010. pii: 379792.
121. Van Mieghem T, Eixarch E, Gucciardo L, Done E, Gonzales I, Van Schoubroeck D, Lewi L, Gratacos E, Deprest J. Outcome prediction in monochorionic diamniotic twin pregnancies with moderately discordant amniotic fluid. Ultrasound Obstet Gynecol. 2011;37(1):15–21. https://doi.org/10.1002/uog.8802.
122. Verbeek LI, Lopriore E. Hemoglobin differences at birth in monochorionic twins. In: Matias A, Blickstein I, editors. Developmental and fetal origins of differences in monozygotic twins: from Genetics to Environmental factors. Elsevier Inc; 2020. (in press).
123. Wittmann BK, Baldwin VJ, Nichold B. Antenatal diagnosis of twin-to-twin transfusion syndrome by ultrasound. Obstet Gynecol. 1981;58:123–7.
124. Wood SL, St. Onge R, Connors G, Elliot PD. Evaluation of the twin peak sign in determining chorionicity in multiple pregnancy. Obstet Gynecol. 1996;88:6–9.
125. Zegers-Hochschild F, Bravo M, Fernandez E, Fabers C, Balmaceda JP, Mackenna A. Multiple gestation as a marker of reproductive efficacy: learning from assisted reproductive technologies. Reprod Biomed Online. 2003;8:125–9.
126. Zosmer N, Bajoria R, Weiner E, Rigby M, Vaughan J, Fisk NM. Clinical and echographic features of in utero cardiac dysfunction in the recipient twin-to-twin transfusion syndrome. Br Heart J. 1994;72:74–9.

GPSR Compliance

The European Union's (EU) General Product Safety Regulation (GPSR) is a set of rules that requires consumer products to be safe and our obligations to ensure this.

If you have any concerns about our products, you can contact us on ProductSafety@springernature.com

In case Publisher is established outside the EU, the EU authorized representative is:

Springer Nature Customer Service Center GmbH
Europaplatz 3
69115 Heidelberg, Germany

Batch number: 10753458

Printed by Printforce, the Netherlands

Renato Augusto Moreira de Sá •
Eduardo Borges da Fonseca
Editors

Perinatology

Evidence-Based Best Practices in Perinatal Medicine

Volume II

Springer

Editors
Renato Augusto Moreira de Sá
Maternal and Child Department
Fluminense Federal University
Niterói, Rio de Janeiro
Brazil

Eduardo Borges da Fonseca
Federal University of Paraíba
João Pessoa, Paraíba
Brazil

ISBN 978-3-030-83436-4 ISBN 978-3-030-83434-0 (eBook)
https://doi.org/10.1007/978-3-030-83434-0

© Springer Nature Switzerland AG 2022
This work is subject to copyright. All rights are reserved by the Publisher, whether the whole or part of the material is concerned, specifically the rights of translation, reprinting, reuse of illustrations, recitation, broadcasting, reproduction on microfilms or in any other physical way, and transmission or information storage and retrieval, electronic adaptation, computer software, or by similar or dissimilar methodology now known or hereafter developed.
The use of general descriptive names, registered names, trademarks, service marks, etc. in this publication does not imply, even in the absence of a specific statement, that such names are exempt from the relevant protective laws and regulations and therefore free for general use.
The publisher, the authors, and the editors are safe to assume that the advice and information in this book are believed to be true and accurate at the date of publication. Neither the publisher nor the authors or the editors give a warranty, expressed or implied, with respect to the material contained herein or for any errors or omissions that may have been made. The publisher remains neutral with regard to jurisdictional claims in published maps and institutional affiliations.

This Springer imprint is published by the registered company Springer Nature Switzerland AG
The registered company address is: Gewerbestrasse 11, 6330 Cham, Switzerland

Rodrigo, Alice, and Isadora, our children and our hope for a better world.

Foreword

As one of the founders of perinatal medicine, it is my particular pleasure to write this foreword and to support the current activities in this fascinating new field of human medicine.

A particular highlight is to do it together with Ana Bianchi, the scientific daughter of my old friend and supporting pioneer in fetal medicine Roberto Caldeyro-Barcia from Uruguay. He in heaven and I still on earth are grateful to the younger, currently so active, and successful generation for continuing what we started and founded decades ago.

Perinatal medicine is very versatile because its main part, the prenatal block – this means everything that happens before birth – was to a high degree, up to the beginning of the 1960s, a medically unexplored space. In the meantime, the evolution has been explosive.

Perinatal medicine is subject to its special characteristics, namely to be interdisciplinary. This means that the cooperation with other important disciplines should be essential. The closest connection exists between obstetrics and neonatology in advanced centres even more than between obstetrics and gynecology.

I wish good success.

Erich Saling
"Professor Emeritus" of Perinatal Medicine at the Charité,
Humboldt-University Berlin - Germany
The Father of Perinatal Medicine

Ana Bianchi
President of Caldeyro-Barcia Foundation - Uruguay

Preface

Perinatal period is defined as *"the period of time between 22 weeks after fertilization and 7 days after parturition."*[1]

Usually, authors specializing in obstetrics and maternal-fetal medicine are invited to write chapters of perinatology books and to express themselves about problems related to perinatology. Consequently, the set of written productions includes strictly obstetric texts, most often intended for prenatal care, or works written by pediatricians and intended for neonatal care.

At the development stage of this book, our desire was to follow the idea of Erich Saling from the book ***The Child in the Field of Obstetrics*** (Das Kind im Bereich der Geburtshilfe) [2]. In the 1950s, "The Father of Perinatal Medicine," exhorts the antenatal care importance, reinforcing the innovative achievement of another pioneer on perinatal care, Roberto Caldeyro-Barcia.

The progressive specialization in the field of medicine has led us to bring two specialties, materno-fetal medicine and neonatology. The improvement in the assessment of fetal well-being and *in-utero* treatment and the advancements in neonatal intensive care have greatly improved the chances of babies' long-term survival. Therefore, to avoid unnecessary confusion for the purposes of this book, the perinatal period will be extended from 20 completed weeks (140 days) of gestation to 28 completed days after birth. This extended definition is accepted by many authors and medical specialty societies.

Keeping in mind the original proposal of the pioneers of perinatology, which correspond with our convictions, we accepted the invitation of Springer to bring together in this book renowned authors of the two great specialties involved in the field of perinatology: obstetrics and neonatology.

---

[1] 1. World Health Organization. ICD-11 for mortality and morbidity statistics. Version: 2020 September. Available from: https://icd.who.int/browse11/l-m/en#/http://id.who.int/icd/entity/914150644. Assessed in February 2021.

[2] Dudenhausen JW. Erich Saling - The Father of Prenatal and Perinatal Medicine-Dedication to his 90th birthday. J Perinat Med. 2015 Jul;43(4):379.

This work was not without its difficulties. The main one comes from the fact that this type of book organization gathers varied chapters in form and content, and is at risk of becoming a "patchwork" that leaves the reader disoriented.

Such inconvenience was overcome by the editors, who were careful to put the texts in consistent thematic blocks, managing to make the book reflect the themes related to pediatrics and obstetrics in an integrated way to allow a better understanding of perinatology. So, our aim was to avoid transmitting an overly integrated and closed view of one of the specialties, leaving to our reader space for their own reflection on the themes and for the development of self-interpretations.

We are grateful to chapter authors and the support by the notable Professors Erich Saling, Asim Kurjak, and Ana Bianchi.

We dedicate this book to our children Rodrigo, Alice, and Isadora, who are the biggest motivation of our lives.

Rio de Janeiro, RJ, Brazil
Niteroi, RJ, Brazil
João Pessoa, Paraíba, Brazil

Renato Augusto Moreira de Sá

Eduardo Borges da Fonseca

Acknowledgement

Prof Asim Kurjak, for supporting the Perinatal Medicine activities all around the world.

Contents

Contributors

Daniela Aires Moreira University of Medical Sciences, João Pessoa, Paraíba, Brazil

Maternal Fetal Medicine Group, Nova Diagnóstico por Imagem, João Pessoa, Brazil

Melania M. Amorim Post-Graduate Program in Instituto de Medicina Integral Professor Fernando Figueira, Recife, Brazil

Obstetrics & Gynecology, Federal University of Campina Grande, Campina Grande, Brazil

Ana Espinosa Institution Matersur, Teaching and Research, Bahía Blanca, Buenos Aires, Argentina

Carla Betina Andreucci Department of Medicine, Center of Biological and Health Sciences, Federal University of São Carlos, São Carlos, Brazil

L. Atzori Clinical Metabolomics Unit, Department of Biomedical Sciences, University of Cagliari, Cagliari, Italy

Diogo Ayres-De-Campos Departamento de Obstetrícia, Ginecologia e Medicina da Reprodução, Faculdade de Medicina da Universidade de Lisboa, Centro Hospitalar Universitário Lisboa Norte – Hospital de Santa Maria, Lisbon, Portugal

Arnaldo Prata Barbosa Instituto D'Or de Pesquisa e Ensino – IDOR, Rio de Janeiro, Brazil

Lara Spalldi Barišić Fetal and Maternal Medicine, Private Clinic Veritas, Zagreb, Croatia

Renato José Bauer Department of Obstetrics, Faculty of Medicine of Pontifical University of Sao Paulo, City of Sorocaba, SP, Brazil

Michael W. Bebbington Washington University School of Medicine in St. Louis, Louis, US

Matheus Cabral L. Beleza Maternal-Fetal Medicine Department, NEXUS Institute, Brasília, Federal District, Brazil

Augusto César Garcia Saab Benedeti FATESA – Faculdade de Tecnologia em Saúde, Ribeirão Preto, SP, Brazil

Leticia Benítez BCNatal - Barcelona Center for Maternal-Fetal and Neonatal Medicine (Hospital Clínic and Hospital Sant Joan de Deu), University of Barcelona, Barcelona, Spain

Lisandra Stein Bernardes Department of Obstetrics and Gynecology, University of São Paulo, São Paulo, Brazil

Sepaco Hospital, São Paulo, Brazil

School of Medicine, Faculdade Israelita de Ciências da Saúde Albert Einstein, São Paulo, Brazil

Carlos A. Bhering Departamento de Neonatologia do Instituto Fernandes Figueira/ FIOCRUZ, Rio de Janeiro, Brazil

Pediatria da Universidade de Vassouras, Vassouras, Brazil

Ana B. Bianchi Perinatal Department, Pereira Rossell Hospital, Montevideo, Montevideo, Uruguay

M. F. Blasina Department of Neonatology, Hospital de Clínicas, Facultad de Medicina, Universidad de la República, Montevideo, Uruguay

Fernando Javier Rojas Bravo Clínica Universidad de los Andes, Las Condes, Chile

Ingrid Schwach Werneck Britto Department of Obstetrics and Gynecology, Faculty of Medical Sciences of Santa Casa of São Paulo, São Paulo, São Paulo, Brazil

Isabela Bussade Pontifícia Universidade Católica (PUC), Rio de Janeiro, RJ, Brazil

Gabriel Martins Cruz Campos Fetal Medicine Residence – Hospital das Clínicas da UFMG, Belo Horizonte, Brazil

José Carlos Carraro-Eduardo Department of Internal Medicine, School of Medicine, Universidade Federal Fluminense (UFF), Niterói, Rio de Janeiro, Brazil

Ricardo Carvalho Cavalli Department of Obstetrics and Gynecology, Ribeirão Preto Medical School, University of São Paulo, São Paulo, SP, Brazil

Department of Obstetrics and Gynecology, Hospital das Clínicas, Faculty of Medicine, University of São Paulo, FMUSP, São Paulo, SP, Brazil

Frank A. Chervenak Department of Obstetrics and Gynecology, Zucker School of Medicine of Hofstra/Northwell, Lenox Hill Hospital, New York, NY, USA

Luciana C. Cima Perinatal/Rede D'or, Rio de Janeiro, RJ, Brazil

V. Corda Department of Prenatal and Preimplantation Genetic Diagnosis and Fetal Therapy, Ospedale Pediatrico Microcitemico "A. Cao", Cagliari, Italy

Egle Couto Department of Obstetrics and Gynecology, University of Campinas (UNICAMP), Campinas, SP, Brazil

Pontifical Catholic University of Campinas, Campinas, Brazil

Antonio José Cunha Faculdade de Medicina da Universidade Federal do Rio de Janeiro, Rio de Janeiro, Brazil

Bartolomeu Expedito da Câmara França Materno-Infantil, Federal Fluminense University, Niteroi, RJ, Brazil

Gisele Passos da Costa Gribel Department of Anesthesiology, Hospital Maternidade Escola, Universidade Federal do Rio de Janeiro (UFRJ), Rio de Janeiro, RJ, Brazil

Eduardo Borges da Fonseca Maternal Fetal Medicine Group - Nova Diagnóstico por Imagem, João Pessoa, PB, Brazil

Ob/Gyn Department, Federal University of Paraiba, João Pessoa, PB, Brazil

Antonio Claudio Lucas da Nóbrega Laboratório de Ciências do Exercício, Instituto Biomédico, Universidade Federal Fluminense, Niterói, RJ, Brazil

Jair Roberto da Silva Braga Maternidade Escola da UFRJ, Universidade Federal do Rio de Janeiro, Rio de Janeiro, RJ, Brazil

Fabrício da Silva Costa Department of Obstetrics and Gynecology, Ribeirão Preto Medical School – University of São Paulo, Ribeirão Preto, São Paulo, Brazil

Fernanda Campos da Silva Department of Obstetrics, Universidade Federal do Estado do Rio de Janeiro (UNIRIO), Rio de Janeiro, RJ, Brazil

Marcos José Burle de Aguiar Medicine School, Federal University of Minas Gerais, Belo Horizonte, Brazil

Regina Amélia Lopes Pessoa de Aguiar Medicine School, Federal University of Minas Gerais, Belo Horizonte, Brazil

João Henrique Carvalho Leme de Almeida Neonatology Department, Instituto Nacional da Saúde da Mulher, da Criança e do Adolescente Fernandes Figueira, Fundação Oswaldo Cruz, Rio de Janeiro, RJ, Brazil

José Maria de Andrade Lopes Perinatal Maternity Hospital, Rio de Janeiro, Brazil

Eduardo Carvalho de Arruda Veiga Department of Obstetrics and Gynecology, Ribeirão Preto Medical School, University of São Paulo, São Paulo, SP, Brazil

Márcia Cristina de Azevedo Gomes Clínica Perinatal, Neonatal Intensive Care, Rio de Janeiro, RJ, Brazil

Mario Henrique Burlacchini de Carvalho Department of Obstetrics and Gynecology, Faculty of Medical Sciences of Santa Casa of São Paulo, São Paulo, São Paulo, Brazil

Paulo Roberto Nassar de Carvalho Instituto Fernandes Figueira, Rio de Janeiro, Fundação Oswaldo Cruz –FIOCRUZ, Rio de Janeiro, Brazil

IETECS – Instituto de Estudos de Tecnologia em Saúde, Rio de Janeiro, Brazil

Grupo Perinatal, Rio de Janeiro, Brazil

Victor Rocha de Castro Alves FATESA – Faculdade de Tecnologia em Saúde, Ribeirão Preto, SP, Brazil

Renata Rodrigues Teixeira de Castro Department of Cardiology, Hospital Naval Marcílio Dias & School of Medicine, Iguaçu University, Rio de Janeiro, RJ, Brazil

Fernando de Freitas Martins Neonatology Department, Fernandes Figueira Institute, Oswaldo Cruz Foundation, Neonatal Intensive Care Unit, Perinatal Clinic, Rio de Janeiro, RJ, Brazil

Guilherme Ramires de Jesús Department of Obstetrics, Universidade do Estado do Rio de Janeiro, Rio de Janeiro, Brazil

Nilson Ramires de Jesús Department of Obstetrics, Universidade do Estado do Rio de Janeiro, Rio de Janeiro, Brazil

José Roberto de Moraes Ramos Departamento de Neonatologia do Instituto Fernandes Figueira/FIOCRUZ, Rio de Janeiro, Brazil

Programa de Reanimação Neonatal da Sociedade Brasileira de Pediatria, Rio de Janeiro, Brazil

Roberto Magliano de Morais Filho Faculdade de Medicina Nova Esperança, Joao Pessoa, Paraiba, Brazil

Roberto Magliano de Morais Universidade Federal da Paraiba, Joao Pessoa, Paraiba, Brazil

Cristiane Alves de Oliveira Federal Fluminense University and Rio de Janeiro Federal University, Niteroi and Rio de Janeiro, Brazil

Elaine de Paula Fiod Costa Medicine Department, Federal University of Maranhão, Maranhão, Brazil

Helenilce de Paula Fiod Costa Neonatology Department, Institution Santa Joana/ Promatre Hospital Group, São Paulo, Brazil

Jorge de Rezende-Filho Maternidade Escola da UFRJ, Universidade Federal do Rio de Janeiro, Rio de Janeiro, RJ, Brazil

Renato Augusto Moreira de Sá Fernandes Figueira Institut - FIOCRUZ, Rio de Janeiro, RJ, Brazil

Danielle Negri de Souza Lopes Neonatology Department, Perinatal Maternity Hospital, Rio de Janeiro, RJ, Brazil

Evaldo Trajano de Souza Silva Filho Maternal-Fetal Medicine Department, NEXUS Institute, Brasília, Federal District, Brazil

J. L. Diaz-Rossello Department of Neonatology, Hospital de Clínicas, Facultad de Medicina, Universidad de la República, Montevideo, Uruguay

Flavia Cunha dos Santos Department of Obstetrics, Universidade do Estado do Rio de Janeiro, Rio de Janeiro, Brazil

Karina dos Santos Research Group on Maternal and Child Health (Grupo de Pesquisa em Saúde Materna e Infantil – GPSMI), Nutrition Institute, Federal University of Rio de Janeiro, Rio de Janeiro, RJ, Brazil

Joachim Dudenhausen Department of Obstetrics and Gynecology, Zucker School of Medicine at Hofstra/Northwell, New York, NY, USA

Siw Helen Westby Eger Department of Pediatrics and Adolescence Medicine, Oslo University Hospital, Oslo, Norway

D. P. Esteves Department of Cardiology, Pregnancy Heart Disease Sector, Hospital Federal dos Servidores do Estado, Rio de Janeiro, RJ, Brazil

Juliana Silva Esteves Hospital Federal dos Servidores do Estado - Ministry of Health, Rio de Janeiro, RJ, Brazil

Carlos Augusto Faria Department of Maternal and Child Health, School of Medicine, Universidade Federal Fluminense (UFF), Niterói, RJ, Brazil

Francesc Figueras BCNatal - Barcelona Center for Maternal-Fetal and Neonatal Medicine (Hospital Clínic and Hospital Sant Joan de Deu), University of Barcelona, Barcelona, Spain

Francisco Mauad Filho FATESA – Faculdade de Tecnologia em Saúde, Ribeirão Preto, SP, Brazil

Mario Julio Franco Florianópolis, SC, Brazil

Amos Grunebaum Department of Obstetrics and Gynecology, Zucker School of Medicine at Hofstra/Northwell, New York, NY, USA

Fernanda Hermeto Neonatology Department, Perinatal Maternity Hospital, Rio de Janeiro, RJ, Brazil

A. Iuculano Department of Prenatal and Preimplantation Genetic Diagnosis and Fetal Therapy, Ospedale Pediatrico Microcitemico "A. Cao", Cagliari, Italy

Edward Araujo Júnior Discipline of Fetal Medicine, Department of Obstetrics, Paulista School of Medicine –Federal University of São Paulo (EPM-UNIFESP), São Paulo, SP, Brazil

Joffre Amim Junior Maternidade Escola da Universidade Federal do Rio de Janeiro, Rio de Janeiro, Brazil

José Eleutério Junior Department of Women's, Child and Teenager Health, Federal University of Ceará, Fortaleza, Brazil

Mário Dias Corrêa Júnior Obstetrics and Gynecology Department – Faculdade de Medicina da UFMG, Belo Horizonte, Brazil

Renato Passini Junior Department of Obstetrics and Gynecology, University of Campinas (UNICAMP), Campinas, SP, Brazil

Leila Katz Catholic University of Pernambuco (UNICAP), Recife, Brazil

Post-Graduate Program in Instituto de Medicina Integral Professor Fernando Figueira, Recife, Brazil

Roxana Knobel Faculty of Medical Sciences, State University of Campinas – UNICAMP, Campinas, Brazil

Department of Obstetrics & Gynecology, Federal University of Santa Catarina (UFSC), Florianópolis, Brazil

Henri Augusto Korkes Department of Obstetrics, Faculty of Medicine of Pontifical University of Sao Paulo, City of Sorocaba, SP, Brazil

Regis Kreitchmann Department of Gynecology and Obstetrics, Federal University of Health Sciences of Porto Alegre, Porto Alegre, Brazil

Asim Kurjak Sarajevo School of Science and Technology, Sarajevo, Bosnia and Herzegovina

Department of Obstetrics and Gynecology, School of Medicine, University of Zagreb, Zagreb, Croatia

Marcela Ignacchiti Lacerda Department of Obstetrics, Universidade do Estado do Rio de Janeiro, Rio de Janeiro, Brazil

Roger Abramino Levy Immunology and Inflammation, GlaxoSmithKline (GSK), Upper Providence, PA, USA

Renata Bastos Lopes Neonatology Department, Perinatal Maternity Hospital, Rio de Janeiro, RJ, Brazil

Jürgen Lüthje Institute of Perinatal Medicine, Berlin-Neukölln, Germany

André Luiz Malavasi Pérola Byington Hospital, São Paulo, Brazil

Hospital do Servidor Público Municipal de São Paulo, São Paulo, Brazil

International Society on Thrombosis and Haemostasis, São Paulo, Brazil

Penélope Saldanha Marinho Maternidade Escola da Universidade Federal do Rio de Janeiro, Rio de Janeiro, Brazil

Judith Martínez BCNatal - Barcelona Center for Maternal-Fetal and Neonatal Medicine (Hospital Clínic and Hospital Sant Joan de Deu), University of Barcelona, Barcelona, Spain

Alexandra Matias Department of Obstetrics, Gynecology and Pediatrics, Faculty of Medicine University of Porto, Centro Hospitalar Universitário Hospital of S. João, Porto, Portugal

Laurence B. McCullough Department of Obstetrics and Gynecology, Zucker School of Medicine of Hofstra/Northwell, Lenox Hill Hospital, New York, NY, USA

Maria Dalva Barbosa Baker Méio Instituto Fernandes Figueira- Fiocruz, Rio de Janeiro, Brazil

Eva Meler BCNatal - Barcelona Center for Maternal-Fetal and Neonatal Medicine (Hospital Clínic and Hospital Sant Joan de Deu), University of Barcelona, Barcelona, Spain

Angelica Espinosa Miranda Department of Social Medicine, Federal Universty of Espírito Santo, Vitória, Brazil

Carolina Carvalho Mocarzel Department of Obstetrics, Hospital Federal dos Servidores do Estado, Rio de Janeiro, Rio de Janeiro, Brazil

G. Monni Department of Prenatal and Preimplantation Genetic Diagnosis and Fetal Therapy, Ospedale Pediatrico Microcitemico "A. Cao", Cagliari, Italy

Viviane P. Monteiro Instituto Fernandes Figueira/Fiocruz, Rio de Janeiro, RJ, Brazil

Maria Elisabeth Lopes Moreira Instituto Fernandes Figueira - Fiocruz, Clinica Perinatal Laranjeiras, Rio de Janeiro, RJ, Brazil

F. Murgia Clinical Metabolomics Unit, Department of Biomedical Sciences, University of Cagliari, Cagliari, Italy

Janaína Luz Narciso-Schiavon Florianópolis, SC, Brazil

Carlos Antonio Negrato Medical school from Faculdade de Odontologia de Bauru (FOB), Universidade de São Paulo, Bauru, São Paulo, Brazil

Antônio Rodrigues Braga Neto Materno-Infantil, Federal Fluminense University, Niteroi, RJ, Brazil

Luiza M. Neves Instituto NAcional de Saude da Mulher, da Criança e do Adolescente, FIOCRUZ, Rio de Janeiro, Brazil

Departamento de Oftalmologia, Universidade do Estado do Rio de Janeiro, Rio de Janeiro, Brazil

Ana Carla Zanchietta Nicolielo Maternidade Perinatal, Department of Obstetrícia, Rio de Janeiro, Rio de Janeiro, Brazil

Rone Peterson Cerqueira Oliveira Department of Gynecology, Obstetrics and Human Reproduction, Federal University of Bahia, Salvador, Bahia, Brazil

Mario S. F. Palermo Diagnomed Affiliated Institution Faculty of Medicine of Buenos Aires, Teaching and Research, Buenos Aires, Argentina

Viral Mahesh Pandya GHU Paris-Centre, Hôpital Necker-Enfants Malades, Paris, France

Mauro Romero Leal Passos Department of Microbiology and Parasitology, Fluminense Federal University, Niterói, Brazil

Alberto Borges Peixoto Department of Gynecology and Obstetrics, University of Uberaba (UNIUBE), Uberaba, Brazil

Department of Gynecology and Obstetrics, Federal University of Triângulo Mineiro (UFTM), Uberaba, Brazil

Fernando Barbosa Peixoto Department of Obstetrics and Gynecology, Ribeirão Preto Medical School, University of São Paulo, São Paulo, SP, Brazil

Fernando Maia Peixoto-Filho Instituto Fernandes Figueira, Rio de Janeiro, Fundação Oswaldo Cruz –FIOCRUZ, Rio de Janeiro, Brazil

IETECS – Instituto de Estudos de Tecnologia em Saúde, Rio de Janeiro, Brazil

Grupo Perinatal, Rio de Janeiro, Brazil

Miguel Pereira-Macedo Centro Hospitalar Universitário Lisboa Central, Lisbon, Portugal

Rafaela Cardoso Gil Pimentel FATESA – Faculdade de Tecnologia em Saúde, Ribeirão Preto, SP, Brazil

Priscila Chaves Pita Ultrasonography Residence – Hospital das Clínicas da UFMG, Belo Horizonte, Brazil

Cristos Pritsivelis Maternidade Escola da UFRJ, Universidade Federal do Rio de Janeiro, Rio de Janeiro, RJ, Brazil

Camila Luiza Meira Pucci Department of Obstetrics and Gynecology, University of São Paulo, São Paulo, Brazil

Sepaco Hospital, São Paulo, Brazil

Conrado Sávio Ragazini Department of Obstetrics and Gynecology, Ribeirão Preto Medical School – University of São Paulo, Ribeirão Preto, São Paulo, Brazil

Gustavo Mourão Rodrigues Department of Obstetrics, Universidade Federal do Estado do Rio de Janeiro (UNIRIO), Rio de Janeiro, Rio de Janeiro, Brazil

Miguel Ruoti University Asuncion, Asunción, Paraguay

Erich Saling Institute of Perinatal Medicine, Berlin-Neukölln, Germany

Susana Santo Departamento de Obstetrícia, Ginecologia e Medicina da Reprodução, Faculdade de Medicina da Universidade de Lisboa, Centro Hospitalar Universitário Lisboa Norte – Hospital de Santa Maria, Lisbon, Portugal

Nelson Sass Department of Obstetrics, Universidade Federal de São Paulo (Federal University of São Paulo) – UNIFESP, City of Sao Paulo, SP, Brazil

Ola Didrik Saugstad Ann & Robert H. Lurie Children's Hospital of Chicago and Prentice Women's Hospital, Division of Neonatology, Feinberg School of Medicine, Northwestern University, Chicago, IL, USA

Department of Pediatric Research, Oslo University Hospital and University of Oslo, Oslo, Norway

Cláudia Saunders Research Group on Maternal and Child Health (Grupo de Pesquisa em Saúde Materna e Infantil – GPSMI), Nutrition Institute, Federal University of Rio de Janeiro, Rio de Janeiro, RJ, Brazil

Matthew A. Shanahan Washington University School of Medicine in St. Louis, Louis, US

Jussara de Lima e Souza Neonatology and Palliative Medicine, University of Campinas – UNICAMP, Clinic of Neonatology, Women's Hospital – CAISM, University of Campinas (UNICAMP), Campinas, Brazil

Milan Stanojevic Clinical Hospital Sveti Duh, Department of Obstetrics and Gynecology Medical School University of Zagreb, Neonatal Unit, Zagreb, Croatia

Mariane T. Tauile Perinatal/Rede D'or, Rio de Janeiro, RJ, Brazil

Julio Cesar Teixeira Department of Gynecology and Obstetrics, Faculty of Medical Sciences, University of Campinas (UNICAMP), Campinas, SP, Brazil

Mónica Trasmonte Hospital Nacional Prof. Dr. A. Posadas, MATERNAL CHILD, Buenos Aires, Argentina

Lucas Trigo Maternal-Fetal Medicine Department, Fetal Medicine Research Center (BCNatal), Hospital Clinic and Hospital Sant Joan de Déu, University of Barcelona, Barcelona, Catalunya, Spain

Shamik Trivedi Ann & Robert H. Lurie Children's Hospital of Chicago and Prentice Women's Hospital, Division of Neonatology, Feinberg School of Medicine, Northwestern University, Chicago, IL, USA

Yves Ville GHU Paris-Centre, Hôpital Necker-Enfants Malades, Paris, France

Liliana Susana Voto Maternal and Childbirth Department, Hospital General de Agudos Dr. Juan A. Fernandez, School of Medicine, University of Buenos Aires, Buenos Aires, Argentina

Masami Yamamoto GHU Paris-Centre, Hôpital Necker-Enfants Malades, Paris, France

Lenita Zajdenverg Internal Medicine Department, Diabetes Division, Hospital Universitário Clementino Fraga Filho, Universidade Federal do Rio de Janeiro, Rio de Janeiro, Brazil

Moises Gabriel Zeitune Maternal and Childbirth Department, Hospital General de Agudos Dr. Juan A. Fernández, School of Medicine, University of Buenos Aires, Buenos Aires, Argentina

Andrea Zin Instituto NAcional de Saude da Mulher, da Criança e do Adolescente, FIOCRUZ, Rio de Janeiro, Brazil

Part VI
Infectious Diseases

Chapter 43
Urinary Tract Infections

Carlos Augusto Faria and José Carlos Carraro-Eduardo

Introduction

The urinary tract is continuously challenged by microbial pathogens ascending from the perineal region across the urethra to bladder, ureters, and kidneys. Thus, to avoid infection, it has developed its mechanisms of defense.

The primary mechanism in the maintenance of the bladder sterility is the continuous flow of urine from the kidneys to the bladder and complete, intermittent emptying across the urethra, resulting in "washout" [1]. Besides, the low pH, the presence of polymorphonuclear cells, the Tamm-Horsfall glycoprotein, the excretion of urea, and the osmolarity are specific antimicrobial urinary characteristics that inhibit bacterial adhesion to the bladder wall [2].

Besides, other characteristics that maintain the urinary sterile are the urothelium layer of glycosaminoglycans, making the surface of the mucosa inappropriate for bacterial adherence, mainly for *E. coli*, and desquamation during infection. Also, the mucosa secretes IgA and IgG, which have an essential role in the prevention of urinary tract infections (UTI). Secretory IgA produced in the posterior urethra and the vesical wall acts to impede bacterial adherence and is an important factor in avoiding the ascension of bacteria into the upper urinary tract [3].

Nonetheless, urinary tract infection, defined as the presence and growth of microbial pathogens in the urinary tract, is one of the most common bacterial infections. They are more frequent in women due to anatomical characteristics, as the shorter urethra, closer proximity of the anus and vagina, as well as easier access of pathogenic microorganisms to the urinary tract during sexual activity [4]. Moreover,

C. A. Faria (✉)
Department of Maternal and Child Health, School of Medicine, Universidade Federal Fluminense (UFF), Niterói, RJ, Brazil

J. C. Carraro-Eduardo
Department of Internal Medicine, School of Medicine, Universidade Federal Fluminense (UFF), Niterói, Rio de Janeiro, Brazil

© Springer Nature Switzerland AG 2022
R. A. Moreira de Sá, E. B. d. Fonseca (eds.), *Perinatology*,
https://doi.org/10.1007/978-3-030-83434-0_43

UTI constitutes one of the most common non-obstetric reasons for hospitalization in pregnant women [5].

Urinary tract infections can be symptomatic (cystitis and pyelonephritis) or asymptomatic (asymptomatic bacteriuria – ABS). When they occur during pregnancy, the maternal and perinatal morbidity varies accordingly to each clinical type of infection.

Influence of Pregnancy on Urinary Tract Infections

The functional and anatomical changes that occur in pregnancy may favor the occurrence of UTI. The kidneys are enlarged in 1–1.5 cm due to renal hypertrophy, increased capacity of the renal collecting system, and augmentation of vascularization. At around 7 weeks, the ureters begin to dilate because of hypotonicity induced by progesterone, also called the physiological hydronephrosis of pregnancy. It reaches a maximum in the second trimester and is more pronounced in the right ureter, probably because of the uterine dextrorotation, which acts as a mechanical compressive factor on the right ureter [3]. Later, mechanical compression from the enlarging gravid uterus further aggravates the phenomenon of hydronephrosis. The urine retained in these ureters varies from 50 to 200 mL.

Hydronephrosis can be observed by ultrasound exam in up to 90% of the pregnancies. The ureters return to normality in 90% of cases until 8 weeks after delivery; however, 6% of patients maintain the dilatation for more than 12 weeks [6].

Furthermore, there is a progressive progesterone-induced bladder relaxation, doubling its storage capacity at the end of the pregnancy. This change may cause incompetence of the vesicoureteral valve, which, combined with decreased intraurethral pressure, could result in intermittent vesicoureteral reflux [4]. Besides, there is an anterior and superior displacement of the bladder base and detrusor hypertrophy; consequently, the bladder shifts from a pelvic to an intraabdominal position [7].

There also maternal adaptations in renal function. Due to the increase in cardiac output and vasodilation of afferent and efferent arterioles, there is an increase in renal plasma flow and glomerular filtration rate, which leads to an increase in the filtrated glucose load. This fact, associated with a decreased proximal tubular glucose reabsorption, results in glycosuria, found in about 50% of pregnant women [8]. Moreover, an increased plasma volume during pregnancy leads to decreased urine concentration (hyposthenuria) and increased bladder volume. Transient diabetes insipidus, secondary to high placental vasopressinase activity, may occur. There is also a decreased fractional reabsorption of amino acids, which results in higher rates of urinary excretion. Thus, pregnant patients may exhibit glycosuria and aminoaciduria in the absence of hyperglycemia or renal disease. Additionally, there are differences in urine pH. Mild compensated respiratory alkalosis resulting from hyperventilation and morning urinary pH tending to alkalinity are common findings in pregnancy [6].

Table 43.1 presents a summary of the most relevant maternal adaptations that can favor UTI in pregnant women.

It is worth noting that the immunosuppression of pregnancy can contribute to UTI. The inflammatory response of the bladder mucosa is decreased due to a decreased serum activity of immunoglobulins IgG, IgA, and IgM. Besides, the lower urinary activity of IgG and IgA and the lower levels of interleukin 6 may be implicated in the frequency and severity of pyelonephritis in pregnancy [9].

Therefore, the association of all these conditions facilitates bacterial growth and UTI during pregnancy. After delivery, unnecessary urethral catheterization, vaginal examinations in excess or performed without adequate care, and genital injuries during childbirth are additional factors that contribute to the increase of UTI in the puerperium [10].

Influence of UTI on Pregnancy

UTI have been associated with various complications and adverse outcomes during pregnancy, because of an elevated risk of a more severe course, with severe consequences for mother and child [5].

Although it is controversial for some of them, UTI, in general, have been implicated as a contributing factor for preeclampsia, premature rupture of membranes, preterm birth, low birth weight infant, and fetal intrauterine growth restriction [4].

If ASB in pregnancy is untreated, it has generally been accepted that up to 20–30% of mothers will develop acute pyelonephritis [11]. When antibiotics were not available, acute pyelonephritis was associated with a 20–50% incidence of preterm birth [12].

Maternal complications include respiratory insufficiency, septicemia, renal dysfunction, anemia, and postpartum endometritis [13]. Morbidity and adverse obstetric outcomes associated with pyelonephritis do not appear to differ by trimester [14].

No correlation has been undoubtedly established between acute cystitis of pregnancy and adverse pregnancy outcomes, probably because pregnant women with symptomatic cystitis usually seek for treatment [15].

Table 43.1 Urinary tract adaptations that can favor UTI in pregnancy

1. Kidney enlargement
2. Dilatation and hypotony of renal collecting system
3. Reduced/absent ureteral peristalsis
4. Increased bladder capacity
5. Vesicoureteral reflux
6. Glycosuria and aminoaciduria
7. Urine alkalization

Etiology

The etiologic agents associated with asymptomatic bacteriuria, cystitis, and pyelonephritis are similar in pregnant and nonpregnant women [16]. Most organisms recovered by routine culture techniques are the coliforms. *E. coli* is the predominant uropathogen, followed by organisms in the *Klebsiella-Enterobacter* group, *P. mirabilis,* and other Gram-negative such as *Pseudomonas* and *Citrobacter* in smaller numbers [4, 7].

Gram-positive organisms, including *Staphylococcus saprophyticus* and group B streptococci, are present in up to 10% of UTI in pregnant women [14]. *Streptococcus agalactiae* is uncommonly seen (<1%) in real infection but is more commonly isolated as a contaminating isolate from the healthy vaginal flora. Enterococci are infrequently associated with symptomatic upper UTI [16].

Many of the Gram-positive isolates have been associated with symptomatic low colony count ($< 10^5$ CFU/mL) infection in nonpregnant women, but the significance of these low colony counts in asymptomatic pregnant women is not well established [16].

More rarely, other microorganisms, like lactobacillus, *M. hominis*, *Ureaplasma parvum*, *G. vaginalis*, and *C. trachomatis*, are identified in urine culture of pregnant women [7]. If bacteria that are not typical uropathogens are isolated, treatment should be reserved if the organism grows as a single isolate on consecutive cultures [14].

Virulence Factors of Uropathogenic Strains

The bacterial virulence has an essential role in the host-pathogen interaction in UTI. Escherichia coli has mechanisms that enhance both colonization and invasion of the urinary tract. Fimbriae are fundamental for adherence to and invasion into the host cells and indispensable for successful infection. It has been well studied that *E. coli* type 1 fimbria is heavily associated with cystitis, and other pathogenic-fimbriated strains are associated with pyelonephritis [17].

Besides, flagella and toxins promote bacterial dissemination, while different iron-acquisition systems allow bacterial survival in the iron-limited environment of the urinary tract [18].

The virulence of *P. mirabilis* depends on the motility, given by bacterial flagella, the presence of fimbriae for adherence, and the property to secrete urease, which catalyzes the hydrolysis of urea to ammonia and carbonic acid, leading to alkalization of urine [19].

Diagnosis

Among the several methods used to detect bacteriuria, the gold standard is urine culture [20]. Cultures are helpful to guide treatment, particularly crucial in pregnancy, when the options of safe antibiotics are reduced.

Ideally, the specimen should be collected in a manner that minimizes contamination. However, a recent study has found no difference in rates of contamination and the levels of diagnostic accuracy for midstream urine specimens collected with or without cleansing. Nonetheless, the authors did not recommend for or against the collection of midstream urine without cleansing [21].

Although the optimal method for collecting voided urine is uncertain, instructing women to perform hygiene of the vestibule region, spread their labia, and collect midstream urine seems most reasonable. Routine catheterization to screen for bacteriuria is not warranted due to the risk of introducing infection [14].

Proper handling at a 4 °C temperature and rapid processing of the specimen aim to avoid false-positive results and contamination (presence of three or more microorganisms isolated from the sample). However, more systematic studies evaluating the utility of these measures are needed [21].

A culture obtained using a midstream, clean-catch urine sample with greater than 10^5 colony-forming units per mL (CFU/mL) of a single uropathogen is considered a positive test result. If the patient is symptomatic, the diagnosis of UTI is confirmed. Otherwise, in asymptomatic women, the diagnosis is ABS [4].

Examination of urinary sediment (urinalysis) in the investigation of a possible UTI can be useful to identify leukocytes, erythrocytes, and cylinders and to detect the presence of bacteria (Table 43.2). However, if a significant amount of squamous epithelial cells (>15–20 per high potency field) is present, the sample is likely to be contaminated, and a new sample should be collected [20].

Findings from urinalysis associated with information obtained using reactive strips (urinalysis dipstick) for pH, nitrites, and leukocyte esterase contribute to the early diagnosis, while the result of the urine culture is not available (Table 43.2).

Positive nitrite is compatible with the presence of Gram-negative bacteria such as *E. coli*, *Klebsiella*, *Proteus*, and *Enterobacter*, as these organisms convert urinary nitrates into nitrites [3]. Urine dipsticks can detect nitrites in the presence of bacteria >10^5 CFU/mL. If the result is negative, it does not necessarily mean that there is no infection [20].

False negatives can be found in the presence of Gram-positive species such as *Staphylococcus* or *Streptococcus*, in very diluted urine samples or after a short period of retention of urine in the bladder before the sample collection [4].

The detection of leukocyte esterase reflects an increased number of leukocytes in the urine and indicates the presence of pyuria. Dipstick testing turns positive in the

Table 43.2 Possible laboratory findings suggestive of UTI before urine culture results

Urinalysis	Dipstick
Pyuria Hematuria Bacteriuria Casts (white and red cells) – not in cystitis Epithelial cells (>15 hpf) indicates contamination	Leukocyte esterase (if >5–15 leukocytes per high-power field) Hematuria Nitrites (if a Gram-negative enterobacterium is the etiology, with >10^5 CFU/mL)

presence of >5–15 leukocytes per high-power field. Therefore, in the early stage of a urinary infection and until this threshold is not reached, the test can be negative [20].

These methods, as well as the interleukin 6 test, although useful in general clinical practice, do not offer adequate sensitivity and specificity for the detection of ABS in pregnant women and should not be used [11].

Asymptomatic Bacteriuria

Asymptomatic bacteriuria (ASB) is defined as persistent colonization of the urinary tract by pathogenic bacteria in at least 10^5 CFU/mL of cultured urine in the absence of signs or symptoms of a UTI. The prevalence is estimated in 2–15% of all pregnancies [4, 7, 11, 22].

In obstetric practice, only one voided urine specimen is typically obtained, and diagnosis (and treatment initiation) is made when there are $\geq 10^5$ CFU/mL in the culture. However, ASB in women is formally defined as two consecutive voided urine specimens with the isolation of the same bacterial strain in quantitative counts of $\geq 10^5$ CFU/mL or a single catheterized urine specimen with one bacterial species isolated in a quantitative count of $\geq 10^2$ CFU/mL [11].

As already mentioned, if ASB in pregnancy is not treated, it has generally been accepted that about 20–30% of mothers will develop acute pyelonephritis; on the other hand, treatment decreases this incidence up to 0.5% [13].

The morbidity of untreated ASB in pregnant women is attributable mainly to acute pyelonephritis occurring in later pregnancy, which may be complicated by severe sepsis or septic shock for some women and may precipitate preterm labor and delivery [23]. One of the hypotheses to explain this fact is that endotoxins released by bacteria trigger inflammatory cascade, resulting in an increased production of cytokines, prostaglandins, and matrix-degrading enzymes. So, uterine contractions are activated, promoting cervical dilatation, preterm rupture of the membranes, and easier entry of pathogens into the uterine cavity and preterm delivery [4, 5]. Antibiotic treatment of ASB is associated with a reduction in the incidence of pyelonephritis and, consequently, of preterm birth and low birth weight [11, 24].

Numerous risk factors for ASB in pregnancy have been identified as low socioeconomic status, higher parity, a history of recurrent UTI, diabetes, and anatomical abnormalities of the urinary tract [24].

Although it is well established that ASB must be screened during pregnancy, there is little evidence on the optimal timing and frequency of screening, and the protocols vary widely following medical societies and countries [22].

The risk of acquiring bacteriuria during pregnancy increases with the duration of pregnancy and is higher between the 9th and 17th weeks of gestation. Thus, screening for ASB during pregnancy may be done with a urine culture at 12–16 weeks of gestation or at the first prenatal visit, if later, because treatment given at that time would provide the highest number of bacteriuria-free gestational weeks [16].

Up to 30% of women receiving a short course of therapy for ASB will not have the urine sterilized. Thus, a repeat culture is generally recommended as a test of cure, which can be performed a week after completion of antibiotic treatment [14].

There are insufficient data informing the utility of repeat testing following an initial episode of ASB, and it is not known whether retreatment of recurrent or persistent bacteriuria improves outcomes. Recommendation for follow-up with monthly urine culture in pregnant women treated for an episode of ASB is based on expert opinions [14].

The treatment of ASB is the same as acute cystitis.

Asymptomatic Group B Streptococcus Bacteriuria

When group B *Streptococcus* is identified in a urine culture of an asymptomatic woman in the pregnancy, it is fundamental to take into consideration the number of CFU/mL to define the adequate approach.

Patients with colony count $\geq 10^5$ CFU/mL should be treated immediately with appropriate antibiotics, but not those with inferior counts. However, regardless of the number of CFU, all patients should be treated at the time of labor or rupture of membranes for the prevention of early onset of neonatal group B streptococcal disease [25].

Acute Cystitis

Acute cystitis is an inflammatory process of the bladder, in most of the cases caused by bacteria. Cystitis complicates 1–4% of pregnancies [3, 7, 26].

Symptoms are the same presented by nonpregnant women: acute onset of dysuria (painful urination), pain (particularly suprapubic), urinary frequency, urinary urgency without systemic symptoms, and fever and chills. Hematuria (blood in urine) may also be present but is more frequently seen in urinalysis [26].

Remarkably, urinary frequency and urgency – the typical symptoms in acute cystitis – frequently occur in pregnant women due to physiological changes in the urinary tract and vaginal infections. However, the probability of cystitis is higher than 50% in women with any symptoms of UTI and greater than 90% in women who have dysuria and frequency without vaginal discharge or irritation [27].

After specimen collection for urinalysis and culture, empirical treatment should be initiated in a patient with consistent symptoms of cystitis and pyuria on urinalysis.

The diagnosis is confirmed when a uropathogenic bacteria is identified in the urine culture of a symptomatic patient, independently of the count of colony-forming units. If a nontypical uropathogens is isolated, the diagnosis of cystitis is made only when the bacterial count is high ($\geq 10^5$ CFU/mL) [14].

Differential clinical diagnosis includes vaginitis and urethritis, responsible for the 10–15% prevalence of pyuria in pregnant women without urinary infection. Vaginitis is generally associated with vaginal irritation and discharge.

As with asymptomatic bacteriuria, a follow-up culture should be obtained as a test of cure, performed a week after completion of therapy [14].

There is no evidence of the association of cystitis with pyelonephritis or adverse gestational outcomes, probably because patients seek treatment, as symptoms are bothersome [14].

Treatment

Antimicrobial treatment for acute cystitis in pregnant women is usually empirical, preferably after specimen collection for urinalysis and culture. Antibiotics for UTI with moderately low risk in pregnancy (category B) include cephalexin, nitrofurantoin, amoxicillin-clavulanate, and fosfomycin [28].

Amoxicillin-clavulanate and fosfomycin are the best options due to the safety profile in pregnancy and the broader spectrum of activity compared to other agents (such as amoxicillin or cephalexin). Nitrofurantoin is another option for the second or third trimester or if other drugs cannot be used for any specific reason, such as drug allergy or gastrointestinal intolerance. The choice must be individualized based on factors such as allergic history, patterns of local practice, the prevalence of resistance from the local community, availability, and cost [28].

Although data on pregnant women are limited, a meta-analysis suggested that there is no significant difference in results between different antibiotic regimens in terms of cure rates, recurrence, the incidence of premature birth, and the need for antibiotic change [29]. However, when there is a presumed infection by *Enterobacteriaceae* producing extended-spectrum beta-lactamase (ESBL), nitrofurantoin and fosfomycin are good options because they are active in vitro against many of these strains [30, 31].

The ideal duration of treatment for acute cystitis during pregnancy is uncertain. As for ASB, short courses of antibiotics are preferred to minimize antimicrobial exposure to the fetus. In acute cystitis, treatment can be done with antibiotics for 3–7 days. Data among nonpregnant women suggest that there is no difference between short (3–7 days) and longer treatments [28]. Single-dose therapy should be limited to fosfomycin, which has an appropriate formulation for this prescription. As proposed in the treatment of ASB, a urine sample should be obtained 1 week after the completion of therapy for culture and antibiotic sensitivity testing.

Alternative treatment options, such as probiotics, herbal products, urinary acidifiers, and vaccines, can help to overcome antibiotic resistance, but further studies are needed to establish their effectiveness in the pregnant population.

Phenazopyridine, an analgesic of the urinary tract, should only be used if the expected benefit outweighs the potential risk. The drug interferes with the dipstick analysis, and there are no well-controlled studies in pregnant women.

Recurrence of UTI, symptomatic or asymptomatic, occurs in approximately 20% of the cases, despite adequate antimicrobial therapy [15]. The approach with prophylactic antimicrobial in a single night dose for a long time is recommended [7]. The drug choice must be supported by in vitro tests. Nitrofurantoin, at a dose of 50–100 mg, and cephalexin, at a dose of 250 mg, are the most used options. Prophylaxis should last for up to 8 weeks after delivery, due to the persistence of anatomical changes in the urinary tract during this period [26].

Women presenting a history of recurrent UTI before pregnancy – defined as two or more episodes in the last 6 months or three or more episodes in the last year [32] – should be treated with suppressive antibiotics (nitrofurantoin 50 mg or cephalexin 250 mg) at bedtime until delivery. If recurrence is related to sexual intercourse, a postcoital dose should be prescribed [14].

Acute Pyelonephritis

Acute pyelonephritis is an infection of the upper urinary tract and kidneys. Histologically, it is characterized by acute interstitial nephritis and clinically by the presence of fever (temperature > 38 °C), chills, nausea, vomiting, flank pain, and costovertebral tenderness at the affected side. Symptoms of cystitis are not always present.

Most cases of this potential severe affection occur during the second and third trimesters [26]. Pyelonephritis may have a catastrophic evolution in approximately 20% of cases, with progression to septic shock syndrome, disseminated intravascular coagulation, renal failure, and acute respiratory distress syndrome (ARDS) [13, 33]. Hence, most of the pregnant patients presenting pyelonephritis, particularly during the third trimester, must be admitted to the hospital [3].

In addition to the already mentioned adverse maternal effects, pregnant women are more likely to have premature delivery and a low birth weight infant [5, 7, 13, 23].

Diagnosis

Laboratory tests for the diagnosis of pyelonephritis may include urinalysis and dipstick urinalysis, but the gold standard is the urine culture.

Findings in urinalysis and dipstick urinalysis are the same described for the diagnosis of UTI in general (Table 43.2). Pyuria is a common finding in urinalysis, where hematuria and the presence of bacterial flora can also be observed. Caution should be taken when evaluating pyuria in cases of higher pH, as in this condition, white cell casts can be broken, impairing the evaluation of the real number of leukocytes. The presence of hyaline and white and red cell casts calls attention to the presence of infection in the upper urinary tract [3].

Even though there is some controversy in the literature if bacteremia portends not a worse prognosis or requires more prolonged therapy in uncomplicated pyelonephritis in pregnancy, it is reasonable to obtain blood cultures in such cases [34].

Moreover, the baseline evaluation of acute pyelonephritis should include a basic metabolic panel, most importantly, to assess renal function [35]. Blood cell counts usually show neutrophilic leukocytosis. A rapid increase in PCR dosage and blood lactate is indicative of the severity of the disease.

Imaging is not routinely used to diagnose pyelonephritis unless there is a history of symptomatic or asymptomatic urolithiasis, diabetes, prior urologic surgery, immunosuppression, repeated episodes of pyelonephritis, or urosepsis [14].

The primary differential diagnosis is nephrolithiasis and intraamniotic infection. Fever is uncommon with uncomplicated stone disease, although significant flank or back pain is the chief complaint in nephrolithiasis. Intraamniotic infection is accompanied by a history of premature rupture of membranes, uterine tenderness and foul odor of the amniotic fluid, and the absence of bacteriuria, in addition to abdominal pain and fever [14].

Potential causes of fever and back or flank pain in the absence of bacteriuria include other infection conditions like influenza, pneumonia, and appendicitis.

Treatment

Pyelonephritis during pregnancy can progress quickly, causing life-threatening complications in the mother and fetus. Consequently, most pregnant women with pyelonephritis, especially during the third trimester, must be hospitalized and receive intravenous therapy [7]. In most cases, the choice of adequate antibiotic therapy is not supported by the identification of the etiologic agent and in vitro sensitivity tests.

The treatment of acute pyelonephritis in pregnant women is particularly challenging because of concerns about the safety of antibiotics. Human data on drug toxicity in pregnancy is limited to studies performed decades ago, so there is little direct information about the safety of many newer antibiotics in pregnancy [14, 36]. Antimicrobial options are limited by the potential toxicity to the fetus of aminoglycosides (during the first trimester), trimethoprim-sulfamethoxazole (near the end of pregnancy), and fluoroquinolones (throughout pregnancy) [37].

An ideal antimicrobial regimen in such cases must meet the following criteria: be proven effective in well-conducted studies, show activity against the most frequent uropathogens in acute pyelonephritis, achieve and maintain adequate serum and tissue concentrations throughout the treatment period, not be associated with the development of resistance, low cost, and good fetal tolerance and safety. As there are few studies comparing the effectiveness of different antimicrobials, there is insufficient data to recommend a specific treatment regimen for pyelonephritis in pregnancy [29].

Penicillins (with or without beta-lactamase inhibitors), cephalosporins, and aztreonam are considered safe. However, ceftriaxone should be avoided near the childbirth, because of its high affinity to proteins and the possibility of displacement of bilirubin and subsequent kernicterus [38].

Thus, broad-spectrum parenteral beta-lactams are the preferred antibiotics for the initial empirical therapy for pyelonephritis (Table 43.3). Penicillin derivatives and cephalosporins reach adequate kidney and parenchymal concentrations shortly after administration and have effective activity against common uropathogens. Ampicillin, for its safety and low-cost characteristics, was, for many years, the first option in the treatment of pyelonephritis in pregnant women. Currently, due to the high prevalence of resistance (e.g., approximately 45–60% of *E. coli* strains are resistant to ampicillin), it has been replaced by first-generation cephalosporins as first-line monotherapy, like cefazolin and cefuroxime [20, 39]. Cefazolin has the same spectrum of activity as broader-spectrum cephalosporins against common causative microbes and is less expensive, but there are concerns about increasing resistance [26, 40]. Although fluoroquinolones reach high renal concentration and

Table 43.3 Treatment options for empirical therapy of UTI in pregnancy, before urine culture results

Cystitis		
Antibiotic/dose	Duration	Comments
Amoxicillin-clavulanate (500 mg or 875 mg)	Every 8 h (500 mg) or 12 h (875 mg), 3–7 days	Class B
Fosfomycin trometamol 3 g	Once (may be repeated in 48 h)	Class B
Cephalexin 500 mg	Every 6 h, 3–7 days	Class B
Nitrofurantoin macrocrystals 100 mg	Every 6 h, 5–7 days	Class B Use in first trimester is appropriate if no other suitable option is available
Nitrofurantoin monohydrate-macrocrystals 100 mg	Every 12 h, 5–7 days	Can cause hemolytic anemia in G6PD Deficiency at term
Pyelonephritis		
Antibiotic/dose	Duration	Comments
Cephalosporins Cefazolin 1–2 g Cefuroxime 0.75–1.5 g Ceftriaxone 1 g	10–14 days Every 6–8 h Every 8 h Once a day	Class B Class B Class B Avoid in the third trimester (kernicterus)
Ampicillin 2 g + Gentamicin 3–5 mg/kg/day	Every 6 h Once a day 10–14 days	Class B No evidence of real teratogenic effects. Use if no other suitable option is available. Class C

are highly recommended in the treatment of UTI in nonpregnant patients, the risk of fetal arthropathy makes its use prohibitive during pregnancy and breastfeeding [7, 40].

The use of aminoglycosides in pregnancy is controversial. Many studies and guidelines do not recommend its use because of the potential risks of ototoxicity and nephrotoxicity in both the mother and the fetus. However, gentamicin has been widely used in pregnancy as first-line therapy for Gram-negative coverage, with no reports of congenital complications [7, 41]. Empirical treatment with gentamicin may be appropriate, provided that monitoring of serum creatinine dosage and adjustments in dose administration are performed [36]. As aminoglycosides are eliminated by renal filtration, dose adjustments of the antibiotic are necessary to avoid nephrotoxicity and ototoxicity. It is worth remembering that the glomerular filtration rate during pregnancy shows a physiological increase of up to 50% over previous values and that an increase in the dose of an aminoglycoside may be necessary to prevent subtherapeutic levels that could compromise the effectiveness of the treatment [42, 43].

Carbapenems are the option for pregnant women with a history of urinary infections by *Enterobacteriaceae* producing extended-spectrum beta-lactamase (ESBL). Meropenem, ertapenem, or doripenem should be the preferred carbapenems for use in such cases, as some animal studies have shown teratogenic effects with imipenem-cilastatin use [44].

Pregnant women generally have definite improvement within 24–48 hours of appropriate antibiotic therapy. Once afebrile for 48 hours, without low back pain, and after laboratory improvement (normalization of the leukogram and decrease in C-reactive protein levels), it is possible to switch to oral therapy. The choice of the antimicrobial agent must be guided by the results of urine culture and antibiogram. If there is good tolerability to the oral antibiotic, the patient can be discharged from the hospital and complete 10–14 days of treatment at home. Oral options such as nitrofurantoin and fosfomycin are not suitable for the treatment of pyelonephritis, as these drugs do not reach adequate serum and tissue levels.

The risk of recurrence of pyelonephritis during pregnancy is 6–8%. Thus, a low-dose antimicrobial prophylactic therapy with an agent to which the original organism is susceptible should be recommended until the end of the pregnancy, at bedtime. Prevention of recurrence should continue after delivery since anatomical changes in the urinary tract persist for up to 8 weeks [45].

References

1. Sobel JD. Pathogenesis of urinary tract infection. Role of host defenses. Infect Dis Clin N Am. 1997;11(3):531–49. https://doi.org/10.1016/s0891-5520(05)70372-x.
2. Neal DE Jr. Host defense mechanism in urinary tract infections. Urol Clin North Am. 1999;26(4):677–86. https://doi.org/10.1016/s0094-0143(05)70210-x.

3. Santos JF, Ribeiro RM, Rossi P, Haddad JM, Guidi HG, Pacetta AM, et al. Urinary tract infections in pregnant women. Int Urogynecol J Pelvic Floor Dysfunct. 2002;13(3):204–9. https://doi.org/10.1007/s192-002-8354-7.
4. Kalinderi K, Delkos D, Kalinderis M, Athanasiadis A, Kalogiannidis I. Urinary tract infection during pregnancy: current concepts on a common multifaceted problem. J Obstet Gynaecol. 2018;38(4):448–53. https://doi.org/10.1080/01443615.2017.1370579.
5. Geerlings SE. Clinical presentations and epidemiology of urinary tract infections. Microbiol Spectr. 2016;4(5). https://doi.org/10.1128/microbiolspec.UTI-0002-2012.
6. Thadhani RI, Maynard SE. Maternal adaptations to pregnancy: renal and urinary tract physiology. In: Post TW, editor. UpToDate. Waltham: UpToDate Inc. https://www.uptodate.com. Accessed on 30 Apr 2020.
7. Glaser AP, Schaeffer AJ. Urinary tract infection and bacteriuria in pregnancy. Urol Clin North Am. 2015;42(4):547–60. https://doi.org/10.1016/j.ucl.2015.05.004.
8. Alto WA. No need for glycosuria/proteinuria screen in pregnant women. J Fam Pract. 2005;54(11):978–83.
9. Petersson C, Hedges S, Stenqvist K, Sandberg T, Connell H, Svanborg C. Suppressed antibody and interleukin-6 responses to acute pyelonephritis in pregnancy. Kidney Int. 1994;45(2):571–7. https://doi.org/10.1038/ki.1994.74.
10. Schwartz MA, Wang CC, Eckert LO, Critchlow CW. Risk factors for urinary tract infection in the postpartum period. Am J Obstet Gynecol. 1999;181(3):547–53. https://doi.org/10.1016/s0002-9378(99)70491-6.
11. Smaill FM, Vazquez JC. Antibiotics for asymptomatic bacteriuria in pregnancy. Cochrane Database Syst Rev. 2019;2019(11) https://doi.org/10.1002/14651858.CD000490.pub4.
12. Nicolle LE. Management of asymptomatic bacteriuria in pregnant women. Lancet Infect Dis. 2015;15(11):1252–4. https://doi.org/10.1016/S1473-3099(15)00145-0.
13. Wing DA, Fassett MJ, Getahun D. Acute pyelonephritis in pregnancy: an 18-year retrospective analysis. Am J Obstet Gynecol. 2014;210(3):219.e1–6. https://doi.org/10.1016/j.ajog.2013.10.006.
14. Hooton TM, Gupta K. Urinary tract infections and asymptomatic bacteriuria in pregnancy. In: Post TW, editor. UpToDate. Waltham, MA: UpToDate Inc. https://www.uptodate.com Accessed on 25 Apr 2020.
15. Millar LK, Cox SM. Urinary tract infections complicating pregnancy. Infect Dis Clin N Am. 1997;11(1):13–26. https://doi.org/10.1016/s0891-5520(05)70339-1.
16. Patterson TF, Andriole VT. Detection, significance, and therapy of bacteriúria in pregnancy. Update in the managed health care era. Infect Dis Clin N Am. 1997;11(3):593–608. https://doi.org/10.1016/s0891-5520(05)70375-5.
17. Abou Heidar NF, Degheili JA, Yacoubian AA, Khauli RB. Management of urinary tract infection in women: a practical approach for everyday practice. Urol Ann. 2019;11(4):339–46. https://doi.org/10.4103/UA.UA_104_19.
18. Lüthje P, Brauner A. Virulence factors of uropathogenic E. coli and their interaction with the host. Adv Microb Physiol. 2014;65:337–72. https://doi.org/10.1016/bs.ampbs.2014.08.006.
19. Armbruster CE, Mobley HLT, Pearson MM. Pathogenesis of Proteus mirabilis infection. EcoSal Plus. 2018;8(1). https://doi.org/10.1128/ecosalplus.ESP-0009-2017.
20. Chu CM, Lowder JL. Diagnosis and treatment of urinary tract infections across age groups. Am J Obstet Gynecol. 2018;219(1):40–51. https://doi.org/10.1016/j.ajog.2017.12.231.
21. LaRocco MT, Franek J, Leibach EK, Weissfeld AS, Kraft CS, Sautter RL, et al. Effectiveness of preanalytic practices on contamination and diagnostic accuracy of urine cultures: a laboratory medicine best practices systematic review and meta-analysis. Clin Microbiol Rev. 2016;29(1):105–47. https://doi.org/10.1128/CMR.00030-15.
22. Henderson JT, Webber EM, Bean SI. Screening for asymptomatic bacteriuria in adults: updated evidence report and systematic review for the US Preventive Services Task Force. JAMA. 2019;322(12):1195–205. https://doi.org/10.1001/jama.2019.10060.

23. Nicolle LE. Updated guidelines for screening for asymptomatic bacteriuria. JAMA. 2019;322(12):1152–4. https://doi.org/10.1001/jama.2019.11640.
24. Wingert A, Pillay J, Sebastianski M, Gates M, Featherstone R, Shave K, et al. Asymptomatic bacteriuria in pregnancy: systematic reviews of screening and treatment effectiveness and patient preferences. BMJ Open. 2019;9(3):e021347. https://doi.org/10.1136/bmjopen-2017-021347.
25. Allen VM, Yudin MH. No. 276-Management of Group B streptococcal bacteriuria in pregnancy. J Obstet Gynaecol Can. 2018;40(2):e181–6. https://doi.org/10.1016/j.jogc.2017.11.025.
26. Mittal P, Wing DA. Urinary tract infections in pregnancy. Clin Perinatol. 2005;32(3):749–64. https://doi.org/10.1016/j.clp.2005.05.006.
27. Hooton TM. Clinical practice. Uncomplicated urinary tract infection. N Engl J Med. 2012;366(11):1028–37. https://doi.org/10.1056/NEJMcp1104429.
28. Gupta K, Hooton TM, Naber KG, Wullt B, Colgan R, Miller LG, et al.; Infectious Diseases Society of America; European Society for Microbiology and Infectious Diseases. International clinical practice guidelines for the treatment of acute uncomplicated cystitis and pyelonephritis in women: a 2010 update by the Infectious Diseases Society of America and the European Society for Microbiology and Infectious Diseases. Clin Infect Dis. 2011;52(5):e103–20. https://doi.org/10.1093/cid/ciq257.
29. Vazquez JC, Villar J. Treatments for symptomatic urinary tract infections during pregnancy. Cochrane Database Syst Rev. 2003;(4):CD002256. Review. Update in: Cochrane Database Syst Rev. 2011;(1):CD002256. https://doi.org/10.1002/14651858.CD002256.
30. Keating GM. Fosfomycin trometamol: a review of its use as a single-dose oral treatment for patients with acute lower urinary tract infections and pregnant women with asymptomatic bacteriuria. Drugs. 2013;73(17):1951–66.
31. Ho PL, Yip KS, Chow KH, Lo JY, Que TL, Yuen KY. Antimicrobial resistance among uropathogens that cause acute uncomplicated cystitis in women in Hong Kong: a prospective multicenter study in 2006 to 2008. Diagn Microbiol Infect Dis. 2010;66(1):87.
32. Soytas M, Kactan C, Guven S. Recurrent bladder cystitis: who takes the role? World J Urol. 2020; https://doi.org/10.1007/s00345-020-03192-1.
33. Cunningham FG, Lucas MJ. Urinary tract infections complicating pregnancy. Baillieres Clin Obstet Gynaecol. 1994;8(2):353–73. https://doi.org/10.1016/s0950-3552(05)80325-6.
34. Gomi H, Goto Y, Laopaiboon M, Usui R, Mori R. Routine blood cultures in the management of pyelonephritis in pregnancy for improving outcomes. Cochrane Database Syst Rev. 2015;(2):CD009216. https://doi.org/10.1002/14651858.CD009216.pub2.
35. Colgan R, Williams M, Johnson JR. Diagnosis and treatment of acute pyelonephritis in women. Am Fam Physician. 2011;84(5):519–26.
36. Jolley JA, Wing DA. Pyelonephritis in pregnancy: an update on treatment options for optimal outcomes. Drugs. 2010;70(13):1643–55. https://doi.org/10.2165/11538050-000000000-00000.
37. Johnson JR, Russo TA. Acute pyelonephritis in adults. N Engl J Med. 2018;378(1):48–59. Review. Erratum in: N Engl J Med. 2018 Mar 15;378(11):1069. https://doi.org/10.1056/nejmcp1702758.
38. Bookstaver PB, Bland CM, Griffin B, Stover KR, Eiland LS, McLaughlin M. A review of antibiotic use in pregnancy. Pharmacotherapy. 2015;35(11):1052–62. https://doi.org/10.1002/phar.1649.
39. Greer LG, Roberts SW, Sheffield JS, Rogers VL, Hill JB, Mcintire DD, et al. Ampicillin resistance and outcome differences in acute antepartum pyelonephritis. Infect Dis Obstet Gynecol. 2008;2008:891426. https://doi.org/10.1155/2008/891426.
40. Bader MS, Loeb M, Brooks AA. An update on the management of urinary tract infections in the era of antimicrobial resistance. Postgrad Med. 2017;129(2):242–58. https://doi.org/10.1080/00325481.2017.1246055.
41. Lamont HF, Blogg HJ, Lamont RF. Safety of antimicrobial treatment during pregnancy: a current review of resistance, immunomodulation and teratogenicity. Expert Opin Drug Saf. 2014;13(12):1569–81. https://doi.org/10.1517/14740338.2014.939580.

42. Carraro-Eduardo JC, Oliveira AV, Carrapatoso ME, Ornellas JF. Effect of sex hormones on gentamicin-induced nephrotoxicity in rats. Braz J Med Biol Res. 1993;26(6):653–62.
43. Graham JM, Blanco JD, Oshiro BT, Magee KP. Gentamicin levels in pregnant women with pyelonephritis. Am J Perinatol. 1994;11(1):40–1. https://doi.org/10.1055/s-2007-994533.
44. Wing DA, Hendershott CM, Debuque L, Millar LK. A randomized trial of three antibiotic regimens for the treatment of pyelonephritis in pregnancy. Obstet Gynecol. 1998;92(2):249–53. https://doi.org/10.1016/s0029-7844(98)00156-2.
45. Sandberg T, Brorson JE. Efficacy of long-term antimicrobial prophylaxis after acute pyelonephritis in pregnancy. Scand J Infect Dis. 1991;23(2):221. https://doi.org/10.3109/00365549109023404.

Chapter 44
Congenital Infection 1 (Syphilis, AIDS, and Viral Hepatitis)

Mauro Romero Leal Passos, José Eleutério Junior, Regis Kreitchmann, and Angelica Espinosa Miranda

Congenital Syphilis

Congenital syphilis (CS) occurs when the *T. pallidum* is transmitted from the mother to the child, usually transplacentally, after a maternal spirochetemia. The transmission also happens by contact with maternal genital lesion [21].

The risk of CS is highest among women with early disease, ranging between 40% and 70% across the trimesters, with a decrease to 10% with late stage in the absence of treatment. About 40% of infected newborns do not present clinical signs [60]. It is estimated that more than 1 million of pregnant women are infected every year worldwide and CS is responsible for 305,000 infant deaths [50].

Despite having a known etiology, having easy diagnosis and treatment, syphilis continues to increase worldwide and the congenital form is a public health problem. From 2012 through 2017, the number of reported CS cases in the United States increased from 334 to 918 (8.4 to 23.8 cases per 100,000 live births), an increase more than 150% [50]. In Brazil, It was reported 158,051 cases of syphilis (detection rate of 75.8 cases/100,000 population) and 26,219 cases of CS (detection rate of 9.0 cases/1000 newborns) in 2018 [13].

M. R. L. Passos (✉)
Department of Microbiology and Parasitology, Fluminense Federal University, Niterói, Brazil

J. E. Junior
Department of Women's, Child and Teenager Health, Federal University of Ceará, Fortaleza, Brazil

R. Kreitchmann
Department of Gynecology and Obstetrics, Federal University of Health Sciences of Porto Alegre, Porto Alegre, Brazil

A. E. Miranda
Department of Social Medicine, Federal Universty of Espírito Santo, Vitória, Brazil

© Springer Nature Switzerland AG 2022
R. A. Moreira de Sá, E. B. d. Fonseca (eds.), *Perinatology*,
https://doi.org/10.1007/978-3-030-83434-0_44

Congenital Syphilis Case Definition [45]

1. First criterion
   - Child whose mother presents, during prenatal care or at the time of delivery, reagent tests for non-treponemic syphilis, with any titration and reagent treponemic test, which has not been treated or has received inadequate treatment
   - Child whose mother was not diagnosed with syphilis during pregnancy and, if the maternity hospital is unable to perform the treponemal test, presents a non-treponemal test reagent with any titration at the time of delivery
   - Child whose mother was not diagnosed with syphilis during pregnancy and, in the impossibility of the maternity hospital to perform the non-treponemal test, presents treponemal test at the time of delivery
   - Child whose mother has a reagent treponemic test and a non-reaponemic non-reactive test at the time of delivery without prior treatment
2. Second criterion
   - Every individual under 13 years of age with at least one of the following serological evidence:
     - Ascending titrations (non-treponemic tests)
     - Reagent non-treponemal tests after 6 months of age (except in the case of therapeutic follow-up)
     - Reagent treponemic tests after 18 months of age
     - Titers in non-treponemal test higher than those of the mother, in lactating women
     - Reagent non-treponemic test, with at least one of the variations: clinical signs and symptoms, cerebrospinal fluid (CSF) abnormalities, or radiological lesions of congenital syphilis
3. Third criterion
   - Miscarriage and stillborn whose mother has tests for non-treponemic reagent syphilis with any titration or reagent treponemic test, performed during prenatal care, at the time of delivery or curettage, that has not been treated or has received inadequate treatment
4. Fourth criterion
   - Any situation of evidence of infection by *T. pallidum* in placenta or umbilical cord and/or sample of the lesion, biopsy, or autopsy of a child, abortion, or stillbirth

Clinical Manifestations

Congenital syphilis is divided into early and late categories.

Congenital syphilis:

- Recent. When it manifests in the first 2 years of the child's life
- Late. When it manifests after the child's second year of life

The findings of congenital syphilis are shown in Table 44.1.

Most cases of CS are seen in women without proper prenatal care or in those who receive improper treatment. Syphilis screening is part of routine standard of care in all pregnant women in Brazil, and continuous monitoring of pregnant women is important to eliminate congenital syphilis [51]. While CS can cause severe illness and fetal demise, most neonates born with CS are asymptomatic at birth [50].

Benzaken et al. [10] observed the correlation between the adequacy of prenatal care and gestational syphilis detection rate. The vulnerability of women receiving inadequate prenatal care and, even worse, when infected with syphilis shows the need of a closer approach on this population, in order to compensate its vulnerability. Other factors associated with vulnerability, such as poverty, violence, and inequality, may be present in different degrees among Brazilian cities, prompting the need of strategies designed to reach those women. In this sense, Family Health Strategy (FHS) is an approach to improve these strategies because it is the main environment for prenatal care in Brazil. Broadening the FHS coverage and quality of care is important because it can provide combining diagnosis and adequate syphilis' treatment for pregnant women and their partners [52].

Recommendations

All pregnant women should be tested for syphilis as early as possible when they first present to care. If they had not received prenatal care prior to delivery, they should be tested in the maternity hospital at labor time [15]. In most cases of congenital syphilis, pregnant women received prenatal care but were not screened and treated for syphilis early enough during the pregnancy to prevent transmission to the fetus [22].

Table 44.1 Mean clinical findings in congenital syphilis [21]

Early congenital syphilis
Preterm, stillborn, nonimmune hydrops fetalis, intrauterine growth restriction, hepatomegaly, jaundice, splenomegaly, skin rash, adenopathy, rhinitis, condyloma lata, pseudoparalysis of parrot, chorioretinitis, cataract, asymptomatic invasion, cranial nerve palsies, seizures
Late congenital syphilis
Hutchinson's teeth, interstitial keratitis, healed chorioretinitis, eighth nerve deafness, rhagades, mental retardation, hydrocephalus, seizures, optic nerve atrophy, juvenile general paresis, cranial nerve palsies, frontal bossing, saddle nose deformity, protuberant mandible, short maxilla, high palatal arch, saber shin, sternoclavicular joint thickening (Higouménakis sign), clutton joints

Treatment

- Regimen recommended by CDC
  1. Primary, secondary, and early latent syphilis (<1 year)
     - Benzathine penicillin G, 2.4 million units IM in single dose
  2. Late latent syphilis (>1 year), latent syphilis of unknown duration, and tertiary syphilis
     - Benzathine penicillin G, 2.4 million units IM for three doses (each 1 week apart)
  3. Neurosyphilis
     - Aqueous crystalline penicillin G, 3–4 million units IV every 4 hours or via continuous infusion for 10–14 days
     - Procaine penicillin, 2.4 million units IM daily plus probenecid 500 mg PO qid both for 10–14 days
  4. Penicillin allergic
     - Confirm allergy and desensitize, and then appropriate treatment as above.

Aids in Pregnancy

Acquired immunodeficiency syndrome (AIDS) is a condition caused by RNA retrovirus called human immunodeficiency virus (HIV). This virus attacks and destroys CD4 T lymphocytes leading to immune depletion and causing the occurrence of opportunistic infections.

The HIV and the AIDS appeared in the last decades of the last century and caused many deaths. However, more recently, its early diagnosis and adequate approach have been shown to be effective in controlling the infection [14]. Sexual intercourse is the major mode of transmission worldwide. The virus can be detected in the blood, semen, vaginal secretion, and breast milk, and infected mothers may transmit to their babies during labor, delivery, or lactation.

Surveillance data from the United Nations Program on HIV/AIDS (UNAIDS) have documented the substantial burden of the disease on mothers and infants living in resource-limited settings [38]. The innovations that occurred in the AIDS research field caused a dramatic reduction in HIV mother-to-child transmission (MTCT) in the last 20 years; still, 160,000 children were infected in 2018 worldwide [1].

The rate of MTCT in developed countries is around 2% or less, but when no intervention is made, this rate can rise to 25%. Risk factors in pregnancy are the absence of prenatal care, injecting drug use, unprotected sex with an HIV-positive partner, and other sexually transmitted infections (STIs) diagnosed in pregnancy [41]. According to the Ministry of Health of Brazil, in the last 10 years, there was an increase of 38.1%

in the rate of HIV detection in pregnant women: in 2008, the observed rate was 2.1 cases/thousand live births and, in 2018, 2.9/thousand live births [14].

MTCT can occur intra utero (indicated by a positive PCR test in the infant within 72 hours after birth), during labor or delivery (indicated by a negative PCR test within the first 72 hours after birth but then positive by 4 weeks of age), or during breastfeeding. In nonbreastfeeding settings, in utero infections were responsible for about one-third of infant HIV infections. At the same time, about two-thirds of the transmissions would have occurred around labor and delivery time.

The mechanisms of in utero transmission seem to be related to the breakdown of the integrity of the placenta, leading to microtransfusions of maternal blood containing virus across the placenta to the fetus and also the occurrence of placental inflammation, especially chorioamnionitis, that has been associated to genital tract infections [31] [32]. Evidence also supports that STI comorbidity may increase MTCT rates [2].

A meta-analysis study showed that the incidence of HIV during pregnancy and peri-delivery was not significantly higher than among nonpregnant women (3.9 per 100 person-years [24]. Thomson et al. [62], however, demonstrated that the risk of acquiring HIV through unprotected intercourse was significantly higher in late pregnancy (3.97 times higher).

The second and third trimesters of pregnancy and the early postpartum period up to 6 months appear to be the periods of greatest risk for acquiring HIV [62]. MTCT among women who contracted the virus during pregnancy or breastfeeding is twice the triple of those who had it before pregnancy [24].

Most cases of transmission occur during childbirth, with an additional risk in breastfeeding. There are better chances of preventing vertical transmission when the diagnosis is early [24].

Management Recommendations [12, 41]

1. Early anti-HIV test in pregnancy (beginning of prenatal care).
2. Repeat the test in the third trimester.
3. Take the test on women in labor not previously tested. If positive, start antiretroviral prophylaxis. The Brazilian Ministry of Health considers testing at the time of delivery regardless of previous testing [15].
4. If not tested before and during labor, it should be tested in the immediate postpartum period. If the test is positive for mother and child, antiretroviral prophylaxis for the newborn should be started. Avoid breastfeeding.

Antiretroviral Therapy

Antiretroviral therapy (ART) is indicated for every pregnant woman infected with HIV, regardless of clinical and immunological criteria. It should not be suspended after delivery, regardless of the LT-CD4+ level at the time of treatment initiation

[15]. Women already taking ART at the onset of pregnancy are encouraged to continue the regimen if viral suppression is reached. Women who are not in ART should receive ART regardless of the trimester and should undergo HIV resistance testing to help guide ART selection. Typically, ART is initiated before obtaining results of these drug-resistance tests and optimized base in their results when strong suppression is not achieved.

The use of ART during pregnancy reduces the rate of HIV MTCT from approximately 30% to less than 1% if suppression of the maternal HIV viral load (plasma HIV viral load <50 copies/mL) is achieved near delivery [15]. Pretreatment genotyping is indicated for all HIV-infected pregnant women to guide the therapeutic scheme [15].

The tenofovir/lamivudine association (TDF/3TC) is the preferred one in HIV-infected pregnant women, as it has an easy dose (single daily dose), in addition to a favorable profile concerning lipoatrophy and hematological toxicity, both associated with zidovudine (AZT) [14]. Data on the use of TDF during the first trimester of pregnancy did not show an increase in birth defects compared to the general population. Besides, this ARV was well tolerated during pregnancy [15].

The goal of elimination of HIV vertical transmission is far to be achieved globally which was defined by the World Health Organization (WHO) as transmission rates of 2% in nonbreastfeeding and 5% in breastfeeding populations [67]. To reach these goals, it is crucial to increase the coverage of HIV tests early in pregnancy in a way to identify HIV-positive women and to start treatment as soon as possible. For those who were tested negative, it is recommended to repeat testing at third trimester (preferably at 34–35 weeks), at the time of delivery, and during lactation [23]. The use of rapid tests for HIV diagnosis is a crucial strategy to obtain immediate access to ART and proper care.

Initial data from an observational study from Botswana suggests a potential association between dolutegravir use at the time of conception and the occurrence of neural tube defects in infants born from HIV-infected mothers. However, in an analysis including a large number of exposures, the magnitude of this risk, although still elevated, has been significantly reduced [33]. The risk period for neural tube defects is limited to the first 28 days of pregnancy, so women at reproductive age should be counseled about the risks and benefits of using this drug or choosing other alternatives. There are advantages and benefits of dolutegravir use in women, including fewer potential of drug interactions, high barrier to resistance development, and rapid viral suppression, outweighing the possible small increased risk of neural tube defects with periconceptional exposure [48, 67].

Observational studies indicated a higher risk of adverse pregnancy outcomes, such as prematurity and low birth weight for gestational age infants in women, who use ART regimens, highlighting the importance of continuous monitoring of these women during pregnancy [4, 35]. During labor and delivery, oral medications can be taken with sips of water. Additionally, IV zidovudine is given to women with HIV viral load >1000 copies/mL or have unknown viral load near delivery.

Delivery and Breastfeeding

In some cases, cesarean delivery lowers HIV transmission, and the American College of Obstetrician and Gynecologists (ACOG) recommends that scheduled cesarean delivery at 38 weeks' gestation should be discussed and recommended for those women with a viral load higher than 1000 copies/mL. For women with HIV viral load lower than 1000 copies/mL, data are insufficient to predict similar benefits, and scheduled cesarean delivery is unlikely to confer additional risk reduction for women already taking ART [16]. If cesarean delivery is chosen or needed for other obstetrical indications in this group presenting a low viral load, it should be performed at 39 weeks whenever possible.

MTCT is increased by breastfeeding, and it is generally not recommended in countries where formula feeding is readily available. ART should not be discontinued postpartum but continued lifelong because of the advantages of viral suppression and avoidance of disease progression. Ideally, all those women who planned their pregnancies should be receiving ART and an undetectable viral load before conception. Also, all infants born to mothers with HIV should receive postexposure antiretroviral prophylaxis.

It is important to take into account the child's perspective to choose the best drugs in terms of its capacity of crossing the placenta (higher with integrase inhibitors or NNRTIs than protease inhibitors), so we can load off the fetus when dosing the medications to the mother. ART, which crosses the placenta, "preloads" the infant for delivery and the first week of life. It is especially important in premature babies who cannot be fed orally.

Infant early diagnosis in the first month of life is crucial for early treatment and to prevent mortality and disease progression [66].

Women presenting viral load >1000 copies/mL within the 4 weeks prior delivery or those who acquired HIV during pregnancy or lactating are considered high risk for transmission, and their infants must receive a more complex regimen [23]. HIV-positive women must keep high adherence to prenatal visits and consultations after delivery to prevent viral resistance, viral rebound, and HIV transmission to their partner and their babies.

Adherence to ARV Treatment

Reduced adherence to ARV treatment has been described at postpartum, and a significant number of women abandon treatment 1 year after delivery. Positive factors that may help women to stay in care include: desire to prevent HIV in the child, wanting to be healthy, to reduce signs of HIV witch might increase stigma, decentralized care, support from clinic staff, partners, and peers [32].

Viral Hepatitis

The most common cause of jaundice in pregnancy is acute hepatitis. Viral hepatitis is meaningful associated to gestational and fetal complications in pregnancy. Following screening guidelines is important to reduce MTCT of viral hepatitis, and a multiprofessional team is essential to provide a complete approach to pregnant women who were exposed or infected with viral hepatitis to accomplish better outcomes. Viral hepatitis can be caused by hepatitis virus A, B, C, D, and E. Clinical course and histological findings are no different between pregnant and nonpregnant women, except for hepatitis E virus [7, 40].

Hepatitis A

The hepatitis A virus (HAV) is a single-stranded RNA virus. There is a single serotype and the infection is self-limiting [7]. It is the most frequent hepatitis, and it can present with or without symptoms, with a variable incubation period of 28 days (mean of 15–50 days). The highest concentration of this virus has been detected in water contaminated with fecal waste. After infection, this virus undergoes a large replication within the hepatocytes, is excreted by the bile into the intestines, and can then be infectious [59]. The main form of transmission is oro-fecal, but sexual transmission had been also described. Transplacental and perinatal transmission are rare [37]. The incidence in pregnancy is considered to be 1:1000, occurring mainly in underdeveloped countries [7].

In children, the infection may be asymptomatic or even undetected, and, depending on climatic conditions, the virus may remain stable for many months in the environment [59]. Serious complications from HAV are rare and occur in less than 1% of cases, and chronicity of this infection does not exist. Immunoglobulin must be given for pregnant women who had contact with an acute viral hepatitis case and for neonates of infected mothers in the third trimester, within 48 hours of life. Breastfeeding is not contraindicated [6, 42].

Hepatitis B

Hepatitis B virus (HBV) infection is a worldwide public health problem [67] due to its high transmissibility, although its epidemiology has been changing over time, due to large-scale vaccination and testing policies for blood banks and general population. HBV is an acute infection that can progress to chronicity, with a significant rate of morbidity and mortality.

HBV can be transmitted parenterally, sexually, and vertically (perinatal and intrauterine). The perinatal route, at the time of delivery, is one of the most important routes of transmission for newborns. In this scenario, the evolution is unfavorable, with a greater chance of chronification. Children born to mothers infected with HBV who are positive for both HBsAg and HBeAg are at higher risk for acquiring the infection – between 70% and 100% – when compared to those born to HBsAg-positive mothers with negative HBeAg (5–30% chance of MTCT). HBV does not cross the placental barrier, unless there is some degree of breakdown of this barrier, such as amniocentesis and chorionic villus biopsy [8, 29, 30, 64].

Chronic HBV infection has little influence on the course of pregnancy, just as pregnancy, in general, does not change the natural history of the infection; however, after delivery, viral reactivation may occur with exacerbation of liver disease in the parturient [44]. Some studies show that women with liver cirrhosis secondary to HBV infection may have impaired fertility due to associated hormonal changes and are at risk of maternal and perinatal death. In addition, gestational hypertension, abortion, preterm birth, and restricted fetal growth can happen due to active infection [36, 65].

Acute HBV infection during pregnancy is not related to an increase in maternal mortality or teratogenic effect on the fetus. However, there are reports of a higher incidence of prematurity, low birth weight, and fetal or perinatal death, possibly due to factors associated with infection [26]. When acute HBV infection occurs in the first trimester of pregnancy, the risk of the infection transmission to the newborn is small, less than 10%; however, when the infection occurs in the second or third trimester of pregnancy, the risk of transmission rises to levels above 60% [58].

In Brazil, despite the introduction of the HBV vaccine since 1999, and progressive efforts for prevention, such as self-sufficient national production of vaccines, MTCT of hepatitis B still occurs. The association of the HBV vaccine with the human anti-hepatitis B immunoglobulin to exposed children, as well as the provision of prophylaxis for pregnant women with antivirals, is an efficient measure to reduce the risk of MTCT of this infection [15, 17].

Prenatal care is important to identify women with chronic HBV, especially those who have high HBV viral load, so that timely prophylaxis can be started in pregnant women when it is necessary and the prophylaxis to exposed newborns in the postpartum period to prevent HBV MTCT. It is important to highlight the significance of the rapid test as a tool for easier and fast access to the HBsAg result [17].

There is no scientific evidence of benefits of performing cesarean section as a preventive measure for MTCT of HBV, which is still a controversial topic in the literature [44, 61, 68]. This procedure should not be performed as the only indication for hepatitis B virus MTCT prevention. Immunoglobulin and vaccine must be given within 12–24 hours of birth to all newborns from HBsAg-positive mothers. In cases where all prophylaxis recommendations have been followed, breastfeeding is not contraindicated [25, 61]. Current guidelines recommend antiviral (nucleotide analog) in the third trimester in highly viremic mothers. The Food and Drug Administration (FDA) recommends lamivudine (LMV; class C) and telbivudine and tenofovir disoproxil fumarate (TDF) (class B) [53].

Hepatitis C

The hepatitis C virus (HCV) is a DNA virus with 11 genotypes and 15 subtypes [57]. Transmission occurs through blood, contaminated needles, sexual intercourse, and MTCT, especially in the last month of pregnancy or childbirth [7]. About 8% of pregnant women in the United States may be infected [55]. A meta-analysis showed a HCV MTCT rate of 5.8% [9], although rates vary depending on geographical factors, disease severity and high CV-HCV titers, comorbidities such as HIV coinfection, or presence of HCV-infected monocytes in peripheral blood.

There is evidence that women with HCV are at risk for worse maternal and neonatal outcomes, such as gestational diabetes, preeclampsia, growth restriction, predelivery bleeding, and preterm delivery ([19]; Huang et al. 2015). Intrahepatic cholestasis is more common in women with positive HCV-RNA, reaching rates of 20% [11, 46]. At the same time, some studies have shown a decrease in transaminase levels during the second and third trimesters of pregnancy, mediated by immunological factors characteristic of pregnancy [20, 27].

There is no scientific evidence to recommend a preferred mode of delivery for preventing MTCT of HCV [3]. The recommendation is to avoid invasive procedures, laborious delivery, and a membrane rupture time greater than 6 hours to minimize the possibility of MTCT. Invasive procedures such as amniocentesis and chronic villus sampling break the maternal-fetal barrier and increase the risk of MTCT of HCV during pregnancy and delivery [39, 63]. There is no evidence that MTCT of HCV can be avoided with the contraindication to breastfeeding [3].

Drugs used to treat acute and chronic hepatitis C are teratogenic or do not have data to prove safety during pregnancy; therefore, they are contraindicated during this period (Spera 2016). With the most modern therapeutic regimens, in the future, women with HCV are expected to be treated before a planned pregnancy.

Hepatitis D

Hepatitis D virus (HDV) is a RNA virus that requires the concomitance of HBV, specifically its surface antigen (HBsAg). Its form of transmission is similar to that of HBV [7]. The parenteral mode is the major mode of transmission, and MTCT during pregnancy is rare. Coinfection of HDV and HBV causes severe acute infection. Superinfection of HDV on chronic HBV leads to higher progression to chronic HDV infection [7].

HDV affects 15–20 million people worldwide with HBV carriers. HDV infection is treated with long-term alpha-interferon and PEGylated interferon. These drugs are contraindicated during pregnancy. HDV transmission has largely decreased due to perinatal prevention and treatment of hepatitis B virus infection [34]. Chronic hepatitis D is associated with a high risk of severe chronic liver disease in pregnant women. Breastfeeding is not contraindicated.

Hepatitis E

Hepatitis E virus (HEV) is an RNA virus that has seven genotypes, and types 1–4 infect humans [47]. Its epidemiological characteristics are similar to those of hepatitis A. Its incubation period is 3–8 weeks, with an average of 40 days [5]. The transmission of this virus also occurs due to inadequate sanitary conditions, such as water contamination by fecal dejects; MTCT of the HEV varies between 23.3% and 50%, and it has not been reported to be transmitted through sexual intercourse [7].

Pregnant women are at high hazard of HEV infection, with an increased risk of complications during pregnancy; it often leads to a fulminant hepatitis and death in some cases. HEV infection can have a serious presentation during pregnancy, particularly in the second and third trimester pregnancies, it may lead to fulminant hepatitis and death in 30%–100% of patients [43, 53]. This infection during the last trimester is associated with severe conditions and maternal death, especially with genotype 1 [18]. Its occurrence during pregnancy may induce a greater risk of fulminant hepatitis, and it is reported that, in a small group of pregnant patients in the third trimester, the death rate conditioned by HEV can reach 20% [28, 54].

There are no studies about the safety and efficacy of the HEV treatment in pregnancy. Obstetric complications include premature rupture of membranes, antepartum and postpartum bleeding, disseminated intravascular coagulation, intrauterine fetal deaths, spontaneous abortions, stillbirths, and complications of fulminant hepatitis [7, 49]. Fetal complications from HEV include preterm and low birth weights. There is no contraindication to breastfeeding in mothers infected with HEV.

Clinical Manifestations

The clinical characteristics do not allow to differentiate the type of hepatitis, which can be asymptomatic, oligosymptomatic, or even present with more intense symptoms. In general, the patient may have some signs and symptoms as jaundice, nausea, anorexia, abdominal pain, adynamia, myalgia, acolia, and choluria. HBV and HCV can progress to decompensation (ascites and encephalopathy, coagulopathy, and esophageal bleeding). HEV can advance with fulminant condition (mortality of up to 25%) [7].

Laboratory Diagnosis

Liver function tests can be used as markers of acute viral hepatitis, such as alanine aminotransferase (ALT), aspartate aminotransferase (AST), and alkaline phosphatase (ALP). Prothrombin time, albumin, and ammonia help in the diagnosis of acute and chronic conditions. The specific diagnosis is made according to Table 44.2.

Table 44.2 Serological diagnostic methods for different types of hepatitis

Hepatitis	Diagnosis
Hepatitis A	Anti-HAV IgM
Hepatitis B	HBsAg B (every pregnant woman should be screened at the beginning of prenatal care)
Hepatitis C	Anti-HCV C (every pregnant woman should be screened at the beginning of prenatal care)
Hepatitis D	Anti-HDAg IgM (should be done in all HBsAg-positive pregnant women)
Hepatitis E	Anti-HEV IgM

References

1. Abuogi LL, Humphrey JM, Mpody C, Yotebieng M, Murnane PM, Clouse K, et al. Achieving UNAIDS 90-90-90 targets for pregnant and postpartum women in sub-Saharan Africa: progress, gaps and research needs. J Virus Erad. 2018;4(Suppl 2):33–9.
2. Adachi K, Xu J, Yeganeh N, Camarca M, Morgado MG, Watts DH, et al. Combined evaluation of sexually transmitted infections in HIV-infected pregnant women and infant HIV transmission. PLoS One. 2018;13(1).
3. Aebi-Popp K, Duppenthaler A, Rauch A, de Gottardi A, Kahlert C. Vertical transmission of hepatitis C: towards universal antenatal screening in the era of new direct acting antivirals (DAAs)? Short review and analysis of the situation in Switzerland. J Virus Erad. 2016;2(1):52–4.
4. Alemu FM, Yalew AW, Fantahun M, Ashu EE. Antiretroviral therapy and pregnancy outcomes in developing countries: a systematic review. Int J MCH AIDS. 2015;3(1):31.
5. Aggarwal R, Krawczynski K. Hepatitis E: an overview and recent advances in clinical and laboratory research. J Gastroenterol Hepatol. 2000;15(1):9–20.
6. ACOG - American College of Obstetricians and Gynecologists. ACOG Practice Bulletin No. 86: viral hepatitis in pregnancy. Obstet Gynecol. 2007;110(4):941–56.
7. Asafo-Agyei KO, Samant H. Pregnancy and viral hepatitis. SourceStatPearls [Internet]. Treasure Island (FL): StatPearls Publishing; 2020.
8. Beasley RP, Trepo C, Stevens CR, et al. The e antigen and vertical transmission of hepatitis B surface antigen. Am J Epidemiol. 1977;105(2):94–8.
9. Benova L, Mohamoud YA, Calvert C, et al. Vertical transmission of hepatitis C virus: systematic review and meta-analysis. Clin Infect Dis. 2014;59:765–73.
10. Benzaken AS, Pereira GFM, Cunha ARCD, Souza FMA, Saraceni V. Adequacy of prenatal care, diagnosis and treatment of syphilis in pregnancy: a study with open data from Brazilian state capitals. Cad Saude Publica. 2019;36(1):e00057219. https://doi.org/10.1590/0102-311X00057219. eCollection 2019.
11. Berkley EMF, Leslie KK, Arora S, et al. Chronic hepatitis C in pregnancy. Obstet Gynecol. 2008;112(2 Pt 1):304–10.
12. Branson BM, Handsfield HH, Lampe MA, Janssen RS, Taylor AW, Lyss SB, Clark JE, Centers for Disease Control and Prevention (CDC). Revised recommendations for HIV testing of adults, adolescents, and pregnant women in health-care settings. MMWR Recomm Rep. 2006;55(RR-14):1–17; quiz CE1-4.
13. BRASIL. Ministério da Saúde. Secretaria de Vigilância em Saúde. Boletim Epidemiológico Sífilis 2019. Available at http://www.aids.gov.br/pt-br/pub/2019/boletim-epidemiologico-sifilis-2019. Accessed 17 May 2020[a].
14. BRASIL. Ministério da Saúde. Secretaria de Vigilância em Saúde. Boletim Epidemiológico de HIV e Aids. Site: file:///F:/Users/Usuario/Downloads/boletim_hivaids_2019%20(2).pdf. Accessed 23 Apr 2020[b].

15. BRASIL. Ministério da Saúde. Secretaria de Vigilância em Saúde. Departamento de Doenças de Condições Crônicas e Infecções Sexualmente Transmissíveis. Protocolo Clínico e Diretrizes Terapêuticas para Prevenção da Transmissão Vertical do HIV, Sífilis e Hepatites Virais 2019 site: http://www.aids.gov.br/pt-br/pub/2015/protocolo-clinico-e-diretrizes-terapeuticas-para-prevencao-da-transmissao-vertical-de-hiv. Acessado em 22 de abril de 2020[c].
16. Briand N, Jasseron C, Sibiude J, Azria E, Pollet J, Hammou Y, et al. Cesarean section for HIV-infected women in the combination antiretroviral therapies era, 2000–2010. Am J Obstet Gynecol. 2013;209(4):335–e1.
17. Brown RS Jr, Mcmahon BJ, Lok AS, Wong JB, Ahmed AT, Mouchli MA, et al. Antiviral therapy in chronic hepatitis B viral infection during pregnancy: a systematic review and meta-analysis. Hepatology. 2016;63(1):319–33.
18. Chaudhry SA, Verma N, Koren G. Hepatitis E infection during pregnancy. Can Fam Physician. 2015;61(7):607–8.
19. Connell LE, Salihu HM, Salemi JL, et al. Maternal hepatitis B and hepatitis C carrier status and perinatal outcomes. Liver Int, [S.l.]. 2011;31(8):1163–70.
20. Conte D, Fraquelli M, Prati D, et al. Prevalence and clinical course of chronic hepatitis C virus (HCV) infection and rate of HCV vertical transmission in a cohort of 15,250 pregnant women. Hepatology. 2000;31:751–5.
21. Cooper JM, Sánchez PJ. Congenital syphilis. Semin Perinatol. 2018;42(3):176–84. https://doi.org/10.1053/j.semperi.2018.02.005. Epub 2018 Apr 5.
22. Curry SJ, Krist AH, Owens DK, et al.; US Preventive Services Task Force. Screening for syphilis infection in pregnant women: US Preventive Services Task Force reaffirmation recommendation statement. JAMA. 2018;320(9):911–7. https://doi.org/10.1001/jama.2018.11785.
23. Updated US HIV Perinatal Guidelines. Available at: https://clinicalinfo.hiv.gov/en/guidelines/perinatal/whats-newguidelines. Accessed on September 20, 2021.
24. Drake AL, Wagner A, Richardson B, John-Stewart G. Incident HIV during pregnancy and postpartum and risk of mother-to-child HIV transmission: a systematic review and meta-analysis. PLoS Med. 2014;11:e1001608.
25. EASL - EUROPEAN ASSOCIATION FOR THE STUDY OF THE LIVER (EASL). EASL clinical practice guidelines: management of chronic hepatitis B virus infection. J Hepatol. 2017;57:167–85.
26. Gambarin-Gelwan M. Hepatitis B in pregnancy. Clinics in liver disease, [S.l.]. 2007;11(4):945–63.
27. Gervais A, Bacq Y, Bernuau J, et al. Decrease in serum ALT and increase in serum HCV RNA during pregnancy in women with chronic hepatitis C. J Hepatol. 2000;32:293–9.
28. Hussaini SH, Skidmore SJ, Richardson P, Sherratt LM, Cooper BT, O'Grady JG. Severe hepatitis E infection during pregnancy. J Viral Hepat. 1997;4(1):51–4.
29. Joshi SS, Coffin CS. Hepatitis B and pregnancy: virologic and immunologic characteristics. Hepatol Commun. 2020;4(2):157–71.
30. Keane E, Funk AL, Shimakaway Y. Systematic review with meta-analysis: the risk of mother-to-child transmission of hepatitis B virus infection in sub-Saharan Africa. Aliment Pharmacol Ther. 2016;44(10):1005–17.
31. King C, Ellington SR, Kourtis AP. The role of co-infections in mother-to-child transmission of HIV. Curr HIV Res. 2013;11(1):10–23.
32. Knettel BA, Cichowitz C, Ngocho JS, Knippler ET, Chumba LN, Mmbaga BT, et al. Retention in HIV care during pregnancy and the postpartum period in the Option B+ era: a systematic review and meta-analysis of studies in Africa. J Acquir Immune Defic Syndr (1999). 2018;77(5):427.
33. Kourtis AP, Bulterys M, Nesheim SR, Lee FK. Understanding the timing of HIV transmission from mother to infant. JAMA. 2001 Fevereiro;285(6):709–12.
34. Krause A, Haberkorn U, Mier W. Strategies for the treatment of HBV/HDV. Eur J Pharmacol. 2018;833:379–91.

35. Kreitchmann R, Li SX, Melo VH, Fernandes Coelho D, Watts DH, Joao E, et al. Predictors of adverse pregnancy outcomes in women infected with HIV in L atin A merica and the C aribbean: a cohort study. BJOG Int J Obstet Gynaecol. 2014;121(12):1501–8.
36. Lao TT, Chan BC, Leung WC, et al. Maternal hepatitis B infection and gestational diabetes mellitus. J Hepatol. 2007;47:46–50.
37. Leikin E, Lysikiewicz A, Garry D, Tejani N. Intrauterine transmission of hepatitis A virus. Obstet Gynecol. 1996;88(4 Pt 2):690–1.
38. Mahy M, Marsh K, Sabin K, Wanyeki I, Daher J, Ghys PD. HIV estimates through 2018: data for decision-making. AIDS. 2019;33 Suppl 3(Suppl 3):S203–11.
39. Mast EE, Hwang LY, Seto DSY, et al. Risk factors for perinatal transmission of hepatitis C virus (HCV) and the natural history of HCV infection acquired in infancy. J Infect Dis. 2005;192:1880–9.
40. Mishra L, Seeff LB. Viral hepatitis, A though E, complicating pregnancy. Gastroenterol Clin N Am. 1992;21(4):873–87.
41. Moore DL, Allen UD. HIV in pregnancy: identification of intrapartum and perinatal HIV exposures. Paediatr Child Health. 2019;24(1):42–9. https://doi.org/10.1093/pch/pxy181.
42. Miller WJ, Clark W, Hurni W, Kuter B, Schofield T, Nalin D. Sensitive assays for hepatitis A antibodies. J Med Virol. 1993;41(3):201–4.
43. Navaneethan U. Seroprevalence of hepatitis E infection in pregnancy – more questions than answers. Indian J Med Res. 2009;130:677–9.
44. Pan CQ, Zou HB, Chen Y, et al. Cesarean section reduces perinatal transmission of hepatitis B virus infection from hepatitis B surface antigen-positive women to their infants. Clin Gastroenterol Hepatol. 2013;11(10):1349–55.
45. Passos MRL, Eleutério JJR, Nahn EP Jr, Giraldo PC, Bravo RS, Varella RQ, et al. Doenças/Infecções Sexualmente Transmissíveis. Cap 62. In: Montenegro CA, Rezende Filho J, editors. Rezende Obstetrícia. 13th ed. Rio de Janeiro: Guanabara Koogan; 2017. p. 615–43.
46. Paternoster DM, Fabris F, Palù G, Santarossa C, Bracciante R, Snijders D, Floreani A. Intrahepatic cholestasis of pregnancy in hepatitis C virus infection. Acta Obstet Gynecol Scand. 2002;81(2):99–103.
47. Pérez-Gracia MT, Suay-García B, Mateos-Lindemann ML. Hepatitis E and pregnancy: current state. Rev Med Virol. 2017;27(3):e1929.
48. Phillips AN, Venter F, Havlir D, Pozniak A, Kuritzkes D, Wensing A, et al. Risks and benefits of dolutegravir-based antiretroviral drug regimens in sub-Saharan Africa: a modelling study. Lancet HIV. 2019;6(2):e116–27.
49. Patra S, Kumar A, Trivedi SS, Puri M, Sarin SK. Maternal and fetal outcomes in pregnant women with acute hepatitis E virus infection. Ann Intern Med. 2007;147(1):28–33.
50. Schmidt R, Carson PJ, Jansen RJ. Resurgence of syphilis in the United States: an assessment of contributing factors. Infect Dis (Auckl). 2019;12:1178633719883282. Published online 2019 Oct 16. https://doi.org/10.1177/1178633719883282.
51. Saraceni V, Pereira GFM, da Silveira MF, Araujo MAL, Miranda AE. Epidemiological surveillance of vertical transmission of syphilis: data from six federal units in Brazil. Rev Panam Salud Publica. 2017;41:e44.
52. Saraceni V, Miranda AE. Coverage by the Family Health Strategy and diagnosis of syphilis in pregnancy and congenital syphilis. Cad Saude Publica. 2012;28(3):490–6.
53. Sarin SK, Kumar M, Lau GK, Abbas Z, Chan HL, Chen CJ, et al. Asian-Pacific clinical practice guidelines on the management of hepatitis B: a 2015 update. Hepatol Int. 2016;10:1–98.
54. Seifoleslami M. An update of the incidence of fulminant hepatitis due to viral agents during pregnancy. Interv Med Appl Sci. 2018;10(4):210–2.
55. Shepard CW, Finelli L, Alter MJ. Global epidemiology of hepatitis C virus infection. Lancet Infect Dis. 2005;5(9):558–67.
56. Shinde N, Patil T, Deshpande A, Gulhane R, Patil M, Bansod Y. Clinical profile, maternal and fetal outcomes of acute hepatitis E in pregnancy. Ann Med Health Sci Res. 2014;4:S133–9.
57. Simmonds P. Viral heterogeneity of the hepatitis C virus. J Hepatol. 1999;31 Suppl 1:54–60.

58. Society for Maternal-Fetal Medicine (SMFM), Dionne-Odom J, Tita AT, Silverman NS. #38: Hepatitis B in pregnancy screening, treatment, and prevention of vertical transmission. Am J Obstet Gynecol. 2016;214(1):6–14.
59. Staes CJ, Schlenker TL, Risk I, et al. Sources of infection among persons with acute hepatitis A and no identified risk factors during a sustained community-wide outbreak. Pediatrics. 2000;106(4):E-54.
60. Stafford IA, Sánchez PJ, Stoll BJ. Ending congenital syphilis. JAMA. 2019. https://doi.org/10.1001/jama.2019.17031. [Epub ahead of print].
61. Terrault NA, Bzowejnh, Chang KM, et al. AASLD guidelines for treatment of chronic hepatitis B. Hepatology. 2016;63(1):261.
62. Thomson KA, Hughes J, Baeten JM, et al. Increased risk of female HIV-1 acquisition throughout pregnancy and postpartum: a prospective per-coital act analysis among women with HIV-1 infected partners. J Infect Dis. 2018;218:16–25.
63. Tovo PA, Calitri C, Scolfaro C, Gabiano C, Garazzino S. Vertically acquired hepatitis C virus infection: correlates of transmission and disease progression. World J Gastroenterol. 2016;22(4):1382–92.
64. Tran TT. Hepatitis B in pregnancy. Clin Infect Dis. 2016;62(Suppl 4):S314–7.
65. Tse K, Siu SL, Yip KT, et al. Immuno-prophylaxis of babies born to hepatitis B carrier mothers. Hong Kong Med J, [S.l.]. 2006;12(5):368–74.
66. Violari A, Cotton MF, Gibb DM, Babiker AG, Steyn J, Madhi SA, et al. Early antiretroviral therapy and mortality among HIV-infected infants. N Engl J Med. 2008;359(21):2233–44.
67. WHO - World Health Organization. Global guidance on criteria and processes for validation: elimination of mother-to-child transmission of HIV and syphilis. 2017.
68. Yang J, Zeng XM, Men YL, et al. Elective caesarean section versus vaginal delivery for preventing mother to child transmission of hepatitis B virus – a systematic review. Virol J, [S.l.]. 2008;5:100.

Chapter 45
Congenital Infection 2 (Toxoplasmosis, CMV, Rubella)

Juliana Silva Esteves, Daniela Aires Moreira, and Eduardo Borges da Fonseca

Toxoplasmosis

Congenital toxoplasmosis is caused by the vertical transmission of the protozoan *Toxoplasma gondii*. Acute infection during pregnancy (first infection) has been associated with miscarriage, prematurity, and low birth weight, as well as disseminated fetal disease.

Congenitally infected infants who are symptomatic at birth may have clinical findings localized to the central nervous system or eye or have generalized manifestations of the disease. Those with mild or subclinical disease at birth may have no manifestations on routine physical examination but remain at risk for long-term sequelae from chorioretinitis.

The rate of vertical transmission of toxoplasma increases in proportion to gestational age, being 15% in the first trimester, 44% in the second, and 77% in the third. At term, this rate is close to 80%. On the other hand, the overall frequency of clinical manifestations during infancy decreases with older gestational age at seroconversion, with a marked reduction in intracranial lesions with older gestational age at seroconversion and a less marked reduction in ocular lesions [1].

J. S. Esteves
Hospital Federal dos Servidores do Estado - Ministry of Health, Rio de Janeiro, RJ, Brazil

D. A. Moreira
University of Medical Sciences, João Pessoa, Paraíba, Brazil

Maternal Fetal Medicine Group, Nova Diagnóstico por Imagem, João Pessoa, Brazil

E. B. d. Fonseca (✉)
Maternal Fetal Medicine Group - Nova Diagnóstico por Imagem, João Pessoa, PB, Brazil

Ob/Gyn Department, Federal University of Paraiba, João Pessoa, PB, Brazil
e-mail: http://novadiagnostico.com.br/

© Springer Nature Switzerland AG 2022
R. A. Moreira de Sá, E. B. d. Fonseca (eds.), *Perinatology*,
https://doi.org/10.1007/978-3-030-83434-0_45

American, British, Canadian, and some European societies recommend against routine universal screening for toxoplasmosis in pregnancy [2–4] because the prevalence of the disease and incidence of maternal infection are very high. Nevertheless, we are in favor of the universal screening at first prenatal visit, and monthly or bimonthly up to 26 weeks for those susceptible. The screening test is not costly and an effective treatment known to decrease vertical transmission [5, 6]. Furthermore, in Latin America, virulent *T. gondii* is prevalent, and many women have risk factors for acquiring the infection because of low sanitation, feeding habits, contact with cats, contact with contaminated soil, and consumption of unboiled, untreated water [7, 8].

Indeed, the balance of risks and benefits of prenatal screening/treatment must be estimated by individual countries/continents/regions because the balance shifts depending on disease prevalence and prevalence of more virulent strains of *T. gondii* (e.g., Western Europe has mostly less virulent strains, and South America has more virulent strains) [9, 10].

In addition, the provision of dietary-hygienic guidelines for susceptible pregnant women (Table 45.1), the availability of spiramycin in health units, the definition of specialized centers, and the diagnosis and treatment of congenital infection are fundamental actions in the control of this disease, and they represent adequate maternal and infant healthcare.

Ultrasound Findings in Congenital Toxoplasmosis

Although fetal ultrasound can provide diagnostic and prognostic information, it is not a useful screening tool as ultrasound changes are observed in approximately 28% of infected fetuses. The sonographic findings have been described in Table 45.2 [10, 11].

The most common sonographic findings in fetal toxoplasmosis are intracranial hyperechogenic foci or calcifications and cerebral ventricular dilation, which often

Table 45.1 Hygienic and dietary actions used in the primary prevention of toxoplasmosis during pregnancy

Do not eat raw or undercooked meat.
Cook the meat and meat products until temperature above 67o or freeze them (−18o for 10 days)
Treat the water or boil it
Wash fruits and vegetables properly with running water
Wear gloves to handle raw meat and avoid contact with any material that may be contaminated with cat feces, such as soil, lawns and litter boxes
Protect food from flies and cockroaches
Boil and pasteurize milk before consumption

Note: Pet cats should be fed meat properly cooked or commercial feed and their faeces should be discarded daily, washing the container with hot water. With this extent, the oocyst does not become infectious, as it needs 24 hours at room temperature to reach this stage

Table 45.2 Ultrasound finding in congenital toxoplasmosis

1. Intracranial hyperechogenic foci (calcifications/densities),
2. Ventricular dilation/hydrocephalus,
3. Echogenic bowel,
4. Hepatosplenomegaly,
5. Intrahepatic calcifications/densities,
6. Fetal growth restriction,
7. Ascites,
8. Pericardial and/or pleural effusions,
9. Hydrops fetalis,
10. Fetal demise,
11. Placental densities and/or increased thickness.

occur together [10–12]. Intracranial calcification or ventricular dilation was found in 6% of infected fetuses in a European prospective cohort study [12]. Ventricular dilation is generally bilateral and can progress rapidly over a period of a few days or weeks [10, 11]. Other brain findings in infected fetuses include periventricular abscesses or, less frequently, periventricular echogenicity, cortical gyration anomalies, lenticulostriate vessels vasculitis, shortened corpus callosum, cerebellar anomalies, and subependymal cysts [10, 11]. Fetal magnetic resonance imaging may add prognostic information to detailed expert ultrasound evaluation in some cases. Extracerebral abnormalities, when present, are usually associated with cerebral abnormalities.

In the absence of maternal serologic screening, one or more of the ultrasound findings described in Table 45.2 may lead to suspicion of congenital toxoplasmosis. However, the sonographic signs are nonspecific, so prenatal ultrasound cannot reliably distinguish between congenital toxoplasmosis and other congenital infections (e.g., cytomegalovirus, Zika virus) or various genetic diseases (e.g., ventricular dilation can be related to trisomy 21; echogenic bowel can be related to cystic fibrosis).

Hence, when toxoplasmosis is suspected because of ultrasound findings rather than a prenatal screening protocol, maternal serology for toxoplasmosis and cytomegalovirus should be performed as these are the two most common infectious causes for these findings. If maternal IgG and IgM antibodies are negative for toxoplasmosis, fetal toxoplasmosis infection is ruled out, and further evaluation can be directed toward other causes for the sonographic findings. If maternal IgG antibodies are positive for toxoplasmosis (even in the absence of IgM), we offer amniocentesis for amniotic fluid analysis for *T. gondii* polymerase chain reaction (PCR) as a component of the work-up of the sonographic findings, guided by the clinical scenario.

In infected fetuses, the prognosis likely depends on the severity of the cerebral damage, and not all abnormal fetal findings lead to serious disabling sequelae, particularly in the presence of early therapy [12, 13]. The probability of serious neurologic sequelae or death for fetuses with abnormal intracranial ultrasound findings was estimated to be 43 percent (95% CI 6–90 percent) [12, 13]. The estimated probabilities were much higher in women infected early in pregnancy and in untreated women [12, 13].

Diagnosis of Fetal Infection

The fetal diagnosis is done by polymerase chain reaction (PCR) in amniotic fluid for *T. gondii*. Amniocentesis is indicated when primary maternal infection during pregnancy is confirmed or is strongly suspected or there are abnormal ultrasound findings.

Amniocentesis is offered to women between 18 and 26 weeks of gestation with serologically confirmed or strongly suspected recent infection for prenatal diagnosis of fetal infection [14]. When possible, amniocentesis is delayed until 2 weeks after documentation of seroconversion (or 4 weeks after the estimated date of maternal primary infection) to improve diagnostic performance.

If fetal infection is diagnosed, maternal drug therapy can be used to mitigate fetal injury. Exclusion of fetal infection can prevent unnecessary treatment of infants without clinical signs of toxoplasmosis and at low risk of congenital infection [15, 16].

Prevention of Fetal Infection

The general approach to treatment of pregnant women in toxoplasmosis screening programs is summarized in the algorithm (Fig. 45.1). In unscreened pregnant women undergoing fetal diagnosis because of abnormal findings on ultrasound, serology would be performed, and if IgG positive, amniotic fluid PCR should be indicated when the timing of maternal seroconversion cannot be determined.

Screening Test

Prenatal routine screening has been encouraged in some parts of Latin America. The Brazilian Ministry of Health recommends serology for toxoplasmosis panel. The interpretation of screening results is summarized bellow [7].

- *Screening performed before 20 weeks* – negative IgM and positive IgG antibodies indicate prior immunity, especially at the first trimester. No further action is recommended.
- *Screening performed after 20 weeks* – negative IgM and positive IgG antibodies. The timing of infection is not clear, and confirmatory testing by an experienced reference laboratory should be recommended.
- *Immunoglobulin M (IgM) is positive or equivocal* – the diagnosis of recent infection should be confirmed by an experienced reference laboratory. To establish if there is a recent or chronic toxoplasmosis infection, confirmatory testing must be obtained with avidity testing (high IgG avidity is a hallmark of chronic infection, more than 4 months). Another possibility is to repeat IgG within 3 weeks. A rising IgG titer of twofold or greater over two sequential samples obtained 3 weeks

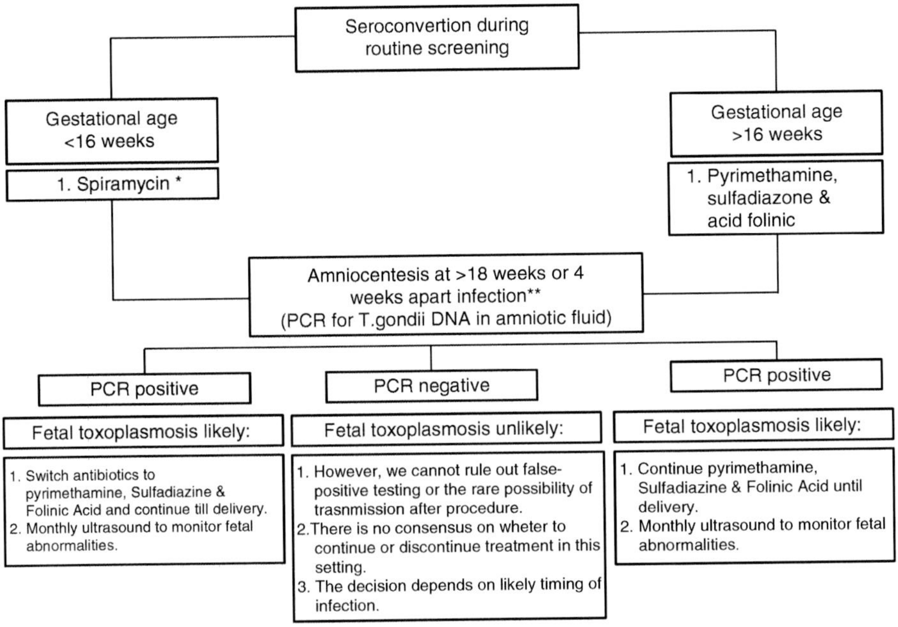

Fig. 45.1 Approach to toxoplasmosis in pregnancies. PCR polymarase chain reaction, *T. gondii Toxoplasma gondii*
* Patients who begin spiramycin <14 weeks can continue this drug until PCR results from amniocentesis at 18 weeks are available to guide further decisions. Alternatively, they can switch to pyrimethamine-sulfadiazine after 14 weeks until PCR is available
** Impossibility for performing amniotic fluid PCR for *T.gondii*. Women may opt to take pyrimethamine, sulfadiazine plus folinic acid from diagnosis of materna toxoplasmosis infection ≥14–16 weeks until delivery since fetal infection cannot be excluded and treatment may improve outcome. If a patient does not want prolonged treatment, it would be mainteined for at least 8 weeks and fetal abnormalities after 22 weeks be ruled out
Amniocentesis should be performed at ≥18 weeks or 2 weeks after documentation of seroconversion to improve PCR accuracy

apart and test simultaneously in the same laboratory with the same technique can also suggest recent infection.

Treatment for Reduction of Congenital Toxoplasmosis

Antimicrobial therapy (Table 45.3) directed against *T. gondii* is indicated to symptomatic and asymptomatic pregnant women diagnosed with recent *T. gondii* infection (acquired during pregnancy) to reduce the risk of congenital toxoplasmosis [1, 7].

There are no direct maternal benefits from treatment. Even for immunocompromised pregnant women with prior toxoplasmosis, there is insufficient evidence to support the routine use of antimicrobial therapy to prevent congenital infection since transmission during reactivation is unlikely and no studies have evaluated this

Table 45.3 Drugs used in prevention of congenital toxoplasmosis

Drug	*Dose*	Contraindications	Side-effects	Monitoring
Spyramicin	1gr (1million IU) orally three times daily	Long QT syndrome	Nausea, vomiting, diarrhea, skin reaction	N.A.
Pyrimethamine	50 mg orally per day (25 mg twice).		Folic acid antagonist (dose-related bone marrow suppression): anemia, leukopenia, and thrombocytopenia	Complete blood count weekly
Sulfadiazine	3 grs orally (500 mg tablets in 3 doses)	Precipitate hemolysis in women with G6PD[a] and Crystaluria		
Folinic acid	10–20 mg per day	–	–	–

[a]*G6PD* glucose-6-phosphate dehydrogenase

strategy. However, some women with HIV may already be on trimethoprim-sulfamethoxazole for Pneumocystis pneumonia and toxoplasmosis prophylaxis.

The initial antimicrobial regimen used for treatment of pregnant women diagnosed with toxoplasmosis is begun as soon as possible upon documentation of probable maternal infection. The therapy should be started before amniocentesis, once the therapeutic "window of opportunity" (when maternal administration of antibiotics may prevent or reduce fetal neurologic damage) is considered to be <3 weeks from seroconversion [1, 17].

There are two antimicrobial regimens that are typically used to reduce the risk of congenital toxoplasmosis: (1) spiramycin and (2) pyrimethamine-sulfadiazine. The choice of drug(s) is based on the gestational age at diagnosis. The Brazilian Ministry of Health agrees with the general consensus to use spiramycin when therapy is begun in early gestational age (<16 weeks) and pyrimethamine-sulfadiazine when therapy is begun thereafter (≥16 weeks) [9].

The rationale for only beginning pyrimethamine-sulfadiazine after first trimester is that any risk of teratogenesis would be lower [18]. Patients who begin spiramycin before 14–16 weeks can continue this drug until PCR results from amniocentesis at 18 weeks are available, or they may switch to pyrimethamine-sulfadiazine at 16 weeks and continue pyrimethamine-sulfadiazine until PCR results from amniocentesis at 18 weeks are available. Some clinicians suggest continuing spiramycin in this setting because no studies have evaluated whether there is any benefit from switching drug regimens at 14–16 weeks, while other clinicians suggest switching to pyrimethamine-sulfadiazine at 14–16 weeks because it has been shown to be more effective than spiramycin in second- and third-trimester pregnancies with recent seroconversion.

If amniotic fluid PCR for *T. gondii* is positive, pyrimethamine-sulfadiazine is indicated until delivery [4, 19]; shorter durations of treatment have not been studied. After birth, the child will be treated with the same regimen. If the patient had been on spiramycin for prophylaxis, the Brazilian Ministry of Health, in accordance with others guidelines, advised that she switch from spiramycin to pyrimethamine-sulfadiazine because it appears to be more effective in treating congenital infection.

If amniotic fluid PCR for *T. gondii* is negative and fetal ultrasound is normal, most authorities, as the Brazilian government, would not continue treatment, whereas some would continue treatment because of concerns about placental transmission occurring after the amniocentesis. If the option is to treat after a negative PCR, there is no worldwide consensus regarding the best regimen for patients, and no data are available on which to base recommendations for the optimal duration of treatment.

In case to continue treatment after negative PCR, an option is spiramycin for those women with periconceptional or first-trimester seroconversion, and for those cases of second- or third-trimester seroconversion, pyrimethamine-sulfadiazine are switched after a total of at least 4 weeks' treatment to spiramycin until delivery.

In case of no amniocentesis is not available or women decline to have it, we suggest treatment with pyrimethamine-sulfadiazine from diagnosis of maternal infection ≥14–16 weeks until delivery since fetal infection cannot be excluded and treatment may improve outcome. If the patient does not want prolonged treatment, we suggest treatment for at least 8 weeks and until results from a fetal ultrasound after 22 weeks are available and negative for anomalies, with the understanding that the risk is not eliminated because a normal ultrasound does not exclude the possibility of congenital toxoplasmosis.

If pyrimethamine-sulfadiazine cannot be obtained expeditiously, trimethoprim-sulfamethoxazole may be used (160 mg trimethoprim and 800 mg sulfamethoxazole, twice daily) until delivery or be switched to pyrimethamine-sulfadiazine when available.

It is important to note that we have not instituted treatment with spiramycin for pregnant women without immunosuppressive diseases with previous immunity to toxoplasmosis because it does not cause fetal involvement. In immunosuppressed pregnant women, who have CD4 <200 cells/mm^3, we recommend the triple treatment illustrated above, starting at 17 weeks.

Rubella

Rubella is an acute exanthematous disease of universal distribution, which occurs predominantly in childhood and adolescence. It is transmitted mainly by direct contact with infected individuals, through droplets of nasopharyngeal secretions. As the disease is asymptomatic in most cases, its diagnosis is serological.

Rubella is an eradication disease in Brazil. Vaccination against this disease has been part of the vaccination schedule since 2000, with the first dose applied to the child at 12 months of age and a boost between 4 and 6 years of life. In Brazil, an outbreak of rubella occurred in young adults in the late 1990s, and, consequently, there were numerous cases of congenital rubella syndrome. This outbreak triggered the first vaccination campaign for women of childbearing age, between 15 and 29 years old, in 2001. As cases continued, mainly in males, in 2008 there was a new campaign, which also immunized men. With these measures, viral circulation was reduced and the number of cases of the disease drastically dropped.

The specific antibodies appear during the rash phase of the disease. Both IgG and IgM antibodies reach their highest levels around 7–10 days after the onset of symptoms. Antibodies of the IgM class disappear around 3–7 weeks after the exanthematic phase, while those of the IgG class remain indefinitely. Currently, using extremely sensitive tests, it is possible to detect IgM after a period of time longer than that previously mentioned, which causes great difficulty in defining the moment of acute disease [20].

Rubella serology is part of the routine examination of the first prenatal consultation, with the aim of detecting patients without immunity. Susceptible people should be vaccinated at the time of discharge from the maternity where they attended, even if they are breastfeeding the newborn. This dose of the vaccine is essential to eradicate the disease.

In prenatal care, for patients with results of serology with IgM and IgG reagents, which configure a possible acute condition, a confirmatory test, such as the IgG avidity test, should be requested in a referral service. We should also search if the pregnant woman has already been vaccinated, if she had possible contact, or if she developed the symptoms of the disease. If the condition is only positive serology, the pregnant woman should be oriented and tranquilized. The most frequent case in this situation is the persistence of IgM or false positive of the test. IgG avidity in infections within 3–4 months is generally low. Asymptomatic disease can rarely have consequences for the fetus, with a lower risk than symptomatic ones [21].

The manifestations of congenital rubella syndrome include deafness, heart defects such as ventricular septal defect, persistence of the ductus arteriosus, pulmonary stenosis and aortic coarctation, retinopathy, and alterations of the central nervous system. These changes are observed in around 50% of the affected children. Other manifestations, such as fetal growth restriction, encephalitis, microcephaly, and mental retardation, are found in 10–20% of cases [22].

Pregnant women infected in the first trimester of pregnancy have a 20% chance of having a newborn with congenital rubella syndrome. The risk of infection and fetal involvement in the first trimester is extremely high, and, after the 17th week, there is theoretically no more risk of serious illness [22].

In the evaluation of suspected cases, ultrasound examination helps, but it is not a sensitive method for detecting affected fetuses. The following changes have already been described: fetal growth restriction, microcephaly, microphthalmia, cardiac malformations (pulmonary stenosis, aortic coarctation, septal defects), echogenic intestine, fetal hydrops, hydrocephalus, cataracts, placental thickening, and changes of the volume of amniotic fluid. Fetal echocardiography is part of the routine screening of congenital infection suspected cases.

Prevention: Vaccine

The rubella vaccine is composed of live attenuated virus, and it was developed over 40 years ago. The seroconversion rate is 95% after one single dose of vaccine. Vaccination of pregnant women is not recommended, even during epidemic periods. Vaccinated women should avoid pregnancy for a period of 30 days after the date of application [23].

In studies and follow-up of cases carried out in the United States with the current vaccine strain of rubella *RA 27/3*, 272 susceptible women were vaccinated before and/or during the beginning of pregnancy, and 272 newborns from these patients were evaluated, with no cases of congenital rubella syndrome detected [23, 24].

The preparation for the vaccination campaign throughout the Brazilian territory, in 2001, involved several sectors, and pregnant women should not receive any vaccination dose. Even with all guidelines, in the State of São Paulo alone, 6473 pregnant women were vaccinated, and, of these, 811 were susceptible at the time of immunization. A multidisciplinary group was organized to follow up these patients with the coordination of the São Paulo Epidemiological Surveillance Center. Of these pregnant women, 20 newborns (4.7%) had IgM in their cord blood. However, all newborns were followed up, and, to date, no signs of congenital rubella syndrome have been observed [25].

It is unacceptable to approach termination of pregnancy for women who have been vaccinated and were unaware of their initial pregnancy status or even who became pregnant before the recommended 30 days' interval of the date of application.

Rubella and congenital rubella syndrome are diseases of compulsory notification. The notification of suspected and / or confirmed rubella cases is important in the characterization of how and where viral circulation occurs, in the effectiveness of the prevention and control actions and in the follow-up of possible susceptible pregnant women and cases of congenital rubella syndrome.

Cytomegalovirus Infection

Cytomegalovirus (CMV) is a herpes virus formed by a double helix of DNA, which is transmitted through contact with blood, saliva, urine, or sexual contact with infected people, and it is one of the most common etiological agents of perinatal and congenital infection in different parts of the world. It occurs in 0.2–2.2% of newborns, with a higher incidence in populations with low socioeconomic status.

About 1% of fetuses born in the USA have congenital CMV infection, 10–15% present symptoms at birth. The most common clinical manifestations are hepatosplenomegaly, periventricular intracranial calcifications, jaundice, growth restriction, microcephaly, chorioretinitis and hearing loss. The most frequent laboratory alterations are thrombocytopenia, hyperbilirubinemia and elevated liver transaminases. Approximately 30% of critically infected newborns die, and 80% of survivors will have severe neurological handicap. About 85–90% of infected fetuses are asymptomatic at birth. Among these, 10–15% will have one or more sequelae up to 2 years of age, such as sensorineural hearing loss, chorioretinitis, dental defects, mental retardation, and optic nerve atrophy. Current studies confirm the old theory that the more premature the infection occurs during pregnancy, the worse the fetal prognosis.

Estimated global CMV seroprevalence in women at childbearing age is about 86%, with the highest seroprevalences in the Eastern Mediterranean, Western Pacific, African, and Southeast Asian regions and the lowest in the European region and the Americas [7]. The CMV seroconversion rates in pregnant women is about 2% as follows [26].

The CMV infection throughout pregnancy is classified as primary (defined as first infection during pregnancy and diagnosed for seroconversion from negative to positive antibodies, with a low avidity of immunoglobulin G) or nonprimary (defined as the first infection occurred before pregnancy and the abnormalities are due to latent infections or virus reactivation).

Primary infection occurs in 25% of all cases of congenital infection. In adults, primary infection is asymptomatic in majority of the cases. Occasionally, patients have a "mononucleosis-like" syndrome, with leukocytosis, lymphocytosis, abnormal liver tests, fever, malaise, myalgia, and chills. After initial infection, CMV remains latent in the host's cells. Reinfection can occur by reactivating the virus in latency, which is a common process in herpesviruses, and occurs in 5–15% of individuals affected by the disease. Viral excretion can last for years after primary infection [27]. However, recurrent maternal infection (nonprimary) has fewer devastating effects, and the fetuses appear to be asymptomatic at birth. In some cases, there may be sequelae up to 5 years of age, and the most common of them is hearing loss. The CMV incubation period is 28–60 days, with an average of 40 days. Primary infections produce a humoral response by IgM that disappears in an average of 30–60 days, which can, in ultra-sensitive kits, remain positive for up to 300 days.

Ultrasound Findings in Congenital CMV

The diagnosis of congenital CMV can be mainly suspected after the detection of ultrasound findings suggestive of infection. These signs are shown in Table 45.4.

In infected fetuses, abnormalities can appear 12 or more weeks after maternal infection, and the most characteristic ultrasound finding is bilateral periventricular hyperechogenicities (calcifications) [28, 29]. These calcifications or hyperechoic foci can be highly reflective and may not cast an acoustic shadow [29]. Branching linear echogenic areas in the thalami also occur and correspond to arteries in the basal ganglia and thalamus [30]. The presence of intraventricular filmy, thin adhesions and linear edges traversing the ventricle is typical in CMV infection of the brain [29, 31, 32].

Table 45.4 Ultrasonographic signs of fetal CMV infection

Central nervous system	Heart	Abdome	Placenta/Amniotic fluid	Other
Cerebral ventriculomegaly	Cardiomegaly	***Hepatomegaly***	***Placental thickening***	Fetal growth restriction
		Splenomegaly		
Periventricular calcifications		Parenchymal calcifications	Small placenta	Hydrops Fetalis
			Oligohydramnios	
Microcephaly		***Ascites***		
			Polyhydramnios	
		Hyperechogenic bowel		

Note: The most frequent signs appear in bold

Diagnosis of Maternal and Fetal Infection

Maternal Infection

The diagnosis of primary maternal infection is currently obtained by seroconversion of IgM anti-CMV, detected using commercial kits of the ELISA test (*enzyme-linked immunosorbent assay*), or by the presence of anti-CMV IgG in patients known to be negative at preconception period. The diagnosis of recurrent infection is suspected when there is an increase in anti-CMV IgG titters, or new IgM seroconversion, in the presence of previously positive IgG [33].

The use of the IgG specific anti-CMV avidity test proved to be effective in dating the primary infection, with the presence of antibodies of low avidity, result of the index examination <30%, present in maternal blood up to 20 weeks after contact with the virus, and high avidity to 80%, to safely exclude CMV infection up to 12 weeks of the exam date. However, this test is not effective for differentiating between recurrent and late infections and, since there is the possibility of fetal involvement in this type of infection, this isolated test is not completely safe to rule out the involvement of the fetus. Therefore, the *gold standard* test for congenital CMV infection is the virus isolation in urine or saliva of the newborn, up to 3 weeks after birth [29, 33, 34].

Fetal Infection

Fetal infection should be diagnosed by detection of CMV DNA on Polymerase Chain Reaction (PCR) analysis of the amniotic fluid. Amniocentesis should be delayed until at least 6–8 weeks after estimated time of maternal infection and after 20 gestational weeks. There are retrospective data showing that the sensitivity of amniotic fluid PCR may be similar at 17 and 20 weeks, provided that there is a time interval of at least 6–8 weeks between maternal infection and amniocentesis. The two most significant risk factors for a false-negative result are time interval <8 weeks and amniocentesis before 18 weeks [35].

Prevention of Fetal Infection

Screening Test

There is no consensus regarding universal screening [29, 34]. Some authors believe that all pregnant women should be screened for primary CMV infection, or all women of childbearing age should know their CMV serostatus since CMV infection is usually asymptomatic, transmissible to the fetus, and knowing that the patient's serology is negative for CMV antibodies, CMV counseling increase patients' motivation to practice good hygiene and thus decrease the risk of seroconversion during pregnancy [36, 37]. Nevertheless, repeated serologic screening during pregnancy to detect seroconversion is not commonly performed because of cost, lack of effective treatment, and generally poor ability of positive serology to predict the fetus's long-term outcome.

Those are against routine serologic screening for CMV, suggest to obtain CMV serology in HIV-infected women at their initial prenatal visit and repeat the serology in screen-negative women who develop signs/symptoms suggestive of CMV infection or have suggestive fetal ultrasound findings. For any woman with a known exposure to CMV, we obtain baseline serology at the time of the exposure and, if negative, repeat serology several weeks later to assess for seroconversion.

Diagnose Fetal Infection

Amniocentesis for fetal diagnosis when fetal infection is suspected due to primary maternal infection or findings on ultrasound should be discussed. The rationale for offering prenatal diagnosis is to determine whether the fetus is infected and prepare the couple for the birth for an infected baby, or possibly affected, infant. Lastly, it may change the intensity of fetal monitoring (eg, frequency of ultrasound examination) and is informative for the pediatricians caring for the child.

Amniocentesis to perform polymerase chain reaction (PCR) for CMV DNA in amniotic fluid is the preferred diagnostic approach for identifying an infected fetus, and can be performed at any time ≥18 weeks, however an interval of at least 8–6 weeks between maternal infection and amniocentesis is desirable to increase diagnostic sensitivity [29].

Treatment for Reduction of Congenital CMV Infection

Antiviral Drug Therapy

Strategies involving antiviral therapy for prevention of vertical transmission are challenging given that most maternal infections are asymptomatic and pregnancy CMV screening is not routinely performed.

Only few data on the effect of such agents on the prevention or outcome of congenital infection is available [29, 38–40]. Strategies for antiviral treatment of infected fetuses identified by ultrasound and diagnostic testing are more promising, but data from randomized trials are not available.

In a multicenter, open-label, phase II study of oral valacyclovir treatment of pregnant women carrying a CMV-infected fetus with measurable extracerebral or mild cerebral ultrasound findings, the intervention improved neonatal outcome of infected fetuses without severe brain abnormalities [38]. Compared with a historical cohort, valacyclovir increased the proportion of asymptomatic neonates from 43% without treatment to 82% with treatment. Valacyclovir 8 g daily was initiated at 25 weeks and continued until delivery or termination of pregnancy.

Hyperimmunoglobulin

Hyperimmunoglobulin therapy of pregnant women with primary CMV infection in early pregnancy is an investigational approach to reducing symptomatic infection in offspring. Four prospective observational studies, administration of CMV-specific hyperimmune globulin to pregnant women with primary CMV infection was associated with a reduction in maternal-to-fetal transmission and severity of congenital infection [41, 42]. However, a randomized trial did not demonstrate such benefit. In the Congenital Human CMV Infection Prevention (CHIP) trial, 124 pregnant women at 5–26 weeks with recent onset of primary CMV infection were randomly assigned to receive hyperimmune globulin or placebo every 4 weeks until 36 weeks or detection of CMV in amniotic fluid [43]. The overall rate of congenital infection was similar for both groups (30% vs 44% in treatment compared to placebo group). The proportion of infected infants symptomatic at birth was also similar for both groups (3/10 CMV-infected newborns in the hyperimmune globulin group [30%] versus 4/17 CMV-infected newborns in the placebo group [24%]). There were also no differences in the viral or immune characteristics of infected infants between the groups. In addition, the number of obstetric adverse events was higher in the hyperimmune globulin group than in the placebo group.

Until more data from randomized trials are available, practitioners should emphasize the simple preventive measures noted above. CMV hyperimmunoglobulin therapy should only be used in a research setting until more data are available.

Post-natal Diagnostic Approach

Laboratory diagnosis of congenital CMV infection should be indicated in five clinical scenarios: (1) newborns with signs and symptoms consistent with congenital CMV disease, (2) newborns with neurological abnormalities consistent with CMV; (3) newborns who have documented sensorineural hearing loss (SNHL), (4) newborns born to mothers with known or suspected CMV infection during pregnancy; and (5) immune-compromised newborns [44].

The diagnosis for congenital CMV infection is based on isolation or molecular detection of CMV from urine or saliva samples collected within the first 3 weeks of life. PCR from urine samples are preferred due to better accurance.

Infants with virologically-confirmed congenital CMV infection should be evaluated for evidence of organ involvement. Comprehensive evaluation should be performed even in infants who appear asymptomatic to detect subtle or subclinical subtle findings. The evaluation includes: (a) a thorough physical, and neurologic and neurodevelopmental examination (b) laboratory testing (complete blood count with differential and platelet count, liver function tests, kidney function tests, coagulation studies in selected cases with liver disease or viral sepsis, hearing evaluation by auditory brainstem response (ABR), ophthalmology evaluation, ultrasound and/or computed tomography (CT) and/or magnetic resonance imaging (MRI) of the brain.

Parvovirus B19 Infection

Discovered casually by Cossart and colleagues in 1975, when researching a hepatitis B surface antigen in blood bags from asymptomatic donors, with a false positive test for hepatitis B, parvovirus B19, also known as erythrovirus, is a single icosahedral, single-stranded DNA helix virus with no envelope, with external capsid containing two structural proteins. The term B19 is due to the fact that this is the number of the bag of blood stock in the laboratory in which this infectious agent was detected. It was later recognized as a causal factor of transient aplastic crisis and implicated as an etiological agent of infectious erythema [45, 46].

Parvovirus B19 presents tropism for erythroid progenitor cells and other cells of the hematological system, such as neutrophils and plaques. After the first infection, the IgM anti-B19 antibody remains undetectable for a few months. The antibodies of the IgG class appear in a few days [46].

Among the viruses of the Parvoviridae family, Parvovirus B19 is the only one that causes the disease in humans. Its asymptomatic form occurs in up to 50% of children and adults, which, obviously, constitutes a real trap during pregnancy, since, if vertical transmission occurs to the fetus, it may suffer serious repercussions, such as the fearful hydrops, which commonly culminates in lethal death of the fetus, in addition to spontaneous abortion in the first trimester of pregnancy [46].

In the symptomatic form, generalized erythema, edema and joint pain, aplastic crisis and severe anemia, possibly associated with prolonged secondary infections, are more commonly observed. In the 1990s, reports began to appear in the medical literature of chronic anemia due to persistent parvovirus B19 infection in patients with the AIDS virus, demonstrating that the immunosuppression caused by this pathology is an important factor for the disease of parvovirus in adults. In patients with sickle cell anemia, it is an important cause for the development of transient aplastic anemia. Despite the transitory character of this disease, some affected individuals may progress to more severe anemia, culminating in congestive heart failure and death.

Diagnosis

Infections with erythro viruses occur more frequently in the form of infectious erythema (fifth childhood disease) during the winter and spring months, although they can also affect several population groups, mainly school-age children, in the other months of the year. year. Not all infected individuals are symptomatic. In about 50% of cases the infection can be asymptomatic [46, 47].

After the first infection, nonspecific symptoms such as headache, myalgia, fever, chills and itchy skin commonly appear, followed by a clinical picture that mimics rheumatoid arthritis.

During pregnancy, parvovirus B19 does not usually have any teratogenic potential. However, the infected fetus often progresses to myocarditis, in addition to a dramatic reduction in its erythropoiesis, which leads to the development of severe anemia and heart failure, culminating in non-immune fetal hydrops, with intrauterine death in around 50% of cases [47].

Serological Diagnosis

The serological diagnosis is usually carried out by searching for specific anti-parvovirus B19 IgG and IgM antibodies, using commercially available kits. The polymerase chain reaction (PCR) can be performed to detect its DNA in the serum or infected tissues of some patients [46, 48, 49].

When facing the diagnosis of primo infection by erythrovirus in pregnancy, the possibility of vertical transmission to the fetus should be considered and, consequently, fetal anemia due to massive hemolysis.

Diagnosis of Fetal Infection

In the fetus, the diagnosis usually occurs with differential diagnosis in cases of non-immune fetal anemia. The quantification of fetal anemia in suspected cases can be done by Doppler evaluation of the peak systolic velocity of the middle cerebral artery of the fetus. Three spectral curves are performed on the Doppler of this artery, and, of the three values chosen, it is considered the largest one to establish the peak systolic velocity as a predictor of fetal anemia. If this parameter exceeds 1.5 multiple of the median of the curve constructed by Mari and collaborators for each gestational age in weeks, a diagnosis of moderate or severe fetal anemia is made, and the concept should preferably be subjected to intrauterine blood transfusion by cordocentesis [48, 49].

An investigation of the parvovirus B19 DNA, in amniotic fluid or fetal blood, detected by the PCR technique, associated with maternal specific IgM antibodies, is important for the search for the causal diagnosis of hydrops of the concept [49].

Treatment of Fetal Infection

The treatment of fetal infection with parvovirus B19, complicated by severe anemia and hydrops, can be done by intrauterine blood transfusion through cordocentesis. It is important to emphasize the great importance of clarifying the pregnant couple and obtaining their consent before carrying out this invasive fetal therapy technique, due to the risk of 1–3% of loss of the fetus due to the procedure itself [49, 50].

References

1. Thiebaut R, Leproust S, Chene G, Gilbert R, Syrocot study group. Effectiveness of prenatal treatment for congenital toxoplasmosis: a meta-analysis of individual patients' data. Lancet. 2007;369:115–22.
2. Gilbert RE, Peckham CS. Congenital toxoplasmosis in the United Kingdom: to screen or not to screen? J Med Screen. 2002;9:135–41.
3. Paquet C, Yudin MH, Society of O, Gynaecologists of C. Toxoplasmosis in pregnancy: prevention, screening, and treatment. J Obstet Gynaecol Can. 2013;35:78–81.
4. American College of O, Gynecologists. Practice bulletin no. 151: cytomegalovirus, parvovirus B19, varicella zoster, and toxoplasmosis in pregnancy. Obstet Gynecol. 2015;125:1510–25.
5. Gilbert R, Gras L, European Multicentre Study on Congenital T. Effect of timing and type of treatment on the risk of mother to child transmission of Toxoplasma gondii. BJOG. 2003;110:112–20.
6. Wallon M, Peyron F, Cornu C, et al. Congenital toxoplasma infection: monthly prenatal screening decreases transmission rate and improves clinical outcome at age 3 years. Clin Infect Dis. 2013;56:1223–31.
7. Costa GB, De Oliveira MC, Gadelha SR, et al. Infectious diseases during pregnancy in Brazil: seroprevalence and risk factors. J Infect Dev Ctries. 2018;12:657–65.
8. Bahia-Oliveira LM, Jones JL, Azevedo-Silva J, Alves CC, Orefice F, Addiss DG. Highly endemic, waterborne toxoplasmosis in north Rio de Janeiro state, Brazil. Emerg Infect Dis. 2003;9:55–62.
9. Maldonado YA, Read JS, Committee On Infectious D. Diagnosis, treatment, and prevention of congenital toxoplasmosis in the United States. Pediatrics. 2017;139:e20163860.
10. Hohlfeld P, MacAleese J, Capella-Pavlovski M, et al. Fetal toxoplasmosis: ultrasonographic signs. Ultrasound Obstet Gynecol. 1991;1:241–4.
11. Malinger G, Werner H, Rodriguez Leonel JC, et al. Prenatal brain imaging in congenital toxoplasmosis. Prenat Diagn. 2011;31:881–6.
12. Cortina-Borja M, Tan HK, Wallon M, et al. Prenatal treatment for serious neurological sequelae of congenital toxoplasmosis: an observational prospective cohort study. PLoS Med. 2010;7:e1000351.
13. McLeod R, Kieffer F, Sautter M, Hosten T, Pelloux H. Why prevent, diagnose and treat congenital toxoplasmosis? Mem Inst Oswaldo Cruz. 2009;104:320–44.
14. de Oliveira Azevedo CT, do Brasil PE, Guida L, Lopes Moreira ME. Performance of polymerase chain reaction analysis of the amniotic fluid of pregnant women for diagnosis of congenital toxoplasmosis: a systematic review and meta-analysis. PLoS One. 2016;11:e0149938.
15. Thalib L, Gras L, Romand S, et al. Prediction of congenital toxoplasmosis by polymerase chain reaction analysis of amniotic fluid. BJOG. 2005;112:567–74.
16. Gilbert RE, Thalib L, Tan HK, et al. Screening for congenital toxoplasmosis: accuracy of immunoglobulin M and immunoglobulin A tests after birth. J Med Screen. 2007;14:8–13.

17. Cornu C, Bissery A, Malbos C, et al. Factors affecting the adherence to an antenatal screening programme: an experience with toxoplasmosis screening in France. Euro Surveill. 2009;14:21–5.
18. Montoya JG, Remington JS. Management of Toxoplasma gondii infection during pregnancy. Clin Infect Dis. 2008;47:554–66.
19. Paquet C, Yudin MH. No. 285-toxoplasmosis in pregnancy: prevention, screening, and treatment. J Obstet Gynaecol Can. 2018;40:e687–e93.
20. Cooper LZ, Prelub SR, Alford CA. Rubella. In: Remington JS, Klein JO, editors. Infectious disease in the fetus and newborn infant. 4th ed. Philadelphia: WB Saunders; 1995.
21. Bos P, Steele D, Alexander J. Prevalence of antibodies to rubella, herpes simplex 2 and cytomegalovirus in pregnant women and in neonates at Ga-Rankuwa. Cent Afr J Med. 1995;41:14–7.
22. Crino JP. Ultrasound and fetal diagnosis of perinatal infection. Clin Obstet Gynecol. 1999;42:71–80.
23. Centers for Disease Control and Prevention. US. Department of health & human services. Guidelines for vaccinating pregnant women from recommendations of the Advisory Comitte on Imunizatio Practices (ACIP).CDC, 2002.
24. Centers for Disease Control and Prevention. Notice to readers: revised ACIP recommendation for avoiding pregnancy after receiving a rubella-containing vaccine. MMWR. 2001;50(49):117.
25. Andrade JQ, Bunduki V, Curti SP, Figueiredo CA, Oliveira MI, Zugaib M. Rubella in pregnancy: intrauterine transmission and perinatal outcome during a Brazilian epidemic. JCV. 2006;35:285–91.
26. Hyde TB, Schmid DS, Cannon MJ. Cytomegalovirus seroconversion rates and risk factors: implications for congenital CMV. Rev Med Virol. 2010;20:311–26.
27. Barber V, Calvert A, Vandrevala T, et al. Prevention of acquisition of cytomegalovirus infection in pregnancy through hygiene-based behavioral interventions: a systematic review and gap analysis. Pediatr Infect Dis J. 2020;39:949–54.
28. Enders G, Bader U, Lindemann L, Schalasta G, Daiminger A. Prenatal diagnosis of congenital cytomegalovirus infection in 189 pregnancies with known outcome. Prenat Diagn. 2001;21:362–77.
29. Khalil A, Sotiriadis A, Chaoui R, et al. ISUOG Practice Guidelines: role of ultrasound in congenital infection. Ultrasound Obstet Gynecol. 2020;56:128–51.
30. Estroff JA, Parad RB, Teele RL, Benacerraf BR. Echogenic vessels in the fetal thalami and basal ganglia associated with cytomegalovirus infection. J Ultrasound Med. 1992;11:686–8.
31. Malinger G, Lev D, Zahalka N, et al. Fetal cytomegalovirus infection of the brain: the spectrum of sonographic findings. AJNR Am J Neuroradiol. 2003;24:28–32.
32. Marques Dias MJ, Harmant-van Rijckevorsel G, Landrieu P, Lyon G. Prenatal cytomegalovirus disease and cerebral microgyria: evidence for perfusion failure, not disturbance of histogenesis, as the major cause of fetal cytomegalovirus encephalopathy. Neuropediatrics. 1984;15:18–24.
33. Kagan KO, Enders M, Schampera MS, et al. Prevention of maternal-fetal transmission of cytomegalovirus after primary maternal infection in the first trimester by biweekly hyperimmunoglobulin administration. Ultrasound Obstet Gynecol. 2019;53:383–9.
34. Kagan KO, Hamprecht K. Cytomegalovirus infection in pregnancy. Arch Gynecol Obstet. 2017;296:15–26.
35. Enders M, Daiminger A, Exler S, Ertan K, Enders G, Bald R. Prenatal diagnosis of congenital cytomegalovirus infection in 115 cases: a 5 years' single center experience. Prenat Diagn. 2017;37:389–98.
36. Vauloup-Fellous C, Picone O, Cordier AG, et al. Does hygiene counseling have an impact on the rate of CMV primary infection during pregnancy? Results of a 3-year prospective study in a French hospital. J Clin Virol. 2009;46 Suppl 4:S49–53.
37. Adler SP, Nigro G. Prevention of maternal-fetal transmission of cytomegalovirus. Clin Infect Dis. 2013;57 Suppl 4:S189–92.

38. Leruez-Ville M, Ghout I, Bussieres L, et al. In utero treatment of congenital cytomegalovirus infection with valacyclovir in a multicenter, open-label, phase II study. Am J Obstet Gynecol. 2016;215:462 e1–e10.
39. Leruez-Ville M, Ville Y. Optimum treatment of congenital cytomegalovirus infection. Expert Rev Anti-Infect Ther. 2016;14:479–88.
40. Jacquemard F, Yamamoto M, Costa JM, et al. Maternal administration of valaciclovir in symptomatic intrauterine cytomegalovirus infection. BJOG. 2007;114:1113–21.
41. Nigro G. Hyperimmune globulin in pregnancy for the prevention of congenital cytomegalovirus disease. Expert Rev Anti-Infect Ther. 2017;15:977–86.
42. Visentin S, Manara R, Milanese L, et al. Early primary cytomegalovirus infection in pregnancy: maternal hyperimmunoglobulin therapy improves outcomes among infants at 1 year of age. Clin Infect Dis. 2012;55:497–503.
43. Revello MG, Lazzarotto T, Guerra B, et al. A randomized trial of hyperimmune globulin to prevent congenital cytomegalovirus. N Engl J Med. 2014;370:1316–26.
44. Adachi K, Xu J, Ank B, et al. Congenital cytomegalovirus and HIV perinatal transmission. Pediatr Infect Dis J. 2018;37:1016–21.
45. Anderson MJ, Higgins PG, Davis LR, Willman JS, Jones SE, Kidd IM, et al. Experimental parvoviral infection in humans. J Infect Dis. 1985;152:257–65.
46. Bond PR, Caul EO, Usher J, et al. Intrauterine infection with human parvovirus. Lancet. 1986;1:448–9.
47. Brown T, Anand A, Ritchie LD, et al. Intrauterine parvovirus infection associated with hydrops fetalis. Lancet. 1984;2:1033–4.
48. Cosmi E, Mari G, Delle Chiaie L, et al. Noninvasive diagnosis by Doppler ultrasonography of fetal anemia resulting from parvovirus infection. Am J Obstet Gynecol. 2002;187:1290–3.
49. De Haan TR, Oepkes D, Beersma MFC, et al. Aetiology, diagnosisand treatment of hydrops foetalis. Curr Pediatr Rev. 2005;1:63–72.
50. Dembinski J, Eis-Hübinger AM, Maar J, et al. Long term follow up of serostatus after maternofetal parvovirus B19 infection. Arch Dis Child. 2003;88:219–21.

Chapter 46
Group B Streptococcus and Pregnancy

Renato Augusto Moreira de Sá, Antônio Rodrigues Braga Neto, and Bartolomeu Expedito da Câmara França

Introduction

The Lancefield group B beta-hemolytic streptococcus infection (*S. agalactiae*) or group B streptococcus (GBS) is the most frequent cause of early neonatal infection (up to the seventh day of life) [1]. It can be manifested by septicemia that develops more frequently up to 72 hours postpartum or by late infections represented by pneumonia or meningitis in the first 4 weeks of life [2]. This microorganism is a β-hemolytic streptococcus of the Lancefield group B and can be further characterized into ten antigenically unique serotypes. GBS is characterized by being a Gram-positive coccus, a negative catalase that can be distributed in chains or in pairs and has the characteristic of complete lysis of red blood cells in blood agar medium (classified as beta-hemolytic) [3]. However, the presence of hemolysis is not mandatory.

It is a commensal of the human gastrointestinal and genitourinary tracts which is thought to be the main source for maternal colonization. Colonization may fluctuate over time and is usually asymptomatic in immunocompetent hosts; however, all serotypes are capable of causing infection [3].

GBS is recognized as the most frequent cause of severe early-onset infection in newborn infants. These infants manifest GBS infection as sepsis, pneumonia, and meningitis. Despite this disease occurring as a continuum over the first 3 months of life, it is commonly divided into early-onset disease, occurring within 0–6 days of birth, or late-onset disease, occurring within 7–90 days of birth [4].

The main route of early-onset neonatal GBS infection is the vertical transmission of mothers colonized during vaginal labor and delivery. Most babies exposed to GBS during delivery become colonized by GBS and do not develop signs or

R. A. Moreira de Sá (✉)
Fernandes Figueira Institut - FIOCRUZ, Rio de Janeiro, RJ, Brazil

A. R. B. Neto · B. E. da Câmara França
Materno-Infantil, Federal Fluminense University, Niteroi, RJ, Brazil

© Springer Nature Switzerland AG 2022
R. A. Moreira de Sá, E. B. d. Fonseca (eds.), *Perinatology*,
https://doi.org/10.1007/978-3-030-83434-0_46

symptoms of GBS infection. The fetus is also susceptible to ascending infection in the amniotic fluid, with or without rupture of membranes [5].

Epidemiology

Colonization by GBS in asymptomatic pregnant women ranges from 15% to 25% in epidemiological studies conducted in industrialized nations. However, substantial variation in incidence of early-onset disease remains in low-income and middle-income countries [4].

Invasive disease incidence varies both within and across geographical regions, ranging from 0.02 per 1000 live births in Southeast Asia to 1.21 per 1000 live births in Africa [6]. The introduction of antibiotic-based interventions may influence geographical variation. Other factors underlying this variation might include differences in case ascertainment and laboratory diagnostics or population differences in exposure and susceptibility [7].

GBS is a frequent cause of asymptomatic bacteriuria, urinary tract infection, upper genital tract infection, postpartum endometritis, pneumonia, puerperal sepsis, and bacteremia without a focus, both in pregnant and postpartum women. It also can cause focal infection such as meningitis and endocarditis, albeit rarely. The serotype distribution of invasive GBS infection in pregnant women is similar to that of early-onset neonatal disease [8].

Maternal Infections

Maternal invasive infection, defined as isolation of GBS from a blood or other usually sterile body site in pregnant women (excluding urinary tract), is not frequent. Upper genital tract infection accounted for approximately one-half of these cases, and isolated bacteremia occurred in one-third of cases [8].

GBS is a frequent cause of asymptomatic bacteriuria, cystitis, and pyelonephritis during pregnancy. GBS accounted for 10% of cases of pyelonephritis [9, 10].

Postpartum endometritis is more frequent in GBS colonized pregnant women. GBS is more commonly a component of polymicrobial infections but has been identified as a single pathogen in 2–14% [11].

Intra-amniotic isolated infection by GBS is not common. Usually, intra-amniotic infection is polymicrobial, often involving vaginal or enteric flora. GBS is one of the pathogens associated with intra-amniotic infection. Diagnosis criteria for GBS intra-amniotic infection include isolation of GBS from culture of placenta, amniotic fluid, or amniotic membranes or from fetal parts in case of pregnancy loss [8, 12].

Unusual peripartum infections such as maternal meningitis, endocarditis, abdominal abscess, and necrotizing fasciitis are rarely associated with GBS [13].

Ascending infection from the maternal genital tract and direct contact during delivery are the methods for vertical transmission to the neonate and account for up to 75% of cases of neonatal GBS colonization. Infants colonized by GBS will develop early-onset GBS infection in 1–2% of these cases, and 11% to almost 50% will develop fatal early-onset GBS neonatal infection [14].

Maternal Colonization

Vertical infection occurs during labor of colonized patients and is associated with high neonatal mortality [3]. Maternal rectovaginal colonization by GBS is therefore a major risk factor for early- and late-onset infant GBS infection [6]. The risk of vertical transmission in the presence of maternal colonization is 40–60%, and of those colonized neonates, about 3% will go on to develop early-onset infant GBS infection [6, 8].

Maternal colonization rates vary depending on population-based differences, as told before [15], and may be transient, intermittent, or persistent [16]. It is important to consider that the intensity of maternal colonization is directly related to the risk of transmission to the baby [17].

GBS bacteriuria occurs in at least 2% of pregnancies and is a surrogate marker of heavy colonization [6, 15]. Babies born to women with GBS bacteriuria (any colony count) during pregnancy are more frequently and more heavily colonized with GBS increasing the risk of early-onset neonatal infection [18].

Neonatal GBS Infection

Neonatal colonization of GBS may occur as a result of in utero ascending infection from the maternal genital tract or direct contact during delivery. Neonatal GBS infection is characterized as early onset if occurring within 7 days of age or late onset if otherwise and involves bacteremia, pneumonia, or meningitis [14].

Prevention Strategies

Several prevention strategies have been adopted to reduce early infection with group B streptococcus. Among them, risk factor detection and universal screening are the most used [3].

In the presence of risk factors, intrapartum antibiotic prophylaxis is recommended. Among the most important risk factors are the following [18, 19]:

- Preterm labor (PTL) at less than 37 + 0 weeks (spontaneous or induced).
- Rupture of membranes (ROM) greater than or equal to 18 hours prior to birth.
- Maternal temperature greater than or equal to 38 °C intrapartum or within 24 hours of giving birth.

- GBS colonization in the current pregnancy.
- GBS bacteriuria in the current pregnancy (any colony count).
- Previous history of a newborn infected with GBS.

By adopting such a conduct, approximately 25% of pregnant women can benefit from antibiotic prophylaxis with a reduction in early neonatal infection by 50–70% [18]. Fig. 46.1 summarizes this strategy.

Universal screening strategy involves swabbing samples obtained from the lower vagina, perineum, and anorectal area and cultured in selective media such as Todd-Hewitt broths. Swabbing must be offered for all women between 35 and 37 weeks of gestation, regardless of the presence of risk factors in the current pregnancy. The detection rate for group B streptococcus is approximately 27%, with a 86% reduction in early neonatal infection [20]. With universal screening, antibiotic prophylaxis is recommended for all pregnant women colonized by the bacteria [21]. Figure 46.2 summarizes universal screening strategy [19].

Despite the studies showing the effectiveness of the procedures recommended by these screening protocols with consequent reductions in the rates of neonatal infection by group B streptococcus, doubts about the screening approach and prevention strategies still persist [3]. There have been no randomized studies addressing whether routine screening has had any impact on all-cause mortality.

The rectovaginal culture strategy has a weakness as the culture is obtained weeks before delivery and changes in GBS status can occur. This fact reduces the sensitivity to about 50% and the positive predictive value to about 60%. Several factors may influence antepartum GBS screening including a low colonization status of the woman, suboptimal timing of specimen collection, and inappropriate transport media for specimens (such as lack of storage at 5 °C if transportation of specimens for culture is delayed or there is inadequate laboratory) [22]. Rapid GBS test strategy can be used intrapartum for better identification of women carrying GBS in the vagina at the time of delivery. The sensitivity of the intrapartum polymerase chain reaction test (PCR) to detect GBS colonization during labor may be superior to antenatal cultures in certain populations [22].

Collection of Specimens

Samples must be collected using nylon flocked swabs submerged into transport medium. Flocked swabs are currently the more efficient to collect larger volume of secretion and to release more easily bacteria in culture. The type of swab used for collection and transport of vaginal-rectal samples may influence sensitivity of culture especially for lightly colonized women with GBS or collection [16, 20].

After proper explanation provided to the patient, swab the lower vagina (vaginal introitus) followed by the rectum (i.e., 2.5 cm beyond the anal sphincter, and gently rotate to sample anal crypts) using the same swab or two different swabs. Cervical, perianal, perirectal, or perineal specimens are not acceptable, and a speculum should not be used for culture collection [16].

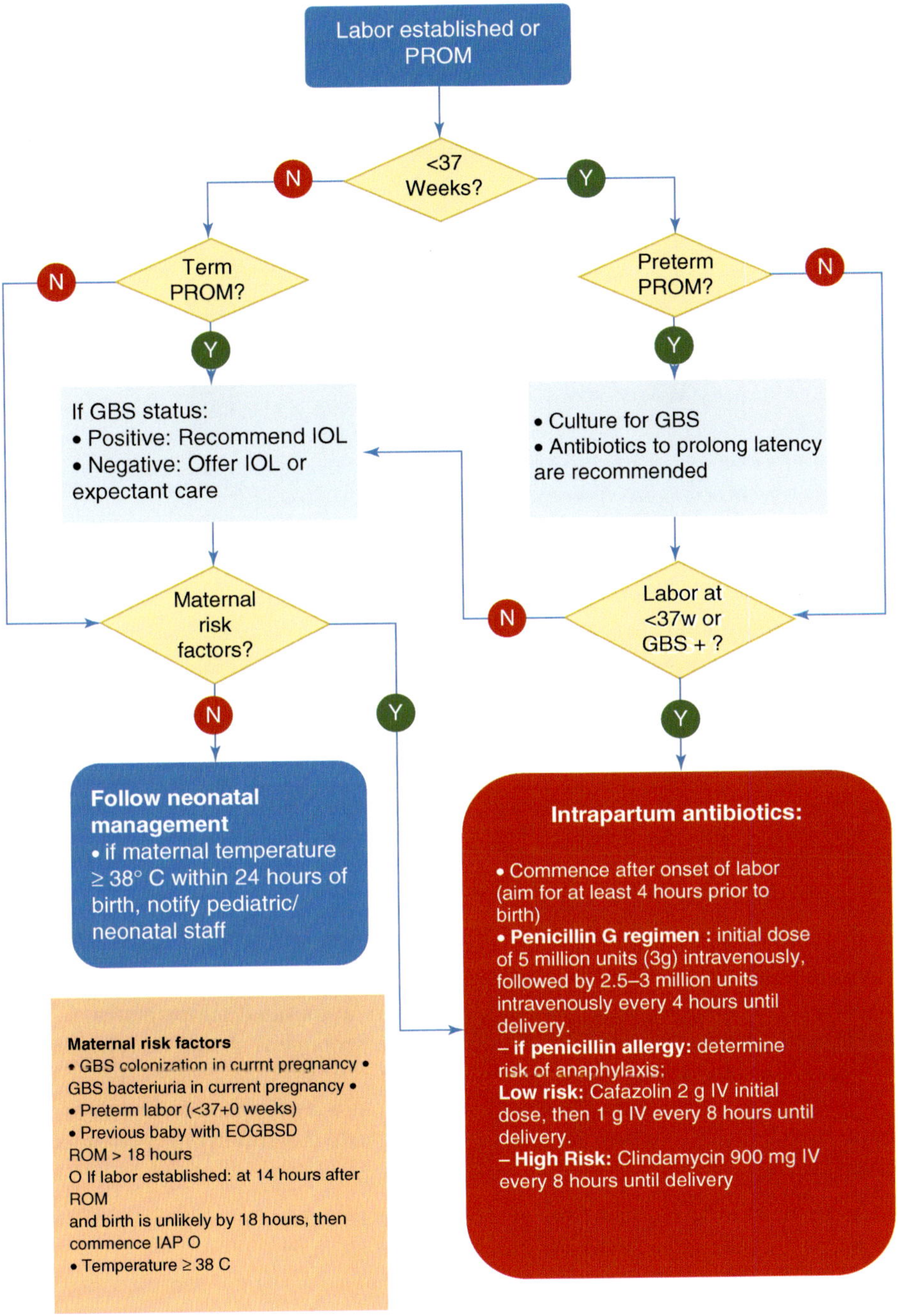

Fig. 46.1 Flowchart of maternal management of early-onset group B streptococcal disease. GBS group B streptococcus, IV intravenous, IOL induction of labor, PROM pre-labor rupture of membranes, > greater than, < less than. (Modified from Queensland Clinical Guidelines. Early onset Group B Streptococcal disease. Guideline No. MN16.20-V4-R21 [8])

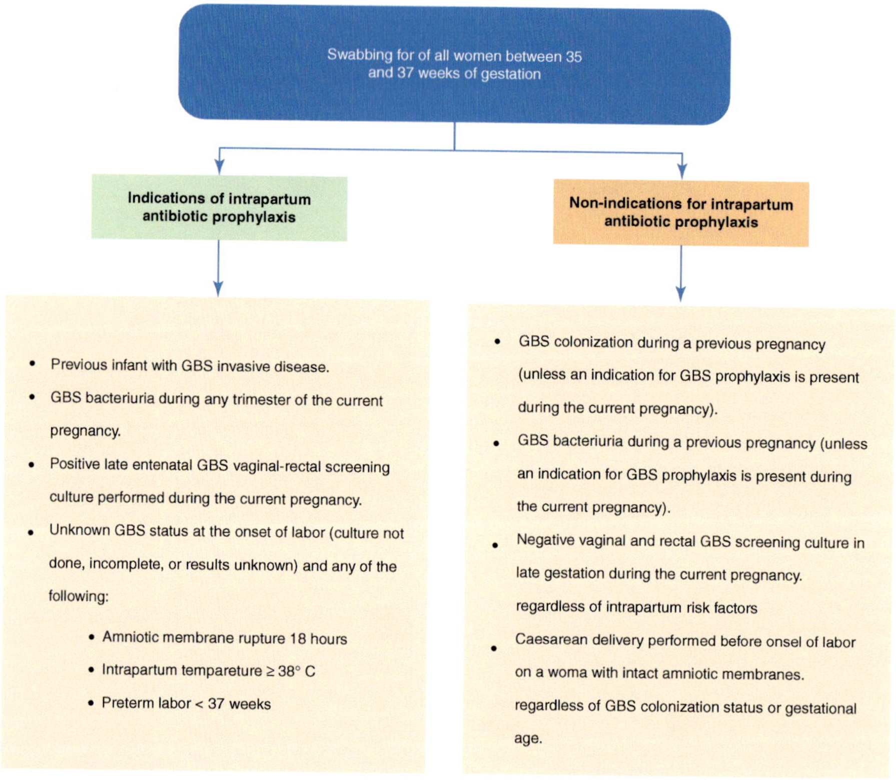

Fig. 46.2 Indications and non-indications for intrapartum antibiotic prophylaxis to prevent early-onset group B streptococcal disease. GBS, group B streptococcal. (Modified from CDC - *MMWR Recomm Rep*. 2010 [19])

Place the swab(s) into a nonnutritive transport medium. GBS isolates can remain viable in transport media for several days at room temperature; however, the recovery of isolates declines over 1–4 days, especially at elevated temperatures, which can lead to false-negative results. When feasible, specimens should be refrigerated before processing [16].

Considering rapid GBS test strategy, commercially available nucleic acid amplification test (NAAT) assay kit must be used with the following recommendations [16]:

1. Wipe away excessive amounts of secretion or discharge.
2. Remove both marked swabs from the transport container.
3. Carefully insert both marked swabs into the patient's vagina. Sample secretions from the mucosa of the lower one-third part of the vagina. Rotate the swabs three times to ensure uniform sample on both swabs.
4. Using the same marked swabs, carefully insert both swabs approximately 2.5 cm beyond the anal sphincter, and gently rotate to sample anal crypts.

5. Place both marked swabs in the transport container.
6. If the specimens will be processed within 24 hours, store at room temperature. If the specimens will be tested after 24 hours, refrigerate until testing is performed. Specimens stored at 2–8 °C are stable for up to 6 days.

Culture-Based Procedure

In the laboratory, the material is inoculated into Todd-Hewitt culture medium enriched with gentamicin (8 mcg/ml) and nalidixic acid (15 mcg/ml) to prevent growth of other microorganisms. After incubating, the material is kept for 18–24 hours at a temperature of 35–37 °C in room air or with 5% CO_2 and subcultured in blood agar medium for approximately 24 hours. Colonies that grew on blood agar medium are selected and analyzed using protein agglutination tests or identification of specific group B streptococcal antigens for isolation [16].

Antibiograms are required for appropriate antibiotic prophylaxis selection for penicillin-allergic women who are at high risk for anaphylaxis because resistance to clindamycin, the most common agent used in this population, is increasing among GBS isolates [16].

Intrapartum Prophylaxis

Figure 46.3 summarizes the prophylactic recommended schemes. Penicillin is the antibiotic of choice because it has a lower spectrum of action and thus presents a lower risk of resistance to other microorganisms [16].

It is very difficult to accurately assess the risk of anaphylaxis in patients who report being allergic to penicillin; the use of clindamycin is recommended due to a well-documented history. In cases where allergy to penicillin is not well documented, cefazolin is recommended [16].

Antibiotic prophylaxis specific for GBS is not required for women undergoing planned caesarean section in the absence of labor and with intact membranes. Although vaginal cleansing with chlorhexidine has been shown to reduce the risk of neonatal GBS colonization, there is no evidence to show that this has any impact on neonatal sepsis.

Secondary Prevention Among Infants

To detect potential sepsis cases in newborns as early as possible, newborns should be managed according to the algorithm provided in Fig. 46.4 [16, 18]. Any newborn with clinical signs of sepsis requires a full diagnostic evaluation and empirical

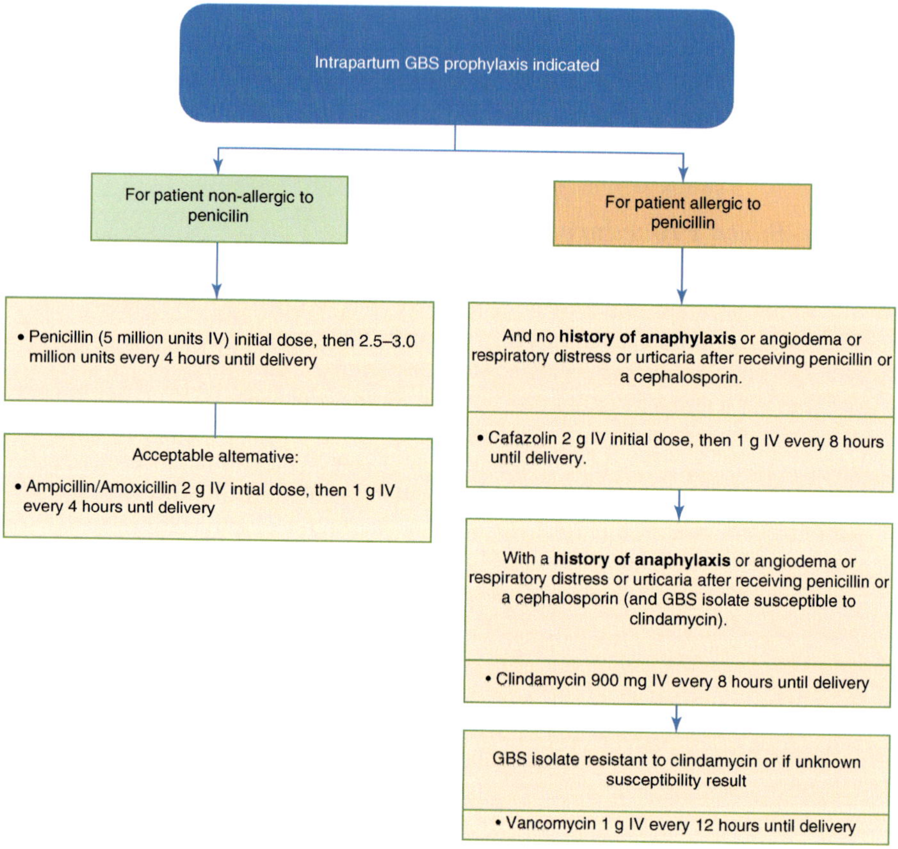

Fig. 46.3 Recommended regimens for intrapartum antibiotic prophylaxis for the prevention of early-onset GBS disease. (Adapted from revised guidelines from CDC 2010 [16])

antibiotic therapy started (within 30 minutes) regardless of adequacy of inadequate intrapartum antibiotic prophylaxis, other obstetrical risk factors, or maternal GBS status [18].

Postnatal antibiotic prophylaxis is not recommended for asymptomatic term infants without known antenatal risk factors.

Indications for Newborn Sepsis Investigation [18]

- Clinical signs of infection.
- Maternal chorioamnionitis is suspected (temperature greater than or equal to 38 °C intrapartum or within 24 hours of birth).
- The woman has had a previous baby with early-onset group B streptococcal disease.

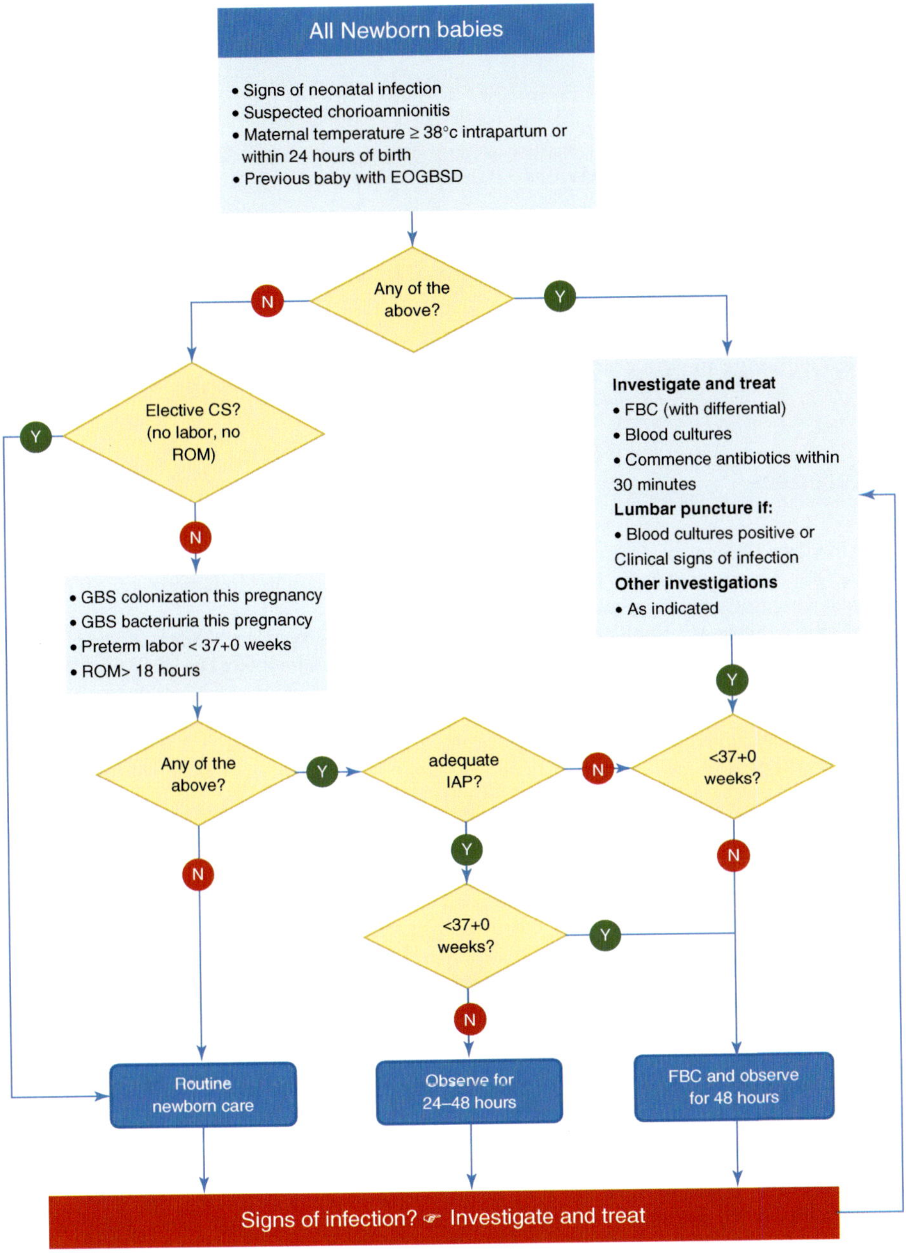

Fig. 46.4 Neonatal management of early-onset group B streptococcal disease. (Modified from Queensland Clinical Guidelines. Early onset Group B Streptococcal disease. Guideline No. MN16.20-V4-R21 [8]). (CS cesarean section, EOGBSD early-onset group B streptococcal disease, FBC full blood count, GBS group B streptococcus, IAP intrapartum antibiotic prophylaxis, IV intravenous, ROM rupture of membranes, > greater than, < less than)

- Gestational age is less than 37 + 0 weeks and there was inadequate intrapartum antibiotic prophylaxis.

Parents and carers should be informed to seek urgent medical advice if they are concerned that the baby [23]:

- Is showing abnormal behavior (e.g., inconsolable crying or listlessness).
- Is unusually floppy.
- Has developed difficulties with feeding or with tolerating feeds.
- Has an abnormal temperature unexplained by environmental factors (lower than 36 °C or higher than 38 °C).
- Has rapid breathing.
- Has a change in skin color.

References

1. American College of Obstetricians and Gynecologists Committee on Obstetric Practice. ACOG Committee Opinion No. 485: prevention of early-onset group B streptococcal disease in newborns. Obstet Gynecol. 2011;117(4):1019–27.
2. Madrid L, Seale AC, Kohli-Lynch M, et al. Infant group B streptococcal disease incidence and serotypes worldwide: systematic review and meta-analyses. Clin Infect Dis. 2017;65:S160–72.
3. Brown AP, Denison FC. Selective or universal screening for GBS in pregnancy (review). Early Hum Dev. 2018;126:18–22.
4. Kwatra G, Cunnington MC, Merrall E, Adrian PV, Ip M, Klugman KP, Tam WH, Madhi SA. Prevalence of maternal colonisation with group B streptococcus: a systematic review and meta-analysis. Lancet Infect Dis. 2016;16(9):1076–84.
5. Morgan JA, Zafar N, Cooper DB. Group B streptococcus and pregnancy. 2020 Aug 23. In: StatPearls [Internet]. Treasure Island (FL): StatPearls Publishing; 2020. PMID: 29494050.
6. Edmond KM, Kortsalioudaki C, Scott S, et al. Group B streptococcal disease in infants aged younger than 3 months: systematic review and meta-analysis. Lancet. 2012;379:547–56.
7. Schrag SJ, Zywicki S, Farley MM, et al. Group B streptococcal disease in the era of intrapartum antibiotic prophylaxis. N Engl J Med. 2000;342:15–20.
8. Puopolo KM, Madoff LC, Baker CJ. Group B streptococcal infection in pregnant women. UpToDate. Available at: https://www.uptodate.com/contents/group-b-streptococcal-infection-in-pregnant-women?search=streptococcus%20agalactiae&source=search_result&selectedTitle=2~150&usage_type=default&display_rank=2. Assessed in 15/11/2020.
9. Romero R, Oyarzun E, Mazor M, et al. Meta-analysis of the relationship between asymptomatic bacteriuria and preterm delivery/low birth weight. Obstet Gynecol. 1989;73:576.
10. Mittendorf R, Williams MA, Kass EH. Prevention of preterm delivery and low birth weight associated with asymptomatic bacteriuria. Clin Infect Dis. 1992;14:927.
11. Zaleznik DF, Rench MA, Hillier S, et al. Invasive disease due to group B Streptococcus in pregnant women and neonates from diverse population groups. Clin Infect Dis. 2000;30:276.
12. Hitti J, Tarczy-Hornoch P, Murphy J, et al. Amniotic fluid infection, cytokines, and adverse outcome among infants at 34 weeks' gestation or less. Obstet Gynecol. 2001;98:1080.
13. Isada NB, Grossman JH. Perinatal infections. In: Gabbe SG, Niebyl JR, Simpson JL, editors. Obstetrics: normal and problem pregnancies. New York: Churchill Livingstone; 1991. p. 1276.
14. Winn HN. Group B streptococcus infection in pregnancy. Clin Perinatol. 2007;34(3):387–92.
15. Colbourn T, Gilbert R. An overview of the natural history of early onset group B streptococcal disease in the UK. Early Hum Dev. 2007;83:149–56.

16. Centers for Diseases Control and Prevention. Prevention of perinatal Group B streptococcal disease; revised guidelines. MMWR. 2010;59 (No. RR-10). [Internet]. 2010 [cited 2015 September 14]. Available from: http://www.cdc.gov.
17. Berardi A, Rossi C, Guidotti I, Vellani G, Lugli L, Bacchi Reggiani ML, et al. Factors associated with intrapartum transmission of group B Streptococcus. Pediatr Infect Dis J. 2014;33(12):1211–5.
18. Queensland Clinical Guidelines. Early onset Group B streptococcal disease. Guideline No. MN16.20-V4-R21. Queensland Health. 2020. Available from: http://www.health.qld.gov.au/qcg.
19. Verani JR, McGee L, Schrag SJ, Division of Bacterial Diseases, National Center for Immunization and Respiratory Diseases, Centers for Disease Control and Prevention (CDC). Prevention of perinatal group B streptococcal disease – revised guidelines from CDC, 2010. MMWR Recomm Rep. 2010;59(RR-10):1–36. PMID: 21088663.
20. Di Renzo GC, Melin P, Berardi A, Blennow M, Carbonell-Estrany X, Donzelli GP, Hakansson S, Hod M, Hughes R, Kurtzer M, Poyart C, Shinwell E, Stray-Pedersen B, Wielgos M, El Helali N. Intrapartum GBS screening and antibiotic prophylaxis: a European consensus conference. J Matern Fetal Neonatal Med. 2015;28(7):766–82.
21. Schrag SJ, Zell ER, Lynfield R, Roome A, Arnold KE, Craig AS, Harrison LH, Reingold A, Stefonek K, Smith G, Gamble M, Schuchat A, Active Bacterial Core Surveillance Team. A population-based comparison of strategies to prevent early-onset group B streptococcal disease in neonates. N Engl J Med. 2002;347(4):233–9.
22. Khalil MR, Uldbjerg N, Thorsen PB, Møller JK. Intrapartum PCR assay versus antepartum culture for assessment of vaginal carriage of group B streptococci in a Danish cohort at birth. PLoS One. 2017;12(7):e0180262.
23. Prevention of early-onset neonatal group B streptococcal disease: green-top guideline no. 36. BJOG. 2017;124(12):e280–e305.

Chapter 47
Arboviruses and Pregnancy (Zika, Dengue, Chikungunya, and Yellow Fever)

Penélope Saldanha Marinho, Antonio José Cunha, Joffre Amim Junior, and Arnaldo Prata Barbosa

Introduction

The spread of arboviruses diseases in the human population occurs through the introduction of the pathogen into the environment, associated with other factors such as ecological changes and human behavior. As the mosquito vectors breed in standing water, events like heavy rain with flooding and construction of dams are associated with the emergence of infections by arboviruses. In addition, urbanization, migration, and international travel are also contributing factors to the transmission of these diseases [1, 2].

The pathogenesis of arboviruses still remains unknown in several respects, but it is recognized that, upon primary inoculation, viral particles infect target cells such as fibroblasts, monocyte, dendritic cells, and host endothelial cells. The viruses then replicate, reaching the regional lymph nodes and, subsequently, the bloodstream [3].

The Zika virus was initially isolated in 1947 from rhesus monkey blood during epidemiological studies on yellow fever in the Zika Forest, in Uganda [4]. This virus was first isolated in humans in 1954, in Nigeria [5], and, in 1969, it was identified outside the African continent, in Malaysia, in the *A. aegypti* mosquito [6]. Throughout the following years, until 2007, the Zika virus was known to cause sporadic infections in both Africa and Asia.

P. S. Marinho (✉) · J. A. Junior
Maternidade Escola da Universidade Federal do Rio de Janeiro, Rio de Janeiro, Brazil
e-mail: penelope@me.ufrj.br

A. J. Cunha
Faculdade de Medicina da Universidade Federal do Rio de Janeiro, Rio de Janeiro, Brazil

A. P. Barbosa
Instituto D'Or de Pesquisa e Ensino - IDOR, Rio de Janeiro, Brazil

© Springer Nature Switzerland AG 2022
R. A. Moreira de Sá, E. B. d. Fonseca (eds.), *Perinatology*,
https://doi.org/10.1007/978-3-030-83434-0_47

The first recognized major outbreak occurred on Yap Island, Micronesia, in 2007 [7], followed by a major outbreak from October 2013 to March 2014 in French Polynesia [8, 9].

In 2015, the Zika virus reached the Americas and was initially identified in Brazil, where a phylogenetic analysis indicated it was the Asian strain of the virus [10]. According to the Pan American Health Organization report of July 2017, cases of autochthonous transmission have been reported at least in 50 other countries or territories of the American continent, totaling more than 200,000 confirmed cases, with approximately 3300 cases of congenital syndrome associated with the Zika infection [11].

The Chikungunya virus was reported for the first time in Tanzania in 1952. After the first epidemic, the virus became endemic in Africa. It reached Asia in 1958 and was responsible for several outbreaks in subsequent years [12].

The virus remained restricted to the African and Asian continents until 2013, when it was introduced in the Latin Caribbean and established the first human cycle in the Americas [13]. Subsequently, cases of autochthonous transmission were reported in South and Central America and in Florida, USA [14].

In September 2014, the first autochthonous case was confirmed in Brazil, in the northern region. After 7 days, new cases were identified in the northeastern region, and, in just 1 month, the Ministry of Health of Brazil had already confirmed 682 cases of this virus infection [15].

Although numerous epidemics with dengue-like characteristics have been described for centuries, the dengue virus was first isolated in 1943 in Japan (DENV1) and in 1945 in Hawaii (DENV2) [16].

The spread of its vector, the *A. aegypti* mosquito, created an environment conducive to the virus transmission, which reached a pandemic status after World War II [17].

In the Americas, dengue was controlled through a campaign conducted by the Pan American Health Organization in 1947 to eliminate mosquitoes. However, in the 1970s, the region was re-infested, and, since then, the incidence of the disease has increased in the Americas, as well as in other regions [18].

Yellow fever originated in Africa and was brought to the Americas in the seventeenth century as a consequence of the slave trade and was responsible for the deaths of thousands of people in the eighteenth and nineteenth centuries. In 1900, transmission was confirmed through the *A. aegypti* mosquito, and, in the 1930s, two live attenuated virus vaccines were developed. The combination of extensive vaccination campaigns and vector control significantly reduced the number of cases of this disease [19].

Over the years, outbreaks in Africa and South and Central America continued to occur [20]. In December 2015, an urban yellow fever epidemic occurred in Angola and expanded to other locations, and in 2017, an outbreak of the disease affected the Brazilian states of Minas Gerais, Espírito Santo, São Paulo, and Rio de Janeiro [21].

Transmission

Arboviruses are thus designated since they are viruses essentially transmitted by arthropods, predominantly mosquitoes. A wide variety of mosquitoes, tick, midge, and sandy species are vectors of arboviruses, although only a few specific vectors are usually implicated for a particular arbovirus. At least 135 types of arboviruses are capable of causing human infection, with the vast majority being RNA viruses [22]. Usually arbovirus transmission involves three factors: a vertebrate reservoir, bloodsucking arthropods that act as biological vectors, and human hosts that can be infected as spillover events and who become a secondary reservoir in urban settings [23].

Considering Zika sexual transmission [24, 25], detected right after the beginning of the outbreak, this brings into question how generalizable these findings are to other arboviruses. More research about the possibility that sexual transmission could be of relevance for other arboviruses would be necessary, especially for other emerging arboviruses [26]. Sexual transmission of the dengue, chikungunya, or yellow fever viruses has not been described.

Arboviruses can also be transmitted by blood transfusion or transplantation of organs or tissues from infected and asymptomatic donors at the time of donation. In the case of yellow fever, transmission is also possible during the viremia period after donor vaccination [27–31].

The occurrence of arboviruses during pregnancy is of additional concern, due to the possibility of vertical transmission and fetal involvement. In addition to the Zika causing intrauterine neurological damage, other arboviruses agents can also promote fetal alterations [32]. Since 2015, there is substantial evidence linking Zika to microcephaly and other central nervous system abnormalities [33, 34]. Many authors demonstrated associations between dengue and chikungunya with neonatal outcomes such as meningoencephalitis, bullous infection, and other clinical manifestations, which reinforce the importance of considering vertical transmission as an important way to arbovirus infections [35–37]. Few studies on yellow fever are available, but perinatal transmission of the disease has been described [38].

Clinical Conditions

The clinical presentation of these arboviruses during pregnancy is supposed to be similar to the general population. However, there is a lack of studies specifically addressing pregnant women.

Zika

The incubation period of this disease is of 4–5 days. The most frequently reported symptoms are a rash, fever, arthritis or arthralgia, and conjunctivitis. Other symptoms include myalgia, headache, retro-orbital pain, edema, and vomiting. It is estimated that only 20% of the people infected with the Zika virus manifest symptoms [39].

In a cohort of pregnant women in Rio de Janeiro, where exanthema was used as the inclusion criterion, in addition to macular or maculopapular exanthema in 100% of the cases, the following symptoms were also observed: pruritus (90%), arthralgia (62%), conjunctivitis (58%), fatigue and malaise (52%), myalgia (41%), and a short mild fever in less than one-third of women with acute infection [40]. Another study, carried out during the outbreak in Micronesia in 2007, found a similar symptom frequency, differing only in the fever incidence, which occurred in 65% of the cases [20].

Chikungunya

Since its discovery, four different genotypes of the chikungunya virus have been identified: East-Central-South African (ECSA), West African, Asian, and Indian Ocean lineage (IOL). The incubation period is usually from 3 to 7 days (ranging from 1 to 12 days) and 80% of the cases are symptomatic [41].

Dengue

Pregnant women are considered a risk group and are more likely to progress to more severe forms of the illness and death [42, 43].

Four serotypes of the dengue virus exist: DENV-1, DENV-2, DENV-3, and DENV-4. Primary infection by one serotype confers immunity against reinfection by the homologous virus, but when infection by another serotype occurs, which is common in endemic areas, the risk of severe disease is increased due to a phenomenon known as antibody-dependent enhancement [44].

The incubation period varies from 4 to 10 days. About 50% of the infections are symptomatic and may present a broad clinical spectrum. The classification for dengue severity is divided into dengue without warning signs, dengue with warning signs, and severe dengue. For the symptomatic patients, three phases may occur:

- First phase – febrile, lasting from 2 to 7 days. The first manifestation is fever, usually high, associated with headaches, myalgia, arthralgia, and retro-orbital pain. The rash, predominantly maculopapular, is present in 50% of the cases. Nausea and vomiting may be present. Most patients present improvements in their general state, but 5% progress to the critical phase.

- Second phase – critical, beginning with the decrease of the fever, between the third and seventh day of the onset of the disease, accompanied by the appearance of one or more warning signs, including:
  - Abdominal pain or tenderness
  - Persistent vomiting
  - Clinical fluid accumulation (i.e., pleural effusion or ascites)
  - Mucosal bleeding
  - Lethargy or restlessness
  - Liver enlargement (≥2 cm)
  - Increases in hematocrit concurrent with rapid decrease in platelet count
- Third phase – recovery, lasting from 3 to 5 days, after which there is progressive clinical improvement of patients who have suffered the critical phase. Severe dengue is defined in the presence of one of the following criteria:
  - Severe plasma leakage, leading to shock or fluid accumulation with respiratory distress
  - Severe bleeding
  - Severe organ involvement (AST or ALT ≥1000, impaired consciousness, failure of heart and other organs)

The process that determines the infection progression to severe forms appears to be multifactorial, involving individual immunological status and virus-related factors.

Yellow Fever

Like other infectious diseases, yellow fever has a wide spectrum of severity, ranging from asymptomatic patients to fatal cases.

The incubation period of the disease ranges from 3 to 6 days. Most symptomatic patients present with fever, headache, chills, muscle aches, and nausea, usually lasting a week. About 10–25% develop hemorrhagic manifestations and hepatic and renal impairment, with mortality occurring in 20–50% of the symptomatic cases [45].

The disease manifests itself in three stages: infection, remission, and intoxication. In milder cases, patients recover without sequelae within a few days. In severe cases, patients develop a more severe form of the disease after the remission period, lasting from 24 to 48 h, called the intoxication period, and may present coagulopathy, hemorrhagic manifestations, jaundice, urinary albuminuria, and acute renal failure [19].

Diagnoses

Clinical Presentation

Due to the similarity between these arboviruses symptoms and the possibility of rapid evolution to severe forms, it is recommended that infection by the dengue virus be considered as the main differential diagnosis in patients who have been in endemic areas. Infections with the Zika and chikungunya virus should also be considered, since they present the same vector and many regions are endemic for different arboviruses. Table 47.1, released by the Fiocruz Agency, summarizes the characteristics and frequencies of symptoms in dengue, Zika, and chikungunya [46].

Laboratory Tests

Some endemic areas display multiple arboviruses which present the same symptoms, such as fever, rash, myalgia, and arthralgia. Therefore, laboratory evaluation of the dengue, Zika, and chikungunya viruses, as well as other TORCH group diseases (toxoplasmosis, rubella, cytomegalovirus, and herpes), is recommended to establish the diagnosis.

In the acute phase, which occurs within the first 7 days after the onset of the symptoms, virus RNA can be identified in the patient's serum, with RT-PCR as the test of

Table 47.1 Comparison of symptoms of symptomatic presentation between dengue, Zika, and chikungunya

Signs/symptoms	Dengue	Zika	Chikungunya
Fever	Above 38 °C (4–7 days)	No fever or subfebrile ≤38 °C (1–2 days)	Above 38 °C (2–3 days)
Rash	Appears from the fourth day 30–50% of the cases	Appears on the first or second day 90–100% of cases	Appears on the second or fifth day 50% of cases
Myalgia	+++/+++	++/+++	+/+++
Arthralgia	+/+++	++/+++	+++/+++
Arthralgia intensity	Slight	Moderate/intense	Moderate/intense
Joint swelling	Rare	Frequent but slight	Frequent but moderate
Conjunctivitis	Rare	50–90% of cases	30%
Headache	+++	++	++
Pruritus	Slight	Moderate/intense	Slight
Adenomegaly	Slight	Intense	Moderate
Blood dyscrasia	Moderate	Absent	Slight
Neurological impairment	Rare	More frequent than dengue and chikungunya	Rare (predominant in neonates)

choice for the diagnosis of dengue, Zika, and chikungunya. In the case of dengue infection, the NS1 antigen can also be detected in the acute phase by the ELISA test. However, this test is not widely available. A negative result, however, does not exclude the infection, and a serological test for IgM antibodies is necessary [46].

In the convalescence phase, the ELISA test for IgM antibodies, which are usually detectable between 2 and 12 weeks after infection, should be performed for dengue, Zika, and chikungunya. However, due to cross-reactions, a positive serology (IgM) for dengue or Zika only indicates a recent flavivirus infection, and it is not possible to distinguish the type of virus in question. In case of positive IgM antibodies, the plaque reduction neutralization test (PRNT), which characterizes and quantifies circulating levels of anti-dengue virus neutralizing antibody, is necessary to confirm the diagnosis. Patients who have received a yellow fever vaccine in the past may also present serology cross-reactivity [47, 48].

The Trioplex RT-PCR is a laboratory test designed to detect Zika, dengue, and chikungunya virus RNA, authorized by the FDA to be used under an Emergency Use Authorization (USA) [49].

The diagnosis of a yellow fever infection follows the same protocol with RT-PCR, and the detection of the NS1 antigen with high sensitivity and specificity is possible during the acute phase. The identification of yellow fever antibodies by IgM ELISA can also be performed. Serology assays, however, present limitations due to the possibility of cross-reactivity with other flaviviruses [20].

In addition to serum, RT-PCR can also be performed on urine and saliva samples. Musso et al. analyzed saliva samples from symptomatic patients during the French Polynesia epidemic from October 2013 to March 2014, and, although there was no increase in the virus detection window, the saliva sample increased the molecular detection rate of viral RNA [50].

Prevention

Vaccines

The dengue vaccine CYD-TDV has recently been licensed but still remains largely unused. It is a tetravalent live attenuated viral vaccine, licensed for the prevention of dengue illness caused by dengue virus serotypes 1, 2, 3, and 4 in individuals ranging from 9 to 45 years old or 9 to 60 years old, depending on the license, living in dengue endemic areas. The vaccination schedule consists of three 0.5 mL injections administered at 6-month intervals, with an average efficiency of approximately 60% [46].

There is no recommendation concerning CYD-TDV during pregnancy and breastfeeding, due to lack of sufficient data in this population. However, the limited data collected during the clinical trials on unintentional immunization in pregnancy have yielded no evidence of harm to the fetus or pregnant women. To date, no studies evaluating the effects of inadvertent use in pregnant women are available [51].

Yellow fever 17D vaccine is widely used for the prevention of yellow fever in travelers, for routine immunization in endemic areas and for emergency response during outbreaks. It is given in a volume of 0.5 ml by the subcutaneous route in a dose of no less than 1000 international units. Approximately 90% of vaccines seroconvert by 10 days and 99% seroconvert by 30 days postimmunization [46].

The yellow fever vaccine is not recommended during gestation or breastfeeding, since it is composed of a live attenuated virus, except in situations of a severe epidemic or unavoidable trip to high-risk locations [37]. However, studies analyzing yellow fever vaccination in pregnant women found no increased risk of adverse events in gestation and newborns, except in a study that presented insufficient statistical power [52, 53]. The risk of miscarriage, malformations, fetal death, and prematurity is similar to that of the general population [54]. It is noteworthy that many of these studies reported small series.

If vaccination is required during pregnancy, it is preferable to be administered during the first trimester, when the immune response appears to be more satisfactory. The vaccine may be administered during breastfeeding, which should be discontinued for 10 days during the post-vaccine viremia phase. Regarding breastfeeding, a case of vaccine-induced encephalitis in one infant was reported 8 days after the mother's primary vaccination [55].

At the time of publication of this article, no vaccines against Zika and chikungunya were available. Future vaccine programs should consider the serological cross-reaction between the Zika virus and dengue virus and the implications for disease pathogenesis [56].

Vector Control

The preventive strategy considered most efficient is vector control, through the use of repellents and long-sleeved clothes, placement of screens in houses, sleeping in rooms with air-conditioning, and avoiding the accumulation of standing water, which serves as a breeding ground for the mosquito vectors. The WHO recommends the use of repellents containing DEET, IR3535, aminopropionic, or icaridin [57].

Other Measures During Pregnancy

The CDC recommends sexual abstinence or condom use for men suspected of contracting a Zika virus infection over a period of 6 months. For those residing or returning from a region with active transmission of the virus but who do not show symptoms, such measures should be adopted for at least 8 weeks after the person's return [46].

Women who are interested in childbearing and pregnant women should not travel to areas with the risk of Zika. If travel is unavoidable, or with regard to pregnant couples living in Zika areas, condoms from start to finish every time sex is performed is recommended, during the entire pregnancy. Populations in endemic areas who have been exposed should conduct early and serial ultrasounds during pregnancy [58].

Management

There is no specific medication for infections caused by dengue, Zika, chikungunya, or yellow fever viruses. The treatment consists in rest, drinking fluids to prevent dehydration, and the use of analgesics, such as acetaminophen. In the presence of warning signs, the patients must be admitted to a hospital where they can receive intensive care. In 2009, the World Health Organization introduced a revised classification scheme consisting of the following categories: dengue without warning signs, dengue with warning signs, and severe dengue (Flowchart 47.1). Gestation, since it is considered a risk condition for dengue infection, should present a follow-up in the maternity hospital or health unit. Pregnant woman is always considered as Group B, despite it has no warning signs [59]. The use of aspirin or other nonsteroidal anti-inflammatory drugs must be avoided. The use of these medicines may aggravate the hemorrhagic condition in case of dengue virus infection [60].

Fetal and Neonatal Outcomes

Mechanisms associated with increased maternal severity in many of arbovirus infection fever are unknown, although the impact of uteroplacental hemorrhages might be involved, especially in low-resources countries where access to transfusion and surgery is limited. Fetal and neonatal complications may result from four complementary processes [23]:

(i) Acute fetal distress in the context of a severe maternal infection impairing maternal hemodynamics and therefore placental/fetal oxygenation
(ii) Placental arbovirus infection with subsequent reduction of the blood flow to the fetus without fetal infection
(iii) Fetal and neonatal infection in the context of virus crossing of the placental barrier
(iv) Neonatal infection in the context of labor-associated placental breaches (Table 47.2)

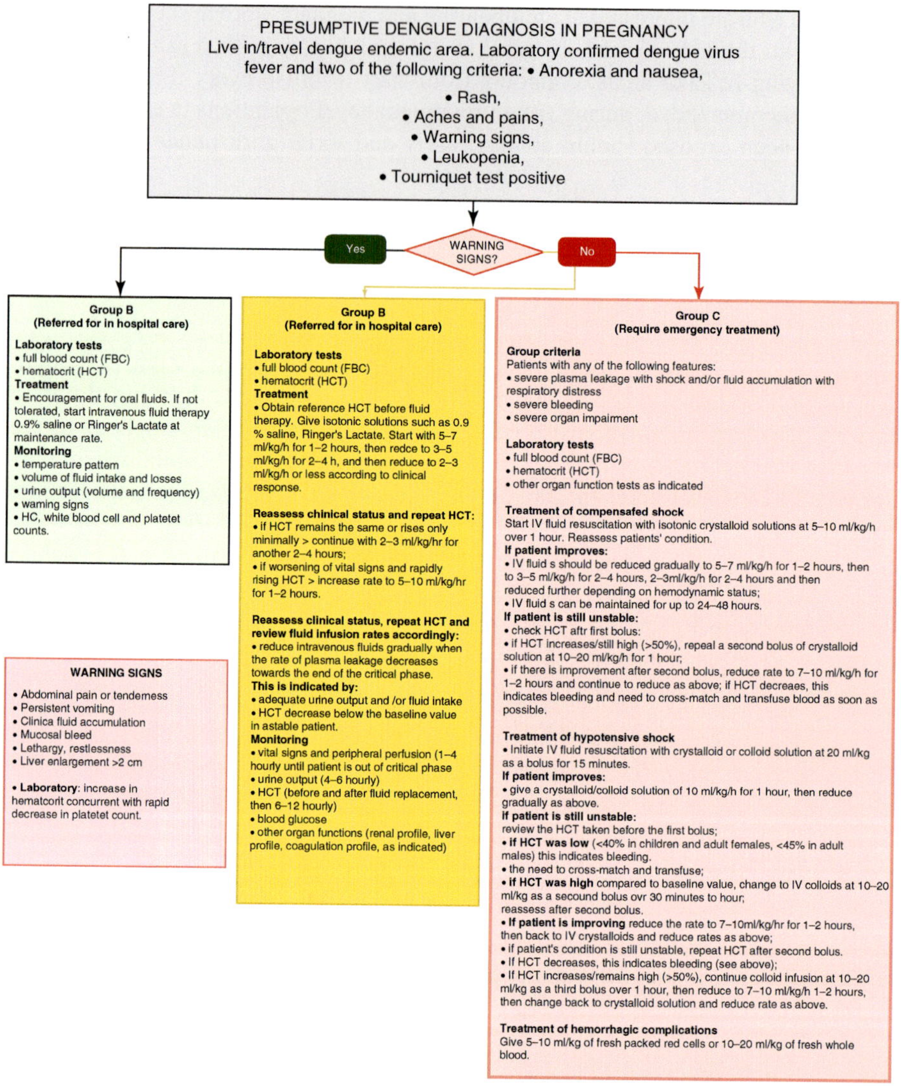

Flowchart 47.1 World Health Organization (2009) revised classification scheme

Zika

A cohort of pregnant women with suspected Zika virus infections was carried out in Rio de Janeiro, between September 2015 and May 2016. Among the 125 pregnant women with confirmed diagnoses, 46.4% presented adverse pregnancy outcomes. Acute infection occurred between 6 and 39 weeks of gestation, and complications were observed in 55% of cases when the infection occurred in the first trimester, 52% when infection occurred in the second trimester, and 29% when the pregnant

Table 47.2 Classification, maternal risk, and consequences of mother-to-child transmission

	Dengue	Zika	Chikungunya	Yellow fever
Main vectors	Mosquito (*Aedes* spp.)	Mosquito (*Aedes* spp.)	Mosquito (*Aedes* spp.)	Mosquito (*Aedes* spp. *or Haemagogus* spp.)
Geographical area	Tropical and subtropical areas worldwide	South Pacific area, Latin America, Caribbean, USA (Florida and Puerto Rico)	America(tropical areas), Africa, Asia, Australia, Indian Ocean	Sub-Saharan Africa, South America
Maternal risk	Severe maternal infection	No increased risk	No increased risk of severe maternal infection	No data
Placenta	Placental infection with or without fetal infection (hypoperfusion/ virus placenta crossing)	Placental infection with fetal infection (virus placenta crossing)	Breaches	Transmission through the placenta
Fetus	Fetal loss Developmental defects	Fetal loss Developmental defects	Transmission documented Low incidence	Transmission documented Extremely rare
Newborn	Prematurity Low birth weight Neonatal infection developmental defects	Neonatal infection developmental defects	Neonatal infection	Neonatal infection

women were infected in the last trimester. Abortion cases accounted for 25% of first trimester outcomes and 3% of second trimester outcomes, with 2 fetal deaths among 34 pregnant women with a positive third trimester examination [40].

Of the 117 neonates, 42% displayed abnormal findings in the first month of life, with almost all cases presenting central nervous system abnormalities. Microcephaly was diagnosed in 3.4% of cases and restriction of fetal growth in 9%. The neurological abnormalities, similar to other studies [61, 62], included cerebral calcification, cerebral atrophy, ventriculomegaly, hypoplasia of the cerebral structures, and hemorrhage of the cerebral parenchyma [60].

The neurological findings, observed even in late infections, result from central nervous system tropism of the virus, leading to the occurrence of fetal microcephaly and Guillain-Barré syndrome in adults [63, 64].

A previous case control study had already established the association of the Zika virus with the occurrence of fetal and neonatal neurological abnormalities. The analysis included 32 neonates with microcephaly, considered cases, and 62 neonates without microcephaly as controls, born in 8 public maternity units in the metropolitan northeastern region of Brazil. Eleven of 32 cases showed severe microcephaly, and significantly higher proportions of cases compared to controls were born with low birth weight and were small for their gestational age. Of the 27 cases investigated by brain imaging, 11 presented 1 or more abnormalities [65].

Another study analyzed the data extracted from the epidemiologic reports published by the Secretary of Health Surveillance of the Brazilian Ministry of Health that monitors cases of microcephaly associated with congenital infection in Brazil. Considering the confirmed cases of microcephaly and related deaths associated with Zika virus in Brazil, from November 2015 to October 2016, the estimated case fatality rate is 8.3% [66].

Chikungunya

Maternal-fetal transmission occurs mainly when there is maternal viremia at the time of delivery, with onset of neonatal symptoms 3–9 days after birth.

The main clinical manifestations in symptomatic newborns are fever, irritability, exanthema, lower or generalized lower limb edema, hyperalgesia, vesicular-bullous dermatosis, meningoencephalitis, and hemodynamic instability [67]. Some cases may progress with neonatal encephalopathy and microcephaly.

A 2-year follow-up of a cohort of children exposed to the virus during the perinatal period showed a delay in global neurodevelopment, with low developmental rates of those exposed compared to negative controls for infections [36].

Dengue

Two possible mechanisms may be responsible for fetal and neonatal morbidity due to dengue virus infection during pregnancy: the presence of maternal hemodynamic changes, which may compromise the placenta and cause fetal hypoxia, and the direct effect of infection on the fetus.

Paixão et al. conducted a systematic review and meta-analysis of adverse fetal outcomes resulting from dengue infection during gestation. Sixteen studies were included in the systematic review and 8 were eligible for the meta-analysis, totaling 292 women exposed to the dengue virus during gestation. The review indicated an association of dengue in pregnancy with abortion (OR 3.51), fetal death (RR 6.7), preterm birth (OR 1.71), and low birth weight (OR 1.41) [68]. Other studies have verified similar results, especially with regard to prematurity and low birth weight [69, 70].

Ribeiro et al. studied the fetal outcome of 24 pregnant women with laboratory-confirmed dengue infections and observed an increase in the incidence of abortions (20.8%), fetal death (8.3%) and prematurity (12.5%). After birth, 29% of the newborns presented symptoms of the disease [69].

The dengue virus is endemic in many localities, and the prevalence of infection during pregnancy, with consequent fetal impairment, may vary according to the local scenario and the cumulative period of exposure to the virus [43, 58]. The analysis of the prevalence and incidence of dengue during pregnancy in a great epidemic in the central region of Brazil indicated an incidence of 2.8%, diagnosed through the presence of maternal IgM, and a prevalence of 53.9% identified by maternal IgG. When umbilical cord blood was analyzed in IgG positive pregnant women, the transfer of maternal antibodies to the fetus was observed to be 99.3% [71].

Yellow Fever

Most studies regarding yellow fever analyzed fetal and neonatal effects after inadvertent vaccinations during pregnancy.

In 2009, a case of perinatal transmission of yellow fever was described during an epidemic in the state of São Paulo, Brazil. The 30-year-old woman presented with fever, headache, and jaundice 3 days before vaginal delivery. The female newborn was discharged after 2 days and on the third day was readmitted with fever and cyanosis, progressing with hemorrhage, liver enzyme alterations, oliguria and death with 12 days of life. The neonate underwent antibiotic therapy, and intensive support during hospitalization. Confirmation of newborn infection was obtained by RT-PCR harvested after 5 days of the onset of symptoms. The maternal infection was confirmed by positive IgM for yellow fever and negative IgM for dengue [38].

References

1. Morse SS. Factors in the emergence of infectious diseases. Emerg Infect Dis. 1999;1(1):7–15.
2. Scrag SJ, Wiener P. Emerging infectious disease: what are the relative roles of ecology and evolution? Trends Ecol Evol. 1995;10(8):319–24.
3. Abushouk AI, Negida A, Ahmed H. An updated review of zika vírus. J Clin Virol. 2016;84:53–8.
4. Dick GW, Cozinha SF, Haddow AJ. Zika virus. I: isolations and serological specificity. Trans R Soc Trop Med Hyg. 1952;46(5):509–20.
5. Macnamara FN. Zika virus: a report on three cases of human infection during an epidemic of jaundice in Nigeria. Trans R Soc Trop Med Hyg. 1954;48(2):139–45.
6. Marchette NJ, Garcia R, Rudnick A. Isolation of zika virus from aedes aegypti mosquitoes in Malaysia. Am J Trop Med Hyg. 1969;18(3):411–5.
7. Duffy MR, Chen TH, Hancock WT, Powers AM, Kool JL, Lanciotti RS, et al. Zika outbreak on Yap Island, Federated States of Micronesia. N Engl J Med. 2009;360:2536–43.
8. Cao-Lormeau VM, Roche C, Teissier A, Robin E, Anne-Laure B, Henri-Pierre M, et al. Zika virus, French Polynesia, South Pacific 2013. Emerg Infect Dis. 2014;20(6):1085–6.
9. Musso D, Nilles EJ, Cao-Lormeau VM. Rapid spread of emerging zika virus in the Pacific area. Clin Microbiol Infect. 2014;20:595–6.
10. Zanluca C, Melo VCA, Mosimann ALP, Santos GIV, Santos CND. First report of autochthonous transmission of Zika virus in Brazil. Mem Inst Oswaldo Cruz. 2015;110(4):569–72.

11. PAHO/WHO. Regional Zika epidemiological. http://www.paho.org/hq/index.php?option=com_content&view=article&id=12390&Itemid=42090&lang=en. 2017. Accessed 16 July 2017.
12. Sudeep AB, Parashar D. Chikungunya: an overview. J Biosci. 2008;33:443–9.
13. Leparc-Goffart I, Nougairede A, Cassadou S, Prat C, Lamballerie X. Chikungunya in the Americas. Lancet. 2014;383(9916):514.
14. Weaver SC, Forrester NL. Chikungunya: evolutionary history and recent epidemic spread. Antivir Res. 2015;120:32–9.
15. Nunes MRT, Faria NR, Vasconcelos JM, Golding N, Kraemer MUG, Oliveira LF, et al. Emergence and potential for spread of Chikungunya virus in Brazil. BMC Med. 2015;13:102.
16. Messina JP, Brady OJ, Scott TW, Zou C, Pigott DM, Duda KA, et al. Global spread of dengue virus types: mapping the 70 year history. Trends Microbiol. 2014;22:138–46.
17. Gubler DJ. Human behaviour and cultural context in disease control. Tropical Med Int Health. 1997;2(11):A1–2.
18. Gubler DJ. The global emergence/resurgence of arboviral diseases as public health problems. Arch Med Res. 2002;33(4):330–42.
19. Gardner CL, Ryman KD. Yellow fever: a reemerging threat. Clin Lab Med. 2010;30:237–60.
20. Monath TP, Vasconcelos PF. Yellow fever. J Clin Virol. 2015;64:160–73.
21. Paules CI, Fauci AS. Yellow fever – once again on the radar screen in the Americas. N Engl J Med. 2017;376(15):1397–9.
22. Dick GW, Kitchen SF, et al. Zika virus. I: isolations and serological specificity. Trans R Soc Trop Med Hyg. 1952;46(5):509–20.
23. Charlier C, Beaudoin MC, Couderc T, Lortholary O, Lecuit M. Arboviruses and pregnancy: maternal, fetal, and neonatal effects. Lancet Child Adolesc Health. 2017;1(2):134–46. https://doi.org/10.1016/S2352-4642(17)30021-4.
24. Kim CR, Counotte M, Bernstein K, Deal C, Mayaud P, Low N, et al. Investigating the sexual transmission of Zika virus. Lancet Glob Health. 2018;6:e24–5.
25. Kumar S. Sexual transmission of Zika virus: more to explore. Lancet Glob Health. 2018;6:e618.
26. Cardona-Ospina JA, Alvarado-Arnez LE, Escalera-Antezana JP, Bandeira AC, Musso D, Rodríguez-Morales AJ. Sexual transmission of arboviruses: more to explore? Int J Infect Dis. 2018;76:126–7.
27. Busch MP, Sabino EC, Brambilla D, Lopes ME, Capuani L, Chowdhury D, et al. Duration of dengue viremia in blood donos and relationships between donor viremia, infection incidence and clinical case reports during a large epidemic. J Infect Dis. 2016;214:49–54.
28. Sabino EC, Loureiro P, Lopes ME, Capuani L, McClure C, Chowdhury D, et al. Transfusion-transmitted dengue and associated clinical symptoms during. The 2012 epidemic in Brazil. J Infect Dis. 2016;231:694–702.
29. Motta IJ, Spencer BR, Silva CSG, Arruda MB, Dobbin JA, Gonzaga YB, et al. Evidence for transmission of Zika virus by platelet transfusion. N Engl J Med. 2016;375(11):1101–3.
30. Lanteri MC, Kleinman SH, Glynn SA, Musso D, Keith HW, Custer BS, et al. Zika virus: a new threat to the safety of the blood supply with worldwide impact and implications. Transfusion. 2016;56:1907–14.
31. Centers for Disease Control and Prevention (CDC). Transfusion-related transmission of yellow fever vaccine vírus – California, 2009. MMWR. 2010;59(2):34–7.
32. Carvalho FR, Medeiros T, Vianna RAO, et al. Simultaneous circulation of arboviruses and other congenital infections in pregnant women in Rio de Janeiro, Brazil. Acta Trop. 2019;192:49–54.
33. Mlakar J, Korva M, Tul N, Popović M, Poljšak-Prijatelj M, Mraz J, et al. Zika virus associated with microcephaly. N Engl J Med. 2016;374(10):951–8.
34. Araújo TVB, Rodrigues LC, Ximenes RAA, Miranda-Filho DB, Souza WV, Montarroyos UR, et al. Association between microcephaly, Zika virus in- fection, and other risk factors in Brazil: nal report of a case-control study. Lancet Infect Dis. 2018;18:328–36.
35. Contopoulos-Ioannidis D, Newman-Lindsay S, Chow C, LaBeaud AD. Mother- to-child transmission of Chikungunya virus: a systematic review and meta-analysis. PLoS Negl Trop Dis. 2018;12(6):e0006510.

36. Gérardin P, Sampériz S, Ramful D, Boumahni B, Bintner M, Alessandri JL, Carbonnier M, Tiran-Rajaoefera I, Beullier G, Boya I, Noormahomed T, Okoï J, Rollot O, Cotte L, Ja ar-Bandjee MC, Michault A, Favier F, Kaminski M, Fourmaintraux A, Fritel X. Neurocognitive outcome of children exposed to perinatal mother-to-child Chikungunya virus infection: the CHIMERE cohort study on Reunion Island. PLoS Negl Trop Dis. 2014;8(7):e2996.
37. Paixão ES, Teixeira MG, Costa MDCN, Barreto ML, Rodrigues LC. Symptomatic dengue during pregnancy and congenital neurologic malformations. Emerg Infect Dis. 2018;24(9):1748–50.
38. Bentlin MR, Almeida RA, Coelho KI, Ribeiro AF, Siciliano MM, Suzuki A, et al. Transmissão perinatal de febre amarela, Brasil, 2009. Infect Emerg Dis. 2011;17(9):1779–80. https://doi.org/10.3201/eid1709.110242.
39. Duffy MR, Chen TH, Hancokc WT, Powers AM, Kool JL, Lanciotti RS, et al. 60. Zika virus outbreak on Yap Island, Federated States of Micronesia. N Engl J Med. 2009;360:2536–43.
40. Brasil P, Pereira JP Jr, Moreira ME, Nogueira RMR, Damaceno L, Pharm LD, et al. Zika virus infection in pregnant women in Rio de Janeiro. N Engl J Med. 2016;375(24):2321–34. https://doi.org/10.1056/NEJMoa1602412.
41. Moro ML, Gagliotti C, Silvi G, Angelini R, Sambri V, Rezza G, et al. Chikungunya virus in north-eastern Italy: a seroprevalence survey. Am J Trop Med Hyg. 2010;82(3):508–11.
42. Adam I, Jumaa AM, Elbashir HM, Karsany MS. Maternal and perinatal outcomes of dengue in PortSudan, Eastern Sudan. Virol J. 2010;7:153.
43. Machado CR, Machado ES, Rohloff RD, Azevedo M, Campos DP, Oliveira RB, Brasil P. Is pregnancy associated with severe dengue? A review of data from. The Rio de Janeiro surveillance information system. PLoS Negl Trop Dis. 2013;7(5):e2217. https://doi.org/10.1371/journal.pntd.0002217.
44. Guzman MG, Alvarez M, Halstead SB. Secondary infection as a risk factor for dengue hemorrhagic fever/dengue shock syndrome: an historical perspective and role of antibody-dependent enhancement of infection. 67. Arch Virol. 2013;158(7):1445–59.
45. Wilder-Smith A, Gubler DJ, Weaver SC, Monath TP, Heymann DL, Scott TW. Epidemic arboviral disease: priorities for research and public health. Lancet Infect Dis. 2017;17:e101–6.
46. Marinho PS, Cunha AJ, Amim Junior J, Prata-Barbosa A. A review of selected Arboviruses during pregnancy. Matern Health Neonatol Perinatol. 2017;3:17. Published 2017 Oct 3. https://doi.org/10.1186/s40748-017-0054-0.
47. World Health Organization (WHO) and the Special Programme for Research and Training in Tropical Diseases (TDR). Dengue: guidelines for diagnosis, treatment, prevention and control. 9a ed. Genebra: WHO; 2009. http://apps.who.int/iris/bitstream/10665/44188/1/9789241547871_eng.pdf.
48. Centers for Disease Control and Prevention (CDC). Guidance for U.S. laboratories testing for zika virus infection. https://www.cdc.gov/zika/laboratories/lab-guidance.html.
49. Centers for Disease Control and Prevention (CDC). Dengue laboratory guidance and diagnostic testing. https://www.cdc.gov/dengue/clinicallab/laboratory.html.
50. Mussoa D, Rocheb C, Tu-Xuan N, Robina E, Teissierb A, Van-Mai CL. Detection of zika virus in saliva. J Clin Virol. 2015;68:53–5.
51. Scott LJ. Drugs. 2016;76:1301. https://doi.org/10.1007/s40265-016-0626-8.
52. Cavalcanti DP, Salomão MA, Lopez-Camelo J, Pessoto MA. Early exposure to yellow fever vaccine during pregnancy. Tropical Med Int Health. 2007;12(7):833–7.
53. D'Acremont V, Tremblay S, Genton B. Impact of vacines given during pregnancy on the offspring of women consulting a travel clinic: a longitudinal study. J Travel Med. 2008;15:77–81.
54. Suzano CE, Amaral E, Sato HK, Papaiordanou PM. The effects of yellow fever immunization (17DD) inadvertently used in early pregnancy during a mass campaign in Brazil. Vaccine. 2006;24:1421–6.
55. Imbert P, Moulin F, Mornand P, Mechai F, Rapp C. Should yellow fever vaccination be recommended during pregnancy or breastfeeding? Med Trop. 2010;70(4):321–4.
56. Dejnirattisai W, Supasa P, Wongwiwat W, Rouvinski A, Barba-Spaeth G, Duangchinda T. Dengue virus sero-cross-reactivity drives antibody-dependent enhancement of infection with zika virus. Nat Immunol. 2016;17:1102–8. https://doi.org/10.1038/ni.3515.

57. WHO. Zika virus fact sheet: World Health Organization; 2016. http://www.who.int/mediacentre/factsheets/zika/en/. Acessado em 08 de abril de 2017.
58. Oster AM, Brooks JT, Stryker JE, Kachur RE, Mead P, Pesik NT, Peterse LR. Interim guidelines for prevention of sexual transmission of Zikavirus_United States. MMWR Morb Mortal Wkly Rep. 2016;5(5):120–1.
59. World Health Organization. Dengue: guidelines for diagnosis, treatment, prevention and control. New ed. Geneva: WHO; 2009. http://www.who.int/tdr/publications/documents/dengue-diagnosis.pdf?ua=1. Accessed on July 2020.
60. Centers for Disease Control and Prevention. Symptoms and what to do if you think you have dengue. https://www.cdc.gov/dengue/symptoms/.
61. Oliveira-Szejnfeld PS, Levine D, Melo ASO, Amorim MMR, Batista AGM, Chimelli L, et al. Congenital brain abnormalities and Zika vírus: what the radiologista can expect to see prenatally and postnatally. Radiology. 2016;281(1):203–18.
62. Honein MA, Dawson AL, Petersen EE, Jones AM, Lee EH, Yazdy MM. Birth defects among fetuses and infants of US women with evidence of possible Zika virus infection during pregnancy. JAMA. 2017;317(1):59–68. https://doi.org/10.1001/jama.2016.19006.
63. Suwanmanee S, Luplertlop N. Dengue and Zika viruses: lessons learned from the similarities between these Aedes Mosquito-vectored arboviruses. J Microbiol. 2017;55(2):81–9. https://doi.org/10.1007/s12275-017-6494-4.
64. França GV, Schuler-Faccini L, Oliveira WK, Henriques CM, Carmo EH, Pedi VD, et al. Congenital zika virus syndrome in Brazil: a case series of the first 1501 livebirths with complete investigation. Lancet. 2016;388:891–7.
65. Araújo TVB, Rodrigues LC, Ximenes RAA, Miranda-Filho DB, Montarroyos UR, Melo APL, et al. Association between Zika virus infection and microcephaly in Brazil, January to May, 2016: preliminary report of a case–control study. Lancet Infect Dis. 2016;16:1356–63.
66. Cunha AJ, de Magalhães-Barbosa MC, Lima-Setta F, Medronho RA, Prata-Barbosa A. Microcephaly case fatality rate associated with Zika virus infection in Brazil: current estimates. Pediatr Infect Dis J. 2017;36(5):528–30.
67. Torres JR, Falleiros-Arlant LH, Dueñas L, Pleitez-Navarrete J, Salgado DM, Castillo JB. Congenital and perinatal complications of chikungunya fever: a Latin American experience. Int J Infect Dis. 2016;51:85–8. https://doi.org/10.1016/j.ijid.57.2016.09.009.
68. Paixão ES, Teixeira MG, Costa MC, Rodrigues LC. Dengue during pregnancy and adverse fetal outcomes: a systematic review and meta-analysis. Lancet Infect Dis. 2016;16:857–65.
69. Friedman EE, Dallah F, Harville EW, Myers L, Buekens P, Breart G, Carles G. Symptomatic dengue infection during pregnancy and infant outcomes: a retrospective cohort study. PLoS Negl Trop Dis. 2014;8(10):e3226.
70. Christiane FR, Lopes VGS, Brasil P, Pires ARC, Rohloffe R, Nogueira RMR. Dengue infection in pregnancy and its impact on the placenta. Int J Infect Dis. 2017;55:109–12.
71. Xiong X, Harville E, Paz-Soldão V, Tomashek KM, Breart L, Buekens P. Maternal dengue and pregnancy outcomes: a systematic review. Obstet Gynecol Surv. 2010;65(2):107–18.

Part VII
Childbirth and Postpartum

Chapter 48
Cervical Ripening and Labor Induction

Renato Augusto Moreira de Sá and Cristiane Alves de Oliveira

Introduction

Induction of labor refers to artificial stimulus for uterine contractions, prior to its spontaneous occurrence, in order to achieve vaginal delivery in medical or surgical means. Augmentation of labor refers to increasing the frequency and the intensity of already existing uterine contractions in a patient in true labor but progressing inadequately [1]. The goal of induction is to achieve a successful vaginal delivery that is as natural as possible [2].

Methods used for induction of labor include mechanical and pharmacologic options (see Fig. 48.1). Oxytocin use was published as a first time by Theobald et al. 1948 describing the use of the posterior pituitary extract – oxytocin – by intravenous drip for labor induction [3].

Over the past several decades, more and more pregnant women around the world have undergone induction of labor [4]. The frequency of induction varies by location and institution. The incidence of labor induction has continued to rise. In developed countries, the number of infants delivered at term following induction of labor can be as high as one in four deliveries. In the United States, around 22% of all gravid women undergo induction of labor [5].

R. A. Moreira de Sá (✉)
Fernandes Figueira Institut - FIOCRUZ, Rio de Janeiro, RJ, Brazil

C. A. de Oliveira
Federal Fluminense University and Rio de Janeiro Federal University, Niteroi and Rio de Janeiro, Brazil

© Springer Nature Switzerland AG 2022

R. A. Moreira de Sá, E. B. d. Fonseca (eds.), *Perinatology*,
https://doi.org/10.1007/978-3-030-83434-0_48

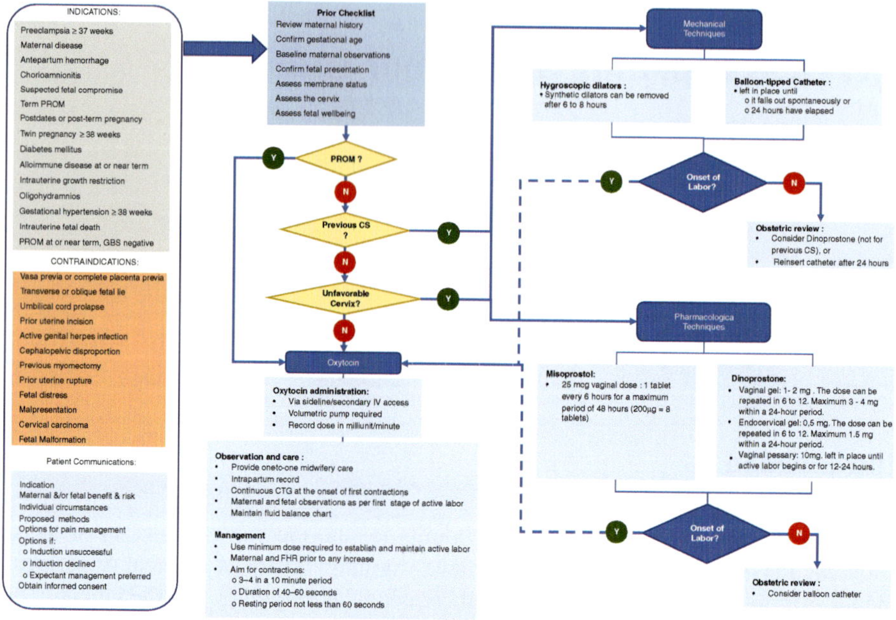

Fig. 48.1 Labor induction flowchart. PROM prelabor rupture of membranes, GBS group B *Streptococcus*, FHR fetal heart rate, CS cesarean section, Y = yes, N - no

Indications

The induction of labor should be performed only when there is a clear medical indication for it, related to maternal and fetal conditions in which the benefit of termination of pregnancy occurs. In other words, induction of labor is indicated when the expected benefits, for the mother or the fetus, exceed the risk associated with induced labor and delivery [2]. Common conditions where induction is often medically/obstetrically indicated include, but are not limited to, the following on Table 48.1.

The indication for induction must be documented, and discussion should include reason for induction, method of induction, and risks, including failure to achieve labor and possible increased risk of cesarean section.

Labor also may be induced for relative indications, for example, risk of rapid labor, distance from hospital, or psychosocial indications. In such circumstances, it is necessary to ensure that the gestational age is correct, preferably with first trimester ultrasound confirmation, supporting gestational age of 39 weeks or greater. A mature fetal lung test result before 39 weeks of gestation, in the absence of appropriate clinical circumstances, is not an indication for delivery [1]. Induction of labor may be associated with an increased risk of the following [2]:

- Failure to achieve labor
- Cesarean section

Table 48.1 Conditions where induction is often medically/obstetrically indicated

High priority
Preeclampsia ≥37 weeks
Significant maternal disease not responding to treatment
Significant but stable antepartum hemorrhage
Chorioamnionitis
Suspected fetal compromise
Term PROM with maternal GBS colonization
Other indications
Postdates (> 41 + 0 weeks) or post-term (> 42 + 0 weeks) pregnancy
Uncomplicated twin pregnancy ≥38 weeks
Diabetes mellitus (glucose control may dictate urgency)
Alloimmune disease at or near term
Intrauterine growth restriction
Oligohydramnios
Gestational hypertension ≥38 weeks
Intrauterine fetal death
PROM at or near term, GBS negative
Relative indications
Logistical problems (history of rapid labor, distance to hospital)
Intrauterine death in a prior pregnancy (induction may be performed to alleviate parental anxiety, but there is no known medical or outcome advantage for mother or baby)
ICP (at 36 + 0 to 36 + 6 weeks of gestation or upon diagnosis if ICP is diagnosed at ≥37 + 0 weeks of gestation)
Polyhydramnios
Fetal anomalies requiring specialized neonatal care

PROM pre-labor rupture of membranes, *GBS* group B *Streptococcus*, *ICP* intrahepatic cholestasis of pregnancy

- Operative vaginal delivery
- Tachysystole with or without fetal heart rate (FHR) changes
- Chorioamnionitis
- Cord prolapse
- Inadvertent delivery of preterm infant in the case of inadequate dating
- Uterine rupture in scarred and unscarred uteri

Contraindications for Labor Induction

Induction should be avoided if there are any contraindications to labor or vaginal delivery. In many conditions, the individual patient and clinical situation should be considered in determining when induction of labor is contraindicated. They include but are not limited to the following in Table 48.2 [6, 7]:

Table 48.2 Conditions where induction is often medically/obstetrically contraindicated

Absolute contraindications
Vasa previa or complete placenta previa
Transverse or oblique fetal lie
Umbilical cord prolapse
Prior classical uterine incision or transfundal uterine surgery or inverted T uterine incision
Active genital herpes infection
Absolute cephalopelvic disproportion, contracted pelvis
Previous myomectomy entering the endometrial cavity
Prior uterine rupture
Fetal distress (Category III fetal heart rate tracing)
Relative contraindications
Malpresentation (breech)
Cervical carcinoma
Fetal malformation (spina bifida, gastroschisis)

Assessment Prior to Labor Induction

Considering that the goal of labor induction is to achieve a successful vaginal delivery, consideration must be given to mother conditions, wishes, and preferences with due emphasis on cervical status, specific method of labor induction, and pregnancy associated conditions. The patient should be counseled regarding the indications for induction, the agents and methods of labor stimulation, and the possible need for repeat induction or cesarean delivery. Take an informed consent form from pregnant woman before labor induction and after explaining her risks and benefits of the procedure [1].

Assessment of gestational age and consideration of any potential risks to the mother or fetus are of paramount importance for appropriate evaluation and counseling before initiating cervical ripening or labor induction. Additional requirements for cervical ripening and induction of labor include assessment of the cervix, pelvis, fetal size, and presentation. An immediately prior checklist to labor induction is presented in Table 48.3 [8].

There are several clinical elements that need to be considered to estimate the success of induction. Factors that have been shown to influence success rates of induction include assessment of cervical mechanical conditions and non-modifiable factors [1, 2].

Cervical mechanical conditions are the physical characteristics (morphology, mechanical resistance) which condition the speed of cervix dilation for a given pattern of uterine contractility [9].

Assessment of cervical status is fundamental for the clinician to estimate the likelihood of a successful vaginal delivery and constitutes one of the essential elements to be analyzed by the clinician [1]. This element becomes secondary compared to the other factors which are the posture of the parturient, the position of the presentation, the weight of the fetus, and the dimensions of the pelvis [2].

Several scoring methods are available to determine the success of induction. The most common is Bishop scores. In 1964, Dr. Edward Bishop developed a scoring system to evaluate multiparous women for elective induction at term. The initial

Table 48.3 Prior checklist to labor induction

Review maternal history
Confirm gestational age
Perform baseline maternal observations (e.g., temperature pulse, respiratory rate, and blood pressure)
Perform abdominal palpation to confirm presentation, attitude, lie, position, and engagement
Assess membrane status (ruptured or intact)
Vaginal examination to assess the cervix
Assess fetal well-being: Fetal heart rate Fetal heart rate tracing (cardiotocography)
Assess for contraindications to labor induction
Consider urgency for labor induction

Table 48.4 Modified Bishop score

Modified Bishop score				
Value	0	1	2	3
Cervical dilatation (cm)	<1	1–2	3–4	>4
Cervical length (cm)	>3	2	1	<1
Station (ischial spines)	−3	−2	−1/0	+1/+2
Cervical consistency	Firm	Medium	Soft	–
Cervical position	Posterior	Mid	Anterior	–

scoring system used five determinants (dilatation, effacement, station, position, and consistency) that attributed a value of zero to two or three points each (for a maximum score of 13). Bishop showed that women with a score of >9 were equally likely to deliver vaginally whether induced or allowed to labor spontaneously [10]. In 1966, Burnett modified the scoring scheme (still in use and still known as the Bishop score) so that each variable was assigned a maximum value of two points (for a maximum score of 10). The higher the Bishop score, the more "ripe" or "favorable" the cervix is for labor induction. A favorable preinduction Bishop score of >6 is predictive of a successful vaginal delivery (Table 48.4). Initial studies were limited to parous women, but the score was later found also to be applicable to nulliparous women [1, 11].

Using the Bishop scoring system, most obstetricians consider a score ≥6 as favorable and a score ≤3 as unfavorable; scores of 4 or 5 are in a gray zone. The most important Bishop score criteria for predicting successful induction are cervical dilatation, effacement, station, and position, with the least important being consistency [12].

In 1967 Friedman developed a score who tries to weigh the relative share of each factor [13]. Indeed, the dilation, the length, and the position of the cervix are probably more dependent on the motor activity of the uterine body than the maturation of the cervical connective (Table 48.5) [9].

Lange et al. (1982) used linear regression to create a new score with the cervical components of dilation and station from the original Bishop score and length measured as centimeters as opposed to percentage, with dilation multiplied by two (Table 48.6) [14].

When the local conditions are unfavorable or intermediate (Bishop score < 5), the only perfusion of oxytocin is insufficient to mature by prostaglandins which will

Table 48.5 Friedman score

Friedman Score	Value				Weighting	
	0	1	2	3	Coefficient	Score
Cervical dilatation (cm)	0	1–2	3–4	5 or +	× 4	0–12
Effacement	0–30%	40–50%	60–70%	80% or +	× 2	0–6
Station (ischial spines)	−3	−2	−1/0	+1/+2	× 2	0–6
Cervical consistency	Firm	Medium	Soft		× 2	0–4
Cervical position	Posterior	Intermediate	Central		× 1	0–2
Total						0–30

Table 48.6 Lange score (score >5 is favorable)

Station (ischial spines)	−3	−2	−1/0	+1/+2
Points	0	1	2	3
Cervical dilatation (cm)	0	1–2	3–4	>4
Points	0	2	4	6
Cervical length (cm)	3	2	1	0
Points	0	1	2	3

improve the local conditions by their direct action on the cervix and sometimes even induce labor by their oxytocic effect [9].

Bishop score was compared with ultrasound assessment of the cervix to predict successful labor induction with conflicting results [1]. None of these tests have been found to be superior to Bishop score. Other methods have been proposed but they have not yet entered daily practice: measurement of cervical compliance, measurement of cervical consistency, or distensibility [9].

Non-modifiable factors in the preinduction period have been shown to increase the cesarean section rate when labor is induced. These are elevated BMI (>40 kg/m^2), maternal age >35 years, estimated fetal weight >4 kg, and diabetes mellitus [15–17]. The presence of these negative predictive factors for a successful induction may play a role in the mutual decision to delay intervention and to allow for the opportunity of a spontaneous labor. These factors should not be used as a deterrent to vaginal delivery. In studies of women with a favorable cervix, the cesarean section rate of induced pregnancies was equivalent to those managed expectantly [1, 18].

Options for Unfavorable Cervix

If the cervical status is unfavorable, effective mechanical and pharmacologic options for cervical ripening can be applied prior to induction to shorten the duration of induction and to increase the success of a vaginal delivery. There is no single clear best practice with respect to the choice of agent used for cervical ripening. Many clinicians consider a Bishop score <6 (Table 48.4) indicative of an unfavorable cervix and the need for a ripening agent, while others use a lower threshold (e.g., ≤3 or 4). Neither amniotomy nor oxytocin are effective cervical ripening agents and should not be used as such [2].

Mechanical Techniques

Mechanical methods, mainly effective in causing cervical dilatation, have been used for many years to induce labor. The more common mechanical methods include balloon-tipped catheters and hygroscopic dilators (laminaria).

Contraindications [19]

Mechanical methods have no absolute contraindications to cervical ripening in women who are candidates for labor and vaginal delivery.

Relative contraindication:

- A low-lying placenta (the edge of the placenta may be disrupted by manipulation during placement of the device) [19]
- Ruptured membranes (there is not total consensus on optimal management in this setting) [19]
- Intraamniotic infection (patients with intact membranes who are undergoing cervical ripening for labor induction; the use of a balloon catheter is not absolutely contraindicated) [19]

Balloon-tipped catheter Balloon catheter is the preferred method for induction of labor in women with prior cesarean section (see Fig. 48.1) [20]. For a single balloon catheter, a no. 18 Foley is introduced under sterile technique into the intracervical canal past the internal os. The bulb is then inflated with 30–60 mL of water. The catheter is left in place until either it falls out spontaneously or 24 hours have elapsed. Some practitioners apply a small degree of traction on the catheter by taping it to the inside of the leg [2].

The double-balloon catheter comprised of two silicone balloons. It was engineered to allow the cervix to naturally and gradually dilate prior to the induction of labor. The first of two balloons is inflated on the uterine side of the cervix; the second is then inflated in the vaginal side of the cervix. The two balloons adapt to the contour of the cervical canal minimizing discomfort for the patient. When the catheter is removed, cervical conditions should have improved to a favorable state to allow for induction of labor and active labor management [20].

Hygroscopic dilators Hygroscopic dilators are more commonly used at early stages for pregnancy termination than for labor induction at term, and it has been reported to be safe and effective [21, 22]. Two mechanisms of action are described: first, hygroscopic dilators gradually expanding within the cervical canal absorbing moisture and second prostaglandin release after disruption of the interface between the fetal membranes and decidua [19].

The cervix and vagina must be prepared with an antiseptic, and then the cervix is held with a nontraumatic clamp, if necessary, and as many dilators as possible are inserted into the endocervical canal without using excessive force. The dilators can be packed in place with two 4 by 4 inch gauze sponges tucked into the fornices. Synthetic dilators can be removed after 6–8 hours, while laminaria are removed 12–24 hours after placement [19]. Dipping the laminaria in a sterile lubricant before insertion may facilitate placement.

Pharmacological Method

Prostaglandins promote cervical ripening and stimulate uterine contractions. They are indicated for unfavorable cervix and may be used following balloon catheter when there has been no/minimal effect on cervical ripening (see Fig. 48.1) [19].

The optimal type, route, frequency, and dose of prostaglandins for cervical ripening have not been determined despite many studies of their use [19].

Contraindications [19, 23]

Absolute contraindications:

- Known hypersensitivity to prostaglandins
- Term pregnancies with a prior cesarean birth or other prior major uterine surgery
- Malpresentation/high presenting part
- Unexplained vaginal bleeding during current pregnancy
- Abnormal CTG/ fetal distress

Relative contraindication:

- Preexisting regular uterine activity (addition of an exogenous uterotonic agent could prompt excessive uterine activity)
- Multiple pregnancy
- Asthma, chronic obstructive pulmonary disease (may cause bronchospasm)
- Epilepsy
- Cardiovascular disease
- Raised intraocular pressure (glaucoma)

1. *Prostaglandin E1 (misoprostol)*. Misoprostol is a prostaglandin E1 analog which can provide 25 or 50 mcg doses. It is rapidly absorbed from both the oral and vaginal routes. Misoprostol seems to have the best efficacy/safety ratio at a dose of 25 mcg every 06 hours per vaginal route (one tablet every 06 hours for a maxi-

mum period of 48 hours 200 mcg = 8 tablets) [24]. When administered orally, the concentration peaks sooner and declines more rapidly than with vaginal administration. Other approaches to use of misoprostol, including buccal and sublingual administration, have been described but are less well studied and should be considered investigational [19].

2. *Prostaglandin E2 (dinoprostone).* Dinoprostone is a prostaglandin E2 and is the most commonly used prostaglandin agent in third trimester for cervical ripening [19]. Dinoprostone preparations include:
   (a) Vaginal gel, 1 mg and 2 mg of dinoprostone gel for vaginal administration. The dose can be repeated in 6–12 hours if cervical change is inadequate and uterine activity is minimal following the first dose. The maximum cumulative dose of dinoprostone does not exceed 3–4 mg within a 24-hour period [25].
   (b) Endocervical gel, 0.5 mg of dinoprostone gel for endocervical administration. The dose can be repeated in 6–12 hours if cervical change is inadequate and uterine activity is minimal following the first dose. The maximum cumulative dose of dinoprostone does not exceed 1.5 mg within a 24-hour period [19].
   (c) Controlled release vaginal pessary containing 10 mg of dinoprostone in a timed-release formulation (the medication is released at 0.3 mg/hour). The insert is left in place until active labor begins or for 12–24 hours [26].

Options for Favorable Cervix

The likelihood that induction will result in vaginal delivery depends on both cervical and noncervical factors. Despite Bishop score limitations, it is the cervical assessment system most commonly used in clinical practice Higher Bishop scores are associated with a higher chance of vaginal delivery, while lower Bishop scores have been associated with a higher chance of cesarean delivery, but there is no universally accepted threshold for a favorable or unfavorable score. It is usually considered a score ≥6 as favorable cervix and if it is unfavorable, cervical ripening is recommended [1, 2].

Amniotomy

Artificial rupture of the membranes may be a simple and effective component of labor induction when the membranes are accessible and the cervix is favorable but the onset of labor is unpredictable and often requires oxytocin [27]. There is insufficient evidence on the efficacy and safety of amniotomy alone for labor induction [28].

Contraindications include placenta previa, vasa previa, and active genital infection except for women colonized with group B *Streptococcus* (GBS), but there are insufficient data to guide the timing of amniotomy in patients who are receiving intrapartum prophylaxis for GBS [1].

Cord prolapse is a risk of amniotomy, especially in case of floating fetal vertex or unstable lie presentation. After the membranes are ruptured, the care provider should continue to palpate the presenting part until it rests against the cervix to ensure there has been no cord prolapse. The amount, color, and consistency of the fluid as well as fetal well-being should be assessed [2].

Oxytocin

Oxytocin is a polypeptide neurohormone originating from the hypothalamus and secreted from the posterior lobe of the pituitary gland. Synthetic oxytocin administration is the most common and proven method of labor induction [6].

Gestational age is a major factor affecting the dose response to oxytocin with the uterus responding to oxytocin at approximately 20 weeks' gestation. The uterus is increasingly responsive to oxytocin as pregnancy progresses (remains quite the same from 34 weeks to term) [6]. The mechanism of action is primarily due to an increase in myometrial oxytocin binding sites, and it has no direct effect on the cervix [2]. When the cervix is unfavorable, it will require previously cervix preparation for cervical ripening. Oxytocin is better in augmenting labor than in inducing labor [4].

Oxytocin can be used in women with a previous cesarean section, but caution, care, and diligence should be used as it has been shown to increase the risk of uterine rupture [2].

Administration

Before prescribing oxytocin, it is necessary to consider the risks and benefits of its use, as well as the contraindications of labor induction. A thorough evaluation of maternal and fetal status is important before undertaking oxytocin administration [2].

- Review the patient's pregnancy and medical history for risk factors for problems that may develop during labor and delivery (previous uterine surgery, fetal macrosomia, shoulder dystocia, or postpartum hemorrhage)
- Perform a cervical examination to decide whether a cervical ripening agent is indicated.
- Determine fetal number and presentation.
- Estimate fetal weight, given risks associated with being small or large for gestational age.

- Review the fetal status and well-being.

Timing of oxytocin administration is only an issue in patients who have received prostaglandins for cervical ripening. In such patients, oxytocin can be initiated, if indicated [7]:

- Six to 12 hours after the final dose of dinoprostone gel
- Thirty minutes after removal of dinoprostone vaginal pessary
- Four hours after the final misoprostol dose

Oxytocin is mainly given by venous infusion (VI). It has a half-life of 5–12 minutes, a time to steady plasma concentration of 30–40 minutes, and a steady-state uterine response of 30 minutes or longer. It is prepared by diluting ten units in 1000 mL of an isotonic solution [2].

Standardized dosing regimen:

- Infusion rate of 2 mU/min or 12 mL/hour.
- Incremental dose of 2 mU/min or 12 mL/hour every 30–45 minutes until contraction frequency is adequate.
- Maximum dose is 16 mU/min or 96 mL/hour.
- Use a volumetric pump to ensure an accurate rate of infusion103.
  - Program delivery pumps for correct infusion concentrations.
  - Administer oxytocin by sideline/secondary VI access (as oxytocin infusion initiated at low volume).
- Record the dose in milliunit per minute.
- Aim for three to four contractions in a 10-minute period with duration of 40–60 seconds and resting period not less than 60 seconds.
- Use the minimum dose required to establish and maintain active labor.
- Register changes to dose clearly and contemporaneously on the intrapartum record and/or electronic monitorization paper.

A high-dose regimen of oxytocin administration may be consider in practical clinic with a starting dose of 6 mU/min and an incremental dose of 3–6 mU/min every 15–40 minutes [2].

Which regimen of oxytocin is superior is debatable; however, both regimens are acceptable for the induction of labor. The high-dose protocol was not only associated with significant shorter induction to delivery time but is also associated with a higher incidence of uterine hyperstimulation and need for oxytocin discontinuation [7].

Side effects [8]:

- Tachysystole or hypertonus with/without signs of FHR abnormalities
- Nausea and vomiting
- Arrhythmias
- Anaphylactoid reaction
- Severe (tetanic) uterine contraction leading to uterine rupture
- Flushing
- Electrocardiograph (ECG) changes (including prolonged QT interval)

- Transient hypotension
- Reflex tachycardia (common with rapid VI)
- Hyponatremia
- Hypotension

Other Drugs and Techniques

There is limited data regarding safety and/or efficacy of glucocorticoids, castor oil, hyaluronidase, isosorbide mononitrate, evening primrose oil, herbal preparations, breast stimulation, or sexual intercourse for labor induction or cervical ripening. None of these can be recommended as an evidence-based approach to labor induction [7, 19].

Complications Associated with Induction of Labor

Uterine Overactivity

This is the most frequently encountered complication of oxytocin or prostaglandin administration. Recent recommendations called for obstetricians to abandon the terms of hyperstimulation and hypercontractility in favor of the more rigidly defined term – tachysystole. Tachysystole is defined as an excessive uterine activity, more than five uterine contractions per 10 minutes in at least two consecutive intervals. Hypertonus is described as a single contraction lasting longer than 2 minutes. Hyperstimulation, although the recommendation above to be abandoned, is described as tachysystole or hypertonus associated with fetal heart rate abnormalities [1, 7].

One of the advantages of oxytocin administration is that if uterine hyperstimulation is noticed, the infusion can quickly be stopped. This usually results in the resolution of such uterine overactivity. In addition, placing the woman in the lateral position and administering oxygen and IV fluids may be of benefit. If FHR tracing abnormalities persist and uterine hyperstimulation is ongoing, the use of a tocolytic such as terbutaline may be considered [7].

Failed Induction

There has not been strong consensus as to the standard for defining a failed induction. Cervical ripening itself can take some time, and the establishment of an active labor is important to label labor as failed induction [2, 7].

The term failed inductions would not be used in the latent phase until oxytocin has been administered for at least 12 hours after membrane rupture. About 40% of the women who remained in the latent phase after 12 hours of oxytocin and membrane rupture were delivered vaginally [29].

Failed induction is not necessarily an indication for cesarean section. Other options include a further attempt to induce labor (the timing should depend on the clinical situation and the patient's wishes) or waiting for spontaneous labor [7].

Uterine Rupture

Uterine rupture is a serious emergency in obstetrics. It is a life-threatening situation for both mother and fetus. Uterine rupture is possible during induced labor in the absence of a scarred uterus and is usually associated with injudicious use of uterotonic agents in the presence of obstructed labor [30].

The incidence of uterine rupture is about 1%. The major morbidities include hemorrhage, disseminated intravascular coagulation, renal failure, prolonged anesthesia, postpartum wound infections, sepsis, anemia, vesicovaginal fistula, bladder rupture, and maternal death [31].

Most of the uterine rupture was repairable, and the most common site was transverse at the site of previous cesarean section scar. Surgical decision in case of uterine rupture is influenced by factors such as the patient's age, parity, her desire for more children, and the intraoperative assessment of the rupture [7].

References

1. ACOG Committee on Practice Bulletins -- Obstetrics. ACOG practice bulletin no. 107: induction of labor. Obstet Gynecol. 2009;114:386. Reaffirmed 2019.
2. SOGC CLINICAL PRACTICE GUIDELINE. Induction of labour. J Obstet Gynaecol Can. 2013;35(9):840–57.
3. Theobald GW, Graham A, Campbell J, Gange PD, Driscoll WJ. Use of post-pituitary extract in obstetrics. Br Med J. 1948;2:123–7.
4. WHO recommendations for induction of labour. World Health Organization: Geneva; 2011.
5. Martin JA, Hamilton BE, Sutton PD, Ventura SJ, Menacker F, Kirmeyer S, et al. Births: final data for 2006. Natl Vital Stat Rep. 2009;57:1–102.
6. Goel K, Gedam JK, Rajput DA, Bhalerao MV. Induction of labor: a review. Indian J Clin Pract. 2014;24(11).
7. Grobman W. Induction of labor with oxytocin. UpToDate. https://www.uptodate.com/contents/induction-of-labor-withoxytocin/print?search=labour%20induction&source=search_result&selectedTitle=1~140&usage_type=default&display_rank=1. Assessed in 12 June 2020.
8. Queensland Clinical Guidelines Steering Committee. Queensland clinical guideline: induction of labour. https://www.health.qld.gov.au/__data/assets/pdf_file/0020/641423/g-iol.pdf. Assessed in 13 June 2020.

9. Magnin G. Le déclenchement artificial du travail. In: Lansac J, Descamps P, Goffinet P, editors. Pratique de L'accouchement. 6th ed. Issy-les-Moulineaux: Elsevier-Masson; 2016.
10. Bishop EH. Pelvic scoring for elective induction. Obstet Gynecol. 1964;24:266–8.
11. Burnett JE Jr. Preinduction scoring: an objective approach to induction of labor. Obstet Gynecol. 1966;28:479–83.
12. Crane JM. Factors predicting labor induction success: a critical analysis. Clin Obstet Gynecol. 2006;49:573–84.
13. Friedman EA, Niswander KR, Bayonet-Rivera NP, Sachtleben MR. Prelabor status evaluation. II. Weighted score. Obstet Gynecol. 1967;29:539–44.
14. Lange AP, Secher NJ, Westergaard JG, Skovgard I. Prelabor evaluation of inducibility. Obstet Gynecol. 1982;60:137–47.
15. Ennen CS, Bofill JA, Magann EF, Bass JD, Chauhan SP, Morrison JC. Risk factors for cesarean delivery in preterm, term, and post-term patients undergoing induction of labour with an unfavourable cervix. Gynecol Obstet Investig. 2009;67:113–7.
16. Ehrenthal DB, Jiang X, Strobino DM. Labour induction and the risk of cesarean delivery among nulliparous women at term. Obstet Gynecol. 2010;116:35–42.
17. Coonrod DV, Drachman D, Hobson P, Manriquez M. Nulliparous term singleton vertex cesarean delivery rates: institutional and individual predictors. Am J Obstet Gynecol. 2008;198:694.e1–694.e11.
18. Guinn DA, Davies JK, Jones RO, Sullivan L, Wolf D. Labor induction in women with an unfavorable Bishop score: randomize controlled trial of intrauterine Foley catheter with concurrent oxytocin infusion versus Foley catheter with extra-amniotic saline infusion with concur- rent oxytocin infusion. Am J Obstet Gynecol. 2004;191:225–9.
19. Grobman W. Techniques for ripening the unfavorable cervix prior to induction. UpToDate. https://www.uptodate.com/contents/techniques-for-ripening-the-unfavorable-cervix-prior-to-induction?search=hygroscopic&source=search_result&selectedTitle=1~7&usage_type=default&display_rank=1. Assessed in 12 June 2020.
20. Boisena AB, Løkkegaardb EC, Fuglsanga J. Double-balloon catheter for induction of labor in 362 women with and without prior cesarean. Euro J Obstet Gynecol Reprod Biol. 2019;X 4:100033. https://reader.elsevier.com/reader/sd/pii/S2590161319300687?token=FB79352C2061918A5E01880442A316872C5DB23FE062F9D37319F39E1744E4203375DF87437BCE79E91AA2268DE28A6A. Assessed in 13 June 2020.
21. Gilson GJ, Russell DJ, Izquierdo LA, et al. A prospective randomized evaluation of a hygroscopic cervical dilator, Dilapan, in the preinduction ripening of patients undergoing induction of labor. Am J Obstet Gynecol. 1996;175:145.
22. Saad AF, Villarreal J, Eid J, et al. A randomized controlled trial of Dilapan-S vs Foley balloon for preinduction cervical ripening (DILAFOL trial). Am J Obstet Gynecol. 2019;220:275.e1.
23. Thomas J, Fairclough A, Kavanagh J, Kelly AJ. Vaginal prostaglandin (PGE2 and PGF2a) for induction of labour at term. Cochrane Database Syst Rev. 2014;2014(6):CD003101. Published 2014 Jun 19. https://doi.org/10.1002/14651858.CD003101.pub3.
24. Hofmeyr GJ, Gülmezoglu AM, Pileggi C. Vaginal misoprostol for cervical ripening and induction of labour. Cochrane Database Syst Rev. 2010;2010(10):CD000941.
25. Smith CV, Rayburn WF, Miller AM. Intravaginal prostaglandin E2 for cervical ripening and initiation of labor. Comparison of a multidose gel and single, controlled-release pessary. J Reprod Med. 1994;39:381.
26. Witter FR, Rocco LE, Johnson TR. A randomized trial of prostaglandin E2 in a controlled-release vaginal pessary for cervical ripening at term. Am J Obstet Gynecol. 1992;166:830.
27. Moldin PG, Sundell G. Induction of labour: a randomised clinical trial of amniotomy versus amniotomy with oxy- tocin infusion. Br J Obstet Gynaecol. 1996;103:306–12.
28. Bricker L, Luckas M. Amniotomy alone for induction of labour. Cochrane Database Syst Rev. 2000;(4):CD002862. https://doi.org/10.1002/14651858.

29. Rouse DJ, Weiner SJ, Bloom SL, Varner MW, Spong CY, Ramin SM, et al. Eunice Kennedy Shriver National Institute of Child Health and Human Development (NICHD) Maternal-Fetal Medicine Units Network (MFMU). Failed labor induction: toward an objective diagnosis. Obstet Gynecol. 2011;117(2 Pt 1):267–72.
30. Smith JG, Mertz HL, Merril DC. Identifying risk factors for uterine rupture. Clin Peinatol. 2008;35(1):85–90.
31. Jain R. Rupture of pregnant uterus: incidence, risk factors, maternal and fetal outcome. Int J Med Res Rev. 2016;4(6):1035–41.

Chapter 49
Analgesia and Anesthesia at Birth

Gisele Passos da Costa Gribel

Abbreviations

ADP	Accidental dural puncture
AOR	Adjusted odds ratio
ASA	American Society of Anesthesiology
CEI	Continuous epidural infusion
CI	Confidence interval
CS	Cesarean section
DPE	Dural puncture epidural technique
E	Ephedrine
EPL	Epidural technique
FB	Fentanyl and low-dose bupivacaine
KLB	Low-dose ketamine, midazolam, and low-dose bupivacaine
LCLAs	Low concentrations of local anesthetics
LRA	Labor regional analgesia
N	Norepinephrine
OR	Odds ratio
P	Phenylephrine
PAC	Preanesthetic consultation
PCEA	Programmed controlled epidural analgesia
PDPH	Postdural puncture headache
PIEB	Programmed intermittent epidural bolus
QLB	Quadratus lumborum block
RR	Risk ratio
TAP	Transversus abdominal plane block

G. P. da Costa Gribel (✉)
Department of Anesthesiology, Hospital Maternidade Escola, Universidade Federal do Rio de Janeiro (UFRJ), Rio de Janeiro, RJ, Brazil

© Springer Nature Switzerland AG 2022

R. A. Moreira de Sá, E. B. d. Fonseca (eds.), *Perinatology*,
https://doi.org/10.1007/978-3-030-83434-0_49

Introduction

Labor regional analgesia is increasingly notorious. It is the most satisfactory method for intense pain control during labor [1]. It has also been proven that there is no influence of LRA on the occurrence of unplanned cesarean section [2]. Therefore LRAs' practice is growing up exponentially in hospital labors, which also is becoming more frequently [3].

Currently, anesthesiologists must reflect upon questions that surround LRA. Many important points related to obstetric care were established in the guidelines of women's perinatal management in the last two decades. Consequently, the contribution of the anesthesiologists is expanding toward other hospital sections. The principal anesthetic interventions and procedures related to women in multidisciplinary obstetric care, labor analgesia including LRA and other techniques, and anesthesia in the perinatal period will be discussed.

Anesthetic Information in Risk Pregnancy

The obstetric practice introduced multidisciplinary routines in prenatal care. They improve the clinical treatment and control for pregnant women with chronic diseases, as gestational diabetes, hypertensive gestational diseases, obesity, and weight gain control, allowing better childbirth outcomes.

Preanesthetic consultation (PAC) during prenatal period is strongly recommended for these women, especially to patients submitted to elective perinatal procedures. It can be also done during hospitalization [4]. During PAC, demographic, obstetric, anesthetic, surgical, and clinical data are collected. Chronic and/or gestational disease data must include medications prescribed and laboratory results. Different body systems are investigated through the clinical exam, including airways. The preanesthetic evaluation includes physical status classification according to the American Society of Anesthesiology (ASA) [5]. Different LRA techniques are explained to patients, including characteristics, contraindications, and possible complications. Psychological tests applied to women can detect anxiety, stress, and depression symptoms and can be accomplished during PAC in a multi-professional environment. These symptoms increase the risk in maternal-fetal outcomes [6]. Literature highlights that the preoperative information can support pregnant women to deal with the hospital anxiety and stress symptoms offering individualized assistance based on information about surgical procedures [7].

Anesthetic Information in Low-Risk Pregnancy

During the prenatal period, labor information, analgesic options, and available interventions are frequently transmitted in a multi-professional way to woman and her companion. The anesthesiologist is also one of the members from this team and can tell the necessary information about LRA to the patient just in prenatal period or during perinatal hospitalization according to need. This care can promote adaptive strategies for women to cope with their pregnancy demands. The prenatal assistance, which included a preanesthetic consultation, is centered on individual needs and can result in the development of positive coping strategies [8].

At the same time, the multi-professional team must talk about the use of non-pharmacological methods to pregnant women, to allow them to choose pain control. Patients who receive complementary therapies do not necessarily refuse pharmacological analgesia [9], but they can use them together and as adjuvants. Both methods can increase maternal satisfaction with the childbirth experience [10, 11].

The Role of LRA in the Current Multi-Professional Childbirth Attention

Pain in Labor

The emotional component of parturient involves psychics, cognitive, cultural, socioeconomic, religious, aspects and influence labor pain perception [12]. This group of factors results in peculiar pain behavior which demands cautious interpretation. Pain score is variable between women and the interpretation should be individualized. In labor, there is not always satisfaction in the absence of pain [13]. Therefore the relation between pain and satisfaction is variable which must be considered in the anesthetic labor management.

LRA and Labor Management

The World Health Organization (WHO) defined the most relevant practices in obstetric care according to the evidence. Also, the companionship and the routine use of non-pharmacological methods were highlighted to keep the patient in control of the parturition process [14].

The parturient regained body control and movement during childbirth, in addition to participating in decisions. Whereas women are allowed to ambulate freely and change positions, the use of diluted local anesthetic-lipophilic opioids increases.

An intravenous catheter is used in case it is necessary to administer even fluids or medications. If the patient remains in starvation for a prolonged period of time intravenous fluids should be considered to help replace losses but do not need to be used continuously on all laboring patients [15].

Oral intake should not be withheld. There is not sufficient evidence to address the safety of any particular fasting period for solids in obstetric patients [16]. Solid food ingestion should be avoided if there is a risk of surgical procedures under anesthesia, especially if the patient is under risk of pulmonary aspiration (morbid obesity, difficult airway).

The most invasive interventions in childbirth, such as the use of oxytocin and maneuvers in the expulsive period, showed considerable decline. Longer periods of labor have become common in hospital births. However, the use of oxytocin to modulate contractility in patients under regional anesthesia continues to be frequent [17].

The use of pharmacological analgesia is indicated from mother's request . However, the parturient or her companion must sign informed consent for regional anesthesia before the procedure. Therefore, LRA must be accomplished considering maternal participation, with the smaller possible doses to achieve her satisfaction. Patients can be evaluated every hour of analgesia using the visual analog scale [18] for pain intensity to adjust the control to the level desired. The Aldrete index [19] can be used in the same way for monitoring other vital functions. The patients who wish and reach index 10 in the evaluation can move and ambulate.

LRA Techniques

This group of techniques is based on blocking, through local anesthetics, the afferent nerve fibers. The painful sensation in childbirth takes on characteristics according to the stage of childbirth. During the first stage, the cervical dilation process triggers impulses in the afferent nerve fibers that, together with the sympathetic fibers, enter the spinal cord in the thoracic (T10, T11, T12) and lumbar (L1) segments. In the second stage, the presence of fetal improve perineal distention, and the painful impulse is taken to the spinal cord through the S2, S3, and S4 segments. Afferent nerve fibers synapse in the posterior horn of the spinal cord and carry painful stimuli to the upper centers, where pain is interpreted and perceived.

In the present days, regional analgesic technique most used is continuous (epidural or combined spinal-epidural) or simple subarachnoid anesthesia, in which only the spinal component is used. For continuous epidural anesthesia, epidural puncture is performed through the L3-L4 vertebral space; after loss of resistance and insertion of the epidural catheter (3 cm) in the epidural space with adequate attachment and negative test dose [1.5% lidocaine (3 ml) and adrenaline 1:200,000], administration of local anesthetic in lower effective doses (bupivacaine, ropivacaine 10 ml) and lipid-soluble opioid (fentanyl or sufentanil) in *bolus* in the lumbar epidural space follows, according to the patient's request. The combined spinal-epidural anesthesia consists of epidural puncture through the L3-L4 vertebral space; and subarachnoid puncture is then performed using an epidural needle with an initial injection (1 ml) containing local anesthetic and lipid-soluble opioid, followed by epidural catheter passage. Later, the same procedure is used, applying a *bolus* of anesthetic solution and lipid-soluble opioid when necessary, in the same way as the isolated epidural technique.

Anesthetic solutions can be administered in *bolus* through the catheter, as prior described or in a continuous epidural infusion modality (CEI). Epidural bolus doses provide better spread as compared to continuous infusions [20]. Recently the bolus technique can be done by a programmed intermittent epidural bolus (PIEB) pump. Patient-controlled epidural analgesia (PCEA) technique is usually accomplished by two modalities: self-application of a bolus dose and a continuous maintenance analgesia by a pump infusion.

Recent studies compared PIEB with PCEA or CEI. A randomized clinical trial [21] compared 150 patients scheduled for labor induction with labor analgesia using bupivacaine with fentanyl at either the PIEB 5 ml every 30 min (5q30), PIEB 10 ml every 60 min (10q60), or 10 ml/h or CEI. The primary outcome was pain score at 30 minutes, 2 h, and every 2 h from then on. The normalized average pain scores did not differ significantly between groups. PIEB group 10q60 had significantly fewer physician-administered boluses as compared to the PIEB group 5q30 and the CEI group (34.9% in 10q60 vs. 61.0% in 5q30 and 61.9% in CEI, $p = 0.022$).The secondary outcomes (dermatomal sensory levels, degree of motor block, and patient satisfaction) did not differ significantly [21].

A new dural puncture epidural technique (DPE) is similar to a needle-through-needle combined spinal-epidural technique, except that after puncturing the dura with the spinal needle, no intrathecal medications are given, and all medications are then administered through the epidural catheter. A randomized controlled trial [22] of 120 patients compared the CSE, DPE, and epidural techniques (EPL) in a continuous infusion with PCA. The primary outcome is time to pain score of ≤1. The median of these outcomes were 2, 11, and 18 minutes for CSE, DPE, and EPL techniques, respectively. It was significantly different for CSE versus DPE (hazard ratio 0.36, 95% CI 0.22–0.59; $p < 0.0001$). There was no significant difference between DPE and EPL techniques (hazard ratio 1.4, 95% CI 0.83–2.4; $p = 0.21$). Secondary outcomes were examined, with significant differences found, including less need for physician top-ups with the DPE compared to the other two techniques (relative risk 0.45, 95% CI 0.23–0.86; $p = 0.01$); less asymmetric block after 30 minutes with the DPE compared with EPL (relative risk 0.19, 95% CI 0.07–0.51; $p < 0.001$); Compared com CSE, DPE had lower incidence of pruritus (relative risk 0.15, 95% CI 0.06–0.38; $p < 0.001$), hypotension (relative risk 0.38, 95% CI 0.15–0.98; $p = 0.03$), combined uterine tachysystole and hypertonia (relative risk 0.22, 95% CI 0.08–0.60; $p < 0.001$) [22].

However, in future studies, the potential benefits of the dural puncture epidural technique need to be confirmed.

Recently, some important evidence about other important outcomes from continuous techniques with low concentrations of local anesthetics (LCLAs) have been studied.

The motor-sparing lower doses used today must not prolong the second stage of labor. A double-blind, randomized, placebo-controlled trial [23] of 400 healthy nulliparous women who were receiving low-dose epidural analgesia with ropivacaine and sufentanil to have their analgesia continued with the same solution in the second stage of labor or switched to a saline solution. The primary outcome of the mean duration of the second stage of labor was not significantly different between the groups epidural and saline (epidural 52 ± 27 versus saline 51 ± 25; 95% CI −3.5 – 7 minutes; $p = 0.52$). There were also no significant differences between the groups in the rate of spontaneous vaginal delivery (epidural 96.5% vs. saline 99%; 95% CI −0.1% —−0.3%; $p = 0.17$) [23].

A systematic review [24] included 1809 women and compared the effects of epidural (epidural or combined spinal-epidural) analgesia with LCLAs (using ropivacaine, levobupivacaine, or bupivacaine) with those of non-epidural (systemic opioids, nitrous oxide, or non-pharmacological analgesia) analgesia on obstetric outcomes. The primary outcomes were the duration of the second stage of labor and the instrumental birth rate. Regarding the duration of the second stage of labor, there was no significant difference between the groups (mean difference = 5.71 minutes, 95% CI −6.14–17.83; $p = 0.36$) as the instrumental birth rate (RR = 1.52, 95% CI 0.97–2.4; $p = 0.07$). There was no significant difference between groups in the cesarean delivery rate (RR = 0.8, 95% CI 0.6–1.05; $p = 0.11$), the spontaneous vaginal delivery rate (RR = 0.98, 95% CI 0.91–1.06; $p = 0.62$), or the duration of the first stage of labor (mean difference = 17.34 minutes, 95% CI −5.89–40.56; $p = 0.14$). However the authors recommended future studies because the meta-analysis was based in small trials of low quality [24].

A population-based retrospective cohort study using data from the Perinatal Registry of the Netherlands between 2000 and 2009 evaluated RLA in women to know whether labor analgesia increased the risk of instrumented deliveries. These data showed that among nulliparous women ($n = 616{,}063$), the rate of epidural labor analgesia use increased over the study period from 7.7% to 21.9%. Although the cesarean delivery rate increased by 2.8% during the study period, the instrumented vaginal delivery rate decreased by 3.3%. In parous women ($n = 762{,}395$), epidural analgesia use increased from 2.4% to 6.8%, whereas absolute rates of cesarean delivery increased by 0.8% and instrumented vaginal delivery decreased by 0.7% [25].

Other benefits obtained from RLA are reduction of circulating catecholamines, hyperventilation prevention, and facilitation of management of the unplanned cesarean section [26].

Among regional techniques' complications are hypotension, pruritis, nausea, urinary retention, total failure or inadequate anesthesia, high/prolonged neuromuscular block, accidental dural puncture, non-intentional intravascular injection, respiratory depression, sensory alterations, back pain, and postdural puncture headache. A recent cross-sectional study [27] evaluated RLA practice among 1351 Indian anesthesiologists [27]. Among complications, hypotension, bradycardia, and pruritis were the most common complications and the rarest were high block and prolonged motor block by hematoma. Management of complication includes checking the availability of adequate basic and advanced life-support equipment and medical team support [16].

The postdural puncture headache (PDPH) can occur following spinal anesthesia and with inadvertent dural puncture during epidural anesthesia. Obstetric patients are considered at risk for this complication. During epidural catheter placement, inadvertent puncture of the dura mater occurs at a rate of 1.5% (95% CI 1.5–1.5%), and more than half (52.1%; 95% CI: 51.4–52.8%) of these patients develop PDPH [28]. PDPH can cause morbidity in obstetric patients and difficult lactation and breastfeeding too. When diagnosing PDPH in this group, it is important to exclude other causes of headache, such as functional headaches. Conservative initial actions should be started immediately. Oral or intravenous hydration, oral caffeine, and analgesics. The majority of patients will be not required other treatments and will be healed in 48 hours.

A multidisciplinary staff must be necessary in persistent cases. Among the invasive treatment, blood-patch is the gold standard. Other invasive treatments like occipital nerve [29] and sphenopalatine nerve [30] blocks are promising treatments after consistent future studies.

Inhaled Analgesia

This modality has been used in low-risk labor. The agents (sevoflurane and/or nitrous oxide) are self-administered when the patient desires. The inhaled agent concentration is established in fixed values. However, epidural analgesia is the most commonly used and the most complete method of pain relief available in the United States [31]. Inhaled nitrous oxide provides less complete pain relief than an epidural but is more potent than IV opioids, making it a viable option for patients who do not wish to have an epidural or are unable to receive one. In addition to providing analgesia in labor, nitrous oxide also has anxiolytic properties.

A Chinese study showed no significant differences in postpartum bleeding volume, neonatal Apgar score, and blood gas analysis between 658 women who inhaled nitrous oxide for labor analgesia and 642 women who inhaled oxygen only [32]. There are common adverse reactions: nausea, vomiting, dizziness, and sedation. Continuous monitoring of oxygen saturation is required for all patients and for respiratory depression in patients who also were given opioids. A scavenger equipment is used to protect healthcare staff [31].

A study [33] compared sevoflurane at 0.8% and Entonox (nitrous oxide 50%/oxygen 50%) for analgesia in 29 parturients during labor. Each mother underwent two open-label three-part sequences in random order, Entonox-sevoflurane-Entonox or sevoflurane-Entonox-sevoflurane. In each part, the agent was self-administered during ten contractions. A 100 mm visual analog score was proceeded for pain relief and sedation after each contraction and the results (median) were compared. Pain relief scores were higher for sevoflurane than Entonox (67.55 and 51.40 mm, respectively; $p < 0.03$). Nausea and vomiting were more common in the Entonox group (RR 2.7, 95% CI 1.3–5.7; $p = 0.0040$. There was significantly more sedation with sevoflurane than with Entonox (74, 66 and 51, 41 mm, respectively; $p < 0.001$) [33].

Parenteral Analgesia

The most common kinds of this modality of opioid analgesia are intramuscular and intravenous (including PCEA). They are used for labor pain relief in many countries.

A systematic review (Cochrane 2018) analyzed around 8000 women to the effectiveness, safety, and acceptability of different types, doses, and modes of administration of parenteral opioid for labor analgesia. Also the effects of opioids on the baby were evaluated. Overall, the evidence was graded as low- or very-low-quality regarding the analgesic effect of opioids and satisfaction with analgesia. No consistent differences were found in maternal satisfaction with intramuscular analgesia with pethidine versus placebo measured during labor (number of women satisfied or very satisfied after 30 minutes: 50 women; 1 trial; RR 7.00, 95% CI 0.38–128.87) or number of women requesting an epidural (50 women; 1 trial; RR 0.50, 95% CI 0.14–1.78; very low-quality evidence). Pain scores (reduction in visual analog scale (VAS) score of at least 40 mm: 50 women; 1 trial; RR 25, 95% CI 1.56–400; low-quality evidence) and pain measured in labor (women reporting pain relief to be "good" or "fair" within 1 hour of administration: 116 women; 1 trial; RR 1.75, 95% CI 1.24–2.47; low-quality evidence) were both reduced in the pethidine group, and fewer women requested any additional analgesia (50 women; 1 trial; RR 0.71, 95% CI 0.54–0.94; low-quality evidence). There was limited information on adverse effects and harm to women and neonates. There were few results that clearly showed that one opioid was more effective than another. Overall, findings indicated that parenteral opioids provided some pain relief and moderate satisfaction with analgesia in labor. Opioid drugs were associated with maternal nausea, vomiting, and drowsiness, although different opioid drugs were associated with different adverse effects. There was no clear evidence of adverse effects of opioids on the newborn [34].

Regional Analgesia Versus Other Techniques

A recent systematic review (Cochrane 2018) compared safety in labor analgesia, including continuous CEI, opioid analgesia, no-analgesia, needle stimulation, inhaled analgesia, and continuous support or another modality of analgesia. Pain scores were lower in women with epidural analgesia when compared to women who received opioids (standardized mean difference −2.64, 95% CI −4.56–−0.73; 1133 women; studies = 5; $I^2 = 98\%$; low-quality evidence), and a higher proportion was satisfied with their pain relief, reporting it to be "excellent or very good" (RR 1.47, 95% CI 1.03–2.08; 1911 women; studies = 7; $I^2 = 97\%$; low-quality evidence). There was substantial statistical heterogeneity in both these outcomes. There was a substantial decrease in the need for additional pain relief in women receiving epidural analgesia compared with opioid analgesia (RR 0.10, 95% CI 0.04–0.25; 5099 women; studies = 16; $I^2 = 73\%$; $Tau^2 = 1.89$; $Chi^2 = 52.07$, $p < 0.00001$). More women in the epidural group experienced assisted vaginal birth (RR 1.44, 95% CI 1.29–1.60; 9948 women; studies = 30; low-quality evidence). A post hoc subgroup analysis of trials conducted after 2005 showed that this effect is negated when trials before 2005 are excluded from this analysis (RR 1.19, 95% CI 0.97–1.46). There was no difference between caesarean section rates (RR 1.07, 95% CI 0.96–1.18;

10,350 women; studies = 33; moderate-quality evidence) and maternal long-term backache (RR 1.00, 95% CI 0.89–1.12; 814 women; studies = 2; moderate-quality evidence). There were also no differences between groups for the neonatal outcomes, admission to neonatal intensive care unit (RR 1.03, 95% CI 0.95–1.12; 4488 babies; studies = 8; moderate-quality evidence), and Apgar score less than 7 at 5 minutes (RR 0.73, 95% CI 0.52–1.02; 8752 babies; studies = 22; low-quality evidence). There were also no clear differences between groups for the neonatal outcomes. Women with epidural experienced more hypotension, motor blockade, fever, and urinary retention. They also had longer first and second stages of labor and were more likely to have oxytocin augmentation than women in the opioid group. Women receiving epidurals had less risk of respiratory depression requiring oxygen and were less likely to experience nausea and vomiting than women receiving opioids [1].

A recent labor pain research [35] used questionnaires to interview 258 women and analyzed pain intensity during labor and the effectiveness of its relief through inhaled or epidural analgesia, the use of complementary therapies, and multiple management (inhaled analgesia and one modality of complementary therapy). Epidural analgesia was comparable to inhaled analgesia in the first stage and was the most effective in the second stage [35].

RLA and Quality

Whether the use of regional labor analgesia is increasing around the world, obstetric patients are each more interested in good-quality obstetric care. Regional labor analgesia currently reflects obstetric analgesia guidelines that focus on the quality of the parturition process and its outcomes.

The recent innovations in obstetric regional analgesia were introduced from clinical research. They improved safety and maternal satisfaction [36]. Balanced analgesia using a low concentration of local anesthetic and lipid-soluble opioid mixture, the combined spinal-epidural technique, and devices for patient-controlled analgesia have all contributed to innovation in obstetric analgesia [21].

Nowadays the parturient is on childbirth control, making decisions about her pain relief methods and ready for emergencies as non-planned cesarean section or operative delivery. But whether they are making decisions in the appropriated moment must be better investigated. A qualitative study [37] evaluated 13 primiparous and 10 multiparous women at 36 weeks of pregnancy and within 6 weeks postnatally. Semi-structured interviews were conducted to know how women could be better supported in preparing for, and making, decisions during pregnancy and labor regarding pain management. During pregnancy, women expressed doubtfulness about the level of pain they would experience in labor and the effect of different methods of pain relief. Also, women reflected on how decisions had been made regarding pain management in labor and the degree of security they had felt making these decisions. Regarding the level of control, women discussed the degree of decision desired and experienced during labor. The authors concluded that in the antenatal preparation, it would be better to concentrate efforts in better informing and engaging women in discussions about their values, expectations, and preferences rather than making firm decisions in advance of labor as it is an unpredictable event [37].

Quality care is a complex and hard phenomenon to define [38], but this involves the woman's perception of herself in the care. In order to achieve quality, healthcare needs to be safe, effective, timely, efficient, equitable, and people-centered [39].

This can highlight the importance of women's expectations, participation in decisions, and satisfaction with the process of childbirth. Overall, expectation and satisfaction are commonly associated factors in psychological maternal outcomes, such as postpartum depression [40], anxiety [41], and post-traumatic syndrome [42]. A quality study [43] evaluated satisfaction on 248 women during postpartum period in a multicenter observational longitudinal study using the Intrapartal-Specific Quality from the Patient's Perspective Questionnaire at three time points: 3 days, 15 days, and 1 year of postpartum. They concluded that the mean scores for satisfaction at each time point were high and lowered with time. The bivariate analysis showed an association between satisfaction and the following variables: "mother's place of birth," "level of education," "type of labor onset," "type of birth," and "type of perineal trauma." For the multivariate analysis, women who gave birth vaginally, began labor spontaneously, and had an epidural were more satisfied than those who did not [43].

However, discrepancies about satisfaction with epidural occur in literature. Instead, some authors reported no relationship between satisfaction and epidural [44], and others described epidural use as a worse experience [45]. The best point to evaluate women's satisfaction is also controversy. A study [46] described how women are more critical with the procedures related to their labor with time [46]. Another study [47] highlighted that the importance of negative events during labor grows up with time [47]. A study [48] involving 2428 patients compared the women opinion about childbirth 2 months and one ear after birth and conclude that there were no differences in 60% of cases. He also avoids to consider early opinions after childbirth because in this moment the patients were euphoric [48].

A qualitative descriptive study [49] explored 25 childbearing women's experiences and perspectives, as the first step in developing an instrument to quantitatively measure quality neuraxial analgesia. Their findings suggest that this outcome involves physical, cognitive, and emotional dimensions that must be measured. The findings further suggest an important relationship between each of these dimensions and perceptions of control [49].

About effectiveness of and satisfaction with LRA with LCLAs, a prospective observational study [50] evaluated this regimen provided at a tertiary care teaching hospital. A total of 294 parturients were managed as per departmental routine based on a PCEA regimen with a maintenance dilute local anesthetic-opioid solution. After delivery, patients completed a satisfaction questionnaire. A large number of women reported having experienced pain during the first or second stages of labor (38% and 26%, respectively). Most women (92%) were satisfied with the quality of analgesia. Overweight women (AOR = 2.56; 95% CI 1.1–5.97), those undergoing induced labor (AOR = 2.4, 95% CI 1.2–5.2), and those requiring top-ups by the anesthesiologist (AOR = 5.08, 95% CI 2.31–11.11) were associated with more dissatisfaction with pain control during the first stage of labor [50].

Anesthesia

Cesarean section (CS) has been a frequent intervention around the world. There are factors associated with the current CS rates, and anesthesiologists must be aware of them. Obesity is an important maternal factor [51] and has become an epidemic and been linked to the prevalence of diabetes mellitus and hypertension in the female population in the reproductive age range. Also maternal age is increasing and nulliparity is becoming more frequent [17]. Fetal, medicolegal, and obstetric factors are also involved and can result in local significant differences in cesarean rates [17].

The Robson classification [52] was developed in 2001 to identify institutional groups with significant differences in CS rates. Patients are classified for one from ten groups based in five parameters: parity, fetal number and presentation, previous cesarean section, gestational age, and labor (induction, spontaneous labor, or no labor). Whereas this classification optimizes the evaluation of CS, anesthetic management will also benefit from the data obtained.

To clarify the differences among emergency and planned CS rates, a retrospective cohort study [53] was conducted from 1989 to 2016 to analyze the indications and rates of planned and emergency CS. The total births in the study were 147,722, and CS occurred in 37,309 patients (total rate of 25%). The rate of CS in 1989–1994 was 18.7% (8.7% emergency, 10% planned) and in 2010–2016 grows up to 30.4% (11.4% emergency, 19% planned). Emergency CI had a relative increase of 62% for slow progress and of 8% for fetal concern. Previous uterine surgery (CS in the majority) was the largest contributor to the increase in planned CS (3.8–9.0 of all births and 29% of overall CS). Primary CS for fetal concern, pregnancy problems, and maternal desire increased from 0.7% to 4.9%. Regarding Robson classification, 6, 7, and 8 groups had the most increase [53].

The most frequent indications in this study were slow labor progress and previous CS. Robson classification was breech presentation and multiple gestation, including nulliparous or multiparous. It can be postulated that regional labor analgesia can be included in the efforts to optimize the childbirth of nulliparous women that have slow labor.

A study [54] analyzed 5400 CS in 2016 and found an overall incidence of 64% of vaginal birth and 33% of CS. The largest Robson classification groups were 5, 8, and 9. Similar to Morton's [53] find, the most common indication was repeated CS [54].

Guideline Before Anesthetic Procedure

Preanesthetic consultation can be also done during hospitalization or during prenatal to patients submitted to elective perinatal procedures. Informed consent is mandatory. Also, it is necessary to include information about postoperative analgesia and transfusion therapy when appropriate. Some clinical situations have a higher risk for hemorrhage, as the presence of coagulopathies, genital trauma and instrumentation, uterine surgery or overdistension, tocolytic agents, abnormal placenta or fetus presentation, and chorioamnionitis. In the occurrence of hemorrhage, multidisciplinary protocols can optimize management.

All operating rooms must be equipped with monitors: noninvasive arterial pressure, pulse oximeter, capnography, electrocardiography, and gas analyzer, as the adequate ventilator. All usual airways material must be available and checked and equipment for difficult airways should be available. Emergency medication solutions must be prepared for each patient, which also must have venous access for fluid infusions and medications. The prophylactic antibiotic is usually implemented before incision, and uterotonics are prepared for intravenous bolus and/or infusion.

A systematic review (Cochrane 2018) about postpartum hemorrhage prevention, in the context of cesarean deliveries, analyzed the effectiveness of carbetocin compared to oxytocin in 2012 patients. There was a significant reduction in the rates of postpartum hemorrhage (RR 0.79; 95% CI 0.66–0.94; $p = 0.009$), use of additional uterotonics (RR 0.57; 95% CI 0.49–0.65; $p < 0.001$), and transfusion (RR 0.31; 95% CI 0.15–0.64; $p = 0.002$). There was significant heterogeneity across studies for the use of additional uterotonics outcome. The study highlights that the protocol must be analyzed before adopting because of the cost disparity between carbetocin and oxytocin [55].

Bronco Aspiration Prophylaxis

Pregnant women must stop drinking 2 hours before elective procedures and to eat solids up to 6–8 hours before, depending on concomitant clinical situations [16].

The use of particulate antacids like sodium citrate is associated with higher gastric pH without change in gastric volume [56]. The use of H2 receptor antagonists, like ranitidine, and proton-bomb inhibitors, like omeprazole, is associated with higher gastric pH without reducing gastric volume [57]. The use of metoclopramide reduces peripartum nausea and vomiting [58]. These medications must be considered in peripartum management, but literature is not clear about the association between reduced gastric acidity to prevent aspiration of acidic stomach contents.

More recently, a study [59] evaluated diabetes and hypertension influence on ranitidine's placental permeation in pregnant women. They examined 40 patients scheduled for elective cesarean section: healthy control ($n = 15$), with hypertension ($n = 16$), and with gestation diabetes ($n = 10$). The parturients received the same dose of intravenous ranitidine. The ranitidine concentration in maternal plasma and umbilical cord samples was analyzed. Ranitidine maternal and umbilical cord (arterial and venous) concentrations were similar in all three groups, and there was no difference between fetuses: maternal ratios nor volume of distribution, clearance, and half-life between the groups. They concluded that hypertension and diabetes did not influence ranitidine placental permeation [59].

Anxiety and Sedation

Although the multidisciplinary approach to parturients and companionship can enhance women's control during the cesarean section, they can still feel stress and anxiety. It is important to discuss the use of low-dose anxiolytics in the obstetric patient in CS. However, studies about the effects of sedatives used in parturients during CS are rare because women have fair to this medication. They desire to see the baby being born and remember that moment.

The effect of low dose of midazolam as premedication on the Amsterdam Preoperative Anxiety and Information Scale (APAIS) scores, the Neonatal Neurologic and Adaptive Capacity Score (NACS), and the Apgar score of the newborn was evaluated in a randomized controlled study [60] of 50 parturients in cesarean section under spinal anesthesia. Patients receiving midazolam as premedication had significantly low anxiety scores ($p = 0{,}0001$), without any adverse effects on the newborns [60].

The sedative effect of venous midazolam before the deliveries was analyzed in a randomized blind controlled study [61]. The neonatal Apgar, umbilical venous pH, maternal hypotension, and incidence of discomfort in 40 patients were evaluated in elective cesarean section performed under spinal anesthesia. Ninety percent of midazolam group felt asleep smoothly before the operation started. There were no differences between the groups in Apgar scores, maternal hypotension, or umbilical venous pH. Intraoperatory maternal discomfort was 11-fold more often in control group [61].

Regional Anesthesia Techniques

Spinal anesthesia is preferentially performed during CS. It is simple and secure, but it is associated with hypotension in about 60% of cases or more [62]. It is recommended to move the uterus to the left in women from 20 weeks and over, after return to supine position during spinal anesthesia for CS.

Some studies evaluated the use of low doses of local anesthetic with adjuvants, to reduce hypotension and obtain an accelerated recovery.

A systematic review with meta-analysis [63] with a total of 693 women demonstrated that intrathecal low doses of bupivacaine with fentanyl significantly reduced the incidence of hypotension and bradycardia in cesarean section, but with insufficient intraoperative analgesia [63].

Other intrathecal adjuvants have been evaluated in some studies. Midazolam improves local anesthetic effect without hemodynamic influence [64], and ketamine stabilizes hemodynamic but is associated with a higher incidence of dissociative manifestations with limited analgesic [65].

Fifty patients were evaluated [66] in a randomized controlled trial for the intrathecal combination of low-dose ketamine, midazolam, and low-dose bupivacaine (KMB), compared with fentanyl and low-dose bupivacaine (FB) to postoperative analgesia during CS. The KMB group presented higher sensory level (p = 0,006), rapid sensor (p = 0,001) and motor (p = 0,005) onsets, prolonged sensory (p = 0,008) and motor (p = 0,002) blocks, and prolonged pain-free period (p = 0,002). KMB group reduced significantly the incidence of hypotension (p = 0,002) and vomiting (p = 0,019). Apgar score in 5 min was comparable in both groups (p = 0,64). Patients' VAS score satisfaction was significantly higher in KMB group (p = 0,001). There were no patients in KMB group presenting neurotoxic or dissociative manifestations [66]. However, the results and safety must be confirmed in the future.

A recent systematic review and meta-analysis [67] analyzed the use of clonidine as an adjuvant for regional anesthesia during 1254 cesarean section. Clonidine prolonged the duration of sensory block by 128.2 min (95% CI 81.7–174.8) as much as motor block by 44.7 min (95% CI 8.7–80.7) significantly. Clonidine increased sedation (RR 3,92; 95% IC 1.17–13.14) without increasing risk of nausea and vomiting and hypotension and with no influence on Apgar score at 1 or 5 min [67].

The use of dexmedetomidine as an adjuvant for regional anesthesia was studied in another systematic review and meta-analysis [68] as an adjuvant for regional anesthesia during cesarean section of 278 patients. The incidence of shivering was significantly lower than in the placebo group (RR 0.40., 95% CI 0.25–0.65, p = 0.0002). There was no effect on nausea and vomiting (RR 1.08, 95% IC 0.68–1.71, p = 0.74), bradycardia (RR 1.33, 95% IC 0.31–5.76, p = 0.7), or hypotension (RR 0.78, 95% IC 0.59–1.03, p = 0,08) [68].

Management of Hypotension

The management of hypotension is based on maintenance of systolic arterial pressure (SAP) at ≥90% of an accurate baseline obtained before spinal anesthesia, and avoid a decrease to <80% baseline [69]. Hypotension induces maternal nausea, vomiting, bradycardia, and also adverse neonatal effects. The best management of hypotension is the use of crystalloid and/or colloid solutions combined with vasopressors. Hypotension degree is lower in patients with preeclampsia than healthy pregnant women. However, they must use lower doses of vasopressor than in normal patients. The use of vasopressors to hypotension control must be individualized in the presence of cardiac diseases. Vasopressors must be prepared to be used in all patients, either as a treatment or prophylactic. Today, phenylephrine is commonly used for preventing maternal spinal hypotension, but the reduction in cardiac output with reflex bradycardia can occur.

Recently, studies compared hemodynamic control obtained with this alpha-agonist to others that have also some beta-adrenergic activity, like norepinephrine. A randomized double-blind controlled trial of 102 women [70] compared the use of phenylephrine (P) or norepinephrine (N) as intermittent bolus administration to maintenance maternal blood pressure during cesarean section over than 80% of baseline value. Compared to group P, women in group N had a higher CO (standardized CO 5.8 ± 0.9 vs. 5.3 ± 1.0L/min, $t = 2.37$, $p = 0.02$). The incidence of bradycardia was lower in group N than in group P (2% vs. 14%, $p = 0.023$), along with an overall higher standardized heart rate (78.8 ± 11.6 vs. 75.0 ± 7.3 beats/min, $p = 0.049$). However, the findings did not present clinical significance [70].

Ephedrine, a beta-agonist agent, is also used in prophylactic infusion for preventing maternal spinal anesthesia hypotension. However, tachycardia is common and can be an adverse outcome. A randomized double-blind controlled trial of 97 patients [71] compared norepinephrine (N) with ephedrine (E) in prophylactic infusion for preventing maternal hypotension during elective cesarean section under spinal anesthesia. Women in group N experienced fewer cases of tachycardia (4.2% vs. 30.6%, $p = 0.002$, OR 0.11, 95% CI 0.02–0.47) [71]. These results must be confirmed in future studies.

Other Regional Techniques

Other regional techniques are described in the literature and in some situations can be chosen.

Epidural anesthesia is used currently to perform regional anesthesia to unplanned CS during labor analgesia. This technique uses greater doses and has a slow installation when compared with spinal anesthesia.

Continuous spinal anesthesia is performed when an accidental dural puncture (ADP) during a difficult region occurs, and to proceed another epidural involves a risk of another ADP.

The combined spinal-epidural anesthesia is appropriated to obese women or when a precise regional block is necessary. It also is appropriate when the low spinal anesthetic local dose is necessary.

General Anesthesia

Today, whereas the safety of general anesthesia was improved, there was a reduction in the frequency of use of general anesthesia to perform a cesarean section [72]. Anesthetic technique was improved. Supraglottic airway devices can be used in the presence of a difficult intubation.

During induction, the rapid sequence with thiopental and suxamethonium that results in inadequate anesthetic plane, tachycardia, and hypertension includes propofol rocuronium and remifentanil currently. To use opioids adequately, the presence of neonatologist during delivery is important to provide adequate management of the baby. Inhaled anesthetics in low doses has limited effects on the uterus response to the oxytocin [73], and prostaglandins enhance uterine contraction during inhaled agent use [74]. Cesarean section is considered to be one of the surgeries in which patients are the most prone to be aware during anesthesia [75], and adequate bispectral index monitoring is mandatory.

Postoperative Analgesia

The parturients, which use regional anesthetic techniques for cesarean section, can have pain control by intrathecal morphine with adjuvants, patient-controlled epidural analgesia, and nonsteroidal anti-inflammatory drugs, choosing that with little breast-milk concentration. Opioids increase the risk of nausea and vomiting, sedation, pruritus, and respiratory depression [72]. Patient-controlled epidural analgesia with low local anesthetic doses combined with opioids or other adjuvants is the best control pain device. However the use of this device difficult patient free mobility and involves learning about and dealing with the use of the equipment.

To control pain in patients submitted to general anesthesia during delivery, intravenous patient-controlled anesthesia can be effective. This modality also has the same morbidity and difficulty to use as patient-controlled epidural analgesia.

Transversus abdominal plane (TAP) block can be used after the general anesthesia with a limited duration of analgesia. In general, it is used as a part of multimodal analgesia [76]. It is accomplished with low local anesthetic doses combined with adjuvants. Some studies discuss the use of the technique after spinal anesthesia instead of intrathecal morphine.

A meta-analysis [77] involving 312 patients concluded that TAP block can provide effective analgesia when spinal morphine is contraindicated or not used in patients undergoing lower segment cesarean section under spinal anesthesia [77].

A study [78] evaluated 92 parturients submitted to spinal anesthesia to the cesarean section in a randomized controlled trial. The duration of postoperative analgesia after using TAP block with low-dose levobupivacaine without (B) or with (BC) clonidine was analyzed. Duration of analgesia was significantly longer in Group BC (17.94 ± 0.76 h) compared to Group B (7.16 ± 0.41 h) ($p < 0.001$). Mean consumption of tramadol was 197.77 ± 14.90 mg and 8.889 ± 28.77 mg in Groups B and BC ($p < 0.001$), respectively. All patients in Group BC were extremely satisfied while those in Group B were satisfied ($p < 0.01$). None of the patients experienced hypotension or bradycardia [78]. However, a study describing two cases of generalized tonic-clonic seizures attributed to local anesthetic systemic toxicity in obstetric patients who received ultrasound-guided TAP blocks for postcesarean analgesia was reported [79].

Other abdominal block has been performed for postoperative analgesia after cesarean section, but future studies must confirm the results. A randomized controlled trial of 90 patients compared postoperative analgesia with quadratus lumborum block (QLB) versus spinal morphine and control group and found that the two techniques were compared but in QLB group, time to the first morphine request was significantly longer, and also there was a sparing effect in morphine postoperative consumption [80].

Regarding the last advances discussed in this chapter, analgesia and anesthesia at birth have amplified resources to control pain, optimize obstetric care, and improve quality of the childbirth process.

References

1. Anim-Somuah M, Smyth RM, Cyna AM, Cuthbert A. Epidural versus non-epidural or no analgesia for pain management in labor. Cochrane Database Syst Rev. 2018;5:CD000331. https://doi.org/10.1002/14651858.CD000331.pub4.
2. Cambic CR, Wong CA. Labor analgesia and obstetrics outcomes. Br J Anaesth. 2010;105:i50–60. https://doi.org/10.1093/bja/aeq311.
3. Marmor TR, Krol DM. Labor pain management in the United States: understanding patterns and the issue of choice. Am J Obstet Gynecol. 2002;186:S173–80. https://doi.org/10.1067/mob.2002.121258.
4. Society of Obstetricians and Gynaecologysts of Canada (SOGC). Clinical practice guideline. No. 239. Obesity in pregnacy. Int J Gynaecol Obstet. 2010;110:167–73. https://doi.org/10.1016/j.ijgo.2010.03.008.
5. Doyle DJ, Garmon EH. American Society of Anesthesiologists. Classification (ASA Class) [Update 2017 Oct 6]. In: StatPearls. Treasure Island: Stat Pearl Publishing; 2018.
6. Sanchez SE, Puente GC, Atencio G, Qiu C, Yanez D, et al. Risk of spontaneous preterm birth in relation to maternal depressive, anxiety, and stress symptoms. J Reprod Med. 2013;58:25–33.
7. Sjöling M, Nordahl G, Olofsson N, Asplund K. The impact of preoperative information on state anxiety, postoperative pain and satisfaction with pain management. Patient Educ Couns. 2003;51:169–76. https://doi.org/10.1016/s0738-3991(02)00191-x.
8. Cunha ACB, Gribel GPC, Akermann LPF, Rocha AC. Pre-anesthetic consultation, stress and preoperative anxiety in risk pregnant woman. Gynecol Obstet Case Report. 2018;4:63. https://doi.org/10.21767/2471-8165.1000063.
9. Gentz BA. Alternative therapies for the management of pain in labor and delivery. Clin Obstet Gynecol. 2001;44:704–32. https://doi.org/10.1097/00003081-200112000-00010.
10. Hodnett ED. Pain and women's satisfaction with the experience of childbirth: a systematic review. Am J Obstet Gynecol. 2002;186:S160–72. https://doi.org/10.1067/mob.2002.121141.
11. Karlsdottir SI, Sveinsdottir H, Kristjansdottir H, Aspelund T, Olafsdottir OA. Predictors of women's positive childbirth pain experience: findings from an Icelandic national study. Women Birth. 2018;31:e178–84. https://doi.org/10.1016/j.wombi.2017.09.007.
12. Tournaire M, Theau-Yonneau A. Complementary and alternative approaches to pain relief during labor. eCAM. 2007;4:409–17. https://doi.org/10.1093/ecam/nem012.
13. Simkin P, Bolding A. Update on nonpharmacologic approaches to relieve labor pain and prevent suffering. J Midwifery Womens Health. 2004;49:489–504. https://doi.org/10.1016/j.jmwh.2004.07.007.
14. The World Health Organization. Care in normal birth: a practical guide. Birth. 1997;24:121–3.
15. Hutchison J, Mahdy H, Hutchison J. Stages of labor. In: Stat Pearls [Internet]. Treasure Island: Stat Pearls Publishing; 2020.

16. Practice guidelines for obstetric anesthesia: an updated report by the American Society of Anesthesiologists Task Force on Obstetric Anesthesia and the Society of Obstetric Anesthesia and Perinatology. Anesthesiology. 2016;124:270–300. https://doi.org/10.1097/ALN.0000000000000935.
17. Hung T-H, Hsieh T-T, Liu H-P. Differential effects of epidural analgesia on modes of delivery and perinatal outcomes between nulliparous and multiparous women: a retrospective cohort study. PLoS One. 2015;10:e0120907. https://doi.org/10.1371/journal.pone.0120907.
18. Huskisson EC. Measurement of pain. Lancet. 1974;304:1127–31.
19. Aldrete JA. The post-anesthesia recovery score revisited. J Clin Anesth. 1995;7:89–91.
20. Kaynar AM, Shankar KB. Epidural infusion: continuous or bolus? Anesth Analg. 1999;89:534.
21. Fidkowiski CW, Shah S, Alsaden M-H. Programed intermittent epidural bolus as compared to continuous epidural infusion for the maintenance of labor analgesia: a prospective randomized single-blinded controlled trial. Korean J Anesthesiol. 2019;72:472–8. https://doi.org/10.4097/kja.19156.
22. Chau A, Bibbo C, Huang C-C, Elterman KG, Cappiello EC, Robinson JN, et al. Dural puncture epidural technique improves labor analgesia quality with fewer side effects compared with epidural and combined spinal epidural techniques: a randomized clinical trial. Anesth Analg. 2017;124:560–9. https://doi.org/10.1213/ANE.0000000000001798.
23. Shen X, Li Y, Xu S, et al. Epidural analgesia during the second stage of labor: a randomized controlled trial. Obstet Gynecol. 2017;130:1097–103. https://doi.org/10.1097/AOG.0000000000002306.
24. Wang T-T, Sun S, Huang S-Q. Effects of epidural labor analgesia with low concentrations of local anesthetics on obstetric outcomes: a systematic review and meta-analysis of randomized controlled trials. Anesth Analg. 2017;124:1571–80. https://doi.org/10.1213/ANE.0000000000001709.
25. Wassen MM, Hukkelhoven CW, Scheepers HC, Smits LJ, Nijhuis JG, Roumen FJ. Epidural analgesia and operative delivery: a ten-year population-based cohort study in The Netherlands. Eur J Obstet Gynecol Reprod Biol. 2014;183:125–31. https://doi.org/10.1016/j.ejogrb.2014.10023.
26. Mhyre JM. What's new in obstetric anesthesia? Int J Obstet Anesth. 2011;20:149–59. https://doi.org/10.1213/ANE.0b013e3181f8e4e9.
27. Narayanappa A, Gurulingaswamy S, Prabhakaraiah U, Kempegowda K, Hanumantharayappa NB. Practice of labor analgesia among anesthesiologists across India: cross-sectional study. Anesth Essays Res. 2018;12:651–6. https://doi.org/10.4103/aer.AER_74_18.
28. Choi PT, Galinski SE, Takeuchi L, Lucas S, Tamayo C, Jadad AR. PDPH is a common complication of neuraxial blockade in parturients: a meta-analysis of obstetrical studies. Can J Anaesth. 2003;50:460–9. https://doi.org/10.1007/BF03021057.
29. Uyar Turkyilmaz E, Camgoz Eryilmaz N, Aydin Guzey N, Moraloğlu O. Bilateral greater occipital nerve block for treatment of post-dural puncture headache after caesarean operations. Braz J Anesthesiol. 2016;66:445–50. https://doi.org/10.1016/j.bjane.2015.03.004.
30. Cohen S, Levin D, Mellender S, Zhao R, Patel P, Grubb W, Kiss G. Topical sphenopalatine ganglion block compared with epidural blood patch for postdural puncture headache management in postpartum patients: a retrospective review. Reg Anesth Pain Med. 2018;43:880–4. https://doi.org/10.1097/AAP.0000000000000840.
31. Hellams A, Sprague T, Saldanha C, Archambault M. Nitrous oxide for labor analgesia. JAAPA. 2018;31:41–4. https://doi.org/10.1097/01.JAA.0000527700.00698.8c.
32. Su F, Wei X, Chen X, et al. Clinical study on efficacy and safety of labor analgesia with inhalation of nitrous oxide in oxygen. Zhonghua Fu Chan Ke Za Zhi. 2002;37:584–7.
33. Yeo ST, Holdcroft A, Yentis SM, Stewart A, Bassett P. Analgesia with sevoflurane during labor: ii. Sevoflurane compared with Entonox for labor analgesia. Br J Anesth. 2007;98:110–5. https://doi.org/10.1093/bja/ael327.
34. Smith LA, Burns E, Cuthbert A. Parenteral opioids for maternal pain management in labor. Cochrane Database Syst Rev. 2018;6:CD007396. https://doi.org/10.1002/14651858.CD007396.pub3.

35. Czech I, Fuchs P, Fuchs A, Lorek M, Tobolska-Lorek D, Drosdzol-Cop A, et al. Pharmacological and non-pharmacological methods of labour pain relief-establishment of effectiveness and comparison. Int J Env Res Pub He. 2018;15:2792. https://doi.org/10.3390/ijerph15122792.
36. Mauricci M. Women in labor and the quality obstetric care system: the hole of evidence-based neuraxial analgesia. Minerva Anestesiol. 2009;75:99–101.
37. Lally JE, Thompson RG, MacPhail S, Exley C. Pain relief in labor: a qualitative study to determine how to support women to make decisions about pain relief in labor. BMC Pregnancy Childbirth. 2014;14:6. http://www.biomedcentral.com/1471-2393/146. Accessed 23 Jan 2020.
38. Lavender DT. Improving quality of care during labor and childbirth and in the immediate postnatal period. Best Pract Res Clin Obstet Gynaecol. 2016;36:57–67. https://doi.org/10.1016/j.bpogyn.206.05.011.
39. Tunçalp Ö, Were W, MacLennan C, Oladapo O, Gülmezoglu A, Bahl R. Quality of care for pregnant women and newborns-the WHO vision. BJOG. 2015;122:1045–9. https://doi.org/10.1111/1471-0528.13451.
40. Bell AF, Andersson E. The birth experience and women's postnatal depression: a systematic review. Midwifery. 2016;39:112–23. https://doi.org/10.1016/j.midw.2016.04.014.
41. Bell AF, Carter CS, Davis JM, Golding J, Adejumo O, Pyra M. Childbirth and symptoms of postpartum depression and anxiety: a prospective birth cohort study. Arch Womens Ment Health. 2016;19:219–27. https://doi.org/10.1007/s00737-015-0555-7.
42. Sentilhes L, Maillard F, Brun S, Madar H, Merlot B, Goffinet F. Risk factors for chronic post-traumatic stress disorder development one year after vaginal delivery: a prospective, observational study. Sci Rep. 2017;7:8724. https://doi.org/10.1038/s41598-017-09314-x.
43. Donate-Manzanares M, Rodríguez-Cano T, Gómez-Salgado J, Rodríguez-Almagro J, Hernández-Martínez A, Barrilero-Fernández E, et al. Quality of childbirth care in women undergoing labor. Satisfaction with care received and how it changes over time. J Clin Med. 2019;8:pii: E434. https://doi.org/10.3390/jcm8040434.
44. Floris L, Irion O, Courvoisier D. Influence of obstetrical events on satisfaction and anxiety during childbirth: a prospective longitudinal study. Psychol Health Med. 2017;22:969–77. https://doi.org/10.1080/13548506.2016.1258480.
45. Nystedt A, Hildingsson I. Women's and men's negative experience of child birth—a cross-sectional survey. Women Birth. 2018;31:103–9. https://doi.org/10.1016/j.wombi.2017.07.002.
46. Bennett A. The birth of a first child: do women's reports change over time? Birth. 1985;12:153–8. https://doi.org/10.1111/j.1523-536x.tb00954.x.
47. Simkin P. Just another day in a woman's life? Part II: nature and consistency of women's long-term memories of their first birth experiences. Birth. 1992;19:64–81. https://doi.org/10.1111/j.1523-536x.1992.tb00382.x.
48. Waldenström U. Women's memory of childbirth at two months and one year after the birth. Birth. 2003;30:248–54. https://doi.org/10.1046/j.1523-536x.2003,00254.x.
49. Angle P, Landy CK, Charles C, Yee J, Watson J, Kung R, et al. Phase 1 development of an index to measure the quality of neraxial labor analgesia: exploring the perspectives of child-bearing women. Can J Anesth. 2010;57:468–78. https://doi.org/10.1007/s12630-010-9289-1.
50. Clivatti J, Siddiqui N, Goel A, Shaw M, Crisan I, Carvalho JC. Quality of labor neuraxial analgesia and maternal satisfaction at a tertiary care teaching hospital: a prospective observational study. Can J Anesth. 2013;60:787–95. https://doi.org/10.1007/s12630-013-9976-9.
51. World Health Organization, "Obesity: preventing and managing the global epidemic. Report of a WHO consultation", WHO Technical Report Series 894, World Health Organization, Geneva, Switzerland; 2000.
52. Robson MS. Classification of cesarean sections. Fetal Matern Med Rev. 2001;12:23–39. https://doi.org/10.1016/j.ajog.2018.05.026.
53. Morton R, Burton AE, Kumar P, Hyett JA, Phipps H, McGeechan K et al. Cesarean delivery: trend in indications over three decades within a major city hospital network. Acta Obstet Gynecol Scand. 2020. https://doi.org/10.1111/aogs.13810.
54. Abdulrahman M, Abdullah SS, Alaani AFK, AlAbdool NH, Sherif FEY, Ahmed ZS, et al. Exploring obstetric interventions and stratified cesarean section rates using Robson clas-

sification in tertiary care hospitals in the United Arab Emirates. Rev Bras Ginecol Obstet. 2019;41:147–54. https://doi.org/10.1055/s-0038-1676524.
55. Voon HY, Suharjono HN, Shafie AA, Bujang MA. Carbetocin versus oxytocin for the prevention of postpartum hemorrhage; a meta-analysis of randomized controlled trials in cesarean deliveries. Taiwan J Obstet Gynecol. 2018;57:332–9. https://doi.org/10.1016/j.tjog.2018.04.002.
56. Dewan DM, Floyd HM, Thistlewood JM, Bogard TD, Spielman FJ. Sodium citrate pretreatment in elective cesarean section patients. Anesth Analg. 1985;64:34–7.
57. Lin CJ, Huang CL, Hsu HW, Chen TL. Prophylaxis against acid aspiration in regional anesthesia for elective cesarean section: a comparison between oral single-dose ranitidine, famotidine and omeprazole assessed with fiberoptic gastric aspiration. Acta Anaesthesiol Sin. 1996;34:179–84.
58. Pan PH, Moore CH. Comparing the efficacy of prophylactic metoclopramide, ondansetron, and placebo in cesarean section patients given epidural anesthesia. J Clin Anesth. 2001;13:430–5.
59. Lalic-Popovic M, Paunkovic J, Grujic Z, Golocorbin-Kon S, Vasovic V, Al-Salami H, et al. The effect of diabetes and hypertension on the placental permeation of the hydrophilic drug ranitidine. Placenta. 2016;48:144–50. https://doi.org/10.1016/j.placenta.2016.11.001.
60. Senel AC, Mergan F. Premedication with midazolam prior to cesarean section has no neonatal adverse effects. Braz J Anesthesiol. 2014;64:16–21. https://doi.org/10.1016/j.bjane.2012.08.005.
61. Fung BK, Gislefoss AJ, Ho ES. The sedative effect of intravenous injection of low dose midazolam during spinal anesthesia in cesarean section. Ma Zui Xue Za Zhi. 1992;30:159–62.
62. Bryson GL, Macneil R, Jeyaraj LM, Rosaeg OP. Small dose spinal bupivacaine for Cesarean delivery does not reduce hypotension but accelerates motor recovery. Can J Anaesth. 2007;54:531–7. https://doi.org/10.1007/BF03022316.
63. Arzola C, Wieczorek PM. Efficacy of low-dose bupivacaine in spinal anaesthesia for Caesarean delivery: systematic review and meta-analysis. Br J Anaesth. 2011;107:308–18. https://doi.org/10.1093/bja/aer200.
64. Bharti N, Madan R, Mohanty PR, Kaul HL. Intrathecal midazolam added to bupivacaine improves the duration and quality of spinal anaesthesia. Acta Anaesthesiol Scand. 2003;47:1101–5. https://doi.org/10.10034/j.1399-6576.2003.00186.x.
65. Kathirvel S, Sadasivam S. Effect of intrathecal ketamine added to bupivacaine for spinal anaesthesia. Anaesthesia. 2000;55:899–910.
66. Basuni AS. Addition of low-dose ketamine to midazolam and low-dose bupivacaine improves hemodynamics and postoperative analgesia during spinal anesthesia for cesarean section. J Anaesthesiol Clin Pharmacol. 2016;32:44–8. https://doi.org/10.4103/0970-9185.173322.
67. Crespo S, Dangelser G, Haller G. Intrathecal clonidine as an adjuvant for neuraxial anaesthesia during caesarean delivery: a systematic review and meta-analysis of randomized trials. Int J Obstet Anesth. 2017;32:64–76. https://doi.org/10.1016/j.ijoa.2017.06.009.
68. Wang YQ, Zhang XJ, Wang Y. Effect of intrathecal dexmedetomidine on cesarean section during spinal anesthesia: a meta-analysis of randomized trials. Drug Des Devel Ther. 2019;13:2933–9. https://doi.org/10.2147/DDDT.S207812.
69. Kinsella SM, Carvalho B, Dyer RA, Fernando R, McDonnell N, Mercier RJ, et al. International consensus statement of the management of hypotension with vasopressors during cesarean sections under spinal anesthesia. Anaesthesia. 2018;73:72–92. https://doi.org/10.1111/anae.14080.
70. Wang X, Mao M, Zhang SS, Wang ZH, Xu SQ, Shen XF. Bolus norepinephrine and phenylephrine for maternal hypotension during elective cesarean section with spinal anesthesia: a randomized, double-blinded study. Chin Med J (Engl). 2020;133:509–16. https://doi.org/10.1097/CM9.0000000000000621.
71. Xu S, Mao M, Zhang S, Qian R, Shen X, Shen J, et al. A randomized double-blind study comparing prophylactic norepinephrine and ephedrine infusion for preventing maternal spinal

hypotension during elective cesarean section under spinal anesthesia: a CONSORT-compliant article. Medicine. 2019;98:e18311. https://doi.org/10.1097/MD.0000000000018311.
72. Sumikura H, Niwa H, Sato M, Nakamoto T, Asai T, Hagihira S. Rethinking general anesthesia for cesarean section. J Anesth. 2016;30:268–73. https://doi.org/10.1007/s00540-015-2099-4.
73. Yildiz K, Dogru K, Dalgic H, Serin IS, Sezer Z, Madenoglu H, et al. Inhibitory effects of desflurane and sevoflurane on oxytocin-induced contractions of isolated pregnant human myometrium. Acta Anaesthesiol Scand. 2005;49:1355–9. https://doi.org/10.1111/j.1399-6576.2005.00804.x.
74. Ohashi Y, Sumikura H, Tateda T. Inhibitory effect of alprostadil against sevoflurane-induced myometrial relaxation in rats. J Anesth. 2007;21:361–6. https://doi.org/10.1007/s00540-007-0536-8.
75. Bogod D, Plaat F. Be wary of awareness--lessons from NAP5 for obstetric anaesthetists. Int J Obstet Anesth. 2015;24:1–4. https://doi.org/10.1016/j.ijoa.2014.12.006.
76. John R, Ranjan RV, Ramachandran TR, George SK. Analgesic efficacy of transverse abdominal plane block after elective cesarean delivery - bupivacaine with fentanyl versus bupivacaine alone: a randomized, double-blind controlled clinical trial. Anesth Essays Res. 2017;11:181–4. https://doi.org/10.4103/0259-1162.186864.
77. Abdallah FW, Halpern SH, Margarido CB. Transversus abdominis plane block for postoperative analgesia after Caesarean delivery performed under spinal anaesthesia? A systematic review and meta-analysis. Br J Anaesth. 2012;109(5):679–87. https://doi.org/10.1093/bja/aes279.
78. Acharya R, Baksi R, Mohapatra P. Comparative analysis of duration of postoperative analgesia between levobupivacaine and levobupivacaine with clonidine after ultrasound-guided transversus abdominis plane block in patients undergoing lower segment cesarean section. Anesth Essays Res. 2018;12:943–8. https://doi.org/10.4103/aer.AER_163_18.
79. Weiss E, Jolly C, Dumoulin JL, et al. Convulsions in 2 patients after bilateral ultrasound-guided transversus abdominis plane blocks for cesarean analgesia. Reg Anesth Pain Med. 2014;39:248–51. https://doi.org/10.1097/AAP.0000000000000088.
80. Salama ER. Ultrasound guided bilateral quadratus lumborum block vs. intrathecal morphine for postoperative analgesia after cesarean section: a randomized controlled trial [published online ahead of print, 2019 Mar 8]. Korean J Anesthesiol. 2019. https://doi.org/10.4097/kja.d.18.00269.

Chapter 50
Cesarean Delivery

Roberto Magliano de Morais Filho and Roberto Magliano de Morais

Introduction

Cesarean delivery is defined as the delivery of a fetus through surgical incisions made through the abdominal wall (laparotomy) and the uterine wall (hysterotomy). This definition is not applied to removal of the fetus from the abdominal cavity in the case of uterine rupture or with abdominal pregnancy. Rarely, hysterotomy is performed in a woman who has just died or in whom death is expected soon—postmortem or perimortem cesarean delivery.In some instances, abdominal hysterectomy is indicated following delivery. When performed at the time of cesarean delivery, the operation is termed cesarean hysterectomy (Williams Obstetrics 25 th Edition, p1247 Chap. 30).

In 2014, 32.2% of women who gave birth in the United States did so by cesarean delivery [1]. The rapid increase in cesarean birth rates from 1996 to 2014 without clear evidence of concomitant decreases in maternal or neonatal morbidity or mortality raises significant concern that cesarean delivery is overused. The most common indications for primary cesarean delivery include labor dystocia, abnormal or indeterminate fetal heart rate tracing, fetal malpresentation, multiple gestation, and suspected fetal macrosomia. Safe reduction of the primary cesarean delivery rate will require different approaches for these indications, as well as others. Increasing women's access to nonmedical interventions during labor has also been shown to reduce cesarean birth rates. External cephalic version for breech presentation and a trial of labor for women with twin gestations when the first twin is in cephalic presentation are examples of interventions that can help to safely lower the primary cesarean delivery rate [2]. A practice bulletin from the American College of

R. M. de Morais Filho
Faculdade de Medicina Nova Esperança, Joao Pessoa, Paraiba, Brazil

R. M. de Morais (✉)
Universidade Federal da Paraiba, Joao Pessoa, Paraiba, Brazil

© Springer Nature Switzerland AG 2022
R. A. Moreira de Sá, E. B. d. Fonseca (eds.), *Perinatology*,
https://doi.org/10.1007/978-3-030-83434-0_50

Obstetricians and Gynecologists (ACOG) recommends that all eligible women with breech presentations who are near term should be offered external cephalic version (ECV) to decrease the overall rate of cesarean delivery [3, 4].

ACOG/SMFM Guidelines for the Prevention of Primary Cesarean Delivery

The American College of Obstetricians and Gynecologists (ACOG) and the Society for Maternal-Fetal Medicine (SMFM) released joint guidelines for the safe prevention of primary cesarean delivery. These include the following [5, 6]:

- Prolonged latent (early)-phase labor should be permitted.
- The start of active-phase labor can be defined as cervical dilation of 6 cm, rather than 4 cm.
- In the active phase, more time should be permitted for labor to progress.
- Multiparous women should be allowed to push for 2 or more hours and primiparous women for 3 or more hours; pushing may be allowed to continue for even longer periods in some cases, as when epidural anesthesia is administered.
- Techniques to aid vaginal delivery, such as the use of forceps, should be employed.
- Patients should be encouraged to avoid excessive weight gain during pregnancy.
- Access to nonmedical interventions during labor, such as continuous support during labor and delivery, should be increased.
- External cephalic version should be performed for breech presentation.
- Women with twin gestations should, if the first twin is in cephalic presentation, be permitted a trial of labor.

Indications

Cesarean deliveries were initially performed to separate the mother and the fetus in an attempt to save the fetus of a moribund patient. They subsequently developed to resolve maternal or fetal complications not amenable to vaginal delivery, either for mechanical limitations or to temporize delivery for maternal or fetal benefit.

The leading indications for cesarean delivery (85%) are previous cesarean delivery, breech presentation, dystocia, and fetal distress [7].

Maternal indications for cesarean delivery include the following:

- Previous classic cesarean delivery
- Obstructive lesions in the lower genital tract, including malignancies, large vulvovaginal condylomas, obstructive vaginal septa, and leiomyomas of the lower uterine segment that interfere with engagement of the fetal head

- Pelvic abnormalities that preclude engagement or interfere with descent of the fetal presentation in labor
- Certain cardiac conditions that preclude normal Valsalva done by patients during a vaginal delivery [8]

Fetal indications for cesarean delivery include the following:

- Situations in which neonatal morbidity and mortality could be decreased by the prevention of trauma
- Malpresentations (e.g., preterm breech presentations, non-frank breech term fetuses)
- Certain congenital malformations or skeletal disorders
- Infection
- Prolonged acidemia

A fetus in a nonvertex presentation is at increased risk for trauma, cord prolapse, and head entrapment. Malpresentation includes preterm breech presentations and non-frank breech term fetuses.

The decision to proceed with a cesarean delivery for the term frank breech singleton fetus has been challenged. Although most practitioners will always perform a cesarean delivery in this situation, ACOG has left open the option to consider a breech delivery under the appropriate circumstances, including a practitioner experienced in the evaluation and management of labor and skilled in the delivery of the breech fetus [22]. Some state maternal care collaborative agencies are even implementing tools to decrease the likelihood of cesarean section in the instance of a breech presentation, with guidelines recommending the formation of a team in the hospital that is trained and confortable with breach and operative deliveries [32].

If a patient is diagnosed with a fetal malpresentation (i.e., breech or transverse lie) after 36 weeks, the option for an external cephalic version is offered to try to convert the fetus to a vertex lie, thus allowing an attempt at a vaginal delivery. An external cephalic version is usually attempted at 36–38 weeks with studies underway to establish the use of performing external cephalic version at 34 weeks' gestational age.

Ultrasonography is performed to confirm a breech presentation. If the fetus is still in a nonvertex presentation, an intravenous (IV) line is started, and the baby is monitored with an external fetal heart rate monitor prior to the procedure to confirm well-being. With a reassuring fetal heart rate tracing, the version is attempted.

An external cephalic version involves trying to externally manipulate the fetus into a vertex presentation. This is accomplished with ultrasonographic guidance to ascertain fetal lie. An attempt is made to manipulate the fetus through either a "forward roll" or "backward roll." The overall chance of success is approximately 60% [33]. Some practitioners administer an epidural to the patient before attempting version, and others may give the patient a dose of subcutaneous terbutaline (a betamimetic used for tocolysis) just before the attempt.

Factors that influence the success of an attempted version include multiparity, a posterior placenta, and normal amniotic fluid with a normally grown fetus. In addition, to be a candidate, a patient must be eligible for an attempted vaginal delivery.

Contraindications to external cephalic version include oligohydramnios, intrauterine growth restriction with abnormal Doppler or fetal heart tracing, major uterine anomalies, antepartum hemorrhage, abnormal fetal heart tracing, multiparity, and rupture of membrane [34].

Relative contraindications include poor fetal growth or the presence of congenital anomalies. Risks of an external cephalic version include rupture of membranes, labor, fetal injury, and the need for an emergent cesarean delivery due to placental abruption. A recent review reported a severe complication rate of 0.24% and a cesarean section rate secondary to complications of 0.34% [33].

If the version is successful, the patient is placed on a fetal monitor in close proximity to the labor and delivery unit or in the labor and delivery unit itself. If fetal heart rate testing is reassuring, the patient is discharged to await spontaneous labor, or she may be induced if the fetus is of an appropriate gestational age or the patient has a favorable cervix.

The first twin in a nonvertex presentation is an indication for a cesarean delivery, as are higher order multiples (triplets or greater). A large body of literature supports both outright cesarean delivery and spontaneous breech delivery or extraction of the second twin.

The decision is made in conjunction with the patient after appropriate counseling regarding the risks and benefits as well as under the supervision of a physician experienced in the management of the labor and delivery of a breech fetus [35]. Evidence suggests that the rate of severe complications of the second breech twin is independent of the mode of delivery [36].

Several congenital anomalies are controversial indications for cesarean delivery; these include fetal neural tube defects (to avoid sac rupture), particularly defects that are larger than 5–6 cm in diameter. One study noted no difference in long-term motor or neurologic outcomes [37]. Some authors noted no relationship between mode of delivery and infant outcomes [38], while others have advocated cesarean delivery of all infants with a neural tube defect [39].

Cesarean delivery is indicated in certain cases of hydrocephalus with an enlarged biparietal diameter and some skeletal dysplasias such as type III osteogenesis imperfecta.

Whether or not an outright cesarean delivery should be performed in the setting of a fetal abdominal wall defect (e.g., gastroschisis or omphalocele) remains controversial. Most reviews agree that cesarean is not advantageous unless the liver is extruded, which is a very rare event [40–42]. The overall incidence of cesarean delivery in this group of patients is probably due to an increased incidence of intrauterine growth retardation and fetal distress prior to or in labor.

In the setting of a nonremediable and nonreassuring pattern remote from delivery, a cesarean delivery is recommended to prevent a mixed or metabolic acidemia that could potentially cause significant morbidity and mortality. Electronic fetal monitoring was used in 85% of labors in the United States in 2002 [43]. Its use has increased the cesarean delivery rate as much as 40% [44]. This has occurred without a decrease in the cerebral palsy or perinatal death rate [45].

ACOG has recommended that any facility providing obstetric care has the capability of performing a cesarean delivery within 30 minutes of the decision. Despite this recommendation, a decision to delivery time of more than 30 minutes is not necessarily associated with a negative neonatal outcome [46].

Among patients with first-episode genital herpes infection, the risk of maternal-fetal transmission is 33 times higher than with recurrent outbreaks. The largest population-based study reported that for primary infection, the risk of transmission to the newborn was 35%, compared with a 2% risk for recurrent infection. Among patients with culture-positive herpes, the transmission rate with vaginal delivery was seven times that with cesarean delivery.

Currently, all patients with active or symptomatic herpes infection are candidates for cesarean delivery [47]. Neonatal infection with herpes can lead to significant morbidity and mortality, especially with a primary outbreak. With recurrent outbreaks, the risk to the neonate is reduced by the presence of maternal antibodies. Unfortunately, not all women with active viral shedding can be detected upon admission to labor and delivery.

Treatment of women with HIV infections has undergone tremendous change in the past few years. Women with a viral count above 1000 should be offered cesarean delivery at 38 weeks (or earlier if they go into labor). In women who are being treated with highly active antiretroviral therapy (HAART), cesarean delivery (before labor or without prolonged rupture of membranes) appears to further lower the risk for neonatal transmission, particularly among those with viral counts above 1000.

Among patients with low or undetectable viral counts, the evidence supporting a benefit is not as clear; nevertheless, the patient should be given the option of a cesarean delivery.

Maternal and Fetal Indications

Indications for cesarean delivery that benefit both the mother and the fetus include the following:

- Abnormal placentation
- Abnormal labor due to cephalopelvic disproportion
- Situations in which labor is contraindicated: prior classic cesarean delivery (vertical incision), prior extensive uterine myomectomy, and placenta previa

In the presence of a placenta previa (i.e., the placenta covering the internal cervical os), attempting vaginal delivery places both the mother and the fetus at risk for hemorrhagic complications. This complication has actually increased as a result of the increased incidence of repeat cesarean deliveries, which is a risk factor for placenta previa and placenta accreta. Both placenta previa and placenta accreta carry increased morbidity related to hemorrhage and need for hysterectomy [29, 49, 50].

Cephalopelvic disproportion can be suspected on the basis of possible macrosomia or an arrest of labor despite augmentation. Many cases diagnosed as cephalopelvic disproportion are the result of a primary or secondary arrest of dilatation or arrest of descent. Predicting true primary or secondary arrest of descent due to cephalopelvic disproportion is best assessed by sagittal suture overlap, but not lambdoid suture overlap, particularly where progress is poor in a trial of labor [51].

Continuing to attempt a vaginal delivery in this setting increases the risk of infectious complications to both mother and fetus from prolonged rupture of membranes [52]. Less often, maternal hemorrhagic and fetal metabolic consequences occur from a uterine rupture, especially among patients with a previous cesarean delivery [16]. Vaginal delivery can also increase the risk of maternal trauma and fetal trauma (e.g., Erb-Duchenne or Klumpke palsy and metabolic acidosis) from a shoulder dystocia [53, 54].

Among women who have a uterine scar (prior transmural myomectomy or cesarean delivery by high vertical incision), a cesarean delivery should be performed prior to the onset of labor to prevent the risk of uterine rupture, which is approximately 4–10% [16].

Relative maternal indications include conditions in which the increasing intrathoracic pressure generated by Valsalva maneuvers could lead to maternal complications. These include left heart valvular stenosis, dilated aortic valve root, certain cerebral arteriovenous malformations (AVMs) [8], and recent retinal detachment. Women who have previously undergone vaginal or perineal reparative surgery (e.g., colporrhaphy or repair of major anal involvement from inflammatory bowel disease) also benefit from cesarean delivery to avoid damage to the previous surgical repair.

No clear evidence supports planned cesarean delivery for extreme maternal obesity. A prospective cohort study from the United Kingdom included women with a body mass index of 50 kg/m^2 or more and noted possible increased shoulder dystocia (3% vs. 0%) but found no significant differences in anesthetic, postnatal, or neonatal complications between women who underwent planned vaginal delivery and those who underwent planned caesarean delivery [25]. However, recent studies indicate that obese and extremely obese women have an increased odds ratio of having a cesarean section, 2.05 and 2.89 compared with normal weight women [26].

Dystocia in labor (labor dystocia) is a very commonly cited indication for cesarean delivery, but it is not specific. Dystocia is classified as a protraction disorder or as an arrest disorder. These can be primary or secondary disorders. Most dystocias are caused by abnormalities of the power (uterine contractions), the passage (maternal pelvis), or the passenger (the fetus) [27].

When a diagnosis of dystocia in labor is made, the indication should be detailed according to the previous classification (i.e., primary or secondary disorder, arrest or protraction disorder, or a combination of the above). For further information, see Abnormal Labor.

Recently, debate has arisen over the option of elective cesarean delivery on maternal request (CDMR). Evidence shows that it is reasonable to inform the pregnant woman requesting a cesarean delivery of the associated risks and benefits for the current and any subsequent pregnancies. The clinician's role should be to provide the best possible evidence-based counseling to the woman and to respect her autonomy and decision-making capabilities when considering route of delivery [28].

Contraindications

There are few contraindications to performing a cesarean delivery. In some circumstances, a cesarean delivery should be avoided, such as the following:

- When maternal status may be compromised (e.g., mother has severe pulmonary disease).
- If the fetus has a known karyotypic abnormality or known congenital anomaly that may lead to death (anencephaly).

Cesarean Delivery on Maternal Request

Controversy exists regarding elective cesarean delivery on maternal request (CDMR). Reasons for the request include pelvic floor protection, convenience, fear of childbirth, and reduced risk of fetal injury. The 2013 American College of Obstetricians and Gynecologists (ACOG) Committee on Obstetric Practice [9] and 2006 National Institutes of Health (NIH) consensus committee [10] determined that the evidence supporting this concept was not conclusive and that more research is needed.

Both committees provided the following recommendations regarding CDMR [9, 10]:

- Unless there are maternal or fetal indications for cesarean delivery, vaginal delivery should be recommended.
- CDMR should not be performed before 39 weeks' gestation without verifying fetal lung maturity (due to a potential risk of respiratory problems for the baby).
- CDMR is not recommended for women who want more children (due to the increased risk for placenta previa/accreta and gravid hysterectomy with each cesarean delivery).
- The unavailability of effective analgesia should not be a determinant for CDMR.

The NIH consensus panel on CDMR also noted the following [10]:

- CDMR has a potential benefit of decreased risk of hemorrhage for the mother and decreased risk of birth injuries for the baby.
- CDMR requires individualized counseling by the practitioner of the potential risks and benefits of both vaginal and cesarean delivery.

- CDMR is associated with a longer maternal hospital stay and increasing risk of placenta previa and placenta accreta with each successive cesarean.
- CDMR has a potential risk of respiratory problems for the baby.

The NIH further noted that the procedure requires individualized counseling by the practitioner of the potential risks and benefits of both vaginal and cesarean delivery, and it should not be motivated by the unavailability of effective pain management [10].

Detractors of CDMR argue that the premise of cesarean on request applies to a very small portion of the population and that it should not be routinely offered on ethical grounds [30]. The emerging consensus is that a randomized prospective study is required to address this issue [31].

Preoperative Management

Guidelines recommend a minimum preoperative fasting time of at least 2 hours from clear liquids, 6 hours from a light meal, and 8 hours from a regular meal [11]. However, patients are usually asked not to eat anything for 12 hours prior to the procedure.

Laboratory Testing

The following laboratory studies may be obtained prior to cesarean delivery:

- Complete blood count
- Blood type and screen, crossmatch
- Screening tests for human immunodeficiency virus, hepatitis B, syphilis
- Coagulation studies (e.g., prothrombin and activated partial thromboplastin times, fibrinogen level)

Imaging Studies

In labor and delivery, document fetal position and estimated fetal weight. Although ultrasonography is commonly used to estimate fetal weight, a prospective study reported the sensitivity of clinical and ultrasonographic prediction of macrosomia, respectively, as 68% and 58%.

The following are also included in preoperative management:

- Placement of an intravenous (IV) line
- Infusion of IV fluids (e.g., lactated Ringer solution or saline with 5% dextrose)

- Placement of a Foley catheter (to drain the bladder and to monitor urine output)
- Placement of an external fetal monitor and monitors for the patient's blood pressure, pulse, and oxygen saturation
- Preoperative antibiotic prophylaxis (decreases risk of endometritis after elective cesarean delivery by 76%, regardless of the type of cesarean delivery [emergent or elective]) [12]
- Evaluation by the surgeon and the anesthesiologist

Skin Preparation

Before anesthesia, the surgeon should evaluate the site of the intended skin incision. The intended area need not be shaved automatically unless the hair will interfere with reapproximation of the skin edges. If the hair is to be removed, it should be clipped immediately before surgery. Shaving appears to be associated with a slightly increased risk for infection [61].

Anesthesia

The anesthesiologist will review regional anesthetic techniques. Regional anesthesia is used for 95% of planned cesarean deliveries in the United States. The three main regional anesthetic techniques are spinal, epidural, and combined spinal epidural [63]. Every patient is evaluated for general anesthesia in case an emergency should arise and establishment of an airway becomes necessary.

A review by Afolabi et al. found that patients undergoing local anesthetic techniques were found to have a significantly lower difference between preoperative and postoperative hematocrit levels when compared with patients undergoing general anesthesia. Women having either an epidural anesthesia or spinal have a lower estimated maternal blood loss [64].

After placement of the regional anesthetic, monitor the fetus until an adequate surgical level has been achieved. When the level of anesthesia is adequate, the skin can be prepared either with an iodine scrub or with 4% chlorhexidine. Before making the initial incision, grasp the patient's skin bilaterally with an instrument such as an Allis clamp at the level of and above the incision to confirm anesthesia up to the level of T4. This ensures that the anesthetic level is appropriate.

The dermatomal level of anesthesia required for cesarean delivery is higher than that required for labor analgesia. A sensory block to the tenth thoracic dermatome is sufficient to achieve analgesia for labor, but for cesarean, the anesthetic level must be extended cephalad to at least the fourth thoracic dermatome to prevent nociceptive input from the peritoneal manipulation.

In patients who require a cesarean delivery secondary to a problem arising during labor, the preparation follows essentially the same steps previously outlined. The only major variation occurs if a patient requires general anesthesia prior to the procedure. In that situation, before intubation, the patient should be prepped and draped and the surgical team should be ready to begin as soon as the patient's airway is secured.

The use of chlorhexidine solution rather than a povidone iodine solution is associated with a decrease risk of both superficial and deep wound infection [62].

Cesarean Delivery

The technique for cesarean delivery includes the following:

- Laparotomy via midline infraumbilical, vertical, or transverse (e.g., Pfannenstiel, Maylard, Joel Cohen) incision.
- Hysterotomy via a transverse (Monroe-Kerr) or vertical (e.g., Kronig, DeLee) incision.
- Fetal delivery.
- Uterine repair.
- Closure.
- If patient has been counseled and consented prior to the procedure, an IUD can be placed prior to the repair of the hysterotomy, or a Levonorgestrel subdermal implant can be placed in the patient's arm at this time.

Technique

With minor variations, surgical performance of cesarean delivery is comparable worldwide. Most steps are founded on evidence-based data, and these have been reviewed by Dahlke and associates (2013) [122]. As with all surgery, a clear understanding of relevant anatomy is essential, and this is described and illustrated below.

Laparotomy

In obstetrics, a suprapubic transverse incision or a midline vertical one is chosen for laparotomy. Transverse abdominal entry is by either Pfannenstiel or Maylard incisions. Of all these, the Pfannenstiel incision is selected most frequently for cesarean delivery.

Transverse incisions follow Langer lines of skin tension. Thus, compared with vertical ones, Pfannenstiel incisions offer superior cosmesis and lower incisional hernia rates. Use of the Pfannenstiel incision, however, is often discouraged for cases in which a large operating space is essential or in which access to the upper abdomen may be needed. With transverse incisions, because of the layers created during incision of the internal and external oblique aponeuroses, purulent fluid can collect between these. Therefore, some favor a midline vertical incision for cases with high infection risks. Emergent entry is typically faster with vertical incision during primary and repeat cesarean delivery. Last, neurovascular structures, which include the ilioinguinal and iliohypogastric nerves and superficial and inferior epigastric vessels, are often encountered with transverse incisions. Logically, bleeding, wound hematoma, and neurological disruption may more frequently complicate these incisions compared with vertical ones. The best incision for the morbidly obese parturient is unclear. Our preference with very obese women is a periumbilical midline vertical incision.

The Maylard incision differs mainly from the Pfannenstiel in that the bellies of the rectus abdominis muscle are transected horizontally to widen the operating space. It is technically more difficult due to its required muscle cutting and isolation and ligation of the inferior epigastric arteries, which lie laterally to these muscle bellies.

Once access is gained, metal handheld retractors provide exposure for hysterotomy. A few small randomized studies have evaluated postcesarean wound infection rates with a disposable plastic barrier retractor. Results showing benefit are contradictory.

Transverse Incisions

With the Pfannenstiel incision, the skin and subcutaneous tissue are incised using a low, transverse, slightly curvilinear incision. This is made at the level of the pubic hairline, which is typically 3 cm above the superior border of the symphysis pubis. The incision is extended laterally sufficiently to accommodate delivery—12 to 15 cm is typical.

Sharp dissection is continued through the subcutaneous layer to the fascia. The superficial epigastric vessels can usually be identified halfway between the skin and fascia, several centimeters from the midline, and are coagulated. If lacerated, these may be suture ligated with 3–0 plain gut suture or coagulated with an electrosurgical blade.

The fascia is then incised sharply at the midline. The anterior abdominal fascia is typically composed of two visible layers, the aponeurosis from the external oblique muscle and a fused layer containing aponeuroses of the internal oblique and transverse abdominis muscles. Ideally, the two layers are individually incised during lateral extension of the fascial incision. The inferior epigastric vessels usually lie outside the lateral border of the rectus abdominis muscle and beneath the fused aponeuroses of the internal oblique and transverse abdominis muscles. Thus, although infrequently required, extension of the fascial incision further laterally may cut these vessels. With extension, these vessels are best identified and coagulated or ligated to prevent bleeding and vessel retraction.

Once the fascia is incised, the inferior fascial edge is grasped with Kocher clamps and elevated by an assistant as the operator separates the fascial sheath from the underlying rectus abdominis muscle either bluntly or sharply until the superior border of the symphysis pubis is reached. Next, the superior fascial edge is grasped and again, separation of fascia from the rectus muscle is completed. Blood vessels coursing between the sheath and muscles are clamped, cut, and ligated, or they are coagulated with an electrosurgery blade. Meticulous hemostasis is imperative to lower rates of incisional hematoma and infection. The fascial separation progresses cephalad and laterally to create a semicircular area above the transverse incision with a radius of approximately 8 cm. This will vary depending on fetal size. The rectus abdominis and pyramidalis muscles are then separated in the midline, first superiorly and then inferiorly, by sharp and blunt dissection to expose the transversalis fascia and peritoneum.

The transversalis fascia and preperitoneal fat are bluntly dissected away to reach the underlying peritoneum. The peritoneum near the upper end of the incision is opened carefully, either bluntly or by elevating it with two hemostats placed approximately 2 cm apart. This upper site lowers cystotomy risks. The tented fold of peritoneum between the clamps is examined and palpated to ensure that omentum, bowel, or bladder is not adjacent. The peritoneum is then incised. The peritoneal incision is extended superiorly to the upper pole of the fascial dissection and downward to just above the peritoneal reflection over the bladder. Importantly, in women with prior intraabdominal surgery, including cesarean delivery, omentum or bowel may be adhered to the undersurface of the peritoneum. In women with obstructed labor, the bladder may be pushed cephalad almost to the level of the umbilicus.

Midline Vertical Incision

This incision begins 2–3 cm above the superior margin of the symphysis. It should be sufficiently long to allow fetal delivery, and 12–15 cm is typical. Sharp or electrosurgical blade dissection through the subcutaneous layers ultimately exposes the anterior rectus sheath. A small opening is made sharply with scalpel in the upper half of the linea alba. Placement here helps avoid potential cystotomy. Index and middle fingers are placed beneath the fascia to elevate it, and the fascial incision is extended first superiorly and then inferiorly with scissors. Midline separation of the rectus muscles and pyramidalis muscles and peritoneal entry are similar to those with the Pfannenstiel incision.

Hysterotomy

Most often, the lower uterine segment is incised transversely as described by Kerr in 1921. Occasionally, vertical incision confined solely to the lower uterine segment may be elected (Krönig 1912). In contrast, a classical incision begins as a low-vertical incision, which is then extended cephalad into the active portion of the uterine corpus. Last, a fundal or even posterior incision may be selected for cases with placental accrete syndromes.

Low-Transverse Cesarean Incision

For most cesarean deliveries, this incision is preferred. Compared with a classical incision, it is easier to repair, causes less incision-site bleeding, and promotes less bowel or omentum adherence to the myometrial incision. Located in the inactive segment, it also is less likely to rupture during a subsequent pregnancy.

Before any hysterotomy, the surgeon palpates the fundus to identify degrees of uterine rotation. The uterus may be rotated so that one round ligament is more anterior and closer to the midline. In such cases, the uterus can be manually reoriented and held to permit centering of the incision. This avoids incision extension into and laceration of the adjacent uterine artery. A moist sponge may be used to pack protruding bowel away from the operative field.

The reflection of peritoneum at the upper margin of the bladder and overlying the lower uterine segment is grasped in the midline with forceps and incised transversely with scissors (Fig. 50.1). Following this initial incision, scissors are inserted between peritoneum and lower uterine segment. Open scissors are pushed laterally from the midline on each side. This transverse peritoneal incision extends almost the full length of the lower uterine segment. As the lateral margin on each side is approached, the scissors are directed slightly cephalad (Fig. 50.2). The lower edge of peritoneum is elevated, and the bladder is gently separated from the underlying lower uterine segment with blunt or sharp dissection within this vesicouterine space (Fig. 50.3). This bladder flap creation effectively moves the bladder away from the planned hysterotomy site. It also helps prevent bladder laceration if an unintended inferior hysterotomy extension occurs during fetal delivery.

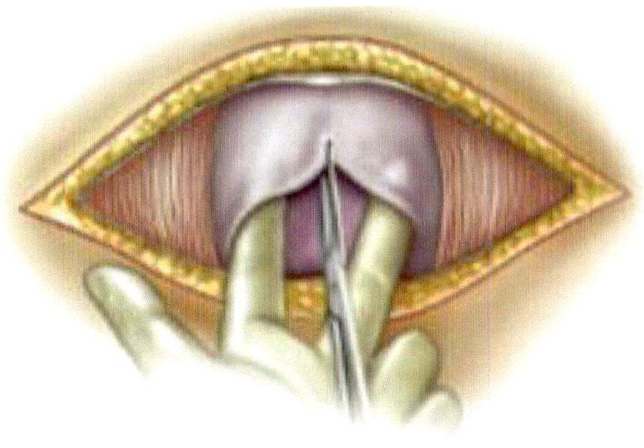

Fig. 50.1 Longitudinal parietal peritoneal incision

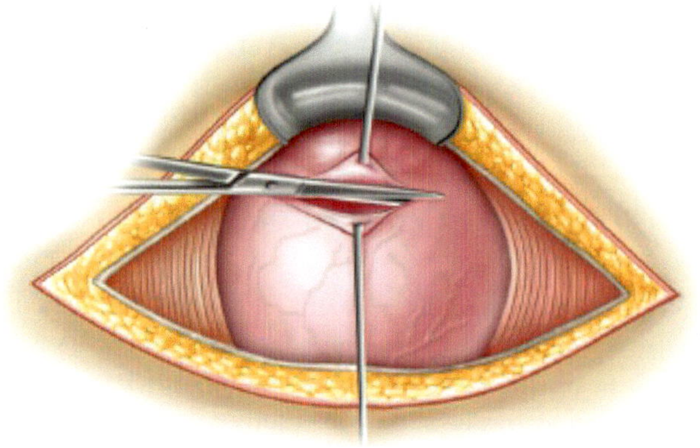

Fig. 50.2 Traverse visceral peritoneal incision on the upper margin of the bladder

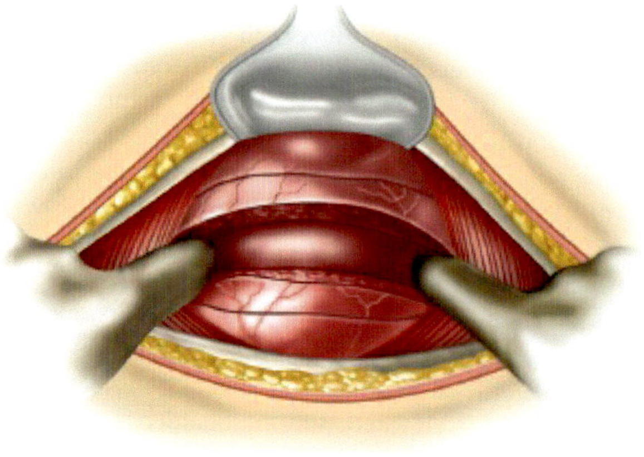

Fig. 50.3 Lower uterine segment hysterotomy by Kocher and Kelly scissors or scalp, followed by bidigital blunt dissection

Uterine Incision

The uterus can be incised by various techniques. Each is initiated by using a scalpel to transversely incise the exposed lower uterine segment for 1–2 cm in the midline. Repetitive shallow strokes avoid fetal laceration. As the myometrium thins, a fingertip can then bluntly enter the uterine cavity. Once the uterus is opened, the hysterotomy is lengthened by simply spreading the incision, using lateral and slightly upward pressure applied with each index finger. Some evidence also supports widening the lower uterine segment incision instead with fingers pulling in opposition in a cephalocaudal direction.

The uterine incision is made large enough to allow delivery of the fetus without tearing into the uterine vessels that course along the lateral uterine margins. If the placenta is encountered in the incision line, it must be either detached or incised. Placental function is thereby compromised, and thus delivery is performed expeditiously.

Delivery of the Fetus

In a cephalic presentation, a hand is slipped into the uterine cavity between the symphysis and fetal head. The head is elevated gently with the fingers and palm through the incision.

After birth, to promote breastfeeding, our practice recommends skin-to-skin contact between newborn and mother in the delivery room following cesarean delivery.

An intravenous infusion containing two ampules or 20 units of oxytocin per liter of crystalloid is infused at 10 mL/min. Some prefer higher infusion dosages; however, nondilute boluses are avoided because of associated hypotension. Once the uterus contracts satisfactorily, the rate can be reduced.

Uterine Repair

Before hysterotomy closure, previously clamped large vessels may be ligated separately or incorporated within the running incision closure. One angle of the uterine incision is grasped to stabilize and maneuver the incision. The uterine incision is then closed with one layer of continuous 0- or no. 1 absorbable suture. Chromic catgut suture is used by many, but some prefer synthetic delayed-absorbable polyglactin 910 (Vicryl). In subsequent pregnancy, neither suture type has been shown superior by mitigating against greater rates of adverse pregnancy outcomes such as uterine incision rupture. Single-layer closure is typically faster and is not associated with higher rates of infection or transfusion [114–116].

Abdominal Closure

The paracolic gutters and cul-de-sac are gently suctioned of blood and amniotic fluid.

Prior to abdominal closure, correct sponge and instrument counts are verified. The rectus abdominis muscle bellies are allowed to fall into place. With significant diastasis, the rectus muscles may be approximated with one or two figure-of-eight sutures of 0 or no. 1 chromic gut suture. The overlying rectus fascia is closed by a continuous, nonlocking technique with a delayed-absorbable suture.

The subcutaneous tissue usually need not be closed if it is less than 2 cm thick. With thicker layers, however, closure is recommended to minimize seroma and hematoma formation, which can lead to wound infection and/or disruption. One recent meta-analysis found lower rates of seroma formation and of developing any wound complication with closure, but hematoma and wound infection rates were unaffected.

Postoperative Management

See the list below:

- Routine postoperative assessment.
- Monitoring of vital signs, urine output, and amount of vaginal bleeding.
- Palpation of the fundus.
- IV fluids; advance to oral diet as appropriate; early feeding has been shown to shorten hospital stay [14].
- IV or intramuscular (IM) analgesia if patient did not receive a long-acting analgesic or had general anesthesia; analgesia is usually not needed if patient received regional anesthesia, with/without a long-acting analgesic.
- Ambulation on postoperative day 1; advance as tolerated.
- If patient plans to breastfeed, initiate within a few hours after delivery; if patient plans to bottle-feed, she may use a tight bra or breast binder in the postoperative period.
- Discharge on postoperative day 2–4, if no complications [15].
- Discuss contraception as well as refraining from intercourse for 4–6 weeks' postpartum, unless the patient had LARC placed at the time of the procedure [13].

Complications

See the list below:

- Approximately twofold increase in maternal mortality and morbidity with cesarean delivery relative to a vaginal delivery [16]: partly related to the procedure itself and partly related to conditions that may have led to needing to perform a cesarean delivery
- Infection (e.g., postpartum endomyometritis, fascial dehiscence, wound, urinary tract)
- Thromboembolic disease (e.g., deep venous thrombosis, septic pelvic thrombophlebitis)
- Anesthetic complications
- Surgical injury (e.g., uterine lacerations; bladder, bowel, ureteral injuries)
- Uterine atony
- Delayed return of bowel function
- Fascial dehiscence

Reasons for Cesarean Rates

The rate of cesarean sections around the world is increasing at an alarming rate, which can contribute to maternal and fetal morbidity when not correctly indicated.

Since 1990, C-sections have more than tripled from about 6 percent of all births to 21 percent, and there are no signs of slowing down. C-sections now outnumber vaginal deliveries in parts of Southeast Europe, Latin America, and China. Even in poor countries, the rates can be extremely high at clinics. For example, in Bangladesh, less than 60 percent of births occur at a clinic, but when they do, about 65 percent of them are C-sections.

The rates can be even higher in private clinics. For example, in Brazil, 80–90 percent of births in private clinics are now C-sections, compared with about 30–40 percent of births in public hospitals.

Such high rates are due mainly to an increase of elective C-sections, among other reasons, as follows:

Decreased frequency of operative vaginal delivery; delay in childbirth and reduced parity; decreased rate of vaginal birth after cesarean delivery; assisted reproductive technology is more widely used than in the past and is associated with greater cesarean delivery rates; decrease in the rate of vaginal breech delivery; decreased perinatal mortality with cesarean delivery; widespread use of electronic fetal monitoring, with concern for an abnormal or nonreassuring fetal heart rate testing; increased incidence of obesity; and fear of malpractice litigation [19].

The risk of having a cesarean delivery is higher in nulliparous patients, and, with increasing maternal age, the risk for cesarean delivery is increased secondary to medical complications such as diabetes and preeclampsia.

By 1985, almost 85% of all breech presentations (3% of term fetuses) were delivered by cesarean. In 2001, a multicenter and multinational prospective study determined that the safest mode of delivery for a breech presentation was cesarean delivery [20]. This study has been criticized for differences in the standards of care among the study centers that do not allow a standard recommendation [30].

The most recent recommendation from the American College of Obstetricians and Gynecologists (ACOG) regarding breech delivery is that planned vaginal delivery may be reasonable under hospital-specific protocol guidelines for both eligibility and labor management [22]. This may lead to a small decrease in breech delivery rates, but the overwhelming majority of cases will probably continue to be delivered by elective cesarean.

A cluster-randomized controlled trial by Chaillet et al. reported a significant but small reduction in the rate of cesarean delivery. The benefit was driven by the effect of the intervention in low-risk pregnancies [23, 24].

Complication Prevention

Perinatal outcome is influenced by gestational age at delivery, the presence of congenital abnormalities and growth abnormalities, and the indication for delivery itself. Improvement in perinatal outcome has been greatly enhanced by improved technology available to neonatologists and by improvements in prenatal care (e.g., identification of patients at high risk; ultrasonography; and increased usage of antenatal steroids, progesterone, and most recently magnesium sulfate cerebral palsy prophylaxis in those at risk for preterm delivery) [64, 65].

Unfortunately, despite the dramatic rise in the rate of cesarean delivery, the overall rate of cerebral palsy has not decreased. The only perinatal intervention for which strong evidence shows a beneficial effect on both mortality and the risk of cerebral palsy is antenatal treatment of the mother with glucocorticoids [66].

A minority of cesarean deliveries are performed for fetal distress, where fetal heart rate tracings are clearly associated with an increased risk of fetal hypoxia and acidosis. Fetal heart rate monitoring has not decreased the overall rate of cerebral palsy; rather, it has decreased the threshold to perform cesarean deliveries for non-reassuring fetal status.

Unfortunately, many obstetricians admit that their practice of medicine has become more defensive. Given the fear of inquiry regarding how a particular patient's labor was managed, many obstetricians may have a lower threshold to perform a cesarean delivery despite the fact that the incidence of neonatal seizures or cerebral palsy has not been affected by increasing cesarean delivery rates [67].

Long-Term Monitoring

After a cesarean delivery, the patient can be observed as a patient who delivered vaginally. The normal recommendation is to have the patient make a follow-up appointment 4–6 weeks after delivery. If bleeding has stopped, a repeat Papanicolaou test as needed based on recent pap screening guidelines is customary. During this visit, review any notable findings from the surgery and discuss delivery options for future pregnancies.

Future and Controversies

Further investigation continues to evaluate which patients should undergo a trial of labor after having a cesarean delivery. Many variables play a role in this discussion and have not been clarified. The NIH held a consensus conference in March 2010 to further discuss the trend in rates of vaginal birth after cesarean (see the image below).

Go to Vaginal Birth After Cesarean Delivery for complete information on this topic.

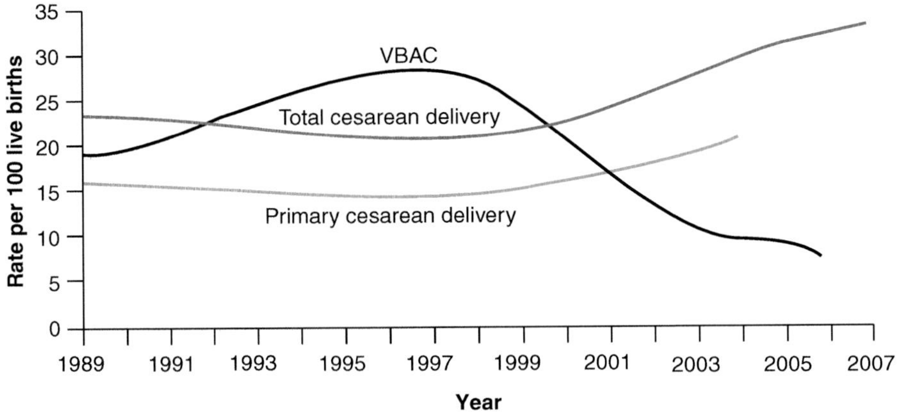

Vaginal birth after cesarean delivery rates

Increased implementation of VBAC is part of a larger movement toward decreasing the cesarean delivery rate in the United States. Recently ACOG and SMFM issued joint guidelines providing a framework for individual organizations and key players at the state and federal level to work with local hospitals to set the agenda to decrease the rate of primary cesarean deliveries. Decreasing the rate of primary cesarean deliveries will result in a decreased number of repeat cesarean deliveries.

A large prospective randomized study is needed to look at single-layer versus double-layer closure and risk of future uterine rupture when a trial of labor is attempted after previous low-transverse cesarean section.

The recommendation that all breech presentations should be delivered by a cesarean delivery is currently a subject of active debate. Additional information is required to address this issue in the setting of appropriately trained physicians and under well-established guidelines.

Urogynecologists suggest that all women should consider outright cesarean delivery to prevent pelvic floor dysfunction. This is an extremely controversial area that continues to receive attention, particularly in that short-term outcomes do not appear to relate to long-term outcomes [112]. Genetic factors appear to play an important role in long-term outcomes, which overshadows the effects that laboring and delivery itself have on short-term outcomes.

Cesarean delivery on maternal request (CDMR) also continues to be an area of debate. A survey of participants in the 2006 state-of-the-science conference revealed that most obstetrician/gynecologists believe that a woman has the right to CDMR, but fewer agree to perform the procedure than they did in 2006. In general, obstetricians/gynecologists associate more risks with cesarean delivery and attribute fewer benefits to it.

Finally, more research evaluating the link between cesarean birth and obesity (in those born by cesarean section) will be needed. A recent article [115] associated cesarean birth with increased risk of obesity later in life. The authors successfully addressed some of the shortcomings of previous studies that analyzed the issue, especially the effects of prepregnancy BMI. However, they also acknowledge that more research is needed to strengthen this relationship as well as to evaluate its generalizability to minorities and the strength of the relationship between cesarean birth, obesity, and increased risk of advanced cardiometabolic outcomes in these individuals. Another study by Cai et al. that included data from 727 infants reported that elective cesarean delivery was associated with high body mass index-for-age z score at 12 months.

References

1. Births - method of delivery. Centers for Disease Control and Prevention. Available at http://www.cdc.gov/nchs/fastats/delivery.htm. July 6, 2016. Accessed: 22 Sept 2016.
2. American College of Obstetricians and Gynecologists, Society for Maternal-Fetal Medicine. Obstetric care consensus no. 1: safe prevention of the primary cesarean delivery. Obstet Gynecol. 2014;123(3):693–711. [Medline].
3. The American College of Obstetricians and Gynecologists. Practice Bulletin No. 161 summary: external cephalic version. Obstet Gynecol. 2016. 127:412–413.
4. Frellick M. ACOG issues guidance on external cephalic version. Medscape Medical News. Available at http://www.medscape.com/viewarticle/858257. February 03, 2016. Accessed: 24 Feb 2016.
5. [Guideline] Barclay L. Longer labor okay to avoid cesarean, new guidelines say. Medscape Medical News from WebMD. 2014 Feb 19. Available at http://www.medscape.com/viewarticle/820842. Accessed: February 23, 2014.
6. [Guideline] Caughey AB, Cahill AG, Guise JM, et al. Safe prevention of the primary cesarean delivery. Am J Obstet Gynecol. 2014;210(3):179–93. [Medline].
7. Notzon FC, Cnattingius S, Bergsjo P, et al. Cesarean section delivery in the 1980s: international comparison by indication. Am J Obstet Gynecol. 1994;170(2):495–504. [Medline].
8. Ruys TP, Cornette J, Roos-Hesselink JW. Pregnancy and delivery in cardiac disease. J Cardiol. 2013;61(2):107–12. [Medline].
9. ACOG Committee on Obstetric Practice. Cesarean delivery on maternal request. Apr 2013. Available at https://www.acog.org/Resources_And_Publications/Committee_Opinions.
10. NIH State-of-the-Science Conference: Cesarean delivery on maternal request; March 27–29, 2006; Bethesda, Md. NIH Consens Sci Statements. 2006. Mar 27–29;23(1):1–29. Available at http://consensus.nih.gov/2006/cesareanstatement.htm. Accessed 30 Oct 2008.
11. Practice guidelines for preoperative fasting and the use of pharmacologic agents to reduce the risk of pulmonary aspiration: application to healthy patients undergoing elective procedures: a report by the American Society of Anesthesiologist Task Force on Preoperative Fasting. Anesthesiology. 1999;90(3):896–905. [Medline].
12. Smaill FM, Gyte GM. Antibiotic prophylaxis versus no prophylaxis for preventing infection after cesarean section. Cochrane Database Syst Rev. 2010:CD007482. [Medline].
13. Weiner Z, Ben-Shlomo I, Beck-Fruchter R, Goldberg Y, Shalev E. Clinical and ultrasonographic weight estimation in large for gestational age fetus. Eur J Obstet Gynecol Reprod Biol. 2002;105(1):20–4. [Medline].

14. Patolia DS, Hilliard RL, Toy EC, Baker B. Early feeding after cesarean: randomized trial. Obstet Gynecol. 2001;98(1):113–6. [Medline].
15. Tan PC, Norazilah MJ, Omar SZ. Hospital discharge on the first compared with the second day after a planned cesarean delivery: a randomized controlled trial. Obstet Gynecol. 2012;120(6):1273–82. [Medline].
16. Landon MB. Vaginal birth after cesarean delivery. Clin Perinatol. 2008;35(3):491–504, ix-x. [Medline].
17. Placek PJ, Taffel SM. Recent patterns in cesarean delivery in the United States. Obstet Gynecol Clin North Am. 1988;15(4):607–27. [Medline].
18. CDC NCHS data brief. Centers for Disease Control and Prevention. Available at http://www.cdc.gov/nchs/data/databriefs/db35.htm. Accessed 7 May 2010.
19. Hamilton BE, Martin JA, Ventura SJ. Births: preliminary data for 2008. National Center for Health Statistics. Available at http://www.cdc.gov/nchs/data/nvsr/nvsr58/nvsr58_16.pdf. Accessed 28 May 2010.
20. Hannah ME, Hannah WJ, Hewson SA, Hodnett ED, Saigal S, Willan AR. Planned caesarean section versus planned vaginal birth for breech presentation at term: a randomised multicentre trial. Term Breech Trial Collaborative Group. Lancet. 2000;356(9239):1375–83. [Medline].
21. Glezerman M. Five years to the term breech trial: the rise and fall of a randomized controlled trial. Am J Obstet Gynecol. 2006;194(1):20–5. [Medline].
22. ACOG Committee Opinion No. 340. Mode of term singleton breech delivery. Obstet Gynecol. 2006;108(1):235–7. [Medline].
23. Chaillet N, Dumont A, Abrahamowicz M, Pasquier JC, Audibert F, Monnier P, et al. A cluster-randomized trial to reduce cesarean delivery rates in Quebec. N Engl J Med. 2015;372 (18):1710–21. [Medline].
24. Barclay L. Unnecessary cesarean deliveries decrease with intervention. Medscape Medical News. Available at http://www.medscape.com/viewarticle/843997. April 30, 2015; Accessed 24 Feb 2016.
25. Homer CS, Kurinczuk JJ, Spark P, Brocklehurst P, Knight M. Planned vaginal delivery or planned caesarean delivery in women with extreme obesity. BJOG. 2011;118(4):480–7. [Medline].
26. Chu SY, Kim SY, Schmid CH, Dietz PM, Callaghan WM, Lau J, et al. Maternal obesity and risk of cesarean delivery: a metaanalysis. Obes Rev. 2007;8(5):385–94. [Medline].
27. ACOG Practice Bulletin Number 49, December 2003: dystocia and augmentation of labor. (Replaces no. 218, December 1995, no. 137, December 1989, and no. 157, July 1991). Reaffirmed 2009. Obstet Gynecol. 2003;102(6):1445–54. [Medline].
28. Hankins GD, Clark SM, Munn MB. Cesarean section on request at 39 weeks: impact on shoulder dystocia, fetal trauma, neonatal encephalopathy, and intrauterine fetal demise. Semin Perinatol. 2006;30(5):276–87. [Medline].
29. Grobman WA, Gersnoviez R, Landon MB, et al. Pregnancy outcomes for women with placenta previa in relation to the number of prior cesarean deliveries. Obstet Gynecol. 2007;110(6):1249–55. [Medline].
30. Schenker JG, Cain JM. FIGO Committee Report. FIGO Committee for the Ethical Aspects of Human Reproduction and Women's Health. International Federation of Gynecology and Obstetrics. Int J Gynaecol Obstet. 1999;64(3):317–22. [Medline].
31. Lee YM, D'Alton ME. Cesarean delivery on maternal request: maternal and neonatal complications. Curr Opin Obstet Gynecol. 2008;20(6):597–601. [Medline].
32. Smith H, Peterson N, Lagrew D, Main E. Toolkit to support vaginal birth and reduce primary cesareans: a quality improvement toolkit. Stanford: California Maternal Quality Care Collaborative; 2016.
33. Grootscholten K, Kok M, Oei SG, Mol BW, van der Post JA. External cephalic version-related risks: a meta-analysis. Obstet Gynecol. 2008;112(5):1143–51. [Medline].
34. Guideline No. 20a. External cephalic version and reducing the incidence of breech presentation. Royal College of Obstetricians and Gynaecologists; December 2006.

35. Cruikshank DP. Intrapartum management of twin gestations. Obstet Gynecol. 2007;109(5):1167–76. [Medline].
36. Alexander JM, Leveno KJ, Rouse D, et al. Cesarean delivery for the second twin. Obstet Gynecol. 2008;112(4):748–52. [Medline]. [Full Text].
37. Sakala EP, Andree I. Optimal route of delivery for meningomyelocele. Obstet Gynecol Surv. 1990;45(4):209–12. [Medline].
38. Preis K, Swiatkowska-Freund M, Janczewska I. Spina bifida--a follow-up study of neonates born from 1991 to 2001. J Perinat Med. 2005;33(4):353–6. [Medline].
39. Luthy DA, Wardinsky T, Shurtleff DB, et al. Cesarean section before the onset of labor and subsequent motor function in infants with meningomyelocele diagnosed antenatally. N Engl J Med. 1991;324(10):662–6. [Medline].
40. How HY, Harris BJ, Pietrantoni M, et al. Is vaginal delivery preferable to elective cesarean delivery in fetuses with a known ventral wall defect?. Am J Obstet Gynecol. 2000;182(6):1527–34. [Medline].
41. Salihu HM, Emusu D, Aliyu ZY, Pierre-Louis BJ, Druschel CM, Kirby RS. Mode of delivery and neonatal survival of infants with isolated gastroschisis. Obstet Gynecol. 2004;104(4):678–83. [Medline].
42. Puligandla PS, Janvier A, Flageole H, Bouchard S, Laberge JM. Routine cesarean delivery does not improve the outcome of infants with gastroschisis. J Pediatr Surg. 2004;39(5):742–5. [Medline].
43. Martin JA, Hamilton BE, Sutton PD, et al. Births: final data for 2002. Natl Vital Stat Rep. 2003;52(10):1–113. [Medline].
44. Alfirevic Z, Devane D, Gyte GM. Continuous cardiotocography (CTG) as a form of electronic fetal monitoring (EFM) for fetal assessment during labour. Cochrane Database Syst Rev. 2006:CD006066. [Medline].
45. Scheller JM, Nelson KB. Does cesarean delivery prevent cerebral palsy or other neurologic problems of childhood? Obstet Gynecol. 1994;83(4):624–30. [Medline].
46. MacKenzie IZ, Cooke I. What is a reasonable time from decision-to-delivery by caesarean section? Evidence from 415 deliveries. BJOG. 2002;109(5):498–504. [Medline].
47. Brown ZA, Wald A, Morrow RA, Selke S, Zeh J, Corey L. Effect of serologic status and cesarean delivery on transmission rates of herpes simplex virus from mother to infant. JAMA. 2003;289(2):203–9. [Medline].
48. Clinical Guidelines Portal. Updated May 24, 2010. Available at http://www.aidsinfo.nih.gov/Guidelines/. Accessed 27 May 2010.
49. Faiz AS, Ananth CV. Etiology and risk factors for placenta previa: an overview and meta-analysis of observational studies. J Matern Fetal Neonatal Med. 2003;13(3):175–90. [Medline].
50. Clark SL, Koonings PP, Phelan JP. Placenta previa/accreta and prior cesarean section. Obstet Gynecol. 1985;66(1):89–92. [Medline].
51. Buchmann EJ, Libhaber E. Sagittal suture overlap in cephalopelvic disproportion: blinded and non-participant assessment. Acta Obstet Gynecol Scand. 2008;87(7):731–7. [Medline].
52. Cheng YW, Hopkins LM, Laros RK Jr, Caughey AB. Duration of the second stage of labor in multiparous women: maternal and neonatal outcomes. Am J Obstet Gynecol. 2007;196(6):585.e1–6. [Medline].
53. Mehta SH, Bujold E, Blackwell SC, Sorokin Y, Sokol RJ. Is abnormal labor associated with shoulder dystocia in nulliparous women? Am J Obstet Gynecol. 2004;190(6):1604–7; discussion 1607–9. [Medline].
54. Gottlieb AG, Galan HL. Shoulder dystocia: an update. Obstet Gynecol Clin North Am. 2007;34(3):501–31, xii. [Medline].
55. Li L, Wen J, Wang L, Li YP, Li Y. Is routine indwelling catheterisation of the bladder for caesarean section necessary? A systematic review. BJOG. 2011;118(4):400–9. [Medline].
56. Mackeen AD, Packard RE, Ota E, Berghella V, Baxter JK. Timing of intravenous prophylactic antibiotics for preventing postpartum infectious morbidity in women undergoing cesarean delivery. Cochrane Database Syst Rev. 2014;12:CD009516. [Medline].

57. Tita AT, Hauth JC, Grimes A, Owen J, Stamm AM, Andrews WW. Decreasing incidence of postcesarean endometritis with extended-spectrum antibiotic prophylaxis. Obstet Gynecol. 2008;111 (1):51–6. [Medline].
58. ACOG Practice Bulletin No. 120: use of prophylactic antibiotics in labor and delivery. Obstet Gynecol. 2011;117(6):1472–83. [Medline].
59. Costantine MM, Rahman M, Ghulmiyah L, et al. Timing of perioperative antibiotics for cesarean delivery: a metaanalysis. Am J Obstet Gynecol. 2008;199(3):301.e1–6. [Medline].
60. Warnes CA, Williams RG, Bashore TM, et al. ACC/AHA 2008 guidelines for the management of adults with congenital heart disease: executive summary: a report of the American College of Cardiology/American Heart Association Task Force on Practice Guidelines (writing committee to develop guidelines for the management of adults with congenital heart disease). Circulation. 2008;118(23):2395–451. [Medline].
61. Hemingway P, Allcock N, Payne H, Tanner J. Pre-operative hair removal to reduce surgical site infection. Joanna Briggs Institute Best Practice Teachnical Report. 2007. Available at http://connect.jbiconnectplus.org/viewsourcefile.aspx?0=4347.
62. Darouiche RO, Wall MJ Jr, Itani KM, Otterson MF, Webb AL, Carrick MM, et al. Chlorhexidine-alcohol versus povidoneiodine for surgical-site antisepsis. N Engl J Med. 2010;362 (1):18–26. [Medline].
63. Bucklin BA, Hawkins JL, Anderson JR, Ullrich FA. Obstetric anesthesia workforce survey: twenty-year update. Anesthesiology. 2005;103(3):645–53. [Medline].
64. Afolabi BB, Lesi FE, Merah NA. Regional versus general anaesthesia for caesarean section. Cochrane Database Syst Rev. 2006:CD004350. [Medline].
65. Rouse DJ, Hirtz DG, Thom E, et al. A randomized, controlled trial of magnesium sulfate for the prevention of cerebral palsy. N Engl J Med. 2008;359(9):895–905. [Medline]. [Full Text].
66. O'Shea M. Cerebral palsy. Semin Perinatol. 2008;32(1):35–41. [Medline].
67. Foley ME, Alarab M, Daly L, Keane D, Macquillan K, O'Herlihy C. Term neonatal asphyxial seizures and peripartum deaths: lack of correlation with a rising cesarean delivery rate. Am J Obstet Gynecol. 2005;192(1):102–8. [Medline].
68. Pritchard JA, Baldwin RM, Dickey JC, et al. Blood volume changes in pregnancy and the puerperium. Am J Obstet Gynecol. 1962;84:1271–82.
69. Hofmeyr GJ, Mathai M, Shah A, Novikova N. Techniques for caesarean section. Cochrane Database Syst Rev. 2008:CD004662. [Medline].
70. Berghella V, Baxter JK, Chauhan SP. Evidence-based surgery for cesarean delivery. Am J Obstet Gynecol. 2005;193(5):1607–17. [Medline].
71. Giacalone PL, Daures JP, Vignal J, Herisson C, Hedon B, Laffargue F. Pfannenstiel versus Maylard incision for cesarean delivery: A randomized controlled trial. Obstet Gynecol. 2002;99(5 Pt 1):745–50. [Medline].
72. Holmgren G, Sjoholm L, Stark M. The Misgav Ladach method for cesarean section: method description. Acta Obstet Gynecol Scand. 1999;78(7):615–21. [Medline].
73. Hohlagschwandtner M, Ruecklinger E, Husslein P, Joura EA. Is the formation of a bladder flap at cesarean necessary? A randomized trial. Obstet Gynecol. 2001;98(6):1089–92. [Medline].
74. Rodriguez AI, Porter KB, O'Brien WF. Blunt versus sharp expansion of the uterine incision in low-segment transverse cesarean section. Am J Obstet Gynecol. 1994;171(4):1022–5. [Medline].
75. Dodd JM, Anderson ER, Gates S. Surgical techniques for uterine incision and uterine closure at the time of caesarean section. Cochrane Database Syst Rev. 2008:CD004732. [Medline].
76. Sung JF, Daniels KI, Brodzinsky L, El-Sayed YY, Caughey AB, Lyell DJ. Cesarean delivery outcomes after a prolonged second stage of labor. Am J Obstet Gynecol. 2007;197(3):306.e1–5. [Medline].
77. Chopra S, Bagga R, Keepanasseril A, Jain V, Kalra J, Suri V. Disengagement of the deeply engaged fetal head during cesarean section in advanced labor: conventional method versus reverse breech extraction. Acta Obstet Gynecol Scand. 2009;88(10):1163–6. [Medline].

78. Lurie S, Sulema V, Kohen-Sacher B, Sadan O, Glezerman M. The decision to delivery interval in emergency and non-urgent cesarean sections. Eur J Obstet Gynecol Reprod Biol. 2004;113(2):182–5. [Medline].
79. Levy R, Chernomoretz T, Appelman Z, Levin D, Or Y, Hagay ZJ. Head pushing versus reverse breech extraction in cases of impacted fetal head during Cesarean section. Eur J Obstet Gynecol Reprod Biol. 2005;121(1):24–6. [Medline].
80. Moertl MG, Friedrich S, Kraschl J, Wadsack C, Lang U, Schlembach D. Haemodynamic effects of carbetocin and oxytocin given as intravenous bolus on women undergoing caesarean delivery: a randomised trial. BJOG. 2011;118(11):1349–56. [Medline].
81. Atkinson MW, Owen J, Wren A, Hauth JC. The effect of manual removal of the placenta on post-cesarean endometritis. Obstet Gynecol. 1996;87(1):99–102. [Medline].
82. Morales M, Ceysens G, Jastrow N, et al. Spontaneous delivery or manual removal of the placenta during caesarean section: a randomised controlled trial. BJOG. 2004;111(9):908–12. [Medline].
83. Coutinho IC, Ramos de Amorim MM, Katz L, Bandeira de Ferraz AA. Uterine exteriorization compared with in situ repair at cesarean delivery: a randomized controlled trial. Obstet Gynecol. 2008;111(3):639–47. [Medline].
84. Bujold E, Goyet M, Marcoux S, Brassard N, Cormier B, Hamilton E, et al. The role of uterine closure in the risk of uterine rupture. Obstet Gynecol. 2010;116 (1):43–50. [Medline].
85. Bujold E, Bujold C, Hamilton EF, Harel F, Gauthier RJ. The impact of a single-layer or double-layer closure on uterine rupture. Am J Obstet Gynecol. 2002;186(6):1326–30. [Medline].
86. Gyamfi C, Juhasz G, Gyamfi P, Blumenfeld Y, Stone JL. Single- versus double-layer uterine incision closure and uterine rupture. J Matern Fetal Neonatal Med. 2006;19(10):639–43. [Medline].
87. Harrigill KM, Miller HS, Haynes DE. The effect of intraabdominal irrigation at cesarean delivery on maternal morbidity: a randomized trial. Obstet Gynecol. 2003;101(1):80–5. [Medline].
88. Duffy DM, diZerega GS. Is peritoneal closure necessary? Obstet Gynecol Surv. 1994;49 (12):817–22. [Medline].
89. Komoto Y, Shimoya K, Shimizu T, et al. Prospective study of non-closure or closure of the peritoneum at cesarean delivery in 124 women: Impact of prior peritoneal closure at primary cesarean on the interval time between first cesarean section and the next pregnancy and significant adhesion at second cesarean. J Obstet Gynaecol Res. 2006;32(4):396–402. [Medline].
90. Chelmow D, Rodriguez EJ, Sabatini MM. Suture closure of subcutaneous fat and wound disruption after cesarean delivery: a meta-analysis. Obstet Gynecol. 2004;103(5 Pt 1):974–80. [Medline].
91. Ramsey PS, White AM, Guinn DA, Lu GC, Ramin SM, Davies JK, et al. Subcutaneous tissue reapproximation, alone or in combination with drain, in obese women undergoing cesarean delivery. Obstet Gynecol. 2005;105(5 Pt 1):967–73. [Medline].
92. Rousseau JA, Girard K, Turcot-Lemay L, Thomas N. A randomized study comparing skin closure in cesarean sections: staples vs subcuticular sutures. Am J Obstet Gynecol. 2009;200(3):265.e1–4. [Medline].
93. Tuuli MG, Rampersad RM, Carbone JF, Stamilio D, Macones GA, Odibo AO. Staples compared with subcuticular suture for skin closure after cesarean delivery: a systematic review and meta-analysis. Obstet Gynecol. 2011;117(3):682–90. [Medline].
94. Basha SL, Rochon ML, Quiñones JN, Coassolo KM, Rust OA, Smulian JC. Randomized controlled trial of wound complication rates of subcuticular suture vs staples for skin closure at cesarean delivery. Am J Obstet Gynecol. 2010;203 (3):285.e1–8. [Medline].
95. Buresch AM, Van Arsdale A, Ferzli M, Sahasrabudhe N, Sun M, Bernstein J, et al. Comparison of subcuticular suture type for skin closure after cesarean delivery: a randomized controlled trial. Obstet Gynecol. 2017. [Medline].

96. Helwick C. Repeat cesarean delivery optimal before 39 weeks. Medscape Medical News from WebMD. Available at http://www.medscape.com/viewarticle/820391. 2014 Feb 10. Accessed 19 Feb 2014.
97. Consortium on Safe Labor, Hibbard JU, Wilkins I, Sun L, Gregory K, Haberman S, et al. Respiratory morbidity in late preterm births. JAMA. 2010;304 (4):419–25. [Medline].
98. Tita AT, Landon MB, Spong CY, et al. Timing of elective repeat cesarean delivery at term and neonatal outcomes. N Engl J Med. 2009;360 (2):111–20. [Medline].
99. American College of Obstetricians and Gynecologists. ACOG Committee Opinion No 579: definition of term pregnancy. Obstet Gynecol. 2013;122 (5):1139–40. [Medline].
100. Barclay DL. Cesarean hysterectomy. Thirty years' experience. Obstet Gynecol. 1970;35(1):120–31. [Medline].
101. Cunningham FG, FLeveno KJ, Bloom S, Hauth JC, Rouse DJ, Spong C. Williams obstetrics. 23rd ed. Norwalk: Appleton & Lange; 2009.
102. Landon MB. Cesarean section. In: Gabbe SG, Niebyl JR, Simpson JL, editors. Obstetrics. 5th ed. New York: Churchill Livingston; 2007.
103. Duff P. Pathophysiology and management of postcesarean endomyometritis. Obstet Gynecol. 1986;67(2):269–76. [Medline].
104. Tipton AM, Cohen SA, Chelmow D. Wound infection in the obese pregnant woman. Semin Perinatol. 2011;35(6):345–9. [Medline].
105. Mowat J, Bonnar J. Abdominal wound dehiscence after caesarean section. Br Med J. 1971;2(5756):256–7. [Medline]. [Full Text].
106. Bonnar J. Venous thromboembolism and pregnancy. Clin Obstet Gynaecol. 1981;8(2):455–73. [Medline].
107. Heit JA, Kobbervig CE, James AH, Petterson TM, Bailey KR, Melton LJ 3rd. Trends in the incidence of venous thromboembolism during pregnancy or postpartum: a 30-year population-based study. Ann Intern Med. 2005;143(10):697–706. [Medline].
108. Brown HL, Hiett AK. Deep vein thrombosis and pulmonary embolism in pregnancy: diagnosis, complications, and management. Clin Obstet Gynecol. 2010;53(2):345–59. [Medline].
109. Witlin AG, Mercer BM, Sibai BM. Septic pelvic thrombophlebitis or refractory postpartum fever of undetermined etiology. J Matern Fetal Med. 1996;5(6):355–8. [Medline].
110. Brown CE, Stettler RW, Twickler D, Cunningham FG. Puerperal septic pelvic thrombophlebitis: incidence and response to heparin therapy. Am J Obstet Gynecol. 1999;181(1):143–8. [Medline].
111. Cunningham FG, Bangdiwala SI, Brown SS, et al. NIH consensus development conference draft statement on vaginal birth after cesarean: new insights. NIH Consens State Sci Statements. 2010;27(3):1–42. [Medline]. [Full Text].
112. Nelson RL, Furner SE, Westercamp M, Farquhar C. Cesarean delivery for the prevention of anal incontinence. Cochrane Database Syst Rev. 2010:CD006756. [Medline].
113. Coleman-Cowger VH, Erickson K, Spong CY, Portnoy B, Croswell J, Schulkin J. Current practice of cesarean delivery on maternal request following the 2006 state-of-the-science conference. J Reprod Med. 2010;55(1–2):25–30. [Medline].
114. Bujold E, Gauthier RJ. Risk of uterine rupture associated with an interdelivery interval between 18 and 24 months. Obstet Gynecol. 2010;115 (5):1003–6. [Medline].
115. Yuan C, Gaskins AJ, Blaine AI, Zhang C, Gillman MW, Missmer SA, et al. Association between cesarean birth and risk of obesity in offspring in childhood, adolescence, and early adulthood. JAMA Pediatr. 2016;170:e162385. [Medline].
116. Cai M, Loy SL, Tan KH, et al. Association of elective and emergency cesarean delivery with early childhood overweight at 12 months of age. JAMA Netw Open. 2018;1(7):e185025.
117. Chapman SJ, Owen J, Hauth JC. One- versus two-layer closure of a low transverse cesarean: the next pregnancy. Obstet Gynecol. 1997;89(1):16–8. [Medline].
118. Durnwald C, Mercer B. Uterine rupture, perioperative and perinatal morbidity after single-layer and double-layer closure at cesarean delivery. Am J Obstet Gynecol. 2003;189(4):925–9. [Medline].

119. Hellums EK, Lin MG, Ramsey PS. Prophylactic subcutaneous drainage for prevention of wound complications after cesarean delivery--a metaanalysis. Am J Obstet Gynecol. 2007;197(3):229–35. [Medline].
120. Beck AC. Observations on a series of cesarean sections done at the Long Island College Hospital during the past six years. Am J Obstet Gynecol. 1919;79:197.
121. Darney BG, Snowden JM, Cheng YW, Jacob L, Nicholson JM, Kaimal A, et al. Elective induction of labor at term compared with expectant management: maternal and neonatal outcomes. Obstet Gynecol. 2013;122(4):761–9. [Medline].
122. Henderson D. Early induction linked to lower odds of cesarean delivery. Medscape Medical News from WebMD. 2013 Sept 09. Available at http://www.medscape.com/viewarticle/810671. Accessed 16 Feb 2014.
123. Kerr JMM. The technic of caesarean section with special reference to the lower uterine segment incision. Am J Obstet Gynecol. 1926;12(5):729–35.
124. Todman D. A history of caesarean section: from ancient world to the modern era. Aust N Z J Obstet Gynaecol. 2007;47(5):357–61. [Medline].
125. Dahlke JD, Mendez-Figueroa H, Rouse DJ, Berghella V, Baxter JK, Chauhan SP. Evidence-based surgery for cesarean delivery: an updated systematic review. Am J Obstet Gynecol. 2013;209(4):294–306. [Medline]. [Full Text].
126. Orji EO, Olabode TO, Kuti O, Ogunniyi SO. A randomised controlled trial of early initiation of oral feeding after cesarean section. J Matern Fetal Neonatal Med. 2009;22(1):65–71. [Medline].

Chapter 51
Perinatal Asphyxia (Acute Fetal Distress)

Fernanda Campos da Silva, Renato Augusto Moreira de Sá, and Cristiane Alves de Oliveira

Introduction

For a long time, perinatal asphyxia was called "acute fetal distress" [1]. It is a severe condition that occurs during labor and childbirth, caused by acute and intense reduction in maternal-fetal exchanges resulting in the lack of oxygen in fetal organs and systems. This reduction leads to an important change in fetal homeostasis characterized by [2]:

- *Hypoxemia* (reduction of circulating O_2)
- *Hypoxia* (decreased tissue O_2)
- *Hypercapnia* (increased CO_2)
- *Acidosis* (accumulation of acidic radicals)
- *Ischemia* (reduction or complete cessation of blood flow to an organ)
- *Asphyxia* (deprivation of enough O_2 to cause neurological damage)

Asphyxia can be prolonged partial, sudden total (due to a sentinel event), or a combination of both. The hypoxic-ischemic neurological damage can occur if perinatal asphyxia's intensity or duration overwhelms the capacity of the fetus to compensate.

F. C. da Silva (✉)
Department of Obstetrics, Universidade Federal do Estado do Rio de Janeiro (UNIRIO), Rio de Janeiro, RJ, Brazil

R. A. Moreira de Sá
Fernandes Figueira Institut - FIOCRUZ, Rio de Janeiro, RJ, Brazil

C. A. de Oliveira
Federal Fluminense University and Rio de Janeiro Federal University, Niteroi and Rio de Janeiro, Brazil

© Springer Nature Switzerland AG 2022
R. A. Moreira de Sá, E. B. d. Fonseca (eds.), *Perinatology*,
https://doi.org/10.1007/978-3-030-83434-0_51

Characterization of Perinatal Asphyxia

The criteria that define perinatal asphyxia as the acute hypoxic-ischemic event are based on the presence of severe metabolic changes (acidosis: pH <7.0; base deficit: ≥12 mmol/L) at birth and in newborns born showing early signs of moderate or severe encephalopathy.

The terms "fetal distress" and "intrapartum fetal asphyxia" should be avoided. The term "possible change in fetal well-being" is preferred or the change found that motivated the suspicion should be described (recurrent variable decelerations, absence of variability, bradycardia, etc.).

The inadequate use of terminology may motivate inadequate actions. A fetus can be characterized as "asphyxic" and be born with good vitality.

The neonatal signs consistent with a peripartum or intrapartum event relating to neonatal encephalopathy have been defined by the *American College of Obstetricians and Gynecologists* (ACOG) and are shown in Table 51.1 [3, 4].

The neonatal encephalopathy caused by acute hypoxia-ischemia is accompanied by abnormal neonatal signals contributing to events and associated in close temporal proximity with labor and childbirth. It is important to determine whether the signals are consistent with acute hypoxia-ischemia and if not can laugh be explained by other causes. Thus, when all criteria are met, it becomes increasingly likely that perinatal hypoxia-ischemia has played a role in the pathogenesis of neonatal encephalopathy [3].

Physiopathology

The process begins with a decrease in the oxygen supply to the fetus. Even with a rise in fetal red cells and the greater capacity of fetal hemoglobin of retaining oxygen, O_2 reserves can be exhausted. The fetus makes use of defensive, metabolic, and cardiovascular mechanisms to adapt to the hypoxemia imposed on it. Acute hypoxemia, detected by the chemoreceptors of the carotid body, stimulates the brain stem to increase parasympathetic and sympathetic stimulation [5].

Table 51.1 Neonatal signs consistent with perinatal asphyxia

Essential criteria for the diagnosis of perinatal asphyxia
1. Fetal metabolic acidosis (cord blood pH <7.0 and baseline deficit ≥12 mmol/L)
2. Apgar score in the fifth and tenth minute <5 (Table 51.2)
3. Neuroimaging evidence of acute brain injury seen on brain magnetic resonance or spectroscopy consistent with hypoxia-ischemia
4. Systemic complications in different organs in the neonatal period (i.e., central nervous, urinary, respiratory, cardiovascular, metabolic, hematological system) – multisystemic dysfunction

Table 51.2 Apgar score

Apgar score			
Points	0	1	2
Heart rate	Absent	<100/minute	> 100/minute
Breath	Absent	Weak, irregular	Strong/crying
Muscle tone	Flaccid	Legs and arms flexion	Active movement/good bending
Color	Cyanotic/pale	Cyanosis of extremities	Pinkish
Reflex Irritability	Absent	Some movement	Sneezing/crying

The consequences of asphyxiation range from no harmful effects to multiple organ damage and death. This enormous variation in the result differs with the severity and duration of the asphyxiation.

In summary, the main fetal adaptations are mentioned:

- ***Fetal heart rate (FHR) deceleration***
  - The initial fetal response to an episode of low oxygen supply is to slow FHR. This bradycardia is a parasympathetic response, seen as a slowdown in CTG [6]. Bradycardia is considered a protective reaction, as it helps to reduce myocardial work and thus decreases the oxygen needs of the heart. In addition, it increases the transit time of red blood cells through tissues (including the placenta), allowing greater extraction of oxygen from HbF and transplacental transfer of oxygen to the fetal circulation [5].
- ***Tachycardia***
  - After the slowdown, the gradually increasing release of catecholamines causes the FHR to return to baseline or even cause a mild tachycardia. This allows cardiac output to contribute to the maintenance of blood pressure.
- ***Selective perfusion*** [5]
  - The peripheral vasoconstriction triggered by the sympathetic nervous system is initially maintained by humoral factors that prolong the redistribution of cardiac output. The vasoconstriction increases the pressure in the descending aorta, increasing the right ventricular afterload, which in turn stimulates the passage of blood from the right atrium, through the foramen ovale, the left atrium, and then to the left ventricle, causing an increase in blood flow in the ascending aorta and in cerebral and coronary circulations, thus maintaining perfusion to critical organs.
  - Vasoconstriction of the fetal intestine causes hyperperistalsis and relaxation of the anal sphincter, changes responsible for the elimination of *meconium.*
- ***Anaerobic breathing*** [5]
  - The fetus anaerobic capacity is increased due to high glycogen stores in the liver and myocardium but also facilitated by the increased release of lactate in fetal circulation primarily by the placenta.
- ***Reduced metabolic rate***
  - Despite the limited supply of oxygen, aerobic metabolism may be able to provide enough power for a longer time, due to the reduction in metabolic rate. The latter, associated with reduced myocardial work and the overall

decrease of fetal activity, including less body and eye movements and a drop in body temperature, are part of this mechanism.
- The reduced metabolic rate also contributes to better fetal gas exchange and oxygen diffusion in the tissues.

In the terminal stage, the fetus loses its ability to compensate for hypoxia, which leads to serious injuries and death.

The hypoxia phase results in further reduction of myocardial glycogen stores, compromised cardiac function, and ultimately profound systemic hypotension and irreversible damage to multiple organs. The systemic hypotension worsens further cardiac function, limiting coronary blood flow and causing subendocardial myocardial lesion.

The selective perfusion, which "protects" the brain, is activated only when the fetal Pa O_2 falls below 37%. However, if Pa O_2 drops below 30% for more than 2 minutes, that response will fail completely and significantly increase the risk of adverse perinatal outcomes.

Finally, the fetus agonizes in bradycardia, that is, a lasting and progressive drop in baseline heart rate.

Etiology

Perinatal asphyxia can be caused by events in the prepartum, intrapartum, or postpartum period or combinations of the three. Asphyxia is related to prepartum events in 50% of cases, intrapartum in 40%, and postpartum in the remaining 10% [7]. In most cases, there is an overlap of intrapartum insults in an already at risk situation. Given the higher incidence of serious complications in labor and the reduced availability of specialized assistance during childbirth, intrapartum causes represent a greater proportion of cases in countries with a lower human development index.

The uteroplacental blood flow depends on the perfusion pressure in relation to maternal hemodynamics and vascular resistance. The factors that modify this flow are numerous, but the role of uterine contraction stands out. However, other factors that reduce the uteroplacental flow or decrease the volume of the intervillous space may contribute to these changes.

Uterine contractions result in a decline in fetal PaO_2 of approximately 25%. Most healthy and properly growing fetuses can tolerate a reduction of 50% in PaO2 (from a Pa O2 of more than 20 mmHg to as low as 10 the 12 mmHg) due to its high glycogen stores in the myocardium, the fetal circulation pattern, to the high oxygen affinity for fetal hemoglobin and the high cardiac output [8].

In face of a reduction in uteroplacental perfusion, peripheral chemoreceptors act in fetal defense against hypoxic injury, by rapidly reducing oxygen consumption and preferentially targeting blood flow to organs sensitive to hypoxic injuries (brain, heart, and adrenal glands) [5]. Fetal adaptations to transient hypoxia are summarized in Fig. 51.1.

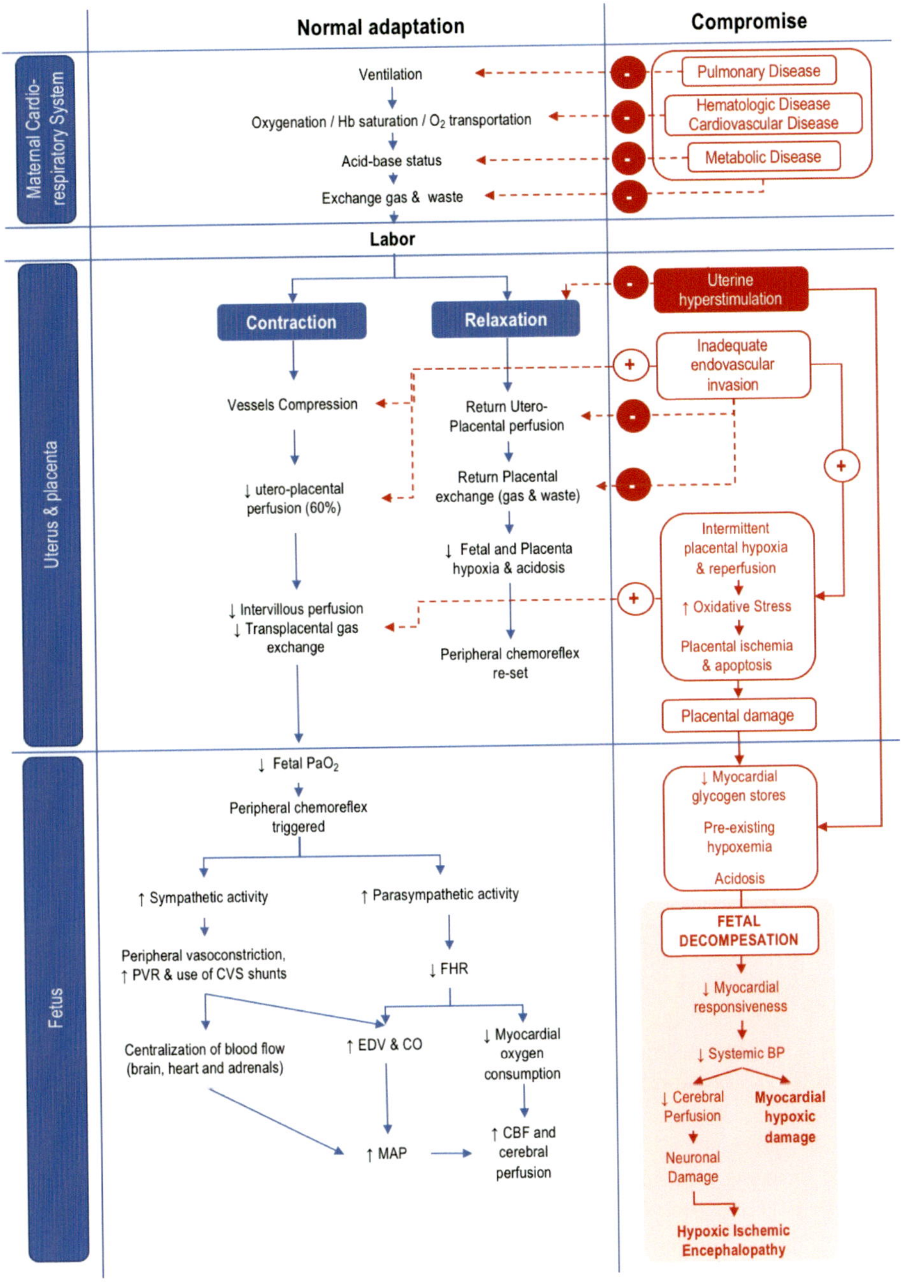

Fig. 51.1 Relationship of uterine contractility with the pathophysiology of perinatal asphyxia. (Modified from Turner 2020) [5]

There are three main mechanisms of perinatal asphyxia [9, 10]:

1. Origin before delivery (prepartum origin):
   (a) Massive fetal-maternal hemorrhage
   (b) Placental lesions that affect oxygen transfer:
      - Preeclampsia
      - Placental infarction
      - Chorioangioma
      - Placental edema in diabetic pregnancy or alloimmunization
2. Decompensation of a previously affected fetus (decompensation of a state of chronic fetal distress aggravated by the interruption of uteroplacental circulation due to uterine contractions):
   (a) At the maternal level:
      - Heart disease
      - Chronic lung diseases
      - Diabetic ketoacidosis
      - Uterine aortic compression, hypotension linked to the supine position
      - Hypotension from too high dosage of antihypertensive drugs for control of preeclampsia
   (b) At the fetal level:
      - Cord compression in case of oligohydramnios, cord knots, or cord circulars
      - Decompensation of severe anemia
3. Occurrence of acute accidents in labor:
   (a) At maternal level:
      - Acute maternal asphyxia by:
         – Convulsions
         – Intubation difficulties
         – Amniotic embolism
      - Sudden fall in uteroplacental perfusion due to:
         – Uterine hypertonia:
            - Retroplacental hematoma
            - Iatrogenic effect of oxytocic use
         – Abrupt hypotension:
            - Hemorrhagic shock because of placenta previa
            - Vasoplegia in epidural analgesia
   (b) At fetal level:
      - During amniotomy:
         – Cord procidence
         – Hemorragia de Benckiser.[1]
      - Prolonged occlusion of the umbilical circulation during:
         – Extraction difficulties
         – Shoulder dystocia

---

[1] It is a fetal hemorrhage after the rupture of one or more vessels whose insertion is abnormal (veined and previous), occurring more frequently during rupture of the membranes. It is a serious complication (fetal mortality rate from 75% to 100%).

Diagnosis

The oxygen concentration in the tissues cannot be quantified; thus, the occurrence of fetal hypoxia can only be assessed by the documentation of metabolic acidosis. The analysis of blood gases and lactate in the umbilical cord or in the circulation of the newborn during the first minutes of life is the only way to objectively quantify the occurrence of hypoxia/acidosis immediately before birth [11].

The vast majority of fetuses born with metabolic acidosis, with or without low Apgar scores (Table 51.2), recover quickly and will not suffer complications in the short or long term [12]. In only a few cases, fetal hypoxia/acidosis will be of sufficient intensity and duration to cause damage to important organs and systems and, thus, put the newborn at risk of death or long-term morbidity [11].

Short-term neurological dysfunction caused by intrapartum hypoxia/acidosis is called hypoxic-ischemic encephalopathy, and this diagnosis requires confirmation of the following:

- Metabolic acidosis
- Low Apgar scores
- Evidence of brain involvement in early imaging
- Appearance of changes in muscle tone, suction movements, convulsions, or coma in the first 48 hours of life [11]

Umbilical Cord Blood Sample

It is necessary to collect blood samples from the umbilical artery and vein right after delivery to objectively document the occurrence of fetal hypoxia/acidosis. Cord clamping is not necessary before collection, but the concentrations of gas and lactate in the umbilical cord blood change rapidly after birth [11]. Table 51.3 presents the reference values for the arterial and venous blood gases of the umbilical cord [13].

Even if double clamping the cord blood is done, collection should be performed as quickly as possible (preferably 15 minutes) because the blood gas values change significantly over time [14].

Blood should be collected in two different pre-heparinized syringes, introducing the least air possible. After blood collection, any existing air bubbles must be removed. Syringes must be covered and rolled between fingers to mix blood with heparin, and blood gas analysis must be performed on a calibrated device within the next 30 minutes [14].

Umbilical arterial blood reflects fetal acid-base status better than venous blood. However, it is important to obtain blood from the artery and vein to validate the arterial sample. The arterial pH is lower than that of the vein. For the sample to be reliable, the difference in pH between the two blood samples should be greater than 0.02 and the difference in pCO_2 greater than 5 mmHg [11]. Similarly, to rule out

Table 51.3 Reference values for arterial and venous blood gas analysis of the umbilical cord [13]

	Premature			Term			
	Umbilical Artery	Percentile 5	95th percentile	Umbilical Artery	Percentile 5	95th percentile	Pathological acidosis
pH	7.28	7.14	7.4	7.27	7.15	7.38	<7.0
PCO_2 (mmHg)	50.2	32	69.2	50.3	32	68	
HCO3 (mEq/L)	22.4	16	27.1	22	15.4	26.8	
BD (mEq/L)	2.5	7.6	1.3	2.7	8.1	0.9	≥12

PCO_2 partial pressure of carbon dioxide, *HCO3* bicarbonate, *BD* base deficit

contamination with the blood of the umbilical vein or air, pCO_2 should be greater than 22 mmHg in the umbilical artery [15].

The "ideal" cutoff point for lactate, arterial, and venous samples, respectively, to predict unfavorable neonatal outcome is 3, 8, and 3.4 mmol/L [16].

When gas exchanges through the placenta are compromised or when there is significant umbilical cord occlusion, an increase in CO_2 and a decrease in O_2 concentrations in the fetus may occur, and, therefore, an acidemia of mixed respiratory and metabolic origin is documented. However, the metabolic component, reflected in the negative base excess (BE) or in the deficit of base, is the one with the greatest potential for damage [11].

Electronic Delivery Monitoring: Intrapartum Cardiotocography

Electronic monitoring of labor is recommended when abnormalities are detected during intermittent fetal auscultation (Table 51.4) [1]. The use of continuous intrapartum cardiotocography (CTG) in low-risk women is controversial. One option is to CTG intermittently, alternating the auscultation of fetal heart rate (FHR) to CTG. Intermittent monitoring must be performed for a sufficient time to allow an adequate assessment of the CTG [11].

Definition of CTG parameters:

- ***Normal baseline***
  Basal fetal heart rate between 110 and 160 bpm. Premature fetuses tend to have values at the upper end of this range and post-term fetuses at the lower end.
- ***Tachycardia***
  Baseline fetal heart rate that persists for more than 10 minutes at levels higher than 160 bpm (*moderate tachycardia*) or 180 bpm (*marked tachycardia*), in particular if there is no other cause and it is associated with other changes FHR such as loss of oscillation or the presence of decelerations. It should alert to the presence of hypoxemia/acidosis [11].

Table 51.4 Cardiotocographic patterns associated with the risk of acidemia

Risk of acidemia	Pattern
Low	Moderate tachycardia (160–180 bpm) Moderate bradycardia (100–110 bpm) Minimum variability (≤5 bpm) for less than 40 min Early decelerations Variable decelerations of less than 3 min or that do not lose the pattern of variability
Moderate	tachycardia>180 bpm isolated Bradycardia of 90–100 bpm Variability ≤5 bpm for more than 40 min Variability>25 bpm Atypical and/or severe variable deceleration Late non-repeated deceleration Variable decelerations of more than 3 min The combination of various abnormalities
High	Decrease without apparent cause of variability (≤5 bpm for more than 60 min) Sinusoidal rhythm[a] greater than 10 min [23] Persistent bradycardia with no variability or sudden bradycardia <90 bpm Atypical and/or severe variable decelerations Repeated late decelerations Prolonged or repeated variable decelerations associated with the absence of accelerations and/or variability ≤5 bpm or even absent

[a]The sinusoidal pattern corresponds to a traction with sinusoidal undulation, with an amplitude of 5–15 bpm and a frequency of three to five cycles per minute, which lasts more than 30 minutes and coincides with the absent accelerations. It occurs in association with severe fetal anemia (anti-D alloimmunization, fetal-maternal hemorrhage, fetal-fetal transfusion syndrome, and vasa-previa rupture). It has also been described in cases of acute fetal hypoxemia, infection, cardiac malformations, hydrocephalus, and gastroschisis

Causes of tachycardia

- Maternal fever: most frequent cause of fetal tachycardia and may be of extra-uterine origin or associated with intrauterine infection.
- Epidural analgesia: can also cause an increase in maternal temperature resulting in fetal tachycardia.
- Early stages of non-acute fetal hypoxemia: catecholamine secretion can result in tachycardia.
- Administration of beta-agonist drugs or parasympathetic blockers (Table 51.5).
- Fetal arrhythmias: such as supraventricular tachycardia and atrial flutter.

- ***Bradycardia***

  Fetal heart rate less than 110 bpm (*moderate bradycardia*) or less than 100 bpm (*marked bradycardia*), maintained for 10 minutes or more

  Causes of bradycardia

  - Fetal hypoxemia
  - Maternal hypothermia [17]
  - Beta-blocker administration [18] (Table 51.2)
  - Fetal arrhythmias, such as atrioventricular block

Table 51.5 Drugs that can affect the tracing in fetal monitoring

Fetal heart rate pattern	Drugs
Tachycardia	Adrenaline Atropine β-Agonist (i.e., ritodrine, terbutaline)
Bradycardia	Anti-titreoidal agents β-Blockers Epidural anesthesia
Sinusoidal pattern	Narcotic pain relievers (i.e., meperidine)
Decreased variability	Atropine Anticonvulsants (except phenytoin) β-Blockers Ethanol General anesthesia Hypnotics (i.e., diazepam) Insulin (if associated with hypoglycemia) Magnesium sulfate Narcotics Promethazine (Fenergam®)

- ***Decreased variability***
  FHR oscillation amplitude below 5 bpm, for more than 50 min or for more than 03 minutes during a declaration in the absence of the use of sedatives or atropine, may be associated with hypoxemia/acidosis [11].
  Causes of decreased variability
  - Hypoxia/acidosis of the central nervous system and decreased sympathetic and parasympathetic activity
  - Infection
  - Administration of central nervous system depressants
  - Parasympathetic blockers
- ***Increased variability***
  FHR oscillation amplitude greater than 25 bpm, for more than 30 min, corresponds to the *saltatory pattern.*
  The cause is not known, but it seems to be associated with fetal autonomic instability, but it can be seen associated with recurrent decelerations, when hypoxemia/acidosis evolves very quickly [19].
- ***Late deceleration***
  FHR reductions below the baseline, over 15 bpm in amplitude and lasting more than 15 seconds. It is motivated by contraction and reflects the fetal chemoreceptor-mediated response hypoxemia. The *intrapartum deceleration* is considered as *late* when the time interval between the onset of the uterine contraction and the beginning of deceleration is greater than 20 seconds (*latency period*). It has U-shaped and/or reduced variability, with a gradual onset and/or a gradual return to baseline and/or reduced variability within the deceleration (Fig. 51.2).
  Late decelerations indicative of fetal distress if they:
  - Are found in more than 20% of contractions.

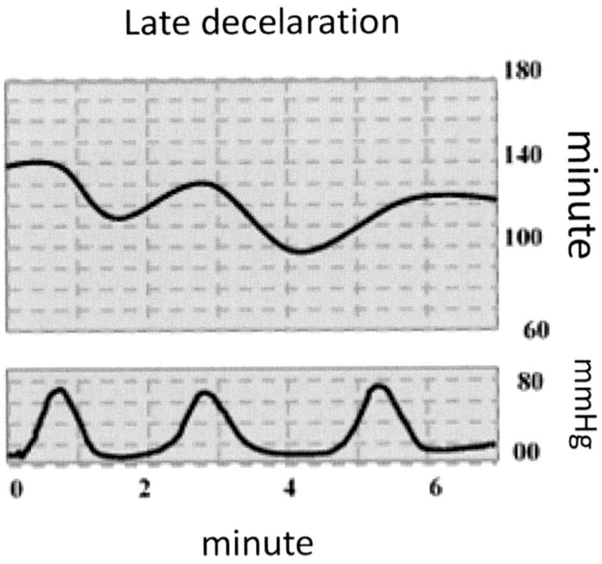

Fig. 51.2 Schematic representation of the late deceleration

  - Do not return to baseline
  - Are not associated with accelerations and have reduced variability (in this case, the definition also includes those late decelerations with amplitude 10 to 15 bpm)
  - Do not improve with the correction of the patient's posture or uterine contractility disorders
- ***Variable decelerations***
  These are decelerations that are not related to uterine contraction and that vary in appearance during the exam. In general, they result from cord compression; hence, they are also called *umbilical decelerations* (Fig. 51.3).
  When a variable deceleration lasts longer than 30 seconds, it can reflect low oxygen concentration when [20]:
  - They feature a "U"-shaped component.
  - They have reduced variability within the deceleration.
  - Its individual duration exceeds 3 minutes.
  - They do not return to the initial *FHR* or recover slowly.
- ***Early deceleration*** features a temporary decrease in the fetal heart rate at the same time as the uterine contraction and results from vagal reflex seen when the head of the fetus is compressed by a uterine contraction. It is more frequent after rupture of membranes, and, in the vast majority of cases, it is not associated with fetal distress [21] (Fig. 51.4).
- ***Complicated deceleration*** characterized by [22]:
  - Failure to return to baseline at the end of the contraction
  - Deceleration lasting ≥60 seconds and up to ≤60 bpm or decrease of ≥60 bpm n the baseline

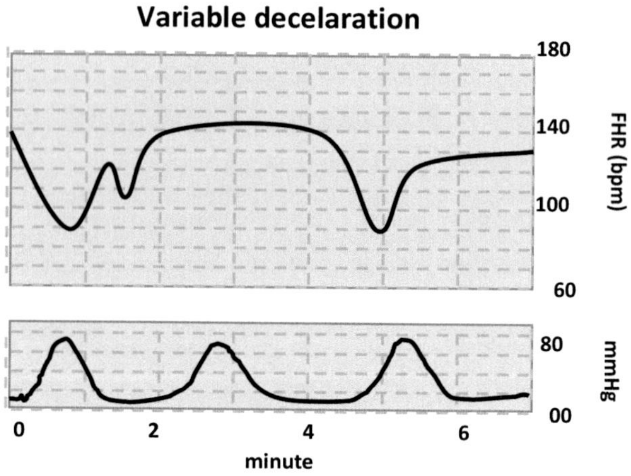

Fig. 51.3 Schematic representation of the variable deceleration

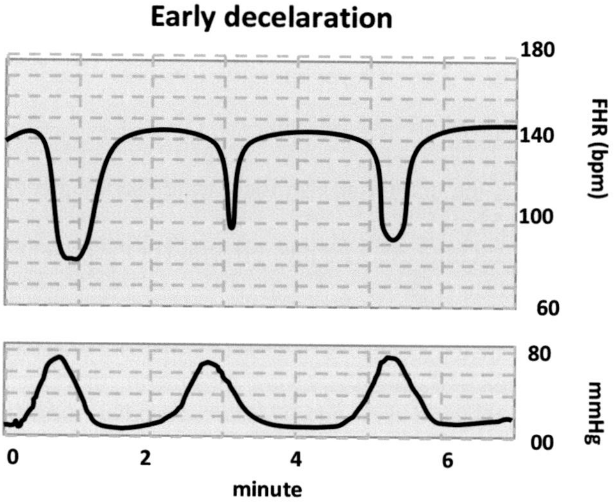

Fig. 51.4 Schematic representation of the early deceleration

- Compensatory tachycardia that crosses the baseline by 20 bpm for 20 seconds after deceleration
- Variable deceleration in the presence of:
  - Minimal or absent variability at baseline
  - Baseline with tachycardia or bradycardia

The classification of electronic fetal monitoring is shown in Table 51.6 [21]. The more atypical or abnormal characteristics that occur simultaneously, the greater the potential for fetal decompensation [21].

Table 51.6 Classification of intrapartum fetal monitoring – cardiotocography intrapartum. (Modified Turner et al. 2020) [22]

	Normal	Suspicious	Pathological
Interpretation	Normal traces, which are strongly predictive of normal fetal acid-base status at the time of observation and can be followed routinely, without any specific action required	Undetermined registry, although not predictive of abnormal fetal acid-base status, cannot be classified as normal. They may correspond to the physiological response. They need continuous assessment and supervision and reassessment	Possible fetal compromise
Uterine activity	Standard contractility pattern ≤5/10 min	Tachysistolia may be present with normal, atypical, or abnormal tracings; closely monitor the characteristics of FHR	
Baseline	110–160 beats per minute	100–110 bpm 160 bpm for 30–80 minutes Ascending baseline Arrhythmia (irregular rhythm)	<100 bpm 160 bpm for >80 minutes Erratic baseline
Variability	Range between 6 and 25 5 bpm	≤5 bpm for 40–80 minutes	≤5 bpm for>80 minutes ≥25 bpm for>10 minutes Sinusoidal
Decelerations	Absence of late decelerations Variable non-repetitive decelerations (sequence of 1 or at most 2) and uncomplicated Early decelerations may or may not be present	Uncomplicated repetitive variables (sequence ≥3) Complicated non-repetitive variables (sequence of 01 or at most 2) Intermittent late decelerations Single prolonged deceleration ≥2 minutes, but <3 minutes	Repetitive complicated variables Recurring late decelerations Single, prolonged deceleration ≥3 minutes but <10 minutes
Accelerations	Accelerations may or may not be present	Absence of induced accelerations after fetal stimulation	Usually absent (accelerations, if present, do not change the classification of the pattern)

Intermittent Fetal Auscultation

Intermittent auscultation (IA) of fetal heartbeats can be used for labor monitoring, especially in low-risk pregnancies (i.e., healthy women between 37 + 0 and 41 + 3 weeks' gestation in spontaneous labor and in the absence of risk factors for adverse perinatal outcomes) [22].

Between 41 + 4 and 42 + 0 weeks of gestation, IA can be used as long as the fetal well-being has been previously assessed by a baseline cardiotocography (CTG) and in the setting of normal amniotic fluid volume [23].

Pregnancies ≤36 + 6 weeks and >42 + 0 weeks are associated with an increased risk of adverse fetal outcome, and continuous electronic monitoring is recommended [24].

IA can be performed through the use of *sonar-Doppler*, and it is recommended that fetal auscultation be initiated during uterine contraction and extended for 1 minute after its end [23].

Recommendations for fetal assessment by IA during labor [22]:

1. Define the pattern of uterine contractions.
   (a) Document uterine activity with the number of contractions present in a 10-minute window and every 30 minutes.
   (b) In the presence of tachysystole, if the fetal heart rate is unusual or abnormal in the first 10 minutes, initiate the intrauterine resuscitation protocol.
2. Determine basal FHR.
   (a) Adequately install the *sonar-Doppler* considering fetal position established by Leopold maneuver, in the absence of fetal activity, acceleration, and deceleration, listening and counting for 60 seconds between uterine contractions.
   (b) Palpate simultaneously maternal pulse and maternal heart rate with FHR.
   (c) Normal basal FHR: between 110 and 160 bpm.
   (d) Fetal tachycardia: >160 bpm per period >10 min.
   (e) Fetal bradycardia: <110 bpm per period >10 min.
3. Determine fetal heart rate.
   (a) Basal heart rate is described as regular or irregular.
   (b) An irregular rhythm occurs when there is an irregular FHR not associated with uterine activity.
   (c) Irregularities in the fetal heart rate demand to a more accurate analysis with other tests (ultrasound or echocardiography) to determine the type of arrhythmia or discard artifact.
4. Evaluate the presence of accelerations and decelerations.
   (a) Record audible increases and decreases that occur at the FHR baseline.
   (b) It is not possible to characterize the amplitude or duration of accelerations and decelerations by IA.

The periodicity of this monitoring depends on the risk level of the fetus, and on the maternal-fetal condition, being recommended [22]:

- Auscultation every hour, during the latent phase, if she is already admitted.
- During the dilation stage, auscultate every 30 minutes or, in high-risk pregnancies, every 15 minutes.
- In the expulsive stage, reduce the intervals to 5 minutes (for low- and high-risk patients).
- Tachycardia, bradycardia, or slowdowns indicate the need for electronic monitoring.

- If a deceleration is perceived by the IA immediately after a contraction, review after a change in position of the pregnant woman or start electronic monitoring immediately.
- If the intrapartum CTG was started because of abnormal IA, the electronic monitoring may be interrupted if it is normal (for a minimum of 20 minutes), after the overall clinical picture is revised and there are no maternal risk factors.

Meconium

The identification of meconium during labor increases the fetal risk for perinatal asphyxia. Thus, monitoring for the presence of meconium, along with the assessment of FHR, can help in diagnosis of asphyxia [1].

Meconium is eliminated early in the uterus by a reflex mechanism secondary to hypoxia by stimulating the parasympathetic system and consists of contraction of the intestine and relaxation of the anal sphincter [9]. Asphyxia is associated with meconium in almost 50% of cases. However, this sign is not absolutely specific, as it is present in 10% of deliveries with normal fetal and neonatal development [25]. It is not, by itself, a sign of fetal asphyxia. For a long time, perhaps reflecting obstetric and neonatal historic customs, the presence of meconium in the amniotic fluid was synonymous of "fetal distress." Reflection of a time when the tendency was to use a single variable or observation for the diagnosis of perinatal asphyxia [26].

In less than 5% of the cases where meconium is present, fetal acidosis will occur in full-term fetuses, so its correlation with acidosis in umbilical cord blood is debatable [9]. The more mature the conceptus is, the greater the chance that it will eliminate meconium, so the meaning of meconium fluid in a full-term pregnancy, in the absence of other risk factors, is different from its occurrence in a premature fetus with growth restriction [1].

In premature infants, the identification of meconium fluid during labor may be less favorable as it is associated with three or four times more periventricular leukomalacia [9].

In the context of prematurity, meconium fluid is associated to an increased risk of infection. This fact can also be considered for term fetuses, if its presence is associated with an absolutely normal FHR record [9].

From the above, in the presence of meconium amniotic fluid, identified after rupture of the membranes or less commonly by amnioscopy, we can infer the following:

- The finding of meconium alone is not a sign of acute fetal distress.
- It requires greater fetal monitoring when it is classified as the recent type, thick, type *pea paste*.
- It represents a greater risk for premature infants than for full-term fetuses.
- It suggests fetal distress when accompanied by changes in fetal heart rate.

Microanalysis of Fetal Blood

- Microanalysis of a drop of blood obtained by incision practiced in the fetal presentation is the only method that diagnoses the biochemical substrate of acute fetal distress: *hypoxemia, hypercapnia*, and *acidosis* [27].
- Its invasive character, its complexity of execution, and its lability, in view of the simplicity, innocuousness, and precision of biophysical methods, limit its routine clinical application [24].
- pH greater than 7.25 shows a healthy fetus and indicates expectant behavior [25].
- pH between 7.20 and 7.25 directs the exam to be repeated in 30 minutes [25].
- pH below 7.20 suggests fetal impairment (acidosis) and indicates termination of pregnancy [25].
- The lactate dosage can be performed by micromethod, with results obtained in 15–60 seconds [28].
- This method has the theoretical advantage of directly evaluating the metabolic share of a possible acidosis [28].
- A lactate level greater than 6 mmol/l is considered abnormal and a severe acidosis if greater than 7.5 mmol/l [28].

Pulse Oximetry

- Fetal oxygen monitoring method, continuous and less invasive when compared to microanalysis of fetal blood, obtained by the intrauterine introduction of a pulse oximeter [28].
- Evaluation of O_2 saturation based on the difference in photometric characteristics of oxyhemoglobin and carboxyhemoglobin.
- Fetal oxygenation is estimated to be adequate if SPO_2 is greater than 30% [29].
- No study has shown any fetal or maternal benefit in terms of reducing interventions or improving neonatal status, so oximetry is no longer available for fetal monitoring [29].

Fetal Electrocardiogram

- Method based on extracting the fetal ECG signal using an electrode on the scalp.
- In the case of hypoxia, the fetus adapts initially by redistributing blood to the vital organs, brain and heart in particular, which makes it possible to preserve myocardial oxygenation and normal ECG [29].
- There is no maternal or fetal benefit to date with the use of fetal ECG [30].
- The only currently accepted benefit of fetal ECG is a reduction in the use of fetal pH microanalysis for teams using this technique [29].

Prophylaxis

Within the current knowledge, it seems clear that the best prenatal surveillance, prevention of preterm birth, and adequate assistance to labor are decisive factors in the prevention of cerebral palsy, a major expression of perinatal asphyxia.

In some pregnancies, the risk factors for perinatal asphyxia identify fetuses that are particularly vulnerable to intrapartum hypoxia before the start of labor: fetal growth restriction, prematurity, congenital malformations, presentation breech, pre-eclampsia, multiple pregnancy, and maternal comorbidities. In others, the risk factors presented after the start of labor are hemorrhage, infection, liquid meconium, premature membrane, prolonged pregnancy, dehiscence of prior uterine scarring, induction, and acceleration of delivery (use of uterotonics) [1].

In the former, chronic fetal distress and therefore the antepartum assessment of fetal well-being are particularly prominent. Uterine contractions reduce uteroplacental perfusion by up to 60%, and, although most fetuses are able to tolerate this reduction in placental perfusion, this group may be unable to adjust to the reduction and is at risk of hypoxic injury [21]. Since not all with fetuses restriction growth is due to some fetal injury, different parameters of biometrics are needed to identify the fetuses' risk before birth, such as first-trimester screening and Doppler assessment of uteroplacental and fetoplacental circulation. Table 51.7 identifies the methods for assessing the fetus well-being of in the perinatal period.

In other pregnancies, identification of intrapartum fetal involvement is not always easy. Although catastrophic, unpredictable, and acute events, such as placental detachment, uterine rupture, or umbilical cord prolapse, are associated with a high risk of severe fetal hypoxia, 75% of cases of intrapartum asphyxia occur gradually as a result of uterine contractions [31]. Despite joint efforts to develop accurate techniques for the identification of intrapartum fetal hypoxia, so far, all techniques have weak positive predictive values. Reviews of conventional antepartum CTG, computerized FHR analysis, or intermittent auscultation concluded that these tests do not result in better perinatal results [31]. The CTG does not perform well as a test, because the interpretation is subjective, has low intra- and interobserver agreement, and lacks discriminatory power to identify truly hypoxic fetuses [32]. Despite these limitations, it remains the basis for intrapartum fetal monitoring, despite the high rate of false-positive results [32].

Table 51.7 Methods for assessing the well-being of the fetus in the perinatal period

Antepartum	Intrapartum	Post childbirth
Cardiotocography (CTG) Fetal biophysical profile (PBF) Fetal Doppler Fetal movement *kick test*	Intermittent auscultation Electronic fetal monitoring (CTG) Microanalysis of fetal blood. Presence of meconium. Pulse oximetry.	Clinical examination of the neonate (convulsions, concussions). Apgar score. Cord blood gas analysis.

Although intrapartum CTG has resulted in a reduction in the incidence of neonatal seizures, there is no improvement in rates of perinatal death or cerebral palsy, despite an increase in operative deliveries [33].

Despite some controversies about the need for electronic monitoring to be included in the routine of monitoring parturition, there is no doubt that the constant presence of a qualified health professional with the parturient significantly reduces the occurrence of perinatal asphyxia.

Acute events in labor and delivery account for about 6–10% of cases of cerebral palsy, justifying special attention for assistance in labor [34]. It is important to note that intrapartum asphyxia may be responsible for other neurological disabilities other than cerebral palsy.

The following are some clinical measures relevant to the prophylaxis of acute fetal distress:

- Do not speed up the delivery that progresses normally.
- Only use oxytocin when the evolution of childbirth is stopped or delayed due to deficiency in uterine contractility.
- If there is a medical indication for inducing labor, it is advisable to use the lowest dose of oxytocin capable of getting you started and progressing.
- Do not induce labor when fetal vitality is compromised.
- In patients with an unfavorable cervix, with fetal well-being proven, labor should be induced after the cervix has matured (*see specific chapter*).
- Monitor all induced births.
- Monitor all high-risk deliveries.
- Promptly correct maternal hypovolemia, hypotension, hypoglycemia, and electrolyte disturbances.

Treatment

Several factors, including gestational age and medications administered to the mother, can alter the FHR pattern. The CTG analysis needs to be integrated with other clinical information for comprehensive interpretation and proper management [22].

The answer will vary according to:

- Clinical situation: gestational age, stage of labor, identification of risk factors.
- Classification of findings.
- Monitoring method used.

As a general rule, if the fetus continues to maintain a stable baseline and adequate variability, the risk of hypoxia is very unlikely [22]. It is worth remembering that premature fetuses, especially between 28 and 32 weeks, tend to have a higher heart rate, less variability, smaller amplitude acceleration, and more variable decelerations.

The initiation of intrauterine resuscitation is usually the first response to atypical or abnormal findings. The main objective is to improve uterine blood flow, umbilical circulation, and maternal-fetal oxygenation. The main actions are to [35]:

- Discontinue prescription of uterotonic agents (excessive uterine activity is the most frequent cause of hypoxia/fetal acidosis).
- Change the position of the woman for lateral decubitus (left preference).
- During the second stage of labor, maternal pulls can contribute to fetal hypoxia/acidosis. Consider asking to stop pulling until the situation is reversed.
- Correct maternal hypotension and hypoglycemia.
- Consider tocolysis in the presence of tachysystole with atypical or abnormal CTG pattern.
- Offer supportive care to reduce maternal anxiety which will decrease the impact of catecholamines.
- Administer oxygen under mask (2–5 l/min) when hypoxia and/or maternal hypovolemia is suspected. Oxygen is reserved for maternal support and not for fetal resuscitation.
- Perform the vaginal exam to assess the presence of cord prolapse, pelvic fetus proportionality, progress of labor, and the conditions of the forceps practicability.
- Shorten the expulsion period, if applicable, with the use of the relief forceps.
- If the measures taken are unsuccessful, indicate an emergency cesarean section.

The changes preceding acidemia are progressive. Most fetuses develop acidemia when the CTG pattern is still atypical but present tachycardia with decelerations and decreased variability. This corresponds to the loss of protection of the adaptation mechanisms and the progression to deterioration (Fig. 51.5) [36]. In the absence of a correctable etiology, this may be the most appropriate time for an intervention. When decelerations (prolonged or not) continue without variability and bradycardia occurs, severe fetal acidemia is likely. Remember that fetuses can be acidemic if they have an atypical CTG pattern, so the transition to the abnormal pattern is not a must for the development of acidemia. Most acidemic fetuses exhibit atypical traces and only 15% exhibit an abnormal pattern [36].

Flowchart 51.1 summarizes the main actions for fetal monitoring in labor.

The key points in assessing fetal well-being during labor are as follows:

- Normal variability: it means that the adaptation mechanisms are ensuring adequate organ perfusion.
- Normal fetal heart rate (with variability also normal baseline) if the deceleration is not accompanied by an increase in the line base FHR (or tachycardia) with reduced variability, they do not represent fetal hypoxia.

Main points – *acute fetal distress*
Acute fetal distress is a severe condition that occurs during labor. It can end up in acidemia and fetal death.

Acute fetal distress can be caused by uteroplacental insufficiency, fetoplacental insufficiency, and also presence of changes in maternal metabolism.
Electronic monitoring of childbirth is a valuable resource for the diagnosis of acute fetal distress.
Intermittent auscultation of the fetus' heartbeat can be used to monitor delivery, especially in low-risk pregnancies.
The presence of meconium, as a unique finding, is not a sign of acute fetal distress.
The constant presence of a qualified health professional with the parturient significantly reduces the occurrence of perinatal asphyxia.

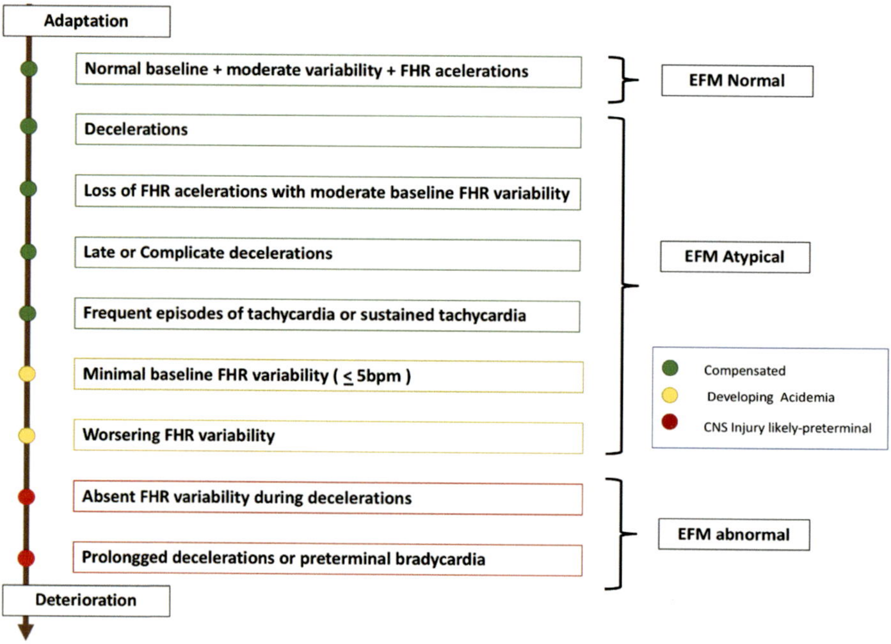

Fig. 51.5 Progression of the fetal heart rate pattern in the deterioration of the fetus until acidemia. (Modified from Vintzileos and Smulian [36])

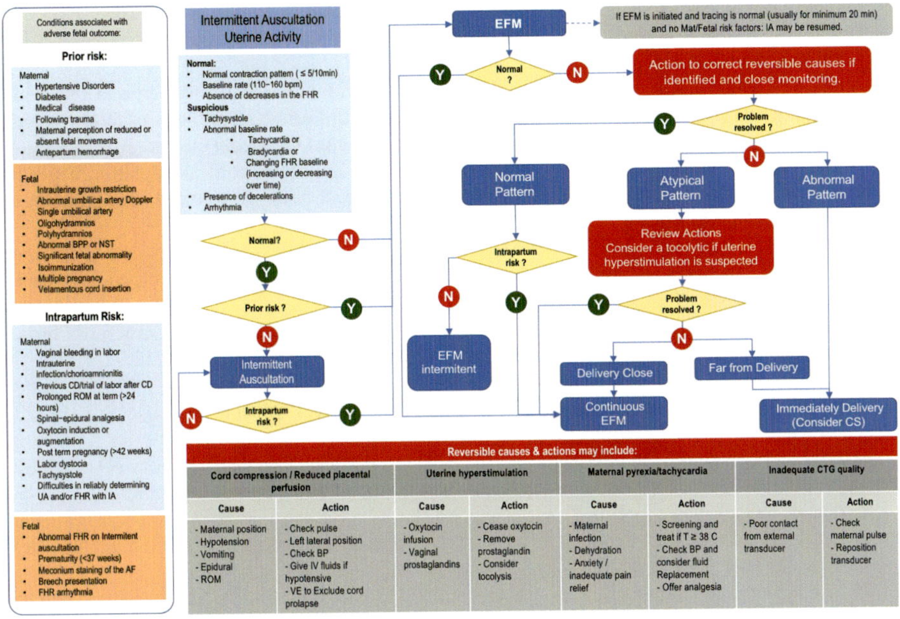

Flowchart 51.1 Evaluation and monitoring of pregnant women in labor to prevent perinatal asphyxia. (Y yes, N no, MF fetal movement, AU umbilical artery, GMP fetal biophysical profile, CTG cardiotocography, MRI membrane rupture, FCF fetal heart rate, AI intermittent auscultation, LA amniotic fluid, bpm beats per minute, DLE left lateral decubitus, EV intravenous, BP blood pressure)

References

1. Langer B. Repérage de l'asphyxie au cours du travail. Rev Méd Périnat. 2013;5:73–80.
2. Groenendaal F, van Bel F. Perinatal asphyxia in term and late preterm infants. In: Martin R. UpToDate. Available at: https://www.uptodate.com/contents/perinatal-asphyxia-in-term-and-late-preterm-infants. Accessed June 2020.
3. Executive summary: neonatal encephalopathy and neurologic outcome, second edition. Report of the American College of Obstetricians and Gynecologists' task force on neonatal encephalopathy. Obstet Gynecol. 2014;123(4):896–901.
4. Locatelli A, Lambicchi L, Incerti M, et al. Is perinatal asphyxia predictable ? BMC Pregnancy Childbirth. 2020;20:186.
5. Turner JM, Mitchell MD, Kumar SS. The physiology of intrapartum fetal compromise at term. Am J Obstet Gynecol. 2020;222(1):17–26.
6. Martin CB Jr. Normal fetal physiology and behavior, and adaptive responses with hypoxemia. Semin Perinatol. 2008;32:239–42.
7. Bhutta ZA. Pediatrics in the tropics. In: Farrar J, Hotez PJ, Junghanss T, et al., editors. Manson's tropical diseases. 23rd ed. Philadelphia: Saunders/Elsevier; 2014. p. 1197–214.
8. Jensen A, Garnier Y, Berger R. Dynamics of fetal circulatory responses to hypoxia and asphyxia. Eur J Obstet Gynecol Reprod Biol. 1999;84:155–72.
9. Boog G. La souffrance foetale aiguë. Journal de Gynécologie Obstétrique et Biologie de la Reproduction. 2001;30:393–429.

10. Gillam-Krakauer M, Gowen CW Jr. Birth asphyxia. [Updated 2020 Apr 23]. In: StatPearls [Internet]. Treasure Island: StatPearls Publishing; 2020. Available from: https://www.ncbi.nlm.nih.gov/books/NBK430782/.
11. Ayres-de-Campos D, Arulkumaran S, FIGO Intrapartum Fetal Monitoring Expert Consensus Panel. FIGO consensus guidelines on intrapartum fetal monitoring: physiology of fetal oxygenation and the main goals of intrapartum fetal monitoring. Int J Gynaecol Obstet. 2015;131:5–8.
12. Andres RL, Saade G, Gilstrap LC, Wilkins I, Witlin A, Zlatnik F, et al. Association between umbilical blood gas parameters and neonatal morbidity and death in neonates with pathologic fetal acidemia. Am J Obstet Gynecol. 1999;181(4):867–71.
13. Simham HN. Umbilical cord blood acid-base analysis at delivery. In: Lockwood CJ, editor. UpToDate. Available at https://www.uptodate.com/contents/umbilical-cord-blood-acid-base-analysis-at-delivery#H4. Accessed on 12/07/20.
14. Mokarami P, Wiberg N, Olofsson P. An overlooked aspect on metabolic acidosis at birth: blood gas analyzers calculate base deficit differently. Acta Obstet Gynecol Scand. 2012;91(5):574–9.
15. ACOG Committee on Obstetric Practice. ACOG Committee Opinion No. 348, November 2006: Umbilical cord blood gas and acid-base analysis. Obstet Gynecol. 2006;108(5):1319–22.
16. Tuuli MG, Stout MJ, Macones GA, Cahill AG. Umbilical cord venous lactate for predicting arterial lactic acidemia and neonatal morbidity at term. Obstet Gynecol. 2016;127(4):674–80.
17. Jadhon ME, Main EK. Fetal bradycardia associated with maternal hypothermia. Obstet Gynecol. 1988;72(3 Pt 2):496–7.
18. Boutroy MJ. Fetal and neonatal effects of the beta-adrenoreceptor blocking agents. Dev Pharmacol Ther. 1987;10(3):224–31.
19. Nunes I, Ayres-de-Campos D, Kwee A, Rosen KG. Prolonged saltatory fetal heart rate pattern leading to newborn metabolic acidosis. Clin Exp Obstet Gynecol. 2014;41(5):507–11.
20. Holzmann M, Wretler S, Cnattingius S, Nordstrom L. Cardiotocography patterns and risk of intrapartum fetal acidemia. J Perinat Med. 2015;43(4):473–9.
21. Turner JM, Mitchell MD, Kumar SS. The physiology of intrapartum fetal compromise at term. Am J Obstet Gynecol. 2020;222(1):17–26. https://doi.org/10.1016/j.ajog.2019.07.032.
22. Dore S, Ehman W. SOGC Clinical Practice Guideline. No. 396-fetal health surveillance: intrapartum consensus guideline. JOGC. 2020;42(3):316–48.
23. Modanlou HD, Murata Y. Sinusoidal fetal heart rate pattern: reappraisal of its definition and clinical significance. J Obstet Gynaecol Res. 2004;30(3):169–80.
24. Guidetti DA, Divon MY, Langer O. Postdate fetal surveillance: is 41 weeks too early? Am J Obstet Gynecol. 1989;161:91–3.
25. Carbonne B. Asphyxie foetale au cours du travail in: Berlan M et al. Practice de lÁccouchement. 2016. Masson, Paris 6th; 185–194.
26. Carter BS, Haverkamp AD, Merenstein GB. The definition of acute perinatal asphyxia. Clin Perinatol. 1993;20:287–304.
27. Carbonne B, Pons K, Maisonneuve E. Foetal scalp blood sampling during labor for pH and lactate measurements. Best Practice Res Clin Obstet Gynaecol. 2015.
28. Ramanah R, Martin ADR, Maillet RJS. Interested in the measurement of lactates on the scalp or on the crossings: comparative nature with the pH on the scalp. J Gynecol Obstet Biol Reprod. 2005;34:311.
29. Carbonne B, Langer B, Goffinet F, et al. Multicenter study on the clinical value of fetal pulse oximetry. II. Compared predictive values of pulse oximetry and fetal blood analysis. The French Study Group on Fetal Pulse Oximetry. Am J Obstet Gynecol. 1997;177(3):593–8.
30. Neilson JP. Fetal electrocardiogram (ECG) for fetal monitoring during labor. Cochrane Database Syst Rev. 2015;(12). Art. No: CD000116. https://doi.org/10.1002/14651858.CD000116.pub5.
31. Devane D, Lalor JG, Daly S, McGuire W, Smith V. Cardiotocography versus intermittent auscultation of fetal heart on admission to labor ward for assessment of fetal wellbeing. Cochrane Database Syst Rev. 2012;(2):CD005122.

32. Ayres-de-Campos D, Bernardes J, Costa-Pereira A, Pereira-Leite L. Inconsistencies in classification by experts of cardiotocograms and subsequent clinical decision. BJOG. 1999;106:1307–10.
33. Alfirevic Z, Devane D, Gyte GML. Continuous cardiotocography (CTG) as a form of electronic fetal monitoring (EFM) for fetal assessment during labor (Review). Cochrane Library; 2007.
34. Bakketeig LS. Only a minor part of cerebral palsy cases begin in labor. But still room for controversial childbirth issues in court. BMJ. 1999;319(7216):1016–7.
35. Ayres-de-Campos D, Spong CY, Chandraharan E; FIGO Intrapartum Fetal Monitoring Expert Consensus Panel. FIGO consensus guidelines on intrapartum fetal monitoring: cardiotocography. Int J Gynaecol Obstet. 2015;131(1):13–24. Screening and treatment if T ≥ 38 C - Check blood pressure and consider fluids Replacement - Providing analgesia.
36. Vintzileos AM, Smulian JC. Decelerations, tachycardia, and decreased variability: have we overlooked significance of longitudinal fetal heart rate changes for detecting intrapartum fetal hypoxia? Am J Obstet Gynecol. 2016;215:261–4.

Chapter 52
Maternal Complications in the Immediate Postpartum Period

Roxana Knobel, Carla Betina Andreucci, Leila Katz, and Melania M. Amorim

Introduction

Postpartum complications can lead to severe maternal morbidity and even mortality. In the period from 2008 to 2018, more than half of maternal deaths that occurred in Brazil occurred during the postpartum period [1]. The main direct causes of maternal death are hypertension, hemorrhage, and sepsis [2, 3]. Embolisms are another complication which can occur postpartum and cause maternal deaths [2].

It is important for obstetrical care teams to follow evidence-based recommendations to prevent or minimize postpartum complications. Recognizing women who are at higher risk of developing complications is also critical. When complications do occur, they must be diagnosed and treated quickly and adequately in order to avoid poor outcomes.

R. Knobel
Faculty of Medical Sciences, State University of Campinas – UNICAMP, Campinas, Brazil

Department of Obstetrics & Gynecology, Federal University of Santa Catarina (UFSC), Florianópolis, Brazil

C. B. Andreucci
Department of Medicine, Center of Biological and Health Sciences, Federal University of São Carlos, São Carlos, Brazil

L. Katz (✉)
Catholic University of Pernambuco (UNICAP), Recife, Brazil

Post-Graduate Program in Instituto de Medicina Integral Professor Fernando Figueira, Recife, Brazil

M. M. Amorim
Post-Graduate Program in Instituto de Medicina Integral Professor Fernando Figueira, Recife, Brazil

Obstetrics & Gynecology, Federal University of Campina Grande, Campina Grande, Brazil

© Springer Nature Switzerland AG 2022
R. A. Moreira de Sá, E. B. d. Fonseca (eds.), *Perinatology*,
https://doi.org/10.1007/978-3-030-83434-0_52

Hypertensive Disorders

Women who develop hypertensive disorders during pregnancy should receive more intense postpartum care. In cases of severe preeclampsia, magnesium sulfate should be continued postpartum or initiated during the postpartum period.

Some women develop hypertensive disorders in the postpartum period – up to 23% of cases of eclampsia occur postpartum. Some medications and substances utilized in the postpartum period may worsen hypertensive disorders, such as non-steroidal anti-inflammatory drugs (NSAIDs) [4].

Although the effectiveness of magnesium sulfate for prophylaxis and treatment of eclampsia has already been established, the ideal protocol for magnesium sulfate use during the postpartum period is unclear [5], and some researchers even question the benefits of magnesium administered postpartum in specific situations [6]. Current recommendations are to follow the same criteria for magnesium administration as during pregnancy – particularly severe headache and/or vision changes [5, 6].

In cases of severe hypertension (more or equal to 160/110) and/or associated symptoms, the use of immediate-acting antihypertensive medications is indicated, such as intravenous hydralazine, labetalol, or nitroprusside. In less severe cases, without symptoms and with lower blood pressure levels (less or equal to 180/120), oral medication may be used, such as captopril or clonidine [7]. Blood pressures must be closely monitored, and oral antihypertensive medications should be adjusted accordingly. In the postpartum period, use of methyldopa should be avoided due to the risk of postpartum depression. Calcium channel blockers such as nifedipine and amlodipine are considered first-line, as are beta-blockers such as labetalol. ACE inhibitors can also be used in the postpartum period; enalapril has been most extensively studied in this context and can be used as long as renal function is preserved. Diuretics are also an option, but they can decrease breast milk production and compromise breastfeeding [4, 8, 9].

A postpartum visit in 2 weeks' time should be scheduled for all these patients in order to check blood pressure control and reassess need for antihypertensive medications [10].

Infectious Complications

Infections that occur during the postpartum period are more likely than others to have severe consequences for several reasons. These include the rapid adaptations of the woman's body to pregnancy and delivery, the tissue trauma that is inflicted during vaginal or Cesarean delivery, and the demands of newborn care and lactation or, in cases of fetal or neonatal demise, the associated grief. It is therefore important to quickly recognize and treat these infections.

On the other hand, healthcare providers should be careful not to abuse of antibiotics, a problem common to all medical specialties and which can lead to multidrug-resistant bacteria. For women who are breastfeeding, antibiotics carry the additional risk of negative effects on the neonate's developing intestinal microbiome [11, 12].

The most important risk factor for postpartum infection is Cesarean delivery. Compared to a vaginal delivery, a Cesarean delivery increases the risk of endometritis between 5 and 30 times; it increases the risk of bacteremia between 2 and 10 times; it doubles the risk of abscess or pelvic thrombophlebitis; and it increases the risk of death due to infection up to 80 times [13]. Emergency Cesarean deliveries carry an increased risk of infection compared to elective ones, with the highest-risk deliveries being Cesareans performed during the second stage of labor.

Other obstetrical procedures also increase the risk of postpartum infection. These include retained placenta and manual extraction, forceps-assisted delivery, prolonged rupture of membranes, prolonged labor, multiple cervical exams during labor, uterine manipulation, and intrauterine fetal monitoring. Chorioamnionitis also increases the risk of postpartum infection [14], as do postpartum hemorrhage and extensive tissue trauma.

Puerperal Infection

The term puerperal infection refers to any infection of the genital tract which occurs during postpartum period. This period lasts from the time of the delivery until 42 days after. According to the World Health Organization (2015), a puerperal infection is diagnosed when two or more of the following criteria are met: pelvic pain, fever, abnormal vaginal discharge, purulent or foul-smelling vaginal discharge, and delay in uterine involution [15].

Puerperal fever is defined as an axillary temperature greater or equal to 38 °C with a minimal duration of 2 days and which started 24 hours to 10 days after delivery.

Clinical Picture and Initial Treatment

Fever, with temperatures typically ranging between 38° and 39 °C, is the most important criterion for diagnosis. Associated chills suggest bacteremia. In general, women complain of abdominal pain, and tenderness is noted on abdominal and bimanual exam. Purulent or foul-smelling lochia may also be seen.

On laboratory analysis, leukocytosis can be a normal finding among postpartum women. Leukocytosis between 15,000 and 30,000 cells/μl and the presence of a left shift are suggestive of infection. Further laboratory evaluation may be necessary to assess end-organ function, especially in patients with severe cases. We recommend checking liver function tests, creatinine, blood gases, and lactate (elevated lactate is a nonspecific finding indicative of severe infections). Additional laboratory evaluation can be considered depending on the specifics of the clinical case.

Cultures are an important step in the diagnosis of the specific site agent of the infection. They should ideally be collected prior to starting antibiotic therapy, but should not be a reason to delay antibiotic initiation. Cultures of the cervicovaginal secretions or of operative wounds that help in the diagnosis, treatment, and follow-up of these cases may be obtained and help in guiding therapy and creating knowledge about the common agents that infect that specific community. Urine culture helps in the diagnosis of urinary tract infections. Blood cultures are only helpful for patients with sepsis without an obvious focal source, since they are often negative and are not predictive of severity in cases of endometritis.

Imaging studies can sometimes help depending on the site and type of infection. Contrast computerized tomography (CT) and magnetic resonance imaging (MRI) are useful to confirm the diagnosis of pelvic thrombophlebitis.

After collecting cultures, initiating empiric antibiotics based on the suspected source of infection is critical. The most prevalent pathogens and their antibiotic resistance patterns may vary based on location and timing. If possible, clinicians should discuss appropriate antibiotic regimens for each clinical scenario according to their practice site.

Analgesics and antipyretics should be prescribed based on the patients' needs and on the severity of the case. In severe cases, patients should receive fluid resuscitation with crystalloids up to 30 ml/kg in addition to broad-spectrum antibiotics, as part of the sepsis treatment protocol. In case of septic shock, vasoactive drugs may be indicated.

Sepsis is a potential and severe complication of any postpartum infection. Genital tract infections include endometritis, infected perineal lacerations or episiotomies, Cesarean wound infections, pelvic thrombophlebitis, adnexal and parametrial infections, and peritonitis. It is very important to pay close attention to the associated clinical signs such as fever, tachycardia, and tachypnea, because symptoms can be more subtle among postpartum women compared to the general population.

Sepsis

Sepsis accounts for around 10% of maternal deaths worldwide and is the third direct cause of maternal mortality, surpassed only by hemorrhage and hypertension [16]. It is estimated that puerperal sepsis is responsible for approximately 75,000 maternal deaths per year, most of which occur in low-income countries [13].

According to The Third International Consensus Definitions for Sepsis and Septic Shock (Sepsis-3), sepsis is defined as "life-threatening organ dysfunction caused by a dysregulated host response to infection." More specifically, sepsis occurs when there is an infection accompanied by acute, life-threatening organ dysfunction [17].

The Consensus document further recommends that sepsis be diagnosed clinically. Severe organ dysfunction occurs when two or more parameters on the SOFA (sepsis-related organ dysfunction assessment) index are altered. These parameters include PaO_2/FiO_2, platelet count, bilirubin levels, blood pressure, creatinine, and Glasgow coma scale (Table 52.1) [18]. In order to use the SOFA parameters, laboratory tests are necessary. However, for a faster diagnosis in resource-limited settings, it is possible to evaluate for organ dysfunction using the quick-SOFA scale, which considers only three variables – altered mental status, increased respiratory rate, and hypotension. Obstetric emergency protocols should be based on the quick-SOFA (qSOFA) scale.

Prevention, early diagnosis, and swift management in cases of sepsis are key to reducing associated morbidity and mortality.

Immediate Management of Sepsis

The immediate management of a postpartum patient in septic shock does not differ from that of any other adult patient [19]. Early diagnosis and rapid initiation of treatment are predictors of a good prognosis, and the goal is to adequately accomplish all the steps included in the 1-hour bundle [20, 21].

As soon as septic shock is diagnosed, the following steps of the 1-hour bundle should be followed: measure the lactate level (blood gas), obtain blood cultures before administering antibiotics (other cultures should also be obtained if there is indication of other possible sites of infection), administer broad-spectrum antibiotics, volume resuscitation should be quickly initiated (20–30 mL/Kg of crystalloid solution, preferably lactated Ringer's), and apply vasopressors if necessary to maintain a mean arterial blood pressure of 65 mmHg.

During the resuscitation laboratory exams should be obtained to evaluate the patient's status and include complete blood count with differential, coagulogram, bilirubin, creatinine, and liver function tests.

Antibiotic initiation within 1 hour of diagnosis is associated with lower morbidity among adults, including pregnant and postpartum women. Septic shock is a serious and potentially fatal condition, and patients should be treated in intensive care units (ICUs) [20–22].

Specific Infections

Endometritis

Endometritis is the most common infection in the postpartum period. It develops in the area of placental implantation and may evolve to in the myometrium or in the parametrial tissues. It occurs after 1–3% of vaginal deliveries [23], but it occurs more commonly (5–6%) after vaginal deliveries with risk factors such as premature rupture of membranes, prolonged labor, and repeated cervical exams. Cesarean delivery is the most significant risk factor for endometritis, and it increases the risk

Table 52.1 The Sequential Organ Failure Assessment (SOFA) score [18]

	SOFA score				
Variable	0	1	2	3	4
Respiratory PaO_2/FiO_2 mm Hg	>400	≤400	≤300	≤200[a]	≤100[a]
Coagulation Platelets × $10^3/\mu L$	>150	≤150	≤100	≤50	≤20
Liver Bilirubin, mg/dL (mg/dL to µmol/L: multiply by 17.1)	<1.2	1.2–1.9	2.0–5.9	6.0–11.9	>12.0
Cardiovascular Hypotension	No hypotension	Mean arterial pressure < 70 mmHg	Dopamine < 5 or dobutamine (any dose)[b]	Dopamine > 5, epinephrine < 0.1, or norepinephrine ≤ 0,1[b]	Dopamine > 15, epinephrine > 0.1, or norepinephrine > 0,1[b]
Central nervous system Glasgow coma score scale	15	13–14	10–12	6–9	< 6
Renal Creatinine, mg/dL, or urine output, mL/d (mg/dL to µmol/L: multiply by 88,4)	<1.2	1.2–1.9	2.0–3.4	3.5–4.9 or <500	> 5.0 or <200

[a]With respiratory support
[b]Adrenergic agents administered for at least 1 hour (doses are in µg/kg per minute)

by tenfold [23]. Intraoperative antimicrobial prophylaxis administered as a single dose during Cesarean delivery reduces the incidence of postpartum endometritis [24].

In any case of postpartum fever, endometritis should be the principal suspected cause. It usually develops in the fourth or fifth day postpartum, but it can occur earlier if it is caused by more virulent pathogens. Fever can be low-grade (in less severe cases restricted to the endometrium and superficial myometrium) or overt (38–39 °C).

The uterine triad characteristic of postpartum endometritis includes:

(a) Subinvolution of the uterus
(b) Lower abdominal pain and uterine tenderness (on abdominal and bimanual exam)
(c) Open and soft cervix

Lochia in cases of endometritis may be odorless (in cases of group A beta-hemolytic strep) or foul-smelling (enterococcus, *E. coli*, *Bacteroides fragilis*).

The diagnosis of endometritis is a clinical diagnosis, but a complete blood count (CBC) can help make the diagnosis and monitor treatment response. Other laboratory studies should be performed depending on the severity of the case (lactate, bilirubin, creatinine, blood gases).

Although it can be difficult to isolate the etiologic agent in cases of endometritis, cervical cultures should be collected. In cases in which group A or B *Streptococcus* or *Neisseria gonorrhoeae* are detected, the pediatricians caring for the newborn should be notified.

Transvaginal pelvic ultrasound can help diagnose retained products of conception, abscesses, and intracavitary and abdominal wall hematomas.

Improvement within 48–72 hours occurs in approximately 90% of women, and treatment should be continued until clinical improvement and until the patient has remained afebrile for 24–48 hours. There is no need to continue antibiotics after hospital discharge. The persistence of fever after 24–48 hours is suspicious for complications, such as a parametrial or abdominal wall abscess or septic pelvic thrombophlebitis. If the symptoms regress but fevers persist, this can be due to bacterial resistance [23, 25].

Surgical intervention in the infected uterine cavity is necessary if retained products of conception are suspected or if there is persistent abnormal bleeding. In these cases, suction D&C is indicated, and uterotonics and antibiotics should also be administered.

In cases of peritonitis or sepsis, hysterectomy can be considered when the uterus is the focus of infection and the clinical picture is severe [15].

The gold standard antibiotic scheme for postpartum endometritis is a short-course intravenous clindamycin and gentamicin. There is no evidence that any one regimen is associated with fewer side effects [23]. If the infection is mild, with low-grade fever after a vaginal delivery, treatment with oral antibiotics such as amoxicillin + clavulanate is usually sufficient [26]. If the infection is severe, other schemes may be initiated, for longer courses of antibiotic therapy.

It is important to remember though that source control is generally as important as the antibiotics and that timely hysterectomy may be more important than changing and amplifying spectrum of the antibiotic drugs.

Surgical Site Infections

A surgical site infection is defined as an infection of the surgical wound or of any part of the anatomy which was manipulated during the surgical process and which occurs in the first 30 postoperative days. These infections are classified according to the depth of infection – they may be superficial (skin and subcutaneous tissue), deep (involvement of the fascia and musculature), or they may involve internal organs such as the uterus and abdominal cavity (Fig. 52.1).

Surgical site infections can develop at the Cesarean section wound or at the episiotomy or perineal laceration site. They are an important risk factor for breastfeeding discontinuation.

The most common infectious agents involved in wound infections are gram-positive rods, group B *Streptococcus*, *Staphylococcus aureus*, and anaerobes. In typical cases fever is low-grade (up to 38.3 °C) and develops between the fourth and the seventh postoperative day (earlier presentations or with higher fever can be seen with infections caused by beta-hemolytic group A or group B *Streptococcus*). Suture dehiscence and pain of variable intensity may also be observed.

In these cases, cultures of wound secretions may be helpful in determining the causative microorganism, but they may also be contaminated by normal skin flora.

Abdominal wall ultrasound can help determine if there are abscesses or hematomas that require drainage. Other imaging studies (such as CT or MRI) are usually unnecessary and should be reserved for specific cases.

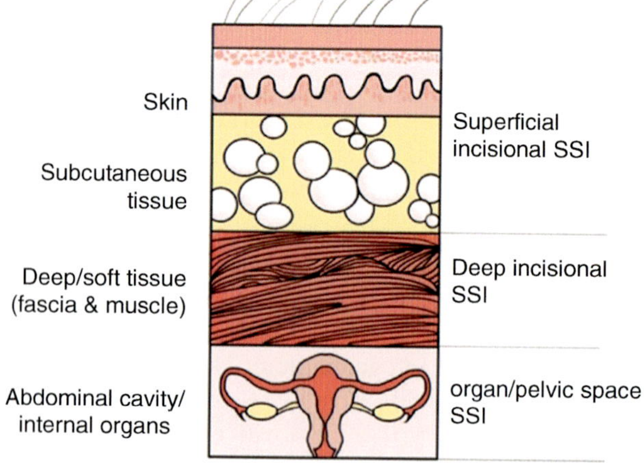

Fig. 52.1 Surgical site infections

Treatment for surgical site infections includes removal of sutures, debridement of devitalized tissue, and extensive irrigation. Wound healing is generally left to occur by secondary intention, but re-suturing may be indicated when the infection is controlled, and healthy granulation tissue is seen. In patients with infected episiotomy sites who do not respond to antibiotic therapy in 24–48 hours and who have edema and erythema beyond the perineal region (abdomen, thighs, gluteal region), surgical exploration is indicated as necrotizing fasciitis is likely. After surgical exploration, most infected episiotomy wounds heal well by secondary intention. Lacerations that involve the external anal sphincter and/or the rectal mucosa should be repaired after resolution of the infection. This is also true for extensive second-degree lacerations, in which re-suturing can be considered after resolution of the infection.

Necrotizing fasciitis is a rare but very serious complication of surgical site infections, with a mortality rate of 13–48%. It is most commonly caused by *Streptococcus* species, anaerobes (*Clostridium perfringens*), and gram-negative rods. It is characterized by progressively high fever which does not respond to antibiotic therapy, and the infected area shows with edema, erythema, fascial induration (with a wood-like consistency), and crepitation. There often are signs of systemic compromise. On evaluation, patients may have severe pain often unilaterally and erythema. Pain can be disproportional to the initial clinical findings. Diagnosis can be made on x-ray, which shows subcutaneous gas. It is important to include wound infection in the differential diagnosis. Treatment is radical surgical debridement of the infected tissue and aggressive antibiotic therapy [27].

Septic Pelvic Thrombophlebitis

Septic pelvic thrombophlebitis (SPT) is one of the least common complications of endometritis. It can also occur after septic abortion. It develops due to the hypercoagulable state typical of the postpartum period, in combination with the presence of bacteria in the bloodstream which cause vascular hyper-reactivity. This can become a starting point for septic emboli which can then cause renal, pulmonary, or other abscesses. However, it does not usually cause massive, fatal pulmonary emboli. Ovarian vein thrombosis complicates less than 0.05% of vaginal deliveries and up to 1–2% of Cesarean deliveries.

Blood cultures are negative in almost all cases of SPT, which is considered to be a diagnosis of exclusion. Infectious agents involved in SPT are similar to those which cause other puerperal infections – streptococcus, *Enterobacteriaceae*, and anaerobes.

The most common symptoms are fever, pelvic pain, and palpable abdominal mass (which is not always present).

There are two clinical presentations which are most common:

- Ovarian vein thrombophlebitis. This presents with fever and abdominal pain. Pain is usually on the affected side, which is the right in 90% of cases, due to the physiologic dextrorotation of the gravid uterus with greater compression of this side. Fever usually develops before the first week after delivery. Nausea and other mild gastrointestinal symptoms may also develop. Physical exam findings are not specific. Usually, ovarian vein thrombophlebitis is only diagnosed in cases of fever which does not respond to antibiotics after 48 hours and which raises suspicion for this condition.

- Deep pelvic thrombophlebitis. This condition presents with milder symptoms, with fever that develops earlier in the postpartum course (3–5 days postpartum up to 3 weeks). The clinical picture is less clear, with persistent fever despite antibiotic therapy in a patient who is ambulatory, who does not have pain or has poorly localized pain. Abdominal exam findings are typically minimal and vague.

Ovarian vein thrombosis is diagnosed with magnetic resonance angiography. Contrast CT can also be used. Ultrasound adds little to the workup, as it only helps eliminate pelvic and tubo-ovarian abscesses. The best treatment for SPT, including ovarian vein thrombosis, is antibiotic therapy (using the same agents as for endometritis), in combination with anticoagulation. Antibiotic therapy is recommended for at least 48–72 hours, and anticoagulation should be continued for a minimum of 7–10 days after resolution of fever. If the thrombosis extends to the renal vein or the inferior vena cava, anticoagulation should be continued for 3 months. Insertion of an inferior vena cava (IVC) filter can be indicated in cases in which a pulmonary embolism develops despite adequate anticoagulation [15, 28].

Salpingitis and Oophoritis

Inflammation and infection of the ovaries (oophoritis) and fallopian tubes (salpingitis) can also occur. Salpingitis is more common than oophoritis and can occur after septic abortions and vaginal deliveries with prolonged labor courses.

Clinically, these conditions present with acute abdominal pain, especially in the iliac fossa, high fever (39–39.5 °C), and discrete abdominal guarding. Bimanual exam reveals significant adnexal tenderness. As the disease progresses, adnexal masses may become palpable.

The treatment consists of antibiotics and analgesics. Although rare, a ruptured pyosalpinx can occur, and in these cases, a salpingectomy is necessary.

Parametritis

Parametritis is the inflammation of the parametrium, the tissue which surrounds the uterus. The most commonly affected part of the parametrium is the lateral cervical portion (unilateral in 70% of cases), although there may also be anterior or posterior invasion, as well as extension into the broad ligament. This condition usually occurs as bacteria spread from cervical and vaginal lacerations to the parametrial fibro-alveolar connective tissue.

Patients typically present with fever which persists for more than 10 days. The fever usually increases gradually and quickly reaches 39–39.5 °C, with decreases in temperature in the morning hours. On bimanual exam exquisite tenderness is detected which reflects hardening of the parametria. If the process is not treated in time, it can progress to an abscess of the parametria or broad ligament. The prognosis is usually favorable. Treatment is with antibiotics and anti-inflammatories. If an abscess forms, drainage may be necessary.

Peritonitis

Peritonitis can develop as a complication of localized puerperal infections such as endomyometritis, salpingitis, and parametritis.

Clinically, it presents with intense pain, abdominal rebound tenderness and guarding, high fever (40 °C), disturbance of bowel function, paralytic ileus, and tachycardia. On bimanual exam, severe pain is noted in the posterior vaginal fossa. If there is a purulent intra-abdominal collection, vaginal bulging may be noted.

Surgical management is indicated if there is an acute abdomen, a worsening in overall clinical status, if the patient meets the criteria for sepsis, if there is an abscess larger than 8 centimeters, and if there is an inadequate response to antibiotic therapy. Surgical drainage can be performed abdominally under ultrasound or CT guidance. Treatment of generalized peritonitis is classically performed via laparotomy, which permits aspiration of the purulent exudate in order to decrease toxic absorption. Prior to closing the abdominal cavity, exhaustive irrigation with physiologic solution is recommended. Depending on the patient's general clinical status, hysterectomy may be needed if the uterus is the source of infection.

Abscess drainage can also be accomplished vaginally and with ultrasound guidance, but this approach should be reserved for localized processes located close to the vaginal apex. Most common bacterial agents and empiric antibiotic therapy for puerperal infections may be seen in (Table 52.2).

Of note, bacteria diagnosed on culture and antibiotics selected based on local antibiograms are always preferable. Local protocols are recommended given the variations in causative agents and bacterial resistance patterns.

Other Infections

Postpartum women may develop infections from sites other than the uterus. These may be community- or hospital-acquired.

Fever in the First 24 Hours After Delivery

Temperature elevations do not always require treatment. In the first 24 hours after delivery, low-grade fever is common and usually self-resolves. In the first 24 hours after vaginal delivery, only 20% of women who have fevers have a puerperal infection. After Cesarean delivery, 70% of febrile women have a puerperal infection. High fevers in the first 24 hours should be investigated and treated because they can be caused by virulent bacteria.

Table 52.2 Most common bacterial agents and empiric antibiotic therapy for puerperal infections

Condition	Most common bacterial agents	Treatment
Endometritis	Polymicrobial – aerobic and anaerobic bacteria of the genital tract	Clindamycin (900mgIV every 8 hours) + gentamicin (5 mg/kg IV every 24 hours) Or Clindamycin (900 mg IV every 8 hours) + gentamicin (5 mg/kg every 24 hours) + ampicillin (2 g IV every 6 hours) Or Ampicillin-sulbactam (3 g–2 g IV every 6 hours) and/or piperacillin-tazobactam (4.5 g–4 g IV every 8 hours)
Surgical wound infection	Gram positives, group B *Streptococcus*, *Staphylococcus aureus*, anaerobes. After surgery, may also be caused by hospital-acquired infections	Suture removal, debridement of devitalized tissue, abscissa drainage **Superficial infection –** cephalexin 500 mg PO every 6 hours Or Amoxicillin+clavulanate (500 + 250 PO every 8 hours) **Deep infection –** clindamycin (900mgIV every 8 hours) and gentamicin (5 mg/kg IV every 24 hours) Or Clindamycin (900mgIV every 8 hours) and ceftriaxone (2 g IV every 24 hours) Or Ampicillin (2 g IV every 4 hours) and gentamicin (5 mg/kg every 24 hours) and metronidazole (500 mg IV every 8 hours) Or Clindamycin (900 mg IV every 8 hours) In case of MRSA – add vancomycin (20 mg/kg every 12 hours – maximum of 2 g per dose)
Necrotizing fasciitis	*Streptococcus* sp., anaerobes (*Clostridium perfringens*), and gram-negative rods	Ceftriaxone (2 g IV every 24 hours), with metronidazole (500 mg IV every 6 hours) Or Piperacillin/tazobactam (4.5 g every 8 hours)
Septic pelvic thrombophlebitis		Anticoagulants and antibiotic (follow endometritis protocol)

Breast Changes

During letdown (the 48–72-h period after delivery during which milk production starts), there can be an increase in axillary temperature which is not a fever. During this period, which lasts 3–4 days on average, breasts increase in size and temperature, and they become painful and engorged. Breast engorgement is common even after letdown. Usually it is bilateral, and it can cause an increase in body temperature, especially if the temperature is measured at the axilla.

Mastitis during breastfeeding usually presents later in the postpartum period. It typically presents with erythema, warmth, and swelling of one breast, accompanied by fever. Generalized malaise, tremors, and myalgias can also occur.

The most common bacterium associated with mastitis is *Staphylococcus aureus*. The prevalence of methicillin-resistant *S. Aureus* is increasing. Mild cases can be treated with oral cephalexin (500 mg every 6 hours) or clindamycin (300 mg every 8 hours). In case of suspected or confirmed MRSA, trimethoprim-sulfamethoxazole (TMP-SMX) can be used (160 mg/800 mg every 12 hours).

Please check sentence starting "For severe cases, abscess..." for completeness.

For severe cases, abscess drainage and intravenous treatment with vancomycin (15–20 mg/kg/dose every 12 hours, with a maximum of 2 g per dose) are recommended.

Respiratory Complications

Respiratory complications are more common among women who undergo general anesthesia as this can lead to atelectasis and aspiration pneumonia. Upper airway infections and community-acquired pneumonia are also on the differential for fever during the postpartum period.

Women who present with flulike symptoms – abrupt onset of fever, malaise, headache, cough, nasal congestion, and sore throat – should be evaluated for possible influenza. Some strains of influenza have worse prognoses among pregnant and postpartum women and should be treated with antiviral medications.

Illness caused by COVID-19 should be suspected and treated as in the nonpregnant population. One important consideration is social isolation to prevent transmission, including as it applies to the newborn. Pregnancy and the postpartum period can be risk factors for severe morbidity and mortality in COVID-19 infection, especially in developing countries [29].

Pyelonephritis

It is rare for pyelonephritis to present for the first time during the postpartum period. That said, a urinary tract infection can be difficult to distinguish from the other infections described earlier. Specific symptoms, urinalysis, and urine culture can help in the diagnosis and treatment.

Hemorrhage

Increased blood loss causing hemodynamic instability during labor, delivery, or the postpartum period is one of the most common life-threatening pregnancy complications.

Maternal deaths due to hemorrhage are considered avoidable, as prompt diagnosis and adequate treatment can prevent serious complications [30].

Postpartum hemorrhage can be acute if it occurs in the first 24 hours after delivery or delayed, if it occurs after this initial period. Delayed postpartum hemorrhage is usually associated with retained products of conception (such as placental remains) and develops slowly.

Hemorrhage is defined as any blood loss that causes hemodynamic instability [31]. Postpartum hemorrhage is the most common situation which leads to hemodynamic instability.

We estimate that acute postpartum hemorrhage occurs in up to 10% of deliveries, independent of preexisting risk factors [32]. These are very frequent events, and the healthcare team has to be ready to promptly diagnose and treat them.

Clinical Picture of Hemorrhage

Careful observation of patients during labor, delivery, and the immediate postpartum period is essential. Women should be closely observed for hemorrhage during the first 24 hours postpartum.

To diagnose acute hemorrhage, we recommend applying the diagnostic clinical criteria for hemorrhagic shock. The Advanced Trauma Life Support (ATLS) classification describes four classes of hemorrhage and emphasizes the progressive signs and symptoms that eventually lead to a state of shock [33]. Although these guidelines were developed for nonpregnant populations, they are applicable to pregnant women. Hemorrhage is divided into four classes:

- Class I: blood loss of up to 15% of blood volume. Heart rate may be slightly increased or normal, and there are no blood pressure, pulse pressure, or respiratory rate changes.
- Class II: blood loss of 15–30% of blood volume; presence of tachycardia (heart rate 100–120), tachypnea (respiratory rate of 20–40), and decreased pulse pressure, although generally the systolic arterial pressure is unchanged. The skin may be cold and humid, and there may be decreased capillary filling. An increase in heart rate and tachypnea with stable systolic blood pressure should be considered as evidence of compensated shock. These findings should prompt further workup and the establishment of a treatment plan, even if only mild vaginal bleeding is observed.
- Class III: blood loss of 30–40% of blood volume, resulting in significant decreases in arterial blood pressures and mental status changes. Any hypotension

(systolic blood pressure less than 90 mmHg) or decreases in blood pressure of more than 20–30% from baseline should raise alerts. In this category, heart rate is increased (≥120), as is respiratory rate. Urinary output is decreased, and capillary filling is slowed.
- Class IV: blood loss of more than 40% of blood volume, leading to significant decreases in blood pressure and altered mental status. The majority of patients in stage IV shock has hypotension (systolic blood pressure below 90 mmHg). Pulse pressure is decreased (≤25 mmHg) and tachycardia is severe (>120). Urine output is minimal or absent, skin is cold and pale, and capillary filling is compromised.

The shock index is calculated as the ratio of the heart rate and systolic blood pressure (SI = HR / SBP) [34]. This is a fast and simple resource to define hemorrhage severity, and it can also help determine treatment. The ratio is equal or lower than 0.8 in cases without hemorrhagic shock. When the SI = 0.9 in the context of blood loss and suspected severe hemorrhage, blood transfusion is indicated. A SI ≥ 1 suggests severe hemorrhage and blood transfusion is required. If the SI is more or equal than 1.4, immediate management via massive transfusion protocol is indicated.

Hemorrhage Etiology

There are four main etiologies for acute postpartum hemorrhage (PPH), which should be considered sequentially from the diagnosis and management standpoint. In order of incidence, the main causes of PPH are uterine atony, trauma (perineal in case of vaginal delivery or abdominal wall or organs in case of Cesarean delivery), retained placenta or retained products of conception, and coagulation disorders (either primary, more rare, or secondary due to the severity and duration of hemorrhage).

The most common cause of PPH is uterine atony, which is due to ineffective uterine contraction after delivery. Atony may or may not be associated with retained products. Abnormal placentation such as placenta accreta or previa and placental disorders such as abruption, retained placenta, and uterine inversion cause PPH because they inhibit effective uterine contraction, either locally or diffusely.

Lacerations lead to trauma-related bleeding. Cervical and vaginal lacerations can occur as a result of natural processes during delivery, or, more commonly, they may be iatrogenic (especially in the cases of forceps-assisted delivery or episiotomy). Lacerations should be suspected if excessive vaginal bleeding is noted postpartum and the uterus is firm. A careful exam of the inferior genital tract should be performed and should also exclude hematomas. In case of women who have had a prior Cesarean delivery, partial or complete uterine ruptures should be excluded by palpating the lower uterine segment.

During Cesarean delivery, hemorrhage is generally caused by the lateral extension of the uterine incision, resulting in spontaneous rupture of the lower uterine section. It may also be caused by the inadvertent transection or laceration of one of the uterine arteries. Retroperitoneal enlargement and bulging of the broad ligament during Cesarean delivery can be signs of retroperitoneal hemorrhage.

Coagulopathy complicates approximately 1 in 500 births and causes less than 7% of PPH cases. Coagulopathy or platelet dysfunction can contribute to PPH in women with hereditary (such as von Willebrand disease) or acquired blood dyscrasias (amniotic fluid embolism, abruption, severe preeclampsia, or HELLP syndrome). More commonly, coagulopathy is a result of massive PPH as the coagulation factors are consumed in the setting of severe persistent bleeding.

Prophylaxis and Treatment of PPH

Pharmacologic prophylaxis with oxytocin 10 IU given intramuscularly is universally recommended for the prevention of PPH. It should be administered to all women immediately after delivery of the infant, even before placental detachment.

Once the diagnosis of hemorrhagic shock is made, the source of bleeding needs to be found and stopped while the hemodynamic instability is also addressed. The primary objective of the therapeutic measures is to avoid inadequate organ and tissue perfusion and the development of the lethal triad of hypothermia, acidosis, and coagulopathy. Management is best accomplished in multidisciplinary teams, with the entire team involved in the patient's care. Simulation training and discussion of hemorrhage protocols are recommended for all healthcare professionals who care for pregnant and postpartum women.

The management steps for PPH are described in the sequence below (all should be performed at the same time):

- Elevation of the inferior limbs to facilitate venous return
- Continuous uterine massage
- Administration of oxygen via face mask (10–15 mL/hr)
- Venous access with two large-bore IVs (arms), laboratory evaluation (CBC, coagulation factors, type and screen, fibrinogen when possible)
- Crystalloid infusion: normal saline or Ringer's lactate bolus up to a maximum of 1500 mL. If hemodynamic instability persists after infusion of 1500 mL of crystalloid, transfusion of blood products is recommended.
- Administration of oxytocin: 10–40 IU diluted in 500–1000 mL of normal saline, infused until atony is controlled. Ten IU can be administered intramuscularly (IM) for improved results (this is in addition to the prophylactic oxytocin administration described above).
- Tranexamic acid: 1 g (10 mL of a 100 mg/mL solution) infused IV for 10–20 minutes. If bleeding persists after 30 minutes, a second dose of 1 g can be administered.

Therapeutic response should occur in 3–5 minutes. If bleeding does not significantly decrease in this interval, all the measures described above should be continued, and, in addition, the following should be implemented:

- Administer methylergonovine: 0.2 mg IM, with the possibility of a second dose after 5 minutes if there is a partial response. Thereafter, it can be re-dosed every 2–4 hours. An alternative is ergometrine 0.5 mg IV or IM or ergonovine 0.25 mg IM or IV every 2 hours. This step should be avoided in patients with hypertensive disorders.
- After 3–5 minutes, if the response is inadequate, administer misoprostol: 800–1000mcg per rectum. If available, other prostaglandins can be utilized, such as carboprost (0.25 mg IM, with maintenance every 15–90 minutes up to eight doses).
- Consider blood transfusion after infusion of 1500 mL of crystalloid solution. Packed red blood cell concentrate is recommended, but platelet and plasma transfusion may be indicated in case of grade III or IV hemorrhagic shock.

At the same time that the medications are administered, uterine massage should be continued, and other causes of hemorrhage should be addressed:

- Suturing of vaginal lacerations and exploration of the birth canal looking for hematomas and cervical lacerations or for vaginal sulcal lacerations (especially after operative deliveries)
- Placental separation if not yet complete, using manual exploration and/or curettage under anesthesia, if necessary

If the patient continues to have hemodynamic instability after 30 minutes of implementing the above, this is considered to be an inadequate treatment response. In these cases, the following invasive measures are indicated:

- Immediate surgical exploration in case of emergency after Cesarean delivery
- Bimanual uterine compression and insertion of a uterine tamponade balloon, in case of vaginal delivery
- Surgical exploration if bleeding is not controlled after inserting the intrauterine tamponade balloon

Surgical treatment consists of exploring the abdominal cavity and suturing any visible lacerations. A B-Lynch hemostatic suture can be performed even with a uterine tamponade balloon in situ. If these measures fail to control the bleeding, hysterectomy and progressive pelvic devascularization with uterine and hypogastric artery ligation are indicated.

Embolism

The postpartum period is a hypercoagulable state. Pregnant and postpartum women are at high risk for thrombosis. The risk of thromboembolism during pregnancy is 4–5 times greater than among nonpregnant women. During the first 6 weeks postpartum, the risk increases 20–80 times [35]. Deep venous thrombosis in the lower extremities can lead to pulmonary emboli, which can be fatal.

Pulmonary emboli can present in a variety of ways, from asymptomatic to respiratory distress to sudden death. They should be suspected if a patient has dyspnea, pleuritic pain, and hemoptysis.

Treatment consists of supportive care, anticoagulation, and, if possible, removal of the clot from the pulmonary arteries. Outside of pregnancy and the postpartum period, the techniques used are thrombolysis, percutaneous embolectomy, and surgical embolectomy. Use of extracorporeal membrane oxygenation (ECMO) is a recent addition to the treatment of pulmonary embolism. In the postpartum period, thrombolysis is associated with an increased risk of hemorrhage, and other therapies are recommended instead [36].

Thromboembolism can be avoided by administering prophylactic measures to high-risk patients. Prophylactic measures include early ambulation (for all women who do not have a contraindication), sequential pneumatic compression of the lower extremities, and use of heparin in a prophylactic dose (especially low-molecular-weight heparin) for patients who have an increased risk of thrombosis. Prophylactic heparin has to be continued for 3–6 weeks postpartum, depending on the patient's risk profile [37].

Amniotic fluid embolism (AFE) occurs when amniotic fluid enters the maternal circulation. This is a potentially fatal event, with mortality rates that range from 10% to 90%. It typically occurs during labor or in the first hours postpartum. Women present with acute respiratory distress and may have cardiac arrest and/or seizures. Disseminated intravascular coagulopathy generally also occurs. This is a diagnosis of exclusion.

Four criteria are present in the majority of cases, though there are atypical forms [38]:

- Cardiopulmonary arrest or hypotension with respiratory insufficiency (dyspnea, cyanosis, or decreased oxygen saturation).
- Presence of disseminated intravascular coagulation.
- Absence of fever.
- Symptoms begin during labor or in the first 30 minutes after delivery.

Treatment of AFE is cardiopulmonary resuscitation, life support (intensive care unit admission, mechanical ventilation, and vasoactive drugs), treatment of hemorrhage, and reversal of coagulopathy [39].

Another important condition that should be on the differential diagnosis for cardiopulmonary insufficiency or shock in the postpartum period is postpartum cardiomyopathy. Although this can happen during pregnancy, most cases are diagnosed postpartum. The predisposing risk factors are multiparity, Black race, smoking, diabetes, preeclampsia, malnutrition, and age extremes (adolescence and advanced age).

Postpartum cardiomyopathy presents with cardiac insufficiency, generally with left ventricle systolic dysfunction with an ejection fraction below 45%. Other causes of cardiac insufficiency have to be eliminated. Mortality rates are high – from 2% to 24% [9].

Pain

Pain during the postpartum period generally is not a life-threatening condition. However, constant or intense pain can make breastfeeding more difficult and can be a barrier to forming a bond with the infant. It can also affect a woman's satisfaction with her birth experience.

The most frequent types of pain experienced by women in the postpartum period are cramping due to uterine contractions or "afterpains," perineal pain in case of a severe perineal laceration or episiotomy, and postoperative pain after Cesarean delivery.

Other types of pain such as pain due to hemorrhoids, musculoskeletal pain, and migraines are not uncommon during the postpartum period.

Pain control is often neglected in this population. Few studies exist about the most effective pain control methods and fewer yet about which medications are safe while breastfeeding.

We recommend using an analgesic such as acetaminophen for mild, tolerable pain levels. Nonsteroidal anti-inflammatory drugs (NSAIDs) may be necessary if the pain is intense, and we recommended using them after Cesarean delivery or after deep or severe perineal lacerations. NSAIDs should be avoided in hypertensive patients. In some situations, opiates are also necessary. In breastfeeding women, morphine is preferable to tramadol or meperidine.

For perineal lesions use of ice or cold compresses can also help control pain.

Intense pain that does not improve with pain medications should be evaluated, and more serious conditions should be excluded, such as postoperative wound infection (perineal or C-section wound) and acute abdomen [40].

Headaches

Postpartum women may develop headaches for a series of reasons, including hormonal changes, lack of sleep, stress and fatigue, administration of spinal or epidural anesthesia or vasoactive drugs during anesthesia for delivery, or postpartum preeclampsia.

Rarely, women experience associated neurologic symptoms, such as visual changes, altered mental status, or loss of balance. In these cases, a neurologic evaluation is warranted to rule out anatomic lesions or other central nervous system etiologies.

If the woman had neuraxial anesthesia for childbirth, evaluation by an anesthesiologist may be necessary. Headaches due to a reduction in spinal fluid caused by spinal anesthesia are very intense and improve when the patient is lying down. Treatment includes massive hydration, analgesics, and in many cases a new lumbar puncture for a blood patch.

Women with history of migraines may develop symptoms in the postpartum period, and in this case they should be treated with specific treatments for migraines [41].

Tension headaches are the most common kinds of headaches. They are characterized by a sensation of pressure or tightness around the head, and they tend to be more or less painful at different time periods.

Urinary Changes

Urinary symptoms can present in the immediate postpartum period after vaginal or Cesarean deliveries. In the first case, these are usually related to microtraumas around the urethra, which may include small bleeding lacerations. In the second case, urinary complaints are related to the urinary catheter used during surgery, which can cause infections, or to administration of neuraxial anesthesia, which may cause urinary retention.

Urinary tract infections are relatively common and were discussed earlier in this chapter. Once infection is excluded, symptoms such as polyuria, burning, bladder tenesmus, or retention should be investigated and managed systematically.

Urethral lacerations which do not require suturing (small extensions or with minimal bleeding) should be treated with analgesics and wound care including cold compresses and local analgesics such as sprays. These usually heal quickly and rarely develop infectious complications.

Urinary retention usually occurs as a complication of spinal anesthesia, due to the large intraoperative volume shifts and/or due to the pharmacologic effects of opiates. Patients often remain partly anesthetized and cannot feel the urge to urinate after removal of the urinary catheter. It is important to monitor for spontaneous micturition during the immediate postpartum period.

In case of urinary distension, intermittent catheterization should be performed until spontaneous micturition resumes, which is usually 24 hours after the surgical procedure [42].

Development of anuria (diuresis of ≤30 mL/h) in the postoperative period after Cesarean delivery (this is less common after vaginal deliveries) should be investigated. Once urinary retention is ruled out, hypovolemic shock should also be ruled out. Once both of these causes are ruled out, possible urinary tract injury during surgery should be considered. In this case, it is necessary to obtain imaging studies (ultrasound, CT, or MRI), and it may be necessary to proceed with exploratory laparotomy.

References

1. Brasil. Ministério da Saúde. Datasus - sistema da informacao de mortalidade [Internet]. Departamento de Informática. 2020. Available from: http://www2.datasus.gov.br/DATASUS/index.php?area=0202&VObj=http://tabnet.datasus.gov.br/cgi/deftohtm.exe?sih/cnv/qi.
2. Say L, Chou D, Gemmill A, Tunçalp Ö, Moller A-B, Daniels J, et al. Global causes of maternal death: a WHO systematic analysis. Lancet Glob Health. 2014;2(6):e323–33.
3. Soares VMN, de Souza KV, de Azevedo EMM, Possebon CR, Marques FF. Causas de mortalidade materna segundo níveis de complexidade hospitalar. Rev Bras Ginecol Obstet. 2012;34(12):536–43.
4. ACOG. ACOG Practice Bulletin No. 202 summary: gestational hypertension and preeclampsia. Obstet Gynecol. 2019;133(1):211–4.
5. Duley L, Gülmezoglu AM, Henderson-Smart DJ, Chou D. Magnesium sulphate and other anticonvulsants for women with pre-eclampsia (Review) Magnesium sulphate and other anticonvulsants for women with pre-eclampsia (Review). Cochrane Database Syst Rev. 2010;nov(11):83.
6. Vigil-De Gracia P, Ludmir J. The use of magnesium sulfate for women with severe preeclampsia or eclampsia diagnosed during the postpartum period. J Matern Neonatal Med. 2015;28(18):2207–9.
7. Noronha Neto CC, Maia SSB, Katz L, Coutinho IC, Souza AR, Amorim MM. Clonidine versus captopril for severe postpartum hypertension: a randomized controlled trial. Fukumoto Y, editor. PLoS One. 2017;12(1):e0168124.
8. Cífková R, Johnson MR, Kahan T, Brguljan J, Williams B, Coca A, et al. Peripartum management of hypertension: a position paper of the ESC Council on Hypertension and the European Society of Hypertension. Eur Hear J Cardiovasc Pharmacother; 2020.
9. Regitz-Zagrosek V, Roos-Hesselink JW, Bauersachs J, Blomström-Lundqvist C, Cífková R, De Bonis M, et al. ESC guidelines for the management of cardiovascular diseases during pregnancy. Eur Heart J. 2018;39:3165–241.
10. Brown MA, Magee LA, Kenny LC, Karumanchi SA, McCarthy FP, Saito S, et al. The hypertensive disorders of pregnancy: ISSHP classification, diagnosis & management recommendations for international practice. In: Pregnancy hypertension, vol. 13. Elsevier B.V.; 2018. p. 291–310.
11. Nogacka A, Salazar N, Suárez M, Milani C, Arboleya S, Solís G, et al. Impact of intrapartum antimicrobial prophylaxis upon the intestinal microbiota and the prevalence of antibiotic resistance genes in vaginally delivered full-term neonates. Microbiome. 2017;5(1):93.
12. Seventieth World Health Assembly Executive Board. Improving the prevention, diagnosis and clinical management of sepsis. World Heal Organ. 2017;(May):1–4.

13. Van Dillen J, Zwart J, Schutte J, Van Roosmalen J. Maternal sepsis: epidemiology, etiology and outcome. Curr Opin Infect Dis. 2010;23:249–54.
14. Chapman E, Reveiz L, Illanes E, Cosp XB. Antibiotic regimens for management of intra-amniotic infection. Cochrane Database Syst Rev. John Wiley and Sons Ltd. 2014;2014.
15. World Health Organization (WHO). WHO recommendations for prevention and treatment of maternal peripartum infections. Geneva: WHO/HRP; 2015. p. 80.
16. Bonet M, Brizuela V, Abalos E, Cuesta C, Baguiya A, Chamillard M, et al. Frequency and management of maternal infection in health facilities in 52 countries (GLOSS): a 1-week inception cohort study. Lancet Glob Health. 2020;8(5):e661–71.
17. Singer M, Deutschman CS, Seymour C, Shankar-Hari M, Annane D, Bauer M, et al. The third international consensus definitions for sepsis and septic shock (sepsis-3). JAMA J Am Med Assoc. 2016;315:801–10.
18. Lopes Ferreira F, Peres Bota D, Bross A, Mélot C, Vincent JL. Serial evaluation of the SOFA score to predict outcome in critically ill patients. JAMA. 2001;286(14):1754–8.
19. Borloz MP, Hamden KE. Sepsis in special populations. In: Emergency medicine clinics of North America, vol. 35. W.B. Saunders; 2017. p. 139–58.
20. Meier B, Staton C. Sepsis resuscitation in resource-limited settings. In: Emergency Medicine Clinics of North America, vol. 35. W.B. Saunders; 2017. p. 159–73.
21. Radbel J, Boutsikaris D. The new usual care. In: Emergency Medicine Clinics of North America, vol. 35. W.B. Saunders; 2017. p. 11–23.
22. Bauer ME, Housey M, Bauer ST, Behrmann S, Chau A, Clancy C, et al. Risk factors, etiologies, and screening tools for sepsis in pregnant women: a multicenter case-control study. Anesth Analg. 2019;129(6):1613–20.
23. Mackeen AD, Packard RE, Ota E, Speer L. Antibiotic regimens for postpartum endometritis. Cochrane Database Syst Rev. John Wiley and Sons Ltd. 2015;2015.
24. American College of Obstetricians and Gynecologists. Clinical management guidelines for obstetricians & gynecologists-use of prophylactic antibiotics in labor and delivery. Obstet Gynecol. 2018;132(3):103–19.
25. Karsnitz DB. Puerperal infections of the genital tract: a clinical review. J Midwifery Womens Health. John Wiley and Sons Inc.; 2013;58:632–42.
26. Meaney-Delman D, Bartlett LA, Gravett MG, Jamieson DJ. Oral and intramuscular treatment options for early postpartum endometritis in low-resource settings. Obstet Gynecol. Lippincott Williams and Wilkins. 2015;125:789–800.
27. World Health Organization. WHO recommendations for prevention and treatment of maternal peripartum infections: Evidence Base. WHO recommendations for prevention and treatment of maternal peripartum infections: Evidence Base. WHO/HRP; 2015.
28. Garcia J, Aboujaoude R, Apuzzio J, Alvarez JR. Septic pelvic thrombophlebitis: diagnosis and management. Infect Dis Obstet Gynecol. 2006;2006:15614.
29. Ramos Amorim MM, Soligo Takemoto ML, Fonseca EB. Maternal deaths with Covid19: a different outcome from mid to low resource countries? Am J Obstet Gynecol. 2020;223:298–9.
30. Alkema L, Chou D, Hogan D, Zhang S, Moller A-B, Gemmill A, et al. Global, regional, and national levels and trends in maternal mortality between 1990 and 2015, with scenario-based projections to 2030: a systematic analysis by the UN Maternal Mortality Estimation Inter-Agency Group. Lancet (London, England). 2016;387(10017):462–74.
31. Committee on Practice Bulletins-Obstetrics. ACOG Practice Bulletin No. 183 Postpartum Hemorrhage. Obstet Gynecol. 2017;130(4):e168–86.
32. Deneux-Tharaux C, Bonnet M-P, Tort J. Epidemiology of post-partum haemorrhage. J Gynecol Obstet Biol Reprod (Paris). 2014;43(10):936–50.
33. American College of Surgeons. Advanced trauma life support (Student Manual); 1997.
34. Lee S-Y, Kim H-Y, Cho G-J, Hong S-C, Oh M-J, Kim H-J. Use of the shock index to predict maternal outcomes in women referred for postpartum hemorrhage. Int J Gynaecol Obstet. 2019;144(2):221–4.

35. Jackson E, Curtis KM, Gaffield ME. Risk of venous thromboembolism during the postpartum period: a systematic review. Obstet Gynecol. 2011;117:691–703.
36. Martillotti G, Boehlen F, Robert-Ebadi H, Jastrow N, Righini M, Blondon M. Treatment options for severe pulmonary embolism during pregnancy and the postpartum period: a systematic review. J Thromb Haemost. 2017;15(10):1942–50.
37. Clinton CM, Kuller JA, James AH. Prevention of postpartum venous thromboembolism. Obstet Gynecol Surv. 2019;74(10):601–6.
38. Stafford IA, Moaddab A, Dildy GA, Klassen M, Belfort MA, Romero R, et al. Evaluation of proposed criteria for research reporting of amniotic fluid embolism. Am J Obstet Gynecol. Mosby Inc. 2019;220:285–7.
39. Pacheco LD, Saade G, Hankins GDV, Clark SL. Amniotic fluid embolism: diagnosis and management. Am J Obstet Gynecol. 2016;215(2):B16–24.
40. Fahey JO. Best practices in management of postpartum pain. J Perinat Neonatal Nurs. 2017;31(2):126–36.
41. Burch R. Headache in pregnancy and the puerperium. In: Neurologic Clinics, vol. 37. W.B. Saunders; 2019. p. 31–51.
42. Mulder FEM, Hakvoort RA, Schoffelmeer MA, Limpens J, Van der Post JAM, Roovers JPWR. Postpartum urinary retention: a systematic review of adverse effects and management. Int Urogynecol J Pelvic Floor Dysfunct. Springer-Verlag London Ltd.. 2014;25:1605–12.

Chapter 53
Care of the Newborn Infant during the Third Stage of Labor

J. L. Diaz-Rossello and M. F. Blasina

Definition

"A live birth is the complete expulsion or extraction from its mother of a product of conception, irrespective of the duration of pregnancy, which, after such separation, breathes or shows any other evidence of life, such as beating of the heart, pulsation of the umbilical cord, or any definite movement of voluntary muscles, whether or not the umbilical cord has been cut or the placenta is attached" [1].

The third stage of labor is the period that starts immediately after delivery of the infant and ends with the completed delivery of the placenta and its attached membranes [2].

Caring the live-newborn infant during the third stage of labor, while the placenta has not yet detached and there is umbilical cord blood flow, is a distinct period in the transition from fetal to extrauterine physiology [3].

The third stage is the shortest of the three stages of labor, and the detachment and expulsion of the "after birth," after 28 weeks of gestation, lasts a median time of 5 minutes (p10 = 2 and p90 = 14–19) increasing significantly at lower gestational ages and also increases the frequency of retained placenta (Table 53.1) [2].

Learning to care for the newborn infant at birth should be based on updated knowledge of this rapidly changing physiology and developing clinical expertise. Trainers should teach how to perform the assessment of the newborn and provide evidence-based interventions to support the infant while still depending on its umbilical-placental circulation. In the past century, training on immediate newborn care was badly influenced by the habit of immediate cord clamping and its adverse consequences.

Initial care requires adaptation of delivery room setting to keep the baby in the "maternal space," constrained by the length of the umbilical cord.

J. L. Diaz-Rossello (✉) · M. F. Blasina
Department of Neonatology, Hospital de Clínicas, Facultad de Medicina, Universidad de la República, Montevideo, Uruguay

© Springer Nature Switzerland AG 2022
R. A. Moreira de Sá, E. B. d. Fonseca (eds.), *Perinatology*,
https://doi.org/10.1007/978-3-030-83434-0_53

Table 53.1 Duration of the third stage of labor in minutes and incidence of retained placenta (after 30 minutes of birth) in vaginal deliveries according to gestational age in weeks

		Percentile			Retained placenta	
Weeks of gestation	N	10th	50th	90th	%	N
20	40	1	15	91	35.0	14
21	68	3	22	122	41.2	28
22	90	2	17	144	35.6	32
23	108	2	15	80	33.3	36
24	118	3	15	55	22.9	27
25	93	2	10	37	14.0	13
26	104	i	7	24	7.7	8
27	88	2	5	16	2.3	2
28	122	2	7	22	3.3	4
29	146	2	5	19	2.7	4
30	219	2	5	19	3.2	7
31	265	2	5	15	2.3	6
32	409	2	5	17	2.0	8
33	583	2	5	19	3.8	22
34	794	2	5	15	1.9	15
35	1147	2	5	15	2.5	29
36	1918	2	5	15	2.3	44
37	3690	2	5	14	2.4	89
38	5893	2	5	13	1.6	94
39	8882	2	5	13	1.7	151
40	13,151	2	5	13	1.5	197
41	5395	2	5	13	1.5	81
42	2212	2	r	14	1.0	23

Adapted with permission from Dombrowski [2]

The major challenge is to overcome previous training and guidelines of neonatal care and to rapidly advance in the de-implementation of the nonevidence-based practice of immediate or early clamping of the umbilical cord.

Umbilical-Placental Circulation and the Cardiopulmonary Switch during the Third Stage of Labor

During the first minutes after birth, there is a redistribution of blood from the placental side to the body of the newborn infant. Although the average final balance of this period results in an increase in neonatal blood volume, the mechanism is not strictly a transfusion because the arterial blood flow from the infant to the placenta continues.

In fetal circulation 30% to 50% of the fetal cardiac output goes to the placenta via the umbilical arteries and returns to the fetus via the umbilical vein. Sixty percent (60%) of this oxygenated blood bypasses (through shunts) the liver, via the ductus venosus, continues via the inferior vena cava, and crosses the right atrium, through the foramen ovale, into the left atrium, and it is pumped into the left ventricle and to the ascending aorta, the heart and brain. Due to the high fetal pulmonary vascular resistance, only 10% of the fetal right ventricle output flows into the lung, and 90% flows through the ductus arteriosus into the descending aorta.

At birth, the sharp decrease in pulmonary resistance reduces the flow through the three shunts that progressively close. Fifty percent (50%) of the cardiac output rapidly irrigates the lungs.

During the third stage, the fetal physiology persists transiently like the mechanisms of an extracorporeal membrane oxygenator, where the placenta is the "membrane," as in fetal life. Postnatal placental respiration has been documented during the first minutes of life before total placental detachment [4].

The obstetric procedure called ex utero intrapartum therapy (EXIT) is a technique used since 1992 to prolong placental function in cesarean sections to gain time to clear the airway of the fetus, in antenatally diagnosed congenital high airway obstruction syndromes [5]. Case series report that, after extracting the fetal head through the incision of the uterus, under induced tocolysis, the placental respiration provides a safe period of an average time of 18 (8–44) minutes, to surgically repair the fetus-neonate airway patency [6]. EXIT experience helps to understand the safety of the support of the placental respiration at birth if the umbilical flow is not interrupted.

While the placenta is not detached and the bidirectional umbilical flow persists, several changes interact to finally achieve neonatal circulatory and ventilatory autonomy.

Initial studies with local thermodilution techniques showed a stable umbilical flow estimated in 75 mL/min/Kg from 20 to100 seconds after birth, decreasing sharply after that [7].

Modern studies using Doppler ultrasound showed that venous and arterial umbilical flow lasts longer than previously described. Venous flow stopped in almost two thirds of vaginal term deliveries at 4:34 min: sec (3:03–7:31) (median (IQR)) before the cord was clamped, and in one third of the cases, the flow continued until cord clamping at 5:13 min: sec (2:56–9:15). Venous flow increased markedly during large breaths and stopped during crying. Arterial flow stopped spontaneously in one half of vaginal deliveries at 4:22 (2:29–7:17) min: sec, even while cord pulsations were still palpable. In the other half of the cases, the cord was clamped before the flow stopped [8].

Using a digital scale with precision of 1 g, the continuous recording of weight shows patterns that suggest variability in the umbilical blood flow that results in neonatal weight (Fig. 53.1). All cases have the largest increase in the first minute, but weight recordings show fluctuations suggesting that blood flow to the infant increases during uterine contractions and decreases between contractions, as if there is a negative balance caused by return of arterial blood to the placenta [9, 10].

Umbilical venous blood flow to the infant may be reinforced by uterine contractions. Uterine contractions during the third stage of labor are painless, but the

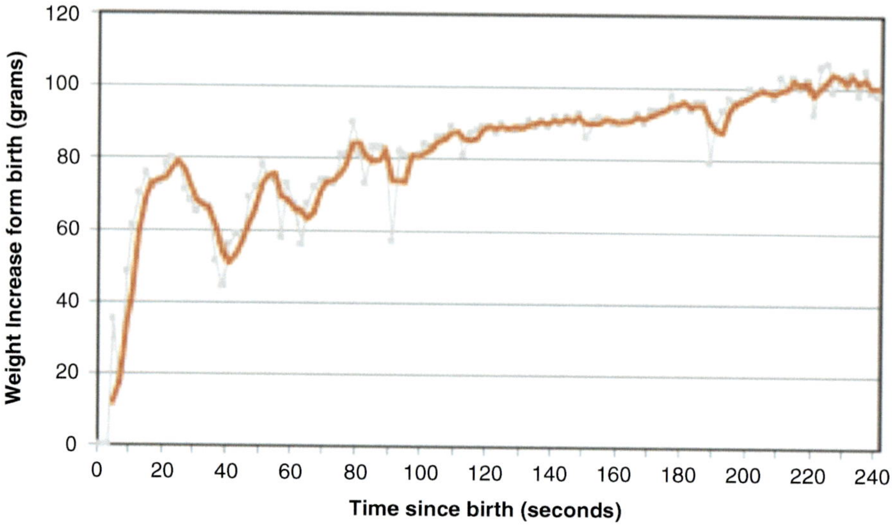

Fig. 53.1 Net weight accumulated from birth, every 2 seconds (smoothed) in an infant of 38 weeks of gestational age whose birthweight was 2865 g before clamping the cord [10]

intrauterine pressure increases in a similar intensity (60–100 mm Hg) to those of the second stage. A simple explanation may be that the intrauterine pressure acts as milking force on the placenta increasing the pressure of the umbilical vein and augmenting its flow to the infant [11]. This, not yet proven, concept of the venous pumping effect of the uterus may explain why the administration of oxytocin to the mother, during the second or third stage of labor, was associated with a smaller residual blood volume in the placenta [12]. This hypothesis was not confirmed in a randomized clinical trial measuring weight gain before cord clamping, and no differences were found between those receiving oxytocin at birth and those receiving placebo [13].

Elective Interruption of Umbilical Blood Flow (Cord Clamping)

Elective interruption of the placental circulation and umbilical blood flow at birth is an obstetric surgical decision that has been debated for decades [14]. This nonevidence practice has extended mainly in hospital deliveries.

The time of clamping became the center of this debate, with poor consideration to the complex physiological events that occur and their variability depending on the gestational age, type of delivery, placental reserve, fetal well-being, etc.

Umbilical cord clamping before completing lung aeration reduces the left ventricle preload and increases its peripheral vascular resistance (post charge), with marked reduction in cardiac output and bradycardia. In preterm infants this elective practice produces a sudden swing in hemodynamic function that has the potential to increase the risk of intraventricular hemorrhage and necrotizing enterocolitis as well as associated mortality and morbidity, further analyzed later in this chapter [15].

If the cord is not clamped, circulation will end in a timely manner when its flow naturally stops. The intact umbilical blood flow during the third stage of labor leads to a more stable neonatal hemodynamic transition.

Many undefined subcategories of cord clamping have been used: immediate, early, delayed, deferred, timely (in Spanish "pinzado oportuno"), and even the oxymoron of "physiologic clamping." If there is umbilical blood flow and it is interrupted, it is not physiologic. After the flow stops, severing, cutting, and tying has been the way for separating the placenta in humans before watches, metal, or plastic clamps were available, just waiting for the flow to stop and the baby breathing.

Assessing Fetal Vitality at Birth

The flow through the umbilical cord is a vital sign to assess the newborn in the first seconds after birth. An engorged blue cord with pulsating arteries is the first sign of vitality to observe (Fig. 53.2). If left intact, it flattens and turns white, bloodless, and cold in a variable time depending on when the umbilical flow ceases. The helicoidal umbilical arterial pulses can be seen or perceived by touch. The pulses cease progressively from the placental side as the arteries begin to close, but the pulses close to the navel may be perceived for minutes and even longer without arterial flow.

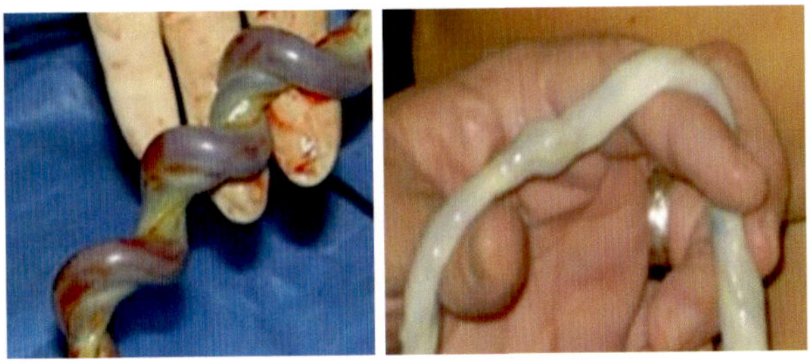

Fig. 53.2 Assessment of umbilical-placental blood flow at birth. Left image shows a normal umbilical cord with a full blue vein and arteries displayed in a helicoid of three loops in 10 cm. Right image shows a flat and white, transparent, bloodless cord

Fetal Asphyxia

Immediate diagnosis of wellbeing or asphyxia is the emergency assessment that has always ruled interventions at the time of birth. When the infant is born with severe fetal asphyxia, professionals have the urge to provide skilled resuscitation and neuroprotective measures to reduce sequelae.

The Greek origin of the word asphyxia is derived from "sphygmus" (pulse) and means "absence of pulse." Virginia Apgar and Erich Saling have proposed scores to quantify this assessment. After Apgar score was published (Table 53.3), Erich Saling proposed a different score of fetal vitality at birth, including the observation of the hemodynamics of the umbilical cord [16]. Virginia Apgar sustained that "Heart rate was the most important diagnostic and prognostic of the five signs" [17], while Saling replaced heart rate by the assessment of the blood flow of the umbilical cord vessels.[1]

An engorged and pulsating cord is an immediate sign of vitality for Saling (Table 53.2). Fetal acidosis is more frequent in those that had a flat umbilical cord at the time of birth [16].

Vitality assessment during the first minute of extrauterine life is so important that has been called the "Golden minute," urging to rush (Time is Gold) to differentiate between the healthy and the asphyxiated fetus with cardiovascular collapse. The benefit of Saling score is that the assessment of the umbilical cord is visible right at the first seconds and provides reassurance by the continuous assessment of the umbilical cord flow before the variable initiation of breathing movements or crying.

Although Apgar score defines a heart rate of less than 100 as the most important diagnostic sign of asphyxia in the first minute, this is not a precise concept. Average heart rate of normal newborn infants at 1 minute of life is less than 100 beats per minute, monitored by pulse oximetry or EKG since the first 15–30 seconds after birth. Assessing heart rate has limitations and should be considered only as part of an overall clinical assessment of an infant [18].

Table 53.2 Vitality score for newborns at birth proposed by E. Saling [16]

Saling score	2	1	0
Umbilical cord	Tense/blue	Half tense	Flat/white
Skin color	Bluish to pink	Bluish and pale	Pale
Tone and move	Active	Reduced	Absent
Breathing	Regular	Irregular	Absent

[1]A feasible explanation is that Dr Virginia Apgar mainly cared for newborn infants with immediate cord clamping. Apgar explains that "If one attends the baby alone, it is easy to learn to look briefly at the epigastrium or precordium for visible heartbeat, while palpation of the cord about 2 inches from the umbilicus is the most satisfactory method for determining the heart rate quickly, and avoids the area of clamping or tying of the cord"17. Apgar V. A proposal for a New Method to Evaluation of the Newborn Infant. Current Researches in Anesthesia and Analgesia 1953;32(4):260–57.

Heart rate <100 bpm, in the first 2 min, when breathing efforts and muscle tone are normal, should not be an indicator for immediate ventilation [19].

The progressive increase in heart rate is now considered the most reliable indicator of normalcy and provides a safety time lapse to avoid rushing to perform unnecessary interventions (Table 53.4).

Severe acidosis in fetal blood gases at the time of birth is the confirmation of fetal asphyxia. Apgar and Saling scores correlate well with abnormal blood gases, low pH, low PaO2, and high PaCO2 in umbilical arterial blood collected in the first seconds of life.

Respiration during the Third Stage of Labor

The respiratory changes of the immediate postnatal period are sufficiently dynamic as to modify blood gases in seconds.

At birth the fetal lung is filled with fluid and the pulmonary vessels offer a high resistance to blood flow.

The first few breaths require a significant respiratory effort producing a high negative pressure (−40 to −50 cm H_2O) and displacement of the alveolar fluid to the

Table 53.3 Vitality score for newborns at birth proposed by V. Apgar [17]

Apgar score	2	1	0
Heart rate	Over 100 bpm	Slow (less than 100 bpm)	Absent
Skin color	Completely pink	Body pink, extremities blue	Blue, pale
Tone and move	Active motion	Some flexion of extremities	Absent
Breathing	Good crying	Slow, irregular	Absent
Reflex irritability	Vigorous cry	Cry	No response

Table 53.4 Five studies of average heart rate during the first minute of life in a total of 2347 newborn infants monitored with pulse oximetry

Author	Gestational Age	Type of Delivery	Number	Heart Rate Trend	Respiratory Support	Average Heart Rate
Gonzalez	Term	VD/CS	380	Increase	Yes	133VD/108CS
Dawson	Preterm	–	126	Increase	Yes	<100
Dawson	Preterm-term	VD/CS	468	Increase	No	96
Smit	Term	VD	109	Increase	No	61
Kc	Late preterm-term	VD	1264	Increase	No	116EC/107 DC

VD Vaginal Delivery, *CS* Cesarean Sectio, *EC* Early Cord Clamping, *DC* Delayed Cord Clamping
Delayed clamping and cesarean sections have lower heart rate [20–23]

interstitium for its reabsorption. The inspired air starts to produce lung distension maintained by the surfactant layer along the alveolar lining.

The initial functional residual lung capacity provides an insignificant amount of pulmonary exchange during the first breaths [24]. Safety of respiration may depend transiently on placental gas exchange that makes a substantial contribution to the infant's oxygen needs during these seconds and minutes of transition to pulmonary respiration [25–27].

Seconds after birth blood gases do not strictly measure the fetal status, because when the umbilical flow is not interrupted, they also change according to postnatal placental and lung functions.

Standard values of blood gases in the umbilical cord blood have been historically obtained with immediate clamping of the cord and may differ from values obtained later in the third stage. Changes occur when placental function and umbilical flow remain during the transition to lung ventilation.

Blood gases may also have a normal rapid change during the first seconds after birth. A drop in pH and base excess (BE) may occur, with an increase in the umbilical artery partial pressures of O_2 (PaO_2) and CO_2 ($PaCO_2$) as well as an increase in lactate concentration in the umbilical artery. This physiological "hidden acidosis" in term vaginal deliveries is considered a consequence of postnatal volume expansion of the less perfused peripheral tissues (acrocyanosis) that trapped metabolites during labor [27, 28]. The blood volume expansion may also be accompanied by changes in hematocrit.

A similar but more severe situation may occur in fetuses with nuchal cord, when a larger blood volume is retained in the placenta by umbilical vein compression during vaginal delivery. In these cases, hypotension may not occur before birth as a consequence of the external pressure supported by the fetus while passing through the birth canal. Hypothetically external forces may act like an anti-shock garment and help to maintain central perfusion of priority organs of the fetus like the brain and the myocardium [29]. Postnatal reperfusion of peripheral tissues, in cases of tight nuchal cord, may increase the magnitude of the postnatal "hidden acidosis."

Elective cesarean sections may have a less pronounced hidden acidosis, as they usually have less acrocyanosis. The caesarean section babies look pinker.

During the Third Stage of Labor, the Baby Turns from Blue to Pink and the Umbilical Cord from Blue to White (Bloodless)

The earliest observation of this rapidly changing condition can be read between lines in the first chapter of the first textbook printed in the history of medicine [30]. Paolo Bagelardo in 1472 describes the management of the umbilical cord: "If the liveborn has a vivid color, then umbilical cord should be cut leaving it with a length of four fingers and tying it with twisted thread of wool or with silk...." The midwife was advised not to cut the cord until the infant was of "lively" color, pink, and then to tie after cutting. No bleeding was expected from the umbilical vessels when cutting the cord before tying, because they waited until the infant was pink, coinciding with time when the umbilical blood flow stops, and the cord is white and bloodless.

Precision pulse oximetry of the infant during the third stage has helped to improve assessment of the infant by providing a safer adaptation without unnecessary and even toxic additional oxygen (Fig. 53.3). In the past, rushing to clamp the cord and moving the baby to a resuscitation table was associated with providing unlimited additional oxygen which has proved to impair outcomes [31].

The Third Stage at Shorter Gestational Ages: No Gestational Week Is Identical to Other Weeks

The shorter the gestational age, the larger the delay in initiating effective breathing because of an immature respiratory drive, poor muscle strength, surfactant deficiency, and high chest compliance. This delay in maintaining a normal functional

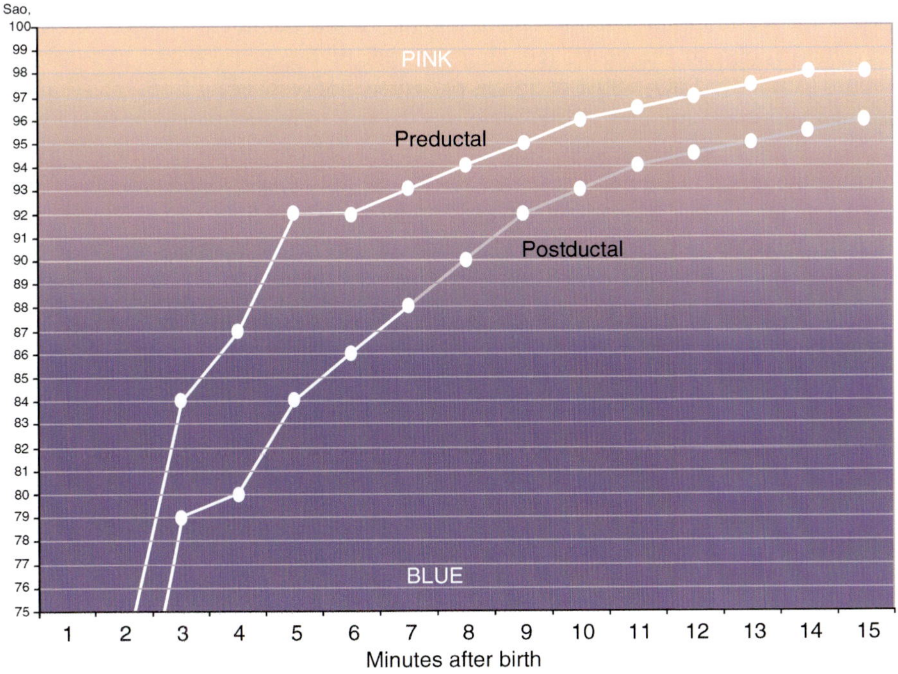

Fig. 53.3 Neonatal oxygen saturation monitored by pulse oximetry at pre- and post-ductal sites during the first minutes of life. Designed with data from Gonzalo Mariani et al. [32]. At birth all babies are blue and turn pink progressively until the end of the third stage. Background color pretends to imitate the color of the skin at each SaO_2

residual capacity produces inefficient gas exchange, increased work of breathing, atelectasis, and hypercapnia with hypoxemia. Placental detachment also takes longer than at term [2].

Nearly all preterm infants start breathing by 60 seconds, spontaneously [33] or when gently stimulated [34].

Caring for the preterm infant with umbilical cord intact and in the "maternal space" allows safe time for assessing the slow initiation of spontaneous breathing. It also allows providing minimally invasive medical support, if needed, avoiding unnecessary and potentially harmful interventions.

The aim of respiratory support at birth is to achieve adequate minute ventilation while the baby is breathing spontaneously. If the infant does not initiate spontaneous breathing, it is urgent to establish and maintain an adequate functional residual capacity. An initial inflating pressure of 20–25 cm H_2O and positive end-expiratory pressure of 6 cm H_2O may be needed to improve lung expansion. However, the shorter the gestational age, the less chances to reach those pressures spontaneously. Supporting ventilation with mask or nasal tube insufflations up to 20–25 cm H_2O and positive end-expiratory pressures of 6 cm is recommended, but mask ventilation before spontaneous inspiratory efforts may be ineffective due to persistence of laryngeal closure [35].

Initial supplementation of oxygen (FiO_2 0,3) in very preterm infants is currently used without confirmation of its benefits and may dilate pulmonary vessels, increasing blood return to the heart, reducing the risk of bradycardia and hypoxemia. Failure to achieve SpO_2 >80% at 5 min, or, worse, not recovering from bradycardia during the initial 5 minutes of life, increases the risk of mortality and/or IVH [36].

New knowledge is available from modern studies comparing the new setting, keeping the infant in the maternal space during the third stage, to old practices rushing the preterm infant to a radiant warmer. Updated systematic reviews of more than 40 randomized clinical trials providing moderate quality of evidence conclude that abandoning clamping in the first minute in preterm infants of less than 34 weeks improves neonatal hematologic measures and may slightly reduce mortality, without increasing any other morbidity [37, 38]. As mentioned above this could be the result of maintaining the umbilical flow intact for a physiological adaptation as well as safe time to assess the infant avoiding unnecessary invasive respiratory support like tracheal intubation in the delivery room [38].

Changes in Blood Volume from Fetal to Neonatal Life

The final balance of admitted blood volume after the completeness of the placental umbilical flow has been subject of research for centuries [14]. During the twentieth century, the total blood volume transfused was also estimated indirectly and invasively measuring blood volume and red cell volumes in neonates with early or delayed clamping. The most precise measurement was obtained by measuring the difference in weight from time 0 when the baby is extracted until the umbilical flow stops. The method consists on placing a scale by the mother's thighs on which to put the newborn at birth and subtracting the initial to the final weight. The difference can only be attributed to the balance of the blood flow, which should be positive if the blood is admitted to the baby side. Term and preterm infants may gain an equivalent of 24 to 40 g per Kg of final weight during the first minutes of life, provided the cord is kept intact [14]. The precision of this method improved to 1 g using digital scales, and recording weight changes continuously [10] (Fig. 53.1).

The progressive amount of blood redistributed from the placenta to the infant was also estimated by measuring the residual blood volume in the placenta, in cases that the umbilical cord was clamped at different times after birth [39].

A systematic review comparing early versus delayed cord clamping in term infants also confirmed that birthweight increases 100 g in term infants when cord clamping is delayed during the third stage of labor [40].

Fetal growth charts built with birthweight at each gestational age need to be updated because they do not describe newborn infants cared with their umbilical cord intact. The magnitude of the change for each gestational may vary, because the size of the placenta and its relation to the fetal body volume and weight changes every week. The relative weight change may be larger in the preterm infants [41].

"The Iron Minutes"

Iron is essential for fetal and neonatal functions, and its deficiency in critical periods may have long-term adverse outcomes in infant development and consequently in adult life [42–44].

Most of the iron needed for hemoglobin and other molecules during the first year of life is daily transferred from maternal reserves through the placenta to the infant, mainly during the third trimester of pregnancy [43].

The large fetal blood volume remaining in the placenta at birth is almost completely transferred to the infant during the third stage of labor and will last for months and is progressively replaced by other dietary sources during infancy. A study was done by transfusion pregnant women with donor blood cells marked with Fe^{55}, prepared in a cyclotron. The study showed that the iron for infant hemoglobin formation during the first 100 days of life was from maternal origin, remained marked with Fe^{55} that, obviously, was not from diet (Fig. 53.4) [45].

Iron deficiency is more frequent in preterm infants due to the shorter duration of pregnancy that limits iron transfer, mostly occurring during the third trimester. Preterm infants also have a larger placenta, and in the case of elective interruption of umbilical flow at birth (clamping), their large placenta retains a relatively larger residual blood volume than in full-term infants [46].

Early and late adverse consequences of cord clamping on infant's hematologic values were initially assessed by hematocrit and hemoglobin level determination. Lower hemoglobin concentration was found in those with early cord clamping [47]. A more precise assessment of iron reserves showed that serum ferritin and total

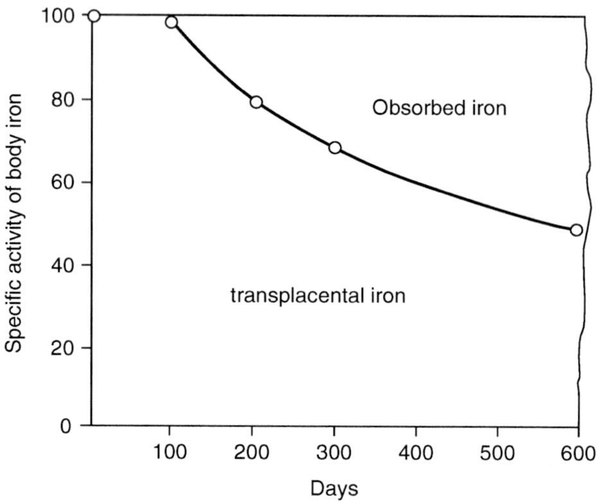

Fig. 53.4 Persistence of specific activity of infant body Fe^{55}, administered to the mother during pregnancy and measured at periodic intervals from birth until 600 days. At the age of 100 days, all hemoglobin was from maternal origin as shown by Clement Smith [45]

body iron levels at 6 months were lower in infants randomly allocated to immediate or early (16 s) compared to delayed (93 s) clamping of the umbilical cord [48]. In another study developmental follow-up at 7 and 18 months showed poorer outcomes in infants assigned to early cord clamping, probably caused by scarcity of iron available for brain growth [49, 50]. New evidence shows that greater ferritin levels are associated with increased brain myelin in important areas for early infant development. Endowment of iron-rich red blood cells obtained by not interrupting umbilical flow at birth may offer a longitudinal advantage for early white matter growth [50].

In the past, pediatricians were concerned about this red cell-enriched early environment with initial higher hematocrit. The risk of adverse consequences of "polycythemia" induced many professionals to clamp the cord immediately as a protective measure. This concept is not supported by systematic reviews confirming that normal physiological values of hematocrit are higher than those with early clamping, but produce no symptoms or late adverse outcomes [51].

A physiologic consequence of the increase in the red blood cell mass is that a larger amount of bilirubin is produced. This condition increases the screening of neonatal jaundice without hemolysis. This higher level of bilirubin is physiologic, needs no treatment, and may be protective because bilirubin is an antioxidant molecule [52].

Fetal Hemoglobin and Stem Cells Load

The complete blood volume redistributed from fetal to neonatal periods also contains the specific fetal hemoglobin adapted to fetal life and initial adaptation, especially in preterm infants. It also increases the availability of more pluripotential stem cells.

Fetal hemoglobin is specific for fetal life and binds oxygen with greater affinity to get it from the low oxygen content environment of the placental intervillous space.

When neonates are born at extremely low gestational age, fetal hemoglobin may protect them from excessive delivery of oxygen to their tissues. During the early postnatal care, many preterm infants receive adult blood transfusions containing adult hemoglobin. Hypothetically, this adult blood will deliver peripherally a non-physiologic higher oxygen supply to the tissues than fetal hemoglobin [53].

The larger admitted blood volume during the complete third stage of labor decreases the need for postnatal adult blood transfusions, also known to increase the risk of necrotizing enterocolitis [37].

Pluripotential stem cells are particularly increased in fetal blood and may have important physiological value [54], provide neuroprotection, and prevent and repair hypoxic-ischemic neural damage at birth [55].

Until recently parents were ill-advised that residual placental blood was useless and discarded and could be banked for later use for stem cell transplants for their own infants in case they developed leukemia or donated to others in public banks. This concept was strictly related to the routine practice of cord clamping immediately, forcing an abnormally large residual placental residual blood volume that could be banked. Delayed clamping was not recommended to the harvesters because less than 70 mL of umbilical cord blood is not accepted by the blood banks. After the complete redistribution of blood to the infant with the intact cord, this volume can seldom be achieved.

The ethics of umbilical cord blood banking were discussed confronting the benefits for the receptors of the banked stem cells versus the adverse effects to the newborn infant by limiting the complete redistribution of its own blood. The concept that "the best bank is the baby" prevailed [10, 56].

Since most of the perinatal professional organizations warned against the adverse effects of immediate clamping and recommended to inform parents on this condition, cord blood banking decreased [57]. Advising families regarding the adverse effects of early clamping also helps them to appreciate the value of waiting, watching, and understanding the safety of completing the third stage with an intact cord.

Heat Loss and Thermal Environment

The fetus in the womb is in a balanced thermal environment. The heat production of its metabolism in a closed milieu is maintained in the normal range by transferring excess of heat to the mother through the placenta and the high conductivity of the liquid interface with the womb.

There is reasonable concern about the best thermal environment at birth. The wet infant at birth is always exposed to a lower environmental temperature. Extreme and even moderate hypothermia put the newborn infant at risk of adverse outcomes. The shorter the gestational, the larger the heat loss, caused by a relatively large skin surface and less heat production.

The umbilical cord temperature depends on the blood flow of warm blood and rapidly cools down to room temperature when the blood flow stops.

All newborn infants need thermal loss protection to prevent from a drop in its axillar temperature to less than 36.5° C. Covering with a cloth, as well as maintaining a room temperature of 25–26 ° C and reducing drifts, has always been recommended and practiced from ancient times [30].

Placing the newborn infants at birth under a radiant warmer, distant from their mothers, has been a practice closely related with immediate cord clamping for more than five decades and should also be de-implemented. Evidence-based care of term infants requires the maternal space during the third stage. After the cord is cut, infants are dressed or wrapped in a towel and held by their mothers or family members. Infants transferred to the NICU for further care do not need to be stationed under the radiant warmer and should be immediately transported in an incubator. Simple dressing items and new materials help to reduce heat loss. Swaddling the infant with a soft cloth, exothermic mattresses, woolen or plastic caps, and polyethylene or polyurethane wraps are currently used to provide a neutral thermal environment. If respiratory support is needed, humidified and heated gases should be available. Normothermia at NICU admission is a relevant quality control check for a neonatal unit and should be recorded as a matter of quality improvement [35].

An unexpected adverse consequence of placing the newborn under the radiant warmer after immediate routine cord clamping was found in infants with severe asphyxia. Resuscitation under a radiant warmer may cause overheating and hyperthermia increasing the risk and severity of ischemic-hypoxic encephalopathy and delaying the initiation of hypothermia as a preventive therapy [58].

Birth of the Microbiome

Another major biological event occurring in the fetal-neonatal transition during the second and third stages of labor is the development of the normal microbiome.

During fetal life, maternal microbiota enhances the generation of innate immune cells in the offspring. After birth, the colonizing microbiota induces the development of intestinal lymphoid tissues and maturation of myeloid and lymphoid cells and imprints the immune system with a reactivity level that persists long after weaning and into adulthood [59].

Although in the fetal environment these processes have begun before birth, a significant exposure to microbes occurs during the passage through the cervix, vagina, and vulva and the initial minutes of life. Microbes in the cervical and vaginal secretions, vernix, and amniotic fluid inoculate the mouth, nose, and skin of the infant. This moment is essential for the establishment of a natural microbiome.

It has been shown that elective cesarean sections deprive the offspring from this natural microbial inoculation occurring during the passage through the birth canal [60].

In the perspective of this new knowledge, it is plausible that the immediate practice of partial or total removal (drying) of this microbial layer, and eventually proceeding to bathe the baby, may modify this physiological process. A warning should be raised about current practices of handling, drying, and dressing this wet newborn infant. More information is needed to decide what benefits the baby.

The Changing Setting for Neonatal Care at Delivery

The assessment and care of a newborn infant during the third stage before cutting the umbilical cord implies a restriction of displacements limited by the length of the intact umbilical cord until the placenta is detached. The length of the cord has been described by Leonardo Da Vinci as equivalent to the length of the newborn infant. The umbilical cord grows continuously, and preterm infants have shorter cords.

The new setting for this initial period, in vaginal and cesarean deliveries, requires keeping the baby in the area, limited by distance, of the "maternal space" [61, 62].

A variety of devices is advancing fast, from simple trays to be used when mothers deliver on a bed (Baby Saver) [63] to more sophisticated designs with the latest monitoring technology and devices for respiratory support for the highest-risk newborn infants (Concord) [64]. These new arrangements (Fig. 53.5) substitute the old setting of the resuscitation table in a corner of the delivery room, far from the mother, under a radiant warmer.

In cesarean sections the setting is the surgical field, the protocol assigns responsibilities, and procedures are adapted to care for term and preterm infants with the cord intact. While there is umbilical cord flow and the placenta has not been detached, the infant is kept on the surgical drapes that cover the mother's thighs or pelvis. Professionals cooperate (Fig. 53.6) ceding space for the care of their respective patients (mother and infant) [65, 66].

Elective detachment of the placenta, milking of the cord, and moving the baby to a resuscitation table interrupt and may interfere with the physiology of the third stage, and there is no evidence yet of advantages to the mother or baby compared to maintaining the cord intact.

Standards of care and guidelines have to adapt to this new setting to be able to provide care for healthy newborn infants or those that need support or resuscitation.

Neonatal Resuscitation Management in Fetal Asphyxia

Resuscitation should be initiated in the maternal space until the umbilical cord flow stops or all its possible benefits have been obtained.

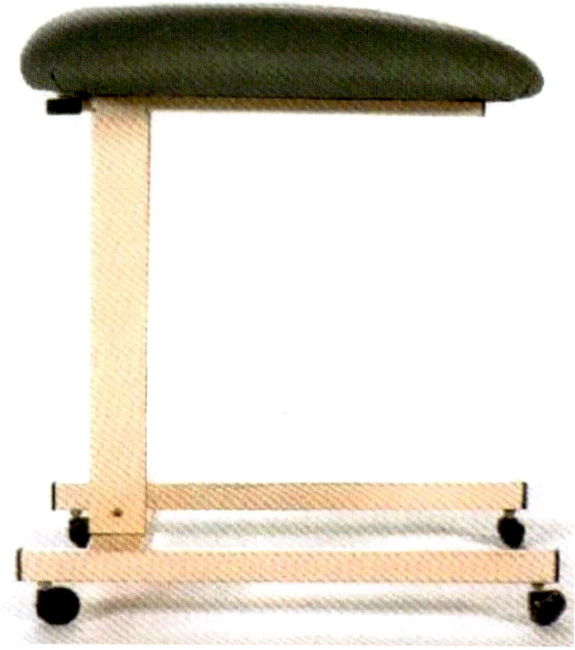

Fig. 53.5 The trolley used in the Glasgow trial in 2006 and debated at the Worcestershire Royal Hospital meeting in 2009. *Photograph courtesy of Anne Marie Heuchan, Consultant Neonatologist, Queen Mother's Hospital, Glasgow*

During resuscitation, ventilatory support insufflates the lungs, increases oxygenation, and produces pulmonary vasodilation increasing blood return by pulmonary veins to the left ventricle. With an intact umbilical cord, there is also increased umbilical venous return from the placenta. Both mechanisms increase the preload of the left ventricle. Patent umbilical arteries irrigating the placenta maintain low the left ventricle afterload. The additional red cell mass transfused, until the blood flow stops, also improves diastolic pressure for better coronary perfusion.

Cord clamping before resuscitation reduces blood volume and red blood cells. Hypovolemia and hypoxia contribute to cerebral hypoperfusion and hypoxic-ischemic encephalopathy (HIE), as well as increase the severity of pulmonary hypoperfusion and persistent pulmonary hypertension (PPHN). Oxidative stress may also increase the severity of HIE and PPHN [67].

As mentioned before during the resuscitation of an infant born with tight nuchal cord, the increased residual blood volume engorging the transiently obstructed venous placental return to the fetus may be recovered avoiding neonatal hypovolemia and its consequences.

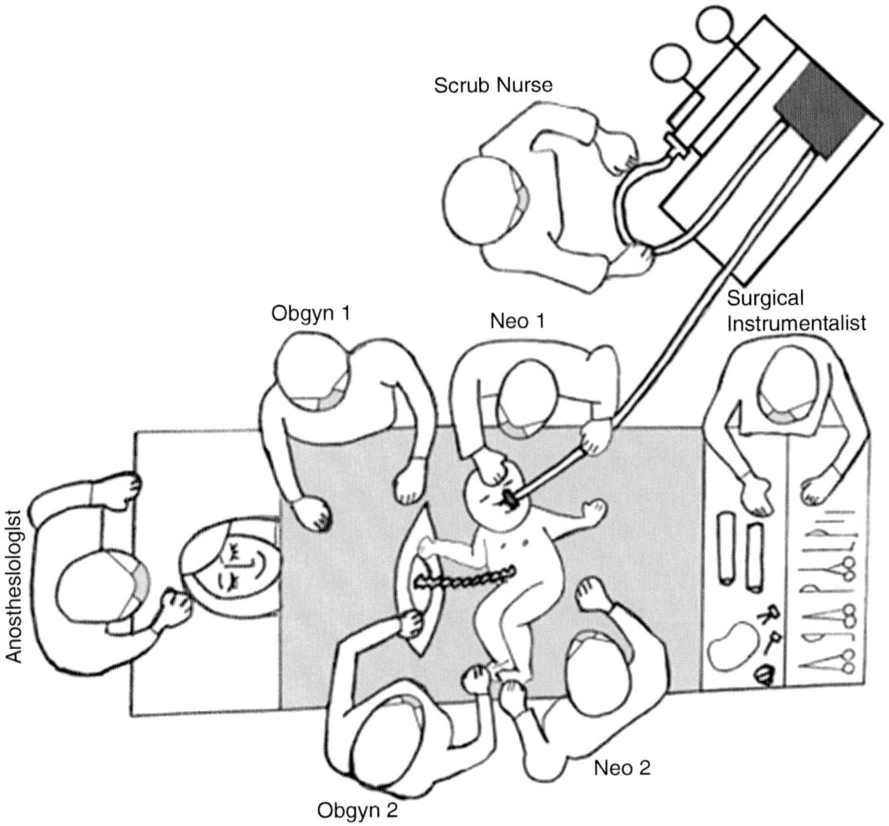

Fig. 53.6 Providing space for neonatal care, during a cesarean section. Neonatal care team (NEO 1–2) access the surgical field at the time the infant is delivered by the obstetrical team (OBGYN 1–2). All equipment needed for respiratory support is available with the same safety and asepsis requirements for any other surgical material used on the surgical field. Anesthesiologists and scrub nurses/surgical instrumentalists remain in the same position and are trained to cooperate in the neonatal care

A Practical Scheme for Special Neonatal Support at Birth

Traditional training on immediate care regarding the initiation of breathing at birth simplified the approach to being prepared for resuscitation and act as soon as possible.

Understanding the basis for the care of the newborn infant, regarding the assessment of the umbilical blood flow and fetal asphyxia, provides a better orientation for caregivers.

Initial care of the transition in a preterm infant may require respiratory support, but it is completely different than the approach when the infant at birth has already the condition of severe fetal asphyxia (Fig. 53.7).

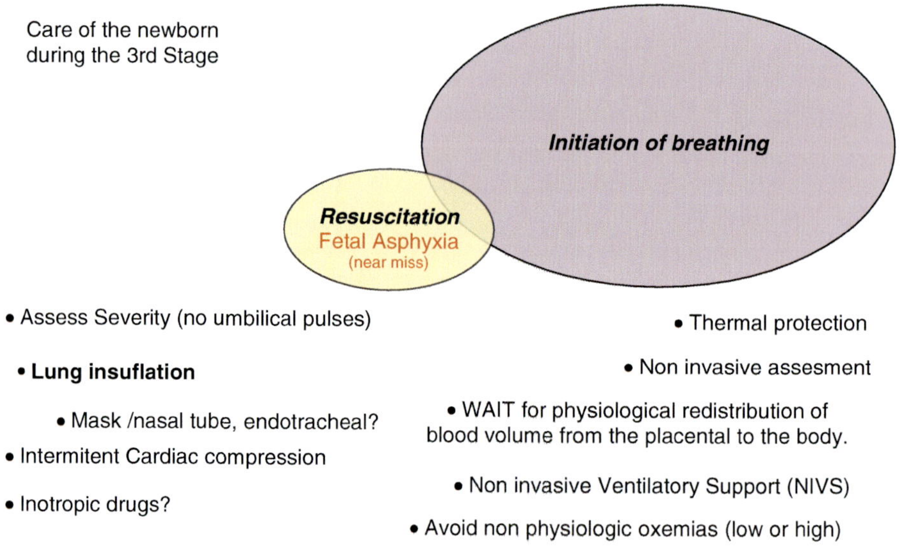

Fig. 53.7 The size of the ovals reminds the relative frequency of the clinical events requiring respiratory support. The order of the texts suggests the timeline of the interventions and its relevancy

The Family at Birth and the Maternal-Infant Space

The marvelous appearance of the amazing newborn creates a euphoric rise in all who are attending birth. The life of both was at risk and there is shared relief when the live baby is out of the womb.

The social value of this moment is attached to the essence of reproduction and is shared by all in every culture. In recent times, hospitals have lifted restrictions to the family to attend this moment. Mothers benefit from familial company during this tense moment, reinforcing their confidence on its safety for both. Cooperation is the great difference in the evolution of humans, and all involved in the birth of a child are eager to help the mother and the baby [68].

Separation of the newborn infant from its mother should only occur transiently, if the infant is transferred to a neonatal intensive care unit (NICU) [69].

In the maternal space, the initial assessment of the baby includes announcing (confirming) its sex, identifying visible anomalies, and assessing vitality.

The mother should be offered a comfortable position to rest and listen or watch the infant and the remarks of the caregiver. After the cord is cut, their care should continue in a calm, safe, and supervised environment where she or a family member holds or watches the infant, according to their preference.

Moving from placental dependence to respiratory autonomy and breastfeeding is a biological transition with evolutionary roots. Dyadic biology will continue, and their autonomy is limited. Parental brain science has shown that infant's needs will stimulate attachment functions aiming to keep parents available full time. The new bonds will persist "life time" because "when a baby is born a mother is born" as the behavioral changes inducing the parental brain are lifelong [70].

After respiratory adaptation, nursing and psychosocial interaction will be key to the transition.

Feeding-related practices and maternal "preoccupation" are the center of initial care. During the third stage, the large volume of blood redistributed to the infant's body could be considered a last boost of "parenteral feed."

Preparation for breastfeeding starts in utero as the fetus may swallow up to 450 mL per day and at term is programmed to feed "ad libitum" with thirst and appetite regulation, showing cues that the mother or other family members respond without any delay [71].

As soon as the umbilical flow stops and the cord is cut, the mother should be helped to reach her baby to the breast. There is evidence that among the many conditions associated with successful breastfeeding, early initiation in the first hour of life may enhance early milk production.

This new setting for the family at birth benefits the sequence of physiological events occurring normally without the need of the "non-evidence-based" rushing practices so common in the delivery room. Families should be informed before labor to understand the value and benefits of non-altering the timing of the physiology of each stage.

Warnings

- Sudden unexpected postnatal collapse (SUPC) is a severe event recently described associated with hospital policies of immediate skin-to-skin contact and breast feeding initiation without adequate supervision of the mother and her newborn infant. Attempts to put the baby on the breast should not start until the cord is cut and only if the mother is comfortable, fully awake, and willing to breastfeed and the institution has taken all preventive measures of education of companions, risk assessment, nursing supervision, and eventually monitoring to prevent SUPC [72, 73].
- Frequently the hospital culture trespasses barriers of modesty regarding nudity. Nurses often help mothers by using hands-on-breast without their permission, and studies show that many women do not like "helpers" to touch their breasts or to be exposed to strangers watching them naked while nursing their infants. Intimacy should prevail as a standard for breastfeeding moments [74].
- When breastfeeding is not feasible during the first 2 postpartum hours, term and preterm mothers should be helped to initiate breast milking with continuous support and comfortable hospital grade breast pumps.

Skin-to-Skin Contact (SSC) during the Third Stage of Labor

There is only one systematic review of "low- and moderate-quality" trials comparing SSC to conventional care. Almost all studies included compared infants placed SSC after the cord was cut. The authors of the review conclude: "We found no clear benefit to immediate SSC rather than SSC after the baby had been washed and examined. Neither did we find any clear advantage of a longer duration of SSC (more than one hour) compared with less than one hour" [75].

There is no evidence that immediate naked ("skin to skin") contact between the infant and the mother may improve or impair outcomes; nevertheless, we should not separate them unless they need special care or treatment that cannot be done in the same space of the mother.

The Perinatal Information System (SIP): Monitoring Quality of Care

The de-implementation of immediate/early clamping requires to collect the timing of cord clamping in every birth, but it is not available in most clinical records [56]. This measure may provide relevant information on how the care of the neonate is managed. The shorter the time, more adverse effects have been found.

The Perinatal Information System (SIP) developed since 1984 by the Latin American Center for Perinatology (CLAP) of the Pan American Health Organization (PAHO) collects information on the time of umbilical cord clamping since 2007 [76] (Fig. 53.8).

A new SIP version in Spanish has added space for recording the time in minutes since birth until cord cutting (Fig. 53.9).

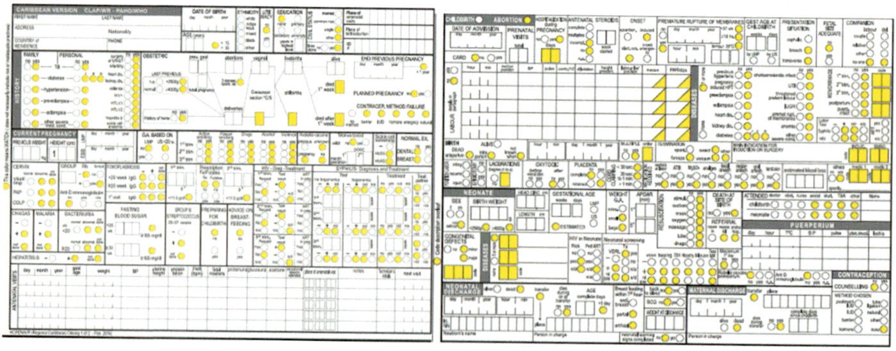

Fig. 53.8 Basic perinatal clinical record of the Perinatal Information System developed by CLAP-PAHO. Demonstration site www.sipplus.org:9000 User: guest. Pass: sipguest

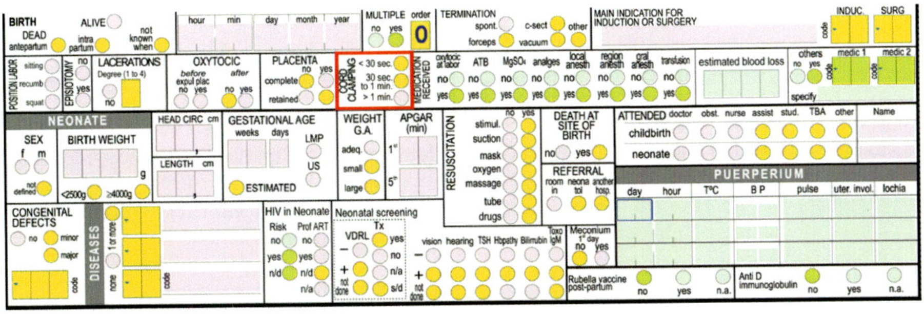

Fig. 53.9 Section of the BPCR customized for Uruguay since 2019, recording the duration until cord clamping in minutes

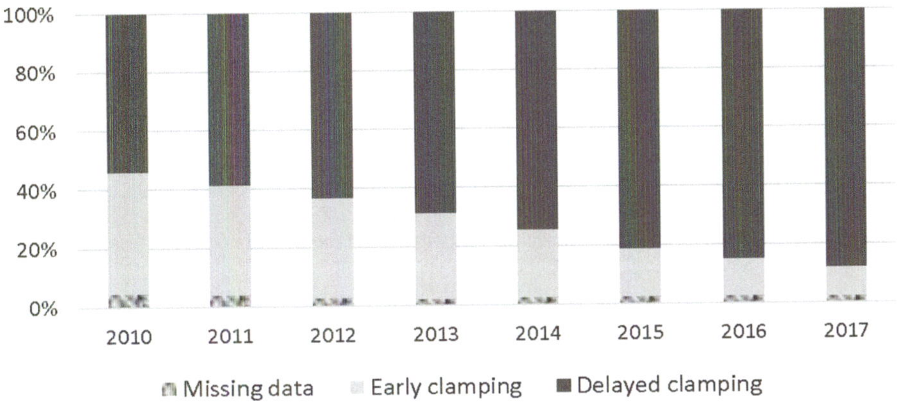

Fig. 53.10 Frequency of early, delayed clamping and missing data frequencies in the total number of live births in Uruguay from January 1, 2010, until December 31, 2017. The practice of delayed clamping increased yearly from 54% to 89%

Knowing the trends of this practice in vaginal or cesarean section deliveries and at different gestational ages will keep institutions aware of how much additional effort is needed to further improve neonatal care during the third stage of labor. Figure 53.10 shows the trend of change of this practice with national figures of Uruguay from 2010 to 2017.

References

1. Zeger HF, Adamson G, De Mouzon J, Ishihara D, Mansour R, Nygren K, et al. International Committee for Monitoring Assisted Reproductive Technology (ICMART) and the World Health Organization (WHO) revised glossary of ART terminology. Fertil Steril. 2009;2009:92.

2. Dombrowski M, Bottoms S, Saleb A, Hurd W, Romero R. Third stage of labor: analysis of duration and clinical practice. Am J Obstet Gynecol. 1995;172:1279–83.
3. Kresch MJ. Management of the third stage of labor: how delayed umbilical cord clamping can affect neonatal outcome. Am J Perinatol. 2017;34(14):1375–81.
4. Dunn P. Postnatal placental respiration. Development Med Child Neurol. 1966;8.
5. Langer J, Tabb T, Thompson P, Paes B, Caco C. Management of prenatally diagnosed tracheal obstruction: access to airway in utero prior to delivery. Fetal Diagn Ther. 1992;7:12–6.
6. Masahata K, Soh H, Tachibana K, Sasahara J, Hirose M, Yamanishi T, et al. Clinical outcomes of ex utero intrapartum treatment for fetal airway obstruction. Pediatr Surg Int. 2019;35(8):835–43.
7. Štembera ZK, Hodr J, Janda J. Umbilical blood flow in healthy newborn infants during the first minutes after birth. Am J Obstet Gynecol. 1965;91(4):568–74.
8. Boere I, Roest AA, Wallace E, Ten Harkel AD, Haak MC, Morley CJ, et al. Umbilical blood flow patterns directly after birth before delayed cord clamping. Arch Dis Child Fetal Neonatal Ed. 2015;100(2):F121–5.
9. Fonseca D, Caldeyro-Barcia R. Importancia del aporte de sangre placentaria al niño recié nacido. Su medida por medio del registro ponderal continuo. Arch Pediatr Uruguay. 1962;7:3.
10. Diaz-Rossello J. Cord clamping for stem cell donation: medical facts and ethics. NeoReviews. 2006;7(11).
11. Alvarez H, Caldeyro-Barcia R. Contractilidad uterina estudiada por nuevos metodos. Terceras Jornadas Chilenas de Obstetricia y Ginecologia 4–9 December, 1949; Santiago de Chile, Chile. Departamento de Obstetricia y Fisiologia de la Facultad de Medicina de Montevideo. Uruguay: Montevideo, Uruguay; 1949.
12. Yao A, Hirvensalo M, Lind J. Placental transfusion-rate and uterine contraction. Lancet. 1968.
13. Vain NE, Satragno DS, Gordillo JE, Fernandez AL, Carrolli G, Romero NP, et al. Postpartum use of oxytocin and volume of placental transfusion: a randomised controlled trial. Arch Dis Child Fetal Neonatal Ed. 2020;105(1):14–7.
14. Limon A. Ventajas que tiene la ligadura tardía del cordón umbilical [Doctoral Thesis in Medicine]. Mexico, Ciudad Mexico: Universidad Autonoma de Mexico; 1895.
15. Te Pas AB, Hooper SB, Dekker J. The Changing Landscape in Supporting Preterm Infants at Birth. Neonatology. 2019;115(4):392–7.
16. Saling E. Zustandsdiagnose beim Neugeborenen unmittelbar nach der geburt. Gynaecologie. 1965;1965(3):133–56.
17. Apgar V. A proposal for a New Method to Evaluation of the Newborn Infant. Current Researches in Anesthesia and Analgesia. 1953;32(4):260–57.
18. Dawson JA, Schmolzer GM, Wyllie J. Monitoring heart rate in the delivery room. Semin Fetal Neonatal Med. 2018;23(5):327–32.
19. Dawson JA, Kamlin CO, Wong C, te Pas AB, Vento M, Cole TJ, et al. Changes in heart rate in the first minutes after birth. Arch Dis Child Fetal Neonatal Ed. 2010;95(3):F177–81.
20. Gonzales GF, A S. Pulse oxygen saturation and neurologic assessment in human neonates after vaginal and cesarean deliveries. International Journal of Gynecology & Obstetrics. 1998;63:63–88.
21. Smit M, Dawson JA, Ganzeboom A, Hooper SB, van Roosmalen J, te Pas AB. Pulse oximetry in newborns with delayed cord clamping and immediate skin-to-skin contact. Arch Dis Child Fetal Neonatal Ed. 2014;99(4):F309–14.
22. Kc A, Singhal N, Gautam J, Rana N, Andersson O. Effect of early versus delayed cord clamping in neonate on heart rate, breathing and oxygen saturation during first 10 minutes of birth - randomized clinical trial. Matern Health Neonatol Perinatol. 2019;5:7.
23. Dawson JA, Kamlin CO, Wong C, te Pas AB, O'Donnell CP, Donath SM, et al. Oxygen saturation and heart rate during delivery room resuscitation of infants <30 weeks' gestation with air or 100% oxygen. Arch Dis Child Fetal Neonatal Ed. 2009;94(2):F87–91.
24. Ullriich J, Ackerman B. Changes in umbilical artery blood gas values with the onset of respiration. Biology Neonate. 1972;20:9.

25. Marquis L, Ackerman BD. Placental respiration in the immediate neonatal period. Am J Obstet Gynecol. 1973;117(3):358–63.
26. Engstrom L, Karlberg P, Rooth G, Tunnel R-AACC, York N. The onset of respiration: a study of respiration and changes in blood gases and acid-base balance, vol. 1966. New York, USA: Association for the Crippled Children; 1966. p. 6.
27. Nudelman M, Belogolovsky E, Jegatheesan P, Govindaswami B, Song D. Effect of delayed cord clamping on umbilical cord gas values in term newborns: a systematic review. Obstet Gynecol. 2020.
28. Mokarami P, Wiberg N, Olofsson P. Hidden acidosis: an explanation of acid-base and lactate changes occurring in umbilical cord blood after delayed sampling. Bjog. 2013;120(8):996–1002.
29. Mercer J, Erickson-Owens DA. Is it time to rethink cord management when resuscitation is needed? J Midwifery Womens Health. 2014;59:9.
30. Bagellardo P. Libellus de infantium aegritudinibus et remediis, per magistrum Paulum Bagellardum: B. de Valdizoccho et M. de Septem arboribus. 1472.
31. Saugstad OD. Take a breath--but do not add oxygen (if not needed). Acta Paediatr. 2007;96(6):798–800.
32. Mariani G, Dik PB, Ezquer A, Aguirre A, Esteban ML, Perez C, et al. Pre-ductal and post-ductal O2 saturation in healthy term neonates after birth. J Pediatr. 2007;150(4):418–21.
33. Odonnell C, Kamlin C, Davis P, Morley C. Crying and breathing by extremely preterm infants immediately after birth. J Aapos. 2010;156:2.
34. Katheria A, Poeltler D, Durham J, Steen J, Rich W, Arnell K, et al. Neonatal resuscitation with an intact cord: a randomized clinical trial. J Pediatr. 2016;178:75–80. e3.
35. The VM. First golden minutes of preterm infants: changing the concepts of resuscitation. innovations and frontiers in neonatology. Pediatric and Adolescent Medicine; 2020. p. 13–24.
36. Oei JL, Finer NN, Saugstad OD, Wright IM, Rabi Y, Tarnow-Mordi W, et al. Outcomes of oxygen saturation targeting during delivery room stabilisation of preterm infants. Arch Dis Child Fetal Neonatal Ed. 2018;103(5):F446–F54.
37. Rabe H, Gyte GM, Diaz-Rossello JL, Duley L. Effect of timing of umbilical cord clamping and other strategies to influence placental transfusion at preterm birth on maternal and infant outcomes. Cochrane Database Syst Rev. 2019;9:CD003248.
38. Fogarty M, Osborn DA, Askie L, Seidler AL, Hunter K, Lui K, et al. Delayed vs early umbilical cord clamping for preterm infants: a systematic review and meta-analysis. Am J Obstet Gynecol. 2018;218(1):1–18.
39. Yao A, Moinian M, Lind J. Distribution of blood between infant and placenta at birth. The Lancet. 1969;3
40. McDonald SJ, Middleton P, Dowswell T, Morris PS. Effect of timing of umbilical cord clamping of term infants on maternal and neonatal outcomes. Cochrane Database Syst Rev. 2013;7:CD004074.
41. Aladangady N. Infants' blood volume in a controlled trial of placental transfusion at preterm delivery. Pediatrics. 2006;117(1):93–8.
42. Georgieff MK. Long-term brain and behavioral consequences of early iron deficiency. Nutr Rev. 2011;69(Suppl 1):S43–8.
43. Hua Y, Kaciroti N, Jiang Y, Li X, Xu G, Richards B, et al. Inadequate iron stores in early term neonates. J Perinatol. 2018;38(8):1017–21.
44. Lozoff B, Beard J, Connor J, Felt B, Georgieff M, Schallert T. Long-lasting neural and behavioral effects of iron deficiency in infancy. Nutr Rev. 2006;64:8.
45. Smith C, Cherry R, Maletskos C, Gibson J, Roby C, Caton W, et al. Persistence and utilization of maternal iron for blood formation during infancy. Journal of Clinical Investigation. 1955;34(9):13.
46. Aladangady N, McHugh S, Aitchison TC, Wardrop CA, Holland BM. Infants' blood volume in a controlled trial of placental transfusion at preterm delivery. Pediatrics. 2006;117(1):93–8.
47. Lanzkowsky P. Effects of early and late clamping of umbilical cord on infant's haemoglobin level. BMJ. 1960;2(5215):6.

48. Chaparro C, Neufeld LM, Tena Alavez G, Eguia-Liz Cedillo R, Dewey KG. Effect if timing of umbilical cord clamping on iron status in Mexican infants: a randomised control trial. The Lancet. 2006;367.
49. Mercer JS, Vohr BR, Erickson-Owens DA, Padbury JF, Oh W. Seven-month developmental outcomes of very low birth weight infants enrolled in a randomized controlled trial of delayed versus immediate cord clamping. Journal of Perinatology. 2009;30(1):11–6.
50. Mercer JS, Erickson-Owens DA, Vohr BR, Tucker RJ, Parker AB, Oh W, et al. Effects of Placental Transfusion on Neonatal and 18 Month Outcomes in Preterm Infants: A Randomized Controlled Trial. J Pediatr. 2016;168:50–5.e1.
51. Rabe H, Mercer J. Early cord clamping protects at-risk babies from polycythemia. Biology Neonate. 2004;86(2).
52. Ceriani Cernadas JM. The effect of timing of cord clamping on neonatal venous hematocrit values and clinical outcome at term: a randomized. Controlled Trial. Pediatrics. 2006;117(4):e779–e86.
53. Del Vecchio A, Henry E, D'Amato G, Cannuscio A, Corriero L, Motta M, et al. Instituting a program to reduce the erythrocyte transfusion rate was accompanied by reductions in the incidence of bronchopulmonary dysplasia, retinopathy of prematurity and necrotizing enterocolitis. J Matern Fetal Neonatal Med. 2013;26:3.
54. Bewley S, Dìaz-Rossello JL, Mercer J. Natural stem cell transplantation: interventions, nuances and ethics. J Cell Mol Med. 2010;14(12):2840–1.
55. Penny TR, Sutherland AE, Mihelakis JG, Paton MCB, Pham Y, Lee J, et al. Human umbilical cord therapy improves long-term behavioral outcomes following neonatal hypoxic ischemic brain injury. Front Physiol. 2019;10:283.
56. Díaz-Rossello JL. Early umbilical cord clamping and cord-blood banking. The Lancet. 2006;368(9538):840.
57. Mancuso S. Controversy on the timing of the clamping and cutting of the umbilical cord at birth, with particular reference to the collection of cord blood for the donation of stem cells. In: Life PAF, editor. . Rome: Vatican: Banks of Umbilical Cord Blood. Appendix; 2014. p. 81–8.
58. Baumgart S. Iatrogenic hyperthermia and hypothermia in the neonate. Clin Perinatol. 2008;35(1):183–97. ix-x.
59. Al Nabhani Z, Eberl G. Imprinting of the immune system by the microbiota early in life. Mucosal Immunol. 2020.
60. Dominguez-Bello MG, De Jesus-Laboy KM, Shen N, Cox LM, Amir A, Gonzalez A, et al. Partial restoration of the microbiota of cesarean-born infants via vaginal microbial transfer. Nat Med. 2016;22(3):250–3.
61. Hutchon D. Evolution of neonatal resuscitation with intact placental circulation. Infant. 2014;10(2):4.
62. Hutchon D, Bettles N. Motherside care of the term neonate at birth. Matern Health Neonatol Perinatol. 2016;2:5.
63. Weeks A, Dital J, Watt P. Liverpool Professor's invention to save thousands of babies' lives in Uganda Liverpool, United Kingdom: University of Liverpool; 2018. Available from: https://news.liverpool.ac.uk/2018/09/12/liverpool-professors-inventionto-save-thousands-of-babies-lives-in-uganda/.
64. Brouwer E, Knol R, Vernooij ASN, van den Akker T, Vlasman PE, Klumper F, et al. Physiological-based cord clamping in preterm infants using a new purpose-built resuscitation table: a feasibility study. Arch Dis Child Fetal Neonatal Ed. 2018;
65. Winter J, Kattwinkel J, Chisholm C, Blackman A, Wilson S, Fairchild K. Ventilation of preterm infants during delayed cord clamping (VentFirst): a pilot study of feasibility and safety. Am J Perinatol. 2017;34(2):111–6.
66. Gonzalez S, Bustelo E, Vidal G, Keishishian R, Rodriguez M, Blasina F, et al. Intubacion al nacer con tubo nasal corto en la transición a la vida extrauterina en reciѐn nacidos de muy bajo peso. Archivos de Pediatria de Uruguay. 2017;88:5.

67. Katheria AC, Rich WD, Bava S, Lakshminrusimha S. Placental transfusion for asphyxiated infants. Front Pediatr. 2019;7:473.
68. Hrdy SB. Variable postpartum responsiveness among humans and other primates with "cooperative breeding": a comparative and evolutionary perspective. Horm Behav. 2016;77:272–83.
69. Klaus M, Jerauld R, Kreger N, McAlpine W, Steffa M, Kennell J. Maternal attachment. NEJM. 1972;296(9):4.
70. Diaz-Rossello JL, Ferreira-Castro A. Maternology: when a baby is born, a mother is born. NeoReviews. 2008;9(8):e326–e31.
71. El-Haddad M. In utero development of fetal thirst and appetite: potential for programming. J Soc Gynecol Investig. 2004;11(3):123–30.
72. Monnelly V, Becher JC. Sudden unexpected postnatal collapse. Early Hum Dev. 2018;126:28–31.
73. Pearlman SA, Paul DA. Sudden unexpected postnatal collapse during early breastfeeding and skin-to-skin care. J Pediatr. 2020.
74. Weimers L, Svensson K, Dumas L, Naver L, Wahlberg V. Hands-on approach during breastfeeding support in a neonatal intensive care unit: a qualitative study of Swedish mothers' experiences. Int Breastfeed J. 2006;1:20.
75. Moore ER, Bergman N, Anderson GC, Medley N. Early skin-to-skin contact for mothers and their healthy newborn infants. Cochrane Database Syst Rev. 2016;11:CD003519.
76. Diaz-Rossello JL. Health services research, outcomes, and perinatal information systems. Curr Opinion Pediat. 1998;10(2):6.

Part VIII
Neonatal Period

Chapter 54
Breastfeeding

Cristiane Alves de Oliveira

Introduction

Adequate nutrition during infancy and early childhood is essential to ensure the growth, health, and development of children to their full potential. Breastfeeding is one of the most effective ways to ensure child health and survival. In 2002, the World Health Organization and UNICEF adopted the Global Strategy for infant and young child feeding. WHO and UNICEF's global recommendations for optimal infant feeding as set out in the Global Strategy include exclusive breastfeeding for 6 months (180 days) and nutritionally adequate and safe complementary feeding starting from the age of 6 months with continued breastfeeding up to 2 years of age or beyond [1, 2].

Malnutrition has been responsible, directly or indirectly, for 60% of all deaths annually among children under 5. Well over two-thirds of these deaths, which are often associated with inappropriate feeding practices, occur during the first year of life. Although the WHO and UNICEF's global recommendations, globally, no more than 40% of infants under 6 months of age are exclusively breastfed, and complementary feeding frequently begins too early or too late, and foods are often nutritionally inadequate and unsafe [2–4].

Malnourished children who survive are more frequently sick and suffer the lifelong consequences of impaired development. Rising incidences of overweight and obesity in children are also a matter of serious concern [2, 3, 5].

Globally, although more than 80% of neonates receive breast milk in 2012, only 38% of infants aged 0 to 6 months were exclusively breastfed. In 2016 this proportion increased to 40%. Moreover, only about half begin breastfeeding within the first hour of life, even though such recommendation was issued by WHO more than 25 years ago [2, 3].

C. A. de Oliveira (✉)
Federal Fluminense University and Rio de Janeiro Federal University,
Niteroi and Rio de Janeiro, Brazil

© Springer Nature Switzerland AG 2022
R. A. Moreira de Sá, E. B. d. Fonseca (eds.), *Perinatology*,
https://doi.org/10.1007/978-3-030-83434-0_54

In May 2012, the 65th World Health Assembly (WHA) endorsed a Comprehensive Implementation Plan on Maternal, Infant and Young Child Nutrition that included increasing the rate of exclusive breastfeeding among the six global targets. The 2025 target for exclusive breastfeeding is to achieve a rate of 50% at the global level [2, 6] (Fig. 54.1).

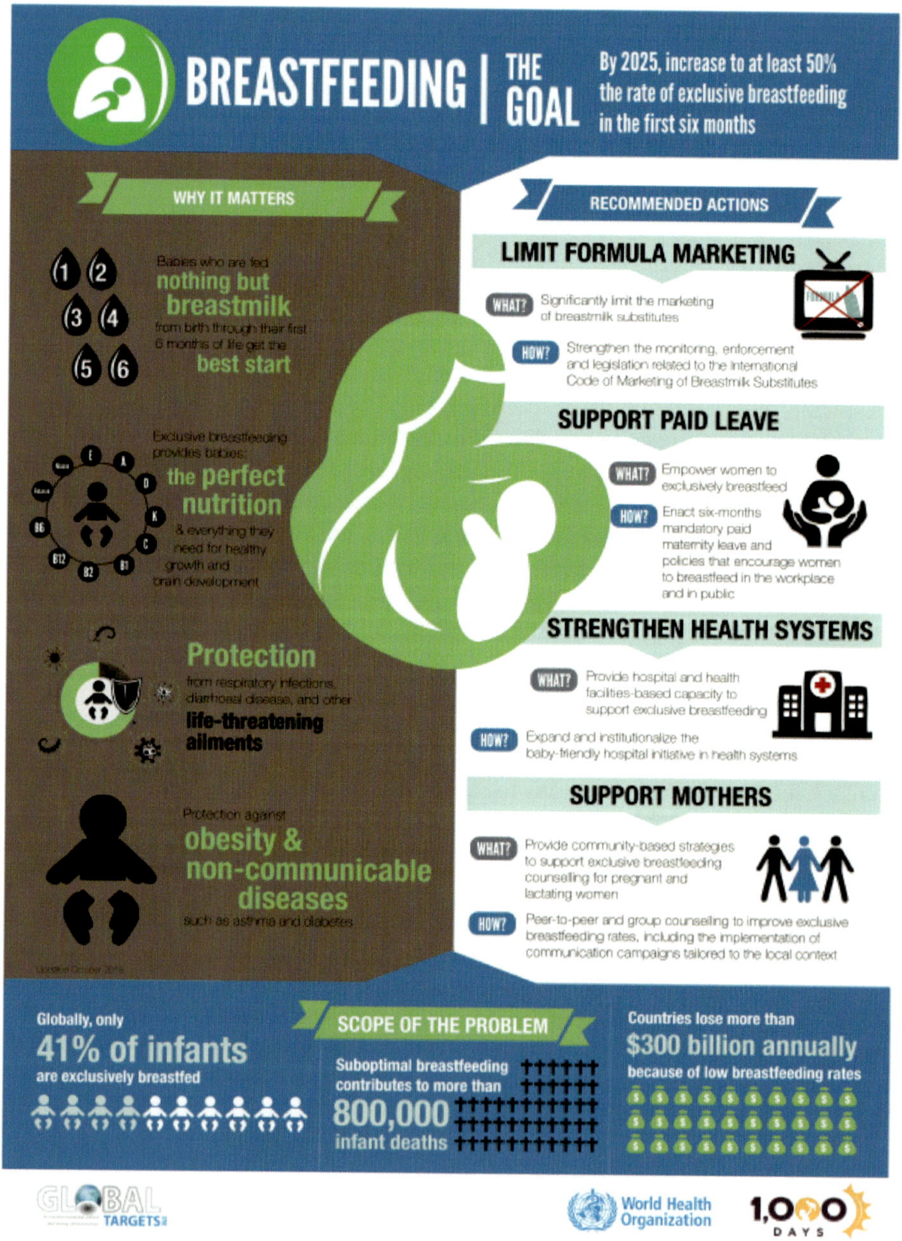

Fig. 54.1 Breastfeeding: Global targets 2025, World Health Organization

Breastfeeding Benefits

Breastfeeding is a way of providing ideal food for the healthy growth and development of infants. Breast milk promotes sensory and cognitive development and protects the infant against infectious and chronic diseases. Exclusive breastfeeding reduces infant mortality due to common childhood illnesses such as diarrhea or pneumonia and helps for a quicker recovery during illness.

Moreover, breastfeeding contributes to the health and well-being of mothers and reduces the risk of ovarian cancer and breast cancer [3]. Frequent breastfeeding can help to delay a new pregnancy, because suckling affects the release of pituitary hormones, which results in suppression of ovulation and menstruation ("Lactational Amenorrhea Method" – LAM – of contraception). Breastfeeding at night is important to ensure this effect. LAM is an effective method of contraception if the woman is amenorrheic and is fully or nearly fully breastfeeding and the infant is less than 6 months of age [1, 7].

Lactation Physiology

The normal physiology of lactation is a process that begins before the initial latch of the newborn infant. It requires the breast to change in composition, size, and shape during each stage of female development. Development includes puberty, pregnancy, and lactation. These stages are influenced by a cascade of physiologic changes that are crucial to successful breastfeeding. The total process of lactation includes the development of the mammary gland (mammogenesis), the process by which the mammary gland develops the ability to secrete milk (lactogenesis), and the process of milk production (lactation) [8].

Cellular Composition of Breast Tissue and Breast Anatomy

The breast structure includes the nipple and areola, mammary tissue, supporting connective tissue and fat, blood and lymphatic vessels, and nerves. The nipple has an average of nine milk ducts passing to the outside and also muscle fibers and nerves. The nipple is surrounded by the circular pigmented areola, in which are located Montgomery's glands. These glands secrete an oily fluid that protects the skin of the nipple and areola during lactation and produce the mother's individual scent that attracts her baby to the breast [1] (Fig. 54.2).

The normal breast consists of two major structures (ducts and lobules), two types of epithelial cells (luminal and myoepithelial), and two types of stroma (interlobular and intralobular). Six to ten major duct orifices open onto the skin surface of the nipple. Large ducts will eventually lead to the terminal duct lobular

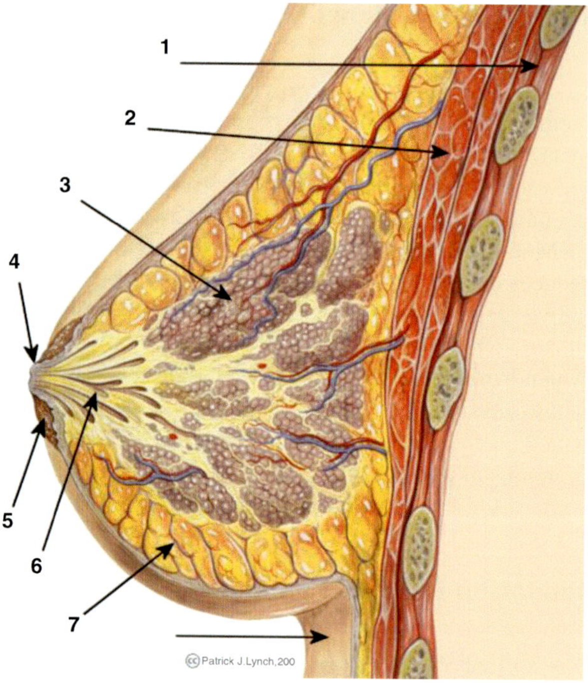

Fig. 54.2 Cross section of the human mammary gland. Patrick J. Lynch, medical illustrator. (From Wikipedia. https://upload.wikimedia.org/wikipedia/commons/thumb/0/0f/Breast_anatomy_normal_scheme.png/800px-Breast_anatomy_normal_scheme.png. Accessed 16 Jan 2020)

unit, and these terminal ducts will then branch into grapelike clusters of small acini to form a lobule. There are three types of lobules, types 1, 2, and 3, which form at different stages in a woman's development. Only with the onset of pregnancy does the breast become completely mature and functional, and by the end of pregnancy, the breast is composed almost entirely of lobules separated by small amounts of the stroma [8].

The nipple has also muscle fibers and nerves. The nipple is surrounded by the circular pigmented areola, in which are located Montgomery's glands. These glands secrete an oily fluid that protects the skin of the nipple and areola during lactation and produce the mother's individual scent that attracts her baby to the breast. The ducts beneath the areola fill with milk and become wider during a feed, when the oxytocin reflex is active [8].

Lactation Hormone Control

Normal lactation involves the female breast, the anterior lobe of the pituitary, and the posterior lobe of the pituitary [8]. Puberty initiates branching morphogenesis, which requires growth hormone and estrogen, as well as IGF1, to create a ductal tree that fills the fat pad. Upon pregnancy the combined actions of progesterone and prolactin generate alveoli, which secrete milk during lactation [9].

There are two hormones that directly affect breastfeeding: prolactin and oxytocin. A number of other hormones, such as estrogen, are involved indirectly in lactation. When a baby suckles at the breast, sensory impulses pass from the nipple to the brain. In response, the anterior lobe of the pituitary gland secretes prolactin and the posterior lobe secretes oxytocin. The ducts beneath the areola fill with milk and become wider during a feed, when the oxytocin reflex is active [1].

Prolactin is necessary for the secretion of milk by the cells of the alveoli. The level of prolactin in the blood increases markedly during pregnancy and stimulates the growth and development of the mammary tissue, in preparation for the production of milk. However, milk is not secreted then, because progesterone and estrogen, the hormones of pregnancy, block this action of prolactin. More prolactin is produced at night, so breastfeeding at night is especially helpful for keeping up the milk supply. Prolactin seems to make a mother feel relaxed and sleepy, so she usually rests well even if she breastfeeds at night [1].

Oxytocin makes the myoepithelial cells around the alveoli contract. This makes the milk, which has collected in the alveoli, flow along and fill the ducts. Oxytocin starts working when a mother expects a feed as well as when the baby is suckling (oxytocin reflex). The reflex becomes conditioned to the mother's sensations and feelings, such as touching, smelling, or seeing her baby, hearing her baby cry, or thinking lovingly about him or her. If a mother is in severe pain or emotionally upset, the oxytocin reflex may become inhibited, and her milk may suddenly stop flowing well. If she receives support, is helped to feel comfortable, and lets the baby continue to breastfeed, the milk will flow again [1].

Lack of demand for milk at weaning initiates the process of involution whereby the gland is remodeled back to its prepregnancy state [9].

Development of the Mammary Gland (Mammogenesis)

During puberty, lobule type 1 is formed, and the changes in the level of estrogen and progesterone during each menstrual cycle stimulate lobule 1 to produce new alveolar buds and eventually evolve to more mature structures, known as type 2 and type 3 lobules (stage I mammogenesis) [8, 9].

During pregnancy, alveolar development and maturation of the epithelium occurs largely in response to higher levels of progesterone (stage II mammogenesis). The proliferation of secretory tissue causes the increased volume of breast tissue during pregnancy. In early pregnancy, lobule type 3 is formed due to the influence of chorionic gonadotropin. These newly formed lobules have larger size and number of epithelial cells composing each acinus. In late pregnancy, the proliferation of new acini is reduced, and the lumen becomes distended with secretory material or colostrum [8, 9].

During labor and lactation, further growth and differentiation can be seen in the lobule along with milk secretion. The glandular component of the breast in this stage is mainly formed of epithelial elements and very little stroma. This will persist throughout lactation [8].

Finally, the involution of mammary glands occurs with the cessation of lactation and requires a combination of lactogenic hormone deprivation and local autocrine signals that signal apoptotic cell death and tissue remodeling. Full regression does not occur, and pregnancy causes a permanent increase in the size and number of lobules. Following lactation, there is always the potential of the glands to produce milk in response to regular stimulation [8].

Development of the Mammary Gland Ability to Secrete Milk (Lactogenesis)

Lactogenesis is the process of developing the ability to secrete milk and involves the maturation of alveolar cells. It takes place in two stages: secretory initiation and secretory activation [8].

Stage I lactogenesis (secretory initiation) takes place during the second half of pregnancy. In this stage, small amounts of milk can be secreted by week 16 gestation. By late pregnancy, some women can express colostrum. The placenta supplies high levels of progesterone which inhibit further differentiation [8].

Stage II lactogenesis (secretory activation) starts after delivery. With the removal of the placenta at delivery, the rapid drop in progesterone and the presence of elevated levels of prolactin, cortisol, and insulin are what stimulate this stage. Usually, at day 2 or 3 postpartum, most women experience swelling of the breast along with copious milk production (lactation) [8].

Process of Milk Production (Lactation)

For the ongoing synthesis and secretion of milk, the mammary gland must receive hormonal signals; and although prolactin and oxytocin act independently on different cellular receptors, their combined action is essential for successful lactation. Lactation is maintained by regular removal of milk and stimulation of the nipple, which triggers prolactin release from the anterior pituitary gland and oxytocin from the posterior pituitary gland [1].

In primiparous women, the secretory activation stage (stage I lactogenesis) is slightly delayed, and early milk volume is lower. Lower milk volume is also observed in women who had cesarean births compared with those who delivered vaginally. Late onset of milk production has also been seen in women who have had retained placental fragments, diabetes, and stressful vaginal deliveries. With retained placental fragments, lactogenesis stage II could be inhibited by the continued secretion of progesterone and would continue to be inhibited until removal of the remaining placental fragments, slowing down the complete process of lactation [8].

Breast Milk Composition

Breast milk contains all the nutrients that an infant need in the first 6 months of life, and it continues to provide up to half or more of a child's nutritional needs during the second half of the first year and up to one-third during the second year of life [1, 3].

Breast milk provides ideal nutrition for infants with fat, carbohydrates, proteins, vitamins, minerals, and water that are more easily digested than formula. The composition of human milk is variable within feeds, diurnally, over lactation, and between mothers and populations. Breast milk contains antibodies from the mother that help babies fight off viruses and bacteria. Other anti-infective factors it provides include immunoglobulin (IgA in particular), white blood cells, whey protein (lysozyme and lactoferrin), and oligosaccharides, which augment the infant's immature immune system, providing protection against infection. Breast milk also contains other factors that help digestion and absorption of nutrients [1, 8, 10] (Table 54.1).

Colostrum and Mature Milk

Colostrum is the special milk that is secreted in the first 2–3 days after delivery. It is produced in small amounts, about 40–50 ml on the first day, but is all that an infant normally needs at this time. Colostrum is rich in white cells and antibodies, especially IgA, and it contains a larger percentage of protein, minerals, and fat-soluble vitamins (A, E, and K) than later milk [1].

Milk starts to be produced in larger amounts between 2 and 4 days after delivery, making the breasts feel full; the milk is then said to have "come in." On the third day, an infant is normally taking about 300–400 ml per 24 hours and on the fifth day 500–800 ml. From days 7 to 14, the milk is called transitional, and after 2 weeks it is called mature milk [1].

Practices to Support Breastfeeding

To enable mothers to establish and sustain exclusive breastfeeding for 6 months, the World Health Organization (WHO) and United Nations Children's Fund (UNICEF) recommend [3]:

- Initiation of breastfeeding within the first hour of life.
- Exclusive breastfeeding – that is, the infant only receives breast milk without any additional food or drink, not even water, except breast milk (including milk expressed or from a wet nurse) for 6 months of life.
- Breastfeeding on demand – that is, as often as the child wants, day and night.
- No use of bottles, teats, or pacifiers.

While breastfeeding is a natural act, it is also a learned behavior. An extensive body of research has demonstrated that mothers and other caregivers require active

Table 54.1 Macronutrient (g/dL) and energy (kcal/dL) composition of human milk from specified references

Author (year), n	Protein mean (± 2 SD)	Fat mean (±2 SD)	Lactase mean (±2 SD)	Energy mean (± 2 SD)
Term infants, 24-hour collection, mature milk				
Nommsen et al. (1991), n = 58	1.2 (0.9, 1.5)	3.6 (2.2, 5.0)	7.4 (7.2, 7.7)	70 (57, 83)
Donor human milk samples				
Wojcik et al. (2009), n = 415	1.2 (0.7, 1.7)	3.2 (1.2, 5.2)	7.8 (6.0, 9.6)	65 (43, 87)
Michaelsen et al. (1990), n = 2553	[a]0.9 (0.6, 1.4)	[a]3.6 (1.8, 8.9)	[a]7.2 (6.4, 7.6)	[a]67 (50,115)
Representative values of mature milk, term infants				
Reference standard	0.9	3.5	6.7	65 to 70
Preterm, 24-hour collection, first 8 weeks of life				
Bauer & Gerss (2011)				
Born <29 weeks, n = 52	2.2 (1.3, 3.3)	4.4 (2.6, 6.2)	7.6 (6.4, 8.8)	78 (61, 94)
Born 32–33 weeks, n = 20	1.9 (1.3, 2.5)	4.8 (2.8, 6.8)	7.5 (6.5, 8.5)	77 (64, 89)
Preterm donor milk				
Hartmann (2012), n = 47	1.4 (0.8, 1.9)	4.2 (2.4, 5.9)	6.7 (5.5, 7.9)	70 (53, 87)

[a]Median (lower sound)
Nommsen et al., 1991: Davis, CA mothers at 3 months postpartum
Wojcik et al., 2909, U.S. milk bank donors
Michaelsen et al., 1990, Danish milk bank donors
Reference standard based on expert review: Pediatric nutrition handbook, sixth edition, table C-1, p. 1201 (mature Milk)
Bauer & Gerss, 2011, preterm infants 23 to 33 weeks gestational age
Hartmann (2012), Australian donor mothers of preterm infants (see article this issue by Landers and Hartmann)
Reference: Ballard and Morrow, 2013 [10]

support for establishing and sustaining appropriate breastfeeding practices. The foundation of the Baby-friendly Hospital Initiative launched by WHO and UNICEF (1992) described the *Ten Steps to Successful Breastfeeding* in order to protect, promote, and support breastfeeding [3, 4, 11] (Fig. 54.3).

- Critical management procedures
  - 1a. Comply fully with the *International Code of Marketing of Breast-milk Substitutes* and relevant World Health Assembly resolutions.
  - 1b. Have a written infant feeding policy that is routinely communicated to staff and parents.
  - 1c. Establish ongoing monitoring and data management systems.
  - 2. Ensure that staff have sufficient knowledge, competence and skills to support breastfeeding

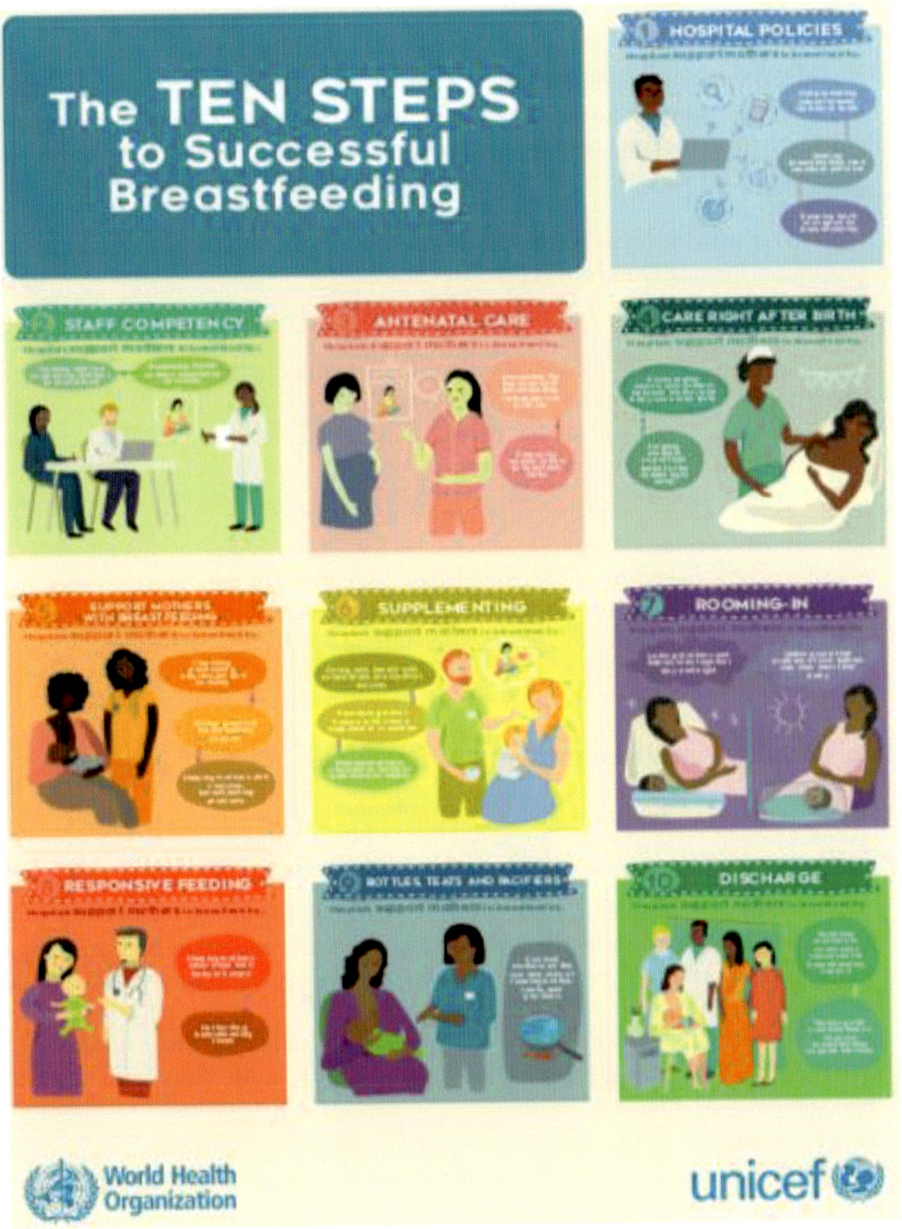

Fig. 54.3 Ten Steps to Successful Breastfeeding described in Protecting, Promoting and Supporting Breastfeeding: a Joint WHO/UNICEF Statement

- Key clinical practices
  3. Discuss the importance and management of breastfeeding with pregnant women and their families.
  4. Facilitate immediate and uninterrupted skin-to-skin contact, and support mothers to initiate breastfeeding as soon as possible after birth.
  5. Support mothers to initiate and maintain breastfeeding and manage common difficulties.
  6. Do not provide breastfed newborns any food or fluids other than breast milk, unless medically indicated.
  7. Enable mothers and their infants to remain together and to practice rooming-in 24 hours a day.
  8. Support mothers to recognize and respond to their infants' cues for feeding.
  9. Counsel mothers on the use and risks of feeding bottles, teats, and pacifiers.
  10. Coordinate discharge so that parents and their infants have timely access to ongoing support and care.

There is substantial evidence that implementing the *Ten Steps* significantly improves breastfeeding rates. A systematic review of 58 studies on maternity and newborn care published in 2016 demonstrated clearly that adherence to the *Ten Steps* impacts early initiation of breastfeeding immediately after birth, exclusive breastfeeding, and total duration of breastfeeding [3].

Breastfeeding and Recommended Practices

Preparation of mothers before they give birth is fundamental to the success of the breastfeeding. During pregnancy, women need information about [1]:

- The benefits of breastfeeding and the risks of artificial or mixed feeding.
- Optimal practices, such as early skin-to-skin contact, exclusive breastfeeding, rooming-in, starting to breastfeed soon after delivery, and why colostrum is important.
- What to expect, including how the milk "comes in" and how a baby suckles.
- What they will need to do: skin-to-skin contact, putting the baby to the breast, and appropriate patterns of feeding.

The key points of contact to support optimal feeding practices include [1]:

- During antenatal care.
- At the time of childbirth and in the immediate postpartum period.
- In the postnatal period (for healthy term babies on days 2–3, days 5–7, and around 3–4 weeks; for low-birth-weight babies more frequently on day 2, day 3, days 5–7, day 14, and day 28; at 6 weeks postpartum for all mothers and babies during immunization contacts).

- During well-baby clinics and/or growth assessment visits during sick child visits and their follow-up.

WHO and UNICEF's global recommendations for optimal infant feeding as set out in the Global Strategy are exclusive breastfeeding for 6 months (180 days) and nutritionally adequate and safe complementary feeding starting from the age of 6 months with continued breastfeeding up to 2 years of age or beyond [1–3].

There is not anything special to do for the breasts when breastfeeding. Practice good hygiene (wash hands before touching the breasts, and keep the breasts and nipples clean by washing them with water in the shower or bath) and wear a supportive bra are common recommendations. To increase milk supply, nursing mothers should seek consultation with a lactation specialist and use nonpharmacologic measures, such as ensuring proper technique, using massage therapy, increasing the frequency of milk expression, prolonging the duration of pumping, and maximizing emotional support [12].

Feeding a baby from a bottle with an artificial teat may make it more difficult for the baby to learn to attach well at the breast and may make it more difficult to establish breastfeeding satisfactorily. If an infant cannot feed from the breast, then the safest alternative is to feed from a cup [1].

Full breasts occur from 3–5 days after delivery when the breast milk "comes in." The breasts became heavy, hot, and hard. The milk flows well during full breasts. This is normal fullness. The management includes to breastfeed frequently to remove the milk and to put the baby well attached to suckle. The fullness decreases after a feed, and after a few days, the breasts become more comfortable as milk production adjusts to the baby's needs [1].

Current recommendations for lactating women are to have a minimum excess of 500 calories per day to meet the caloric demands for milk production. Women are also encouraged to empty the breast as often as possible, typically every 2 to 3 hours to maintain milk supply [8].

Reflexes in the Baby

The baby's reflexes are important for appropriate breastfeeding. The main reflexes are rooting, suckling, and swallowing. When something touches a baby's lips or cheek, the baby turns to find the stimulus and opens his or her mouth, putting his or her tongue down and forward. This is the *rooting reflex* and is present from about the 32nd week of pregnancy. When something touches a baby's palate, he or she starts to suck it. This is the *sucking reflex*. When the baby's mouth fills with milk, he or she swallows. This is the *swallowing reflex*. Preterm infants can grasp the nipple from about 28 weeks gestational age, and they can suckle and remove some milk from about 31 weeks. Coordination of suckling, swallowing, and breathing appears between 32 and 35 weeks of pregnancy [1].

How a Baby Attaches and Suckles at the Breast

A baby needs to be well attached to suckle effectively in order to stimulate the nipple and to ensure an adequate supply and a good flow of milk. The points to notice are [1] (Fig. 54.4):

- Much of the areola and the tissues underneath it, including the larger ducts, are in the baby's mouth.
- The breast is stretched out to form a long "teat," but the nipple only forms about one-third of the "teat."
- The baby's tongue is forward over the lower gums, beneath the milk ducts (the baby's tongue is in fact cupped around the sides of the "teat," but a drawing cannot show this).
- The baby is suckling from the breast, not from the nipple.

When a baby is well attached, his mouth and tongue do not rub or traumatize the skin of the nipple and areola.

Different Nipple Shapes

Different nipple shapes are a natural physical feature of the breast. An inverted nipple is held by tight connective tissue that may slacken after a baby suckles from it for a time. Antenatal treatment is not helpful. The babies can often suckle without difficulty from nipples of unusual shapes, and that skilled help after delivery is the most important thing. If a baby cannot attach in the first week or two, the mother can express her breast milk and feed it by cup [1, 8].

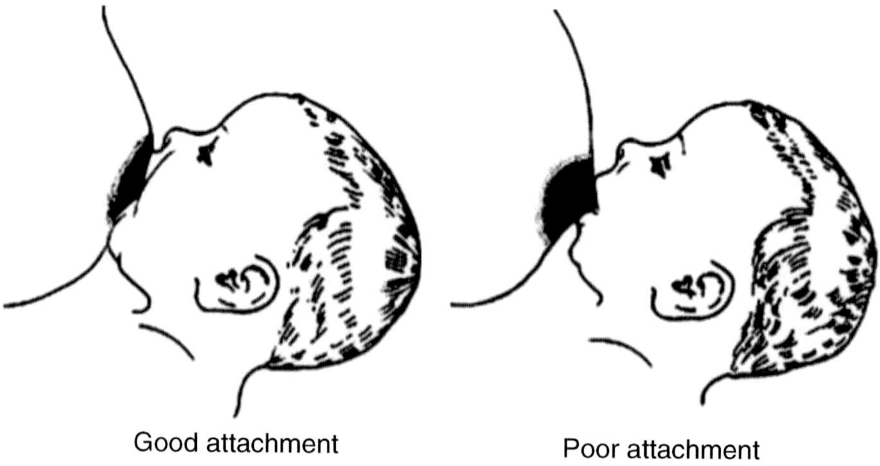

Fig. 54.4 Good and poor attachment to the breast. WHO/UNICEF

Effective Suckling

The baby takes slow, deep suckles followed by a visible or audible swallow about once per second. Sometimes the baby pauses for a few seconds, allowing the ducts to fill up with milk again. When the baby starts suckling again, he or she may suckle quickly a few times, stimulating milk flow, and then the slow deep suckles begin. The baby's cheeks remain rounded during the feed [1].

Positioning the Mother and Baby for Good Attachment

The mother can be sitting or lying down or standing. However, she needs to be relaxed and comfortable, and without strain, particularly of her back. The baby can breastfeed in several different positions in relation to the mother: across her chest and abdomen, under her arm, or alongside her body [1].

Whatever the position of the mother and the baby's general position in relation to her, there are four key points about the position of the baby's body that are important to observe [1]:

1. The baby's body should be straight, not bent or twisted. The baby's head can be slightly extended at the neck, which helps his or her chin to be close into the breast.
2. He or she should be facing the breast. The nipples usually point slightly downward, so the baby should not be flat against the mother's chest or abdomen, but turned slightly on his or her back able to see the mother's face.
3. The baby's body should be close to the mother which enables the baby to be close to the breast and to take a large mouthful.
4. His or her whole body should be supported.

Breastfeeding Pattern

To ensure adequate milk production and flow for 6 months of exclusive breastfeeding, a baby needs to feed as often and for as long as he or she wants, both day and night. This is called demand feeding, unrestricted feeding, or baby-led feeding. The 24-hour intake of milk varies between mother-infant pairs from 440 to 1220 ml, averaging about 800 ml per day throughout the first 6 months [1–3].

It is important not to restrict the duration or the frequency of feeds. Nipple damage is caused by poor attachment and not by prolonged feeds. The baby should be allowed to continue suckling on the breast until he or she spontaneously releases the nipple. After a short rest, the baby can be offered the other side [1].

If a baby stays on the breast for a very long time (more than one-half hour for every feed) or if the baby wants to feed very often (more often than every

1–11/2 hours each time), then the baby's attachment must be checked and improved. Prolonged and frequent feeds can be a sign of ineffective suckling and inefficient transfer of milk to the baby [1].

Breastfeeding during Pregnancy

The consequences of breastfeeding during pregnancy (BDP) have not been clearly established. Since suckling during breastfeeding induces release of oxytocin from the posterior pituitary gland that, theoretically, may cause uterine simulation during pregnancy, there is a concern about a risk of miscarriage and preterm labor in breastfeeding during pregnancy. However, the oxytocin released during breastfeeding is usually released in such a small amount during breastfeeding that is not enough to cause preterm labor, and there are other protective mechanisms against the effective contractions during the pregnancy. Generally, it's safe to continue breastfeeding while pregnant, especially in low-risk pregnancies for preterm labor. Data suggest that BDP does not affect the way pregnancies end or even birth weights [13].

In pregnant women who are breastfeeding, it is important to attempt to maternal nutritional and the calories intake must be adjusted [13].

Although breast milk continues to be nutritionally sound throughout pregnancy, the composition of breast milk will change as well as its tastes. In addition, the milk production is likely to decrease with pregnancy progresses. These factors could lead the nursing child to wean on his or her own before the baby is born [13].

Further studies of BDP are needed with larger samples, adequate methodology, and proper control of the main confounders.

Proper Storage and Preparation of Breast Milk

Before expressing or handling breast milk, it is recommended to wash your hands well with soap and water (if soap and water are not available, use an alcohol-based hand sanitizer that contains at least 60% alcohol). Mothers can express breast milk by hand or with a manual or electric pump. If using a pump, inspect the pump kit and tubing to make sure it is clean. Discard and replace moldy tubing immediately. If using a shared pump kit, clean pump dials, power switch, and countertop with disinfectant wipe [14].

Use breast milk storage bags or clean food-grade containers with tight fitting lids made of glass or plastic to store expressed breast milk. Avoid bottles that may be made of a BPA-containing plastic. Never store breast milk in disposable bottle liners or plastic bags that are not intended for storing breast milk. Table 54.2 shows the storage location and temperatures recommendations for breast milk [14, 15].

There are several ways to thaw your breast milk: in the refrigerator overnight, set in a container of warm or lukewarm water, and under lukewarm running water.

Never thaw or heat breast milk in a microwave. Microwaving can destroy nutrients in breast milk and create hot spots, which can burn a baby's mouth. Use breast milk within 24 hours of thawing in the refrigerator (this means from the time it is no longer frozen or completely thawed, not from the time when you took it out of the freezer). Once breast milk is brought to room temperature or warmed after storing in the refrigerator or freezer, it should be used within 2 hours. Never refreeze breast milk once it has been thawed [14, 15] (Table 54.2).

Twins

Twins who are low birth weight need to be managed according to specific recommendations. For larger twins, management should be as for singletons. Mothers may need help to find the best way to hold two babies to suckle, either at the same time or one at a time. They may like to give each baby its own breast or to vary the side. Holding one or both babies in the underarm position for feeding and support for the babies with pillows or folded clothes are often helpful. Building the mother's confidence that she can make enough milk for two, and encouraging relatives to help with other household duties, may help her to avoid trying to feed the babies artificially [1].

HIV and Infant Feeding

The HIV pandemic and the risk of mother-to-child transmission of HIV through breastfeeding pose unique challenges to the promotion of breastfeeding, even among unaffected families. Complex emergencies, which are often characterized by

Table 54.2 Human milk storage

Storage location and temperatures			
Type of breast milk	Countertop 77 °F (25 °C) or colder (room temperature)	Refrigerator 40 °F (4 °C)	Freezer 0 °F (−18 °C) or colder
Freshly expressed or pumped	Up to 4 hours	Up to 4 days	Within 6 months is best up to 12 months is acceptable
Thawed, previously frozen	1–2 hours	Up to 1 day (24 hours)	Never refreeze human milk after it has been thawed
Leftover from a feeding (baby did not finish the bottle)	Use within 2 hours after the baby is finished feeding		

CDC Guidelines & Recommendations, Proper Storage and Preparation of Breast Milk, revised 2020 [14]

population displacement, food insecurity, and armed conflict, are increasing in number and intensity, further compromising the care and feeding of infants and young children the world over.

The recognition that HIV is transmitted through breast milk raised the important question of whether strategies that promote breastfeeding in areas of high HIV prevalence should be evaluated. This policy decision is particularly difficult, given that breastfeeding provides important protection against infectious diseases.

The United Nations recommendations for feeding of infants by mothers who are HIV- infected include [1]:

- The most appropriate infant feeding option for an HIV-infected mother depends on her individual circumstances, including her health status and the local situation, but should take consideration of the health services available and the counselling and support she is likely to receive.
- Exclusive breastfeeding is recommended for HIV-infected mothers for the first 6 months of life unless replacement feeding is acceptable, feasible, affordable, sustainable, and safe for them and their infants before that time.
- When replacement feeding is acceptable, feasible, affordable, sustainable, and safe, avoidance of all breastfeeding by HIV-infected mothers is recommended.
- All HIV-exposed infants should receive regular follow-up care and periodic reassessment of infant feeding choices, particularly at the time of infant diagnosis and at 6 months.
- At 6 months, if adequate feeding from other sources cannot be ensured, HIV-infected women should continue to breastfeed their infants and give complementary foods in addition and return for regular follow-up assessments. All breastfeeding should stop once an adequate diet without breast milk can be provided.
- Breastfed infants and young children who are HIV-infected should continue to breastfeed according to recommendations for the general population.

The main factors which increase the risk of HIV transmission through breastfeeding include [16]:

- Acquiring HIV infection during breastfeeding, because of high initial viral load.
- The severity of the disease (as indicated by a low CD4+ count or high RNA viral load in the mother's blood or severe clinical symptoms).
- Poor breast health (e.g., mastitis, subclinical mastitis, fissured nipples).
- Possibly, oral infection in the infant (thrush and herpes).
- Nonexclusive breastfeeding (mixed feeding).
- Longer duration of breastfeeding.
- Possibly, nutritional status of the mother.

There is a wide agreement that the final decision on whether or not to breastfeed if a woman is HIV-positive should reside with the mother and the family [1].

Drug Safety during Breastfeeding

Many mothers are inappropriately advised to discontinue breastfeeding or avoid taking essential medications because of fears of adverse effects on their infants. This cautious approach may be unnecessary in many cases, because only a small proportion of medications are contraindicated in breastfeeding mothers or associated with adverse effects on their infants [12].

Healthcare providers should weigh the risks and benefits when prescribing medications to breastfeeding mothers by considering the following [12]:

- Need for the drug by the mother.
- Potential effects of the drug on milk production.
- Amount of the drug excreted into human milk.
- Extent of oral absorption by the breastfeeding infant.
- Potential adverse effects on the breastfeeding infant.
- Age of the infant.
- Proportion of feedings that are breast milk.

The benefits of breastfeeding for both the infant and mother need to be weighed against the risks of drug exposure to the infant (or to the mother, in the case of agents intended to induce lactation). Many factors affect the individual risk/benefit decision, including specific information about chemical and pharmacologic properties of the drug [12].

Antibiotics

Antibiotics are one of the most common medications mothers are prescribed, and all pass in some degree into milk. In general, if the antibiotic would be administered directly to a premature infant or a neonate, then it is safe for the mother to take during breastfeeding. A question arises when sulfa drugs are provided because they compete for albumin-binding sites. Until bound and unbound bilirubin can be measured clinically, sulfa drugs should not be administered during lactation in a jaundiced infant younger than 1 month because the amount of free bilirubin available to cross into the brain would be unmeasurable. Infants with glucose-6-phosphate disease should not be exposed to sulfa drugs at any time. Erythromycin appears in higher amounts in the milk than in the plasma; if provided intravenously to the mother, then the levels in milk are 10 times higher. After 1 month of age, administering erythromycin directly to the infant is usually safe. Another concern with erythromycin is the risk of cross-reaction with other drugs, such as carbimazole, cyclosporin, digoxin, triazolam, theophylline, and anticoagulants [12, 17].

Some medications are classified as contraindicated medications during breastfeeding. Concerns exist for amiodarone (may affect thyroid function in infant), iodine (high doses, >150 micrograms daily, lead to risk of infant hypothyroidism), chemotherapeutic/antineoplastic agents (leukopenia, bone marrow suppression), chloramphenicol, ergotamine, gold salts (rash, nephritis, hematological abnormalities), phenindione, radioactive pharmaceuticals, retinoids, tetracyclines (chronic >3 weeks), and certain psychotropic medications (lithium now can be taken with careful monitoring of blood levels in mother and baby) [12, 17].

The Drugs and Lactation Database (LactMed® database) contains information on drugs and other chemicals to which breastfeeding mothers may be exposed. It includes information on the levels of such substances in breast milk and infant blood and the possible adverse effects in the nursing infant. Suggested therapeutic alternatives to those drugs are provided, where appropriate.

Antidepressants, Anxiolytics, and Antipsychotics

Many antianxiety drugs, antidepressants, and mood stabilizers appear in low concentrations in human milk, with estimated relative infant doses less than 2% of weight-adjusted maternal dose and/or milk-plasma ratios less than 1. However, the percentage of maternal doses that approach clinically significant levels (10% or more) have been reported for bupropion, diazepam, fluoxetine, citalopram, lithium, lamotrigine, sertraline, and venlafaxine. Data on drug excretion in human milk are not available for up to one-third of psychoactive therapies. Because of the long half-life of some of these compounds and/or their metabolites, coupled with an infant's immature hepatic and renal function, nursing infants may have measurable amounts of the drug or its metabolites in plasma and potentially in neural tissue [12].

Drugs of Abuse

Although many women are appropriately advised to refrain from smoking, drinking, and using recreational drugs during and after pregnancy, in part because of adverse effects on their infants (Table 54.3), some are unable to do so and may seek assistance after delivery. Maternal smoking should be strongly encouraged to stop smoking and to minimize secondhand exposure for multiple reasons, including the association of sudden infant death syndrome with tobacco exposure. Exposure to alcohol or recreational drugs may impair a mother's judgment and interfere with her care of the infant and can cause toxicity to the breastfeeding infant [12].

Limited information is available regarding the use of medications in lactating women to treat substance abuse or alcohol dependence or for smoking cessation. Continued breastfeeding by women undergoing such treatment presumes that the patient remains abstinent, is HIV-negative, and is enrolled in and closely monitored by an appropriate drug treatment program with significant social support [12].

Table 54.3 Drugs of abuse for which adverse effects on the breastfeeding infant have been reported[a]

Drug	Reported Effect or Reason for Concern	Reference
Alcohol	Impaired motor development or postnatal growth, decreased milk consumption, sleep disturbances	Koren 2002,[34] Backstrand 2004,[35] Mennella 2007[36]
	Note: Although binge drinking should be avoided, occasional, limited ingestion (0.5 g of alcohol/kg/d; equivalent to 8 oz. wine or 2 cans of beer per day) may be acceptable.	National Academy of Sciences 1991[37]
Amphetamines	Hypertension, tachycardia, and seizures.	Product labeling
	In animal studies of postnatal exposure, long-term behavioral effects, including learning and memory deficits and altered locomotor activity, were observed.	
Benzodiazepines	Accumulation of metabolite, prolonged half-life in neonate or preterm infant is noted; chronic use not recommended	Jain 2005,[38] Malone 2004[39]
	Apnea, cyanosis, withdrawal, sedation, cyanosis, and seizures.	
Cocaine	Intoxication, seizures, irritability vomiting, diarrhea, tremulousness.	Chasnoff 1987,[40] Winecker 2001[41]
Heroin	Withdrawal symptoms, tremors, restlessness, vomiting, poor feeding.	vandeVelde 2007[42]
LSD	Potent hallucinogen.	
Methamphetamine	Fatality, persists in breast milk for 48 h.	Ariagno 1995,[43] Bartu 2009[44]
Methylene dioxy-methamphetamine (ecstasy)	Closely related products (amphetamines) are concentrated in human milk.	
Marijuana (cannabis)	Neurodevelopmental effects, delayed motor development at 1 y, lethargy, less frequent and shorter feedings, high milk-plasma ratios in heavy users.	Djulus 2005,[45] Campolongo 2009,[46] Garry 2010[47]
Phencyclidine	Potent hallucinogen, infant intoxication.	AAP 2001,[6] Academy of Breastfeeding Medicine[48]

[a]Effect an maternal judgment or mood may affect ability to care for infant
Reference: Sachs, 2013 [12]

Pain Medications

When narcotic agents are needed to treat pain in the breastfeeding woman, agents other than codeine (i.e., butorphanol, morphine, or hydromorphone) are preferred, because normal doses of codeine given to lactating women may result in dangerously high levels of its active metabolite morphine in breastfeeding infants. Morphine appears to be tolerated by the breastfeeding infant. Other narcotic agents, such as oxycodone, pentazocine, propoxyphene, and meperidine, are not recommended in the lactating mother [12].

Regardless of the choice of therapy, to minimize adverse events for both the mother and her nursing infant, the lowest dose and shortest duration of therapy should be prescribed [12].

When narcotics are not required to relieve mild to moderate pain, other analgesic agents can be used. Presuming that pain relief is adequate, short-acting agents, such as ibuprofen and acetaminophen, are acceptable. Although the half-life of ibuprofen may be prolonged in neonates, particularly in preterm infants (according to product labeling), minimal amounts of ibuprofen are excreted into human milk. Although all nonsteroidal antiinflammatory drugs (NSAIDs) carry a boxed warning regarding gastrointestinal bleeding and potential long-term cardiac toxicity, celecoxib, flurbiprofen, and naproxen are considered to be compatible with breastfeeding, because less than 1% is excreted into human milk [12].

Galactagogues

Galactagogues (or lactogogues), or agents to stimulate lactation, are often used to facilitate lactation, particularly for mothers of preterm infants. They also may be used to in women inducing lactation when they have not been pregnant with the current child, in women relactating after weaning, or in transgender women. However, evidence to support these agents, including use of dopamine antagonists, such as domperidone and metoclopramide; herbal treatments; and hormonal manipulation, is lacking. These agents have a limited role in facilitating lactation and have not been subject to full assessments of safety for the nursing infant. Nursing mothers should seek consultation with a lactation specialist and use nonpharmacologic measures to increase milk supply, such as ensuring proper technique, using massage therapy, increasing the frequency of milk expression, prolonging the duration of pumping, and maximizing emotional support [12, 18].

Diagnostic Imaging during Breastfeeding

For most radiopharmaceuticals, breastfeeding should be interrupted for a time period based on the rate of decline of the agent and dosimetry to avoid infant exposures greater than 1 mSv (100 mrem). Because there is considerable variability in milk radioactivity and close contact with an infant may result in additional exposure, consultation with a radiologist should be sought. When feasible, elective imaging procedures should be delayed until a woman is no longer breastfeeding. If deemed necessary, individualized testing of expressed milk may be performed to ensure that radioactivity has reached background levels before breastfeeding is resumed [12].

Breastfeeding and Vaccines

With rare exceptions, maternal immunization does not create any problems for breastfeeding infants. Breastfeeding does not interfere with the infant's immune response to most routine immunizations, despite the presence of maternal antibodies in human milk. Seroconversion rates are also similar between breastfed and formula-fed infants. Breastfeeding may decrease the incidence of fever after infant immunization. Therefore, the timing of infant feeding (including human milk) relative to immunization is not restricted, even for live vaccines, such as rotavirus. Inactivated vaccines given to a nursing mother do not pose a risk to the breastfeeding infant, and most live vaccines are not associated with virus secretion in human milk [19, 20].

Although attenuated rubella can be secreted into human milk and transmitted to breastfed infants, infections are usually asymptomatic or mild. In contrast, infants are considered to be at high risk of developing vaccinia after exposure to smallpox vaccine or encephalitis after yellow fever vaccine. Therefore, most vaccines, with the exception of smallpox or yellow-fever vaccine, which are contraindicated in nonemergency situations, may be administered during lactation [19, 20].

Management of Breastfeeding Difficulties

The process of lactation and breastfeeding can be negatively affected by anything that interrupts the normal development of the female breast or that interferes with the production of milk. Women who have had breast augmentation may experience issues with lactation and breastfeeding, but this is dependent on the location of the incision. Incisions made in the armpit are more favorably for normal breastfeeding, whereas the "smile" incision around the areola increases the woman's risk of having breastfeeding issues [8].

In the postpartum period, some women may experience difficulty with lactation if they have inadequate milk production, poor milk extraction, and insufficient caloric intake to meet demands. There are two reliable signs that a baby is not getting enough milk: poor weight gain and/or low urine output (an exclusively breastfed baby who is taking enough milk usually passes dilute urine 6–8 times or more in 24 hours; if a baby is passing urine less than 6 times a day, especially if the urine is dark yellow and strong smelling, then he or she is not getting enough fluid). Passing meconium (sticky black stools) 4 days after delivery is also a sign of the baby not getting enough milk [1]. Current recommendations for lactating women are to have a minimum excess of 500 calories per day to meet the caloric demands for milk production and to empty the breast as often as possible, typically every 2 to 3 hours to maintain milk supply [8].

Other issues of concern regarding lactation include the infant's inability to suckle, nipple pain, mastitis, or plugged ducts [1].

Blocked Duct

The symptoms include a tender, localized lump in one breast, with redness in the skin over the lump. It is caused by failure to remove milk from part of the breast. The management involves to improve removal of milk and correct the underlying cause (infrequent breastfeeds, poor attachment, or trauma to the breast). Feeding from the affected breast frequently, gently massage the breast over the lump while her baby is suckling, to apply warm compresses, and to vary the position of the baby are helpful to manage blocked duct [1].

Breast Engorgement

During the breast engorgement, the breasts are swollen, edematous, and painful, and the skin looks shiny and diffusely red. Usually both breasts are affected. The woman may have a fever that usually subsides in 24 hours. The nipples may become stretched tight which makes it difficult for the baby to attach and remove the milk. The milk does not flow well. Breast engorgement is caused by failure to remove breast milk, especially in the first few days after delivery when the milk comes in. The common reasons why milk is not removed adequately are delayed initiation of breastfeeding, infrequent feeds, poor attachment, and ineffective suckling [1].

The management includes to remove the milk (by breastfeeding as frequently as the baby is willing or expressing the milk by hand or with a pump a few times until the breasts are softer), warm compresses to the breast or take a warm shower before expressing (which helps the milk to flow) and cold compresses after feeding or expressing (which helps to reduce the edema), continuing support for the mothers, and to start breastfeeding soon after delivery [1].

Fissured Nipple

The main cause of sore and fissured nipples is poor attachment. There may be a visible fissure across the tip of the nipple or around the base, and the main symptom is severe nipple pain when the baby is suckling. This may be due to the baby pulling the nipple in and out as he or she suckles and rubbing the skin against his or her mouth; or it may be due to the strong pressure on the nipple resulting from incorrect suckling. The mother should be helped to improve her baby's position and attachment. When the baby is well attached, the pain usually is less. There is no need to rest the breast, because the nipple will heal when it is no longer being damaged [1].

Mastitis

Mastitis is commonest in the first 2–3 weeks after delivery but can occur at any time. When mastitis occurs, there is a hard swelling in the breast, with redness of the overlying skin and severe pain. Usually only a part of one breast is affected, which is different from engorgement, when both breasts are affected. The woman has fever (of 38.5 °C – 101.3 °F – or greater) and feels ill. Important causes are long gaps between feeds, poor attachment, incomplete removal of milk, unrelieved engorgement, frequent pressure on one part of the breast from fingers or tight clothing, and trauma [21].

Mastitis is usually caused by milk stasis, which results in noninfective inflammation. Infection may supervene if the stasis persists or if the woman also has a nipple fissure that becomes infected [21].

The management includes to improve the removal of milk and try to correct any specific cause that is identified, to start breastfeeding the baby with the unaffected breast, to stimulate the oxytocin reflex, and to vary the position of the baby. Breastfeeding should not be stopped. Analgesics helps to handle with the pain (if available, ibuprofen also reduces the inflammation of the breast) [21].

If symptoms are severe, if there is an infected nipple fissure, or if no improvement is seen after 24 hours of improved milk removal, the treatment should then include penicillinase-resistant antibiotics. First-generation cephalosporins are also generally acceptable as first-line treatment, but may be less preferred because of their broader spectrum of coverage. Cephalexin is usually safe in women with suspected penicillin allergy, but clindamycin is suggested for cases of severe penicillin hypersensitivity. However, antibiotics will not be effective without improved removal of milk [1, 21].

Worldwide, the most common pathogen in infective mastitis is penicillin-resistant *S. aureus*. Less commonly, the organism is a *Streptococcus* or *Escherichia coli*. *S. aureus* resistant to penicillinase-resistant penicillins (methicillin-resistant *S. aureus* [MRSA], also referred to as oxacillin-resistant *S. aureus*) has been increasingly isolated in cases of mastitis and breast abscesses. When mastitis is not improving 48 hours after starting first-line treatment, clinicians should be aware of the likelihood of this occurring in their community and should order a breast milk culture and assay of antibiotic sensitivity. Culture and sensitivity testing should be also undertaken if the mastitis recurs, and in cases of hospital-acquired mastitis, presence of allergy to usual therapeutic antibiotics or in severe or unusual cases [21].

Breast Abscess

If a well-defined area of the breast remains hard, red, and tender despite appropriate management, then an abscess should be suspected. This occurs in about 3% of women with mastitis. An abscess needs to be drained and treated with penicillinase-resistant antibiotics [1, 21].

A diagnostic breast ultrasound will identify a collection of fluid. The collection can often be drained by needle aspiration, which itself can be diagnostic as well as therapeutic. Serial needle aspirations may be required. Surgical drainage may be necessary if the abscess is very large or if there are multiple abscesses. When possible, drainage should be guided by ultrasound. A course of antibiotics should follow drainage of the abscess [1, 21].

After drainage, breastfeeding on the affected breast should continue, even if a drain is present, with the proviso that the infant's mouth does not come into direct contact with purulent drainage or infected tissue. However, if suckling is too painful or if the mother is unwilling, she can be shown how to express her milk and advised to let her baby start to feed from the breast again as soon as the pain is less, usually in 2–3 days [1, 21].

Candida Infection (Thrush) in Mother and Baby

Candida infection has been associated with burning nipple pain or radiating breast pain symptoms. This is an infection with the fungus *Candida albicans*, which often follows the use of antibiotics in the baby or in the mother to treat mastitis or other infections. Diagnosis is difficult, as the nipples and breasts may look normal on examination, and milk culture may not be reliable. A trial of antifungal medications (i.e., nystatin), either with or without culture, is the current expert consensus recommendation. If the mother has symptoms, both mother and baby should be treated. If only the baby has symptoms, it is not necessary to treat the mother [1, 21].

In the baby, the candida infection (thrush) presents with white spots inside the cheeks or over the tongue, which look like milk curds, but they cannot be removed easily [1, 21].

References

1. World Health Organization. Infant and young child feeding: model chapter for textbooks for medical students and allied health professionals. World Health Organization; 2009. Available from: https://apps.who.int/iris/handle/10665/44117. Accessed 10 Dec 2019.
2. WHO/UNICEF. Global strategy for infant and young child feeding. Geneva, World Health Organization; 2003.
3. World Health Organization. Fifty-Fifth World Health Assembly. Infant and young child nutrition Global strategy on infant and young child feeding Report by the Secretariat. http://apps.who.int/gb/archive/pdf_files/WHA55/ea5515.pdf?ua=1 Accessed 14 Jan 2020.
4. Academy of Breastfeeding Medicine Protocol Committee. ABM Clinical Protocol #7: Model Maternity Policy Supportive of Breastfeeding. Revised 2018. Breastfeed Med. 2018;13(9):559–74.
5. WHO Collaborative Study Team on the Role of Breastfeeding on the Prevention of Infant Mortality. Effect of breastfeeding on infant and child mortality due to infectious diseases in less developed countries: a pooled analysis. Lancet. 2000;355:451–5.

6. Victora CG, Bahl R, Barros AJD, França GVA, Horton S, Krasevec, et al. Breastfeeding in the 21st century: epidemiology, mechanisms, and lifelong effect. Lancet. 2016;387:475–90.
7. Academy of Breastfeeding Medicine Protocol Committee. ABM Clinical Protocol #13: Contraception During Breastfeeding, Revised 2015. Breastfeed Med. 2015;10:3–12.
8. Pillay J, Davis TJ. Physiology, Lactation. [Updated 2019 Apr 25]. In: StatPearls [Internet]. Treasure Island (FL): StatPearls Publishing; 2020 Jan-. Available from: https://www.ncbi.nlm.nih.gov/books/NBK499981/. Accessed 14 Jan 2020.
9. Macias H, Hinck L. Mammary gland development. Wiley Interdiscip Rev Dev Biol. 2012;1(4):533–57.
10. Ballard O, Morrow AL. Human milk composition: nutrients and bioactive factors. Pediatr Clin North Am. 2013;60:49–74.
11. Shealy KR, Li R, Benton-Davis S, Grummer-Strawn LM. The CDC Guide to Breastfeeding Interventions. U.S. Department of Health and Human Services, Centers for Disease Control and Prevention: Atlanta; 2005.
12. American Academy of Pediatrics. Sachs HC and Committee on drugs. The transfer of drugs and therapeutics into human breast milk: an update on selected topics. Pediatrics. 2013;132:e796–e809.
13. López-Fernández G, Barrios M, Goberna-Tricas J, Gómez-Benito J. Breastfeeding during pregnancy: a systematic review. Woman and birth. 2017;30(6):e292–300.
14. CDC Guidelines & Recommendations. Proper Storage and Preparation of Breast Milk. Revised Jan 2020. https://www.cdc.gov/breastfeeding/recommendations/handling_breastmilk.htm. Accessed 10 Fev 2020.
15. Academy of Breastfeeding Medicine Protocol Committee. ABM clinical protocol #8: human milk storage information for home use for full-term infants, Revised 2017. Breastfeed Med. 2017;7:390–5.
16. WHO/UNICEF/UNAIDS/UNFPA. HIV transmission through breastfeeding: a review of available evidence, 2007 update. Geneva, World Health Organization; 2008.
17. Hotham N, Hotham E. Drugs in breastfeeding. Aust Prescr. 2015;38:156–9.
18. Academy of Breastfeeding Medicine Protocol Committee. ABM clinical protocol #9: use of galactogogues in initiating or augmenting maternal milk production. Revised 2018. Breastfeed Med. 2018;13:307–14.
19. Centers for Disease Control and Prevention (CDC). Transmission of yellow fever vaccine virus through breast-feeding - Brazil, 2009. MMWR Morb Mortal Wkly Rep. 2010;59:130–2.
20. Traiber C, Coelho-Amaral P, Ritter VR, Winge A. Infant meningoencephalitis caused by yellow fever vaccine virus transmitted via breastmilk. J Pediatr (Rio J). 2011;87:269–72.
21. Academy of Breastfeeding Medicine Protocol Committee. ABM Clinical Protocol #4: Mastitis, Revised 2014. Breastfeed Med. 2014;9:239–43.

Chapter 55
Caring for the Normal Newborn

Milan Stanojevic

Introduction

The human birthing process is assisted in modern societies, while in the nature in mammal animals, it is mostly self-regulated, instinctive, and natural process. It is questionable when and why this happened in our species from the evolutionary point of view. The human belongs to the nature, and assisted birth seems to be contradictory procedure in terms of evolution and natural developments. This needs to be investigated and followed and many unanswered questions arise and need to be answered.

Most of the mammals give birth without any assistance from other members of the species, and caring for the offspring is a natural and instinctive activity. Self-assisted birth is usual in most of the primates as well, tending the mothers to guide the fetus in occipito-posterior position, protecting the umbilical cord from entanglement, wrapping around the neck and compression, and sucking the mucus from the nose of the newborn to enable breathing [169, 190]. In the world of some nonhuman primates, assisting of the birthing process by more experienced female animals sometimes happens to the primiparous animals who give birth in unusual occipito-anterior position [86, 169]. Evolution enabled development of the modern pelvis in *Homo sapiens* around 200.000 years ago to improve locomotion, childbirth, and thermoregulation of that species [79]. The evolution of human pelvis and birthing canal resulted in occipito-anterior birth and mandatory rotation of the head during birth in *Homo sapiens*, meaning that assistance of other individuals or midwives during birthing process is needed more often than in other species [79]. It is estimated that the process of helping during childbirth took place between 2 and 3

M. Stanojevic (✉)
Clinical Hospital Sveti Duh, Department of Obstetrics and Gynecology Medical School University of Zagreb, Neonatal Unit, Zagreb, Croatia
e-mail: milan.stanojevic@optinet.hr

© Springer Nature Switzerland AG 2022

R. A. Moreira de Sá, E. B. d. Fonseca (eds.), *Perinatology*,
https://doi.org/10.1007/978-3-030-83434-0_55

million years ago and could be considered as the origin of midwifery [97, 116]. It seems that in *Homo sapiens* assisted birth is prerequisite for survival and/or better outcome, which prompted development of special birthing centers and hospitals in which skilled healthcare providers help mothers and the newborns to survive. In developed countries some 50 years ago (in the 1970s), development of regionalized perinatal care resulted from the understanding that some births are more risky than the others needing more skilled healthcare providers and teamwork approach with better equipment. Such organizational endeavor resulted in better survival and less mortality of mothers and newborn babies in developed countries [23, 85, 249]. This kind of organization needs well-developed and wealthy healthcare system, meaning that in developing countries without such resources, it is not possible to organize regionalized perinatal healthcare [175]. Parallel with the concept of regionalization, the concept of birth medicalization developed as well, with the strong tendency of the healthcare providers to have everything under control during childbirth and to intervene as much as possible [42]. More than 90% of births, 98% of fetal deaths, and 98% of neonatal deaths occur in less developed countries [42]. It is estimated that out of 137 million births in the world in 2012, 48.5 million (35.4%) were not registered, while for 21.5 million (15.7%) births, no data were available [118]. The most disappointing characteristic of perinatal care in the world is inequity, which means that regardless of political proclamation that children and the mothers have the right to be cared for in the best possible conditions, they have not equal chance to survive in developed and in developing countries [221]. This is the reason why in this chapter caring for the normal newborn will be presented from the point of view of developed and developing countries, whenever suitable.

Intrauterine Environment and the Neonate

Intrauterine environment is optimal for growth and development of the human. Although we have learned and investigated many aspects of intrauterine life, still it is not clear why implantation rate in our species is low and that implanted blastocysts have still a 15% of the possibility to be aborted [161]. For embryos which remain implanted and whose development is undisturbed, the whole intrauterine development is the preparation for extrauterine life. Intrauterine milieu is characterized by microgravity in watery environment, the temperature of 37°C, and low oxygen (relative hypoxia) [139, 200, 211]. This is so-called gravity, age, thermoregulation, and oxygenation (GATO) hypothesis [139, 200, 211]. Namely, microgravity, early age, heat, and hypoxia exert the same effect on the fetus motor system with development of fast type muscle fibers enabling proper intrauterine motoric development, stimulating the central nervous system (particularly the brain) to develop properly [211]. Toward the end of gestation, quantity of amniotic fluid is decreasing, buoyancy is decreasing, and microgravity in utero is approaching, but never reaching 1 [139, 200, 211]. After the birth, newborn is experiencing tyranny of gravity, lower environmental temperature, and normoxia with development of slow-type muscle fibers, enabling behavior which is comparable with astronaut returning from the space [139, 200, 211]. The entire postnatal motoric development of the neonate is characterized by struggling against gravity, which will result with the disappearance of the defensive Moro reflex around 4 months of age and by verticalization and independent walking at the age of 1 year. After the birth, the neonate should adjust to the hostile environment of the outer world, and its adjustment should be thoroughly followed and assessed.

Labor and Birthing Process and the Neonate

Human term pregnancy on average lasts 280 days (40 gestational weeks – GW), but the range is from 259 (37 GW) to 294 days (42 GW). When the woman is in labor, many painful contractions are needed to deliver the baby [134, 135, 245]. The contractions are painful, and the pain is producing the stress affecting the mother and the fetus [91]. Toward the end of the labor, the level of the stress hormones (steroids, vasopressin, and catecholamines) is increasing resulting in improved ability of the fetus to pass through the transition from fetal to neonatal life, while for the mother it will shorten the recovery after delivery [91]. In the fetus these hormonal changes are programmed for full expression at term gestation and after spontaneous labor [91]. The first peak of cortisol in fetus happens at 30 to 36 weeks of gestation and then before spontaneous labor at term [151]. If the baby is delivered by Cesarean section (CS) without contractions, the level of stress hormones is lower, than if oxytocin test was performed before the CS, meaning that any uterine activity can produce the stress [228]. Fetus is actively participating in labor, resulting in many changes which are needed to prepare the fetus for extrauterine life [151, 214].

The Transition from Intrauterine to Extrauterine Life

The fetus-to-neonate transition is an overly complex process which should be thoroughly followed and monitored during birth in order to timely intervene if needed [151, 214]. The most important factors affecting the transition from fetus to neonate are maternal health condition, function of the placenta, duration of the gestation, health condition of the fetus and the delivery room care (Table 55.1) [151, 214]. Only those fetuses in whom all the before mentioned factors are uneventful will pass the transition process without need to act, but in 10% of infants, some intervention and assistance will probably be needed to facilitate the process of transition [151, 214]. Transition is a complex physiological process affecting many physiological processes of the fetus which are barely understood [151]. It was pointed out that breathing movements begin at around 10 weeks of gestation and they are important for lung development and preparation for postnatal breathing [151]. However, most of the investigators are focused on the cardiovascular and

Table 55.1 Maternal, placental, fetal/infant conditions and delivery issues affecting neonatal transition [Modified according to [214]]

Possible conditions affecting neonatal transition			
Maternal	Placental	Fetal/infant	Delivery
Hypertensive disorders (primary and secondary hypertension, preeclampsia, hemolysis, elevated liver enzymes, low platelets – HELLP) Diabetes mellitus Perinatal substance abuse Lupus Myasthenia gravis Advanced maternal age Other conditions	Abruption of the placenta Placenta previa Vasa previa	Congenital anomalies (congenital heart defects, diaphragmatic hernia, airway anomalies, pulmonary hypoplasia) Persistent pulmonary hypertension of the newborn Prematurity Sepsis/conatal pneumonia Intrauterine growth restriction/small for gestational age Large for gestational age	Maternal analgesia Meconium stained amniotic fluid Breech and other pathological fetal presentations Instrumentation (forceps, vacuum) Cesarean delivery

pulmonary changes which are particularly important to preserve the most important vital signs with resuscitation procedures if needed. It is well known that transition begins before onset of labor at the end of the third trimester of pregnancy with the increase of cortisol production which is important in preparation of many organ systems for the process of the transition [151, 214]. In the lungs cortisol together with thyroid hormones is enabling onset of the clearance of the lung fluid and production of the surfactant with the decrease of alveolar surface tension [151, 214]. Besides that, cortisol increases the number of beta-adrenergic receptors in the lungs and increases the transcription of the genes producing epithelial sodium channels [214]. Epithelial sodium channels transform the lung from a chloride-secreting organ into one that reabsorbs sodium, thereby pulling fetal lung fluid out of the alveolar air spaces and into the interstitium and intravascular spaces [214]. It is believed that before delivery almost half of the lung fluid is cleared, while after the delivery this process continues for the next 2 hours when it is completed [151]. By increased oxygen saturation after delivery, gene expression of epithelial sodium channels is increased enabling the transport of sodium and water into the lung interstitium [214]. The second important mechanism of driving alveolar fluid to the interstitium is high negative intrapulmonary pressure generated by initial infant's breaths [214]. The third less important mechanism of lung fluid clearance is thoracic squeeze while fetus is passing through the birth canal [214]. In the meantime, due to the decrease of the pulmonary vascular resistance and increase of the systemic vascular resistance, significant increase of the cardiac output by both the right and the left ventricles occurs with increasing blood flow to the lungs, heart, kidneys, and intestines [214]. At the same time, many fetal vascular shunts are closing which is resulting in the increase of the oxygen saturation from the fetal level of the 60% to well above 90% 10 minutes after delivery [151]. Gas exchange

Table 55.2 Targeted preductal oxygen saturation in the first 10 minutes after birth [246]

Time in minutes after birth	Targeted oxygen saturation [%]
2	65
3	70
4	80
5	85
10	90

is stabilized by 2 minutes in most vaginally delivered term neonates [151]. The dynamic changes of the oxygen saturation in healthy term newborn are shown in Table 55.2 [246]. Postductal saturations are on average 8% lower than preductal for the first 15 minutes of life [151]. The process of transition can be disturbed by premature clamping of the umbilical cord which will prevent the blood flow from the placenta to the infant through dilated umbilical vein in the direction of gravity, which will happen if the umbilical cord is clamped before the initial infant breaths [214].

It is very important to assess the process of postnatal transition after delivery in all newborn infants regardless of gestational age and birth weight. The best method to assess the transition was invented by Virginia Apgar almost 70 years ago [5, 12, 46, 152, 204]. Apgar scoring includes assessment of five components: color, heart rate, reflexes, muscle tone, and respiration. For each component one can be scored 0, 1, or 2, with total maximal score of 10 [5, 12, 46, 152, 204]. The score is reported at 1 minute and 5 minutes after birth for all neonates and at 5-minute intervals thereafter until 20 minutes for infants with a score less than 7 [12, 46, 152, 204]. Hemodynamic compromise during transition from intrauterine to extrauterine life such as respiratory depression or apnea, bradycardia hypoperfusion, cyanosis, and hypotonia are assessed by Apgar score [5, 12, 46, 152, 204]. Scores of 7 to 10 are considered reassuring, a score of 4 to 6 as moderately abnormal, and a score of 0 to 3 as low in the term and late-preterm infant [12, 46, 152, 204]. Apgar score should not be used or abused for the purposes for which it has not be designed, such as long-term neurodevelopmental outcome or as a sign of fetal/neonatal peripartum hypoxia causing neonatal encephalopathy [12, 46, 152, 204]. If Apgar score is 5 or less at 5 and 10 minutes after birth, the risk of cerebral palsy is increased, although most of infants with low Apgar scores will not develop cerebral palsy [12, 46, 152, 204]. Individual mortality cannot be predicted based on Apgar scores. Assessment of Apgar score is subjective with low inter-rater reproducibility because it is affected by gestational age, resuscitation, cardiorespiratory and other conditions influencing neonatal muscle tone, resuscitation, maternal medications, experience of the evaluator, and some others [12, 46, 152, 204]. Neonatal encephalopathy caused by peripartum hypoxia-ischemia is unlikely if Apgar score at 5 minutes is 7 or more [12, 46, 152, 204].

It is estimated that 85% of newborns will initiate spontaneous respirations within 15s after delivery, and additional 10% will respond to stimulation and/or suctioning [5, 12, 46, 152, 204]. Positive pressure ventilation will be needed in 3% to 5% of infants, while only 0.1% will need chest compressions and/or medications (cardiopulmonary resuscitation) [5, 46, 152]. Positive pressure ventilation in population of newborns who need it is essential for the recovery of the circulation [5, 46, 152]. Apgar score is used to record response of the newborn to the resuscitative efforts, which is shown in Table 55.3 [5, 46, 152]. Scores should be recorded in the appropriate place at specific time intervals of Table 55.3 [5, 46, 152]. The additional resuscitative measures (if appropriate) are recorded, while the score is reported by using a checkmark in the appropriate box [5]. The comment box is used to list other factors, including maternal medications and/or the response to resuscitation between the recorded times of scoring [5]. It is essential for the survival of the newborn who needs resuscitation to be born in the setting where skilled professionals could deliver it whenever appropriate. Risk-based approach for the resuscitation needs is essential in the medical setting where the baby is delivered [5]. The newborn is at high risk for resuscitation if fetal heart rate abnormalities are present, if there is prolapse of the umbilical cord, or if the baby is born prematurely [5, 46, 152]. If high risk factors are present during delivery, then there should be at least two healthcare providers who are skilled to initiate timely basic stabilization and resuscitation [5, 46, 152]. This prerequisite can be fulfilled in high and middle developed countries, while in less developed countries, even basic equipment and personnel sometimes are not available to initiate neonatal resuscitation [153].

According to the World Health Organization Millennium Development Goal (MDG) report from 2015, still 6 million children under 5 die in 2015 due to preventable causes, which is much less than in 1990 when the number of deaths was 12.7 million [221]. It has been estimated that death rate of under-5 children decreased from 90 to 43 per 1,000 between 1990 and 2015, which is more than 50% in all regions except Oceania [221]. Regardless of such improvements, it will take another 10 years to meet the global MDG target [221]. About 16,000 children under 5 continue to die every day in 2015, and most of them in the first day of life, the first week of life, and the first month of life [221]. In the period from 1990 to 2015, worldwide neonatal mortality decreased from 33 to 19 deaths per 1,000 live births, which was much slower decline than for children aged 1–59 months, which is the reason why in the after-2015 period, every region in the world will have more neonatal deaths within the total under-5 children deaths [221]. Of around 6 million under-5 children who die in 1 year, 1 million die in the first day of life, another 1 million die in the first week, and 0.8 million die after the first week of life, which is 2.8 million neonates who die in the first 4 weeks of life [221]. Most of the neonates die (35%) because of complications of preterm birth, additional 24% because of the complications during birth and delivery, and sepsis is the cause of death for 15% of neonates [221]. Many neonatal deaths are avoidable with simple and cost-effective interventions around the time of birth, which are not available in developing countries [221].

Table 55.3 Expanded Apgar score reporting form for the resuscitative efforts (if appropriate)

Apgar Score								
Sign	0	1	2	1 minute	5 minute	10 minute	15 minute	20 minute
Color	Blue or Pale	Acrocyanotic	Completely Pink					
Hear rate	Absent	<100/minute	>100/minute					
Reflex irritability	No Response	Grimace	Cry or Active Withdrawal					
Muscle tone	Limp	Some Flexion	Active Motion					
Respiration	Absent	Weak Cry: Hypoventilation	Good, Crying					
Total								

Comments:	Resuscitation					
	Minutes	1	5	10	15	20
	Oxygen					
	PPV/NCPAP[a]					
	ETT[a]					
	Chest Compressions					
	Epinephrine					

[a]*ETT* endotracheal tube, *PPV/NCPAP* positive pressure ventilation/nasal continuous positive airway pressure

Promotion of Breastfeeding and Skin-to-Skin Contact

Most of the pregnant women and their babies are healthy, and the main task of perinatal care is to maintain or even enhance this healthy state [178]. In recent research and follow-up of pregnancy and neonatal outcome, the indicators of morbidity and mortality are focused on the risk and adverse outcomes, meaning that maternity care evaluation is pathogenically oriented [178]. In the care for healthy mothers and their children, it seems very important to find the ways how to maintain health and well-being, having on mind concepts of salutogenesis and resilience [11, 49, 178]. This approach includes provision of care minimizing medicalization and iatrogenic intervention, with the promotion and enhancement of positive state of health [11, 49, 178]. Even research of maternity intrapartum care as well as clinical care is focused mostly on the indicators and managements preventing adverse health outcomes, rather than on activities preserving well-being and health (salutogenesis) [208].

Breast milk is a product of evolution which is 200 to 300 million years old, and it is a golden standard of infant feeding [125]. Global promotion of breastfeeding is one of the most important public health interventions, related to more than 130 million of neonates born in 1 year in the world [125].

Teaching skilled health attendants to implement new World Health Organization (WHO) and UNICEF Baby-Friendly Hospital Initiative (BFHI) to strengthen breastfeeding would have short- and long-term benefits on maternal and infant health and breastfeeding rates [19, 179, 239]. New criteria for BFHI are shown in Table 55.4 [239].

Table 55.4 Ten steps to successful breastfeeding (WHO and UNICEF) – new criteria from 2018 [239]

Critical management procedures
1a. Comply fully with the International Code of Marketing of Breast-milk Substitutes and relevant World Health Assembly resolutions
1b. Have a written infant feeding policy that is routinely communicated to staff and parents
1c. Establish ongoing monitoring and data management systems
2. Ensure that staff have sufficient knowledge, competence, and skills to support breastfeeding
Key clinical practices
3. Discuss the importance and management of breastfeeding with pregnant women and their families
4. Facilitate immediate and uninterrupted skin-to-skin contact, and support mothers to initiate breastfeeding as soon as possible after birth
5. Support mothers to initiate and maintain breastfeeding and manage common difficulties
6. Do not provide breastfed newborns any food or fluids other than breast milk, unless medically indicated
7. Enable mothers and their infants to remain together and to practice rooming-in 24 hours a day
8. Support mothers to recognize and respond to their infants' cues for feeding
9. Counsel mothers on the use and risks of feeding bottles, teats, and pacifiers
10. Coordinate discharge so that parents and their infants have timely access to ongoing support and care

The most important procedures supportive to breastfeeding are skin-to-skin contact (SSC) between healthy mother and healthy newborn and keeping them together from birth (so-called rooming-in) [19, 179, 239]. The evidence supports using immediate or early SSC between healthy newborn and healthy mother to promote breastfeeding, helping newborns to stay healthy [148]. It is still not known whether early SSC for healthy infants helps them to go through the transition from intrauterine to the outside world more smoothly [148]. The evidence supports that early SSC should be a normal practice for healthy newborns including those born by Cesarean and babies born prematurely at 35 weeks or more [148].

It is crucial that safe and uninterrupted SSC lasting at least 1 hour begins immediately after birth before any other procedure (like cord clamping and cutting, weighting, giving vitamin K). During this period after birth, the newborn goes through nine instinctive stages: birth cry, relaxation, awakening, activity, rest, crawling, familiarization, suckling, and sleeping (Table 55.5) [232, 233]. In a systematic review, evidence supports recommendations of SSC for all full-term healthy babies [43].

It is crucial not to interrupt the SSC because all nine stages are following one after another and any interruption means that the whole process would begin from the first stage after interruption of the whole process. The ways how to practice safe SSC are shown in Table 55.6 [232, 233].

Table 55.5 Instinctive stages of newborn during skin-to-skin contact [232, 233]

Instinctive stage	Behaviors
1. Birth cry	Intense cry just after birth, transition to breathing air
2. Relaxation stage	Infant rests. No activity of the mouth, head, arms, legs, or body
3. Awakening stage	Infant begins to show signs of activity. Small thrusts of the head: up, down, from side to side. Small movements of limbs and shoulders
4. Active stage	Infant moves the limbs and head, more determined movements. Rooting activity, "pushing" with limbs without shifting body
5. Resting stage*	Infant rests, with some activity, such as mouth activity, sucks on hand
6. Crawling	Could include crawling, leaping, sliding, bulldozing, or many other interesting names of ways to move from the position between the breasts to a position very close to the nipple
7. Familiarization	Infant has reached the areola/nipple with the mouth positioned to brush and lick the areola/nipple
8. Suckling	Infant has taken the nipple in the mouth and commences suckling
9. Sleeping	Infant closes eyes and falls asleep

©2019 The Authors. Acta Pædiatrica published by John Wiley & Sons Ltd on behalf of Foundation Acta Pædiatrica 2019 108, pp. 1192–1204
This is an open-access article under the terms of the Creative Commons Attribution-Non Commercial-No Derivs License, which permits use and distribution in any medium, provided the original work is properly cited, the use is noncommercial, and no modifications or adaptations are made

Table 55.6 Safe skin-to-skin contact in the first hour after birth [232, 233]

Procedure
1. Make sure that the mother is in a comfortable semi-reclined position with support under her arms
2. After drying the newborn infant, lift the newborn infant gently to avoid compression of the thorax when placing the baby skin-to-skin. Put the baby prone, in a lengthwise position with the head on the mother's chest above the breast
3. Cover the baby with a dry blanket/towel. Leave the face visible
4. Make sure that the nose and mouth are not enveloped by the mother's breast or body or obscured by the blanket. Initially, the baby's head should be turned to the side
5. The newborn infant must have the opportunity to use its reflexes to lift the head so the nose and mouth can be free. This is of special concern if the mother has large and/or very soft breasts
6. The nipple must be accessible to the newborn infant. For some mothers, this may require positioning a towel or pillow under or on the side of the mother's breast
7. Show the parents how to support the breast to secure free airways especially during the time the baby starts searching for the breast. Verify understanding
8. Remind the parents to focus on the newborn infant and follow the newborn infant's early behavior, making sure that the parents follow the nine stages. The other parent should be observant, not distracted by mobile phones, etc., during skin-to-skin
9. Extra attention may be required if the mother is affected by sedation after childbirth as well as during possibly postpartum suturing. The other parent should be aware of the situation and watch for the safety of the infant
10. Labor medications can affect the newborn infant and hamper reflexes. The medications may impair the newborn infant's reflexes enough to prevent the ability to lift the head to protect itself from suffocation. Babies affected by labor medications must be constantly monitored
Adapted from The Swedish-American Team for Baby Adapted Care of Health Infants in the First Hours after Birth, Widström, Svensson and Brimdyr, for Kom Ombo Hospital, Egypt, 2007 and from www.lof.se/patientsakerhet

©2019 The Authors. Acta Pædiatrica published by John Wiley & Sons Ltd on behalf of Foundation Acta Pædiatrica 2019 108, pp. 1192–1204
This is an open-access article under the terms of the Creative Commons Attribution-Non Commercial-No Derivs License, which permits use and distribution in any medium, provided the original work is properly cited, the use is noncommercial, and no modifications or adaptations are made

It is important not to separate the mother and the newborn infant after birth. In comparison to separate care, the rooming-in infants were 92% more likely to be exclusively breastfed on day 4 postpartum before hospital discharge (RR 1.92, 95% CI (1.34 to 2.76), $p = 0.00038$; 153 participants) [90].

Globally, the main efforts have been done to preserve and support breastfeeding especially in healthy term and near-term newborn infants from birth and throughout the whole infancy and thereafter for as long as mother and child want it [181, 239]. These efforts have been done to counteract marketing-driven shift to formula feeding especially in developing countries and in mothers of low socioeconomic status, who have lower rates of breastfeeding and higher rates of obesity in childhood and other health concerns connected with low breastfeeding rates [213, 247]. Therefore, in low-resource countries, social policies are needed to support the initiation and maintenance of breastfeeding, among which WHO and UNICEF BFHI plays a central role [213].

Microbiome and the Neonate

Gut microbiome plays a crucial role in health and disease of every human individual but also of the entire mankind [157]. The fetus is included to the ecological system of the Earth through the colonization from the maternal organism and by sharing symbiont genetic material from maternal blood [142, 157, 193]. According to the holobiont theory, not only eukaryotic body is reproduced but also its symbiotic microorganisms, meaning that there are three interconnected components: the mother, the fetus, and maternal microbiome [142]. Fetus is not free from the maternal symbiont associations even if assumed that intrauterine environment is sterile [142]. Maternal microbiome is actively metabolizing nutrients, while maternal blood may be modified by maternal microbiota [133, 234]. After the birth infant is moving from prenatal set of symbiont assemblies to transitioning form of microbiota, which is composed of maternal and environmental microbiota, becoming original neonatal microbiota [234]. The vertical mother-to-infant transmission of microbes plays a crucial role in normal development and maturation of immune, metabolic, and neurological system of the neonate [234]. It is speculated that besides vertical, mother-to-infant transmission of microbiome could be hematogenous and ascendant and horizontal from the surrounding environment to the infant [142, 157]. Microbes have been detected in healthy human placenta and amniotic fluid even after Cesarean section [45, 193]. Besides bacteria, microbiome consists of viruses, protozoa, and other microorganisms [142]. It is estimated that human gut is colonized with 10^{12} bacteria and their bacteriophages, with the ratio of bacteria to viruses 10:1 [142]. Postnatal colonization with microbiota is influenced by many factors like birth and feeding mode, gestational age, surrounding environment, exposure to the antibiotics, geography, and many others [157]. If the process of microbial colonization is disturbed, this may result in higher risk for some diseases like asthma, inflammatory bowel disease, obesity, type 2 diabetes, systemic connective tissue disorders, juvenile arthritis, immune deficiencies, leukemia, and many others [142, 157]. It is important for the infant and for the mother that the baby is vaginally born, exclusively breastfed, and in skin-to-skin contact with the mother to enable desirable microbiome colonization and to avoid health risks later in life [157].

Vaginally delivered infants come in the contact with vaginal and fecal microbiome of their mothers with prevailing bacteria from vaginal flora like *Lactobacillus* and *Prevotella* [142]. In contrast, CS-delivered babies are colonized with bacteria from the mother's skin and hospital environment with *Clostridium* and *Clostridium difficile* as prevailing bacteria, while *Bifidobacterium* and *Bacteroides* are less frequent in those infants [142]. Besides that, their microbial gut flora shows less complexity [142, 234]. Persistent differences between gut microflora of infants born by CS and vaginally remain till the age of 7 years [142, 234]. Natural birth has protective effect on health throughout life because in CS-born infants, the concentrations of some cytokines are reduced, while the risk of development of some immune disorders like asthma, allergy, and type 1 diabetes and obesity is increased in CS-born infants [142, 234]. CS rate increased six times in the last 30 years and is increasing up to 80% in some countries, which may have long-term health consequences for mothers and for their offspring [194].

After the first month of age, the gut microbiome consists of hundreds of different species interacting with each other and with the host [213]. Low rates of breastfeeding and radical increase in formula feeding together with evolutionary mismatch of diet low in fibers, high in fat and sugar, provided to global disturbance of the human gut microbiome in terms of its proportions and diversity [213]. It is claimed that mismatch in human gut microbiome could relate to the epidemic of noncommunicable diseases like obesity, type 2 diabetes, childhood allergies, celiac disease, and autism [213]. This is one of the reasons to preserve natural ways of the colonization of human offspring with microbiome beginning with pregnancy, birthing process, infancy, and childhood and continuing during the whole life.

Assessment of Healthy Term Newborn After Birth and Preventive Methods in the Early Neonatal Period

Assessment of Healthy Term Newborn

Assessment of the newborn begins in pregnancy and during labor by identifying the risk factors for assigning the pregnancy and the labor to the high, intermediate, or low risk, to determine the need for equipment, personnel, and other resources which may be required immediately after delivery to resuscitate the baby [23, 85, 249]. The term infants are those between 37 and 42 weeks of gestation, while within the group are infants between 37+0 and 38+6 days defined as early-term infants, while term infants are those above 39 completed weeks of gestation [249]. Most of the well late-preterm infants (34+0 to 36+6 gestational weeks) who are above 35 weeks of gestation could be included in this group for assessment, although it is expected that this group of infants will be those with higher risk and higher morbidity rate [134, 135, 245]. Who should make initial assessment of well baby? In developed countries it would be a midwife who is attending birth, sometimes residents in obstetrics and gynecology, rarely pediatricians or neonatologists, while in developing countries it would be person attending birth (midwife, birth attendant, traditional birth attendant, other people attending birth, rarely physicians) [245]. It should be pointed out that according to the data from 2014, in low-income countries 29% of births are not attended by skilled health personnel [221].

At initial assessment immediately after birth, the following questions concerning the infant should be asked [134, 135, 245]:

1. Is the infant above 35 weeks of gestation?
2. Does infant have a good muscular tone (moving extremities and other body parts vigorously)?
3. Is the infant breathing or crying (some infants born after water birth do not cry)?

After the first 60 seconds and 5 minutes, the Apgar score should be noted (look above) [5, 12, 46, 152, 204]. If the answer to all the questions is positive, then the infant should be given to the mother in SSC, as described previously, with the continuous care at well-baby nursery for low-risk neonates [5, 12, 46, 152, 204]. If the answer to any of the questions is negative, then some resuscitation measures are indicated, which is described elsewhere in the book [5, 12, 46, 152, 204]. During the SSC the baby should be monitored every 30 to 60 minutes without disturbing SSC, as described before [5, 12, 46, 152, 204].

Infants with Apgar score 7 and above after 5 minutes, whose gestation is 35 weeks and above, with good muscle tone, spontaneously breathing, and of pink tongue and mouth mucosa, can continue to be in SSC for at least 60 minutes continually without interruption [232, 233]. During SSC and during the next 4 to 6 hours, the transitional processes between intrauterine and extrauterine life are taking place with decreasing pulmonary vascular resistance, clearance of the alveolar fluid, and functional closure of the arterial duct and other fetal shunts [232, 233]. The following parameters are monitored beginning in the delivery room and continuing to the place where the mother and infant are being together [134, 135, 232, 233, 245]:

1. Body axillary temperature which should be between 36.5 and 37.5°C, while the temperature in the room should be from 23°C to 25°C. Initial hyperthermia may be due to maternal fever and high temperature in utero, while hypothermia may be a sign of inappropriate technique of SSC, and sometimes also of hypoglycemia, and some metabolic and other disorders. Hyper- and hypothermia may be signs of sepsis.
2. Respiratory rate is 40 to 60 per minute counted over a full minute. Increased or decreased respiratory rate may relate to severe disease in neonatal period, and the neonate should be carefully monitored.
3. Heart rate is 120 to 160 beats per minute, with as low as 85 per minute in some term infants while asleep.
4. Color of the tongue, lips, and central trunk should be pink, while the hand and feet may be cyanotic in the first hours after birth. Central cyanosis is always a warning sign of potentially severe condition.
5. Muscle tone – usually there is a good tone with prevailing flexors in the neonate after delivery. Some of term neonates may be exhausted after birth and may be hypotonic needing some time to recover usually during SSC. Neonatal hypoto-

nia may be secondary to maternal medications or epidural analgesia. Neonatal hypotonia in term neonates may be indicative of some underlying conditions like infection, hypoglycemia, congenital defects, neurologic conditions, and many others.

After SSC thorough evaluation of the newborn should follow with the detailed history, physical examination, and postnatal preventive and screening procedures [134, 135, 232, 233, 245]. The aim of the evaluation is to detect congenital defects, birth injuries, or other health conditions like infection or jaundice [134, 135, 232, 233, 245]. The second postnatal detailed evaluation should take place after SSC and within 24 hours after birth in the presence of parents or at least the mother [134, 135, 245]. The third evaluation of healthy newborn is performed before discharge from the maternity care unit [134, 135, 245].

The evaluation of the neonate after SSC is as detailed as possible with the aim to detect all conditions which may put the newborn under increased risk of disease [134, 135, 245]. Before the physical evaluation of the newborn, detailed family history, history of previous pregnancies and actual pregnancy, and course of delivery should be taken to detect possible risks of congenital defects and inherited conditions, infections, jaundice, and other health conditions which may be of significance during physical examination of the neonate [134, 135, 245]. The most important issues from the history before physical examination of the newborn after birth are shown in Table 55.7 [134, 135, 245].

The risk factors for perinatal infection of the newborn from the course of delivery are [134, 135, 245]:

Table 55.7 The most important issues from the history before physical examination of the newborn after birth [134, 135, 245]

Mother's and father's history	Mother's and father's family history	Review of previous pregnancies	Review of actual pregnancy and labor and delivery
Age of the parents Medical and genetic history Maternal medications Cigarette smoking, alcohol, illicit drug use Substance use disorder Epidemiologic history Social status of the family	Medical and genetic history of close family members (father, mother, siblings)	Number of pregnancies and their outcome Complications in previous pregnancies Live births and stillbirths (sex, gestation, and birth weight) Health conditions of the live-born and cause of death of stillborn babies Epidemiologic history of live-born babies (attendance of day care center for children or school)	Was it spontaneous pregnancy or after assisted reproduction? Last menstrual period Course of pregnancy with all screening tests and ultrasound exams (anomaly scan and gestational age determination in the first trimester, fetal growth) Any illness during pregnancy (pregnancy-induced hypertension, gestational diabetes, infections, etc.) Mode of delivery Course of delivery Medications during delivery Membrane rupture

- Mother's intrapartal body temperature ≥ 38.0°C
- Rupture of amniotic membranes ≥ 18 hours
- Chorioamnionitis
- Maternal Group B streptococcus colonization
- Delivery before 37 completed weeks of gestation (early-term infants are at increased risk compared to full-term infants)

After the history, postnatal gestational age assessment is sometimes performed in term newborns if there is discrepancy between the estimated date of delivery (EDD) based on the last menstrual period (LMP) and ultrasound determination of gestation if performed before 22+0 weeks of gestation, if there is obvious discrepancy between the orientational clinical assessment of the newborn and EDD based on the LMP and/or ultrasound, or if the data on the LMP and/or ultrasound are not available [134, 135, 245]. When maternal history is reliable, a simple method of pregnancy dating by counting back 3 months from the LMP and adding 7 days remains an accepted standard for calculating gestational age and EDD known as Naegele's rule [134, 135, 245]. The clinical postnatal assessment of gestational age is made based on neuromuscular signs of maturity and physical examination. Many methods of postnatal gestational age assessment are available like Farr, Dubowitz, new Ballard, and others [18, 56, 66]. Recently, new methods of estimation of gestational age from dried blood spots used for metabolic neonatal screening purposes by using metabolomics were emerging and tried to be implemented in the developed countries [237]. Another method developing in high-technology settings was estimation of gestational age via image analysis of anterior lens capsule vascularity in preterm infants [172]. The most accurate method of gestational age assessment is prenatal ultrasound performed in the first trimester or maximum till 22+0 weeks of gestation in the second trimester in developed and developing countries, while all other clinical methods are not so reliable and accurate [31, 224]. In recently published systemic review, the results revealed that compared to ultrasound, Dubowitz score accurately dated 95% of pregnancies within ± 2.6 weeks, while compared to LMP within ± 2.9 weeks. For new Ballard score, the numbers were ± 3.8 weeks for ultrasound and ± 4.2 weeks for LMP [119]. The authors concluded that new more specific and simpler methods of gestational age assessment should be developed either by finding some new signs or by applying new technology [119]. New Ballard score is shown in Fig. 55.1 [18].

Physical Examination of the Newborn

Thorough physical examination should be performed after SSC in the delivery room in front of parents or after the mother is transferred from the delivery room to the nursery in the warm and quiet place with good lightening and naked newborn baby with diaper [134, 135, 245]. Before the physical examination, the following measurements are performed: birth weight, birth length, and head circumference [134, 135, 245]. The measurements should be compared with intrauterine growth of the fetus and ultrasound estimation of fetal weight. This will give the opportunity to the

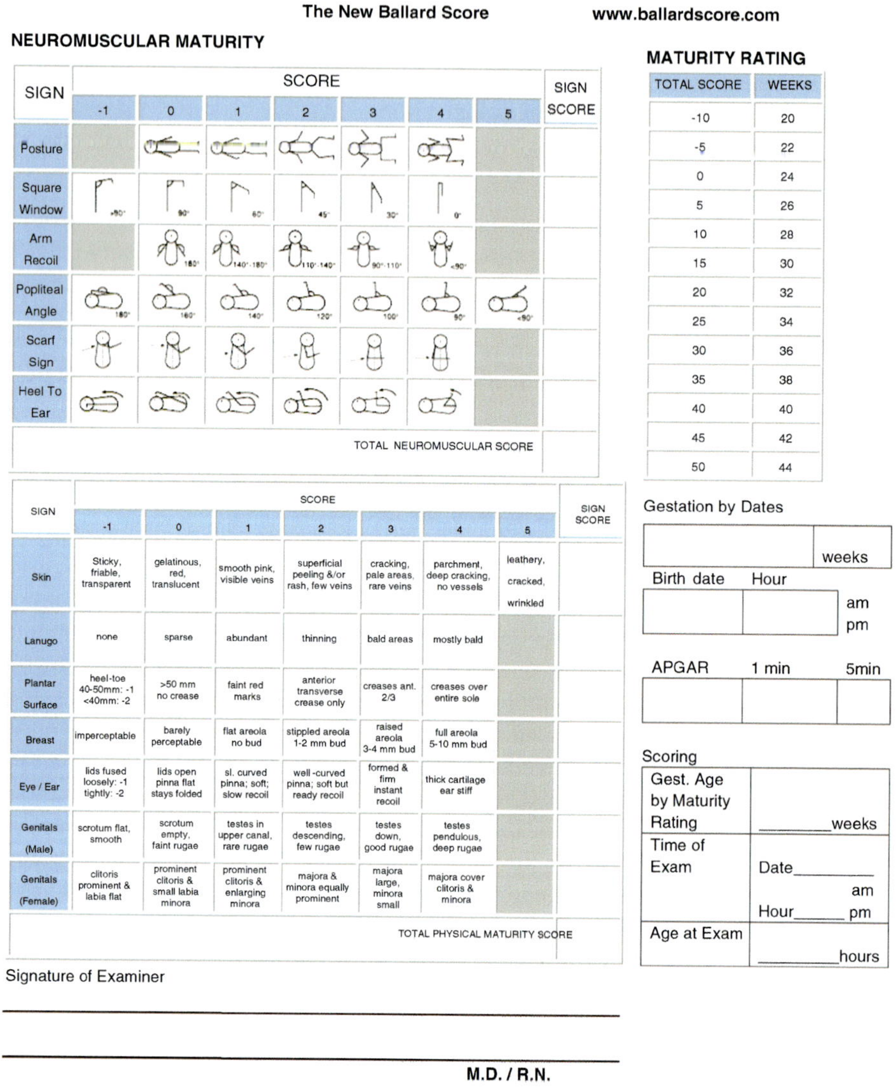

The New Ballard Score www.ballardscore.com

NEUROMUSCULAR MATURITY

SIGN	-1	0	1	2	3	4	5	SIGN SCORE
Posture								
Square Window	>90°	90°	60°	45°	30°	0°		
Arm Recoil		180°	140°-180°	110°-140°	90°-110°	<90°		
Popliteal Angle	180°	160°	140°	120°	100°	90°	<90°	
Scarf Sign								
Heel To Ear								
						TOTAL NEUROMUSCULAR SCORE		

MATURITY RATING

TOTAL SCORE	WEEKS
-10	20
-5	22
0	24
5	26
10	28
15	30
20	32
25	34
30	36
35	38
40	40
45	42
50	44

PHYSICAL MATURITY

SIGN	-1	0	1	2	3	4	5	SIGN SCORE
Skin	Sticky, friable, transparent	gelatinous, red, translucent	smooth pink, visible veins	superficial peeling &/or rash, few veins	cracking, pale areas, rare veins	parchment, deep cracking, no vessels	leathery, cracked, wrinkled	
Lanugo	none	sparse	abundant	thinning	bald areas	mostly bald		
Plantar Surface	heel-toe 40-50mm: -1 <40mm: -2	>50 mm no crease	faint red marks	anterior transverse crease only	creases ant. 2/3	creases over entire sole		
Breast	imperceptable	barely perceptable	flat areola no bud	stippled areola 1-2 mm bud	raised areola 3-4 mm bud	full areola 5-10 mm bud		
Eye / Ear	lids fused loosely: -1 tightly: -2	lids open pinna flat stays folded	sl. curved pinna; soft; slow recoil	well-curved pinna; soft but ready recoil	formed & firm instant recoil	thick cartilage ear stiff		
Genitals (Male)	scrotum flat, smooth	scrotum empty, faint rugae	testes in upper canal, rare rugae	testes descending, few rugae	testes down, good rugae	testes pendulous, deep rugae		
Genitals (Female)	clitoris prominent & labia flat	prominent clitoris & small labia minora	prominent clitoris & enlarging minora	majora & minora equally prominent	majora large, minora small	majora cover clitoris & minora		
						TOTAL PHYSICAL MATURITY SCORE		

Gestation by Dates ______ weeks

Birth date ______ Hour ______ am pm

APGAR 1 min ______ 5min ______

Scoring

Gest. Age by Maturity Rating	________weeks
Time of Exam	Date________ Hour______ am pm
Age at Exam	________hours

Signature of Examiner

____

______________________________ M.D. / R.N.

Fig. 55.1 New Ballard score for the estimation of gestational age in newborn infants postnatally [18]

examiner to estimate whether the baby is growth restricted or overweight, which are the conditions with increased short-term and long-term health risks for the baby. There are many growth charts used for the assessment of neonatal growth. Before assessment of the growth, neonatal sex should be determined, and the baby should have identification sign (usually bracelet) [134, 135, 245]. The Fenton growth charts (Figs. 55.2 and 55.3) are proposed to be used for postnatal growth assessment of newborn babies of different gestations [68], because they are connected with postnatal child growth standards of the World Health Organization, available online at https://www.who.int/childgrowth/standards/en/.

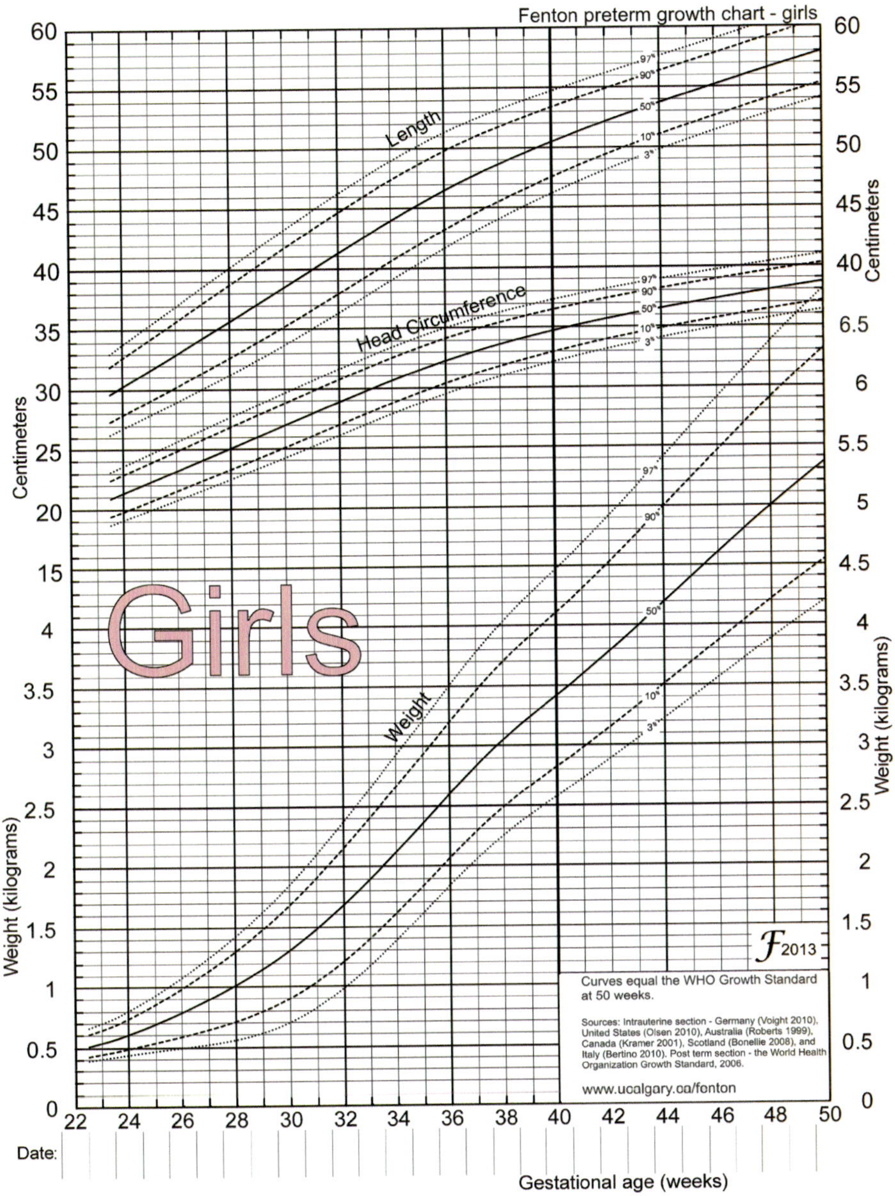

Fig. 55.2 Fenton growth chart girls [68]

Now the physical examination of the newborn can begin with the observation of previously described vital signs, followed by the general appearance of the baby, with the impression if the baby looks healthy or sick [134, 135, 245]. The general position of the body is reflecting baby's position in the uterus with flexed hips,

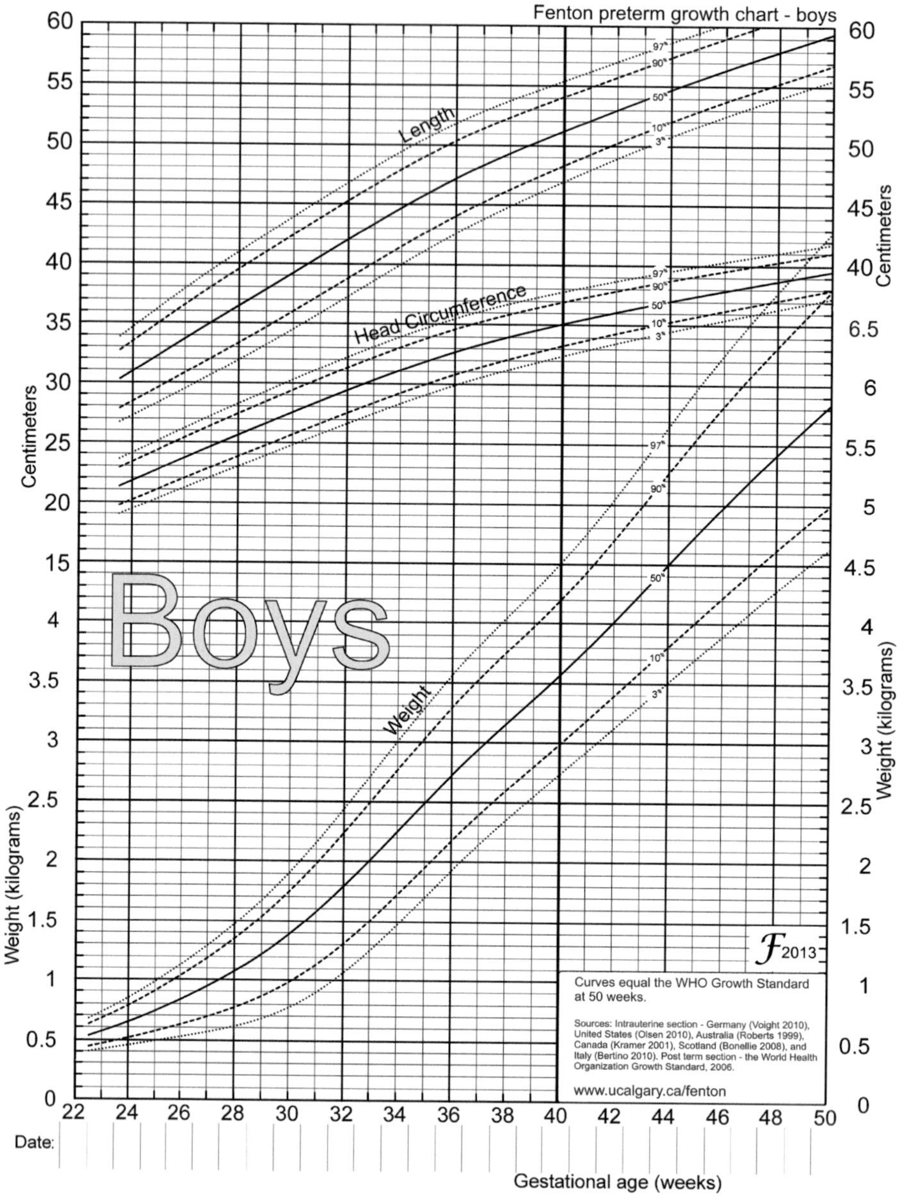

Fig. 55.3 Fenton growth charts boys [68]

knees, and ankles if the baby was in the vertex presentation and with extended legs in breech presentation (Fig. 55.4 in child with arthrogryposis multiplex congenita after breech presentation) [134, 135, 245]. It is particularly important to check if the baby is moving vigorously; and symmetrically; can some primitive reflexes be detected; does the baby vigorously cry; what is the color of the body, tongue, and

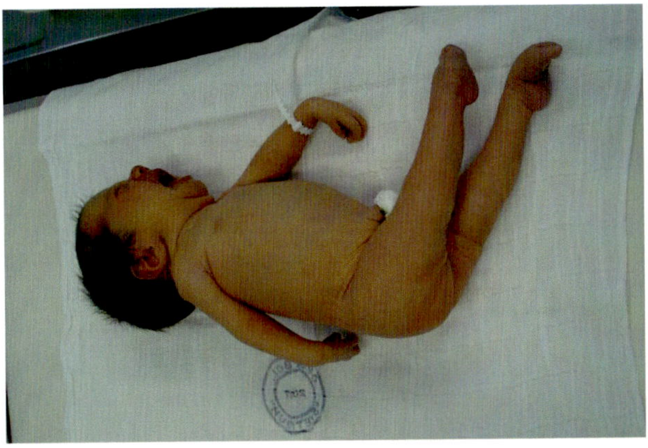

Fig. 55.4 Neonate with arthrogryposis multiplex congenital after breech presentation with extended legs and multiple contractures

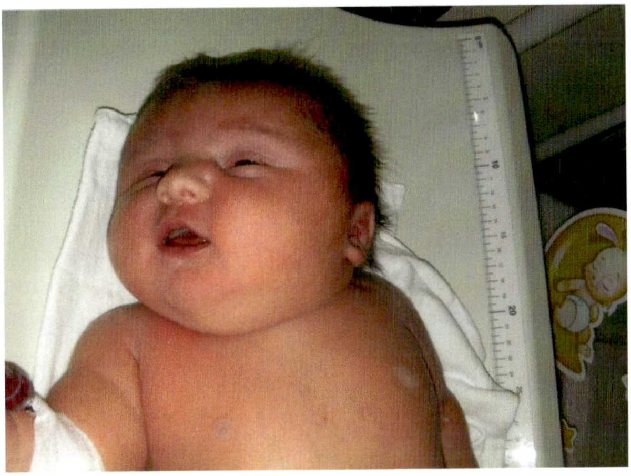

Fig. 55.5 The newborn of diabetic mother showing overdeveloped subcutaneous fat, giving the face cushingoid appearance

lips; is the respiratory effort normal or increased; and how the voice of the baby sounds [134, 135, 245]. The examination should be very systematic and thorough from the head to the toe and from the front to the back. While the baby is quiet, the heart and lungs should be auscultated, but sometimes it is not easy to calm down the baby. Usually at the end of checkup, the spine and the hips are examined because maneuvers used to check the hips are unpleasant and sometimes painful for the newborn, which is the reason why most of the newborns cry during hip assessment [39].

By observation of the baby, much can be learned, which is the opportunity to look at the naked baby in resting state without stimulation. The first impression about the appearance of the baby is the most important and should answer the question does the baby look healthy or sick? Does it look dysmorphic or normal? If it looks dysmorphic, then the first thing is to look at the parents to get the impression are there any similarities between the baby and the parents. By all occasions remember the data from the history because some of the physical signs should be interpreted in relation to the data from the history. It is important to compare the data from the growth curves with appearance of the baby: is the newborn subcutaneous fat well developed, under-, or overdeveloped? Fig. 55.5. shows the newborn of diabetic mother showing overdeveloped subcutaneous fat, giving the face cushingoid appearance. If the umbilical cord in term baby is thin with less Warthon's jelly, it could be a sign of growth restriction.

Color of the baby should be checked several times after delivery and during the SSC and at the beginning of the physical examination as well. The term well baby should be pink. Acrocyanosis (cyanotic hands, feet, peroral area) is normal in the first days of life [134, 135, 245]. Pallor in term well baby may indicate severe anemia caused by chronic blood loss prenatally or acute blood loss intrapartally [134, 135, 245]. Plethoric infant may indicate neonatal polycythemia [134, 135, 245]. The yellow color of the skin, sclera, and mucous membranes (soft palate) is best to be assessed at natural light and in the first 24 hours of life is indicative of pathologic hyperbilirubinemia [134, 135, 245]. The term neonate with early jaundice should be evaluated for the cause [134, 135, 245]. Some babies with meconium-stained amniotic fluid may look grayish, with yellow or grayish vernix caseosa [134, 135, 245].

Assessment of respiratory effort is important, and isolated paradoxical breathing movements could be a normal finding in term neonates, but if the breathing is above 60 (counted over a full 60 seconds) and if there are a nasal flaring, grunting, and significant intercostal, subcostal, supraclavicular, and suprasternal retractions, it suggests respiratory distress due to different causes from the pulmonary to cardiac or metabolic and other reasons [134, 135, 245]. Vital signs should be evaluated every 30 to 60 minutes in the first 4 to 6 hours after birth and every 8 to 12 hours subsequently till discharge [134, 135, 245].

Skin of the term newborn should be evaluated for the lesions which are mostly benign and transitory, but in rare occasions they may be suggestive of congenital skin abnormality or other underlying disease [111, 216]. The skin of the newborn is covered with vernix caseosa, cottage cheese resembling substance protecting the skin from amniotic fluid, disappearing with gestational age, and in term infants usually located in the neck skin folds, in the inguinal region (Fig. 55.6) or axillae, on the back of the knees, and in front of ankles [134, 135, 245]. Lanugo hair can be seen on the back of the baby (Fig. 55.7), also disappearing with gestational age [134, 135, 245]. Sometimes, to visualize the lanugo, it is necessary to lift the baby in front of the examiner's eyes and expose the baby's back toward the natural light.

Temporary skin lesion in the first few days to weeks of life is skin desquamation appearing on the hands, feet, and ankles, usually accompanied with post maturity [134, 135, 245]. The most often appearing benign skin lesions are pink-red vascular malformations called naevus simplex or salmon patch, angel kiss, or stork bite, located on the upper eyelids, upper lip, middle of the forehead (between the eyebrows at the base of the nose – Fig. 55.8), or the nape of the neck. The lesions are benign and most of them fade in early childhood [111, 216]. Milia are small white papules on the nose or cheeks (Fig. 55.9) with the retention of sebaceous material and keratin in the pilaceous follicles, resolving in the neonatal period [111, 216]. Miliaria look similar to the milia, but they are caused by obstruction of the eccrine

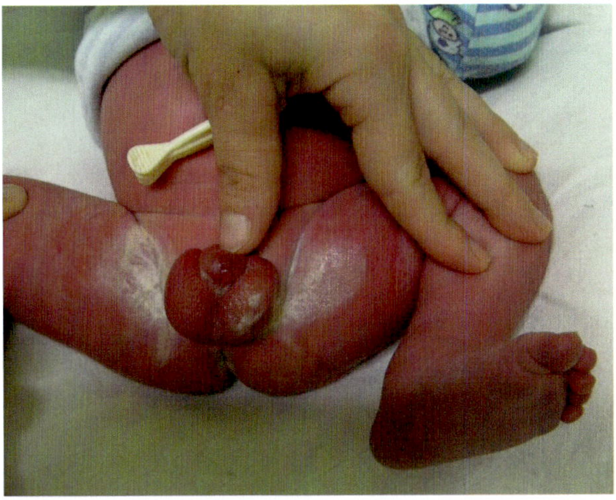

Fig. 55.6 Vernix caseosa in the inguinal region in male newborn with glandular hypospadia

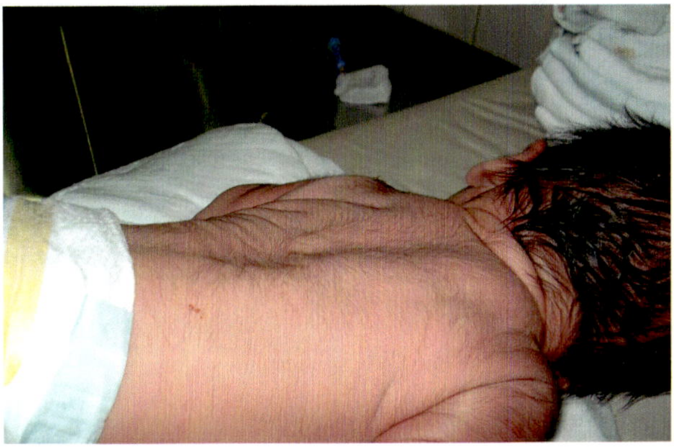

Fig. 55.7 Lanugo hair on the back of term baby

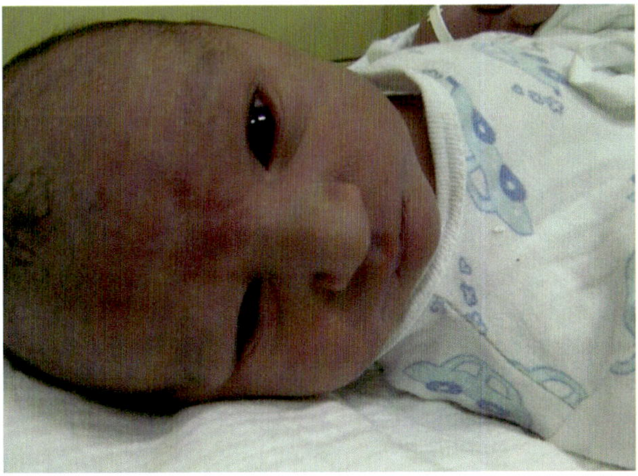

Fig. 55.8 Naevus simplex, salmon patch, angel kiss, or stork bite on neonate's forehead

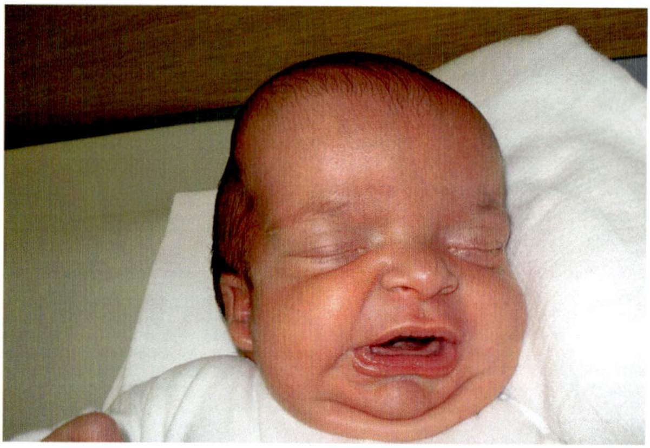

Fig. 55.9 Milia on the tip of the nose and cheeks in baby with large head

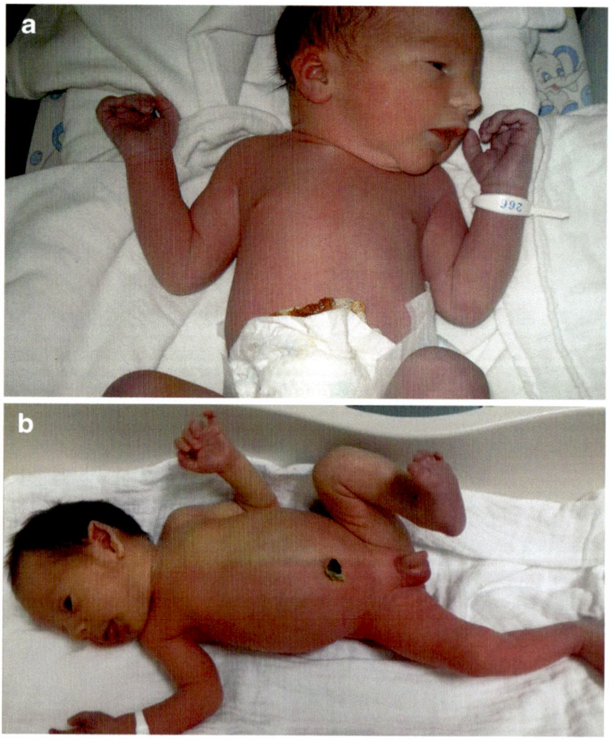

Fig. 55.10 Harlequin baby with clear demarcation line between the left and right side of the body in the middle (**a**) term and (**b**) preterm newborn baby

gland duct, appearing as vesicles located in the intertriginous areas (neck, axillae, cloth-covered truncal areas) which have a tendency to rupture with the following desquamation [111, 216]. No treatment is needed for milia and miliaria as self-limited conditions. Cutis marmorata appears like red-blue reticulated cyanosis of the extremities and trunk, as a response to temperature changes caused by immature autonomic control of the vascular plexus [111, 216]. Harlequin baby is a transient erythema on one side of the baby (most often premature), with clear demarcation line, disappearing within few minutes and sometimes repeating in the next days or weeks (Fig. 55.10a and b) [111, 216]. Infection should be excluded. Erythema toxicum appears on the second to the third day of life in 30% to 70% of term babies. Usually, it appears as small white papules 1 to 2 mm in diameter with erythematous halo located on the trunk and proximal extremities (never on soles and palms), rarely on the cheek or other parts of the face [111, 216]. They are appearing on one location of the body and fading at the other. Mongolian spots are blue gray, blue green, or brown congenital pigmented macules appearing probably due to the disturbed melanocytes migration more often in swarthy newborn babies like Roma or the babies of African or Asian origin [111, 216]. They are located most often at the sacrogluteal area but can appear anywhere on the body as benign skin lesions usually disappearing within several years after birth [111, 216]. Transient pustular melanosis is an idiopathic benign skin condition appearing most often in black newborns, located on the forehead, neck, chest, sacrum, and thighs [111, 216]. They appear as small vesicles, superficial pustules, and hyperpigmented macules, but in post-term infants, only macules without pustules or vesicles can be present [111, 216]. Vesicles and pustules disappear within the first week of life, while the macules can be present several months. No treatment is necessary, as this is a self-limited condition. Neonatal acne typically appear like comedones, inflammatory papules, and pustules most often located on the forehead, nose, and cheeks, which may be connected with the colonization of *Malassezia* spp. [111, 216]. If they fade away in neonatal period, there is no need to investigate for the cause and the treatment is also not necessary, but if persistent, then the investigation and the treatment may be needed [111, 216].

Naevus flammeus, or port wine stain, is a vascular malformation of the skin and can be isolated (Fig. 55.11a) or connected with some syndromes (Fig. 55.11b) [111, 216]. Usually, some treatment may be necessary if the location of the naevus flammeus is on the face.

Capillary hemangioma (Fig. 55.12) is a vascular anomaly appearing in 4 to 5% neonates, which may be located anywhere on the body, and they have variable size [109]. In 60% of cases, they are located on the neck and the head, 25% on the trunk, and 15% on the extremities [109]. The girls are more often affected than the boys, and premature infants more often than term, in white more common than in black infants [109]. They can be isolated or appear as a part of other underlying condition. They should be followed in the postnatal period, but in 50% of cases, complete involution appears in the first 5 years of age [109].

Skin tags can be present anywhere, but most often in front of the outer ear [2, 195]. It is important to decide whether tag or pit is an isolated finding or is it connected with other health conditions or congenital malformations (Fig. 55.13) [2, 195]. Follow-up of the infant is advisable during infancy, and sometimes surgical removal of the tag will be indicated.

Lumbosacral and/or coccygeal hairiness could be found in some neonates, together with dimples and deviated or duplicated gluteal creases, which may be insignificant findings in low-risk newborns but should be of some concern in

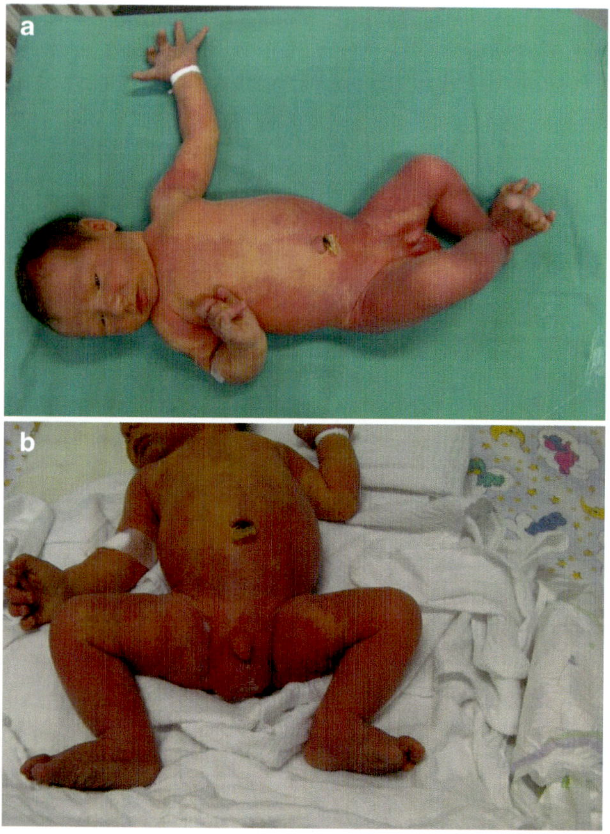

Fig. 55.11 Naevus flammeus or port-wine stain in term newborn (**a**) isolated. (**b**) with right-sided hemihypertrophy (Klippel-Trenaunay-Weber syndrome)

Fig. 55.12 Capillary hemangioma of the capillitium

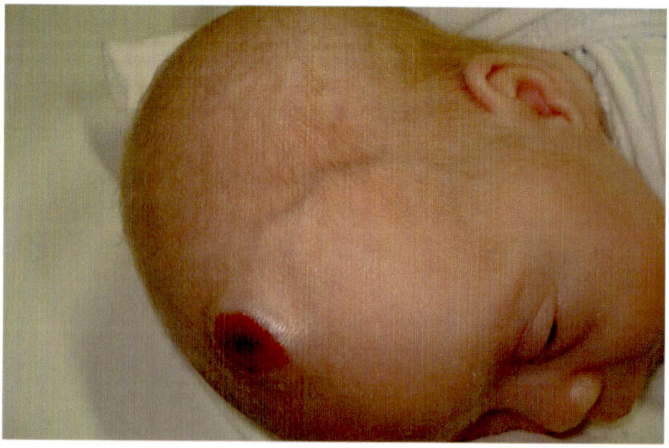

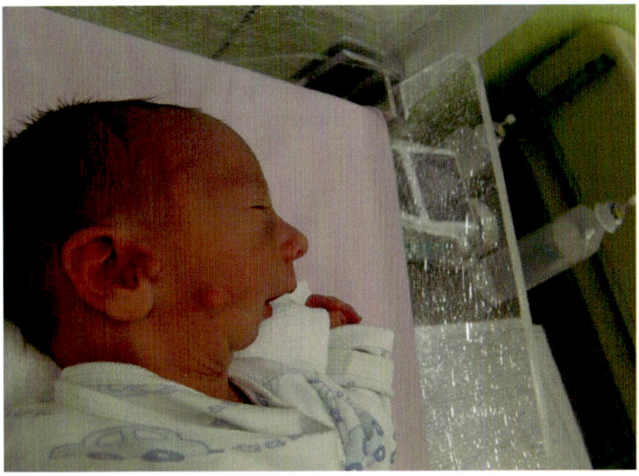

Fig. 55.13 Ear and facial tags in Goldenhar syndrome (note severe microretrognathia and dysmorphic face)

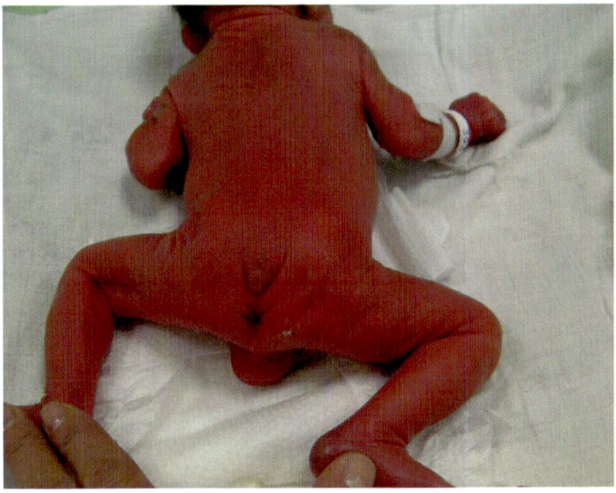

Fig. 55.14 Sacral dimple suspicious for spinal dysraphism

high-risk infants who should be further evaluated for exclusion of underlying conditions like spinal dysraphism (Fig. 55.14) [2, 14].

The head should be inspected first, with head circumference measured and plotted on the growth curve to see whether the head was growing normally. Prenatal ultrasound findings of head growth could be informative for assessing head growth postnatally. In babies born after vertex delivery, the head is shaped differently than in the babies after breech presentation: based on the shape of the head, one can assume type of the birth [41, 79, 134, 135, 245]. Molding of the fetal head is happening during labor, which is also influencing the neonatal head shape [8]. The shape and the head circumference are expectedly changing during the first week of life, with shrinkage and biparietal flattening of the skull in preterm and term infants born by caesarean section and in preterm infants born vaginally [209]. Fontanelles should be soft and flat while palpated, preferably with the infant in sitting position. All sutures (sagittal, coronal, metopic, and lambdoid) of the head should be palpated. The rhomboid anterior fontanelle of variable size is at the juncture of the metopic, sagittal, and coronal sutures [134, 135, 245]. The triangular soft and flat posterior fontanelle, usually smaller than anterior, is located at the juncture of lambdoid and the sagittal sutures [134, 135, 245]. If asymmetry of the head after labor persists for longer than several days, with persistent palpable ridge, craniosynostosis should be suspected and excluded [40, 47]. Bulging fontanelles with widely split sutures, prominent forehead, and large head may be indicative of hypertensive hydrocephaly (Fig. 55.15) [108]. Small head (microcephaly) is presented in Fig. 55.16. Craniotabes can be sometimes palpated in term infants in the parietal regions giving sensation of a ping-pong ball when depressed [134, 135, 245]. The most frequent cause is head rest on the maternal pelvic ridge during the last weeks of gestation, although it can be caused by vitamin D deficiency, syphilis, and other causes [248].

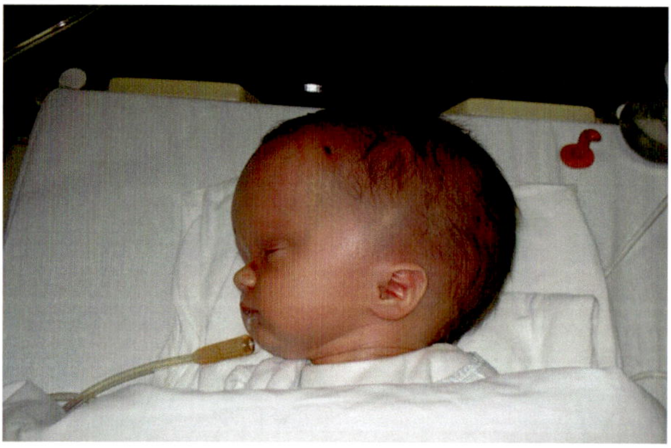

Fig. 55.15 Hydrocephalic configuration of the head (prominent forehead with large neurocranium)

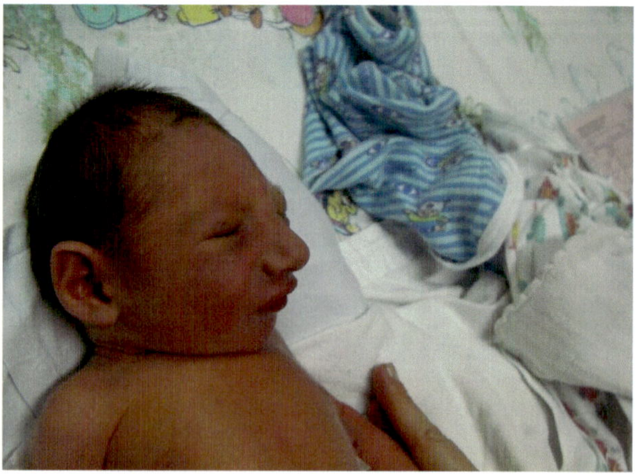

Fig. 55.16 Microcephalic configuration of the head

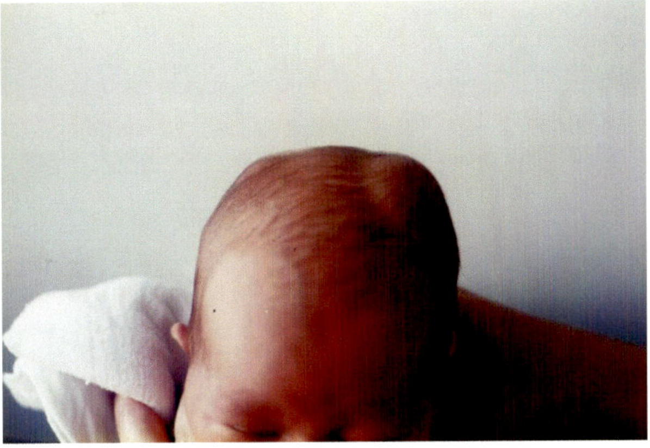

Fig. 55.17 Cephalohematoma

Birth injuries can be detected as extracranial injuries, such as caput succedaneum, cephalohematomas, and subgaleal hemorrhage [134, 135, 245]. All three birth injuries are usually benign self-limited conditions. Soft edema over the presenting part of the head crossing the sutures and resolving within few days after birth is caput succedaneum [34, 73]. Cephalohematoma is a subperiostal collection of blood, usually fluctuating, not crossing the sutures; could be bilateral, but mostly unilateral; and may increase in size after birth, resolving within few weeks or months after birth (Fig. 55.17) [188]. Cephalohematoma is present in 0.4 to 2.5% of newborns [188].

Subgaleal hemorrhage is a fluctuant collection of blood between the aponeurosis covering the scalp and periosteum extending across the sutures [120]. Usually most of the infants were born by vacuum-assisted vaginal or cesarean delivery. Accompanied intracranial lesions were subdural hemorrhage, subarachnoid hemorrhage, intraventricular hemorrhage, cerebral infarct, skull fracture, and cephalohematoma [120]. More than half of infants require blood transfusion, some have seizures, and some may die [120].

Neonatal face is examined for dysmorphic signs, birth trauma, asymmetry, and facial expression. From the face assessment of the newborn, much can be learned because the face is the mirror of the brain, while many dysmorphic signs have been described, and just by looking at the face, the diagnosis can be suspected or even made. Sometimes the blue skin color of the neonatal face after birth looks scary, with bruising (Fig. 55.18). Immediate look at the tongue and oral mucosa can be informative, because pink color indicates that the cyanosis of the face is not central. It is important to examine the face symmetry while the newborn is crying, because peripheral facial palsy can be diagnosed especially after forceps or prolonged delivery [34, 103]. While crying "dropping" mouth appearance is the most informative for facial palsy in neonate together with the loss of nasolabial fold, inability to close the eye or closing the eyelid is not that strong as on the unaffected side, and forehead scowling is asymmetrical (Fig. 55.19) [34, 103]. Most of the facial palsies recover spontaneously within a few days, while those which do not recover or are associated with other neurologic signs should always be evaluated in the neonatal

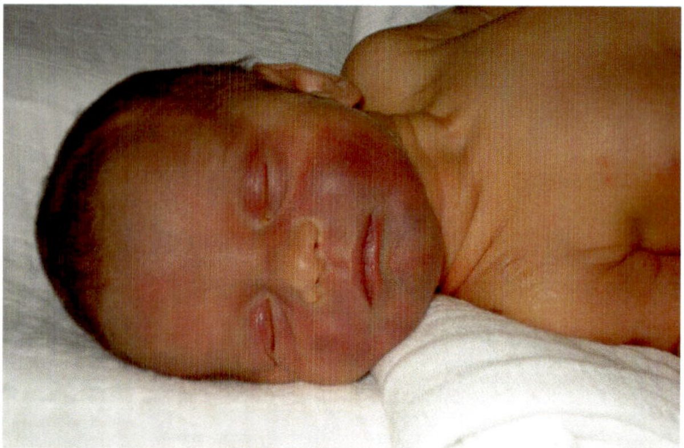

Fig. 55.18 Bruising and hematoma of the face (birth trauma)

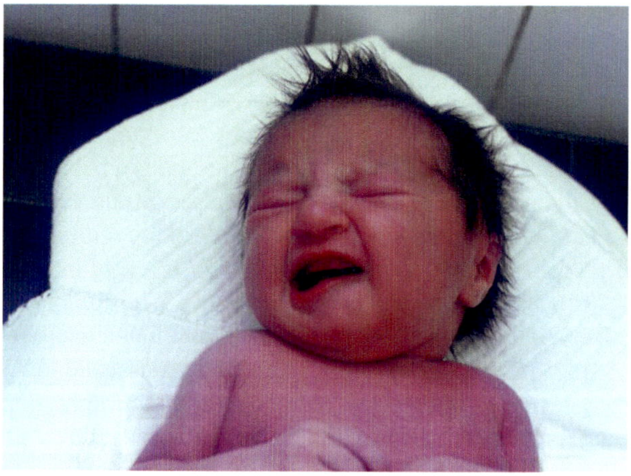

Fig. 55.19 Left-sided peripheral facial paresis

period to exclude severe conditions [96, 106, 170]. Asymmetric crying may sometimes relate to rare congenital condition absence or hypoplasia of the depressor anguli oris muscle which can be associated with other congenital malformations [113].

Eyes should be examined during the first postnatal checkup, but examination can be difficult due to eyelid swelling and very narrow eye opening particularly while the baby cries [15, 54, 122, 203]. Eye opening may be obtained if the infant is raised in sitting position during traction if the ambient light is low. The examiner should note if all anatomical parts of the eyes are present including eyebrows, eyelashes, eyelids, and lacrimal glands (Fig. 55.20 left dacryocystocele), are both eyes symmetrical, what is the width of palpebral fissures, how are they positioned, and is the space between the eyes of normal size (as one palpebral fissure), narrowed, or widened [15, 54, 122, 203]. The color of the eyes, appearance of the sclera and conjunctiva, corneal size, pupillary size and reaction to the light, transparency of both corneas, and red reflex are examined by direct ophthalmoscopy of both eyes (Fig. 55.21 dermoid of the right eyeball) [126]. Movement of both eyeballs should be examined to exclude pathology. Presence of tears should also be noted [15, 54, 122, 203]. Very often the subconjunctival hemorrhage can be observed close to the cornea as a result of birth trauma, resolving spontaneously by several days after delivery [15, 54, 122, 203].

The nose should be examined for symmetry, shape, and patency. Sometimes there is slight asymmetry of the nose because of the septum deviation caused by compression in pregnancy or during birth [189]. Nasal bridge can be concave, nares openings can be more laterally positioned, and tip of the nose may be deformed [134, 135]. Patency of the nose is decreased after birth, because of the congestion of the nasal mucosa, and some neonates may have difficulties to breath, with loud breath sounds during the first hours to days after birth. If the patency of the nose is decreased, this can be a serious problem for the newborns as they are obligatory nose breathers. If there are any doubts about the patency of the nose, it should be checked by placing a suction catheter or a feeding tube through the nose [37].

The ears are inspected for the appearance, symmetry, position, size, and patency of external ear canal opening (Fig. 55.22 malformed pinna with atretic outer opening of hearing canal) and existence of preauricular cutaneous tags and pits or branchial cleft cysts [50]. The ear position is examined by the position of the helix in relation to the horizontal line drawn from the outer canthus of the eye perpendicular to the vertical axis of the head [134, 135]. If the line is intersecting the helix, then the position of the ear is correct, while if the helix is below the line, the auricle is considered low set. The auricle is considered posteriorly rotated if its vertical axis deviates more than 10 degrees from the vertical axis of the head [134, 135]. If ears look dysmorphic, they can indicate possibility of other congenital malformations [50].

The examination of the mouth should begin with the lips, and then the symmetry, shape, and the size of the mouth should be examined [134, 135]. The philtrum, a midline groove from the tip of the lip toward the nose, should be examined and could be absent or abnormal in some conditions like fetal alcohol syndrome [72, 138]. Upper and lower jaws should be in congruent position, which will enable to close the mouth. If there is micrognathia (small jaw), the Goldenhar syndrome (Fig. 55.13), Pierre Robin sequence, or other conditions can be suspected [88]. There is a possibility of slight asymmetry of the mouth because of the birthing process, which usually does not have any repercussion on the function and resolves within the next days. If there is any swelling of the mandible, then birth trauma may be suspected, especially in infants after obstetric maneuvers or trauma [74]. The tongue, gingiva, palate, and uvula should be included in the examination of the mouth. The tongue should not deviate during examination, and the movement should not be restricted by a tongue tie or short tongue frenulum. Tongue tie is not significant if breastfeeding is successful without sore or cracked nipples if the technique of the sucking is appropriate [166].

Neonatal teeth can be found in the mouth, which should be treated with caution to avoid tracheal aspiration [30]. The palate should be without clefts, and uvula should not be bifid [78, 196]. Figure 55.23 shows bilateral cleft lip without cleft palate.

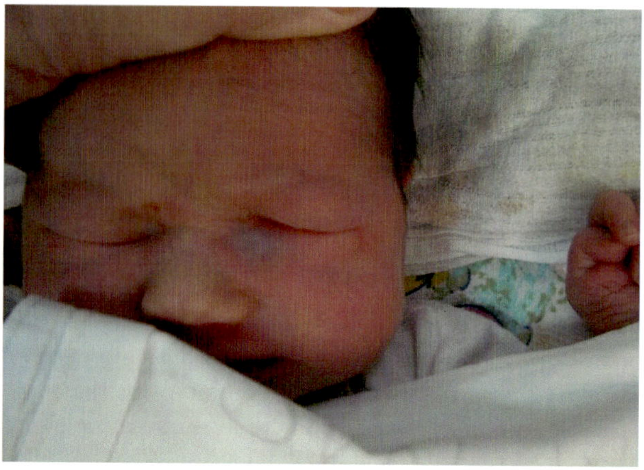

Fig. 55.20 Left dacryocystocele

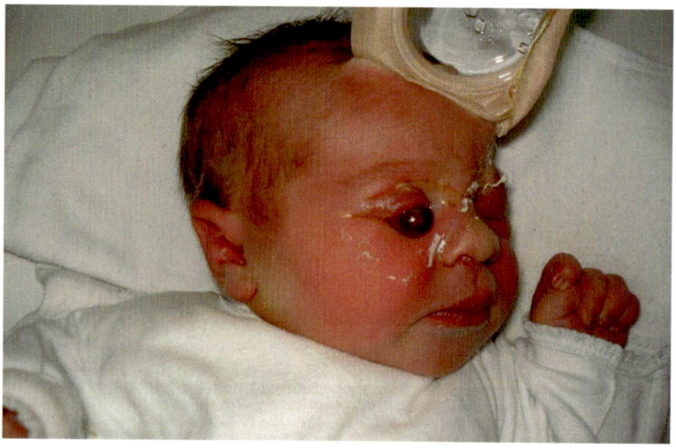

Fig. 55.21 Dermoid of the right eyeball

Sometimes small, white cysts like pearls are seen medially on the palate usually at the junction between hard and soft palate. Some parents are confusing them with thrush. They are known as Epstein's pearls [134, 135]. On the gums (usually lower), mucocele or retention cyst can be seen, while if it is located at the floor of the mouth (under the tongue), then it is called ranula [64, 223].

The neck should be examined for morphology, function, and symmetry. While undisturbed infant is laying down, the neck symmetry could be assessed by position of infant's head. Although the neck in newborns is short and not easy to observe, this simple observation during examination can be informative. One should search for the skin folds with redundant skin at the base of the neck in some chromosomopathies like Down syndrome [143]. Webbed neck is present in Turner and Noonan syndrome, but it may be present in some other rare conditions too [25, 76]. Torticollis is most often caused by intrauterine malposition of the head and neck, and this asymmetry resolves in several weeks [160]. Trauma to the sternocleidomastoid muscle can cause tumor (hematoma or swelling) within the muscle, which is mostly self-limited, but in some cases the torticollis may be caused by the malformations of the cervical spine, and the diagnostic procedure and the treatment may

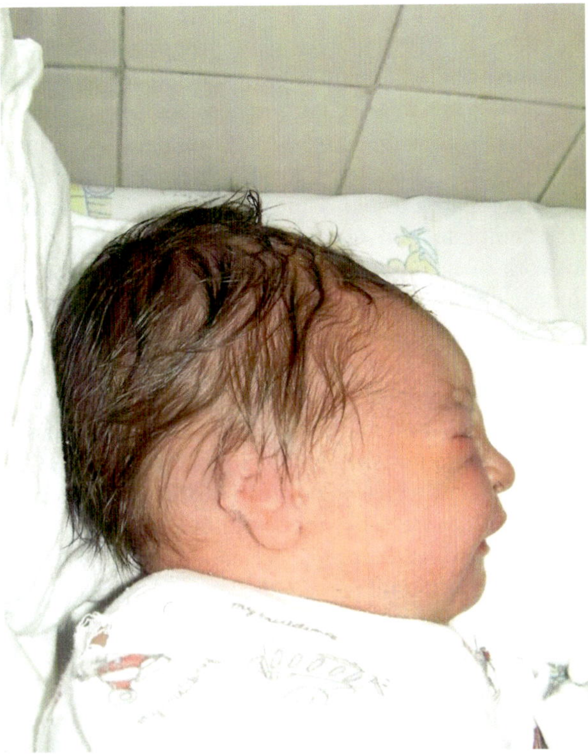

Fig. 55.22 Absent external auditory canal and malformed pinna with preauricular tag

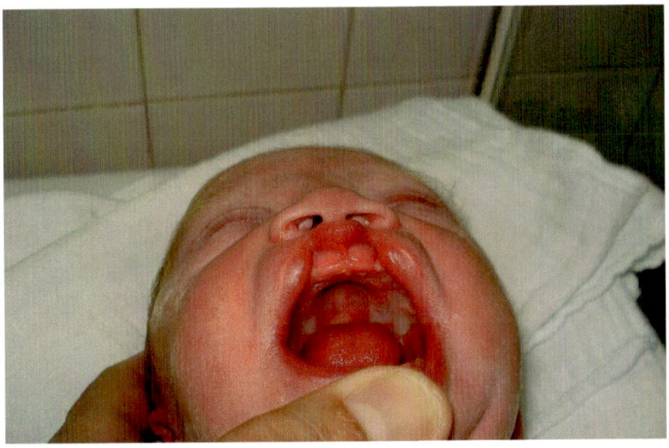

Fig. 55.23 Bilateral cleft lip without cleft palate

be necessary [134, 135]. Cystic hygroma and lymphangioma are sometimes diagnosed prenatally and if they are large should be evaluated and treated [95, 165]. Sometimes the tumors may be dermoid cysts, teratomas, and vascular lesions like hemangioma [186]. Cervical lymphadenopathy is common in healthy newborns, although they can be indicative of congenital infection [20]. They are up to 12 mm in size and resolve spontaneously in several weeks to months postnatally. Branchial cleft cysts are located laterally along the anterior margin of sternocleidomastoid muscle, while midline cysts are thyroglossal duct cysts [55, 186].

Neonatal thorax should be inspected for size, shape, symmetry, anatomy, and function. While newborn is lying on the back, frontal part of the thorax is examined, while the back will be assessed during the spine examination if the baby is well and asymptomatic. Usually, neonatal chest has a rounder circumference (barrel-like) when compared to the adult more flattened appearance [115]. Neonatal thorax is very compliant and susceptible to collapse during negative intrathoracic pressure, so work of breathing in neonates is normally increased [115]. Pectus excavatum (funnel chest) and pectus carinatum (pigeon breast) can be present in neonatal period as isolated findings or connected with the syndrome [29, 162].

By inspection clavicles and supraclavicular spaces should be checked for symmetry, breast nipples for the position and presence of accessory nipples alongside the milk line (from axillae to the pubis), and pectoral muscles should be present on both sides. Sternum and xiphoid process should be present, with sometimes protuberant xiphoid which is normal [115]. Clavicles should be palpated either one by one or both at the same time with index finger of the examiner through the whole length to confirm their presence and birth injury. If the clavicle is fractured, then by palpation one should palpate the crepitation or palpable spongy mass over the fracture [3, 38]. The palpation may be painful as well as the spontaneous movements of the arm of affected side. Sometimes the asymmetric Moro reflex can be the sign of the fractured clavicle, but also the brachial plexus Erb's palsy (Fig. 55.24) [3, 38]. Usually, the fractured clavicle is present in 0.41% of vaginal and 0.05% of cesarean deliveries [3, 38]. The risk factors for clavicle fracture are instrumental delivery (vacuum, forceps), shoulder dystocia, big baby weighing at birth above 4500 g, prolonged second stage of labor, high maternal weight and age, vaginal breech birth, and use of oxytocin [3, 38]. The clavicle fracture is usually incomplete (greenstick fracture), while complete fractures are rare [3, 38]. The clavicle fracture is usually self-limited and heals without intervention. Palpable lump over collar bone

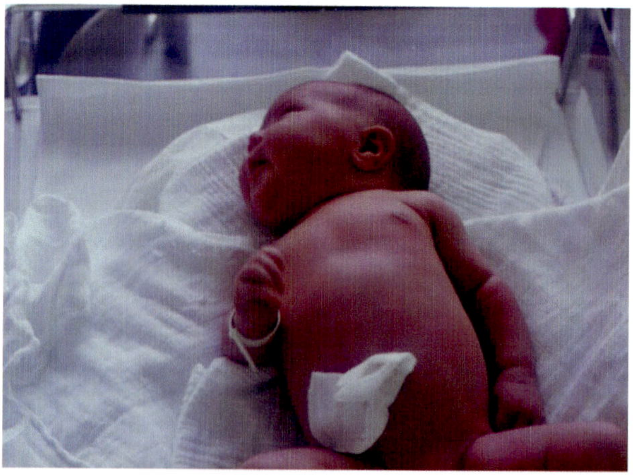

Fig. 55.24 Lift-sided Erb's brachial paresis

may be present when callus formation of the fractured clavicle occurs. Callus formation over the fracture may occur even on the third day of life. Less than half of the clavicle fractures can be detected by the first physical exam, while at discharge on the third day of life, it can increase to about 80% [3, 38].

Absent pectoralis muscle can be present in Poland syndrome and other congenital syndromes which may be present with absent or hypoplastic pectoralis muscle [16].

Breast should be palpated for the determination of the gestational age, and size and location of the nipples should be evaluated. Hypertrophy of the breasts may be present in baby boys and baby girls, with the milk production (witch milk), which should not be expressed to avoid infection [134, 135].

Lungs should be examined beginning with the inspection of breathing, as described before [62]. Respiratory rate counted through the whole minute should be performed, and the decision should be made whether the baby is stable or sick. Auscultation should be performed when the neonate is in quiet state, bat mostly this is almost impossible [62, 134]. If auscultation of the baby is performed immediately after delivery, scattered rales can be heard in the period of even few hours after delivery [62, 134]. The breath sounds are bronchovesicular and are heard equally on both sides of the chest. If the baby is grunting, sometimes it can be detected only by auscultation with the stethoscope [62, 134].

The examination of cardiovascular system can begin with the inspection for the central cyanosis and then inspection of the heart beats at the chest wall, then palpation, and the location of the heart apex, with the possibility to palpate heave, tap, or thrill, if present [132, 156, 180]. Auscultation of the heart can be more informative if the infant is quiet. Number of heart beats per second should be counted, with noting the rhythm. The first and second heart sounds should be heard, and examiner should look for the presence of murmurs [227]. The auscultation should be performed alongside the left sternal border, and at all typical places on both sides of the sternum, continuing with the auscultation between the scapulae on the back and in axillary areas [134]. Murmurs should be characterized for the intensity from I to VI, quality, appearance in relation to the cardiac cycle, location where they are best heard, and whether and where they are transmitted [140]. On the first exam and during the first days of life, innocent murmurs can be heard, mostly related to patent arterial duct. Sometimes it is not easy to determine whether the murmur is innocent or organic, and if it persists, then pediatric cardiologist consultation should be asked for [134]. In every well baby after 24 hours of age, postductal oxygen saturation will be checked as the screening for congenital heart defects, which will be later described. The femoral pulses should be checked in inguinal region for the diagnosis of patent ductus arteriosus (if increased) or coarctation of the aorta (if decreased) [134, 140]. When pulses are pathological, then brachial, radial, and pedal pulses should be palpated on the periphery [134].

The abdomen on the first examination should be also assessed in a quiet neonate. During the exmination the abdominal shape should be checked, position of umbilical cord, and relation of the abdomen and the chest. Normally, the abdomen in neonate is slightly distended, while if it is markedly protuberant, then the cause should be searched for (intestinal obstruction, organomegaly, ascites, tumor) [134]. The palpation of the abdomen is easier if legs are flexed and/or the infant sucks examiner, attending nurse, or mother finger. Most of the times, the abdomen in neonate is soft by palpation, and the liver may be palpated 1 to 3 cm under the right costal margin [134]. The spleen is usually not palpated (although the tip of the spleen can be palpated), while in some infants lower poles of kidneys may be palpated [134]. The presence of the two rectus muscles should be confirmed, with the possibility of small diastasis present along the white line. Small umbilical or paraumbilical hernia can be present in term neonates, which usually resolves spontaneously after several months [134]. If the abdomen is scaphoid, then diaphragmatic hernia may be suspected. Sometimes by suprapubic palpation, full urinary bladder can be found in term neonates.

The umbilical cord is placed in the lower third of the abdomen, and usually it is about 2 cm wide and has Warthon's jelly and three umbilical vessels which should be counted. Single umbilical artery (SUA) may be indicative of associated congenital malformations [59, 60]. If isolated in term healthy newborns, SUA is indicative of higher risks in the third stage of labor and adverse perinatal outcome [59, 60]. Thin umbilical cord is present in growth-restricted newborns. Umbilical cord clamping and care will be discussed later.

Genitalia are inspected immediately after birth to identify and confirm prenatal diagnosis of infant gender. In term female infants, the anatomy of external genitalia is inspected. The labia majora in term infants are almost closed and wrinkled resembling scrotum in male infants. Labia minora and clitoris are also visualized while labia majora are gently opened, and then external opening of the urethra and hymen can be visualized. Most of baby girls have annular hymen, while in very few hymen could be closed and bulging (imperforate hymen – Fig. 55.25), which may cause hydrometrocolpos [134]. Many baby girls have vaginal skin tags which are presenting as the protrusion of vaginal epithelium in the posterior part of vulva, because of maternal

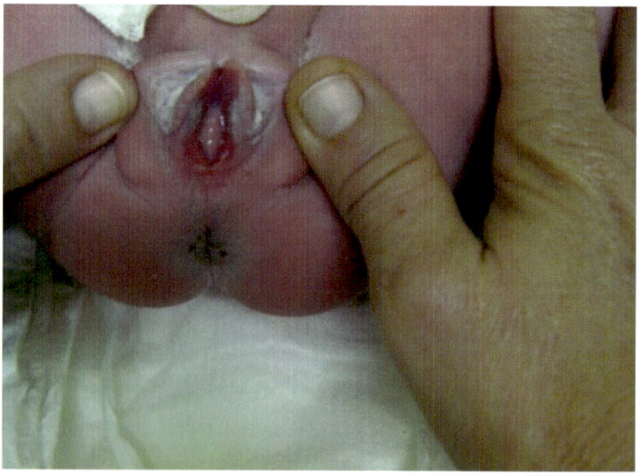

Fig. 55.25 Imperforate hymen

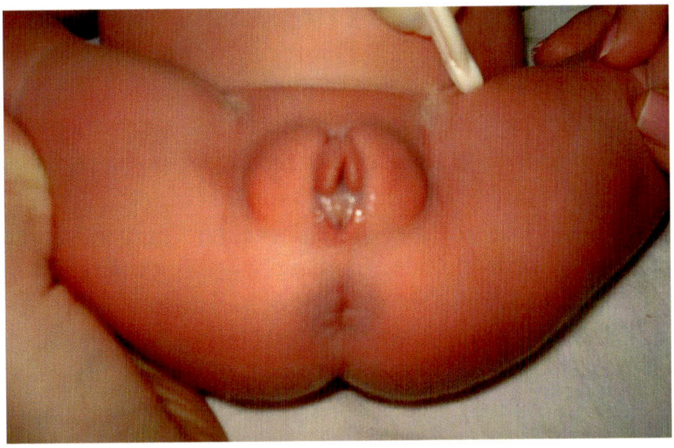

Fig. 55.26 Milky vaginal discharge

hormones [134]. Some baby girls have milky vaginal discharge (Fig. 55.26), which is normal and will fade in several days to weeks after withdrawal of maternal hormones.

Assessment of male genitalia in term newborns includes size and appearance of the penis and testes which should be descended, appearance of the scrotum, and the position and appearance of external urethral opening. The penis should be evaluated for the anatomy, with raphe penis continuing to raphe scroti, physiological phimosis, with barely seen external opening of the urethra. The length of the penis is usually 2.5 to 4.5 cm, which could be plotted on the centile curve [36, 82]. The penile length in term newborn infants is gestational age dependent [82]. The scrotum in term infants should be rugated and pigmented especially in swarthy White newborns and most of the Black infants. The testes should be descended, although in 3.5% to 5% of term infants, cryptorchidism can be present, and the testes could be palpated in the inguinal canal or absent [205]. Size of the testes could be equal, or one testis could be larger than the other mostly due to the hydrocele caused by pregnancy hormones [163]. Hydrocele does not need any treatment, and postnatal follow-up is warranted. There is a need to make a differential with inguinal hernia, which can be made by palpation and by transillumination of the scrotum or ultrasound [197]. If the testis is enlarged, sore, and sometimes of different color, the torsion or other causes of acute scrotum should be suspected, and surgical consultation is urgently needed [27]. In case of prenatal testicular torsion, the atrophy of affected testis may be present, while sometimes it can resemble cryptorchidism, but with careful palpation it can be ruled out [146]. The foreskin is tight and adherent in most of the term neonates with physiological phimosis [137]. Small sebaceous cyst at the tip of the foreskin may be present, which will fade in several days to weeks spontaneously and does not need to be treated [137]. As pointed out before, the urethral opening should be determined. The most common placement of urethral meatus is in the middle of the glans. If urethral meatus is positioned anywhere at the ventral part of the penis, scrotum, or perineum, the condition is called hypospadias (Fig. 55.6) [24]. If the urethral opening is on the dorsal part of the penis, the condition is called epispadia (Fig. 55.27), which is usually associated with the bladder exstrophy (Fig. 55.28 Exstrophy of the urinary bladder with associated anomalies: omphalocele-exstrophy-imperforate anus-spinal defects (OEIS) complex) [104].

Ambiguous genitalia (virilized female genital) and/or dark scrotum in male neonates are usually suspected of congenital adrenal hyperplasia (CAH); however many other conditions can be assumed (Fig. 55.29) [63]. In phenotypic female newborns, enlarged clitoris, fused labia, and palpable gonads in inguinal canal can be observed, while in phenotypic male usually micropenis, bifid scrotum, severe hypospadias or epispadias, and cryptorchidism could be found [51]. If CAH is suspected, urgent postnatal evaluation is justified, because of the possibility of life-threatening salt-wasting form of CAH [63].

The anus which is inspected after genital examination should be located properly and patent. Imperforate anus sometimes is not easy to recognize if very close observation with moving apart one gluteus from another and observing if there is some meconium appearing (Fig. 55.30a and b imperforate anus with rectovaginal fistula) [206]. If there is membrane at the skin level, then the diagnosis is obvious, but if a bit deeper, then the diagnosis is difficult. More than 90% of neonates pass

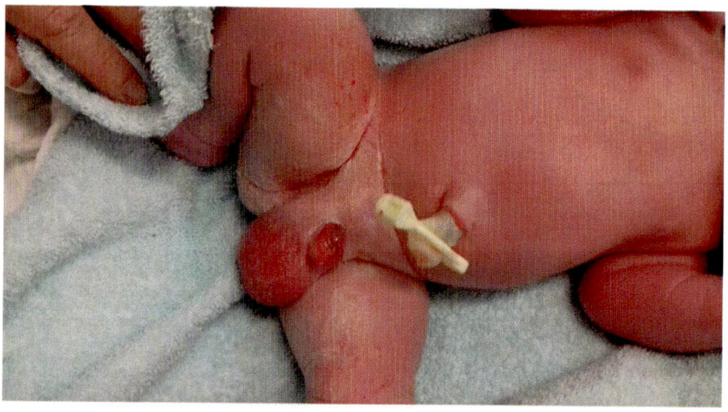

Fig. 55.27 Epispadia

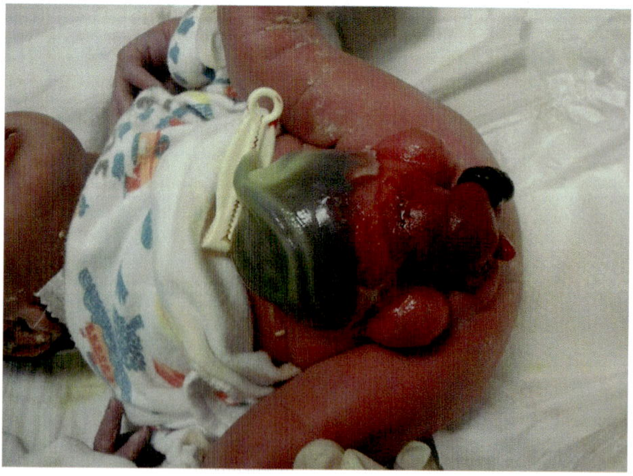

Fig. 55.28 Exstrophy of the urinary bladder with associated anomalies (omphalocele-exstrophy-imperforate anus-spinal defects (OEIS) complex)

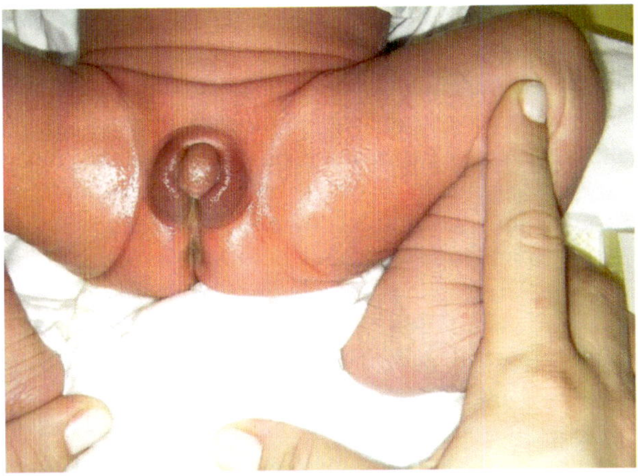

Fig. 55.29 Ambiguous genital

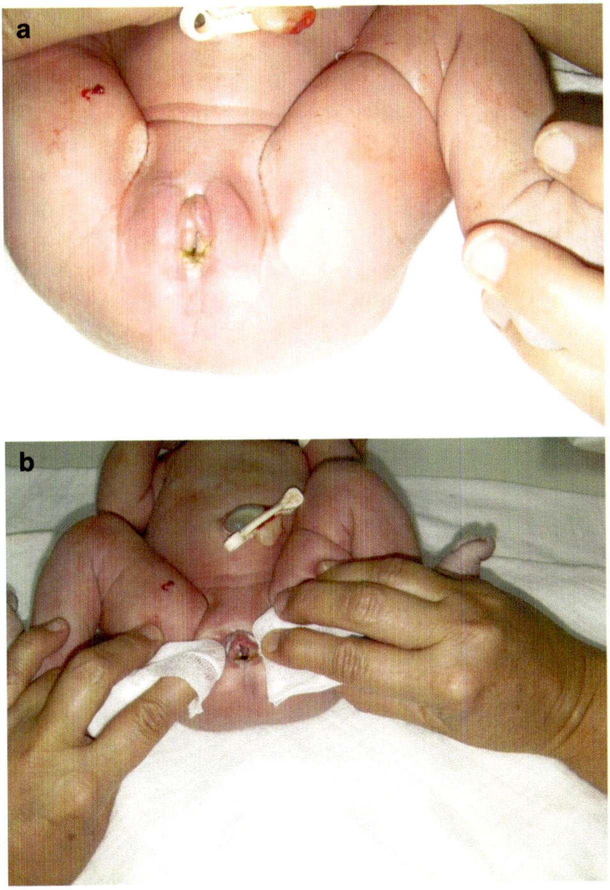

Fig. 55.30 (**a** and **b**) Imperforate anus with rectovaginal fistula

meconium within 48 hours of life [65]. If the anus is not patent, accompanied anomalies should be looked for like vertebral defects, cardiac defects, tracheoesophageal fistula, renal anomalies, and limb anomalies (VACTERL association) [206].

The trunk and spine should be inspected for any asymmetry, deviation of spine and presence of sacral dimples with or without hair [2]. The neonate should be turned face down to lie on the belly, or the examiner should hold the newborn with the newborn's face turned down. Both scapulae should be visualized, together with normal spine without gibbus deformity present and with all ribs inspected [168, 207]. Sacral simple and single dimples are usually placed in the midline above the coccyx at the tip of the gluteal cleft, with intact visible base, usually 0.5 cm or less in diameter [168, 207]. They are insignificant, and there is no need for further investigation. If they are more than 0.5 cm in diameter, placed more than 2.5 cm above the anus, and are excessively hairy, with changed color, then neural tube defects should be suspected, and ultrasound following with magnetic resonance (if indicated) should be performed [14, 112].

Extremities should be visualized for anatomy, deformity, function (motility), and symmetry. All fingers should be counted on the hand and feet, together with the visualization of their motility and position of the thumb and toe and little finger. Syndactyly should be searched for on hands (Fig. 55.31) and feet, and occasionally the family history may be helpful not to miss the condition. If syndactyly or polydactyly (Fig. 55.32) is isolated, they are not part of the syndrome, but always during the life, infant should be observed for presence of other malformations. Single or simian palmar crease may be a normal finding if unilateral but can be present bilaterally in most of the babies with Down syndrome [134]. Equal motility should be present on upper and lower extremities. Birth injuries like fractures or paresis of the nerves are among the causes. Brachial plexus palsy, depending on the level of injury, can be upper (injury of C-5 to C-7 roots) or Erb's and lower (injury of C-8 to Th-1 roots) Klumpke's palsy. Injury of C-7 to Th-1 may be connected with the Horner syndrome (ptosis and myosis on affected site) [57]. Erb's paresis is prognostically better than Klumpke's [184].

At the end, the hips should be checked for signs which can indicate the risk for developmental dysplasia of the hip (DDH) [39, 110, 173, 201]. The hip stability

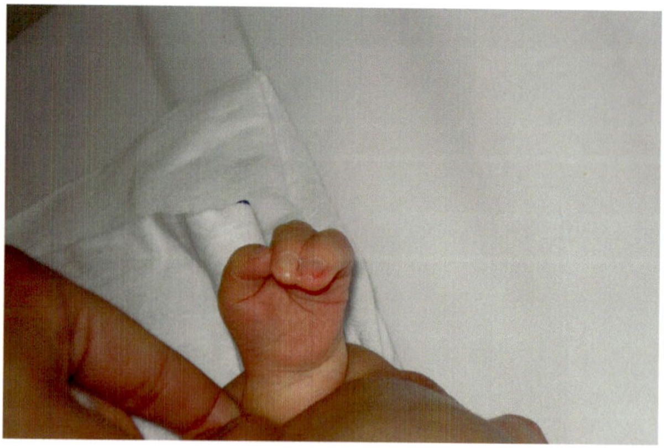

Fig. 55.31 Hand oligodactyly and syndactyly

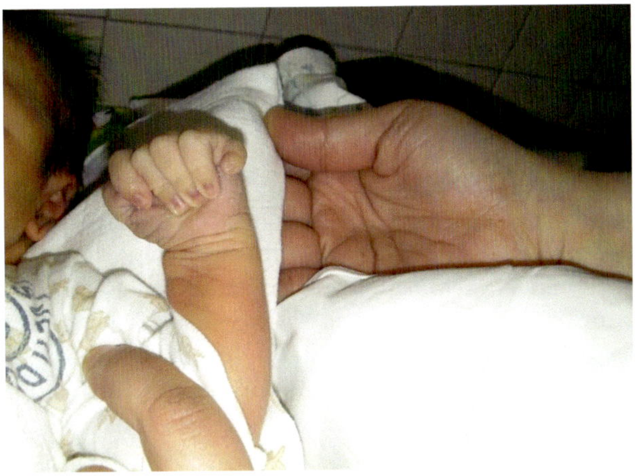

Fig. 55.32 Hand polydactyly

should be checked gently but according to the techniques described by Ortolani (in which a subluxated or dislocated femoral head is reduced into the acetabulum with gentle hip abduction by the examiner, usually negative after 3 months of age) and Barlow and/or Palmén (reduced femoral head is gently adducted until it becomes subluxated or dislocated) [39, 110, 173, 201]. Sometimes the hips are only instable without DDH [39, 110, 173, 201]. Risk factors for DDH are breech position (2% to 27% have DDH), female sex (female sex alone accounts for 75% of DDH cases), incorrect lower-extremity swaddling (maintaining the hips in an adduction and extension), and positive family history (first-line relative increases the risk by 12 times) [201]. Restricted, asymmetric hip abduction of the involved hip becomes the most important finding by the age of 3 months [201]. "Hip clicks" without the sensation of hip instability are clinically insignificant [201]. Other low sensitive signs of possible DDH may be limb length discrepancy, asymmetric thigh, or buttock (gluteal) creases [201].

Neurologic examination of the newborn includes posture, level of consciousness and alertness, spontaneous and elicited motor activity, muscle tone, muscle strength, and primitive reflexes. It is important to determine head (brain) growth, cranial nerves, and the defense against gravity. By assessment of fontanelles and sutures, many important information can be gained and some conditions excluded and some confirmed.

Clinical neurological assessment proposed by Amiel-Tison could be very useful in the early detection of newborns at risk for neurodevelopmental disabilities from the first days of life till the age of 6 years [9, 75, 202, 210, 226]. Development of the central nervous system (CNS) is a complex and long-lasting process. Therefore, the evaluation of its developmental optimality should be assessed to investigate whether the infant is neurologically normal or abnormal. Neurological assessment at term by Amiel-Tison (ATNAT) is considering neurological maturation exploring so-called lower subcortical system, developing earlier from the reticular formation, vestibular nuclei, and tectum, and upper cortical system, developing from the corticospinal pathways [9, 75, 202, 210, 226]. The role of lower system is to maintain posture against gravity, while the upper system is responsible for the control of erect posture and for the movements of the extremities [9]. Neurologic assessment of the term neonate consists of head circumference measurement, assessment of cranial sutures, visual pursuit, social interaction, sucking reflex, raise-to-sit and reverse, passive tone in the axis, passive tone in the limbs, fingers and thumbs outside the fist, and autonomic control during assessment [9]. The ATNAT has increasing accuracy in assessing CNS function in the neonate by using simple scoring system, focusing on the most meaningful items, promoting a clinical synthesis at term, for term and preterm infants [9]. It was recognized that clinico-anatomic correlations using high-resolution neuroimaging techniques could be helpful in the neurological assessment of newborns, while the neurological examination and the functional assessment of the developing CNS are bringing a new perspective of CNS status in neonatal period [9]. According to the investigation of very low birth weight infants, ATNAT at 40 weeks had a positive predictive value of 33% and negative predictive value of 88%, respectively, with similar results for neurodevelopmental assessment at the age of 3 months [171, 210].

Routine Prophylactic Procedures in the Immediate Postnatal Care

After postnatal assessment, the following procedures are performed in the early postnatal period:

- Cord clamping and cord care to prevent infection
- Prophylactic care to prevent neonatal gonococcal ophthalmia
- Prevention of vitamin K deficiency bleeding
- Vaccination in the early neonatal period
- Screening in the early neonatal period
- Monitoring for hypoglycemia and hyperbilirubinemia
- Breastfeeding follow-up

Umbilical Cord Clamping and Core Care to Prevent Infection

Umbilical Cord Clamping

After the birth, the blood from the placenta continues to flow to the newborn, especially if the infant is below the level of the placenta and if vigorously crying [52, 99, 241]. It is estimated that about 80 ml of blood is transfused from the placenta to the newborn after 1 minute and 100 ml after 3 minutes [52]. Early cord clamping is considered when the cord is clamped in the first 60 seconds after birth [52]. If the cord is clamped more than 1 minute after birth or the cord pulsation has ceased, it is considered late [52, 121, 241]. Delayed cord clamping is important for the mother and for term and preterm infants [52, 121, 241]. Late cord clamping is improving iron status in infant in the first 6 to 12 months, which is decreasing the incidence of anemia and better neurodevelopmental outcome in term infants, while blood transfusions, necrotizing enterocolitis, and intracranial hemorrhage are less frequent in premature infants [102]. Risk of postpartum hemorrhage and anemia in mother are not increased [185]. All term infants who do not need positive pressure ventilation or resuscitation after birth are the candidates for the late cord clamping; however there are studies proving that it is better to resuscitate the newborn if the cord is not clamped [10]. If the mother has HIV, late cord clamping can be practiced as well because the benefits of the late cord clamping overweight the risks of HIV vertical transmission [52, 241]. The World Health Organization recommends intrapartum HIV testing (if not done before), and all HIV-positive pregnant and breastfeeding women and their infants should receive appropriate antiretroviral (ARV) drugs to prevent mother-to-child transmission of HIV [183, 241]. If cord blood is collected for stem blood cells, late cord clamping may decrease the appropriate volume of cord blood for stem cell separation [52, 155]. In the absence of directed donation of stem cells from cord blood, the benefits to the infant of transfusion of additional blood volume at birth after late cord clamping likely exceed the benefits of banking that volume for possible future use [52, 155]. Maternal conditions in which late cord clamping should be individualized or immediate cord clamping performed are intrapartum hemorrhage, hemodynamic instability, or both and if there is abnormal placentation (placenta previa or abruption) [52]. Fetal and neonatal conditions in which late cord clamping should be individualized or immediate cord clamping performed are need for immediate resuscitation and placental circulation not intact (abruption, previa, cord avulsion, IUGR with abnormal cord Doppler evaluation) [52]. Delayed cord clamping is indicated in vaginally born term neonates and those born by cesarean section [229]. In term infants with delayed cord clamping, neonatal jaundice requiring phototherapy is slightly increased [52]. Currently, there is insufficient evidence to either support or refute umbilical cord milking in term infants [52, 99, 100].

Umbilical Cord Care

Umbilical cord care is different in developed and developing countries due to increased infection hazard in developing countries. The World Health Organization recommends for developing countries with high neonatal mortality rate [245]:

"Daily chlorhexidine (7.1% chlorhexidine digluconate aqueous solution or gel, delivering 4% chlorhexidine) application to the umbilical cord stump during the first week of life is recommended for newborns who are born at home in settings with high neonatal mortality (30 or more neonatal deaths per 1000 live births)."

Inappropriate cord care in developing countries is connected with the increased incidence of sepsis and deaths in neonatal period [148, 149]. Recommendation of WHO is not followed in developing countries, which has been shown in systematic review showing that cord-care practices vary by country and by regions or cultural groups within a country and employ a wide range of substances [44]. The desire to promote healing and hasten cord separation is the underlying beliefs related to application of substances to the umbilical cord [44]. In low-income countries, application of chlorhexidine to umbilical cord stump compared to dry cord care reduced the incidence of sepsis by 32% and neonatal mortality by 13%, as recently published in meta-analysis [71].

"Clean, dry cord care is recommended for newborns born in health facilities and at home in low neonatal mortality settings. Use of chlorhexidine in these situations may be considered only to replace application of a harmful traditional substance, such as cow dung, to the cord stump" [245].

Clean dry cord care in developed countries was associated with low incidence of omphalitis (3.8%) and umbilical granuloma (8.6%) and appropriate time of the cord separation in the first week of life (6.61 days) [123].

Prophylactic Care to Prevent Neonatal Gonococcal Ophthalmia

Historically, prevention of gonococcal ophthalmia was developed by Credé at the end of the nineteenth century, and that is why this procedure was named after him Credé prophylaxis [47, 58, 215]. Gonococcal ophthalmia neonatorum is still the cause of blindness in developed countries, which is the reason for antibiotic treatment [215, 244]. Sight-threatening disease is almost eradicated in developed countries, thanks to the eye prophylaxis in neonatal period, which is mandatory for all neonates in many countries, recommended by WHO [244]. According to the data from the USA, estimated rate of gonococcal ophthalmia was 0.4 per 100,000 live births, with the transmission rate without prophylaxis of 30% to 50%, which may cause blindness in affected neonate as quickly as in 24 hours [222].

Nowadays *Chlamydia*-caused neonatal conjunctivitis is more prevalent, and WHO by its recommendations claims that eye prophylaxis in newborns is used for the prevention of gonococcal and chlamydial infection [215, 244]. They suggest the following options for topical application to both eyes immediately after birth [244]:

- Tetracycline hydrochloride 1% eye ointment
- Erythromycin 0.5% eye ointment
- Povidone iodine 2.5% water-based solution
- Silver nitrate 1% solution
- Chloramphenicol 1% eye ointment

Other options like fusidic acid were also proposed but still not accepted for topical prophylaxis [98, 250]. According to the recent data from the systematic review, the procedure is effective, safe, harmless, and low risk for development of antibiotic resistance and chemical conjunctivitis [80].

Prevention of Vitamin K Deficiency Bleeding

Vitamin K deficiency bleeding (VKDB) can occur in neonatal period due to the insufficient transplacental passage of vitamin K from the mother to the fetus, low concentrations of vitamin K in the breast milk, and insufficient production of vitamin K by intestinal bacterial flora [32]. According to the time of occurrence, VKDB or hemorrhagic disease of newborn may occur in the first 24 hours of life (early VKDB), between 1 and 7 days of life (classic VKDB), and after the first week throughout the infancy (late VKDB) [32]. VKDB can be idiopathic (of unknown cause) and secondary, connected with underlying condition of the mother (maternal antibiotic, warfarin or antiepileptic drugs used in pregnancy, vitamin K deficiency in the mother of other causes) and the infant (late initiation of breastfeeding, infant antibiotic treatment for any cause, cholestasis, malabsorption of vitamin K, diarrhea longer than 7 days, prolonged jaundice, warfarin treatment) [136]. Healthy term newborns should receive vitamin K1 immediately after birth (within 1 hour after birth, but skin-to-skin contact should not be postponed) with the dose of 0.5 to 1.0 mg intramuscularly as a single dose, while those whose parents refuse intramuscular application should get three per oral doses of vitamin K (2.0 mg at birth, repeated at 2 to 4 and 6 to 8 weeks of age) [4, 159]. The first recommendation of vitamin K1 prophylaxis was published by the American Academy of Pediatrics in 1961 [6]. In developed countries it is well established, and recently even the most populated countries India and China adopted national policy for prevention of VKDB [187]. In some European countries, it was investigated that parenteral dose of vitamin K1 is the most efficient in the prevention of late VKDB, but still the late VKBD was not eradicated (severe forms of late VKDB as severe intracranial hemorrhage were published), which was the reason for introduction of prolonged oral prophylaxis after intramuscular prophylaxis immediately after birth [4, 105, 141]. There were two strategies: weekly doses of 1 mg of vitamin K1 or small daily doses from 25 to 150 μg from the second week to the age of 3 months in exclusively breastfed infants [105, 141]. Both strategies resulted in decreased incidence of late VKDB, although it seems like the first strategy is more efficient [105]. Parents are sometimes refusing vitamin K prophylaxis, which is the reason for increased risk of late VKDB [124, 130]. In Australian recently published study in the period from 1993 to 2017 (24 years), 58 cases of VKD bleeding were found of which 5 (9%) were early, 11 (19%) were classic, and 42 (72%) were late VKDB, of which 53 (91%) were exclusively breastfed [251]. Seven (12%) out of 58 received oral vitamin K1 prophylaxis [251]. Rates of VKDB were higher in the period from 1993 to 1994 (2.46 95% CI 1.06 to 4.85 per 100,000 live births) when oral prophylaxis was recommended, while with current recommendations overall incidence of VKDB was 0.84 (95% confidence interval (CI), 0.64 to 1.08) per 100,000 live births [251]. Incidence of the late VKDB was 0.61 (95% CI, 0.44 to 0.82) per 100,000 live births [252]. Vitamin K was not given in 33 (57%) out of 58 patients due to parental refusal, and 6 infants died due to the late VKDB of whom 3 were delivered home and parents refused vitamin K1 prophylaxis [251].

Vaccination in the Early Neonatal Period

The vaccination in neonatal period is different than in any other age group due to at least two reasons: the first is passive immunity from maternal antibodies and the second is inadequate stimulation of type 1 immunity in neonates and impaired humoral immunity resulting in poorer antibody response than later in life [150, 198]. Besides mentioned reasons related to the host, other factors include intrinsic immunoregulatory mechanisms, host genetic factors, prematurity, infant comorbidities, chronic maternal conditions, and environmental factors which are affecting response of the neonate to the vaccines [198]. Regardless of mentioned barriers, there are currently at least three vaccines which are used in neonates proved to be effective: Bacillus Calmette-Guérin (BCG), oral polio vaccine, and hepatitis B vaccine [1, 21, 198, 242, 243]. All healthy newborns should receive BCG vaccine in the first days of life, before discharge in the regions where tuberculosis is highly endemic or there is a high risk of exposure to tuberculosis [240]. In HIV-positive children, BCG vaccine should not be given because of the increased risk of severe and often fatal disseminated BCG disease [240]. In infants whose HIV status is unknown and who are born to HIV-positive mothers and who lack symptoms suggestive of HIV, BCG vaccine should be given after considering local factors [240].

Hepatitis B vaccine should be given to all term newborns with a birth weight of above 2000g as soon as possible after birth (preferably not later than 24 hours of life) [1, 242]. If infant of HBsAg-negative mother is below 2000g, then hepatitis B vaccine should be given at 1 month of age or at discharge (whichever comes first) [1]. All newborns at all birth weights of hepatitis B surface antigen (HBsAg)-positive mothers should receive within 12 hours of life hepatitis B immunoglobulin (HBIG) and hepatitis B vaccine [1, 242]. All infants above 2000g of the mothers of unknown HBsAg status should receive hepatitis B vaccine within 12 hours after birth, and HBIG should be given within 7 days if HBsAg status is positive or by 7 days of life or by hospital discharge if HBsAg remains unknown [1]. If infant is below 2000g and the HBsAg status of the mother is not known, it should receive within 12 hours of life hepatitis B vaccine and HBIG, unless maternal HBsAg status is negative by that time [1].

Oral polio vaccine (OPV) is recommended in newborns who live in all polio endemic countries and in countries at high risk for occurrence of imported polio cases with the possibility to spread [243]. The birth dose, which does not count toward the primary series, should be administered at birth or as soon as possible after birth [243]. OPV consists of three strains of polio viruses (Sabin1, Sabin 2, and Sabin 3). Data on seroconversion following this individual dose of trivalent OPV vary greatly, from 10% to 15% in India to 76% in South Africa [231]. Suboptimal responses to OPV in developing countries are determined by a complex array of factors related to vaccine, host, and environment [243]. Factors that have been shown to negatively influence the response to OPV in developing countries include high levels of maternal antibody, vaccination during the rainy season, diarrhea at the time of vaccination, household exposure to other OPV recipients, and breastfeeding [243].

Other vaccines like heptavalent conjugated pneumococcal vaccine, whole cell pertussis vaccine, and *Haemophilus influenzae* type B vaccine have also been used in neonatal period, but there is lack of consensus to begin vaccination in neonatal period due to previous mentioned factors affecting immune response of neonates [21, 198, 231].

Newborn Screening

Newborn screening **(NBS)** is an important preventive public health program developed about 60 years ago for early detection of asymptomatic newborns with rare congenital conditions, with the main aim to early intervene to prevent severe health consequences for the individual, family, and entire society [81, 219, 220]. The screening begun with Robert Guthrie from the USA who developed simple method for the detection of phenylketonuria (PKU), so even nowadays in medical slang, biochemical screening in some countries is called PKU screening. The condition is considered as rare disease in the USA if affecting 200,000 people or more, while in European Union the definition of rare disease is prevalence of the condition 1 to 2000 [191, 192]. It is estimated that there are about 6,000 to 7,000 rare diseases, and in the USA there are 25 to 30 million people living with rare diseases, while the estimation in European Union is 30 million [191, 192]. The World Health Organization in 1948 set the criteria for screening health problems, which are shown in Table 55.8 [236].

It is estimated that about 6% or eight million of annual births worldwide are affected with congenital disorders, of which top 5 contribute 25% to the global burden of these disorders, among them three which can be identified by newborn screening program. In some countries of Latin America, sub-Saharan Africa, and the Asia Pacific region, partnership among governments, nongovernmental organizations, universities, and private and civil sector organized newborn screening programs to save lives and prevent disabilities [87]. Five conditions contributing to 25% to the global burden of congenital disorders, with world number of annually affected births in brackets, are (1) congenital heart defects (1,040,835 births); (2) neural tube defects (323,904 births); (3) the hemoglobin disorders, thalassemia, and sickle cell disease (307,897 births); (4) Down syndrome (trisomy 21) (217,293 births); and (5) glucose-6-phosphate dehydrogenase (G6PD) deficiency (178,032 births) [40].

The stakeholders for newborn screening are scientists, physicians, policymakers, bioethicists, parents, and government [33]. The process of screening consists of the

Table 55.8 World Health Organization criteria for screening for health problems [236]

1. The condition should be an important health problem
2. There should be a treatment of the condition
3. Facilities for the diagnosis and treatment should be available
4. There should be a latent stage of the disease
5. There should be a suitable test or examination for the condition
6. The test should be acceptable to the population
7. The natural history of the disease should be adequately understood
8. There should be an agreed-on policy on whom to treat
9. The total cost of finding a case should be economically balanced in relation to medical expenditures as a whole
10. Case finding should be a continuous process

Copyright permission not needed: https://www.who.int/about/who-we-are/publishing-policies/copyright

following levels: sampling, transportation, laboratory screening, diagnosis, follow-up, treatment, and education [33]. Even if there is a political will to organize and finance the screening, usually there is a lack of consensus concerning the number and type of disorders to screen for [33].

The following screening programs are available in the newborn period [87]:

- Screening for metabolic and genetic disorders
- Hearing screening
- Screening for congenital heart defects
- Other screening programs

Screening for Metabolic and Genetic Disorders

There are more than 60 metabolic and genetic disorders which may belong to the following groups: amino acid disorders, organic acid disorders, hemoglobinopathies, and other metabolic and genetic disorders, which are prone to be included in the newborn screening program [33]. From dried blood Guthrie test almost 60 years ago and TSH test about 30 years ago, metabolic and genetic newborn screening evolved to tandem mass spectrometry screening and next-generation gene sequencing, mostly from the same sample as from Guthrie's times [33]. In the USA 35 conditions are in the recommended panel of screening disorders (9 organic acidemias, 5 fatty acids oxidation disorders, 6 amino acid disorders, 2 other inborn errors of metabolism, 2 endocrine disorders, 3 hemoglobinopathies, hearing loss, severe combined immunodeficiency, lysosomal storage disorders, congenital heart disease using pulse oximetry, cystic fibrosis, and spinal muscular atrophy), while some states are screening for lysosomal storage diseases, for example, Krabbe disease, Fabry disease, Gaucher disease, Niemann-Pick disease, and Hurler disease as well as adrenoleukodystrophy [33]. The use of genome sequencing for newborn screening presents an opportunity to detect and prevent or treat many more serious early-onset health conditions than is possible today [70]. It is not expected that genome sequencing due to high costs would be included for screening purposes yet [33].

Hearing Screening

Hearing impairment is an important public health issue in developed and developing countries. It is estimated that prevalence of sensorineural hearing impairment is 6 per 1,000 live births in low- and middle-income countries, while it is 2 per 1,000 live births in high-income countries, which gives annually the number of about 740,000 children with hearing impairment in the world [164]. The World Health Organization estimates that around 7.5 million of children under 5 years have disabling hearing impairment worldwide of which at least 80% live in low- and middle-income countries [164]. Without hearing screening program, the condition was diagnosed in most of the affected children after the second year of life, which was too late for any intervention to overcome severe adverse consequences on their psychomotor development [164]. Usually, children with severe hearing impairment are faced with deficits in speech and language development, psychosocial development, fine and gross motor skills, and cognition [164]. From the socioeconomic point of view, hearing impairment is not only affecting the child but also the family and entire society [164]. Benefits of early detection of hearing impairment through newborn screening program are [164]:

- Timely information about hidden and imminent disability.
- Associated conditions can be diagnosed more promptly with appropriate treatment.
- Misdiagnosis of developmental delay instead of hearing impairment is avoided.
- Timely engagement of professional support, with early intervention possible from 3 months of age.
- Enables as normal as possible development of auditory system, allowing better speech and language outcome, with the commencement of other communication options.
- Long-term benefits for the child, family, and community.

There are two main tests used for neonatal hearing screening: transient evoked optoacoustic emission (TEOAE) and auditory brainstem response (ABR) [164]. The TEOAE is a physiological test for measuring the integrity of the hearing function of the outer hair cells of the cochlea in response to audible sounds [164]. During the test clicks are presented to the ear through a small probe placed into the external auditory canal [164]. The probe consists of the transducer and receiver to elicit low-intensity sounds of OAE generated by hair cells in the cochlea. The results of the test are "pass" or "fail" [164]. It can be performed by personnel without audiological expertise and is quick and noninvasive, and infant does not need sedation, although they should not cry or produce sounds while sucking the pacifier, which may affect the results of the test [164]. Ambient noise and obstructed external ear canal by amniotic fluid or vernix caseosa can affect the result of the OAE test adversely, which means that the test should not be performed in the first day of life [164]. Any retrocochlear dysfunction of the inner hair cells and beyond like auditory neuropathy spectrum disorders will not be detected by OAE [164].

Electrophysiological response of the auditory pathway from the eighth cranial nerve through the brainstem can be measured by auditory brainstem response (ABR) [164]. The response is correlated with the degree of hearing loss and can be obtained in sedated or sleeping baby [164]. The click-evoked threshold predicts the behavioral audiometric threshold in the 1,000 to 4,000 Hz range within 10–15 dB (HL) [164]. The automated version of ABR is designed for screening purposes producing a "pass" or "fail/refer" result [164].

In order to have the impact on infant health and to fulfill screening aims, at least 95% of infants should be covered by hearing screening before discharge, with less than 4% of infants referred for diagnostic evaluation, while the mean age at which the hearing loss is confirmed should not exceed 3 months [164].

Recommended framework for early hearing detection and intervention in well-developed healthcare system in the USA is described elsewhere [94].

Postnatal Screening for Congenital Heart Defects (CHD)

The outcome of critically sick newborns is better if they can obtain ultimate care at hospital of birth without need to be transported to obtain required care, which also refers to infants with CHD [167, 199]. Therefore, prenatal diagnosis of CHD is important for the newborn, parents, and healthcare providers, because treatment plan can be made prenatally with improved short- and long-term outcome [167]. Prenatal detection rate of CHD is estimated to range from 13% to 87%, not exceeding in unselected population 45.1% (95% confidence interval 33.5%–57.0%) [17, 225]. The detection rate of univentricular defects and heterotaxy was 64% to 87%, while it was not satisfactory for conotruncal defects and total anomalous pulmonary venous return [17, 225]. This is the reason why postnatal screening for critical CHD (CCHD) is needed. The screening of CCHD is based on the preductal pulse oximetry in all infants after the first 24 hours of age [17, 225]. According to the meta-analysis, the overall sensitivity of pulse oximetry for detection of critical congenital heart defects was 76.5% (95% CI 67.7–83.5), and the specificity was 99.9% (99.7–99.9), with a false-positive rate of 0.14% (0.06–0.33) [218]. The targets of CCHD screening include seven primary targets (hypoplastic left heart syndrome, pulmonary atresia with intact septum, tetralogy of Fallot, total anomalous pulmonary venous return, transposition of the great arteries, tricuspid atresia, and truncus arteriosus) and five secondary targets (coarctation of the aorta, double outlet right ventricle, Ebstein anomaly, interrupted aortic arch, and single ventricle) [128, 218]. A screening is considered positive if [128]:

- Any oxygen saturation measure is <90% in the initial screen or in repeat screens.
- Oxygen preductal saturation is <95% (in the right hand or foot) on three measures, each separated by 1 hour.
- A >3% absolute difference exists in oxygen saturation between the right hand and foot on three measures, each separated by 1 hour.

Any screening result that is ≥95% in the right hand or foot with a ≤3% absolute difference in oxygen saturation between the right hand and foot is considered a negative screen, and screening would end [128]. Pulse oximetry screening is cost-effective in high-income countries [154]. The problem with pulse oximetry screening is that noncardiac causes (pulmonary causes or sepsis) can be connected with false-positive screening which might be missed without screening [83, 217]. The sensitivity and specificity of pulse oximetry screening for noncardiac diseases were 42% and 99.9%, respectively [92]. According to the current meta-analysis, pulse oximetry is a highly specific and moderately sensitive test for detection of CCHD with very low false-positive rates [182]. Current evidence supports the introduction of routine screening for CCHD in asymptomatic newborns before discharge from the well-baby nursery or better after the age of at least 24 hours [182].

Other Screening Programs

Among other screening programs in neonatal period, ultrasound screening for the developmental dysplasia of the hip was mentioned before as controversial issue due to low sensitivity and low positive predictive value [173]. According to some data, there is a significant risk of overdiagnosis and overtreatment, and main claim was that ultrasound screening is expensive and did not affect the incidence of the late-diagnosed DDH, which is the reason that there is no international consensus on DDH screening [173]. Regardless of these claims which come mainly from the USA and Canada, in some European countries, ultrasound screening for DDH is well recognized [110]. In the recently published study from Sweden, it was concluded that the incidence of late-diagnosed hip dislocation in Swedish-born children appears to have decreased substantially since the screening program was initiated, and they advised to institute the ultrasound screening of DDH in upper-middle- and lower-middle-income countries [230].

Newborn infants should be examined using inspection and red reflex testing to detect structural ocular abnormalities, such as cataract, corneal opacity, and ptosis [7, 54]. The red reflex test uses transmission of light from an ophthalmoscope through transparent parts of the eye: the tear film, cornea, aqueous humor, crystalline lens, and vitreous humor [7]. Abnormality of the red reflex is detected in the presence of any factor that blocks this optical pathway [7]. An abnormal red reflex can result from mucus or other foreign bodies in the tear film, corneal opacities, aqueous opacities, iris abnormalities affecting the pupillary aperture (pupil), cataracts, vitreous opacities, and retinal abnormalities including tumors or chorioretinal colobomata, high refractive errors, and strabismus [7]. Children from different racial or ethnic groups may have significant variation in the red reflex related to different levels of pigmentation of the ocular fundus [7].

Neonatal Screening in Developing Countries

According to the criteria issued by the WHO, screening should not be expensive, but in the last 60 years of its development, screening is using more sophisticated and technologically advanced methods, making screening more expensive than at the beginning of its development [81, 236]. Low-income and middle-income countries with underdeveloped healthcare system cannot fulfill all requirements for the screening like the diagnosis, treatment, and long-term follow-up after the screening. Besides that, the diseases which are screened for are not healthcare priorities in low-income countries, because in those countries many preventable conditions with high prevalence rate like infections and maternal and infant deaths should be solved first [145]. Underdeveloped screening programs in low-income countries are also reflecting inequality and injustice between poor and wealthy countries.

Congenital hypothyroidism is the most cost-effective screened condition in most countries. In sub-Saharan Africa, India, and some parts of Asia, screening for hemoglobinopathies and glucose-6-dehydrogenase deficiency are also important [219]. Expanded screening for metabolic conditions is most needed in areas of high consanguinity [219]. Screening for hearing disorders and critical congenital heart defects is increasing globally [219]. The largest birth cohorts are India and China, but only China has successful newborn screening (NBS) [219]. Reports from completed government research projects in India support initiation of NBS [26, 127, 219].

Breastfeeding Assessment and Follow-Up

Women in labor and their families should be treated with dignity, respecting their human rights. Implementing Mother Friendly Hospital Initiative either 10 steps launched by International Federation of Gynecology and Obstetrics (FIGO) and partners or 12 steps introduced by International Childbirth Initiative is helpful in finding the ways how to implement safe and respectful care in birthing facilities [89, 114, 211, 212]. Both initiatives are in close relation with Baby-Friendly Hospital Initiative (BFHI) launched by WHO and UNICEF, which are protecting, preserving, and promoting breastfeeding [89, 114, 211, 239]. Implementation of BFHI is a prerequisite to implement Mother friendly initiative [77]. Promotion and protection of breastfeeding begins with the support to the mother, using her intrinsic capacity to preserve breastfeeding, but also by ongoing support which should continue at home after discharge from maternity center, through breastfeeding support groups [176, 177]. Prenatal classes and other steps of BFHI, which has been recently revised, have positive impact on breastfeeding initiation and dealing with complications connected with the initiation of breastfeeding [13, 101, 131].

It is expected that newborn will latch on within the first hour after birth, and after that the breastfeeding should be as frequent as the baby is demanding it, or in other words neonatal feeding cues should be recognized and followed by the mother [61]. The term newborn baby is tired after birth, and after skin-to-skin contact which is calming him/her down, newborn fell asleep and continues to do so for the next several hours, giving very mild signs of hunger, which firstborn mothers usually do not recognize [61]. It is particularly important to teach the mothers when to put newborn on the breast and to increase their self-confidence that they are competent mothers who are capable of taking care for their infants [61]. All mothers should be encouraged to breastfeed their babies with strong support by healthcare providers [61]. The risks of formula feeding should be presented to all mothers as well as the benefits of breastfeeding [13, 101]. Only those infants whose mothers do not want to breastfeed or for whom breastfeeding is contraindicated should get breastfeeding supplements. All breastfeeds as well as supplement feeds should be noted. Breastfeeding could be followed by the mother who should be instructed how to record breastfeeding or alternative feeding methods duration and frequency. The mothers are usually concerned about the weight gain of the baby. They should be informed that the baby should lose weight during the first few days after birth, and nomograms published for the follow-up of the weight loss in the first days of life are available and helpful particularly for early identification of neonates on a trajectory for greater weight loss and related morbidities [69]. The nadir of lost birth weight occurs on days 2 to 4, and on day 3 mean weight loss was 7% to 8% sometimes even more than 10% in exclusively breastfed infants [53]. With increasing weight loss, rates of exclusive breastfeeding are decreasing [53]. Most of the newborns regain their birth weight by the age 10 to 14 days [53].

Assessment of Hyperbilirubinemia in Low-Risk Term Newborns

Hyperbilirubinemia in neonatal period has passed the way from unrecognized problem to overestimated condition with many controversies producing anxiety in parents and healthcare providers. Why has Mother Nature endowed human neonates with jaundice? From the evolutionary point of view, this was a purposeful phenomenon protecting a neonate from hyperoxia by increasing its antioxidant capacity by higher than later in life bilirubin production and at the same time to get rid of the high amounts of unnecessary red blood cells [28]. Everyone is afraid of severe hyperbilirubinemia in term and late-preterm infants because it can increase the risk for development of bilirubin-induced neurologic dysfunction previously known as kernicterus [28]. Incidence of hyperbilirubinemia at the age of >72 hours in term and late-preterm infants is as follows [93, 129]:

- 290 μmol/L 1 in 10 infants
- 342 μmol/L 1 in 70 infants
- 428 μmol/L 1 in 700 infants
- 513 μmol/L 1 in 10,000 infants

Visual assessment of jaundice should be done whenever vital signs of newborn are assessed, but no less than every 6 to 12 hours [158]. The most appropriate is daylight for the assessment of jaundice, which is done on the forehead, the mid-sternum, or the knee/ankle after the digital pressure of the skin and subcutaneous tissue [107, 129]. Jaundice is seen first on the head, spreading to the trunk and at the end to hands and feet, but also sclera, gums, and palate should be checked [107, 129]. The jaundice is more intensive if the skin color is orange. It is useful to use Kramer scheme for clinical assessment of jaundice, which however is not very sensitive and reliable [107, 129]. The baby should be naked and examined in the bright natural light [158, 238]. One should not rely on the visual inspection without checking total serum bilirubin if needed [158]. In well babies who are not jaundiced, routine bilirubin checking should not be performed [158]. All the newborn babies should be checked all the times by parents or healthcare providers, particularly within 72 hours of life [158]. The babies with risk factors, and in particular if the baby is less than 38 weeks of gestation and has a previous sibling with the significant neonatal hyperbilirubinemia requiring phototherapy, if the mother expressed desire to exclusively breastfeed, and if the baby is jaundiced in the first 24 hours, might need serum bilirubin checked [158, 238].

When measuring bilirubin level using a transcutaneous bilirubinometer, the baby's gestational age should be 35 weeks or more, while chronological age should be 24 hours and more [158]. In case that transcutaneous bilirubinometer is not available, serum bilirubin should be checked. If transcutaneous bilirubin is above 250 μmol/L, serum bilirubin should be asked for [158]. Serum bilirubin should be measured if the jaundiced baby is less than 24 hours old, if it is below 35 weeks of gestation, or for babies with bilirubin levels at or above the relevant treatment threshold for their postnatal age and for all subsequent measurements [158].

Transcutaneous or serum bilirubin levels should be checked in all babies of 38 weeks of gestation and above [158]. Total bilirubin level together with risk factors should be plotted on the treatment threshold curve which might be found at https://www.nice.org.uk/guidance/cg98/resources/treatment-threshold-graphs-excel-544300525 , and those who need should be treated accordingly [158]. Preferable treatment is phototherapy, while exchange transfusion is rarely needed [84].

The parents of children who are checked and/or treated for hyperbilirubinemia should get the information about hyperbilirubinemia, possibilities of treatment, and anticipated duration of treatment, reassuring them that breastfeeding and diaper changing can usually continue, together with holding and cuddling the baby [158]. Lactation and breastfeeding support to the mothers of jaundiced babies may be needed, because hyperbilirubinemia may cause sleepiness and less frequent and inadequate breastfeeding.

Safety Issues in Term Neonate

As it was stressed before, SSC and rooming-in are two out of ten very important steps in the WHO and UNICEF "Baby-Friendly Hospital Initiative" improving patient safety and postnatal outcomes by improving infant postnatal transition to extrauterine life, decreasing the risk of infection and sepsis, decreasing stress responses by the mother and her neonate, and improving postnatal sleep patterns in the mother [67, 239]. Keeping mothers and newborns together in a hospital setting which is defined as rooming-in is connected with better overall and exclusive breastfeeding rates, but this kind of care is consistent with the family-centered care as well. Both SSC and rooming-in are facing patients and healthcare providers with some safety concerns. SSC in the immediate postnatal period may be connected with sudden unexpected postnatal collapse (SUPC), which includes any condition resulting in temporary or permanent cessation of breathing or cardiorespiratory failure, which may occur if neonate is not appropriately monitored. In a retrospective study from Japan, it was concluded that unsupervised breastfeeding during early SSC resulting in SUPC was found in 10 out of 45 children diagnosed with severe cerebral palsy from the population of 1,182 patients [144]. Some neonates who experienced the SUPC may end up with death or severe disability. In the recent study from the USA on sudden unexpected infant death syndrome (SUID), two categories were found: sudden unexpected early neonatal deaths (SUENDs; days 0–6) and postperinatal SUIDs (days 7–364) which should be separated to study epidemiology and causes of these two entities [117]. Epidemiological study revealed that after introducing a safe infant sleeping recommendation in the USA, SUID in the early neonatal period (0 to 6 days of life) due to unsafe sleep position increased, while it decreased in postneonatal period (7 to 364 days of life) [22, 147]. Rooming-in was connected with the increased prevalence of unexpected falls and suffocation of the newborns while co-sleeping with the mother who unintentionally fell asleep [67]. The rate of unintentional falls of term neonates increased after the introduction of rooming-in to 3.94 per 10,000 births, while it was 1.6 per 100,000 births in the period before the introduction of rooming-in [67]. All these facts were the reason to propose the procedures to increase patient safety and decrease the risk of severe disability or dying [67, 174]. These recommendations are more oriented toward the developed countries, although patient safety issues are being recognized as important in developing countries as well [35]. To improve the safety of two important steps of the BFHI which are SSC and rooming-in, the following is proposed by AAP [67, 174]:

- Standardized procedures should be developed for SSC with attention to continuous monitoring and assessment, with good results accomplished in one study [175].

- Standardized observation procedures of postnatal transition of the newborn and the mother, with direct observation of the first breastfeeding session during SSC.
- All observations of the mother and the baby should be documented, especially the changes in their conditions.
- Position the newborn in manner that provides an unobstructed airway (face can be seen, head aside, nose not covered, sniffing position, neck is straight, legs flexed, back covered).
- Monitor frequently mother-infant dyad while roomed-in, especially during nighttime and early morning.
- Ask mother if she is tired or sleepy and move the infant to a separate sleep surface next to the mother's bed.
- Avoid bed-sharing in the immediate postpartum period, and if it is practiced, educate the mother when and how to use separate sleep surface for the infant.
- Supine infant sleeping should be promoted. The mother or the father who is in SSC with baby who is in a prone position should be awake and alert during the whole procedure.
- To decrease the risk of SUID, at discharge the parents should be educated that infants should sleep in supine position, in the nonsmoking environment, parents should not drink alcohol, mother should exclusively breastfeed, and infant should not be placed to sleep on arm chairs or sofas alone or with other person [148].

Discharge Home of Well Term Newborn

The length of hospital stay of well newborn baby depends on the delivery mode, health stability of the mother and the baby, initiation and establishment of breastfeeding, self-confidence of the mother to take the responsibility for the infant care, socio-economic situation of the family, organization and availability of post-discharge care, support, and follow-up. After discharge mother and infant should continue to be together, so bonding process can continue after discharge. The decision concerning discharge should be made jointly with the obstetric and neonatal team and the family to decrease the possibility of readmission rate. First-time mothers, with chronic illness; who have breastfeeding difficulties, inadequate prenatal care, and poor social support; or whose newborns are sick and treated, may need a longer hospital stay. It is expected that approximately after 48 hours, all discharge criteria should be met. The following discharge criteria were developed and proposed by the American Academy of Pediatrics for term infants (gestation from 37+0 days and 41+6 days) [235]:

- At follow-up examinations and at discharge, while in the facility, the newborn does not have congenital abnormality, birth trauma, or other disease requiring hospitalization.
- The infant is stable, with vital signs stable for at least 12 hours before discharge (respiratory rate < 60 per minute, heart rate between 120 and 160 beats per min-

ute, with resting heart rate as low as 85 which is acceptable, axillary temperature from 36.5 to 37.5°C).

- The infant has passed one stool and urinated at least once while in the facility.
- It had at least two successful feedings in the facility which were recorded in the medical records. Breastfeeding is successful, mother understands the importance of continuing breastfeeding on demand and who should she contact if any problem arises, and the infant is well latching on, sucking, swallowing, and showing signs of hunger, calming down while on the breast. Formula fed mothers were taught how to prepare formula and how to bottle feed the baby, and the baby has a good coordination between sucking, swallowing, and breathing.
- In case the infant was circumcised, there were no signs of bleeding within 2 hours before discharge after circumcision.
- If the infant had hyperbilirubinemia, clinical significance with risk factors determined, with appropriate treatment if needed, and appropriate follow-up plans at discharge.
- Infant has been screened and monitored for sepsis based on maternal risk factors from the pregnancy and birth, the appropriate workup and the treatment performed, if needed.
- Maternal prenatal tests on syphilis screening, HBs antigen, HIV infection screening, and other tests recommended by healthcare authority were reviewed at discharge. When indicated, infant blood type and direct Coombs test were performed and checked.
- All vaccines in concordance with the recommendation of healthcare authority were given to the newborn at discharge, and appropriate protection of infants of HBsAg-positive mothers with hepatitis B immunoglobulin and hepatitis B vaccine was completed.
- Maternal and family member vaccination status should be checked, and members of the family counselled concerning the vaccinations against tetanus, diphtheria, pertussis, and influenza during influenza season, and all other vaccines recommended by local healthcare authority.
- Mother's health condition should be checked at discharge, especially for infection, postpartum bleeding, and problems with breasts (particularly if breastfeeding), and attention should be addressed to the detection of postpartum depression. Mothers at high risk for health problems at discharge are the firstborn mothers, adolescent mothers, socially deprived mothers, and those with chronic or acute health problems before and during pregnancy.
- All screening tests performed in neonate should be checked and in line with the local recommendations. If there is a need to repeat the test, appropriate information should be given to the family.
- Mother has been appropriately trained to care for her infant (appropriate hygiene of infant, care of umbilical cord stump, skin care, genital and diaper region care, temperature assessment), being competent, self-confident, skilled, and informed whom to call in the case of emergency.

- All safety issues like prone sleeping position, use of car seats, and smoking-free environment should be discussed with the parents. Availability of the transportation from the birthing facility to home should be checked.
- Social and environmental risk factors of the family should be addressed and in particular the barriers to follow-up care, shelter for the family, the communication with the local healthcare provider, availability of the food and water for the family if appropriate, and availability of infant formula if the baby is formula fed. The first follow-up visit at home, healthcare, or other facility after discharge should take place within 48 hours after discharge.

References

1. AAP Committee on Infectious Diseases and AAP Committee on Fetus and Newborn. Elimination of perinatal hepatitis B: providing the first vaccine dose within 24 hours of birth. Pediatrics. 2017;140(3):e20171870. https://doi.org/10.1542/peds.2017-1870.
2. Aby J, Kim JL. A cross-sectional assessment of cutaneous lumbosacral and coccygeal physical examination findings in a healthy newborn population. Glob Pediatr Health. 2018:5;2333794X18756133. https://doi.org/10.1177/2333794X18756133. eCollection 2018.
3. Ahn ES, Jung MS, Lee YK, Ko SY, Shin SM, Hahn MH. Neonatal clavicular fracture: recent 10 year study. Pediatr Int. 2015;57(1):60–3. https://doi.org/10.1111/ped.12497.
4. American Academy of Pediatrics Committee on Fetus and Newborn. Controversies concerning vitamin K and the newborn. American Academy of Pediatrics Committee on Fetus and Newborn. Pediatrics. 2003;112(1 Pt 1):191–2.
5. American Academy of Pediatrics Committee on Fetus and Newborn; American College of Obstetricians and Gynecologists Committee on Obstetric Practice. The Apgar Score. Pediatrics. 2015;136(4):819–22. https://doi.org/10.1542/peds.2015-2651.
6. American Academy of Pediatrics. Committee on Nutrition Vitamin K compounds and the water-soluble analogues: use in therapy and prophylaxis in pediatrics. Pediatrics. 1961;28:501–7.
7. American Academy of Pediatrics, Section on Ophthalmology, American Association for Pediatric Ophthalmology and Strabismus, American Academy of Ophthalmology, American Association of Certified Orthoptists. Red reflex examination in neonates, infants, and children. Pediatrics Dec. 2008;122(6):1401–4. https://doi.org/10.1542/peds.2008-2624.
8. Ami O, Maran JC, Gabor P, Whitacre EB, Musset D, Dubray C, et al. Three-dimensional magnetic resonance imaging of fetal head molding and brain shape changes during the second stage of labor. PLoS One. 2019;14(5):e0215721. https://doi.org/10.1371/journal.pone.0215721. eCollection 2019.
9. Amiel-Tison C. Update of the Amiel-Tison Neurological assessment for the term neonate or at 40 weeks corrected age. Pediatr Neurol. 2002;27:196–212.
10. Andersson O, Rana N, Ewald U, Målqvist M, Stripple G, Basnet O, et al. Intact cord resuscitation versus early cord clamping in the treatment of depressed newborn infants during the first 10 minutes of birth (Nepcord III) - a randomized clinical trial. Matern Health Neonatol Perinatol. 2019;5:15. https://doi.org/10.1186/s40748-019-0110-z. eCollection 2019.
11. Antonovsky A. The structure and properties of the sense of coherence scale. Soc Sci Med. 1993;368(6):725–33.
12. Apgar V. A proposal for a new method of evaluation of the newborn infant. Curr Res Anesthe Analg. 1953;32(4):260–7. https://doi.org/10.1213/00000539-195301000-00041.
13. Aryeetey R, Dykes F. Global implications of the new WHO and UNICEF implementation guidance on the revised Baby-Friendly Hospital Initiative. Matern Child Nutr. 2018;14(3):e12637. https://doi.org/10.1111/mcn.12637.

14. Ausili E, Maresca G, Massimi L, Morgante L, Romagnoli C, Rendeli C. Occult spinal dysraphisms in newborns with skin markers: role of ultrasonography and magnetic resonance imaging. Childs Nerv Syst. 2018;34(2):285–91. https://doi.org/10.1007/s00381-017-3638-0.
15. Axer-Siegel R, Herscovici Z, Davidson S, Linder N, Sherf I, Snir M. Early structural status of the eyes of healthy term neonates conceived by in vitro fertilization or conceived naturally. Invest Ophthalmol Vis Sci. 2007;48(12):5454–8.
16. Baas M, Burger EB, Sneiders D, Galjaard RH, Hovius SER, van Nieuwenhoven CA. Controversies in Poland Syndrome: Alternative Diagnoses in Patients With Congenital Pectoral Muscle Deficiency. J Hand Surg Am. 2018;43(2):186.e1–16. https://doi.org/10.1016/j.jhsa.2017.08.029.
17. Bakker MK, Bergman JEH, Krikov S, Amar E, Cocchi G, Cragan J, et al. Prenatal diagnosis and prevalence of critical congenital heart defects: an international retrospective cohort study. BMJ Open. 2019;9(7):e028139. https://doi.org/10.1136/bmjopen-2018-028139.
18. Ballard JL, Khoury JC, Wedig K, Wang L, Eilers-Walsman BL, Lipp R. New Ballard Score, expanded to include extremely premature infants. J Pediatr. 1991;119(3):417–23. https://doi.org/10.1016/s0022-3476(05)82056-6. https://www.ballardscore.com/files/BallardScore_scoresheet.pdf.
19. Balogun OO, O'Sullivan EJ, McFadden A, Ota E, Gavine A, Garner CD, Renfrew MJ, MacGillivray S. Interventions for promoting the initiation of breastfeeding. Cochrane Database Systemat Rev. 2016;11:Art. No. CD001688. https://doi.org/10.1002/14651858.CD001688.pub3.
20. Bamji M, Stone RK, Kaul A, Usmani G, Schachter FF, Wasserman E. Palpable lymph nodes in healthy newborns and infants. Pediatrics. 1986;78(4):573–5.
21. Basha S, Surendran N, Pichichero M. Immune responses in neonates. Expert Rev Clin Immunol. 2014;10:1171–84.
22. Bass JL, Gartley T, Lyczkowski DA, Kleinman R. Trends in the incidence of sudden unexpected infant death in the newborn: 1995-2014. J Pediatr. 2018;196:104–8. https://doi.org/10.1016/j.jpeds.2017.12.045.
23. Berger GS, Gillings DB, Siegel E. The evaluation of regionalized perinatal health care programs. Am J Obstet Gynecol. 1976;125(7):924–32.
24. Bergman JE, Loane M, Vrijheid M, Pierini A, Nijman RJ, Addor MC, et al. Epidemiology of hypospadias in Europe: a registry-based study. World J Urol. 2015;33(12):2159–67. https://doi.org/10.1007/s00345-015-1507-6.
25. Bhambhani V, Muenke M. Noonan syndrome. Am Fam Physician. 2014;89(1):37–43.
26. Bhatia V. Reporting units of thyroid stimulating hormone in newborn thyroid screening. Indian Pediatr. 2019;56(12):1063.
27. Bhatt S, Ahmad M, Batra P, Tandon A, Roy S, Mandal S. Neonatal adrenal hemorrhage presenting as "Acute Scrotum"-looking beyond the obvious: a sonographic insight. J Ultrasound. 2017;20(3):253–9. https://doi.org/10.1007/s40477-017-0248-3. eCollection 2017 Sep
28. Bin-Nun A, Mimouni FB, Kasirer Y, Schors I, Schimmel MS, Kaplan M, et al. Might bilirubin serve as a natural antioxidant in response to neonatal encephalopathy? Am J Perinatol. 2018;35(11):1107–12. https://doi.org/10.1055/s-0038-1641746.
29. Blanco FC, Elliott ST, Sandler AD. Management of congenital chest wall deformities. Semin Plast Surg. 2011;25(1):107–16. https://doi.org/10.1055/s-0031-1275177.
30. Bulut G, Bulut H, Ortac R. A comprehensive survey of natal and neonatal teeth in newborns. Niger J Clin Pract. 2019;22(11):1489–94. https://doi.org/10.4103/njcp.njcp_152_19.
31. Butt K, Lim KI. Guideline No. 388-determination of gestational age by ultrasound. J Obstet Gynaecol Can. 2019;41(10):1497–507. https://doi.org/10.1016/j.jogc.2019.04.010.
32. Centers for Disease Control and Prevention (CDC). Notes from the field: late vitamin K deficiency bleeding in infants whose parents declined vitamin K prophylaxis–Tennessee, 2013. MMWR Morb Mortal Wkly Rep. 2013;62(45):901–2.
33. Chan K, Petros M. Simple test, complex system: multifaceted views of newborn screening science, technology, and policy. Glob Pediatr Health. 2019;6:2333794X19894812. https://doi.org/10.1177/2333794X19894812. eCollection 2019.

34. Chaturvedi A, Chaturvedi A, Stanescu AL, Blickman JG, Meyers SP. Mechanical birth-related trauma to the neonate: an imaging perspective. Insights Imaging. 2018;9(1):103–18. https://doi.org/10.1007/s13244-017-0586-x.
35. Chawla D, Darlow BA. Development of quality measures in perinatal care - priority for developing countries. Indian Pediatr. 2018;55(9):797–802.
36. Chikani UN, Chinawa JM, Ikefuna AN, Ibekwe MU. Stretched penile length of healthy term neonates: normative values among Igbo babies in southeastern Nigeria. J Trop Pediatr. 2015;61(1):69–73. https://doi.org/10.1093/tropej/fmu064.
37. Chirico G, Beccagutti F. Nasal obstruction in neonates and infants. Minerva Pediatr. 2010;62(5):499–505.
38. Choi HA, Lee YK, Ko SY, Shin SM. Neonatal clavicle fracture in cesarean delivery: incidence and risk factors. J Matern Fetal Neonatal Med. 2017;30(14):1689–92. https://doi.org/10.1080/14767058.2016.1222368.
39. Chow YW, Turner I, Kernohan WG, Mollan RA. Measurement of the forces and movements involved in neonatal hip testing. Med Eng Phys. 1994;16(3):181–7. https://doi.org/10.1016/1350-4533(94)90036-1.
40. Christianson A, Howson CP, Model B. March of dimes global report on birth defects. White Plains, New York: The Hidden Toll of Dying and Disabled Children. March of Dimes Birth Defects Foundation; 2006. https://www.marchofdimes.org/global-report-on-birth-defects-the-hidden-toll-of-dying-and-disabled-children-full-report.pdf (Accessed 1 Jan 2020).
41. Ciurea AV, Toader C, Mihalache C. Actual concepts in scaphocephaly: (an experience of 98 cases). J Med Life. 2011;4(4):424–31.
42. Clesse C, Lighezzolo-Alnot J, de Lavergne S, Hamlin S, Scheffler M. The evolution of birth medicalisation: a systematic review. Midwifery. 2018;66:161–7. https://doi.org/10.1016/j.midw.2018.08.003.
43. Cleveland L, Hill CM, Pulse WS, DiCioccio HC, Field T, White-Traut R. Systematic review of skin-to-skin care for full-term, healthy newborns. J Obstet Gynecol Neonatal Nurs. 2017;46(6):857–69. https://doi.org/10.1016/j.jogn.2017.08.005.
44. Coffey PS, Brown SC. Umbilical cord-care practices in low- and middle-income countries: a systematic review. BMC Pregnancy Childbirth. 2017;17(1):68. https://doi.org/10.1186/s12884-017-1250-7.
45. Collado MC, Rautava S, Aakko J, Isolauri E, Salminen S. Human gut colonization may be initiated in utero by distinct microbial communities in the placenta and amniotic fluid. Sci Rep. 2016;6:23129.
46. Committee on Obstetric Practice American Academy of Pediatrics - Committee on Fetus and Newborn. Committee Opinion No. 644: The Apgar Score. Obstet Gynecol. 2015;126(4):e52–5. https://doi.org/10.1097/AOG.0000000000001108.
47. Credé CSE. Die Verhürtung der Augenentzündung der Neugeborenen. Archiv für Gynaekologie. 1881;17:50–3.
48. Cunningham ML, Heike CL. Evaluation of the infant with an abnormal skull shape. Curr Opin Pediatr. 2007;19(6):645–51. https://doi.org/10.1097/MOP.0b013e3282f1581a.
49. d'Alessio PA. Salutogenesis and beyond. Dermatol Ther. 2019;32(1):e12783. https://doi.org/10.1111/dth.12783.
50. Daniali LN, Rezzadeh K, Shell C, Trovato M, Ha R, Byrd HS. Classification of newborn ear malformations and their treatment with the ear well infant ear correction system. Plast Reconstr Surg. 2017;139(3):681–91. https://doi.org/10.1097/PRS.0000000000003150.
51. Davies JH, Cheetham T. Recognition and assessment of atypical and ambiguous genitalia in the newborn. Arch Dis Child. 2017;102(10):968–74. https://doi.org/10.1136/archdischild-2016-311270.
52. Delayed umbilical cord clamping after birth. Committee Opinion No. 684. American College of Obstetricians and Gynecologists. Obstet Gynecol. 2017;129:e5–10. https://www.acog.org/Clinical-Guidance-and-Publications/Committee-Opinions/Committee-on-Obstetric-Practice/Delayed-Umbilical-Cord-Clamping-After-Birth (Accessed January 20, 2020).

53. DiTomasso D, Cloud M. Systematic review of expected weight changes after birth for full-term, breastfed newborns. J Obstet Gynecol Neonatal Nurs. 2019;48(6):593–603. https://doi.org/10.1016/j.jogn.2019.09.004.
54. Donahue SP, Baker CN Committee on Practice and Ambulatory Medicine, American Academy of Pediatrics; Section on Ophthalmology, American Academy of Pediatrics; American Association of Certified Orthoptists; American Association for Pediatric Ophthalmology and Strabismus; American Academy of Ophthalmology. Procedures for the Evaluation of the Visual System by Pediatricians. Pediatrics. 2016;137(1). https://doi.org/10.1542/peds.2015-3597.
55. D'Souza JN, Valika T, Maddalozzo J. Surgical management of midline cervical cleft. Int J Pediatr Otorhinolaryngol. 2019;127:109657. https://doi.org/10.1016/j.ijporl.2019.109657.
56. Dubowitz LM, Dubowitz V, Goldberg C. Clinical assessment of gestational age in the newborn infant. J Pediatr. 1970;77(1):1–10. https://doi.org/10.1016/s0022-3476(70)80038-5.
57. Duff SV, DeMatteo C. Clinical assessment of the infant and child following perinatal brachial plexus injury. J Hand Ther. 2015;28(2):126–33.; quiz 134. https://doi.org/10.1016/j.jht.2015.01.001.
58. Dunn PM. Dr Carl Credé (1819-1892) and the prevention of ophthalmia neonatorum. Arch Dis Child Fetal Neonatal Ed. 2000;83(2):F158–9. https://doi.org/10.1136/fn.83.2.f158.
59. Ebbing C, Kessler J, Moster D, Rasmussen S. Isolated single umbilical artery and the risk of adverse perinatal outcome and third stage of labor complications: a population-based study. Acta Obstet Gynecol Scand. 2019; https://doi.org/10.1111/aogs.13747.
60. Ebbing C, Kessler J, Moster D, Rasmussen S. Single umbilical artery and risk of congenital malformations: a population-based study in Norway. Ultrasound Obstet Gynecol. 2019; https://doi.org/10.1002/uog.20359.
61. Edwards ME, Jepson RG, McInnes RJ. Breastfeeding initiation: An in-depth qualitative analysis of the perspectives of women and midwives using Social Cognitive Theory. Midwifery. 2018;57:8–17. https://doi.org/10.1016/j.midw.2017.10.013.
62. Edwards MO, Kotecha SJ, Kotecha S. Respiratory distress of the term newborn infant. Paediatr Respir Rev. 2013;14(1):29–36.; quiz 36-7. https://doi.org/10.1016/j.prrv.2012.02.002.
63. El-Maouche D, Arlt W, Merke DP. Congenital adrenal hyperplasia. Lancet. 2017;390(10108):2194–210. https://doi.org/10.1016/S0140-6736(17)31431-9.
64. Ercan F, Sarikaya M, Toprak E, Findik S, Arbag H, Acar A. Prenatal diagnosis and intrapartum management of congenital ranula. Z Geburtshilfe Neonatol. 2018;222(6):262–5. https://doi.org/10.1055/a-0660-9808.
65. Ezomike UO, Ugwu EO, Ezomike NE, Eke CB, Ekenze SO. Evaluation of impact of perinatal factors on time to first meconium passage in nigerian neonates. Malawi Med J. 2019;31(2):150–4. https://doi.org/10.4314/mmj.v31i2.8.
66. Farr V, Mitchell RG, Neligan GA, Parkin JM. The definition of some external characteristics used in the assessment of gestational age in the newborn infant. Dev Med Child Neurol. 1966;8(5):507–11. https://doi.org/10.1111/j.1469-8749.1966.tb01796.x.
67. Feldman-Winter L, Goldsmith JP; Committee on Fetus and Newborn; Task force on sudden infant death syndrome. Safe sleep and skin-to-skin care in the neonatal period for healthy term newborns. Pediatrics. 2016;138(3):e20161889. https://doi.org/10.1542/peds.2016-1889.
68. Fenton TR, Nasser R, Eliasziw M, Kim JH, Bilan D, Sauve R. Validating the weight gain of preterm infants between the reference growth curve of the fetus and the term infant. BMC Pediatr. 2013;13(1):92. https://doi.org/10.1186/1471-2431-13-92.
69. Flaherman VJ, Schaefer EW, Kuzniewicz MW, Li SX, Walsh EM, Paul IM. Early weight loss nomograms for exclusively breastfed newborns. Pediatrics. 2015;135(1):e16–23. https://doi.org/10.1542/peds.2014-1532.
70. Friedman JM, Cornel MC, Goldenberg AJ, Lister K, Sénécal K, Vears DF, et al. Genomic newborn screening: public health policy considerations and recommendations. BMC Med Genomics. 2017;10(1):9. Published 2017 Feb 21. https://doi.org/10.1186/s12920-017-0247-4.

71. Gelano TF, Bacha YD, Abate D. Effect of chlorhexidine cord application on prevention of neonatal sepsis in developing countries: systematic review and meta-analysis. Int J Health Sci (Qassim). 2019;13(1):40–51.
72. Georgieff MK, Tran PV, Carlson ES. Atypical fetal development: fetal alcohol syndrome, nutritional deprivation, teratogens, and risk for neurodevelopmental disorders and psychopathology. Dev Psychopathol. 2018;30(3):1063–86. https://doi.org/10.1017/S0954579418000500.
73. Gilboa Y, Kivilevitch Z, Kedem A, Spira M, Borkowski T, Moran O, et al. Caput succedaneum thickness in prolonged second stage of labour: a clinical evaluation. Aust N Z J Obstet Gynaecol. 2013;53(5):459–63. https://doi.org/10.1111/ajo.12104.
74. Gopalakrishnan V, Sahoo NK, Roy ID. Mandibular fracture in a neonate. Int J Oral Maxillofac Surg. 2017;46(1):59–61. https://doi.org/10.1016/j.ijom.2016.08.009.
75. Gosselin J, Gahagan S, Amiel-Tison C. The Amiel-Tison neurological assessment at term: conceptual and methodological continuity in the course of follow-up. Mental Retardation and Developmental Disabilities Research Reviews. 2005;11:34–51.
76. Gravholt CH, Andersen NH, Conway GS, Dekkers O, MGeffner ME, Klein KO, Lin AE, Mauras N, Quigley CA, Karen R. Clinical practice guidelines for the care of girls and women with Turner syndrome: proceedings from the 2016 Cincinnati International Turner Syndrome Meeting. Europ J Endocrinol. 2017;177:G1–G70. https://doi.org/10.1530/EJE-17-0430.
77. Grguric J, Zakarija Grkovic I, Pavicic Bosnjak A, Stanojevic M. A multifaceted approach to revitalizing the Baby-Friendly Hospital Initiative in Croatia. J Hum Lact. 2016;32(3):568–73.
78. Grill FD, Rau A, Bauer FX, Hellmundt F, Hilmer B, Roth M, et al. The absolute and relative effects of presurgical nasoalveolar moulding in bilateral cleft lip and palate patients compared with nasal growth in healthy newborns. J Craniomaxillofac Surg. 2019;47(7):1083–91. https://doi.org/10.1016/j.jcms.2019.01.044.
79. Gruss LT, Schmitt D. The evolution of the human pelvis: changing adaptations to bipedalism, obstetrics and thermoregulation. Philos Trans R Soc Lond B Biol Sci. 2015;370(1663):20140063. https://doi.org/10.1098/rstb.2014.0063.
80. Guirguis-Blake JM, Evans CV, Rushkin M. Ocular prophylaxis for gonococcal ophthalmia neonatorum: updated evidence report and systematic review for the us preventive services task force. JAMA. 2019;321(4):404–6. https://doi.org/10.1001/jama.2018.17847.
81. Guthrie R, Susi A. A simple phenylalanine method for detecting phenylketonuria in large populations of newborn infants. Pediatrics. 1963;32:338–43.
82. Halil H, Oğuz ŞS. Establishment of normative data for stretched penile length in Turkish preterm and term newborns. Turk J Pediatr. 2017;59(3):269–73. https://doi.org/10.24953/turkjped.2017.03.006.
83. Hamilçıkan Ş, Can E. Critical congenital heart disease screening with a pulse oximetry in neonates. J Perinat Med. 2018;46(2):203–7. https://doi.org/10.1515/jpm-2017-0006.
84. Hansen TWR, Maisels MJ, Ebbesen F, Vreman HJ, Stevenson DK, Wong RJ, et al. Sixty years of phototherapy for neonatal jaundice – from serendipitous observation to standardized treatment and rescue for millions. J Perinatol. 2020;40:180–93. https://doi.org/10.1038/s41372-019-0439-1.
85. Hein HA. Regionalized perinatal care in North America. Semin Neonatol. 2004;9(2):111–6. https://doi.org/10.1016/j.siny.2003.08.009.
86. Hirata S, Fuwa K, Sugama K, Kusunoki K, Takeshita H. Mechanism of birth in chimpanzees: humans are not unique among primates. Biol Lett. 2011;7(5):686–8. https://doi.org/10.1098/rsbl.2011.0214.
87. Howson CP, Cedergren B, Giugliani R, Huhtinen P, Padilla CD, Palubiak CS, et al. Universal newborn screening: a roadmap for action. Mol Genet Metab. 2018;124(3):177–83. https://doi.org/10.1016/j.ymgme.2018.04.009.
88. Hsieh ST, Woo AS. Pierre robin sequence. Clin Plast Surg. 2019;46(2):249–59. https://doi.org/10.1016/j.cps.2018.11.010.
89. International Federation of Gynecology and Obstetrics, International Confederation of Midwives, White Ribbon Alliance, International Pediatric Association, World Health

Organization. FIGO GUIDELINES. Mother–baby friendly birthing facilities. Inter J Gynecol Obstet 128. 2015;128:95–9. https://doi.org/10.1016/j.ijgo.2014.10.013.
90. Jaafar SH, Ho JJ, Lee KS. Rooming-in for new mother and infant versus separate care for increasing the duration of breastfeeding. Cochrane Database Systemat Rev. 2016;8:Art. No. CD006641. https://doi.org/10.1002/14651858.CD006641.pub3.
91. Jain L. Stress at birth and its inextricable link to the neonatal transition. Obstet Gynecol. 2016;128(4):685–7. https://doi.org/10.1097/AOG.0000000000001657.
92. Jawin V, Ang HL, Omar A, Thong MK. Beyond critical congenital heart disease: newborn screening using pulse oximetry for neonatal sepsis and respiratory diseases in a middle-income country. PLoS One. 2015;10(9):e0137580. Published 2015 Sep 11. https://doi.org/10.1371/journal.pone.0137580.
93. Johnson L, Bhutani VK, Karp K, Sivieri EM, Shapiro SM. Clinical report from the pilot USA kernicterus registry (1992–2004). J Perinatol. 2009;29(Suppl 1):S25–45.
94. Joint Committee on Infant Hearing. Year 2007 Position Statement: Principles and Guidelines for Early Hearing Detection and Intervention Programs. Pediatrics Oct. 2007;120(4):898–921. https://doi.org/10.1542/peds.2007-2333.
95. Jun Ha J, Yu YC, Lannigan F. A review of the management of lymphangiomas. Curr Pediatr Rev. 2014;10(3):238–48.
96. Karaaslan B, Doğan E, Börcek AÖ. Management of neonatal facial paralysis due to cerebellopontine angle arachnoid cyst: a case report. Pediatr Neurosurg. 2019;54(4):253–7. https://doi.org/10.1159/000500762.
97. Karasavvas T. The Evolution of Human Birth: An Incredible Story a Million Years in the Making. https://www.ancientorigins.net/news-evolution-human-origins/evolution-human-birth-incredible-story-million-years-making-007976 (Accessed 15 Jan 2020).
98. Kaštelan S, Anić Jurica S, Orešković S, Župić T, Herman M, Gverović Antunica A, et al. A survey of current prophylactic treatment for ophthalmia neonatorum in croatia and a review of international preventive practices. Med Sci Monit. 2018;24:8042–7. https://doi.org/10.12659/MSM.910705.
99. Katheria A, Hosono S, El-Naggar W. A new wrinkle: Umbilical cord management (how, when, who). Semin Fetal Neonatal Med. 2018;23(5):321–6. https://doi.org/10.1016/j.siny.2018.07.003.
100. Katheria AC. Umbilical cord milking: a review. Front Pediatr. 2018;6:335. https://doi.org/10.3389/fped.2018.00335. eCollection 2018.
101. Kavle JA, LaCroix E, Dau H, Engmann C. Addressing barriers to exclusive breast-feeding in low- and middle-income countries: a systematic review and programmatic implications. Public Health Nutr. 2017;20(17):3120–34. https://doi.org/10.1017/S1368980017002531.
102. Kc A, Rana N, Målqvist M, Jarawka Ranneberg L, Subedi K, Andersson O. Effects of delayed umbilical cord clamping vs early clamping on anemia in infants at 8 and 12 months: a randomized clinical trial. JAMA Pediatr. 2017;171(3):264–70. https://doi.org/10.1001/jamapediatrics.2016.3971.
103. Khair AM, Ibrahim K. Idiopathic non-traumatic facial nerve palsy (bell's palsy) in neonates; an atypical age and management dilemma. Oman Med J. 2018;33(1):65–8. https://doi.org/10.5001/omj.2018.12.
104. Ko JS, Lue K, Friedlander D, Baumgartner T, Stuhldreher P, DiCarlo HN, et al. Cystectomy in the pediatric exstrophy population: indications and outcomes. Urology. 2018;116:168–71. https://doi.org/10.1016/j.urology.2017.09.009.
105. Koletzko B, Buonocore G, Zimmermann L, Hellstrom-Vestas L, Fewtrell M, Perrone S, Verkade H. Prevention of vitamin K deficiency bleeding (VKDB) at birth. 2019. https://newborn-health-standards.org/prevention-vkdb/ (Accessed 16 Jan 2020).
106. Kouri I, Mathews K, Joshi C. Facial weakness and ophthalmoplegia in a 4-day-old infant. Semin Pediatr Neurol. 2018;26:63–6. https://doi.org/10.1016/j.spen.2017.03.008.
107. Kramer LI. Advancement of dermal icterus in the jaundiced newborn. Am J Dis Child. 1969;118(3):454–8.

108. Krishnan P, Raybaud C, Palasamudram S, Shroff M. Neuroimaging in pediatric hydrocephalus. Indian J Pediatr. 2019;86(10):952–60. https://doi.org/10.1007/s12098-019-02962-z.
109. Krowchuk DP, Frieden IJ, Mancini AJ, Darrow DH, Blei F, Greene AK, et al. Clinical practice guideline for the management of infantile hemangiomas. Pediatrics. 2019;143(1):e20183475. https://doi.org/10.1542/peds.2018-3475.
110. Kural B, Devecioğlu Karapınar E, Yılmazbaş P, Eren T, Gökçay G. Risk factor assessment and a ten-year experience of DDH screening in a well-child population. Biomed Res Int. 2019;2019:7213681. https://doi.org/10.1155/2019/7213681. eCollection 2019.
111. Kutlubay Z, Tanakol A, Engýn B, Onel C, Sýmsek E, Serdaroglu S, Tuzun Y, Yilmaz E, Eren B. Newborn Skin: common skin problems. Maedica (Buchar). 2017;12(1):42–7.
112. Ladino Torres MF, DiPietro MA. Spine ultrasound imaging in the newborn. Semin Ultrasound CT MR. 2014;35(6):652–61. https://doi.org/10.1053/j.sult.2014.08.001.
113. Lahat E, Heyman E, Barkay A, Goldberg M. Asymmetric crying facies and associated congenital anomalies: prospective study and review of the literature. J Child Neurol. 2000;15(12):808–10.
114. Lalonde A, Herschderfer K, Pascali-Bonaro D, Hanson C, Fuchtner C, Visser GHA. The International Childbirth Initiative: 12 steps to safe and respectful MotherBaby-Family maternity care. Int J Gynaecol Obstet. 2019;146(1):65–73. https://doi.org/10.1002/ijgo.12844.
115. Lander A, Newman J. Pediatric anatomy. Surgery. 2013;31(3). https://www.surgeryjournal.co.uk/article/S0263-9319(13)00003-3/pdf. (Accessed 18 Jan 2020).
116. Laudicina NM, Rodriguez F, DeSilva JM. Reconstructing birth in Australopithecus sediba. PLoS One. 2019;14(9):e0221871. https://doi.org/10.1371/journal.pone.0221871. eCollection 2019.
117. Lavista Ferres JM, Anderson TM, Johnston R, Ramirez JM, Mitchell EA. Distinct populations of sudden unexpected infant death based on age. Pediatrics. 2020;145(1):e20191637. https://doi.org/10.1542/peds.2019-1637.
118. Lawn JE, Blencowe H, Oza S, You D, Lee ACC, Waiswa P, Lalli M, Bhutta Z, Barros AJD, Christian P, et al. Every Newborn: progress, priorities, and potential beyond survival. Lancet. 2014;384(9938):189–205. Published online 2014 May 19. https://doi.org/10.1016/S0140-6736(14)60496-7.
119. Lee AC, Panchal P, Folger L, Whelan H, Whelan R, Rosner B et al. Diagnostic accuracy of neonatal assessment for gestational age determination: a systematic review. Pediatrics [Internet]. 2017;140:e20171423. Available from: http://pediatrics.aappublications.org/lookup/doi/10.1542/peds.2017-1423. (Accessed 19 Jan 2020).
120. Lee SJ, Kim JK, Kim SJ. The clinical characteristics and prognosis of subgaleal hemorrhage in newborn. Korean J Pediatr. 2018;61(12):387–91. https://doi.org/10.3345/kjp.2018.06800.
121. Leslie MS, Greene J, Schulkin J, Jelin AC. Umbilical cord clamping practices of U.S. obstetricians. J Neonatal Perinatal Med. 2018;11(1):51–60. https://doi.org/10.3233/NPM-181729.
122. Li LH, Li N, Zhao JY, Fei P, Zhang GM, Mao JB, Rychwalski PJ. Findings of perinatal ocular examination performed on 3573, healthy full-term newborns. Br J Ophthalmol. 2013;97(5):588–91. https://doi.org/10.1136/bjophthalmol-2012-302539.
123. López-Medina MD, López-Araque AB, Linares-Abad M, López-Medina IM. Umbilical cord separation time, predictors and healing complications in newborns with dry care. PLoS One. 2020;15(1):e0227209. https://doi.org/10.1371/journal.pone.0227209. eCollection 2020.
124. Loyal J, Taylor JA, Phillipi CA, Goyal NK, Wood KE, Seashore C, et al. Factors associated with refusal of intramuscular vitamin K in normal newborns. Pediatrics. 2018;142(2):e20173743. https://doi.org/10.1542/peds.2017-3743.
125. Lucas A. Scientific evidence for breastfeeding. N Nutr Inst Workshop Ser. 2019;90:1–12. https://doi.org/10.1159/000490290.
126. Ludwig CA, Callaway NF, Blumenkranz MS, Fredrick DR, Moshfeghi DM. Validity of the red reflex exam in the newborn eye screening test Cohort. Ophthalmic Surg Lasers Imaging Retina. 2018;49(2):103–10. https://doi.org/10.3928/23258160-20180129-04.
127. Ma S, Guo Q, Zhang Z, He Z, Yue A, Song Z, et al. Expanded newborn screening for inborn errors of metabolism by tandem mass spectrometry in newborns from Xinxiang city in China. J Clin Lab Anal. 2020;8:e23159. https://doi.org/10.1002/jcla.23159.

128. Mahle WT, Martin GR, Beekman RH 3rd. Morrow WR; Section on Cardiology and Cardiac Surgery Executive Committee. Endorsement of Health and Human Services recommendation for pulse oximetry screening for critical congenital heart disease. Pediatrics. 2012;129(1):190–2. https://doi.org/10.1542/peds.2011-3211.
129. Maisels MJ, Kring E. Transcutaneous bilirubin levels in the first 96 h in a normal newborn population of 35 or more weeks' of gestation. Pediatrics. 2006;117(4):1169–73. https://doi.org/10.1542/peds.2005-0744.
130. Marcewicz LH, Clayton J, Maenner M, Odom E, Okoroh E, Christensen D, et al. Parental refusal of vitamin K and neonatal preventive services: a need for surveillance. Maternal Child Health J. 2017;21(5):1079–84. https://doi.org/10.1007/s10995-016-2205-8.
131. Marinelli A, Del Prete V, Finale E, Guala A, Pelullo CP, Attena F. Breastfeeding with and without the WHO/UNICEF baby-friendly hospital initiative: a cross-sectional survey. Medicine (Baltimore). 2019;98(44):e17737. https://doi.org/10.1097/MD.0000000000017737.
132. Masic I, Begic Z, Naser N, Begic E. Pediatric cardiac anamnesis: prevention of additional diagnostic tests. Int J Prev Med. 2018;9:5. https://doi.org/10.4103/ijpvm.IJPVM_502_17. eCollection 2018.
133. McFall-Ngai M, Hadfield MG, Bosch TC, Carey HV, Domazet-Loso T, Douglas AE, et al. Animals in a bacterial world, a new imperative for the life sciences. Proc Natl Acad SciUSA. 2013;110:3229–36. https://doi.org/10.1073/pnas.1218525110.
134. McKee-Garrett TM. Assessment of the newborn infant. https://www.uptodate.com/contents/assessment-of-the-newborn-infant (Accessed 13 Jan, 2020).
135. McKee-Garrett TM. Overview of the routine management of the healthy newborn infant. https://www.uptodate.com/contents/overview-of-the-routine-management-of-the-healthy-newborn-infant?topicRef=4984&source=see_link (Accessed 13 Jan 2020).
136. McNinch A. Vitamin K deficiency bleeding: early history and recent trends in the United Kingdom. Early Hum Dev. 2010;86(Suppl 1):63–5. https://doi.org/10.1016/j.earlhumdev.2010.01.017.
137. McPhee AS, McKay AC. Phimosis. (Updated 2019 Jan 30). In: StatPearls (Internet). Treasure Island (FL): StatPearls Publishing; 2019 Jan-. Available from: https://www.ncbi.nlm.nih.gov/books/NBK525972/ (Accessed 19 Jan 2020).
138. Medeiros AMC, Santos KCF, Santi VDN, Santos FB, Sereno BRS, Santana ARS, et al. Orofacial anthropometric measures in fullterm newborns. Codas. 2019;31(6):e20180261. https://doi.org/10.1590/2317-1782/20192018261. eCollection 2019.
139. Meigal AY. Synergistic action of gravity and temperature on the motor system within the lifespan: a "Baby Astronaut" hypothesis. Med Hypotheses. 2013;80(3):275–83. https://doi.org/10.1016/j.mehy.2012.12.004.
140. Mesropyan L, Sanil Y. Innocent heart murmurs from the perspective of the pediatrician. Pediatr Ann. 2016;45(8):e306–9. https://doi.org/10.3928/19382359-20160720-09.
141. Mihatsch WA, Braegger C, Bronsky J, Campoy C, Domellöf M, Fewtrell M, et al. Prevention of vitamin K deficiency bleeding in newborn infants: a position paper by the ESPGHAN committee on nutrition. J Pediatr Gastroenterol Nutr. 2016;63(1):123–9. https://doi.org/10.1097/MPG.0000000000001232.
142. Milani C, Duranti S, Bottacini F, Casey E, Turroni F, Mahony J, et al. The first microbial colonizers of the human gut: composition, activities, and health implications of the infant gut microbiota. Microbiol Mol Biol Rev. 2017;81(4):e00036-17. https://doi.org/10.1128/MMBR.00036-17.
143. Mircher C, Toulas J, Cieuta-Walti C, Marey I, Conte M, González Briceño L, et al. Anthropometric charts and congenital anomalies in newborns with Down syndrome. Am J Med Genet A. 2017;173(8):2166–75. https://doi.org/10.1002/ajmg.a.38305.
144. Miyazawa T, Itabashi K, Tamura M, Suzuki H, Ikenoue T; Prevention Recurrence Committee, Japan Obstetric Compensation System for Cerebral Palsy. Unsupervised breastfeeding was related to sudden unexpected postnatal collapse during early skin-to-skin contact in cerebral palsy cases. Acta Paediatr. 2019. https://doi.org/10.1111/apa.14961.
145. Mohapatra A, Gomare M. A critical appraisal of the maternal and child health scenario in a metropolitan city in India with reference to achievements of millennium develop-

ment goals. J Family Med Prim Care. 2019;8(3):995–1001. https://doi.org/10.4103/jfmpc.jfmpc_379_18.
146. Monteilh C, Calixte R, Burjonrappa S. Controversies in the management of neonatal testicular torsion: a meta-analysis. J Pediatr Surg. 2019;54(4):815–9. https://doi.org/10.1016/j.jpedsurg.2018.07.006.
147. Moon RY, Task Force on Sudden Infant Death Syndrome. SIDS and other sleep related infant deaths: expansion of recommendations for a safe infant sleeping environment. Pediatrics. 2011;128(5). Available at: www. pediatrics. org/c gi/c ontent/f ull/128/5 /e 1341.
148. Moore ER, Bergman N, Anderson GC, Medley N. Early skin-to-skin contact for mothers and their healthy newborn infants. Cochrane Database Systemat Rev. 2016;11. Art. No.: CD003519. https://doi.org/10.1002/14651858.CD003519.pub4.
149. Moraa PK, Mweu MM, Njoroge PK. Association between umbilical cord hygiene and neonatal sepsis among neonates presenting to a primary care facility in Nairobi County, Kenya: a case-control study. F1000Res. 2019;8:920. Published 2019 Jun 21. https://doi.org/10.12688/f1000research.19544.2.
150. Morris MC, Surendran N. Neonatal vaccination: challenges and intervention strategies. Neonatology. 2016;109(3):161–9. https://doi.org/10.1159/000442460.
151. Morton SU, Brodsky D. Fetal Physiology and the Transition to Extrauterine Life. Clin Perinatol. 2016;43(3):395–407. https://doi.org/10.1016/j.clp.2016.04.001.
152. Moshiro R, Mdoe P, Perlman JM. A global view of neonatal asphyxia and resuscitation. Front Pediatr. 2019;7:489. https://doi.org/10.3389/fped.2019.00489.
153. Moshiro R, Perlman JM, Mdoe R, Kidanto H, Kvaløy JT, Ersdal HL. Potential causes of early death among admitted newborns in a rural Tanzanian Hospital. PLoS ONE. 2019;14:e0222935. https://doi.org/10.1371/journal.pone.0222935.
154. Mukerji A, Shafey A, Jain A, Cohen E, Shah PS, Sander B, Shah V. Pulse oximetry screening for critical congenital heart defects in Ontario, Canada: a cost-effectiveness analysis. Can J Public Health. 2020. https://doi.org/10.17269/s41997-019-00280-7.
155. Munro A, Corsi DJ, Martin L, Halpenny M, Dibdin N, Elmoazzen HE, et al. Obstetrical and neonatal factors associated with optimal public banking of umbilical cord blood in the context of delayed cord clamping. Clin Invest Med. 2019;42(3):E56–63. https://doi.org/10.25011/cim.v42i3.33093.
156. Murphy MC, De Angelis L, McCarthy LK, O'Donnell CPF. Comparison of infant heart rate assessment by auscultation, ECG and oximetry in the delivery room. Arch Dis Child Fetal Neonatal Ed. 2018;103(5):F490–2. https://doi.org/10.1136/archdischild-2017-314367.
157. Nagpal R, Yamashiro Y. Gut microbiota composition in healthy Japanese infants and young adults born by C-section. Ann Nutr Metab. 2018;73(suppl 3):4–11. https://doi.org/10.1159/000490841.
158. National Institute for Health and Care Excellence Neonatal jaundice [homepage on the Internet]. Clinical guideline 98. London: Royal College of Obstetricians and Gynaecologists; 2010. Available from: https://www.nice.org.uk/guidance/cg98/evidence/fullguideline-pdf 245411821 (Accessed 23 Jan 2020).
159. Ng E, Loewy AD. Position Statement: Guidelines for vitamin K prophylaxis in newborns: A joint statement of the Canadian Paediatric Society and the College of Family Physicians of Canada. Can Fam Physician. 2018;64(10):736–9.
160. Nichter S. A clinical algorithm for early identification and intervention of cervical muscular torticollis. Clin Pediatr (Phila). 2016;55(6):532-6. https://doi.org/10.1177/0009922815600396.
161. Norwitz ER, Schust DJ, Fisher SJ. Implantation and the survival of early pregnancy. N Engl J Med. 2001;345(19):1400–8. https://doi.org/10.1056/NEJMra000763.
162. Nuss D, Obermeyer RJ, Kelly RE Jr. Pectus excavatum from a pediatric surgeon's perspective. Ann Cardiothorac Surg. 2016;5(5):493–500. https://doi.org/10.21037/acs.2016.06.04.
163. Ogundoyin OO, Atalabi OM. Comparison between testicular volumes as measured with prader orchidometer and ultrasonography in Healthy Nigerian Newborns. Afr J Paediatr Surg. 2018;15(2):93–6. https://doi.org/10.4103/ajps.AJPS_32_17.

164. Olsunya B. Screening for neonatal deafness in resource - poor countries: challenges and solutions. Res Rep Neonatol. 2015;5:51–64.
165. Orgul G, Ozyuncu O, Oktem A, Beksac MS. Management and outcomes of cystic hygromas: experience of a tertiary center. J Ultrasound. 2017;20(2):127–31. https://doi.org/10.1007/s40477-017-0251-8.eCollection 2017.
166. O'Shea JE, Foster JP, O'Donnell CP, Breathnach D, Jacobs SE, Todd DA, et al. Frenotomy for tongue-tie in newborn infants. Cochrane Database Syst Rev. 2017;3:CD011065. https://doi.org/10.1002/14651858.CD011065.pub2.
167. Pace ND, Oster ME, Forestieri NE, Enright D, Knight J, Meyer RE. Sociodemographic factors and survival of infants with congenital heart defects. Pediatrics. 2018;142(3): e20180302. https://doi.org/10.1542/peds.2018-0302.
168. Pahys JM, Guille JT. What's New in Congenital Scoliosis? J Pediatr Orthop. 2018;38(3):e172–9. https://doi.org/10.1097/BPO.0000000000000922.
169. Pan W, Gu T, Pan Y, Feng C, Long Y, Zhao Y, Meng H, Liang Z, Yao M. Birth intervention and non-maternal infant-handling during parturition in a nonhuman primate. Primates. 2014;55(4):483–8. https://doi.org/10.1007/s10329-014-0427-1.
170. Pandita A, Mishra N, Gupta G, Shukla A. Neonatal facial palsy, a case series: is CPAP the culprit? BMJ Case Rep. 2018;2018: bcr-2018-224842. https://doi.org/10.1136/bcr-2018-224842.
171. Paro-Panjan D, Neubauer D, Kodric J, Bratanic B. Amiel-Tison Neurological Assessment at term age: clinical application, correlation with other methods, and outcome at 12 to 15 months. Dev Med Child Neurol. 2005;47(1):19–26.
172. Patel M, Mukherjee D, Farsiu S, Munoz B, Blood AB, Wilson CG, et al. Estimation of gestational age via image analysis of anterior lens capsule vascularity in preterm infants: a pilot study. Front Pediatr [Internet]. 2019;7. Available from: https://www.frontiersin.org/article/10.3389/fped.2019.00043/full. (Accessed 19 Jan 2020).
173. Paton RW. Screening in Developmental Dysplasia of the Hip (DDH). Surgeon. 2017;15(5):290–6. https://doi.org/10.1016/j.surge.2017.05.002.
174. Paul DA, Johnson D, Goldstein ND, Pearlman SA. Development of a single-center quality bundle to prevent sudden unexpected postnatal collapse. J Perinatol. 2019;39(7):1008–13. https://doi.org/10.1038/s41372-019-0393-y.
175. Paul VK, Singh M. Regionalized perinatal care in developing countries. Semin Neonatol. 2004;9(2):117–24. https://doi.org/10.1016/j.siny.2003.08.010.
176. Pavicic Bosnjak A, Grguric J, Stanojevic M, Sonicki Z. Influence of sociodemographic and psychosocial characteristics on breastfeeding duration of mothers attending breastfeeding support groups. J Perinat Med. 2009;37:185–92.
177. Pavicic Bosnjak A, Rumboldt M, Stanojevic M, Lee DC. Psychometric assessment of the croatian version of the breastfeeding self-efficacy scale-short form. Journal of Human Lactation. 2012;25(10):565–9. https://doi.org/10.1177/0890334412456240.
178. Perez-Botella M, Downe S, Magistretti CM, Lindstrom B, Berg M. The use of salutogenesis theory in empirical studies of maternity care for healthy mothers and babies. Sex Reprod Healthc. 2015;6(1):33–9. https://doi.org/10.1016/j.srhc.2014.09.001.
179. Pérez-Escamilla R, Martinez JL, Segura-Pérez S. Impact of the Baby-friendly Hospital Initiative on breastfeeding and child health outcomes: a systematic review. Maternal & Child Nutrition. 2016;12:402–17. https://doi.org/10.1111/mcn.12294.
180. Phillipos E, Solevåg AL, Pichler G, Aziz K, van Os S, O'Reilly M, Cheung PY, Schmölzer GM. Heart rate assessment immediately after birth. Neonatology. 2016;109(2):130–8. https://doi.org/10.1159/000441940.
181. Piwoz EG, Huffman SL. The impact of marketing of breast-milk substitutes on WHO-recommended breastfeeding practices. Food Nutr Bull. 2015;36(4):373–86.
182. Plana MN, Zamora J, Suresh G, Fernandez-Pineda L, Thangaratinam S, Ewer AK. Pulse oximetry screening for critical congenital heart defects. Cochrane Database Syst Rev. 2018;3(3):CD011912. Published 2018 Mar 1. https://doi.org/10.1002/14651858.CD011912.pub2.

183. Pogliani L, Erba P, Nannini P, Giacomet V, Zuccotti GV. Effects and safety of delayed versus early umbilical cord clamping in newborns of HIV-infected mothers. J Matern Fetal Neonatal Med. 2019;32(4):646–9. https://doi.org/10.1080/14767058.2017.1387896.
184. Pondaag W, Malessy MJA. Outcome assessment for Brachial Plexus birth injury. Results from the iPluto world-wide consensus survey. J Orthop Res. 2018;36(9):2533–41. https://doi.org/10.1002/jor.23901.
185. Purisch SE, Ananth CV, Arditi B, Mauney L, Ajemian B, Heiderich A, et al. Effect of delayed vs immediate umbilical cord clamping on maternal blood loss in term cesarean delivery: a randomized clinical trial. JAMA. 2019;322(19):1869–76. https://doi.org/10.1001/jama.2019.15995.
186. Quintanilla-Dieck L, Penn EB Jr. Congenital neck masses. Clin Perinatol. 2018;45(4):769–85. https://doi.org/10.1016/j.clp.2018.07.012.
187. Rai RK, Luo J, Tulchinsky TH. Vitamin K supplementation to prevent hemorrhagic morbidity and mortality of newborns in India and China. World J Pediatr. 2017;13(1):15–9. https://doi.org/10.1007/s12519-016-0062-6.
188. Raines DA, Jain S. Cephalohematoma. [Updated 2019 Dec 9]. In: StatPearls [Internet]. Treasure Island (FL): StatPearls Publishing; 2019 Jan-. Available from: https://www.ncbi.nlm.nih.gov/books/NBK470192/ (Accessed 16 Jan 2020).
189. Rajan R, Tunkel DE. Choanal Atresia and Other Neonatal Nasal Anomalies Clin Perinatol. 2018;45(4):751–67. https://doi.org/10.1016/j.clp.2018.07.011.
190. Rane A, Iyer J, Ananthram H, Currie T. Can We Deliver Better? J Obstet Gynaecol India. 2017;67(3):157–61. https://doi.org/10.1007/s13224-017-0981-8.
191. Rare disease. https://www.eurordis.org/about-rare-diseases (Accessed 22 Jan 2020).
192. Rare disease: frequently asked questions. https://rarediseases.info.nih.gov/diseases/pages/31/faqs-about-rare-diseases (Accessed 22 Jan 2020).
193. Rautava S. Probiotic Intervention through the pregnant and breastfeeding mother to reduce disease risk in the child. Breastfeeding Medicine. Apr 2018. ahead of: https://doi.org/10.1089/bfm.2018.29076.sjr.
194. Rautawa S, Cerebral Palsy Alliance Research Institute. Australian Cerebral Palsy Register. Report 2013. Available at: https://www.cpregister.com/pubs/pdf/ACPR-Report_Web_2013.pdf. (Accessed 10.12.2018).
195. Roth DA, Hildesheimer M, Bardenstein S, Goidel D, Reichman B, Maayan-Metzger A, Kuint J. Preauricular skin tags and ear pits are associated with permanent hearing impairment in newborns. Pediatrics. 2008;122(4):e884–90. https://doi.org/10.1542/peds.2008-0606.
196. Sales SAG, Santos ML, Machado RA, Dias VO, Nascimento JE, Swerts MSO, et al. Incidence of bifid uvula and its relationship to submucous cleft palate and a family history of oral cleft in the Brazilian population. Braz J Otorhinolaryngol. 2018;84(6):687–90. https://doi.org/10.1016/j.bjorl.2017.08.004.
197. Sameshima YT, Yamanari MG, Silva MA, Neto MJ, Funari MB. The challenging sonographic inguinal canal evaluation in neonates and children: an update of differential diagnoses. Pediatr Radiol. 2017;47(4):461–72. https://doi.org/10.1007/s00247-016-3706-8.
198. Saso A, Kampmann B. Vaccine responses in newborns. Semin Immunopathol. 2017;39(6):627–42. https://doi.org/10.1007/s00281-017-0654-9.
199. Savoie KB, Huang EY, Aziz SK, Blakely ML, Dassinger S, Dorale AR, et al. Improving gastroschisis outcomes: does birth place matter? J Pediatr Surg. 2014;49(12):1771–5. https://doi.org/10.1016/j.jpedsurg.2014.09.019.
200. Sekulić SR, Lukac DD, Naumović NM. The fetus cannot exercise like an astronaut: gravity loading is necessary for the physiological development during second half of pregnancy. Med Hypotheses. 2005;64(2):221–8. https://doi.org/10.1016/j.mehy.2004.08.012.37.
201. Shaw BA, Segal LS, AAP Section on Orthopaedics. Evaluation and Referral for Developmental Dysplasia of the Hip in Infants. Pediatrics. 2016;138(6):e20163107.
202. Simard MN, Lambert J, Lachance C, Audibert F, Gosselin J. Stability of neurocranial signs in the first two years of life in infants at risk. Early Hum Dev. 2010;86(8):473–8. https://doi.org/10.1016/j.earlhumdev.2010.06.007.

203. Simkin SK, Misra SL, Battin M, McGhee CNJ, Dai S. Prospective observational study of universal newborn eye screening in a hospital and community setting in New Zealand. BMJ Paediatr Open. 2019;3(1):bmjpo-2018-000376. https://doi.org/10.1136/bmjpo-2018-000376. eCollection 2019.
204. Simon LV, Hashmi MF, Bragg BN. APGAR Score. (Updated 2019 Sep 29). In: StatPearls (Internet). Treasure Island (FL): StatPearls Publishing; 2019 Jan. Available from: https://www.ncbi.nlm.nih.gov/books/NBK470569/. (Accessed 15 Jan 2020).
205. Simpson M, Sundaram V. Urologic conditions in infants and children: inguinal hernia, hydrocele, and Cryptorchidism. FP Essent. 2020;488:16–20.
206. Singh M, Mehra K. Imperforate Anus. [Updated 2019 Nov 3]. In: StatPearls (Internet). Treasure Island (FL): StatPearls Publishing; 2019 Jan-. Available from: https://www.ncbi.nlm.nih.gov/books/NBK549784/. (Accessed 19 Jan 2020).
207. Smith JT. Bilateral rib-based distraction to the pelvis for the management of congenital gibbus deformity in the growing child with myelodysplasia. Spine Deform. 2016;4(1):70–7. https://doi.org/10.1016/j.jspd.2015.07.004.
208. Smith V, Daly D, Lundgren I, Eri T, Begley C, Gross MM, Downe S, Alfirevic Z, Devane D. Protocol for the development of a salutogenic intrapartum core outcome set [SIPCOS]. BMC Med Res Methodol. 2017;17(1):61. https://doi.org/10.1186/s12874-017-0341-5.
209. Souza SW, Ross J, Milner RD. Alterations in head shape of newborn infants after caesarean section or vaginal delivery. Arch Dis Child. 1976;51(8):624–7. https://doi.org/10.1136/adc.51.8.624.
210. Stahlmann N, Härtel C, Knopp A, Gehring B, Kiecksee H, Thyen U. Predictive value of neurodevelopmental assessment versus evaluation of general movements for motor outcome in preterm infants with birth weights <1500 g. Neuropediatrics. 2007;38:91–9.
211. Stanojevic M, Zaputovic S, Pavicic BA. Continuity between fetal and neonatal neurobehavior. Semin Fetal Neonatal Med. 2012;17:324–9. https://doi.org/10.1016/j.siny.2012.06.006.
212. Stanojevic M. Implementation of FIGO Mother Friendly Hospital Initiative in Croatia – Role of neonatologist. J Neonatal Perinatal Med. 2017;10(2):224.
213. Swain Ewald HA, Ewald PW. Natural selection, the microbiome, and public health. Yale J Biol Med. 2018;91(4):445–55. eCollection 2018 Dec.
214. Swain Ewald HA, Ewald PW. Natural selection, the microbiome, and public health. Yale J Biol Med. 2018;91(4):445–55. eCollection 2018 Dec.
215. Tan AK. Ophthalmia Neonatorum. N Engl J Med. 2019;380(2):e2. https://doi.org/10.1056/NEJMicm1808613.
216. Techasatian L, Sanaphay V, Paopongsawan P, Schachner LA. Neonatal birthmarks: a prospective survey in 1000 Neonates. Glob Pediatr Health. 2019;6:2333794X19835668. https://doi.org/10.1177/2333794X19835668. eCollection 2019.
217. Tekleab AM, Sewnet YC. Role of pulse oximetry in detecting critical congenital heart disease among newborns delivered at a high altitude setting in Ethiopia. Pediatric Health Med Ther. 2019;10:83–88. Published 2019 Aug 15. https://doi.org/10.2147/PHMT.S217987.
218. Thangaratinam S, Brown K, Zamora J, Khan KS, Ewer AK. Pulse oximetry screening for critical congenital heart defects in asymptomatic newborn babies: a systematic review and meta-analysis. Lancet. 2012;379(9835):2459–64. https://doi.org/10.1016/S0140-6736(12)60107-X.
219. Therell BL, Buechner C, Lloyd-Puryear MA, van Dyck PC, Mann MY. What's new in newborn screening? Pediatr Health. 2008;2(4):411–29. https://www.medscape.com/viewarticle/580450 (Accessed 1 Jan 2020).
220. Therrell BL Jr, Padilla CD. Newborn screening in the developing countries. Curr Opin Pediatr. 2018;30(6):734–9. https://doi.org/10.1097/MOP.0000000000000683.
221. United Nations. Millennium Development Goals Report, 2015. New York: United Nations; 2015. https://www.un.org/millenniumgoals/2015_MDG_Report/pdf/MDG%202015%20rev%20[July%2015].pdf (Accessed 4 Jan 2020).
222. Preventive Services Task Force US, Curry SJ, Krist AH, Owens DK, Barry MJ, Caughey AB, Davidson KW, et al. Ocular prophylaxis for gonococcal ophthalmia neonatorum: US Preventive

services task force reaffirmation recommendation statement. JAMA. 2019;321(4):394–8. https://doi.org/10.1001/jama.2018.21367.
223. Valerio E, Cutrone M, Chiandetti L, Trevisanuto D. Exuberant upper gum lesions in a neonate. J Pediatr. 2013;163(5):1521.e1. https://doi.org/10.1016/j.jpeds.2013.06.017.
224. van den Heuvel TLA, de Bruijn D. Moens-van de Moesdijk D, Beverdam A, van Ginneken B, de Korte CL. Comparison study of low-cost ultrasound devices for estimation of gestational age in resource-limited countries. Ultrasound Med Biol. 2018;44(11):2250–60. https://doi.org/10.1016/j.ultrasmedbio.2018.05.023.
225. van Velzen CL, Ket JCF, van de Ven PM, Blom NA, Haak MC. Systematic review and meta-analysis of the performance of second-trimester screening for prenatal detection of congenital heart defects. Int J Gynaecol Obstet. 2018;140(2):137–45. https://doi.org/10.1002/ijgo.12373.
226. Volpe JJ. Neurological examination: Normal and abnormal fetuses. In. Neurology of the newborn, 4th ed. Philadelphia: WB Saunders, 2001:127.
227. Warriner D, Michaels J, Morris PD. Cardiac auscultation: normal and abnormal. Br J Hosp Med (Lond). 2019;80(2):C28–31. https://doi.org/10.12968/hmed.2019.80.2.C28.
228. Wellmann S, Koslowski A, Spanaus K, Zimmermann R, Burkhardt T. Fetal release of copeptin in response to maternal oxytocin administration: a randomized controlled trial. Obstet Gynecol. 2016;128(4):699–703. https://doi.org/10.1097/AOG.0000000000001594.
229. Welsh S, Elwell J, Manister NN, Gildersleeve RK. Implementing delayed umbilical cord clamping in cesarean birth using a novel method: a pilot study of feasibility and safety. J Midwifery Womens Health. 2020; https://doi.org/10.1111/jmwh.13075.
230. Wenger D, Düppe H, Nilsson JÅ, Tiderius CJ. Incidence of late-diagnosed hip dislocation after universal clinical screening in Sweden. JAMA Netw Open. 2019;2(11):e1914779. https://doi.org/10.1001/jamanetworkopen.2019.14779.
231. Whittaker E, Goldblatt D, McIntyre P, Levy O. Neonatal immunization: rationale, current state, and future prospects. Front Immunol. 2018;9:532. Published 2018 Apr 4. https://doi.org/10.3389/fimmu.2018.00532.
232. Widström AM, Brimdyr K, Svensson K, Cadwell K, Nissen E. Skin-to-skin contact the first hour after birth, underlying implications and clinical practice. Acta Paediatr. 2019;108:1192–204. https://doi.org/10.1111/apa.14754.
233. Widström A-M, Lilja G, Aaltomaa-Michalias P, Dahllöf A, Lintula M, Nissen E. Newborn behaviour to locate the breast when skin-to-skin: a possible method for enabling early self-regulation. Acta Paediatr Oslo Nor. 2011;1992:79–85.
234. Wikoff WR, Anfora AT, Liu J, Schultz PG, Lesley SA, Peters EC, Siuzdak G. Metabolomics analysis reveals large effects of gut microflora on mammalian blood metabolites. Proc Natl Acad SciUSA. 2009;106:3698–703. https://doi.org/10.1073/pnas.0812874106.
235. William E. benitz, committee on fetus and newborn. Hospital stay for healthy term newborn infants. Pediatrics May. 2015;135(5):948–53. https://doi.org/10.1542/peds.2015-0699.
236. Wilson JMG, Junger G. Principles and practice of screening for disease. Geneva: World Health Organization; 1968. https://www.who.int/ionizing_radiation/medical_radiation_exposure/munich-WHO-1968-Screening-Disease.pdf. (Accessed 1 Jan 2020).
237. Wilson LA, Murphy MS, Ducharme R, Denize K, Jadavji NM, Potter B, et al. Postnatal gestational age estimation via newborn screening analysis: application and potential. Expert Rev Proteomics. 2019;16(9):727–31. https://doi.org/10.1080/14789450.2019.1654863.
238. Wong RJ, Bhutani VK. Unconjugated hyperbilirubinemia in term and late preterm infants: Management. https://www.uptodate.com/contents/unconjugated-hyperbilirubinemia-in-term-and-late-preterm-infants-management#subscribeMessage. (Accessed 24 Jan 2020).
239. World Health Organization, UNICEF. Protecting, promoting, and supporting breastfeeding in facilities providing maternity and newborn services: the revised Baby-friendly Hospital Initiative, 2018. Implementation guidance. World Health Organization: Geneva, 2018. https://www.who.int/nutrition/publications/infantfeeding/bfhi-implementation/en/. (Accessed 9 Jan 2020).

240. World Health Organization. Guidance for national tuberculosis programmes on the management of tuberculosis in children. 2nd ed. Geneva: WHO; 2014. https://apps.who.int/iris/bitstream/handle/10665/112360/9789241548748_eng.pdf?sequence=1 (Accessed 20 Jan 2020).
241. World Health Organization. Guideline: Delayed umbilical cord clamping. World Health Organization: Geneva, 2014. http://www.who.int/elena/titles/cord_clamping/en/ (Accessed 20 Jan 2020).
242. World Health Organization. Hepatitis B vaccine. WHO position paper. Weekly Epidemiological Record. 2009;84(40):405–20. http://www.who.int/wer. (Accessed 20 Jan 2020).
243. World Health Organization. Polio vaccines and polio immunization in the pre-eradication era: WHO position paper. Weekly Epidemiological Record. 2010;85(23):213–28. http://www.who.int/wer. (Accessed 20 Jan 2020).
244. World Health Organization. WHO guidelines for the Treatment of Neisseria gonorrhoeae. World Health organization: Geneva, 2016. https://apps.who.int/iris/bitstream/handle/10665/246114/9789241549691-eng.pdf?sequence=1 (Accessed 20 Jan 2020).
245. World Health Organization. WHO Recommendation on postnatal care of the mother and the newborn. World Health organization: Geneva, 2014. https://apps.who.int/iris/bitstream/handle/10665/97603/9789241506649_eng.pdf?sequence=1 (Accessed 20 Jan 2020).
246. Wyllie J, Bruinenberg J, Roehr CC, Rüdiger M, Trevisanutoc D, Urlesberger B. European Resuscitation Council Guidelines for Resuscitation 2015 Section 7. Resuscitation and support of transition of babies at birth. Resuscitation. 2015;95:249–63. https://doi.org/10.1016/j.resuscitation.2015.07.029.
247. Yan J, Liu L, Zhu Y, Huang G, Wang PP. The association between breastfeeding and childhood obesity: A meta-analysis. BMC Public Health. 2014;14:1267.
248. Yorifuji J, Yorifuji T, Tachibana K, Nagai S, Kawai M, Momoi T, et al. Craniotabes in normal newborns: the earliest sign of subclinical vitamin D deficiency. J Clin Endocrinol Metab. 2008;93(5):1784–8. https://doi.org/10.1210/jc.2007-2254.
249. Yu VY, Dunn PM. Development of regionalized perinatal care. Semin Neonatol. 2004;9(2):89–97. https://doi.org/10.1016/j.siny.2003.08.011.
250. Zuppa AA, D'Andrea V, Catenazzi P, Scorrano A, Romagnoli C. Ophthalmia neonatorum: what kind of prophylaxis? J Matern Fetal Neonatal Med. 2011;24(6):769–73. https://doi.org/10.3109/14767058.2010.531326.
251. Zurynski Y, Grover CJ, Jalaludin B, Elliott EJ. Vitamin K deficiency bleeding in Australian infants 1993-2017: an Australian Paediatric Surveillance Unit study. Arch Dis Child. 2019:archdischild-2018-316424. https://doi.org/10.1136/archdischild-2018-316424.

Chapter 56
Palliative Care in Perinatology

Jussara de Lima e Souza

Definition of Pediatric Palliative Care

According to the World Health Organization (WHO), palliative care for children is the total active care of the child's body, mind, and spirit and involves supporting the family. It begins when the disease is diagnosed and continues regardless of whether treatment is directed at the disease. Healthcare providers should assess and alleviate the child's physical, psychological, and social suffering. Hence, curative and palliative care are complementary [1–3].

When to Take Care

During Pregnancy

With technological developments, many diagnoses of life-threatening diseases are already made during pregnancy. Therefore, care for these children and their families should be initiated during prenatal care.

After the detection of fetal malformation, it is necessary for the professional to make a careful assessment of the diagnosis and its prognosis, in order to start the discussion with the family about the possible treatments and care to be proposed for the child, pregnant woman, and other family members.

Some of these defects may present benign changes and, even without intrauterine treatment, they may even disappear. Other pathologies may require treatment even

J. d. L. e. Souza (✉)
Neonatology and Palliative Medicine, University of Campinas – UNICAMP, Clinic of Neonatology, Women's Hospital – CAISM, University of Campinas (UNICAMP), Campinas, Brazil

© Springer Nature Switzerland AG 2022

R. A. Moreira de Sá, E. B. d. Fonseca (eds.), *Perinatology*,
https://doi.org/10.1007/978-3-030-83434-0_56

before birth, with a high risk of complications or, in some cases, which may bring future complications to the functional and/or aesthetic health of these children [4].

Some of these changes may even be incompatible with life, and death may occur in the fetal phase or shortly after birth [5].

When a family "gets pregnant," there is an expectation for that life to come. Sometimes, these dreams existed before pregnancy. The diagnosis of a life-threatening disease of the fetus can bring disorders to the family, with the need to monitor an interdisciplinary care team [6].

The family will need guidance to understand the child's condition, to understand future needs and support to deal with the differences between the "idealized baby" and the "real baby."

In addition to this care for the family, in relation to their needs, there is a need for individualized therapeutic planning in relation to the child. In this planning, the team and family must define what is the best treatment to be given to the child and a birth plan, in which it is defined: place of birth, indication of delivery, who will accompany the delivery (team and family), indication or not of resuscitation procedures, and referral to intensive care units [7].

This integrated care will enable the construction and maintenance of the bond with the fetus, even for short survival [8–10].

Eligible Patients: malformed fetuses diagnosed with diseases with high morbidity and/or high mortality or with lethal disease [4] see Table 56.1.

Delivery Room

When the birth of an extreme premature child (less than 23 weeks and less than 400 g) or who presents potentially lethal malformations is expected, together with the family, exclusive comfort measures can be chosen, without a proposal for intensive treatment.

And, in this situation, promoting symptom control and maintaining the family-newborn bond in the delivery room [11].

Thus, according to the symptoms presented, the child may need analgesia or sedation or the association of both [12–14]:

(a) Analgesia

- Morphine – 0.05 mg/kg/dose subcutaneous (SC) or
- Fentanyl

Initial dosage of 1 to 2 mcg/kg intranasal (IN).

With recommendation of 0.1 to 0.3 mL IN per dose in a single nostril (larger volumes would be divided between the nostrils).

(b) Sedation

- Midazolam – 0.1 mg/kg/dose SC or IN.

The doses of drugs should be repeated as the evolution of the framework and continuous reassessment.

Table 56.1 Pathologies with high mortality and/or high morbidity or lethal disease [4]

	Fetal diagnosis	
Classification	Group	Pathology
Lethal anomalies	Genetic diseases	Trisomy 13, 15, or 18 Triploidy
	Nervous system malformations	Anencephaly/acrania Holoprosencephaly Large encephaloceles
	Cardiac malformations	Acardia Inoperable cardiac malformations
	Kidney malformations	Potter syndrome Renal agenesis Multicystic or dysplastic kidney, bilaterally Polycystic kidney disease with early onset
Uncertain diagnosis, but certain prognosis	Genetic diseases	Thanatophoric dwarfism Lethal forms of osteogenesis imperfecta
	Early-onset anhydramnia (pulmonary hypoplasia)	Potter syndrome with unknown etiology
	Nervous system malformations	Hydranencephaly
	Prematurity	Prematurity below 22 weeks
Uncertain diagnosis and prognosis	Genetic diseases	Metabolism errors that can be lethal even with available therapy
	Oligomania and anhydramnia starting in the third quarter	Dialysis renal failure
	Nervous system malformations	Complex or severe cases of meningomyelocele Neurodegenerative diseases, such as spinal muscular atrophy Severe congenital hydrocephalus with minimal brain growth
	Cardiac malformations	Some cases of left heart hypoplasia syndrome Cantrell pentalogy (*ectopia cordis*)
	Other structural abnormalities	Some cases of giant omphalocele Severe congenital diaphragmatic hernia with hypoplastic lungs Idiopathic nonimmune hydrops Inoperable united twins Multiple severe anomalies
	Prematurity	Viability limit (23–24 weeks)

Modified from: Oliveira et al. [4]

According to family acceptance and maternal conditions, keep the child in skin-to-skin contact.

Postnatal Period: During Hospitalization [15]

The planning of care to be offered to newborns should be based on their clinical condition and perspective of survival. Some children may be cured of their pathologies, others will die while still hospitalized, and some will become chronically ill.

As the focus of care is the individual and not the disease, the conduct should always be individualized.

Childcare

In general, children should receive symptomatic treatment in the face of apparent discomfort, as needed.

A. **Analgesia.**

Newborns admitted to intensive neonatal care units (NICU) are exposed daily to numerous painful procedures [16, 17].

Severely ill newborns can also have illnesses that are accompanied by painful conditions.

A.1. **Scales**

To assess the need for pain treatment and the effectiveness of the treatment instituted, systematic use of pain assessment scales is necessary.

Although there are several scales for pain assessment, only five have been validated [18]. The validated scales are Neonatal Facial Coding System [19]; Premature Infant Pain Profile (PIPP) [20]; Neonatal Pain, Agitation, and Sedation Scale (N-PASS) [21]; Behavioral Infant Pain Profile [22]; and Douleur Aiguë du Nouveau-né [23].

A.2. **Treatment**

There are controversies regarding complications related to the effect that opioids have on neurological development, but there is also evidence of how much stress can compromise the development of patients [24].

A.2.1. **Non-pharmacological Treatment**

- **Breastfeeding.**
  In a systematic study was observed that breastfeeding was as effective in controlling pain in single procedures in neonates [25].
- **Skin-to-Skin Contact.**
  Skin-to-skin contact seems to improve pain indicators in the newborn [26, 27].

- **Therapeutic Massage.**
  In a study that evaluated patients undergoing heel puncture, there was an improvement in pain assessment according to the NIPS scale [28].
- **Sensory Stimulation.**
  The association of simultaneous stimuli of the four elements (touch, taste, hearing, and vision) seems to be more efficient than the use of sucrose alone [18].
- **Pharmacological Treatment.**
- **Sucrose.**
  The use of sucrose was effective in decreasing the pain of newborns in single events (e.g., venipuncture) and is indicated in premature or term children [29].
  Suggested dose: 0.2 to 0.5 mL/kg of 25% sucrose (use 2 minutes before the procedure) [30, 31].

Non-opioid Analgesics

The use of non-opioid analgesics may decrease the use of the opioid. Nonhormonal anti-inflammatory drugs should only be used to close the ductus arteriosus [18].

- **Paracetamol.**

  Dose:
  Term: 10 to 15 mg/kg every 6 hours.
  Premature: 10 mg/kg every 6 hours.

- **Dipyrone.**

  Dose: 10 to 15 mg/kg every 6 hours.
- **Lidocaine.**

  Dose: 5 mg/kg in local infiltration.
- **EMLA.**

  Dose: one application (once a day) – 30 to 60 minutes before the procedure.

Opioid Analgesics

They are the most used agents for persistent pain, although there is still a need for studies to define adequate doses and long-term effects [18].

- **Morphine**

  Dose:
  Intravenous intermittent: 0.05 to 0.20 mg/kg every 4–6 hours (infusion – 30 minutes).

Continuous infusion, with the following dosage:

Term: 0.005 to 0.010 mg/kg per hour
Premature: 0.002 to 0.005 mg/kg per hour
Intermittent orally: 0.30 to 0.60 mg/kg.

- **Tramadol**

  Dose: 0.1 to 1 mg/kg IV or PO every 4 to 6 hours, in slow infusion.

- **Fentanyl**

  Dose:
  Intermittent: 1 to 4 mcg/kg IV every 2–4 hours (slow infusion – 30 minutes).

Continuous infusion, with the following dosage:

Term: 0.5 to 1.0 mcg/kg per hour
Premature: 0.5 mcg/kg per hour

- **Other Drugs**

  Other medications have been proposed for use, such as ketamine, requiring further studies for the neonatal population [32].

B. **Palliative Sedation**

  Palliative sedation is indicated to control symptoms that do not respond to other symptomatic treatments, such as dyspnea.

- **Midazolam**

  Dose: 0.03 to 0.1 mg/kg per hour, continuous IV.
- **Other Drugs**

  Other medications have been proposed for use, such as clonidine, propofol, and dexmedetomidine, with studies that have shown good results but need to be expanded [33–36].

Care for Family Members After the Loss

Because grief does not end after death, parents will still need care after the loss.

The legal procedures for burial are usually not known to people. Therefore, there is a need for information [15].

Surveys of parents' opinions have emphasized the importance of a meeting to discuss death with the neonatologist. This usually occurs a few weeks or months later [2].

In the case of necropsies, the results can be reported at this time. At these meetings parents may want to address the implications for future pregnancies [15].

Bioethics and Decision-Making

Therapeutic Adequacy

Much has been discussed about the futility of some procedures and the need to create adequate parameters for limiting life-sustaining treatments.

With the increase in rates of extreme prematurity and prenatal diagnoses of conditions that limit life, it is necessary to pay attention to the discussions about individualized treatment. Thus, we must discuss what is the most appropriate treatment for that patient, according to their diagnosis and evolution. From there, it can be considered that, in that condition, the most appropriate would be the limitation of intensive treatment, or even the adoption of palliative care, with comfort measures [2].

There are situations in which there is greater agreement between team members and family members on the best way forward. However, there are conditions in which there is disagreement regarding the best treatment to be instituted. The different opinions are legally correct and ethically defensible. This is the gray zone [37].

Decision-Making

Decision-making in relation to the treatment of critically ill newborns should be based on the discussion between health team professionals and parents. But, usually, the way these groups perceive the child's condition is different. Parents tend to accept frames of severe future disabilities better. Conflicts usually arise when parents want treatments that professionals consider futile [37].

In this discussion, the relationship between doctors and parents is unbalanced, due to the difference in knowledge that exists regarding the topic discussed. In addition, the emotions that parents experience in this process make it difficult for them to understand the information given.

There is yet another aspect. The way information is transmitted shapes its content and, consequently, the decision to be made. This process is known as "choice architecture" [38].

Professionals must be aware of the ethical role they play in this process. They must be able to assist parents not only in understanding their clinical condition and prognosis but also in the consequences of their choices [37].

For this process some steps must be followed [39].

Health Team Discussion

The team's discussion should be based on the analysis of the patient's conditions, considering their diagnosis, evolution, previous complications, dependence on technology, and prognosis.

Deliberation

Respect for the patient's right to autonomy is essential, which, in the case of neonates, is delegated to parents [40].

End-of-life discussions with parents should be individualized and personalized. Parents are not prepared to deal with difficult situations, and each will react in a different way.

For parents to be able to contribute to decision-making, professionals need to be aware of their expectations and desires [2].

Parents must be involved in the deliberation, and, together with the team, they must determine their child's best interest, building a life and end-of-life project for them.

Parents' views can vary widely from previous pregnancy experiences: mothers with healthy previous children may consider the risk of disability differently than a mother with multiple losses [2].

Ethnicity and religion also influence acceptance of withdrawal from intensive care.

A model was created with criteria to be valued by the team in order to individualize this communication: SOBPIE [41].

- *Situation*: what is the situation, and how it should occur communication with family.
- *Opinions and options*: what are the alternatives and biases.
- *Basic interactions*: thinking about the "meeting" between professionals and family.
- *Parents*: what is the information about parents.
- *Information*: what information parents need.
- *Emotions*: which emotions, paternal and team, are permeating the discussion.

In conflict situations, when parents insist on interventions that professionals consider inadequate, the team must [42]:

- Identify, for the family, the damage and suffering inflicted on the patient.
- Promote intense emotional support.
- Maintain a good relationship with the family despite the disagreement of opinions.

Applying Decisions

Some attitudes can be taken in order to improve decision-making: greater education of professionals and family members about the palliative care (CP) process, improved support for professionals, improved communication in the NICU, adoption of a PC protocol, and involvement of the Ethics Committee.

As for the parents' hope, the team can work on its reformulation, moving from the hope of a cure to the hope that the child and family will have their suffering relieved [43].

All discussions held must be recorded in the medical record, informing who was present and how the decision was made [39].

Eligible Patients

The most severely ill patients, hospitalized in the NICU, are severe extreme premature or malformed.

The issues regarding malformed children were discussed in item 2.1.

Extreme Prematurity

The World Association of Perinatal Medicine considers that life support treatments should not be initiated or continued if the physician cannot expect the prevention of imminent death or minimization of morbidity and maximization of functional status [39].

The British Association of Perinatal Medicine has created a guide for the management of children under 26 weeks [2, 44]. The guideline is that in cases <23 weeks, usually do not resuscitate; 23 to 24 weeks, assess parents' wishes; 24 to 25 weeks, resuscitate and reassess; and 25 weeks resuscitate and refer for intensive care.

Despite technological development, the viability limits, between 22 and 23 weeks, have remained stable among developed countries [45].

References

1. Feudtner C. Collaborative communication in pediatric palliative care: a foundation for problem-solving and decision-making. Pediatr Clin North Am. 2007;54(5):583–607.
2. Warrick C, Perera L, Murdoch E, Nicholl RM. Guidance for withdrawal and withholding of intensive care as part of neonatal end-of-life care. Br Med Bull. 2011;98:99–113.
3. Organization WH. WHO definition of palliative care for children. Accessed on January 30, 2020. Available from: https://www.who.int/cancer/palliative/definition/en/.
4. Oliveira FF, Nascimento NB, Benute G, Barbosa T, Bolibio R, Gomes ALH, et al. Cuidados Paliativos no Período Pré-Natal. In: Rubio AV, Souza JL, editors. Cuidado Paliativo Pediátrico e Perinatal. Rio de Janeiro: Editora Atheneu; 2018.
5. Farraposo S, Montenegro N, Matias A. Evaluation of the role of first-trimester obstetric ultrasound in the detection of major anomalies: a systematic review. J Perinat Med. 2014;42(2):141–9.
6. Titapant V, Chuenwattana P. Psychological effects of fetal diagnoses of non-lethal congenital anomalies on the experience of pregnant women during the remainder of their pregnancy. J Obstet Gynaecol Res. 2015;41(1):77–83.
7. Leuthner S, Jones EL. Fetal concerns program: a model for perinatal palliative care. MCN Am J Matern Child Nurs. 2007;32(5):272–8.
8. Hoeldtke NJ, Calhoun BC. Perinatal hospice. Am J Obstet Gynecol. 2001;185(3):525–9.
9. Calhoun BC, Napolitano P, Terry M, Bussey C, Hoeldtke NJ. Perinatal hospice. Comprehensive care for the family of the fetus with a lethal condition. J Reprod Med. 2003;48(5):343–8.

10. Fisher M, Ridley S. Uncertainty in end-of-life care and shared decision making. Crit Care Resusc. 2012;14(1):81–7.
11. Garbi LR, Shah S, La Gamma EF. Delivery room hospice. Acta paediatrica (Oslo, Norway: 1992). 2016;105(11):1261–5.
12. Chaudhary R, Silwal A, Gupta A, Kelsall W. Drugs used for comfort care after withdrawal of intensive treatment in tertiary neonatal units in the UK. neonatal units in the UK. Arch Dis Child Fetal Neonatal Ed. 2012;97(6):F487.
13. Harlos MS, Stenekes S, Lambert D, Hohl C, Chochinov HM. Intranasal fentanyl in the palliative care of newborns and infants. J Pain Symptom Manage. 2013;46(2):265–74.
14. Parravicini E. Neonatal palliative care. Curr Opin Pediatr. 2017;29(2):135–40.
15. Marba STM, Costa SMM, Souza JL, Bianchi MO. Cuidado Paliativo em Neonatologia. In: Marba STM, Mezzacappa Filho F, editors. Manual de Neonatologia UNICAMP. 2nd ed. Rio de Janeiro: Revinter; 2009. p. 425–9.
16. Anand KJ, Aranda JV, Berde CB, Buckman S, Capparelli EV, Carlo W, et al. Summary proceedings from the neonatal pain-control group. Pediatrics. 2006;117(3 Pt 2):S9–S22.
17. Carbajal R, Rousset A, Danan C, Coquery S, Nolent P, Ducrocq S, et al. Epidemiology and treatment of painful procedures in neonates in intensive care units. JAMA. 2008;300(1):60–70.
18. Lim Y, Godambe S. Prevention and management of procedural pain in the neonate: an update, American Academy of Pediatrics, 2016. Arch Dis Child Fetal Neonatal Ed. 2017;102(5):254–6.
19. Grunau RE, Oberlander T, Holsti L, Whitfield MF. Bedside application of the Neonatal Facial Coding System in pain assessment of premature neonates. Pain. 1998;76(3):277–86.
20. Stevens B, Johnston C, Petryshen P, Taddio A. Premature infant pain profile: development and initial validation. Clinical J Pain. 1996;12(1):13–22.
21. Deindl P, Unterasinger L, Kappler G, Werther T, Czaba C, Giordano V, et al. Successful implementation of a neonatal pain and sedation protocol at 2 NICUs. Pediatrics. 2013;132(1):e211–e8.
22. Holsti L, Grunau RE. Initial validation of the Behavioral Indicators of Infant Pain (BIIP). Pain. 2007;132(3):264–72.
23. Carbajal R, Paupe A, Hoenn E, Lenclen R, Olivier-Martin M. APN: evaluation behavioral scale of acute pain in newborn infants. Arch Pediatr. 1997;4(7):623–8.French.
24. Doesburg SM, Chau CM, Cheung TPL, Moiseev A, Ribary U, Herdman AT, et al. Neonatal pain-related stress, functional cortical activity and visual-perceptual abilities in school-age children born at extremely low gestational age. Pain. 2013;154(10):1946–52.
25. Shah PS, Herbozo C, Aliwalas LL, Shah VS. Breastfeeding or breast milk for procedural pain in neonates. Cochrane Database Syst Rev. 2012;12:Cd004950.
26. Johnston C, Campbell-Yeo M, Disher T, Benoit B, Fernandes A, Streiner D, et al. Skin-to-skin care for procedural pain in neonates. Cochrane Database Syst Rev. 2017;2:Cd008435.
27. Olsson E, Ahlsen G, Eriksson M. Skin-to-skin contact reduces near-infrared spectroscopy pain responses in premature infants during blood sampling. Acta Paediatr. 2016;105(4):376–80.
28. Jain S, Kumar P, McMillan DD. Prior leg massage decreases pain responses to heel stick in preterm babies. J Paediatr Child Health. 2006;42(9):505–8.
29. Stevens B, Yamada J, Ohlsson A, Haliburton S, Shorkey A. Sucrose for analgesia in newborn infants undergoing painful procedures. The Cochrane database of systematic reviews. 2016;7(7):CD001069-CD.
30. Committee on fetus and newborn and section on anesthesiology and pain medicine. Prevention and management of procedural pain in the neonate: an update. Pediatrics. 2016;137(2):e20154271.
31. Harrison D, Beggs S, Stevens B. Sucrose for procedural pain management in infants. Pediatrics. 2012;130(5):918–25.
32. Elalouf C, Le Moing AG, Fontaine C, Leke A, Kongolo G, Gondry J, et al. Prospective follow-up of a cohort of preterm infants<33 WG receiving ketamine for tracheal intubation in the delivery room: neurological outcome at 1 and 2 years. Arch Pediatr. 2018;25(4):295–300.
33. Romantsik O, Calevo MG, Norman E, Bruschettini M. Clonidine for sedation and analgesia for neonates receiving mechanical ventilation. The Cochrane database of systematic reviews. 2017;5(5):CD012468-CD.
34. van Hoorn CE, Hoeks SE, Essink H, Tibboel D, de Graaff JC. A systematic review and narrative synthesis on the histological and neurobehavioral long-term effects of dexmedetomidine. Paediatr Anaesth. 2019;29(2):125–36.

35. Chrysostomou C, Schulman SR, Herrera Castellanos M, Cofer BE, Mitra S, da Rocha MG, et al. A phase II/III, multicenter, safety, efficacy, and pharmacokinetic study of dexmedetomidine in preterm and term neonates. J Pediatr. 2014;164(2):276–82.e823.
36. Thewissen L, Caicedo A, Dereymaeker A, Van Huffel S, Naulaers G, Allegaert K, et al. Cerebral autoregulation and activity after propofol for endotracheal intubation in preterm neonates. Pediatr Res. 2018;84(5):719–25.
37. Lantos JD. Ethical problems in decision making in the Neonatal ICU. The New England journal of medicine. 2018;379(19):1851–60.
38. Thaler RH, Sustein CR, Balz JP. Choice Architecture. Accessed on January 30, 2020. Available from: https://poseidon01.ssrn.com/delivery.php?ID=390114006122096109073074102096079112056050065027039051078098006067064087112072120109005035107005061025044073075018123127065094038037078052000086108023102005109029090033033078082120080082081020020017111093002120112026075093111109003107092020113085064098&EXT=pdf.
39. Dageville C, Betremieux P, Gold F, Simeoni U. The French Society of Neonatology's proposals for neonatal end-of-life decision-making. Neonatology. 2011;100(2):206–14.
40. Bellieni CV, Buonocore G. Flaws in the assessment of the best interests of the newborn. Acta Paediatr. 2009;98(4):613–7.
41. Janvier A, Barrington K, Farlow B. Communication with parents concerning withholding or withdrawing of life-sustaining interventions in neonatology. Semin Perinatol. 2014;38(1):38–46.
42. Workman S, McKeever P, Harvey W, Singer PA. Intensive care nurses' and physicians' experiences with demands for treatment: some implications for clinical practice. J Crit Care. 2003;18(1):17–21.
43. Catlin A. Transition from curative efforts to purely palliative care for neonates: does physiology matter? Adv Neonatal Care. 2011;11(3):216–22.
44. Kaempf JW, Tomlinson MW, Campbell B, Ferguson L, Stewart VT. Counseling pregnant women who may deliver extremely premature infants: medical care guidelines, family choices, and neonatal outcomes. Pediatrics. 2009;123(6):1509–15.
45. Berger TM. Guidelines for the management of extremely preterm deliveries in the grey zone of viability between 23 and 24 weeks' gestation vary widely in developed countries. Evid Based Med. 2015;20(6):227.

Chapter 57
Hypoxic-Ischemic Encephalopathy

Maria Elisabeth Lopes Moreira

Introduction

Hypoxic-ischemic encephalopathy (HIE) or perinatal asphyxia occurs in one to three per thousand live births at term. Of the newborns who suffered perinatal asphyxia, 15–20% will die in the postnatal period, and an additional 25% will develop severe and permanent neuropathological sequelae, including mental retardation, motor deficits, perceptual visual dysfunction, increased hyperactivity, cerebral palsy, and epilepsy [1].

The results of HIE are devastating and permanent, making it a great burden for the patient, family, and society. The pathophysiology underlying perinatal HIE is difficult to study in humans; thus, most of the knowledge produced in relation to this pathophysiological condition is derived from animal studies. Rodents are the animals most used in SHI research, followed by pigs and sheep [2].

The neuropathological characteristics of perinatal asphyxia can vary considerably with the child's gestational age, the nature of the insult, vascular territories, and the types of intervention. It is impossible to generalize the different injury profiles seen after a hypoxic-ischemic insult, and several factors can influence the type of brain injury, such as gestational age, cell susceptibility, vascular territories, and type of insult [1–3].

Gestational Age Maturity plays an important role in the susceptibility of brain structures to hypoxic-ischemic insults. Neuropathological studies indicate that many critical neuronal groups are more vulnerable to injury in immature animals, especially related to a higher density and function of excitatory amino acid recep-

M. E. L. Moreira (✉)
Instituto Fernandes Figueira - Fiocruz, Clinica Perinatal Laranjeiras,
Rio de Janeiro, RJ, Brazil
e-mail: elisabeth.moreira@iff.fiocruz.br

© Springer Nature Switzerland AG 2022
R. A. Moreira de Sá, E. B. d. Fonseca (eds.), *Perinatology*,
https://doi.org/10.1007/978-3-030-83434-0_57

tors and a greater vulnerability to attack by reactive oxygen species (ROS) and reactive nitrogen species (RNS). Hypoxic-ischemic insults that occur before 20 weeks resulting from serious maternal diseases can lead to heterotopy or polymicrogyria because in this gestational period, the neuronal migration that happens until the 21st week of gestation is still occurring. Insults affecting the brain between 26 and 36 weeks of gestational age predominantly damage white matter causing periventricular leukomalacia, and insults that happen after 35 weeks result predominantly in damage to the gray substance (posterior putamen, ventrolateral nucleus, and thalamus). There is a long-standing general notion that the perinatal brain is more tolerant of asphyxia than that of the adult [3].

Cell Susceptibility Neurons are more susceptible to hypoxic damage than are glial cells, and the most susceptible neurons are the pyramidal cells of the hippocampus and neocortex and Purkinje cells of the cerebellum [1, 3].

Vascular Territories Injury to vascular beds occurs in regions that are more vulnerable to reduced cerebral perfusion in places where the blood supply is weaker. These tissues are at the most distant points of an arterial anastomosis and are exposed to damage when the perfusion pressure drops, usually as a result of compromised cardiac output and low blood pressure. These vulnerable areas change with advancing development. Between 26 and 34 weeks, the periventricular white matter may be vulnerable due to its position between the ventriculopetal and ventriculofugal arterioles [3, 4].

At term, the cortical vascular bed (parasagittal region) is present between the three main arteries that irrigate each hemisphere. The paracentral gyrus appears to be more vulnerable, with less sensitivity in the posterior parietal region. The motor cortex is particularly susceptible to injuries, which corroborates the observation that spastic cerebral palsy is the main sequel to the term hypoxic-ischemic insult. As a corollary, the hippocampus and temporal and occipital lobe are more resistant to this type of insult. Volpe and colleagues, using positron emission tomography to measure regional cerebral blood flow in 17 full-term asphyxiated newborns, found a consistent decrease in blood flow to the parasagittal region of both cerebral hemispheres in most children. The groove bases are also sensitive to hypoxic-ischemic insult. Reduced perfusion in small vessels at the base of the grooves during hypoxia-ischemia leads to columnar necrosis and can lead to ulegyria in the older child's brain [1–3].

Type of Insult In studies on primate animals, two different patterns of hypoxic-ischemic insult were modeled, which have shown different patterns of neuronal damage, depending on the type of insult. Acute asphyxia was produced in fetal monkeys by clamping the umbilical cord. This produced lesions in the thalamus, brain stem, and spinal cord structures. The longer the duration of the acute attack was, the more extensive the damage was in these regions. Little damage has been reported in larger structures [4, 5].

The second model was the attempt to imitate an insult by partial asphyxia lasting 1–5 hours. This damage produced insults predominantly in the cerebral hemispheres, usually with preservation of the brain stem, hippocampus, and temporal and occipital lobes. Damage was also seen in the basal ganglia and cerebellum. In half of the animals studied, significant asymmetry was observed between the damage to both hemispheres [4–6].

Clinical Features

The clinical picture is variable and depends on the degree of cerebral insult. It can vary from mild hypotonia to hypertonia, weak or high-pitched crying, stupor, and coma, and convulsions are frequent. aEEG is an important ally in making decisions about the treatment of seizures. In addition to brain injury, other organs may be affected, such as the kidney and heart. Neonates with suspected HIE are classified according to the Sarnat staging system, which evaluates the level of consciousness, muscle tone, tendon reflexes, complex reflexes, and autonomic function. The Sarnat stage classifies neonatal hypoxic-ischemic encephalopathy into the following three categories: stage I (mild), stage II (moderate), and stage III (severe) [7].

Potential Therapies for Neonatal Hypoxic-Ischemic Encephalopathy

Intensive Supportive Care

In most cases, admission to intensive care units will be necessary for monitoring and addressing potential complications. The use of the Sarnat and Sarnat scale can help in the monitoring of brain impairment as well as transfontanelle ultrasound, EEG, and NIRS. Other organs can be affected such as the heart, kidney, and intestines. Perinatal asphyxia is a major cause of death and disability worldwide, and intensive supportive care in general is the main handling to be done. These precautions include the correction of hemodynamic and respiratory disorders (hypotension, metabolic acidosis, and maintenance of adequate ventilation); correction of metabolic disorders of glucose, calcium, magnesium, and electrolytes; treatment of seizures if present; and monitoring for other system dysfunctions organic, such acute renal failure [8].

Maintaining adequate ventilation and adequate perfusion is a central aspect of supportive care. Oxygen deprivation can lead to disorders of cerebrovascular self-regulation and increase white matter damage. On the other hand, severe hyperoxia in the first hours of life can contribute to increased oxidative stress, with long-term neurological consequences [1, 8].

Seizures Control

The presence of seizures, which occur practically in the first hours, is generally a predictor of a worse prognosis. Therefore, anti-seizure drugs are among the most commonly used drugs after an episode of hypoxic-ischemic syndrome. Energy metabolism may be compromised by hyperactive neurons and, along with acute energy deprivation after seizures, may be implicated in the occurrence of excitotoxicity. Thus, the therapeutic value of anti-seizure drugs can include not only controlling seizure activity itself but also potentially bringing benefits to compromised cellular energy metabolism. Phenobarbital and topiramate are the drugs most used to treat seizures [1, 8, 9].

Renal Function

Abnormalities in renal function can occur in 23 to 70% in newborns with severe asphyxia. Water restriction is necessary in children with inappropriate antidiuretic hormone secretion and in those with alterations in tubular renal function. The water supply, in these cases, must be based on the dosages of blood and urinary electrolytes.

Acute renal failure should be handled carefully with daily dosages of plasma and urinary creatinine, plasma and urinary electrolytes, and daily weight gain. Kidney failure usually lasts a few days and must be handled conservatively. Chronic kidney failure and the need for dialysis are rare.

Cardiovascular System

Hypotension is a common complication after a hypoxic-ischemic insult, and volume supply is often ineffective in restoring blood pressure. The use of dopamine (5 to 15 μg/kg/minute) has been shown to be more effective in restoring blood pressure. Other changes in the cardiovascular system described are acute cardiac dilation with tricuspid regurgitation, myocardial ischemia, and ischemic necrosis of the papillary muscle [1, 8].

Troponin measurements and electrocardiographic assessment can be used to assess myocardial damage as well as echocardiogram.

Neuroimaging

Initial transfontanelle ultrasonography is the most used imaging test in neonatal units. Cerebral edema may be frequent after an insult but later the MRI is the test to be used. The ideal would be to do it in the first week of life as soon as the newborn has clinical possibilities of being transported to the examination site. Bedside resonances are generally available at research sites. Magnetic resonance imaging (MRI) can provide detail of the soft tissues of the fetal and neonatal brain that cannot be obtained by any other imaging modality. Conventional T1- and T2-weighted sequences provide anatomic detail of the normally developing brain and can demonstrate lesions, including those associated with preterm birth, hypoxic-ischemic encephalopathy, perinatal arterial stroke, infections, and congenital malformations. Specialized imaging techniques can be used to assess cerebral vasculature (magnetic resonance angiography and venography), cerebral metabolism (magnetic resonance spectroscopy), cerebral perfusion (arterial spin labeling), and function (functional MRI) [10].

Neuroprotective Strategies

Therapeutic Hypothermia

Hypothermia has been effective in reducing neurological sequelae, particularly in newborns with moderate HIE, and in improving the long-term prognosis of newborns with HIE. Meta-analysis studies have shown that the use of therapeutic hypothermia decreases mortality and improves prognosis regarding the neurodevelopment of infants with HIE [1, 11].

There is evidence from large randomized trials and meta-analysis demonstrating that induced hypothermia (33.5–34.5 °C), when started within the 6-h window after the birth of full-term asphyxiated newborns, is beneficial in reducing mortality and neurodevelopmental delay in the follow-up at 3–5 years of life [11–15] Well-organized protocols for hypothermia indication as well as adequate rewarming are necessary.

The neuroprotective strategy of therapeutic hypothermia involves the modulation of some irreversible injury mechanisms, such as inflammatory cascade inhibition, reduced production of reactive oxygen species, reduction in the metabolic rate with reduced oxygen consumption and carbon dioxide production, and an endogenous neuroprotective effect. There are two therapeutic hypothermia methods: selective head cooling and total body cooling. The target body temperature is 34.5 °C for selective head cooling and 33.5 °C for total body cooling. Temperatures lower than 32 °C are less neuroprotective, and temperatures below 30 °C are very dangerous, with severe complications. Therapeutic hypothermia must start within the first 6 h after birth, as studies have shown that this represents the therapeutic window for the hypoxic-ischemic event. Therapy must be maintained for 72 h, with very strict control of the newborn's body temperature. It has been shown that therapeutic hypothermia is effective in reducing neurologic impairment, especially in full-term or near-term newborns with moderate hypoxic-ischemic encephalopathy [11–16]. However there is no current evidence about to recommend routine therapeutic hypothermia for babies with mild encephalopathy, and significant benefits or harm cannot be excluded [17].

The indication of therapeutic hypothermia under clearly defined protocols for newborns follows the recommendations from ILCOR and protocols from clinical trials: newborns with gestational age >35 weeks, with birth weight >1800 g, who have fewer than 6 h of life, and who meet the following criteria: umbilical cord blood gas analysis or in the first hour of life with pH <7.0 or base excess (BE) <−16 or history of perinatal acute event (placental abruption, cord prolapse), Apgar score of 5 or less in the tenth minute of life, need for mechanical ventilation beyond the tenth minute of life, or any of the following associated with evidence of moderate to severe encephalopathy before 6 h of life: seizure, level of consciousness, spontaneous activity, posture, tone, reflexes, and autonomic system [18].

Drugs

At the moment, no individual neuroprotective agent is considered to be proven safe and effective for the prevention of neurological sequelae in newborns after hypoxic-ischemic insults. Knowledge about the biochemical and cellular mechanisms of neuronal injury after a hypoxic-ischemic episode has helped in the search for interventions to interrupt these deleterious cascades, mainly focusing on the potential effects of free radical scavengers, such as N-acetylcysteine (NAC) and allopurinol, magnesium, glutamate receptor blockers, erythropoietin (Epo), and melatonin [1, 11, 19, 20].

NAC is a free radical scavenger and has been studied to minimize hypoxia induced by brain ischemia injury in several acute models. The combined therapy of NAC and systemic hypothermia would decrease the volume of infarction and the expression of myelin after focal HI injury [20].

Treatment with allopurinol, a xanthine oxidase inhibitor and responsible for washing free radicals, also has a benefit in reducing cerebral edema and neuropathological damage after neonatal HIE. However, a randomized, controlled, blinded study using it did not show a reduction in mortality or morbidity [20].

Erythropoietin, the main hematopoietic growth factor, has been considered to have beneficial effects on various diseases of the nervous system based on the effects of preventing metabolic breakdown, neuronal and vascular degeneration, and activation of inflammatory cells. Gonzalez et al. demonstrated that the treatment of Epo preserves hemispheric brain volume after an occlusive brain injury in P10 rats. There are several studies underway on the use of erythropoietin associated with hypothermia after a perinatal asphyxia with promising results. Initial phase I clinical trials of monotherapy with Epo (i.e., without TH) administered in the first week of life to full-term newborns with asphyxia showed viability, safety, and improvements in neurological outcome. However, studies are still limited by the small sample size. In a larger randomized, phase III, placebo-controlled study, monotherapy with Epo has been shown to decrease the combined risk of death or moderate to severe condition, with an average age of 19 months in treatment (40%)

compared to placebo (70%). However, in the era of therapeutic hypothermia, clinical trials began to investigate Epo as an adjunct to neonatal asphyxia [19–22].

Other experimental studies on the potential value of magnesium sulfate reveal that glutamate receptor blockers have contradictory results. Some studies show a significant reduction in cerebral palsy, but others report the association of high doses with neonatal hypotension, which can cancel out its beneficial effects [1, 19].

Conclusion

Hypoxia-ischemia in the perinatal period is a major cause of neonatal death and long-term disability. There have been advances in the investigation of cellular processes and molecular mechanisms underlying HIE in the past two decades. Hypothermia is the only effective treatment for neonatal HIE at present. The combined therapy of hypothermia and other neuroprotective strategies, with a focus on preventing acute injuries, increasing the therapeutic window of time and improving neural repair can help improve the neurological results of HIE. The next phase of clinical trials in neonatal encephalopathy focuses on adjuvant therapies for hypothermia aimed at alternative recovery mechanisms during the process of hypoxic brain injury. The identification of babies eligible for neuroprotective therapies begins with the clinical detection of brain injury and the classification of severity. The combination of a variety of biomarkers with clinical examination, EEG, and movement patterns with study designs and innovative analysis of clinical trials can help target children with the most appropriate and timely treatments. The timing of magnetic resonance imaging (MRI) and MRI spectroscopy after hypoxic-ischemic encephalopathy helps to identify the acute perinatal nature of the lesion (days 3 to 7) and assesses the complete extent and evolution of the lesion (days 10 to 21). The early intermediate outcome of neuroprotective interventions can best be defined by neuroimaging 21 days after injury, but the recognition of changes in the complete path of neurological development is not yet defined. Functional recovery can be assessed using a trajectory of assessments of neurological development in childhood [23].

References

1. Volpe JJ, Inder TE, Darras BT, de Vries LS, du Plessis AJ, Neil JJ, Pearlman J. Volpe's neurology of the newborn. 6th ed. Elsevier; 2017.
2. Graham EM, Ruis KA, Hartman AL, Northington FJ, Fox HE. A systematic review of the role of intrapartum hypoxia-ischemia in the causation of neonatal encephalopathy. Am J Obstet Gynecol. 2008;199(6):587–95.
3. Johnston MV, Trescher WH, Ishida A, Nakajima W, Zipursky A. Neurobiology of hypoxic-ischemic injury in the developing brain. Pediat Res. 2001;49(6):735–41.

4. Lai MC, Yang SN. Perinatal hypoxic-ischemic encephalopathy. J Biomed Biotechnol. 2011;2011:609813.
5. de Vries LS, Groenendaal F. Patterns of neonatal hypoxic-ischaemic brain injury. Neuroradiology. 2010;52(6):555–66.
6. Goriely A, Geers MGD, Holzapfel GA, Jayamohan J, Jerusalem A, Sivaloganat S, et al. Mechanics of the brain: perspectives, challenges, and opportunities. Biomech Model Mechanobiol. 2015;14:931–65.
7. Sarnat HB, Sarnat MS. Neonatal encephalopathy following fetal distress: a clinical and electroencephalographic study. Arch Neurol. 1976;33(10):696–705.12.
8. Douglas-Escobar M, Weiss MD. Hypoxic-ischemic encephalopathy a review for the clinician. JAMA Pediatr. 2015. Available https://www.perinatal.com.br/simposio2016/pdf/aula04-asfixia-review.pdf.
9. Glass HC. Neonatal seizures. Advances in mechanisms and management. Clin Perinatal. 2014;41:177–90.
10. Counsell SJ, Arichi T, Arulkumaran S, Rutherford MA. Fetal and neonatal neuroimaging. Neonatal Neurol. 2019:67–103.
11. Levene MI, de Vries LS. Hypoxic-Ischemic Encephalopathy. In: Martin RJ, Fanaroff AA, Walsh M, editors. Neonatal-perinatal medicine: diseases of fetus and infant. 11th ed. Elsevier; 2019.
12. Azzopardi DV, Strohm B, Edwards AD, Dyet L, Halliday HL, Juszczak E, Kapellou O, Levene M, Marlow N, Porter E, Thoresen M, Whitelaw A, Brocklehurst P, TOBY Study Group. Moderate hypothermia to treat perinatal asphyxial encephalopathy. N Engl J Med. 2009;361(14):1349–58. https://doi.org/10.1056/NEJMoa0900854. Erratum in: N Engl J Med. 2010 Mar 18;362(11):1056.
13. Laptook AR, Shankaran S, Tyson JE, Munoz B, Bell EF, Goldberg RN, Parikh NA, Ambalavanan N, Pedroza C, Pappas A, Das A, Chaudhary AS, Ehrenkranz RA, Hensman AM, Van Meurs KP, Chalak LF, Khan AM, Hamrick SEG, Sokol GM, Walsh MC, Poindexter BB, Faix RG, Watterberg KL, Frantz ID 3rd, Guillet R, Devaskar U, Truog WE, Chock VY, Wyckoff MH, McGowan EC, Carlton DP, Harmon HM, Brumbaugh JE, Cotten CM, Sánchez PJ, Hibbs AM, Higgins RD; Eunice Kennedy Shriver National Institute of Child Health and Human Development Neonatal Research Network. Effect of therapeutic hypothermia initiated after 6 hours of age on death or disability among newborns with hypoxic-ischemic encephalopathy: a randomized clinical trial. JAMA. 2017;318(16):1550–60.
14. Azzopardi D, Strohm B, Marlow N, Brocklehurst P, Deierl A, Eddama O, Goodwin J, Halliday HL, Juszczak E, Kapellou O, Levene M, Linsell L, Omar O, Thoresen M, Tusor N, Whitelaw A, Edwards AD, TOBY Study Group. Effects of hypothermia for perinatal asphyxia on childhood outcomes. N Engl J Med. 2014;371(2):140–9.
15. Campbell H, Eddama O, Azzopardi D, Edwards AD, Strohm B, Rivero-Arias O. Hypothermia for perinatal asphyxia: trial-based quality of life at 6–7 years. Arch Dis Child. 2018;103(7):654–9.
16. Jacobs SE, Berg M, Hunt R, Tarnow-Mordi WO, Inder TE, Davis PG. Cooling for newborns with hypoxic ischaemic encephalopathy. Cochrane Database Syst Rev. 2013;1:CD003311.
17. Kariholu U, Montaldo P, Markati T, Lally PJ, Pryce R, Teiserskas J, Liow N, Oliveira V, Soe A, Shankaran S, Thayyil S. Therapeutic hypothermia for mild neonatal encephalopathy: a systematic review and meta-analysis. Arch Dis Child Fetal Neonatal Ed. 2020;105(2):225–8.
18. Wyllie J, Perlman JM, Kattwinkel J, et al. Part 7. Neonatal resuscitation: 2015 international consensus on cardiopulmonary resuscitation and emergency cardiovascular care science with treatment recommendations. Resuscitation. 2015;95:e169–201.
19. Gunn AJ, Thoresen M. Neonatal encephalopathy and hypoxic-ischemic encephalopathy. Handb Clin Neurol. 2019;162:217–37.
20. McNally MA, Soul JS. Pharmacologic prevention and treatment of neonatal brain injury. Clin Perinatol. 2019 Jun;46(2):311–25.

21. Oorschot DE, Sizemore RJ, Amer AR. Treatment of neonatal hypoxic-ischemic encephalopathy with erythropoietin alone, and erythropoietin combined with hypothermia: history, current status, and future research. Int J Mol Sci. 2020;21(4):1487.
22. Wu YW, Mathur AM, Chang T, et al. High-dose erythropoietin and hypothermia for hypoxic-ischemic encephalopathy: a phase II trial. Pediatrics. 2016;137:e20160191.
23. Benninger KL, Inder TE, Goodman AM, Cotten CM, Nordli DR, Shah TA, Slaughter JC, Maitre NL. Perspectives from the society for pediatric research. Neonatal encephalopathy clinical trials: developing the future. Pediatr Res. 2020;

Chapter 58
Neonatal Complications of Prematurity

Helenilce de Paula Fiod Costa and Elaine de Paula Fiod Costa

Introduction

The World Health Organization (WHO) defines preterm birth as those occurring before 37th completed week (less than 259 days) of pregnancy. In 2010, approximately 15 million babies, 1 in 10 live births, were born preterm, and more than one million of these children died due to complications in first month of life [1]. In 2013, 11.4% of live births in the United States of America (USA) were preterm, and 0.7% born before 28 weeks; this proportion had remained the same since 2000. In Brazil, 300,000 births are preterm, which represents 11.2% of all births [2, 3].

Prematurity is also potentially related to short- and long-term morbidity accounting for almost 45% of children with cerebral palsy, 35% with visual impairment, and 25% with cognitive or hearing impairment in the US [3–5].

Neonatal complications and outcomes vary according to gestational age (GA) and birth weight (BW), place of birth, perinatal care, and best practices implementation in the neonatal period and at the long term. In 2005, the National Institute of Health (NIH) and the National Institute of Child Health and Development (NICHD) classified different degrees of prematurity according with the birth weight (BW) [6, 7]:

- Low birth weight (LBW) – BW < 2500 g
- Very low birth weight (VLBW) – BW < 1500 g
- Extremely low birth weight (ELBW) – BW < 1000 g

H. de Paula Fiod Costa (✉)
Neonatology Department, Institution Santa Joana/Promatre Hospital Group, São Paulo, Brazil

E. de Paula Fiod Costa
Medicine Department, Federal University of Maranhão, Maranhão, Brazil

© Springer Nature Switzerland AG 2022

R. A. Moreira de Sá, E. B. d. Fonseca (eds.), *Perinatology*,
https://doi.org/10.1007/978-3-030-83434-0_58

And also according to the gestational age (GA):

- Late preterm (LPT) – GA 34 to 36^{+6} weeks
- Moderate preterm (MPT) – GA 32 to 33^{+6} weeks
- Very preterm (VPT) – GA 28 to 31^{+6} weeks
- Extremely preterm (EPT) – GA <28 weeks

In 2012, the American College of Obstetrics and Gynecology and the Society of Maternal Fetal Medicine recommended designating 37 to 38 completed weeks gestation as "early term" newborns, because this group has higher rates of neonatal morbidity, particularly respiratory disorders, than "full term" newborns born at 39 to 41 weeks [8].

Small for gestational age newborns are those smaller in size than normal for their gestational age, most commonly defined as a weight below the 10th percentile for the gestational age. A baby is also called "large for gestational age" if its weight is greater than the 90th percentile at birth. A 1995 World Health Organization (WHO) expert committee originally developed this classification, and the definition is based on a BW for GA measure compared to a gender-specific reference population [1].

Complications of prematurity infants are divided into short term or neonatal (e.g., respiratory and cardiovascular disorders) and long term (e.g., neurodevelopmental disorders, cerebral palsy, and others). Survival rates are directly proportional to GA and risk of complications is inversely proportional [9].

Epidemiology

Over the previous two decades, the NICHD and Human Development Neonatal Research Network have monitored trends in morbidity and mortality rates among VLBW infants born at the university centers. According to the report published in 2010, the following morbidities were observed in 8515 newborns with VLBW [10]:

- Respiratory Syndrome Disease (RDS) – 93%
- Retinopathy of prematurity (ROP) – 59%
- Patent duct arteriosus (PDA) – 46%
- Bronchopulmonary dysplasia (BPD) – 42%
- Late-onset sepsis – 36%
- Necrotizing enterocolitis (NEC) – 11%
- Grade III/IV perintraventricular hemorrhage (IVH) – 7 and 9%
- Periventricular leukomalacia (PVL) – 3%

In a British population–based study (EPI Cure 2 Study) [11], the survival and morbidity of 3378 extreme premature infants with GA between 22 and 26 weeks born in 2006 were reported [3]. In this cohort, 83% of live births were admitted to a neonatal intensive care unit (NICU) and 9% died in the delivery room. Survival to hospital discharge was 62%. Among the 1041 patients who survived discharge, 59% had serious morbidity reported:

- BPD with supplemental oxygen at 36 weeks of post menstrual age (PMA) – 68%
- Abnormal brain ultrasound – 13%
- Laser treatment for ROP – 16%
- Laparotomy for NEC – 8%

In 2012, the European Neonatal Network evaluated newborns in 38 neonatal units in 11 countries. MPT had 90% of survival and morbidities reported were BPD = 12%, IVH = 7%, PVL = 1%, and severe ROP = 1% [12].

According to the WHO, Brazil ranks 10th among countries with the highest number of PTB and 16th in deaths from complications of prematurity [1, 13]. From three million children born in Brazil in 2012, 350,000 (11.6%) had PTB, 45,000 (1.5%) with GA <32 weeks, and 40,000 (1.37%) of VLBW. In 2017–2018, the PTB prevalence was 11.5%, about 52% were LBW, 1.37% VLBW, and 0.51% EBW [13]. Survival data of VLBW with higher morbidities are limited.

Guinsburg et al. [13] published data from Brazilian Network of Neonatal Research. The prospective cohort included PTB with GA from 23 0/7 to 33 6/7 weeks without congenital malformation, born in 20 university hospitals between January 2012 and December 2013. The primary endpoint was death and secondary outcome was at least one of the following major morbidity: BPD, grade III and IV IVPH, and severe ROP. It was included 2646 infants, which corresponded to 4.8% of the total VLBW born in Brazil. Mortality rate was 30% and survival with severe morbidity was 53%. At discharge from hospital, 29% the babies had BPD, 8% had IVH grade III or IV, 5% had PVL, and 5% had surgically treated ROP. The major risk factors related to morbidity and mortality were GA < 30 weeks, perinatal asphyxia, hypothermia at the time of admission to the NICU, RDS, generalized infections, NEC, and PDA requiring surgical intervention [13].

Neocosur Network in 2014 published data on 8234 VLBW infants from 15 neonatal units in Latin America (Argentina, Chile, Paraguay, Uruguay, and Peru). The mortality rate was 25.8% and 53% had higher morbidities (25% BPD, 7% for IVH grades III / IV, 5% for PVL, 31% for any stage of ROP and 10.9% for NEC). Only 21.2% survived without major morbidities [14].

The lowest VLBW mortality rate was reported in a 2008 Japanese study. From 3806 only 8.7% died but Asians were at higher risk for ROP [15].

The Neonatal Research Network evaluated how care practices, major morbidities, and mortality have evolved over a 20-year period [16]. An important finding was that the increased adherence to care practices such as antenatal steroids, antenatal antibiotics, cesarean delivery, delivery room resuscitation, surfactant therapy, and respiratory support has been associated with improved neonatal outcomes. Antenatal corticosteroids were one of the most effective interventions.

There was a significant increase in survival rates without major neonatal morbidity for infants born at 25–28 weeks' GA. Although overall survival rates increased for infants born at 23–24 weeks' GA, few infants less than 25 weeks' GA survived without major neonatal morbidity, underscoring the continued need for interventions to improve outcomes for the most immature infants [16].

Despite increased use of maternal antibiotics over the years, rates of early-onset sepsis did not change significantly. Strategies to reduce lung injury, including less aggressive ventilation, were increasingly embraced. There was a decreased intubation in the delivery room but increased surfactant use, suggesting an increase in selective use of surfactant [16]. ROP rates decreased for infants born at 25–28 weeks and may be related to changes in oxygen use in the delivery room and oxygen saturation targets or to improved adherence to oxygen targets during and after the SUPPORT trial (2005–2009) [17].

Among infants who survived to 36 weeks PMA age, BPD rates increased from 2009 to 2012 for infants born at 26 and 27 weeks, with significant increases for infants 22–27 weeks born in the eight centers in 20 years. This may partly be explained by increased active resuscitation and intensive care and increased survival, especially for the most immature infants.

Although the risk of mortality decreases with increasing GA, moderate PT are at significant risk of morbidities. In a Swedish study with 6674 PT infants between 2004 and 2008, the major complications were hyperbilirubinemia (59%), acute RDS (28%), hypoglycemia (16%), and bacterial infection (15%) [18].

In late PTB, the transition from the fetal to the neonatal period is usually slower and may cause lower Apgar scores at birth, thermal instability, early respiratory distress, and apnea. The pulmonary maturation process is still evolving toward alveolar phase. Vascular development has not been completed, which interfere in pulmonary fluid absorption. Subsequently, insufficient surfactant and impaired gas exchange manifest as early and progressive respiratory failure [19, 21].

The most frequent lung disease in this group is the Transient Tachypnea or Wet Lung Syndrome. RDS may be present, especially in the offspring of diabetic mothers. Metabolic disorders such as hypoglycemia and disorders of calcium and magnesium are common. Infectious risk and neonatal sepsis are aggravating factors, which may lead to intravenous antibiotic therapy. Hyperbilirubinemia is frequent; bilirubin level usually rise between the fifth and seventh day, and may remain high until the second week of life. This is a risk group for bilirubin encephalopathy usually related to early discharge, with less than 48 hours, and difficulties in breastfeeding and/or feeding [20].

Studies have considered whether the etiology of early term birth is similar to PTB [21, 22, 39, 42]. It is suggested that there could be shared mechanisms, with some differences. In spontaneous deliveries, diabetes mellitus was a strong determinant of late PTB and early term birth (odds ratio > 2), as well polyhydramnios, oligohydramnios, placental ischemia, other hypoxia, and a previous PT birth. Infection and inflammation, on the other hand, were risk factors for spontaneous PTB but not early term birth.

The contribution of late PTB and early term births to the overall burden of infant mortality, according to data from US in 2013 and 23 European countries in 2010 revealed that about 22% of the total of infant mortalities occur among late PTB or early term births in the USA, and 26% in Europe [22]. In countries where there is a relatively high proportion of early term births (> 30%), such as the USA, Portugal, and Brazil, there has been a recent push by professional societies to reduce the number of elective obstetric deliveries before 39 weeks, and in the USA financial incentives are used to limit these births based on Medicaid policy [21].

Short-Term Neonatal Complications

Despite all advances in perinatal care, some prematurity complications remain as overcoming challenges. Newborns, especially VLBW, are more likely to have severe or major clinical complications requiring intensive and advanced care soon after birth and during hospitalization [13]. In this chapter we will briefly address some complications of prematurity due to their relevance and frequency.

Perinatal Asphyxia

Neonatal asphyxia accounts for 20.9% of neonatal deaths. Although the vast majority of newly born infants (90%) do not require intervention to breathe during transition from intrauterine to extrauterine life, approximately 10% of the newborns require some assistance to begin breathing at birth, and about 1% require extensive resuscitative measures.

The incidence of perinatal depression is markedly increased among preterm neonates because of the complications associated with preterm labor and the physiological immaturity and lability of the preterm infant. Most VLBW require fast and effective resuscitation at birth. Diminished lung compliance, respiratory musculature, and respiratory drive may contribute to the need for assisted ventilation.

All material necessary to assist the PTB must be available prepared in an easily accessible place before birth. Two health professionals must be present in the delivery room and at least one of them trained and qualified to perform all resuscitation maneuvers according to the recommendation of the International Liaison Committee on Resuscitation (ILCOR) and Neonatal Resuscitation Program [23, 24].

At birth it is important to avoid hypothermia (axillary temperature < 36.5 °C). In PTB, especially in extremes, hypothermia is associated with increased mortality and complications such as IVH, respiratory failure, pulmonary hemorrhage, and metabolic disorders. Risk factors for hypothermia include room temperature < 25 °C, maternal temperature < 36 °C, lack of preventive measures for heat loss, and use of respiratory support with cold gas at birth.

To prevent hypothermia, it is recommended: Use heated cradle with radiant heat, keep delivery room temperature at least 26 °C, welcome the newborn in heated fields, wrap the body with polyethylene plastic bag or chemical thermal mattress, use a plastic cap and tubular mesh or wool, and heated humidified air for initial respiratory support. Immediately after stabilization, transfer the newborn to double-wall transport incubator previously heated at 37 to 37.5 °C. Strive to maintain the newborn's temperature from 36.5 to 37.5 °C, avoiding hyperthermia (> 37.5 °C) [25–28].

The first hour ("Golden Hour") is a critical time window for newborn ready stabilization. Initial first hour of neonatal life includes neonatal resuscitation, post-resuscitation care, transportation of sick newborn to neonatal intensive care unit, respiratory and cardiovascular support, and initial course in nursery. Studies that evaluated the concept of golden hour in preterm neonates showed marked reduction in hypothermia, hypoglycemia, PIVH, BPD, and ROP [29].

Respiratory Disorders

Respiratory Distress Syndrome (RDS)

RDS is a common breathing disorder that affects newborns. RDS occurs most often in babies born with VLBW or GA < 32 weeks. RDS is more common in premature newborns because their immature lungs are not able to make enough alveolar surfactant. Surfactant is a foamy substance that keeps the lungs fully expanded so that newborns can breathe in air once they are born. Without enough surfactant, the lungs collapse and the newborn has to work hard to breathe.

RDS may be prevented or its severity decreased with the use of antenatal steroid therapy, early administration of positive airway pressure and, in some cases, exogenous surfactant therapy. Despite the use of preventive interventions, RDS may still develop and be associated with both acute and chronic complications [10]. Frequency and severity are directly related to the degree of prematurity [30, 31].

Treatments for RDS include surfactant replacement therapy in the first 2 hours of life, breathing support from a ventilator or continuous positive airway pressure (CPAP) machine. Studies suggest that INSURE strategy (INtubate-SURfactant) administration and extubate to CPAP is better than mechanical ventilation (MV) with rescue surfactant, for the management of RDS in VLBW neonates, as it has a synergistic effect on alveolar stability. The INSURE strategy reduces the need and duration of MV, length of oxygen therapy, the need of additional surfactant doses, and length of hospitalization in the NICU [32].

Minimally invasive surfactant therapy (MIST) is another technic to administrate exogenous surfactant with a thin catheter, which allows spontaneously breathing neonates to remain on CPAP in the first week after birth without intubation [32].

Transient Tachypnea of the Newborn (TTN)

TTN is a benign, self-limited condition that can present in infants of any gestational age, shortly after birth. It is the main cause of respiratory failure in late preterm and early term born from an elective cesarean delivery without labor. And it occurs due to delay in clearance of fetal lung fluid after birth, which leads to ineffective gas exchange, respiratory distress, and tachypnea. The onset of respiratory distress occurs in the first hours of life, with a predominance of tachypnea and expiratory moan. Usually the evolution is good and the preventive measure in these cases is to avoid the resolution of the pregnancy by elective cesarean section without labor, and before GA = 39 weeks [33].

Persistent Pulmonary Hypertension of Newborn (PPHN)

PPHN occurs when pulmonary vascular resistance remains abnormally elevated after birth, resulting in right-to-left shunting of blood through fetal circulatory pathways. This in turn leads to severe hypoxemia that may not respond to conventional respiratory support [36]. This condition can result from intrinsic changes in pulmonary vessels or from a wide variety of neonatal cardiorespiratory diseases such as RDS, congenital pneumonia, pulmonary hemorrhage, and TTN. PPNH is almost always present in cases of PT infants <28 weeks with prolonged amniorrhexis associated or not with chorioamnionitis and/or pulmonary hypoplasia. PPHN should always be considered in newborns with severe hypoxemic respiratory failure [34].

Bronchopulmonary Dysplasia (BPD)

BPD is the result of a complex process in which several prenatal or postnatal factors interfere with respiratory tract development and growth. It is thought to be a combination of pulmonary immaturity, injury, inflammation, and scarring [35, 36]. Currently, the risk population for BPD is the PT newborn with GA < 32 weeks. The lungs of these newborns are in the transition from the canalicular to saccular stage, that is, still in the pre-alveolar phase. This development process may be interrupted or changed by premature delivery, prenatal and postnatal events. Prenatal events include intrauterine growth restriction and exposure to inflammatory mediators. Postnatal events are related to neonatal resuscitation, oxygen administration, mechanical ventilation, PDA, and pulmonary and systemic infections [36–38].

BPD has been classified into two clinical forms: classical BPD or severe lung injury and atypical form or "new BPD" [37]. The classical form was more commonly observed before the introduction of corticosteroid therapy in pregnancy and the surfactant replacement therapy. The proposed triggering factors were high oxygen concentrations and high pressures on mechanical ventilation, pulmonary edema in the first week of life, PDA, air leak syndrome, such as pneumothorax and/or pulmonary interstitial emphysema, and genetic predisposition. And, it is characterized by inflammatory process, emphysematous areas alternating with areas of atelectasis, squamous metaplasia of the respiratory epithelium, alveolar and peribronchial fibrosis, necrotizing bronchiolitis, hypertrophy and hyperplasia of the smooth muscles of the airways and pulmonary arteries [37]. As a result, these infants develop chronic respiratory condition characterized by pulmonary edema, bronchospasm attacks, recurrent lung infections, atelectasis, chronic respiratory failure, pulmonary hypertension, right ventricular failure and *cor pulmonale*. The patients may need ventilatory support for months and sometimes tracheostomy.

The atypical form is observed in PT with VLBW or ELBW whose mothers received steroids before birth, which are between the canalicular (GA = 16–23 weeks) and saccular (GA = 23–32 weeks) stage of pulmonary development. They usually have a mild form of RDS and respond favorably to surfactant replacement therapy, requiring more non-invasive support, and more "gentle" mechanical ventilation. "New BPD" is characterized by a stop in alveolar septation and vascular development, reduction gas exchange surface, alveolar hypoplasia, distal airspaces dilation, and vascular dysmorphism. Abman et al. suggested that abnormal vascular endothelial growth factor (VEGF) signaling would lead to pulmonary vascular development interruption, similar to what occurs in ROP, and the association of PPH would support this concept [37].

The lung lesion is lighter and more uniform. There is a minimal respiratory epithelium metaplasia and hyperplasia and areas with emphysema, atelectasis, and fibrosis are not usually observed. However, long-term functional pulmonary changes are similar in both clinical forms, which means they exhibit similar clinical patterns that persist in childhood and adulthood [37].

BPD may also be categorized according to its severity, established by NICHD in 2001 (Table 58.1).

A new proposed scheme for a revised BPD definition considers newer modes of noninvasive ventilation that were not included in the previous definitions (Table 58.2). Grade III would refer to the most severe form of BPD. Continuation of the 36-week PMA time point was suggested because most infants remain in the hospital at this time point, which makes ascertainment of a diagnosis of BPD possible for many patients.

BPD persists as one of the main sources of short- and long-term morbidities newborns with BPD (classic or atypical form). These babies are at high risk for

Table 58.1 Bronchopulmonary dysplasia severity criteria [38]

Gestational age	<32 weeks	≥ 32 weeks
Time point of assessment	36 weeks PMA or discharge to home, whichever comes first	<56 days postnatal age or discharge to home, whichever comes first
	Treatment with >21% oxygen for ≥28 days	
Mild BPD	Breathing room air at 36 weeks PMA or discharge to home, whichever comes first	Breathing room air at <56 days postnatal age or discharge to home, whichever comes first
Moderate BPD	Need for <30% oxygen and/or positive pressure (PPV or CPAP) 36 weeks PMA or discharge to home, whichever comes first	Need for <30% oxygen and/or positive pressure (PPV or CPAP) < 56 days postnatal age or discharge to home, whichever comes first
Severe BPD	Need for ≥30% oxygen and/or positive pressure (PPV or CPAP) 36 weeks PMA or discharge to home, whichever comes first	Need for ≥30% oxygen and/or positive pressure (PPV or CPAP) < 56 days postnatal age or discharge to home, whichever comes first

PMA postmenstrual age, *BPD* bronchopulmonary dysplasia, *PPV* positive pressure ventilation, *CPAP* continuous positive airway pressure

Table 58.2 Suggested refinements to the classification and definition of BPD proposed by Higgins et al. [38]

A premature infant (<32 weeks gestational age) with BPD has persistent parenchymal lung disease, radiographic confirmation of parenchymal lung disease, and at 36 weeks PMA requires of the following FiO_2 ranges/oxygen levels/O_2 concentrations for ≥3 consecutive days to maintain arterial oxygen saturation in the 90%–95% range

Grades	Invasive IPPV[a]	N-CPAP, NIPPV, or nasal cannula ≥ 3 L/min	Nasal cannula nasal flow of 1– < 3 L/min	HoodO_2	Nasal cannula flow of 1 L/min
I	–	21%	22–29%	22–29%	22–70%
II	21%	22–29%	≥30%	≥30%	>70%
III	>21%	≥30%			
III (A)	Early death (between 14 days of postnatal age and 36 weeks) owing to persistent parenchymal lung disease and respiratory failure that cannot be attributable to other neonatal morbidities (e.g., necrotizing enterocolitis, peri-intraventricular hemorrhage, redirection of care, episodes of sepsis, etc.).				

[a]Excluding infants ventilated for primary airway disease or central respiratory control conditions
CPAP continuous positive airway pressure, *IPPV* intermittent positive pressure ventilations, *N-CPAP* nasal continuous positive airway pressure, *NIPPV* noninvasive positive pressure ventilation

chronic lung disease, adverse results in neurological development and frequent hospital readmissions in the first year of life.

Pulmonary Hemorrhage (PH)

Pulmonary hemorrhage is usually sudden and catastrophic, occurring between second and fourth days of life. It is characterized by hemorrhagic secretion discharge from the upper respiratory tract or tracheal cannula. It usually occurs in newborns with GA < 28 weeks in mechanical ventilation with PDA and intrauterine growth retardation. The cause is a combination of factors cardiac dysfunction and severe hemodynamic deterioration, where left ventricle has a limited capacity to respond, to increased afterload and preload, along with respiratory failure. This is fast and is often associated with high mortality rates [39].

Apnea of Prematurity

Apnea of prematurity is defined as respiratory pause for more than 15–20 seconds, or when associated with bradycardia (≤ 80 beats minute) and desaturation (SpO2 ≤ 80%) for a period ≥4 seconds in PT newborn. Apneas for more than 15–20 seconds with SpO2 ≤ 80% can lead to short- and long-term complications.

PT newborns with GA <32 weeks are a group of risk [3]. In short term, these episodes may decrease systemic blood pressure and cerebral perfusion causing hypoxemia and ischemia to the brain. Hypoxemia episodes can damage the immature and affect the developing brain. Although sudden death is three times more frequent in preterm infants, the current literature does not show a direct relationship with apnea of prematurity [3].

Cardiovascular Disorders

Arterial Hypotension

Arterial hypotension is considered one of clinical practice parameters for hemodynamic support. Approximately 25% of the PT admitted in NICU has arterial hypotension in the first 24 hours of life, and half receive some type of hemodynamic support to treat hypotension [40]. This is largely due to the difficulties in properly monitoring hemodynamic conditions. In most neonatal units, normal blood pressure is defined when the mean pressure is equal the GA. PT newborn with low blood pressure may have systemic perfusion reduction, decreased cerebral oxygen supply, increased brain injury, and elevated acute complications of prematurity [40].

Patent Duct Arteriosus (PDA)

PDA is the most common cardiovascular disorder in PT infants [41]. The ductus arteriosus serves as a shunt between the pulmonary artery and the aorta. During fetus development, the ductus arteriosus is normally open and allows for oxygenated blood to bypass the pulmonary circulation (since breathing is not yet possible) and enter directly into the systemic circulation. Shortly after birth and the first breath, the lungs are filled with oxygen, and the pulmonary arterioles dilate. This change in pulmonary-arteriole resistance allows for a significant increase in pulmonary blood flow. The ductus arteriosus responds to these changes by closing in the first 72 hours of life and becoming the ligamentum arteriosum.

In PT newborns, particularly in the VLBW, the duct remains patent after the first week of life in more than 30–65% of cases. The main factors contributing to keeping the duct open in this population are low blood oxygen partial pressure, as well as the endogenous production of prostaglandins and nitric oxide. PDA results in an excessive blood flow in the pulmonary circulation and a concomitant hypoperfusion in the systemic one. In these cases, the ductus arteriosus is considered hemodynamically significant and the infants may present a variety of symptoms, including apnea, breathing difficulties, or heart failure. Several adverse neonatal outcomes, such as pulmonary hemorrhage, BPD, NEC, PIVH, and death, are associated with PDA [42, 43].

Infections

Sepsis

In preterm infants, early-onset sepsis is defined as occurring in the first 3 days of life and is caused by bacterial pathogens transmitted vertically from mother to infant before or during delivery. Late-onset sepsis occurs after 72 h in NICU infants and usually has hospital origin. Although advances in neonatal care have improved survival and reduced complications in preterm infants, sepsis still contributes significantly to mortality and morbidity among VLBW and extremes infants in NICU.

Precise estimates of neonatal sepsis occurrence vary by setting, population type and perinatal care. In NICHD data, 20% of VLBW newborns presented blood culture–confirmed sepsis, 70% were caused by Gram-positive microorganisms and in 48% by coagulase-negative Staphylococci [3]. Fungal infection, mainly candidiasis, was responsible for 9% of late-onset sepsis cases and was associated with high mortality rate (28%) [9].

In Brazil, data from the Neonatal Research Network in 2014 showed a 27.5% of sepsis confirmed with blood culture with a large variation between member centers. Premature infants who developed late-onset sepsis were more likely to die than those who were not infected, and survivors had longer hospital stays (79 versus 60 days). Other complications associated with an increased risk of infection were increased likelihood of poor neurological development and growth impairment [44].

Necrotizing Enterocolitis (NEC)

NEC is a gastrointestinal disease characterized by ischemic necrosis of the intestinal mucosa, which is associated with severe inflammation, invasion of enteric gas-forming organisms, and dissection of gas into the bowel wall and portal venous system. The etiology is complex and multifactorial, including genetic predisposition, intestinal immaturity, imbalance in microvascular tone, abnormal microbial colonization, and highly immunoreactive intestinal mucosa. Although early recognition and aggressive treatment of this disorder has improved clinical outcomes, NEC accounts for substantial long-term morbidity in survivors of NCIU. It affects especially VLBW (2 to 10%), GA < 31 weeks, small for GA, PT newborns with perinatal asphyxia, PDA, hemodynamic instability, and intrauterine growth retardation [45, 46].

Mortality rates ranging from 15% to 30% have been reported. Surgical treatment is often needed, and survivors are at increased risk for poor long-term growth and neurodevelopmental impairment, gastrointestinal difficulties such as short bowel syndrome, and malabsorption. Preventive strategies include prenatal glucocorticoid administration, breastfeeding or use of donor milk, and probiotic supplementation [45, 46].

Germinal Matrix Hemorrhage/Intraventricular Hemorrhage (IVH)

IVH is the most common of intracranial hemorrhages in PT newborns. It typically initiates in the germinal matrix, which is a richly vascularized collection of neuronal–glial precursor cells in the developing brain, and located in the caudal sulcus on the floor of the lateral ventricles, the place of brain support tissue origin. The brain support tissue has its maximum development between 23–24 weeks, and then it starts to evolve in such a way that after 36 weeks it becomes practically nonexistent [47].

The etiology of IVH is multifactorial and is primarily attributed to the intrinsic fragility of the germinal matrix vasculature, disturbance in the cerebral blood flow, inflammatory mediators and angiogenic factors, changes in coagulation factors, and genetic predisposition. When hemorrhage in the germinal matrix is extensive, rupture of the ependyma occurs, and blood leaks into the ventricles and intraventricular hemorrhage [48].

IVH is classified into degrees according (Table 58.3). Grades III and IV are the most severe, with an increased risk to post-hemorrhagic hydrocephalus, hemorrhagic lesion of the cerebellum, atrophy of the gray matter cerebellar and supratentorial, cystic periventricular leukomalacia with white matter injury, epilepsy, cerebral palsy, and mental retardation [48].

IVH is more frequent in preterm infants with GA < 30 weeks, VLBW (20–25%) and in extreme preterm infants around 45%. Differences may occur according with the population served, perinatal care, and diagnostic methods (ultrasound or magnetic resonance imaging). Preventive strategies include prenatal tocolytics, corticosteroids and magnesium sulfate, antibiotics in premature amniorrhexis and transfer the pregnant mother to a tertiary care center [49].

Retinopathy of Prematurity (ROP)

ROP is the main cause of preventable blindness in childhood. The incidence of ROP is closely correlated with the weight and the gestational age at birth. Pathophysiology of ROP is related to the interruption of the normal retinal vascularization process. Vascular development comprises two phases: vasculogenesis and angiogenesis [50]. The former phase is characterized by the formation of blood vessels from

Table 58.3 Intraventricular hemorrhage classification

Grade	Brain lesion
I	Hemorrhage restricted to the germinal matrix
II	Hemorrhage without ventricular dilation
III	Hemorrhage with ventricular dilation
IV	Parenchymal hemorrhage

endothelial precursor cells within the central retina, whereas the latter phase is characterized by the development of new blood vessels that bud from existing blood vessels. Angiogenesis is responsible for increasing the vascular density and peripheral vascularization of the superficial retina and for forming the outer plexus and radial peripapillary capillaries. The retinal vessels' progress from the optic nerve toward the peripheral retina around the 16th week of pregnancy, reaching the nasal retina around the 39th week, and the temporal peripheral retina around the 42nd week of GA. The mechanisms underlying the generation of the retinal vasculature have been found to be similar to those of the central nervous system [50].

With PTB, a vasoconstriction reflex occurs due to changes in oxygen extrauterine concentration and may be worsen by acid–base imbalances, congenital heart diseases, and septic conditions. Retinal vessels stop developing, while neuronal cells continue to proliferate, differentiate, and increase their metabolic activity. Thus, after a few weeks, the avascular retina becomes critically hypoxic and angiogenic factors and erythropoietin begin to be secreted in an attempt to end normal angiogenesis. The recovery of vascularization causes the formation of more fragile abnormal vessels, called neovessels, which are susceptible to bleeding and may cause vitreous hemorrhage, retinal detachment, and blindness.

ROP is classified into stages and zones according to the way the vascular growth happen [51, 52]. In the vast majority of newborns, ROP regresses spontaneously with minor deficits in photoreceptors function. ROP involution usually occurs in PMA from 35 to 44 weeks. Currently, in USA the screening protocol involves newborns GA < 30 weeks, or BW < 1500 grams or newborns with clinical instability in neonatal period. In Brazil, it is also recommend the examination in newborns between 32 and 30 weeks.

Oxygen saturation should also be monitored to avoid the consequences of hypoxia or hyperoxia. The target saturation currently recommended by neonatologists, ophthalmologists, and pediatricians specialized in child development is 90–95%. The Neonatal Oxygen Prospective Meta-analysis (Neo Pro M) continues to select studies (the goal is to include 5000 infants with GA < 28 weeks) to make available and recommend, after a final analysis, the target saturation levels for PT newborns in NICUs [17].

Extrauterine Growth Restriction (EUGR)

Premature newborns with GA < 30 weeks have cumulative protein and calorie deficiency, which starts in the first days and is accentuated due to the nutritional limitations. Neonatal morbidities and digestive tract immaturity result in delay to start feeding with nutritional deficit and, consequently, slow BW recovery (12 to 20 days of life) and growth rate [53]. EUGR is typically defined as a growth measurement (weight, length, or head circumference) that is <tenth percentile of the expected intrauterine growth for the PMA at the time of discharge; 36 weeks' PMA or 40 weeks' PMA (term-equivalent age) [54].

A NICHD study evaluating PT infants with VLBW found that 22% were small for GA at birth and 97% were below the tenth percentile at 36 weeks of PMA by the intrauterine growth curve [55]. Besides morbidities and immaturity other risk factors were cited: invasive ventilatory support for more than 28 days, prolonged duration of parenteral nutrition and late start of enteral feeding, hypomotility of the gastrointestinal tract, use of postnatal corticosteroids, and being small for age gestational age at birth. Longitudinal follow-up studies of VLBW PT newborn with assessment at 18–22 months of PMA have shown that children with EUGR have lower neurodevelopment scores [56].

Pediatric Complications in Long-Term Prematurity

Premature survivors have a higher rate of recurrent hospitalizations during childhood and adolescence. Recurrent hospitalizations rates increase with the decrease in GA, being greater in the VLBW and ELBW. Infants who have had BPD are more likely to have respiratory disorders as respiratory syncytial virus infection, pneumonia, pulmonary hypertension, bouts of bronchial hyperactivity, asthma, and gastrointestinal problems as gastroesophageal reflux, food intolerances and malabsorption syndrome. Children or adolescents who were born before 28 weeks or ELBW may present lung function impairment and difficulties in physical exercise. On the other hand, moderate and late PTB there is minimal or no effect on the respiratory function in adolescence [10].

Chronic health problems presented by the most immature are asthma, high blood pressure, chronic kidney disease, heart disease, post-hemorrhagic hydrocephalus, porencephaly, underweight, or overweight. VLBW preterm infants are more likely to show low growth compared to those born at term. PT with restricted intra and extrauterine growth, may also have low length/height, weight, body mass index, and head circumference [10].

Neurologic deficiencies increase with the decrease in GA. They include fine and gross motor delays, spastic diplegia and cerebral palsy, impaired and subnormal cognitive abilities, sensory impairment, including vision and hearing loss, refractive problems with severe myopia and amblyopia behavioral problems, autistic spectrum, psychiatric disorders, and psychological disorders. Cerebral palsy is a non-progressive motor disability that results in movement disorders, such as plegias, spasticity, and dystonia. The exact cause is still unknown, but 8–9% of PT newborn with GA between 22 and 32 weeks has cerebral palsy [3, 10].

Premature infants with BW between 1500 and 2499 g may also have more health needs such as chronic conditions, intellectual, vision, difficulties in learning and/or attention disorder, and asthma than term newborn.

Qualified medical professionals for clinical follow-up, multidisciplinary health team and education services (individualized education programs), and financial resources support are essential for improving survival and quality of life in long term.

Impact of Prematurity on Adult Health

Long-term complications seen in adult survivors include insulin resistance, diabetes mellitus, arterial hypertension, ischemic heart disease, obesity or overweight. LBW was associated with primary high blood pressure and prematurity with lower reproductive rate in adulthood. Also, premature women were at greater risk of having premature children. Neurodevelopment, psychological, behavioral, functional, and caregiver dependencies were observed. The increased risk of early death for individuals between 30 and 45 years of age was inversely associated with GA [57].

As the preterm survival rate improves, the potential impact of prematurity on long-term health in adulthood becomes more apparent. Even thought, most individuals born prematurely survive adulthood without major comorbidities. This was illustrated by a Swedish study of all births (2,566,699 individuals) between 1973 and 1997 [18]. At follow-up (mean age 29.8 years), 54.6% of PTB (5.8% of the entire cohort) were alive without significant morbidity. Survival without morbidity was lower in those born with GA < 28 weeks: and increased from 22.3% to 48.5% in those with GA from 28 to 33 weeks. And in late preterm infants, survival in adulthood without morbidity was 61% [18].

More longitudinal studies with follow-up in adulthood are needed to determine the impact of the extremely PT infants on the limit of fetal viability with the advances in current perinatal care and to identify the impact of good clinical practice as antenatal corticosteroids, magnesium sulfate for neuroprotection, effective initial resuscitation, the principles for maintaining normal cardiopulmonary function and hemodynamic stability, early surfactant, currently recommended oxygen saturation levels, gentle ventilation, prevention of intracranial hemorrhage, early or late infection and ROP will translate into better results throughout life [57].

Understanding the short- and long-term results can help us to take better care of these newborns and to inform families more objectively. A recent consensus statement from the American College of Obstetricians and Gynecologists and the Society of Maternal–Fetal Medicine recommends that obstetricians should provide accurate, balanced, and impartial guidance when advising families on fetuses care and newborn with GA close to fetal viability [58]. The information should include survival and mortality estimates and the use of available resources and strategies for the proposed treatment. The statement also suggests that institutions develop their own consensus guidelines on viability limits, survival without major morbidities, and mortality according with GA or BW.

Conclusions

In the last 20 years, there have been changes in perinatal care practices with prematurity. A small decrease in severe morbidities among extreme PT newborns has been reported, although BPD has increased. There was less mortality among those born with GA between 23 and 24 weeks and longer survival without severe morbidity among newborns with GA from 25 to 28 weeks. In addition to increasing survival, an important goal of perinatal care was reducing neonatal morbidities. In very low GA, the decision to provide active obstetric care and neonatal intensive care is complex and requires a multi-professional approach with discussions between the obstetric and neonatal teams and families. The evaluation of morbidity and mortality data among PT newborns, in particular those with GA <32 weeks, of each hospital is important for counseling families and implementing best practices in care.

References

1. Howson CP, Kinney MV, Mc Dougall L, Lawn JE, Born Too Soon Preterm Birth Action Group. Born too soon: preterm birth matters. Reprod Health. 2013;10(Suppl 1):S1.
2. Blencowe H, Cousens S, Oestergaard MZ, Chou D, Moller A-B, Narwal R, et al. National, regional, and worldwide estimates of preterm birth rates in the year 2010 with time trends since 1990 for selected countries: a systematic analysis and implications. Lancet. 2012;379(9832):2162–72.
3. Glass HC, Costarino AT, Stayer SA, Brett CM, Cladis F, Davis PJ. Outcomes for extremely premature infants. Anesth Analg. 2015;120(6):1337–51.
4. Matthews TJ, MacDorman MF, Thoma ME. Infant mortality statistics from the 2013 period linked birth/infant death data set. Natl Vital Stat Rep. 2015;64(9):1–30.
5. Hamilton BE, Martin JA, Ventura SJ. Births: preliminary data for 2012. Natl Vital Stat Rep. 2013;62(3):1–20.
6. Raju TNK. Epidemiology of late preterm (near-term) births. Clin Perinatol. 2006;33(4):751–63. abstract vii
7. Engle WA. A recommendation for the definition of "late preterm" (near-term) and the birth weight-gestational age classification system. Semin Perinatol. 2006;30(1):2–7.
8. ACOG. Committee opinion no 579: definition of term pregnancy. Obstet Gynecol. 2013;122(5):1139–40.
9. Stoll BJ, Hansen NI, Bell EF, Shankaran S, Laptook AR, Walsh MC, et al. Neonatal outcomes of extremely preterm infants from the NICHD Neonatal Research Network. Pediatrics. 2010;126(3):443–56.
10. Patel RM. Short- and long-term outcomes for extremely preterm infants. Am J Perinatol. 2016;33(3):318–28.
11. Costeloe KL, Hennessy EM, Haider S, Stacey F, Marlow N, Draper ES. Short term outcomes after extreme preterm birth in England: comparison of two birth cohorts in 1995 and 2006 (the EPICure studies). BMJ. 2012;345:e7976.
12. EuroNeoNet. General report for very-low-birth-weight/very–low gestational-age infants. Bizkaia(Spain)2012.
13. Guinsburg R, de Almeida MFB, de Castro JS, Silveira RC, Caldas JP de S, Fiori HH, et al. Death or survival with major morbidity in VLBW infants born at Brazilian neonatal research network centers. J Matern Fetal Neonatal Med. 2016;29(6):1005–9.
14. Fernández R, D'Apremont I, Domínguez A, Tapia JL. Red neonatal Neocosur. Survival and morbidity of very low birth weight infant in a south American neonatal network. Arch Argent Pediatr. 2014;112(5):405–12.
15. Kusuda S, Fujimura M, Uchiyama A, Totsu S, Matsunami K. Neonatal research network, Japan. Trends in morbidity and mortality among very-low-birth-weight infants from 2003 to 2008 in Japan. Pediatr Res. 2012;72(5):531–8.
16. Stoll BJ, Hansen NI, Bell EF, Walsh MC, Carlo WA, Shankaran S, et al. Trends in care practices, morbidity, and mortality of extremely preterm neonates, 1993-2012. JAMA. 2015;314(10):1039–51.

17. SUPPORT Study Group of the Eunice Kennedy Shriver NICHD Neonatal Research Network, Carlo WA, Finer NN, Walsh MC, Rich W, Gantz MG, et al. Target ranges of oxygen saturation in extremely preterm infants. N Engl J Med. 2010;362(21):1959–69.
18. Altman M, Vanpée M, Cnattingius S, Norman M. Neonatal morbidity in moderately preterm infants: a Swedish national population-based study. J Pediatrics. 2011;158(2):239–44.e1.
19. Wang ML, Dorer DJ, Fleming MP, Catlin EA. Clinical outcomes of near-term infants. Pediatrics. 2004;114(2):372–6.
20. WHO recommendations on interventions to improve preterm birth outcomes. Geneva: World Health Organization. 2015.
21. Martin JA, Hamilton BE, Osterman MJK. Births in the United States, 2018. NCHS Data Brief. 2019;346:1–8.
22. Martin JA, Hamilton BE, Osterman MJK, Driscoll AK, Drake P. Births: final data for 2017. Natl Vital Stat Rep. 2018;67(8):1–50.
23. Perlman JM, Wyllie J, Kattwinkel J, Wyckoff MH, Aziz K, Guinsburg R, et al. Part 7: neonatal resuscitation: 2015 international consensus on cardiopulmonary resuscitation and emergency cardiovascular care science with treatment recommendations (Reprint). Pediatrics. 2015;136(Suppl 2):S120–66.
24. Wyllie J, Perlman JM, Kattwinkel J, Wyckoff MH, Aziz K, Guinsburg R, et al. Part 7: neonatal resuscitation: 2015 international consensus on cardiopulmonary resuscitation and emergency cardiovascular care science with treatment recommendations. Resuscitation. 2015;95:e169–201.
25. Laptook AR, Bell EF, Shankaran S, Boghossian NS, Wyckoff MH, Kandefer S, et al. Admission temperature and associated mortality and morbidity among moderately and extremely preterm infants. J Pediatrics. 2018;192:53–59.e2.
26. de Almeida MFB, Guinsburg R, Sancho GA, Rosa IRM, Lamy ZC, Martinez FE, et al. Hypothermia and early neonatal mortality in preterm infants. J Pediatr. 2014;164(2):271.
27. Ting JY, Synnes AR, Lee SK, Shah PS, Canadian Neonatal Network and Canadian Neonatal Follow-Up Network. Association of admission temperature and death or adverse neurodevelopmental outcomes in extremely low-gestational age neonates. J Perinatol. 2018;38(7):844–9.
28. McCall EM, Alderdice F, Halliday HL, Vohra S, Johnston L. Interventions to prevent hypothermia at birth in preterm and/or low birth weight infants. Cochrane Database Syst Rev. 2018;2:CD004210.
29. Sharma D. Golden hour of neonatal life: need of the hour. Matern Health Neonatol Perinatol. 2017;3:16.
30. Beltempo M, Isayama T, Vento M, Lui K, Kusuda S, Lehtonen L, et al. Respiratory management of extremely preterm infants: an international survey. Neonatology. 2018;114(1):28–36.
31. Committee on Fetus and Newborn, American Academy of Pediatrics. Respiratory support in preterm infants at birth. Pediatrics. 2014;133:171–4.
32. Sweet DG, Carnielli V, Greisen G, Hallman M, Ozek E, Plavka R, et al. European consensus guidelines on the management of respiratory distress syndrome – 2016 Update. Neonatology. 2017;111:107–25.
33. Buchiboyina A, Jasani B, Deshmukh M, Patole S. Strategies for managing transient tachypnoea of the newborn - a systematic review. J Matern Fetal Neonatal Med. 2017;30(13):1524–32.
34. de Waal K, Kluckow M. Prolonged rupture of membranes and pulmonary hypoplasia in very preterm infants: pathophysiology and guided treatment. J Pediatr. 2015;166(5):1113–20.
35. Guaman MC, Gien J, Baker CD, Zhang H, Austin ED, Collaco JM. Point prevalence, clinical characteristics, and treatment variation for infants with severe bronchopulmonary dysplasia. Am J Perinatol. 2015;32(10):960–7.
36. Donn SM. Bronchopulmonary dysplasia: myths of pharmacologic management. Semin Fetal Neonatal Med. 2017;22(5):354–8.
37. Abman SH, Collaco JM, Shepherd EG, Keszler M, Cuevas-Guaman M, Welty SE, et al. Interdisciplinary care of children with severe bronchopulmonary dysplasia. J Pediatr. 2017;181:12–28.e1.
38. Higgins RD, Jobe AH, Koso-Thomas M, Bancalari E, Viscardi RM, Hartert TV, et al. Bronchopulmonary dysplasia: executive summary of a workshop. J Pediatr. 2018;197:300–8.

39. Ahmad KA, Bennett MM, Ahmad SF, Clark RH, Tolia VN. Morbidity and mortality with early pulmonary haemorrhage in preterm neonates. Arch Dis Child Fetal Neonatal Ed. 2019;104(1):F63–8.
40. Barrington KJ. Low blood pressure in extremely preterm infants: does treatment affect outcome? Arch Dis Child Fetal Neonatal Ed. 2011;96(5):F316–7.
41. Kluckow M, Jeffery M, Gill A, Evans N. A randomised placebo-controlled trial of early treatment of the patent ductus arteriosus. Arch Dis Child Fetal Neonatal Ed. 2014;99(2):F99–F104.
42. Clyman RI, Couto J, Murphy GM. Patent ductus arteriosus: are current neonatal treatment options better or worse than no treatment at all? Semin Perinatol. 2012;36(2):123–9.
43. Rozé J-C, Cambonie G, Marchand-Martin L, Gournay V, Durrmeyer X, Durox M, et al. Association between early screening for patent ductus arteriosus and in-hospital mortality among extremely preterm infants. JAMA. 2015;313(24):2441–8.
44. de Souza Rugolo LMS, Bentlin MR, Mussi-Pinhata M, de Almeida MFB, Lopes JM de A, Marba STM, et al. Late-onset sepsis in very low birth weight infants: a Brazilian Neonatal Research Network Study. J Trop Pediatr. 2014;60(6):415–21.
45. Sharma R, Hudak ML. A clinical perspective of necrotizing enterocolitis: past, present, and future. Clin Perinatol. 2013;40(1):27–51.
46. Faa G, Gerosa C, Fanni D, Nemolato S, van Eyken P, Fanos V. Factors influencing the development of a personal tailored microbiota in the neonate, with particular emphasis on antibiotic therapy. J Matern Fetal Neonatal Med. 2013;26(Suppl 2):35–43.
47. Papile LA, Burstein J, Burstein R, Koffler H. Incidence and evolution of subependymal and intraventricular hemorrhage: a study of infants with birth weights less than 1,500 gm. J Pediatr. 1978;92(4):529–34.
48. Volpe JJ. The encephalopathy of prematurity--brain injury and impaired brain development inextricably intertwined. Semin Pediatr Neurol. 2009;16(4):167–78.
49. Wei JC, Catalano R, Profit J, Gould JB, Lee HC. Impact of antenatal steroids on intraventricular hemorrhage in very-low-birth weight infants. J Perinatol. 2016;36(5):352–6.
50. Hughes S, Yang H, Chan-Ling T. Vascularization of the human fetal retina: roles of vasculogenesis and angiogenesis. Invest Ophthalmol Vis Sci. 2000;41(5):1217–28.
51. International Committee for the Classification of Retinopathy of Prematurity. The international classification of retinopathy of prematurity revisited. Arch Ophthalmol. 2005;123:991–9.
52. Early Treatment For Retinopathy Of Prematurity Cooperative Group. Revised indications for the treatment of retinopathy of prematurity: results of the early treatment for retinopathy of prematurity randomized trial. Arch Ophthalmol. 2003;121(12):1684–94.
53. Embleton NE, Pang N, Cooke RJ. Postnatal malnutrition and growth retardation: an inevitable consequence of current recommendations in preterm infants? Pediatrics. 2001;107(2):270–3.
54. Shan HM, Cai W, Cao Y, Fang BH, Feng Y. Extrauterine growth retardation in premature infants in Shanghai: a multicenter retrospective review. Eur J Pediatr. 2009;168(9):1055–9.
55. Lemons JA, Bauer CR, Oh W, Korones SB, Papile LA, Stoll BJ, et al. Very low birth weight outcomes of the National Institute of child health and human development neonatal research network, January 1995 through December 1996. NICHD Neonatal Research Network. Pediatrics. 2001;107(1):E1.
56. Dusick AM, Poindexter BB, Ehrenkranz RA, Lemons JA. Growth failure in the preterm infant: can we catch up? Semin Perinatol. 2003;27(4):302–10.
57. Cheong JLY, Wark JD, Cheung MM, Irving L, Burnett AC, Lee KJ, et al. Impact of extreme prematurity or extreme low birth weight on young adult health and well-being: the Victorian Infant Collaborative Study (VICS) 1991-1992 Longitudinal Cohort study protocol. BMJ Open. 2019;9(5):e030345.
58. American College of Obstetricians and Gynecologists, Society for Maternal-Fetal Medicine. ACOG Obstetric Care Consensus No. 3: Periviable Birth. Obstet Gynecol. 2015;126:e82–94.

Chapter 59
Small for Gestational Age

Maria Elisabeth Lopes Moreira and Maria Dalva Barbosa Baker Méio

Definitions

Small for gestational age (SGA) infants have been classically defined as having birth weight less than two standard deviations below the mean or less than the tenth percentile of a population-specific birth weight for specific gestational age. SGA is a statistical definition of a deviation of size measurement, with the tenth percentile as the most used threshold. An SGA fetus may be healthy, whereas pathology of growth is implicit in a diagnosis of fetal growth restriction. Studies often do not differentiate between small-for-gestational age (SGA) fetuses and fetal growth restriction, even though the two terms are not synonymous. Not all newborns that are SGA are pathologically growth restricted and, in fact, may be constitutionally small [1, 2, 3].

The definition of fetal growth restriction (FGR) is also a controversial issue. There is inconsistency in terminology, definition, monitoring, and clinical management, both in clinical practice and in the existing literature. This impairs interpretation and comparison of rates and related clinical results. However, with the incorporation in the obstetric care of higher-resolution ultrasound machines, the knowledge about fetal growth has been in a constant state of evolution. FGR is pathological state and courses with poor somatic growth and compensated umbilical/cerebral blood flow. Recently, however, additional parameters such as placental biomarkers, hormones, biochemical factors, markers of inflammation in the mother and biometrics including skinfold thickness, and other anthropometric parameters of the neonate have been added to assess this condition [2, 3].

M. E. L. Moreira (✉)
Instituto Fernandes Figueira - Fiocruz, Clinica Perinatal Laranjeiras, Rio de Janeiro, RJ, Brazil
e-mail: elisabeth.moreira@iff.fiocruz.br

M. D. B. B. Méio
Instituto Fernandes Figueira- Fiocruz, Rio de Janeiro, Brazil

© Springer Nature Switzerland AG 2022

R. A. Moreira de Sá, E. B. d. Fonseca (eds.), *Perinatology*,
https://doi.org/10.1007/978-3-030-83434-0_59

Other terms that are often used as synonyms for small for gestational age are low birth weight (LBW) and very low birth weight (VLBW). Low birth weight is a name used only for those who are born weighing less than 2500 g and very low birth weight for those who are born weighing less than 1500 g at birth. Both terms (LBW and VLBW) use a single dimension for the denomination – the birth weight. However, the definition of SGA considers two dimensions: birth weight and gestational age. The term low birth weight fetus is described as birth weight < 2.5 kg irrespective of gestational age, gender, ethnicity, and other associated clinical conditions. It includes constitutionally small, premature, SGA, and intrauterine growth restriction (IUGR) babies [1].

Fetal Growth

Fetal growth is a complex and ill-understood interplay of (a) genetic factors; (b) maternal metabolism or substrate availability; (c) placental functions and inflammation, and fetal adaptability to both. Normal fetal growth up to 20 weeks of gestation mainly occurs by cellular hyperplasia; from 20th to 28th weeks it occurs by hyperplasia and hypertrophy; and from 28 weeks onwards, by hypertrophy with rapid accumulation of fat, muscles, and connective tissues. Fetal growth accelerates from about 5 g per day at 14–19 weeks of gestation to 10 g per day at 20–29 weeks, peaks at 25–35 g per day at 30–36 weeks, and afterwards growth rate decreases to 15 g per day. Almost 90% of fetal weight gain happens in later half of pregnancy [1, 4, 5, 6].

Growth of the fetus is dependent on various factors. It includes the interplay of hormones (insulin; hormones secreted by the thyroid, adrenal, and pituitary glands; and others). Among these, insulin-derived growth factor-I (IGF-I) is probably the most significant. IGF-1 influences amino acid and glucose transport across the placenta [5, 6] and plays a role in neurodevelopment of the fetus by promoting brain growth, by increasing the number of oligodendrocytes, neuronal number, and increasing fine branching of axons at their terminal ends [5, 6, 7]. Some other factors proven to influence the pathogenesis of FGR are vasoactive intestinal polypeptide (VIP), insulin-like growth factor-II, and insulin-like growth factor binding proteins-2 and 3 [6, 7, 8].

Fetal Growth Restriction

Fetal growth restriction (FGR) occurs when the fetus does not reach its intrauterine potential for growth and development as a result of compromise in placental function. Fetuses with FGR present with a greater risk of perinatal morbidity and mortality and long-term health defects. These include impaired neurological and cognitive development and cardiovascular or endocrine diseases in adulthood. FGR is an intercurrence in 5–10% of pregnancies [1, 2, 8]. It is the second leading cause of perinatal mortality and is responsible for 30% of stillborn infants; it is also the most common cause of premature births and intrapartum asphyxia [1, 7, 8].

At present, there is no gold standard for the diagnosis of FGR. It is generally defined by a statistical deviation from fetal size in the population of reference, with percentile limits of 10, 5, or 3. These limits, however, are better understood as indicative of fetuses that are small for gestational age (SGA). In clinical practice, FGR is defined on the basis of the weight percentile relative to the gestational age. There are different definitions: The World Health Organization (WHO) defines FGR as an estimated fetal weight below the third percentile and the American College of Obstetrics and Gynecology (ACOG) defines FGR as an estimated fetal weight below the tenth percentile for gestational age and states that it is frequently associated with placental insufficiency [1, 3]. This is the most commonly used classification [1, 9, 10].

Classification

FGR is classified in various and different ways [1, 3].

1. According to fetal biometry [1]
   (a) Type I/symmetric:
   Usually, early onset with intrinsic genetic disorders or infections to fetus. Ponderal index is normal, whereas biparietal diameter (BPD), femur length (FL), head and abdominal circumference (HC and AC) are proportionally reduced. Often the prognosis is poor. Incidence is 20–30%.
   (b) Type II/asymmetric
   Usually, later onset and occurs by uteroplacental insufficiency. Ponderal index is low (< 3), whereas BPD, HC, and FL are normal. Abdominal circumference is often decreased. Brain growth is often preserved. Prognosis is better. Incidence 70–80%.
2. According to etiological factors
   - Intrinsic due to fetal factors
   - Extrinsic due to placental/maternal/environment factors
   - Combined
   - Idiopathic
3. According to gestational age:
   - Early onset – onset is early in pregnancy, usually before 32 weeks. Usually the disease is of genetic or fetal origin. Hypoxia is present and significant; however, fetus tolerates the hypoxia due to cardiovascular adaptations. It is associated with high mortality. Management is relatively more complex.
   - Late onset – onset is later in pregnancy (more than 32 weeks), placental/maternal disease, or idiopathic hypoxia may be present. The adaptive mechanisms are mainly by the cardiovascular system, but tolerance to hypoxia is low. The mortality rates are lower; however, the morbidity is high and is associated with poor long-term outcomes.

Maternal Causes Associated with High Risk of Fetal Growth Restriction

There are several causes or pathologies associated with fetal growth restriction. Some of these causes are listed below: [9, 10]

- Maternal hypertension (chronic hypertension and preeclampsia)
- Chronic maternal diseases
- Diabetes with vascular injury
- Autoimmune maternal diseases
- Severe maternal malnutrition
- Smoking and use of alcohol or other drugs
- Congenital infections (TORCH, Syphilis, and Zika)

Neonatal Consequences of SGA

The birth of a SGA newborn implies in many risks, not only during the postnatal period but on infancy and adulthood. And these risks are not restricted to neurodevelopment. It is well known that adult diseases, such as hypertension, diabetes, metabolic abnormalities, have their origin in the restriction of fetus growth. So, the correct identification of these newborns are essential to foresee the outcome of a specific newborn. It is also important to consider which SGA one is facing: a term born SGA or a preterm born SGA newborn? There are differences between these newborns. In a term SGA newborn the organs have completed the development, although with a smaller size, and adapted to survive in utero until term. The preterm SGA newborns are smaller compared to their counterparts at the same gestational age and the organs are still under development, even considering that the intrauterine adaptation have accelerated the development of some of them. Moreover, the growth after birth is also extremely important to anticipate or predict the life course of that baby. But how can the neonatologist evaluate this growth trajectory? This has become a challenge, as many concepts are being questioned [11, 12].

First comes the decision on which growth neonatal chart to use when we are dealing with preterm newborn infants. Actually, there are two neonatal charts that are recommended: the Fenton 2013 neonatal growth reference [13] and the Intergrowth-21 growth standards, which has two modalities: the neonatal standard and the preterm longitudinal standard [14, 15]. Both neonatal reference charts, Fenton 2013 and Intergrowth-21, reflect the intrauterine growth; the Intergrowth-21 preterm longitudinal standard reflects the growth of preterm newborns after birth, considering the physiological weight loss and the postnatal nutritional challenges. Two studies compared these three charts: at birth the Fenton 2013 and Intergrowth-21 neonatal reference, and at discharge the Fenton 2013 and the preterm longitudinal Intergrowth-21; both used the tenth percentile to define IUGR and EUGR, and used the Fenton 2013 at birth and the neonatal Intergrowth-21 at birth and the longitudinal preterm Intergrowth-21 at discharge. Both reported a higher incidence of IUGR at birth and a lower incidence of EUGR at discharge with the Intergrowth-21, compared to the Fenton 2013 [16, 17].

The definition of SGA is also still controversial considering the neonatal reference used. In 2003, an international consensus defined SGA as those newborns with a birthweight less than 2 SD from the reference neonatal chart [18]. In spite of this consensus, some studies recommend the tenth percentile [19, 20], while other studies consider the third percentile of the reference neonatal growth chart [21, 22] to define SGA. However, the definition of intrauterine growth restriction based solely on a predetermined cut-off point can be misleading as it does not account for the growth potential of the fetus; the obstetric evaluation of fetal growth and well-being is fundamental [23–25].

Another important issue is the concept of extrauterine growth restriction (EUGR). As it is used it refers to the weight below the tenth percentile of the reference neonatal chart at a specific time point, set at 36 weeks postmenstrual age, term age, or at discharge from hospital. A recent review of this concept, as well as the concept of postnatal growth failure, questions these definitions and the reasoning under them [11]. The experts recommendations are that the preterm newborn infant should grow at the intrauterine growth rate [25–27]. The evidences point to the importance of a postnatal growth pattern for the preterm newborns, as showed by Rochow et al. [28]. In this review [11], the experts question the belief that the failure to reach a predetermined percentile at a specific time point could represent a growth deficit, as it does not account for the physiological weight loss. Moreover, SGA newborn infants would be classified as EUGR more frequently, since they start their catch up growth in a lowest level. More comprehensive would be the notion of postnatal altered growth, considering the weight gain, calculated as the difference in score Z for weight from birth to at least term age. They also question the guidance to contemplate solely the weight to define growth failure. It is important to consider, as well, the increases in length and head circumference to determine the adequacy of postnatal growth, which means finding how well these babies are able to grow, increasing weight, length, and head circumference. A classification of growth restriction is proposed by a consensus of experts, considering weight, length, and nutrient intake [29]. Considering the changes in Z scores, for all anthropometric measurements, appears to be more comprehensive, inclusive to evaluate the SGA born infants.

References

1. Shrivastava D, Master A. Fetal growth restriction. J Obstet Gynaecol India. 2020 Apr;70(2):103–10.
2. Gordijn SJ, Beune IM, Ganzevoort W. Building consensus and standards in fetal growth restriction studies. Best Pract Res Clin Obstet Gynaecol. 2018;49:117–26.
3. Beune IM, Bloomfield FH, Ganzevoort W, Embleton ND, Rozance PJ, van Wassenaer-Leemhuis AG, Wynia K, Gordijn SJ. Consensus based definition of growth restriction in the newborn. J Pediatr. 2018;196:71–6.
4. Avagliano L, Garo C, Marconi AM. Placental amino acids transport in intrauterine growth restriction. J Pregnancy. 2012;972562

5. Chen YY, Gupta MB, Grattton R, Powell TL, et al. Down-regulation of placental folate transporters in intrauterine growth restriction. J Nutr Biochem. 2018;59:136–41.
6. Murphy VE, Smith R, Giles WB, Clifton VL. Endocrine regulation of human fetal growth: the role of the mother, placenta, and fetus. Endocr Rev. 2006;27(2):141–69.
7. Sharma D, Farahbakhsh N, Shastri S, Sharma P. Intrauterine growth restriction—part 2. J Matern Fetal Neonatal Med. 2016;29(24):4037–48.
8. Singh M. Disorders of weight and gestation. In: Singh M, editor. In care of the newborn. 5th ed. New Delhi: Sagar Publications; 1999. p. 224–45.
9. Fleiss B, Wong F, Brownfoot F, Shearer IK. Knowledge gaps and emerging research areas in intrauterine growth restriction associated brain injury. Front Endocrinol. 2019;10:188.
10. Sharma D, Shastri S, Sharma P. Intrauterine growth restriction: antenatal and postnatal aspects. Clin Med Insights Pediatr. 2016;10:67–83.
11. Fenton TR, Cormack B, Goldberg D, Nasser R, Alshalkh B, Eliasziw M, Hay WW, Hoyos A, Anderson D, Bloomfield F, Griffin I, Embleton N, Rochow N, Taylo S, Senterre T, Schanler RJ, Elmrayed S, Groh-Wargo S, Adamkin D, Shah OS. "Extrauterine growth restriction" and "postnatal growth failure" are misnomers for preterm infants. J Perinatol. 2020;40:704–14.
12. Chou FS, Pandey V, Yeh HW. Postnatal growth in extremely low birth weight newborns: nature or nurture? J Perinatol. 2021;41(3):648–49.
13. Fenton TR, Kim JH. A systematic review and meta-analysis to revise the Fenton growth chart for preterm infants. BMC Pediatr. 2013;13:59.
14. Villar J, Giuliani F, Fenton TR, Ohuma EO, Ismail LC, Kennedy SH. For the INTERGROWTH-21st consortium. INTERGROWTH-21st very preterm size at birth reference charts. Lancet. 2016;387:844–5.
15. Villar J, Giuliani F, Bhutta ZA, Bertino E, Ohuma EO, Ismail LC, Barros FC, Altman DG, Victora C, Noble JA, Gravett MG, Purwar M, Pang R, Lambert A, Papageorghiou AT, Ochieng R, Jaffer YA, Kennedy SH. For the international fetal and newborn growth consortium for the 21st century (INTERGROWTH-21st). Postnatal growth standards for preterm infants: the preterm postnatal follow-up study of the INTERGROWTH-21st project. Lancet. 2015;3:e681–91.
16. Tuzun F, Yucesoy E, Baysal B, Kumral A, Duman N, Oskan H. Comparison of Intergrowth-21 and Fenton growth standards to assess size at birth and extrauterine growth in very preterm infants. J Matern Fetal Neonatal Med. 2018;31:2252–7.
17. Reddy KV, Sharma D, Vardhelli V, Bashir T, Deshbotla SK. Comparison of Fenton 2013 growth curves and the Intergrowth-21 growth standards to assess the incidence of intrauterine growth restriction and extrauterine growth restriction in preterm neonates ≤ 32 weeks. J Matern Fetal Neonatal Med. 2019;27:1–8.
18. Lee PA, Chernausek SD, Hokken-Koelega ACS, Czernichow P. International small for gestational age advisory board consensus development conference statement: Management of Short Children Born Small for Gestational Age, April 24-October 1, 2001. Pediatrics. 2003;111:1253–61.
19. Radmacher PG, Looney SW, Rafait ST, Adamki DH. Prediction of extrauterine growth retardation (EUGR) in VVLBW infants. J Perinatol. 2003;23:392–5.
20. Feldman R, Eidelman AI. Neonatal state organization, neuromaturation, mother-infant interaction, and cognitive development in small-for-gestational-age premature infants. Pediatrics. 2006;118:e869–78.
21. Finken MJJ, Dekker FW, de Zegher F, Wit JM. The Dutch Project on Preterm and Small-for-gestational-age-19 Collaborative Study Group. Long-term height gain of prematurely born children with neonatal growth restraint: parallelism with growth pattern of short children born small for gestational age. Pediatrics. 2006;118:640–3.
22. Pierrat V, Marchand-Martin L, Guemas I, Matis J, Burguet A, Picaud JC, Fresson J, Albrge C, Marret S, Roze JC, Kaminski M, Larroque B, Ancel PY, the EPIGAGE Study Group. Height at 2 and 5 years of age in children born very preterm: the EPIPAGE Study. ADC-FNN Online First 2011.

23. Mamelle N, Boniol M, Rivière O, Joly MO, Mellier G, Maria B, Rousset B, Claris O. Identification of newborns with fetal growth restriction (FGR) in weight and/or length based on constitutional growth potential. Eur J Pediatr. 2006;165:717–25.
24. Mayer C, Joseph KS. Fetal growth: a review of terms, concepts and issues relevant to obstetrics. Ultrasound Obstet Gynecol. 2013;41:136–45.
25. Figueras F, Gratacós. Update on the diagnosis and classification of fetal growth restriction and proposal of stage-based management protocol. Fetal Diagn Ther. 2014;36:86–98.
26. Committee on Nutrition American Academy of Pediatrics. Assessing nutrition status. In: Pediatric Nutrition Handbook. 8th ed. Elk Grove Village II: American Academy Pediatrics; 2020.
27. Agostoni C, Buonocore G, Carnielli VP, De Curtis M, Darmaun D, Decsi T, Domellöf M, Embleton ND, Fusch C, Genzel-Boroviczeny O, Goulet O, Kalhan SC, Kolacek S, Koletzko B, Lapillonne A, Mihatsch W, Moreno L, Neu J, Poindexter B, Puntis J, Putet G, Rigo J, Riskin A, Salle B, Sauer P, Shamir R, Szajewska H, Thureen P, Turck D, van Goudoever JB, Ziegler EE, ESPGHAN Committee on Nutrition. Enteral nutrient supply for preterm infants: commentary from the European Society of paediatric gastroenterology, hepatology and nutrition committee on nutrition. J Pediatr Gastroenterol Nutr. 2010;50(1):85–91.
28. Rochow N, Raja P, Liu K, Fenton T, Landau-Crangle E, Göttler S, Jahn A, Lee S, Seigel S, Campbell D, Heckmann M, Pöschl J, Fusch C. Physiological adjustments to postnatal growth trajectories in healthy preterm infants. Ped Research. 2016;79:870–879 29.
29. Goldberg DL, Becker PJ, Brigham K, Carlson S, Fleck L, Gollins L, Sandrock M, Fullmer M, Van Poots HA. Identifying malnutrition in preterm and neonatal populations: Recommended indicators. J Acad Nutr Diet. 2018;118:1571–82.

Chapter 60
Respiratory Distress Syndrome in the Newborn

José Roberto de Moraes Ramos and Carlos A. Bhering

Introduction

Respiratory diseases are the main responsible for morbidity and mortality during the neonatal period, representing the most common cause of hospitalization in this age group. Respiratory distress syndrome (RDS) is the most frequent cause of respiratory failure in the neonatal period [1]. It is associated with primary deficiency or surfactant dysfunction and particularly affects the preterm newborn (PTNB; <37 weeks).

The estimated global preterm birth rate was 10.6%, equating to an estimated 15 million live preterm births approximately. 12 million (81.1%) of these preterm births occurred in Asia and sub-Saharan Africa. Regional preterm birth rates for 2014 ranged from 13.4% (6.3–30.9) in North Africa to 8.7% (6.3–13.3) in Europe. In Brazil, 300,000 births are preterm which represents 11.2% of all birth and represents 2.2% of all preterm birth in the world [2].

The incidence of RDS is inversely proportional to gestational age and birth weight, affecting about 5% of late preterm infants (34–36 weeks of gestational age), 30% of those under 30 weeks, and 60% of those under 28 weeks.

J. R. de Moraes Ramos (✉)
Departamento de Neonatologia do Instituto Fernandes Figueira/FIOCRUZ, Rio de Janeiro, Brazil

Programa de Reanimação Neonatal da Sociedade Brasileira de Pediatria, Rio de Janeiro, Brazil

C. A. Bhering
Departamento de Neonatologia do Instituto Fernandes Figueira/FIOCRUZ, Rio de Janeiro, Brazil

Pediatria da Universidade de Vassouras, Vassouras, Brazil

© Springer Nature Switzerland AG 2022

R. A. Moreira de Sá, E. B. d. Fonseca (eds.), *Perinatology*,
https://doi.org/10.1007/978-3-030-83434-0_60

The incorporation of technological advances in the care provided to critically ill newborns, as well as the use of new diagnostic and therapeutic approaches in the management of neonatal respiratory disease, contributed to the increase in the survival rates of premature babies, particularly those born with very low birth. Data from literature demonstrate that in the last years, the administration of antenatal corticosteroids and the replacement of exogenous surfactant reduced the incidence and severity of RDS and significantly improved survival [1, 3]. However, with the improvement of intensive care, especially in extremely preterm infants, RDS still remains an important cause of neonatal morbidity since newborns who survive may present complications such as intracranial hemorrhage (ICH), persistence of the ductus arteriosus (PCA), sepsis, and bronchopulmonary dysplasia (BPD), among others [3].

Prenatal and Perinatal Care

Interventions to improve outcomes and prevent RDS should be started before birth. It is currently agreed that the quality of prenatal care performed by the family can have a positive impact on the birth conditions of newborns. In the imminence of a premature birth, it is necessary to consider interventions that can prolong pregnancy to decrease the risk of an adverse unfavorable outcome. Currently, obstetric studies have sought biomarkers that can determine which women is at the highest risk of preterm birth in the next 7 days and thus allow the more judicious use of prenatal treatments. The use of these markers associated with the measurement of uterine cervical length can be especially useful in such process (Table 60.1).

Pathophysiology

Initially, RDS was called "asphyxia neonatorum" due to the presentation and clinical evolution of the condition, mainly due to progressive hypoxia. Later, it came to be called "hyaline membrane disease" (DMH), well translating the anatomopathological picture found: Presence of a characteristic membrane (giving rise to the name "hyaline membrane disease") formed by a fibrinous matrix, the result of a massive exudation of plasma proteins, in association with cell debris from epithelial injury, located mainly at the junction of respiratory bronchioles and alveolar ducts. It was observed that these anatomopathological findings were secondary to the deficiency of the surfactant, a phospholipid substance produced by type II pneumocytes after the 20th week of pregnancy and peaked around the 35th week. In addition to prematurity, other factors such as hypoxia, acidosis, and hypovolemia can interfere with surfactant synthesis. The lack of surfactant and/or its dysfunction causes an increase in the alveolar surface tension and the elastic retraction force, leading to alveolar instability, progressive atelectasis, with a consequent decrease in lung compliance. The tendency for alveolar collapse in the absence of surfactant is due to the increased attraction between hydrogen molecules, at the water and air interface, inside the alveolus. This whole process triggers an inflammatory response with the

Table 60.1 Recommendations for antenatal care in the management of RDS

Recommendations	Grade evidence
Mothers at high risk of preterm birth <28–34 weeks of gestation should be transferred to tertiary centers	C1
Healthcare provider should offer a single course of antenatal steroids for lung maturation to all women at risk of preterm delivery from 24 to 34 weeks, ideally at least 24 h before birth	A1
A single repeated course of steroids can be given in a threatened preterm birth before 32–34 weeks of gestation if the first course was administered at least 1–2 weeks earlier	A2
$MgSO_4$ should be administered to women in imminent labor before 32 weeks of gestation	A2
In women with symptoms of preterm labor, measurements of cervical length, and fibronectin should be considered to avoid the unnecessary use of tocolytic drugs and/or antenatal steroids	B2
Doctors should consider the short-term use of tocolytic drugs in very preterm pregnancies to allow course of steroids for lung maturation and/or transfer in the uterus to the tertiary center	B1

Modified from European Consensus [4]

release of cytokines that can cause serious damage to the capillary endothelium and alveolar epithelium, further increasing the leakage of fluid, rich in proteins, into the alveoli. Factors such as hyperoxia, barotrauma, and volutrauma contribute to the increase in the inflammatory response, reducing the synthesis and function of the surfactant. This entire process results in an increase in total lung water, making the lungs hepatized, poorly aerated, and with reduced compliance.

Therefore, it is possible to understand the nonuniform distribution of air in the lungs affected by RDS, since there are areas of atelectasis (alveolar collapse) and well-aerated areas. In fact, during the respiratory cycle, there are fixed collapsed areas – during inspiration and expiration, mixed areas – ventilated on inspiration with subsequent atelectasis during expiration, and pulmonary areas or regions that remain stable throughout the respiratory phase. The distribution of these compartments is influenced by a number of factors, especially with the treatment with pressure of continuous distension in the airways and/or exogenous surfactant. The use of continuous distension pressure in the airways increases the functional residual capacity (FRC) and lung volume, and promotes recruitment of new terminal air spaces with improved compliance and tidal volume. This pulmonary effect reduces the venous mixture, decreasing the D-E shunt.

Clinical Manifestation

The manifestations are variable according to the degree of deficiency and/or dysfunction of surfactant and the immaturity of the newborn. Gas exchange that occur in utero are mediated exclusively by placental diffusion, since the lungs are not yet functional. The process of lung expansion that occurs at birth, associated with other adaptive physiological phenomena, leads to a reduction in pulmonary vascular resistance, with a consequent increase in the blood flow that reaches the lungs, so that the newborn starts the gas exchange directly with the external environment. Most babies start breathing in the delivery room (physiological transition period, from intrauterine to extrauterine life) and symptoms may only appear in the first hours of life with mild clinical signs and symptoms initially progressing both in intensity and severity. Chest auscultation may show decreased breath sounds and low intake of air. In very low-birth-weight preterm infants, the clinical expression of respiratory distress may be unclear, with the early appearance of apnea and cyanosis being frequent. We can observe the progression of respiratory discomfort mainly due to the presence of tachypnea, expiratory grunts, cyanosis, nasal flaring, intercostal and/or subcostal retractions, and sternal retraction. The infant may be restless and agitated, depending on the degree of hypoxia. As symptoms worsen, the need for supplemental oxygen increases. This clinical condition if left untreated can lead to respiratory failure and/or death in the first 72 hours of life.

Diagnosis

The diagnosis is based on the presence of significant respiratory distress in a premature newborn, in the first hours after birth. The radiological analysis shows variable changes, according to the degree of deficiency and/or dysfunction of the pulmonary surfactant. Usually, the lung volume is decreased and there are granular reticular condensations (ground glass), due to the aeration of the respiratory bronchioles contrasting with the atelectasis alveoli (Fig. 60.1). The presence of air bronchograms is important for determining the degree of impairment and classification of radiological changes. These changes are generally asymmetrical since RDS is a nonhomogeneous lung disease. Despite this typical radiological pattern, the infection caused by

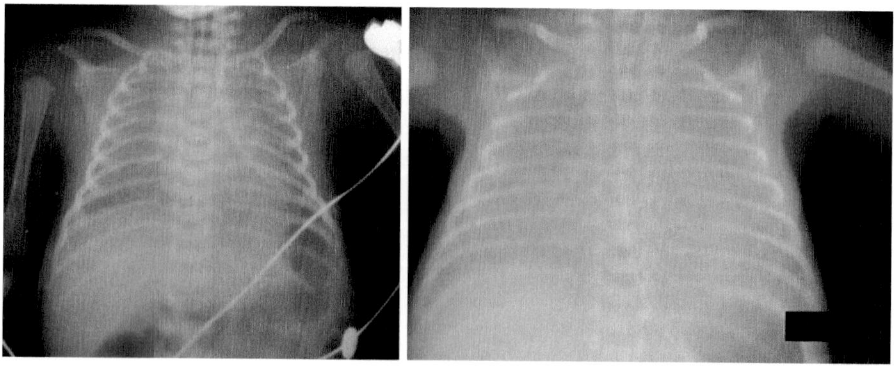

Fig. 60.1 Radiological aspects of the newborn's respiratory distress syndrome: Presence of reticulogranular condensations and atelectatic alveoli

Table 60.2 Radiological differences in neonatal respiratory diseases

Gestional age	X-ray changes	Possible diagnosis
Term infants	Reinforcement of the vascular network, especially on the right	Transient tachypnea of the newborn
Preterm newborn	Hypotransparency, reticulogranular aspect, ground glass image	Hyaline membrane disease
Very low-birth-weight newborn	Decreased volume without hypotransparency	Pulmonary immaturity
Sudden worsening at any gestational age	Air outside lung parenchyma	Pulmonary Emphysema Pneumothorax

Modified from Moreira and Lopes [5]

group B hemolytic streptococcus has a very similar appearance and is sometimes difficult to differentiate. Table 60.2 shows some radiological differences of hyaline membrane disease and other respiratory pathologies. Arterial blood gases are important to assess the severity of respiratory failure, response to supportive therapy, and therapeutic measures. Other tests, such as complete blood count, blood culture, C-reactive protein, and others, contribute to the assessment of the patient in general and to help in the differential diagnosis, mainly of pulmonary infection secondary to group B hemolytic beta streptococcus.

Treatment

The treatment of RDS includes the use of different methods of noninvasive or invasive ventilatory assistance; administration of exogenous surfactant; and general measures of thermal, metabolic, water, and hemodynamic control, when necessary.

Methods of Ventilatory Assistance

Maintaining good oxygenation is the primary goal. For this to happen, it is necessary to use oxygen therapy as early as recommended by the neonatal resuscitation program [6] and in newborns with spontaneous breathing and respiratory distress, use continuous positive airway pressure (CPAP) in order to keep them open and ventilated, promoting early lung recruitment (preventing alveolar collapse). The prophylactic use of CPAP is generally recommended in premature infants younger than 30 weeks [7, 19]. The intention of using CPAP early is to decrease the need for invasive ventilatory support. Therefore, adequate resuscitation with the use of CPAP via a manual T-shaped ventilator or in water seal still in the delivery room, should be the initial treatment of choice in the vast majority of cases, regardless of gestational age or birth weight. With adequate ventilation and oxygenation from the first minutes of life, changes in the ventilation–perfusion relationship, atelectasis, and pulmonary vasoconstriction can be avoided, which are responsible for aggravating the condition of RDS. In fact, multicenter clinical studies have shown that the use of CPAP in the delivery room reduces the need for intubation and the use of exogenous surfactant, in addition to decreasing mortality in extremely premature infants (24–25 weeks) [7–10, 23]. Therefore, delaying the administration of surfactant in premature infants who may need it later does not harm these patients. Even with this less invasive approach, a significant number of premature newborns still end up being intubated during resuscitation in the delivery room.

In the neonatal ICU, the type of ventilatory assistance to be used will be determined by the severity of the condition and may change according to the evolution of each case. CPAP is usually applied through the use of a nasal interface (nasal prong or mask), with an initial pressure of 5 cm H_2O (maximum of 8 cm H_2O), continuous flow of a mixture of air and oxygen of 5–10 l / min, through the respirator or in water seal.

Some studies have evaluated a combination of strategies such as INSURE (Intubation– Surfactant–Extubation). This strategy showed less need for mechanical ventilation, less pneumothorax, and less retreatment with surfactant when compared to the CPAP group (42). However, the studies were small, subject to bias, included patients of more advanced gestational age, and used criteria for intubation and mechanical ventilation different from multicenter clinical studies on the use of CPAP [11–14].

Invasive mechanical ventilation (IMV) has been used for a long time and has increased the survival of preterm newborns with more severe RDS. Despite this, IMV have deleterious effects on the lungs. Therefore, during IMV it is important to use efficient and protective strategies, such as synchronized modes and guaranteed volume ventilation [15, 16]. Table 60.3 shows the 2019 European Consensus

Table 60.3 Recommendations for mechanical ventilation strategies: European Consensus –2019 [4]

Recommendations	Grade evidence
After stabilization, MV should be used in babies with RDS when other methods of respiratory support have failed (A1). The duration of the VM should be minimized	B2
The primary choice of ventilation mode is at the discretion of the clinical team; however, if conventional MV is used, the target tidal volume should be used (TO 1)	A1
When weaning from MV, it is reasonable to tolerate a modest degree of hypercarbia as long as the pH remains above (7.22)	B2
Caffeine should be used to facilitate MV weaning (A1). Early caffeine should be considered for babies at high risk of needing MV, such as those on noninvasive respiratory support	C1
A short course of low dose or very low dexamethasone should be considered to facilitate extubation in babies who remain on MV after 1–2 weeks	A2
Inhaled budesonide can be considered for babies at very high risk of BPD	A2
Opioids should be used selectively when indicated by clinical judgment and assessment of pain indicators (D1). Routine use of infusions of morphine or midazolam in ventilated preterm babies is not recommended	A1

recommendations for mechanical ventilation strategies for the management of newborn respiratory distress syndrome.

Administration of Exogenous Surfactant

The surfactant is a complex substance whose composition comprises about 90–95% of lipids, 5–10% of apoproteins (SP-A, SP-B, SP-C, and SP-D) and a small percentage of carbohydrates. Phosphatidylcholine, in saturated form, is the most important phospholipid. Replacement therapy with exogenous surfactant has been tested in several controlled clinical trials that have shown a 30–40% reduction in the mortality rate. In newborns intubated and submitted to IMV, the administration of surfactant with up to 2 hours of life is more effective due to a better distribution of the surfactant in the lungs that still have a greater number of aerated bronchiolar units [17].

There are several recommendations on how to administer the surfactant into the lungs. The goal is to promote a homogeneous distribution of the drug to fully exercise its lung function. The ideal method of instillation is still widely discussed. A recent literature review highlighted some relevant points and recommended bolus instillation associated with ventilatory strategies before, during, and after drug instillation [17] (Table 60.4).

The slow infusion of surfactant in order to mitigate side effects can result in poor distribution in the lungs. Some side effects may occur during instillation: transient drop in oxygen saturation, bradycardia, airway obstruction, pulmonary hemorrhage, and pulmonary hypertension. Pulmonary hemorrhage is generally rare and more common in the first 72 hours of life [20].

The initial dose ranges from 100 to 200 mg/kg [18]. After administration, there is usually a progressive reduction in O_2 requirements and respiratory effort due to an improvement in respiratory mechanics and lung volume. With this, it is possible to actively decrease the parameters used by mechanical ventilation. Initially, the inspired fraction of O_2 (FiO_2) should be reduced, followed by a reduction in inspiratory pressure when FiO_2 is less than 50%. An additional dose (100 mg/kg) can be

Table 60.4 Suggested surfactant instillation method

Keep the newborn in the supine position
Increase pressure by 1–2 cm H_2O in the respirator, 5 minutes before instillation, or use a manual ventilator with 1–2 cm H_2O above the pressure previously used
Disconnect the orotracheal tube (TOT) from the respirator circuit
Instill the surfactant in the middle third of the trachea, in bolus (in 10″ to 20″). Divide the total dose into 1 to 2 aliquots with an interval of 30″ to 60″ between them
Ventilate with a frequency of 60 IPM and enough pressure to push the liquid column of the drug into the airways
Try not to suck the TOT in the next 2 hours, unless you have signs of airway obstruction

taken 6 hours after the first dose if the newborn continues on mechanical ventilation and with high FiO_2.

Prevention

The best way to prevent DMH and its complications is adequate antenatal care, in order to avoid preterm labor. Regular prenatal evaluation, periodic examinations of low complexity, and serology can indicate preventable causes of spontaneous and medically indicated preterm birth. Another important measure is the administration of steroids to pregnant women between 24 and 34 weeks when there is a risk of preterm delivery. It is most effective when administered before 34 weeks of gestational age and at least 24 hours up to 7 days before birth. Its use before 24 and after 34 weeks of gestational age is controversial, but very frequent. The combination of antenatal corticosteroids and exogenous surfactant is highly positive, because while corticoids induce structural maturation in the lung, the surfactant causes a functional improvement in it.

References

1. Polin RA, Carlo WA, Committee on Fetus and Newborn, American Academy of Pediatrics. Surfactant replacement therapy for preterm and term neonates with respiratory distress. Pediatrics. 2014;133:156–63.
2. Chawanpaiboon S, Vogel JP, Moller AB, Lumbiganon P, Petzold M, Hogan D, Landoulsi S, et al. Global, regional, and national estimates of levels of preterm birth in 2014: a systematic review and modelling analysis. Lancet Glob Health. 2019;7(1):e37–46. https://doi.org/10.1016/S2214-109X(18)30451-0.
3. Soll RF. Synthetic surfactant for respiratory distress syndrome in preterm infants. Cochrane Database Syst Rev. 2000;2:CD001149. pmid:10796417.
4. Sweet DG, Carnielli V, Greisen G, Hallman M, Ozek E, Te Pas A, Plavka R, Roehr CC, Saugstad OD, Simeoni U, Speer CP, Vento M, Visser GHA, Halliday HL. European consensus guidelines on the management of respiratory distress syndrome - 2019 Update. Neonatology. 2019;115(4):432–50. https://doi.org/10.1159/000499361. Epub 2019 Apr 11
5. Lopes JMA, Moreira MEL. Patologias respiratórias. In: Moreira MEL, Lopes JMA, Carvalho M, editors. O recém-nascido de alto risco: teoria e prática do cuidar. Rio de Janeiro: Fiocruz; 2004. p. 109–38.
6. Programa de reanimação neonatal da SBP. https://www.sbp.com.br/fileadmin/user_upload/DiretrizesSBPReanimacaoPrematuroMenor34semanas26jan2016.pdf.
7. Schmölzer GM, Kumar M, Pichler G, Aziz K, O'Reilly M, Cheung PY. Non-invasive versus invasive respiratory support in preterm infants at birth: systematic review and meta-analysis. BMJ. 2013;347:f5980.
8. Dunn MS, Kaempf J, de Klerk A, de Klerk R, Reilly M, Howard D, Ferrelli K, O'Conor J, Soll RF, Vermont Oxford Network DRM Study Group. Randomized trial comparing 3 approaches to the initial respiratory management of preterm neonates. Pediatrics. 2011;128(5):1069–76.
9. Rojas-Reyes MX, Morley CJ, Soll R. Prophylactic versus selective use of surfactant in preventing morbidity and mortality in preterm infants. Cochrane Database Syst Rev. 2012;3(3):CD000510pmid:22419276.

10. Wright CJ, Polin RA. Noninvasive support: does it really decrease bronchopulmonary dysplasia? Clin Perinatol. 2016;43(4):783–98. https://doi.org/10.1016/j.clp.2016.07.012. Review. PMID:27837759.
11. Stevens TP, Harrington EW, Blennow M, Soll RF. Early surfactant administration with brief ventilation vs. selective surfactant and continued mechanical ventilation for preterm infants with or at risk for respiratory distress syndrome. Cochrane Database Syst Rev. 2007;4:CD003063. pmid:17943779.
12. Dunn MS, Kaempf J, de Klerk A, et al. Randomized trial comparing 3 approaches to the initial respiratory management of preterm neonates. Pediatrics. 2011;128(5):e1069–76.
13. Finer NN, Carlo WA, Walsh MC, et al. Early CPAP versus surfactant in extremely preterm infants. N Engl J Med. 2010;362(21):1970–9.
14. Morley CJ, Davis PG, Doyle LW, et al. Nasal CPAP or intubation at birth for very preterm infants. N Engl J Med. 2008;358(7):700–8.
15. Jensen EA, DeMauro SB, Kornhauser M, Aghai ZH, Greenspan JS, Dysart KC. Effects of multiple ventilation courses and duration of mechanical ventilation on respiratory outcomes in extremely low-birth-weight infants. JAMA Pediatr. 2015;169(11):1011–7.
16. Miller JD, Carlo WA. Pulmonary complications of mechanical ventilation in neonates. Clin Perinatol. 2008;35(1):273–81.
17. Horbar JD, Carpenter JH, Buzas J, Soll RF, Suresh G, Bracken MB, Leviton LC, Plsek PE, Sinclair JC. Timing of initial surfactant treatment of infants 23 to 29 weeks' gestation: is routine practice evidence based? Pediatrics. 2004;113:1593.
18. Ramanathan R, Rasmussen MR, Gerstmann DR, Finer N, Sekar K. A randomized, multicenter masked comparison trial of poractant alfa (Curosurf) versus beractant (Survanta) in the treatment of respiratory distress syndrome in preterm infants. Am J Perinatol. 2004;21:109–19.
19. Soll RF, Morley CJ. Prophylactic versus selective use of surfactante in prevening morbidity and mortality in preterm infants. Cochrane Database Syst Rev. 2001;2:CD000510. SUPPORT Study Group of the Eunice Kennedy Shriver NICHD Neonatal Research Network Early CPAP versus surfactant in extremely preterm infants, N Eng J Med 2010; 362:1970.
20. Tarawneh A, Kaczmarek J, Bottino MN, Sant'Anna GM. Severe airway obstruction during surfactant administration using a standardized protocol: a prospective, observational study. J Perinatol. 2012;32:270–5.

Chapter 61
Transient Tachypnea of the Newborn

Carlos A. Bhering and José Roberto de Moraes Ramos

Transient tachypnea of the newborn (TTN) is a benign and self-limited condition that can present in babies of any gestational age, shortly after birth. It is related to a delay in the absorption of pulmonary fluid after birth, which leads to ineffective gas exchange, respiratory discomfort, and tachypnea.

During birth, significant changes occur due to the transition from fetal to neonatal circulation, characterized by the end of the production of pulmonary fluid and its replacement by ambient air. The absorption of the liquid begins before birth, already occurring during labor and by mechanisms still largely unknown. It is estimated that 60–70% is reabsorbed before birth, 5–10% in the birth canal, and the remainder in the first hours of life by the pulmonary capillaries.

It usually presents as a benign and self-limited disease, but some babies evolve develop severe respiratory distress and require the admission to a neonatal intensive care unit (NICU). There is often a doubt in the diagnosis, and it is necessary to exclude other causes of respiratory disorder in the neonatal period.

C. A. Bhering
Departamento de Neonatologia do Instituto Fernandes Figueira/FIOCRUZ, Rio de Janeiro, Brazil

Pediatria da Universidade de Vassouras, Vassouras, Brazil

J. R. de Moraes Ramos (✉)
Departamento de Neonatologia do Instituto Fernandes Figueira/FIOCRUZ, Rio de Janeiro, Brazil

Programa de Reanimação Neonatal da Sociedade Brasileira de Pediatria, Rio de Janeiro, Brazil

© Springer Nature Switzerland AG 2022

R. A. Moreira de Sá, E. B. d. Fonseca (eds.), *Perinatology*,
https://doi.org/10.1007/978-3-030-83434-0_61

Etiology

Maternal risk factors include delivery before the end of 39 weeks of gestation, an elective cesarean section without labor, gestational diabetes, and maternal asthma. [1, 2] Some authors call attention to the fact that the risk of TTN increases two to six times if we compare those born with normal delivery and elective cesarean section, especially when there is hypotension in the predelivery period [3].

Fetal risk factors include male gender, perinatal asphyxia, prematurity, small for gestational age, and large for gestational age [4].

Epidemiology

The incidence is inversely proportional to the gestational age and affects approximately 10% of babies born between 33 and 34 weeks, approximately 5% between 35 and 36 weeks, and less than 1% in term babies [5].

Pathophysiology

In the fetal lung, the pulmonary epithelium secretes alveolar fluid at around 6 weeks of gestation. The chloride ions, in the pulmonary interstitium, enter the epithelial cell through the active transport of sodium, potassium, and chloride (Na–K–2Cl transporter), which, in turn, are secreted in the alveolus through various chloride channels. Chloride ions via paracellular pathways and water is transported through protein channels in the cell membrane. The volume of the fetal lung is maintained by the larynx, which acts as a unidirectional valve, allowing only fluid to escape [6].

The main mechanism of reabsorption of fetal pulmonary fluid is believed to be the passive movement of sodium through the epithelial sodium channels (CENa), with chest compression playing a minor role in clearance. With the onset of labor, epinephrine maternal and glucocorticoids, released in greater quantity during stress, activate CENa in apical membranes of type II pneumocytes. In this way, alveolar sodium is passively transported through these channels and, in turn, is actively transported back to the interstice by the Na + / K + -ATPase pump [6]. In this way, an osmotic gradient is created that allows chloride and water to also be absorbed by the pulmonary circulation and by the lymphatics [6].

The study by Atasay et al. found an association between low levels of some hormones (cortisol, free ACTH eT3) in the umbilical cord with TTN and the authors believe that there is a relationship between these and the clearance of fetal pulmonary fluids and in postnatal pulmonary adaptation through its modulating effect on the sodium epithelial channel and Na–K–ATPase [7]. Tsuda et al. also found an association between low levels of cortisol in the umbilical cord and TTN between twins who developed or not a respiratory disorder [8].

History and Physical Examination

The condition starts within the first minutes to hours after birth and the findings of the physical examination may include signs of respiratory distress, such as follows:

- Tachypnea (respiratory rate greater than 60 per minute)
- Nasal flaring
- Grunting
- Intercostal, subcostal, and suprasternal retractions
- Crackling, decreased breath, and normal breath sounds or auscultation

Other occasional findings in the exam:

- Tachycardia
- Cyanosis
- Increased chest diameter due to hyperinflation

Diagnostic Approach

The duration of respiratory distress is the main determinant for the diagnosis of TTN. If the distress improves within the first 1 to 2 hours of birth, it can be labeled as a transient condition. It is often a diagnosis of exclusion and, therefore, any persistent tachypnea should be investigated to rule out other causes of respiratory distress.

In the initial approach, we must measure pre- and post-ductal saturations and assess the need for complete blood count, blood culture, C-reactive protein (CRP). It is important to rule out the possibility of early neonatal sepsis.

Arterial blood gases may show hypoxemia and hypocapnia due to tachypnea. Hypercapnia is a sign of fatigue or some possible complication.

The chest X-ray can be quite variable, showing from normal X-rays to changes such as pulmonary hyperinflation with rectification of the diaphragm, diffuse and homogeneous infiltration of pulmonary edema, peri-hilar congestion, and thickening or cisural effusion [9].

The echocardiogram can be considered to rule out congenital heart defects in patients with cyanosis or persistent tachypnea for more than 4 to 5 days.

Treatment

As it is a self-limited condition, supportive care is the basis of treatment. The child should be placed in the NICU, where he should receive routine care, including continuous cardiopulmonary monitoring, thermoneutral environment, blood glucose control, and minimal handling.

The water and nutritional support will be according to the respiratory condition. If the respiratory rate is greater than 80 rpm or there is an increase in respiratory work, we should consider oral fasting and beginning of venous hydration (60–80 ml/kg/day), with an adequate glucose infusion speed (VIG) (4–6 mg/kg/minute). The beginning of the diet should be evaluated as early as possible according to the clinical and hemodynamic conditions.

Oxygen therapy is necessary, and it may generally be necessary to use it through a nasal or labial catheter, and in some places even through the use of oxyhood or a helmet. If the child's condition does not improve or worsen, or if the required fraction of inspired O_2 (FiO_2) is greater than 40%, the use of continuous positive airway pressure (CPAP) should be considered.

TTN can be difficult to distinguish from early neonatal sepsis and pneumonia and, therefore, we should be carefully evaluated and empirical antibiotic therapy should also be considered when deemed necessary.

Randomized clinical trials on the efficacy of furosemide [10] or racemic adrenaline [11] on TTN showed no significant difference in the duration of tachypnea or length of hospital stay compared to controls.

Salbutamol (inhaled beta2-agonist) has been shown to decrease the duration of symptoms and length of hospital stay. However, they call attention to the need for further studies to confirm its effectiveness and safety [12]. A systematic review has shown that current evidence is insufficient to determine the efficacy and safety of salbutamol in the handling of TTN [13].

Differential Diagnosis

- Pneumonia
- Respiratory distress syndrome
- Aspiration syndromes: meconium, blood, or amniotic fluid
- Pneumothorax
- Congenital heart disease
- Persistent pulmonary hypertension
- Central nervous system (CNS): subarachnoid hemorrhage, hypoxic-ischemic encephalopathy
- Inborn errors of metabolism
- Congenital malformations: congenital diaphragmatic hernia, cystic adenomatoid malformations

Prognosis

The overall prognosis is excellent, with most symptoms resolving within 48 hours of onset.

Complications

Air leaks, such as pneumothorax, are rare complications.

Longitudinal studies have shown an association between TTN and the subsequent development of wheezing in the future [14].

References

1. Badran EF, Abdalgani MM, Al-Lawama MA, Al-Ammouri IA, Basha AS, Al Kazaleh FA, Saleh SS, Al-Katib FA, Khader YS. Effects of perinatal risk factors on common neonatal respiratory morbidities beyond 36 weeks of gestation. Saudi Med J. 2012;33(12):1317–23.
2. Brown MJ, Olver RE, Ramsden CA, Strang LB, Walters DV. Effects of adrenaline and of spontaneous labour on the secretion and absorption of lung liquid in the fetal lamb. J Physiol Lond. 1983;344:137–52.
3. Singh S, et al. Transient tachypnea of newborns is associated with maternal spinal hypotension during elective cesarean delivery: A retrospective cohort study. Anesth Analg. 2019;129:162–7.
4. Morrison JJ, Rennie JM, Milton PJ. Neonatal respiratory morbidity and mode of delivery at term: influence of timing of elective caesarean section. Br J Obstet Gynaecol. 1995;102(2):101–6.
5. Zanardo V, Simbi AK, Franzoi M, Soldà G, Salvadori A, Trevisanuto D. Neonatal respiratory morbidity risk and mode of delivery at term: influence of timing of elective caesarean delivery. Acta Paediatr. 2004;93(5):643–7.
6. Jain L. Alveolar fluid clearance in developing lungs and its role in neonatal transition. Clin Perinatol. 1999;26(3):585–99.
7. Atasay B, et al. The association between cord hormones and transient tachypnea of newborn in late preterm and term neonates who were delivered by cesarean section. J Matern Fetal Neonatal Med. 2013;26(9):877–80.
8. Tsuda H, et al. Relationship between the cortisol levels in umbilical cord blood and neonatal RDS/TTN in twin pregnancies. J Matern Fetal Neonatal Med. 2016;29(13):2151–6.
9. Kurl S, Heinonen KM, Kiekara O. The first chest radiograph in neonates exhibiting respiratory distress at birth. Clin Pediatr. 1997;36(5):285–9.
10. Kassab M, Khriesat WM, Anabrees J. Diuretics for transient tachypnoea of the newborn. Cochrane Database Syst Rev. 2015;11:CD003064.
11. Kao B, Stewart de Ramirez SA, Belfort MB, Hansen A. Inhaled epinephrine for the treatment of transient tachypnea of the newborn. J Perinatol. 2008;28(3):205–10.
12. Armangil D, Yurdakök M, Korkmaz A, Yiğit S, Tekinalp G. Inhaled beta-2 agonist salbutamol for the treatment of transient tachypnea of the newborn. J. Pediatr. 2011;159(3):398–403.e1.
13. Moresco L, Bruschettini M, Cohen A, Gaiero A, Calevo MG. Salbutamol for transient tachypnea of the newborn. Cochrane Database Syst Rev. 2016;5:CD011878.
14. Birnkrant DJ, Picone C, Markowitz W, El Khwad M, Shen WH, Tafari N. Association of transient tachypnea of the newborn and childhood asthma. Pediatr Pulmonol. 2006;41(10):978–84.

Chapter 62
Bronchopulmonary Dysplasia

José Maria de Andrade Lopes and Danielle Negri de Souza Lopes

Introduction

BPD was first described by Northway et al. in 1967 as a disease in premature babies with severe respiratory distress syndrome (RDS) subjected to mechanical ventilation and high inspiratory pressures, breathing high oxygen concentrations, characterized by cystic changes and fibrosis in the lung, with high mortality rates [1].

In the last 50 years with the development of NICU, progress in technology of mechanical ventilators, incorporation of several therapies as antenatal steroids (ANS), artificial surfactant, nasal continuous positive airway pressure (CPAP), we have witnessed a major increase in survival of premature babies shifting the limits of viability from 32–34 weeks at that time to 23–24 weeks in the present days [2].

The survival of extreme preterm infants is now very high and with more effective prevention (ANS), respiratory therapies (surfactant) lung disease is now much more a process of arrested development with damage and repair producing a different clinical picture most of the time with a mild chronic lung disease. Major risk factors are still the same, being the most important today the degree of prematurity, followed by supplemental oxygen, mechanical ventilation, intrauterine or extrauterine infection. Genetic factors may play a role and research with new biomarkers are in the pipeline to contribute to our understanding and treatment of BPD [2].

J. M. de Andrade Lopes (✉) · D. N. de Souza Lopes
Perinatal Maternity Hospital, Rio de Janeiro, RJ, Brazil
e-mail: jlopesma@perinatal.com.br

© Springer Nature Switzerland AG 2022
R. A. Moreira de Sá, E. B. d. Fonseca (eds.), *Perinatology*,
https://doi.org/10.1007/978-3-030-83434-0_62

Definition

Eduardo Bancalari has first defined BPD as the need of oxygen at 28 days. However, due to the increasing survival rate of extreme VLBI, such definition was not suitable for most cases. Nevertheless, it is still a criterion used in many studies [3]. In 1988, Shennan et al. described a good correlation of oxygen at 36 weeks and abnormal pulmonary outcomes which derived another commonly used criterion to define BPD – the need of oxygen at 36 correct gestational age [4]. The current definition was proposed in 2001 by Eunice Kennedy Shriver National Institute of Child Health and Human Development (NICHD)–sponsored workshop (Table 62.1), based on the need of supplemental oxygen, respiratory support, at 36 weeks gestational age and also stratifying for BPD severity. This definition was revised in 2018 (Table 62.2), addressing the broadly definition of severe BPD which combined infants on low flow devices, receiving 21% oxygen and infants on high ventilator settings [3].

Incidence

The BPD incidence is higher the lower is gestational age. The Vermont Oxford Network reports rates of 70%, 57%, 50%, 25%, and 17% at 24, 25, 26, 27, and 28 weeks' gestation. Israeli Neonatal Network recently published data on 12,139 babies weighting less than 1500 g, based on the use of oxygen at 36 weeks PMA [5]. The rates for very low birth weight (VLBW) were 13.7% and for extremely low birth

Table 62.1 Definition of bronchopulmonary dysplasia

GESTATIONAL age	< 32 weeks	≥ 32 weeks
Time point of assessment	36 weeks PMA or discharge to home, whichever comes first. Treatment with oxygen >21% for at least 28 days plus	28 days but <56 days postnatal age or discharge to home, whichever comes first
Mild BPD	Breathing room air at 36 weeks PMA or discharge, whichever comes first	Breathing room air by 56 days postnatal age or discharge, whichever comes first
Moderate BPD	Need[a] for <30% oxygen at 36 weeks PMA or discharge, whichever comes first	Need[a] for <30% oxygen at 56 days postnatal age or discharge, whichever comes first
Severe BPD	Need[a] for ≥30% oxygen and/or positive pressure, (PPV or NCPAP) at 36 weeks PMA or discharge, whichever comes first	Need[a] for ≥30% oxygen and/or positive pressure, (PPV or NCPAP) at 56 days postnatal age or discharge, whichever comes first

BPD bronchopulmonary dysplasia, *NCPAP* nasal continuous positive airway pressure, *PMA* post-menstrual age, *PPV* positive pressure ventilation.
[a]A physiologic test confirming that the oxygen requirement at the assessment time point remains to be defined

Table 62.2 Suggested improvements to the definition of BPD

A premature infant (<32 weeks' gestational age) with BPD has persistent parenchymal lung disease, radiographic confirmation of parenchymal lung disease, and at 36 weeks PMA requires one of the following FiO2 ranges/oxygen levels/O2 concentrations for ≥ 3 consecutive days to maintain arterial oxygen saturation in the 90%–95% range

Grades	Invasive IPPV	N-CPAP, NIPPV, or nasal cannula ≥ 3 L/min	Nasal cannula flow of 1–<3 L/min	Hood O2	Nasal cannula flow of <1 L/min
I	–	21	22–29	22–29	22–70
II	21	22–29	≥30	≥30	>70
III	≥21	≥30			
III(A)	Early death (between 14 days of postnatal age and 36 weeks) owing to persistent parenchymal lung disease and respiratory failure that cannot be attributable to other neonatal morbidities (e.g., necrotizing enterocolitis, intraventricular hemorrhage, redirection of care, episodes of sepsis, etc.) [11]				

CPAP continuous positive airway pressure, *IPPV* intermittent positive pressure ventilation, *N-CPAP* nasal continuous positive airway pressure, *NIPPV* noninvasive positive pressure ventilation

weight (ELBW) were 31%. The NICHD Network reported rates of 68% in extreme preterm infants (22–28 weeks gestation). In USA 50,000 ELBW are born every year and about 31% of them will develop BPD [6].

Neonatal Networks from the USA, Canada, Korea, Switzerland, and even China demonstrate a BPD prevalence of 11–50%, with large variability among different centers due to differences in birth weight, gestational age, or diagnostic criteria [7–9].

In 2015, the NIHCD reported data from 1993 to 2012 looking at survival, use of therapies and major neonatal morbidities including BPD. After a period without any change rates of BPD increased from 2009 to 2012 for infants in the 26–27 week range from 50% to 55%. Among extremely preterm infants born at the US academic centers over the last 20 years, changes in maternal and infant care practices and modest reductions in several morbidities were observed, although bronchopulmonary dysplasia increased. Survival increased most markedly for infants born at 23 and 24 weeks and survival without major morbidity increased for infants 25–28 weeks. These findings are important and may be valuable in counselling families and developing novel interventions [7].

Risk Factors

Several risk factors have been described for BPD, but preterm birth and low birth weight are the strongest predictors. In the NICHD Network, the reported incidence of BPD at 23 weeks is close to 70% and at 28 weeks not more than 25% confirming the strong role of prematurity. Similar data has been described by other Neonatal

Networks in Canada, Israel, and Europe. Fetal growth restriction and small for gestational age are also known prenatal risk factors, the odds for BPD being two- or threefold higher than AGA babies [10–12].

The use of antenatal steroids, known to decrease the incidence and severity of respiratory distress syndrome, as well as other neonatal morbidities and mortality, has not been consistently associated with the reduction in BPD rates [13].

Chorioamnionitis association with BPD has also been controversial and inconsistent mainly due to diagnostic criteria (clinical or histological) and confounding effects of gestational age and birth weight [14, 15]. Among other perinatal risk factors, sex and maternal smoking has also been related to BPD .

Genetic risk factors may be implicated to the development of BPD as demonstrated in twin studies and also by observation of several different phenotypes of the disease in babies with very similar gestational age, birth conditions, and neonatal morbidities [16].

Mechanical Ventilation Nasal CPAP and Supplemental Oxygen

Mechanical ventilation and supplemental oxygen were the main factors implicated in the original description of BPD but no doubt they still play a major role today. Both animal and human studies show pathologic structural changes similar to BPD induced by mechanical ventilation. Both lung distension named "Volutrauma" and lung poor aeration followed by repeated collapse and recruitment of lung units named "Atelectotrauma" can cause injury to the lungs. These episodes often lead to release of inflammatory mediators characterizing what is known as "VILI" – ventilation-induced lung injury [17, 18].

In recent years, several publications have addressed the benefits of Continuous Positive Airway Pressure (CPAP), noninvasive positive pressure ventilation (NIPPV), and high flow nasal canula in the prevention of lung injury and reduction in the incidence of BPD. Although most studies show benefits in the short-term outcomes, the effect on BPD has been only modest [19–22].

Supplemental oxygen has an important role in the genesis of BPD, together with immature lungs and a poorly developed antioxidant system. Very preterm infants are especially vulnerable to oxidative damage. Exposure to increased inspired oxygen (FiO_2) for several days or weeks causes lesions that mimic BPD in experimental animal models and the same is true for the human neonate [23–25].

Evidence from studies of saturation targeting has shown conflicting results regarding the effect of different levels of oxygen and incidence of BPD. Although in only two out of eight trials, the reduction achieved statistical significance, most studies showed some reduction of BPD when infants were kept in lower target groups 85–89% versus 90–95%. The other side is that mortality was also increased in low target saturation groups [26].

Clinical Management and Profiles

Management of the VLBW and ELBW is very important regarding the prevention of BPD since the very first minutes of life. In the last decade, we have witnessed a dramatic change in the approach of resuscitation, with decrease in the rates of endotracheal intubation and use of nasal continuous positive airway pressure (CPAP) since birth.

Several clinical trials have tried to relate this change in practice to rates of BPD alone or the composite outcome of BPD and death. The use of prophylactic surfactant is decreasing with the best evidence today of an early therapeutic approach [27].

In the NICU, most babies with birth weight > 1250 g, will receive surfactant by intubation–surfactant–extubation (INSURE), minimally invasive surfactant treatment (MIST), less-invasive surfactant administration (LISA), or other noninvasive approach. Mechanical ventilation, noninvasive ventilation, and other approaches will be covered in a latter topic of this chapter [28–31].

Fluid administration and maintenance of cardiovascular homeostasis is a major challenge specially in the micro preemies with birth weight below 500–600 g. Not infrequent today is to look after babies with less than 500 g. To little fluid will make them dehydrate and too much will lead to overhydration, lung edema, PDA, and worsening of respiratory condition with requirements of higher ventilatory support, which is a risk factor for BPD.

Once BPD is established, some infants will require continuous diuretic use in order to maintain cardiovascular equilibrium and prevent fluid retention.

Treatment of Patent Ductus Arteriosus (PDA) is one of the most controversial issues in NICU care today. We have shifted from a very aggressive approach with prophylactic treatment at the NICU admission to no-treatment at all and observation of the clinical course with intervention if cardiovascular symptoms become important. Nevertheless, the association of a PDA and BPD have been not confirmed in several recent reviews [32, 33].

Many ELBW will require ventilatory assistance since birth. They may progress to distinct patterns of disease which will give some insight about the development of BPD. Some will have a mild disease and improvement after surfactant administration, tolerating extubation, a second group will improve initially but get worse in 1 or 2 weeks progressing to ventilator dependence and a very sick group from the beginning. The second and third group will certainly be babies with mild-to-severe BPD.

There have been some attempts to predict BPD based on physiological parameters and ventilatory requirement in the first days or weeks of life. The NICHD Neonatal Network has developed a risk estimator (http://neonatal.rti.org/index.cfm) that accurately estimate the risk of developing BPD by postnatal day of age [34]. The use of nitric oxide and steroids are some of the drugs used early in life trying to prevent or decrease BPD severity (see latter in the chapter).

The general supportive measures for sick infants are applicable to BPD. These infants need a special attention to nutritional support because of high caloric expenditure and use of multiple drugs that may compromise metabolic homeostasis. A common gastrointestinal complication is reflux, leading many times to gastrostomy and fundoplication in the sicker and chronically ventilated babies.

It is important also to emphasize airway care, physiotherapy, and individualized nursing attention. Cyanotic and or hypoxemic spells may occur in some of the sicker infants, requiring continuous surveillance and prompt reversal to avoid prolonged hypoxemia. These infants are prone to develop pulmonary hypertension which will further compromise recovery and may lead to a severe cardiovascular compromise.

Chronically ventilated babies may present bronchospasm requiring beta-agonist therapy. It may be clinically apparent or only detectable with pulmonary function tests. When starting bronchodilators is important to evaluate the efficacy, plan the route of administration (inhaled or intravenous), and reach the desired dose, in order to obtain a prompt reversal of the symptoms and correctly titrate medications [35].

Pulmonary Hypertension

Pulmonary hypertension (PH) has been identified in 15–35% of chronically ventilated BPD babies. A recent meta-analysis of over 1400 patients from 25 publications confirmed the association of PH with severity of pulmonary disease with cumulative prevalence of PH in 6%, 12%, and 39% of infants with mild, moderate, and severe BPD, respectively [36]. Several drugs are currently used to treat pulmonary hypertension, being Sildenafil the most common (Table 62.3).

Recent studies have reported changes not only in lung parenchyma but also the effects of postnatal insults into vascular bed remodeling and development. The elevated pulmonary resistance will lead to pulmonary hypertension, followed by compensatory right ventricular hypertrophy, further complicating clinical management. The presence of PH will affect outcome with a mortality rate ranging from 16% to 38%. Some of the infant characteristics associated with the presence of PH are SGA, severe BPD, and surprisingly NEC [36].

Long-Term Outcome

The discharge of a BPD baby demands for a close follow-up due to the high frequency of respiratory symptoms in the first year of life. Up to 50% of these infants are rehospitalized in the first 2 years of life, with viral infections, asthma, bronchiolitis, which will occur in an infant recovering from severe pulmonary disease [37].

Longitudinal studies show persistent pulmonary abnormalities into adolescence and even adult age.

While pulmonary disease improves with growth, long-term follow-up studies raise concerns for persistent pulmonary dysfunction, asthma-like symptoms, and exercise intolerance in young adults after BPD. Abnormal ventilatory responses and

Table 62.3 Pharmacotherapy of pulmonary hypertension in BPD

Names	Dose/titration	Side Effects	Comments
Sildenafil phiosphodiesterase-5 inhibitor	PO: 1 mg/kg 6–8 h; start with low dose (0.3–0.5 mg/kg/dose) and increase gradually to 1 mg/kg/ dose as tolerated; slower as outpatient. Maximal dose of 10 mg q 8 h per EMA guidelines for infants	Hypotension, GER, irritability (headache), bronchospasm, nasal stuffiness, fever, rarely priapism	Monitor for adverse effects, lower the dose or switch to alternate therapy if not tolerated
Bosentan (endothelin receptor antagonist)	Intravenous: 0.25–0.5 mg/kg/dose q 6–8 h (titrate slowly and administer over 60 min.) 1 mg/kg PO q 12 h as starting dose; may increase to 2 mg/kg BID in 2–4 weeks, if tolerated and liver enzymes stable	Liver dysfunction especially during viral infections, VO mismatch, hypotension, anemia (edema and airway issues rare in infants)	Monitor LFTs monthly (earlier with respiratory infections), monitor CBC quarterly. Teratogenicity precautions for caregivers
Inhaled iloprost	2.5–5 mcg every 2–4 h. can be given as continuous inhalation during mechanical ventilation. Can titrate dose from 1 to 5 mcg and frequency from 1 to 5 mcg and frequency from every 4 h to continuous	Bronchospasm, hypotension, ventilator tube crystallization and clogging, pulmonary hemorrhage, prostanoid side effects (Gi disturbances), may be teratogenic to caregivers	Need close monitoring for clogged tubing, may need further dilution. May need bronchodilators or inhaled steroid pretreatment with bronchospasm
Intravenous epoprostenol (Flolan)	Start at 1–2 ng/kg/min, titrate up slowly every 4–6 h to 20 ng/kg/min; need to increase dose at regular intervals because of tachyphylaxis. Further increases as guided by clinical targets	Hypotension, VO mismatch, GI disturbances. Needs dedicated line, very short half-life with high risk for rebound PH with brief interruption of therapy; line-related complications include infection, clogging, breaks in line, thrombosis, arrhythmia)	Monitor closely if added to other vasodilator therapies, such as milrinone; careful attention to line care is essential
Treprostinil (Remodulin) IV or subcutaneous	Start at 2 ng/kg/min and titrate every 4–6 h up to 20 ng/kg/min, then slow increase dose as tolerated (dose often 1.5–2 times greater than equivalent epoprostenol dose, if switching medications)	SO: Local site pain; IV: Similar risks as with epoprostenol, but Treprostinil has a longer half-life, which reduces risk for severe PH with interruption of infusion	Pain can be managed with local and systemic measures
Milrinone (IV) (phosphodiesterase −3 inhibitor)	0.15–0.5 mcg/kg/min – Careful with loading dose	Arrhythmogenic; systemic	May need to add a vasopressor

pulmonary hypertension can further complicate disease. These pulmonary morbidities, combined with environmental and infectious exposures, may result in significant long-term pulmonary sequalae and represent a growing burden on health system [37–39].

Pharmacologic Treatment

Postnatal Steroids

There has been many changes in the recommendations of postnatal steroids for infants with BPD in the last two decades. The use of dexamethasone became very popular in the 1990s due to its potent anti-inflammatory effect which usually decreased respiratory assistance allowing extubation of chronically ventilated babies. Many clinical trials confirmed the improvement in clinical condition and ventilator settings, but most failed to demonstrate improved survival with many different dosages and treatment duration [40–42].

In early 2000s, concerns about neurodevelopment impairment led the American Academy of Pediatrics – Committee on Fetus and Newborn publish recommendations against its use [40]. Steroid use decreased dramatically but in many centers 8–10% use of admitted VLBW infants were still reported.

In 2006, Doyle et al. published the "Dart Trial," using low-dose dexamethasone to facilitate extubation among chronically ventilated dependent infants and subsequently the follow-up with 2 years of age which did not show neurodevelopment impairment. Later in 2014, Doyle and Halliday et al. revised the available evidence about the impact of postnatal steroids on mortality and cerebral palsy in preterm infants and the modification by the risk of BPD. They pointed out that the earlier use of steroids in very sick infant at a very high risk of BPD would decrease disease severity and the subsequent the risk of cerebral palsy instead of increasing CP [42, 43].

Current practice is more liberal today, trending to the use steroids (dexamethasone) after 2 weeks of age in infants at risk for BPD, dependent on mechanical ventilation in order to decrease lung injury and prevent severe BPD.

At the same time, a prophylactic approach has been attempted with hydrocortisone with the rationale that BPD has an important inflammatory component and VLBW and ELBW may have an immature adrenal function and low cortisol levels. After a small single-center placebo-controlled trial, showing positive effects. Waterberg et al. conducted a randomized controlled trial of low-dose hydrocortisone to increased survival without BPD. The study was showing results in the right direction but has to be stopped because a high incidence of gastrointestinal perforations in the treatment group. Similar findings were described in two other small trials.

More recently, Baud et al. conducted the PREMILOC trial with premature babies born at 24–27 weeks' gestation and found that a positive safety and efficacy profile for hydrocortisone, despite a significant increase in late-onset sepsis, as there were no negative effects on neonatal mortality and neurodevelopmental outcomes. Survival without BPD was 60% versus 51% with placebo [44].

In 2017, based on four randomized controlled trials and more than 1000 babies, Baud and Waterberg concluded that there are beneficial effects of early low-dose hydrocortisone and make a strong case for its use in extremely preterm infants at high risk for BPD. There were no cases of intestinal perforation in the absence of indomethacin. Hydrocortisone to improve survival without BPD still need further discussion in order to become current best evidence [44].

Nitric Oxide

Nitric oxide (NO) is a potent pulmonary vasodilator and very effective in the treatment of pulmonary hypertension in many different pulmonary diseases of the newborn. Preterm infants with BPD who develop this complication usually benefit from NO and the dependency of minimal doses in not rare. NO also has anti-inflammatory actions and may play a role in normal pulmonary development, as demonstrated in animal models [45, 46].

The question whether early NO treatment could improve survival without BP was addressed in several trials, with more than 3000 babies enrolled so far. However, none of these trials has been able to conclusively show significant effects. Recently, Shabih et al. published a multicenter, randomized, controlled trial with 451 preterm infants with less than 30 weeks, on mechanical ventilation or positive airway pressure that received NO (20 ppm) or placebo from 5 to 14 days of life NO (20 ppm) or placebo from 5 to 14 days of life.

Although NO appears to be safe with no adverse effects on neurodevelopment, no effect could be demonstrated on survival without BPD [47].

Caffeine

In 2006, Schmidt et al. published a very important randomized clinical trial to test long-term effect of caffeine for apnea of prematurity. More than 2000 infants from 500 to 1250 g were enrolled. The use of caffeine during the first 10 days of life was associated with better neurodevelopment outcome at 2 years of age. It also demonstrated that the drug reduces the risk of BPD and shortens the duration of ventilation with an endotracheal tube and exposure to supplemental oxygen. Several subsequent publications have confirmed the effect on BPD [48, 49].

In 2015, a systematic review and meta-analysis was undertaken to document the effect of early (0–2 days) versus late (>3 days) caffeine administration in very low birth weight babies on neonatal outcomes, including BPD. More than 50,000 VLBW infants were included from five studies. It was shown that the risk of bronchopulmonary dysplasia (OR, 0.507; 95% CI, 0.396–0.648; $P < 0.001$), and BPD or death (OR, 0.526; 95% CI, 0.384–0.719; $P < 0.001$) were lower in the early caffeine group [50].

Early caffeine administration is now standard therapy in the clinical practice in most NICU around the world.

Stem Cell

Mesenchymal stem cells (MSC) offer very promising therapeutic options for the prevention of BPD. The documented safety of MSCs in adults and children, and the dramatic benefits observed in experimental models, has prompted the clinical translation of this promising therapy. Selection of patients, timing and route of administration, source of cells, and protocols for MSC manufacturing can determine success or failure of this therapy and indelibly influence further research. During the next 5 years, well-designed trials will indicate whether MSC therapy can become a novel breakthrough in neonatal medicine [51].

Within less than 10 years from the initial proof-of-concept studies promising preclinical data with MSCs have led to phase I clinical trials [51, 52]. Two trials have shown that administration of a single intratracheal dose of allogeneic cord blood–derived MSCs in extreme preterm infants during the first week of life is feasible and without severe adverse events attributable to the intervention [53, 54]. Similarly, the successful off-label use of repeated intravenous injections of bone marrow–derived MSCs in two extreme preterm infants with severe and advanced BPD supports the feasibility of this therapy.

Ongoing phase II trials will indicate whether MSC therapy is safe and effective. Numerous other types of repair cells are being investigated in the clinic [54] and in the laboratory for use in BPD therapy. Despite rapid clinical translation, cell-based therapies for regenerative indications are still in their infancy and major knowledge gaps remain. A better understanding of the biology and mechanism of action of MSCs and other repair cell types and the link between resident stem or progenitor cells and disease pathogenesis, together with technological advances, will allow the development of potency assays and manufacturing processes to yield superior cell products that may truly curb complications of prematurity and improve outcomes.

References

1. Northway WH Jr, Rosan RC, Porter DY. Pulmonary disease following respiratory therapy of hyaline membrane disease. Bronchopulmonary dysplasia. N Engl J Med. 1967;276:357–86.
2. Abman SH, Bancalari E, Jobe A. The evolution of bronchopulmonary dysplasia after 50 years. Am J Respir Crit Care Med. 2017;195:421–4.
3. Jobe AH, Bancalari E. Bronchopulmonary dysplasia. Am J Respir Crit Care Med. 2001;163:1723–9.

4. Shennan AT, Dunn MS, Ohlsson A, Lennox K, Hoskins EM. Abnormal pulmonary outcomes in premature infants: prediction from oxygen requirement in the neonatal period. Pediatrics. 1988;82:527–32.
5. Horbar JD, Carpenter JH, Badger GJ, et al. Mortality and neonatal morbidity among infants 501 to 1500 grams from 2000 to 2009. Pediatrics. 2012;129:1019–26.
6. Stoll BJ, Hansen NI, Bell EF, et al. Neonatal outcomes of extremely preterm infants from the NICHD neonatal research network. Pediatrics. 2010;126:443–56.
7. Lapcharoensap W, et al. Hospital variation and risk factors for bronchopulmonary dysplasia in a population-based cohort. JAMA Pediatr. 2015;169:e143676.
8. Adams M, et al. Variability of very low birth weight infant outcome and practice in Swiss and US neonatal units. Pediatrics. 2018;141:e20173436.
9. Bhunwal S, Mukhopadhyay K, Bhattacharya S, Dey P, Dhaliwal LK. Bronchopulmonary dysplasia in preterm neonates in a level III neonatal unit in India. Indian Pediatr. 2018;55:211–5.
10. Bose C, et al. Fetal growth restriction and chronic lung disease among infants born before the 28th week of gestation. Pediatrics. 2009;124:e450–8.
11. Isayama T, et al. Revisiting the definition of bronchopulmonary dysplasia: effect of changing panoply of respiratory support for preterm neonates. JAMA Pediatr. 2017;171:271–9.
12. Stoll BJ, Hansen NI, Bell EF, Shankaran S, Laptook AR, Walsh MC, Hale EC, Newman NS, Schibler K, Carlo WA, Kennedy KA, Poindexter BB, Finer NN, Ehrenkranz RA, Duara S, Sánchez PJ, O'Shea TM, Goldberg RN, Van Meurs KP, Faix RG, Phelps DL, Frantz ID 3rd, Watterberg KL, Saha S, Das A, Higgins RD, Eunice Kennedy Shriver National Institute of Child Health and Human Development Neonatal Research Network. Neonatal outcomes of extremely preterm infants from the NICHD Neonatal Research Network. Pediatrics. 2010;126(3):443–56.
13. Van Marter LJ, Allred EN, Leviton A, et al. Antenatal gluco-corticoid treatment does not reduce chronic lung disease among surviving preterm infants. J Pediatr. 2001;138:198–204.
14. Jobe AH. Effects of chorioamnionitis on the fetal lung. Clin Perinatol. 2012;39:441–57. [PubMed: 22954262].
15. Redline RW, Faye-Petersen O, Heller D, et al. Amniotic infection syndrome: nosology and reproducibility of placental reaction patterns. Pediatr Dev Pathol. 2003;6:435–48.
16. Parker RA, Lindstrom DP, Cotton RB. Evidence from twin study implies possible genetic susceptibility to bronchopulmonary dysplasia. Semin Perinatol. 1996;20:206–9. [PubMed: 8870123].
17. Dreyfuss D, Saumon G. Ventilator-induced lung injury: les- sons from experimental studies. Am J Respir Crit Care Med. 1998;157:294–323.
18. Mokres LM, Parai K, Hilgenforff A. Prolonged mechanical ventilation with air induces apoptosis and causes failure of alveolar septation and angiogenesis in lungs of newborn mice. Am J Phys. 2010;298:L23–35.
19. Schmolzer GM, et al. Non-invasive versus invasive respiratory support in preterm infants at birth: systematic review and meta-analysis. BMJ. 2013;347:f5980. [PubMed: 24136633].
20. Lemyre B, Davis PG, De Paoli AG, Kirpalani H. Nasal intermittent positive pressure ventilation (NIPPV) versus nasal continuous positive airway pressure (NCPAP) for preterm neonates after extubation. Cochrane Database Syst Rev. 2017;2:CD003212. [PubMed: 28146296].
21. Lemyre B, Laughon M, Bose C, Davis PG. Early nasal intermittent positive pressure ventilation (NIPPV) versus early nasal continuous positive airway pressure (NCPAP) for preterm infants. Cochrane Database Syst Rev. 2016;12:CD005384. [PubMed: 27976361].
22. Wilkinson D, Andersen C, O'Donnell CP, De Paoli AG, Manley BJ. High flow nasal cannula for respiratory support in preterm infants. Cochrane Database Syst Rev. 2016;2:CD006405. [PubMed: 26899543].
23. Bonikos DS, Benson KG, Northway WHJ. Oxygen toxicity in the newborn. The effect of chronic continuous100 percent oxy- gen exposure on the lung of newborn mice. Am J Pathol. 1976;85:623–50.
24. Delacourt C, d'Ortho MP, Macquin-Mavier I, et al. Oxidant–antioxidant balance in alveolar macrophages from newborn rats. Eur Respir J. 1996;9:2517–24.

25. Saugstad OD. Chronic lung disease: the role of oxidative stress. Biol Neonate. 1998;74:21–8.
26. Darlow AB, Morley C. Oxygen saturation targeting and bronchopulmonary dysplasia. Clin Perinatol. 2015;42:807–23.
27. Thebaud B, Goss KN, Laughon M, Whitsett JA, et al. Bronchopulmonary dysplasia. Nat Rev Primers. 2020;5(1):781–53.
28. Kribs A, et al. Nonintubated surfactant application vs conventional therapy in extremely preterm infants: a randomized clinical trial. JAMA Pediatr. 2015;169:723–30. [PubMed: 26053341].
29. Dargaville PA, et al. Minimally-invasive surfactant therapy in preterm infants on continuous positive airway pressure. Arch Dis Child Fetal Neonatal Ed. 2013;98:F122–6. [PubMed: 22684154].
30. Aldana-Aguirre JC, Pinto M, Featherstone RM, Kumar M. Less invasive surfactant administration versus intubation for surfactant delivery in preterm infants with respiratory distress syndrome: a systematic review and meta-analysis. Arch Dis Child Fetal Neonatal Ed. 2017;102:F17–23.). [PubMed: 27852668].
31. Dargaville PA, et al. The OPTIMIST-A trial: evaluation of minimally-invasive surfactant therapy in preterm infants 25–28 weeks gestation. BMC Pediatr. 2014;14:213. [PubMed: 25164872].
32. Ohlsson A, Walia R, Shah SS. Ibuprofen for the prevention of patent ductus arteriosus in preterm and/or low birth weight infants. Cochrane Database Syst Rev. 2013;4:CD003481.
33. Cooke L, Steer P, Woodgate P. Indomethacin for asymptomatic patent ductus arteriosus in preterm infants. Cochrane Database Syst Rev. 2003;1:CD003745.
34. Laughon MM, et al. Prediction of bronchopulmonary dysplasia by postnatal age in extremely premature infants. Am J Respir Crit Care Med. 2011;183:1715–22. [PubMed: 21471086].
35. Clouse BJ, Jadcherla SR, Slaughter JL. Systematic review of inhaled bronchodilator and corticosteroid therapies in infants with bronchopulmonary dysplasia: implications and future directions. PLoS One. 2016;11(2):e0148188. https://doi.org/10.1371/journal.pone.0148188. eCollection (2016).
36. Sara K. Berkelhamer MD, Karen K. Mestan, Robin Steinhorn. An update on the diagnosis and management of bronchopulmonary dysplasia (BPD)-associated pulmonary hypertension. Semin Perinatol.
37. Smith VC, Zupancic JAF, McCormick MC, et al. Rehospitalization in the first year of life among infants with bronchopulmonary dysplasia. J Pediatr. 2004;144:799–803.
38. Fawke J, Lum S, Kirkby J, et al. Lung function and respiratory symptoms at 11 years in children born extremely preterm. Am J Respir Crit Care Med. 2010;182:237–45.
39. Vollsæter M, Roksund OD, Eide GE, et al. Lung function after preterm birth: development from mid-childhood to adult- hood. Thorax. 2013;68:767–76.
40. Committee on Fetus and Newborn. Postnatal corticosteroids to treat or prevent chronic lung disease in preterm infants. Pediatrics. 2002;109:330–8. [PubMed: 11826218].
41. Doyle LW, Halliday HL, Ehrenkranz RA, Davis PG, Sinclair JC. An update on the impact of postnatal systemic corticosteroids on mortality and cerebral palsy in preterm infants: effect modification by risk of bronchopulmonary dysplasia. J Pediatr. 2014;165:1258–60. [PubMed: 25217197].
42. Doyle LW, et al. Outcome at 2 years of age of infants from the DART study: a multicenter, international, randomized, controlled trial of low-dose dexamethasone. Pediatrics. 2007;119:716–21. [PubMed: 17403842].
43. Doyle LW, et al. Low-dose dexamethasone facilitates extubation among chronically ventilator- dependent infants: a multicenter, international, randomized, controlled trial. Pediatrics. 2006;117:75–83. [PubMed: 16396863].
44. Baud O, et al. Effect of early low-dose hydrocortisone on survival without bronchopulmonary dysplasia in extremely preterm infants (PREMILOC): a double-blind, placebo-controlled, multicentre, randomised trial. Lancet. 2016;387:1827–36. [PubMed: 26916176].

45. Bland RD, Albertine KH, Carlton DP, MacRitchie AJ. Inhaled nitric oxide effects on lung structure and function in chronically ventilated preterm lambs. Am J Respir Crit Care Med. 2005;172:899–906. [PubMed: 15976381].
46. Cotton RB, et al. Inhaled nitric oxide attenuates hyperoxic lung injury in lambs. Pediatr Res. 2006;59:142–6. [PubMed: 16327001].
47. Hasan SU, Potenziano J, Konduri GG, Perez JA, Van Meurs KP, Walker MW, Yoder BA. For the newborns treated with nitric oxide (NEWNO) trial group. Effect of inhaled nitric oxide on survival without bronchopulmonary dysplasia in preterm infants. JAMA Pediatr. 2017;71:1081–9.
48. Schmidt B, et al. Caffeine therapy for apnea of prematurity. N Engl J Med. 2006;354:2112–21. [PubMed: 16707748].
49. Schmidt B, et al. Long-term effects of caffeine therapy for apnea of prematurity. N Engl J Med. 2007;357:1893–902. [PubMed: 17989382] References 173 and 174 report results of the CAP trial in 2,000 infants and its long-term follow-up study, which convincingly demonstrated the pathway between shortened exposure to assisted ventilation, reduced rates of BPD, and improved neurodevelopmental outcomes.
50. Kua KP, Lee SW. Systematic Review and Meta-analysis of clinical outcomes of early caffeine therapy in preterm neonates. Br J Clin Pharmacol. 2017;83(1):180–91.
51. Chang YS, et al. Mesenchymal stem cells for bronchopulmonary dysplasia: phase 1 dose-escalation clinical trial. J Pediatr. 2014;164:966–972.e6. [PubMed: 24508444] This is the first phase I trial showing the feasibility and no short-term toxicity of a single intratracheal administration of allogeneic cord-blood-derived mesenchymal stromal cells in extreme preterm infants at risk of developing BPD.
52. Powell SB, Silvestri JM. Safety of intratracheal administration of human umbilical cord blood derived mesenchymal stromal cells in extremely low birth weight preterm infants. J Pediatr. 2019;210:209–213.e2. [PubMed: 30992220].
53. Alvarez-Fuente M, et al. Off-label mesenchymal stromal cell treatment in two infants with severe bronchopulmonary dysplasia: clinical course and biomarkers profile. Cytotherapy. 2018;20:1337–44. [PubMed: 30327248].
54. Lim R, et al. First-in-human administration of allogeneic amnion cells in premature infants with bronchopulmonary dysplasia: a safety study. Stem Cell Transl Med. 2018;7:628–35.

Chapter 63
Retinopathy of Prematurity

Luiza M. Neves and Andrea Zin

Introduction and Epidemiology

Retinopathy of prematurity (ROP) is a vasoproliferative condition affecting retinal vessels of preterm infants and can lead to retinal detachment and blindness. The World Health Organization (WHO) classifies childhood blindness causes as avoidable and non-avoidable [1]. The avoidable ones comprise preventable etiologies (vitamin A deficiency and congenital infections) and treatable causes (congenital cataract, congenital glaucoma, and ROP) [1].

Indeed, ROP represents the leading cause of treatable childhood visual impairment and blindness worldwide [2–4]. Childhood blindness constitutes a priority for the WHO Vision 2020 effort [WHO 1997] for several reasons: visual loss irreversibility as a result of a late treatment, many years lived with visual impairment and morbidity, associated global motor development delay, and, additionally, social and economic implications [1, 5, 6].

ROP was first described in 1942 by T. L. Terry as a bilateral retrolental fibroplasia in infants born extremely premature [7]. He observed that this disorder was similar to the fibroblastic sheath behind the crystalline lens in persistent tunica vasculosa lentis but related to prematurity. In 1952, Hugh Ryan studied histopathological specimens and noted that the disease could initiate with folds in peripheral retina and progress centrifugally with retinal detachment [8].

L. M. Neves
Instituto Nacional de Saúde da Mulher, da Criança e do Adolescente, FIOCRUZ, Rio de Janeiro, Brazil

Departamento de Oftalmologia, Universidade do Estado do Rio de Janeiro, Rio de Janeiro, Brazil

A. Zin (✉)
Instituto NAcional de Saude da Mulher, da Criança e do Adolescente, FIOCRUZ, Rio de Janeiro, Brazil
e-mail: andrea.zin@iff.fiocruz.br

© Springer Nature Switzerland AG 2022

R. A. Moreira de Sá, E. B. d. Fonseca (eds.), *Perinatology*,
https://doi.org/10.1007/978-3-030-83434-0_63

Historically, there have been three ROP epidemics. The first epidemic occurred in the 1940s/1950s and was related to unmonitored oxygen use for treatment of respiratory distress in preterm infants [3]. Infants born with a birth weight (BW) under 1000 g exhibited a survival rate of 5–8% [9]. The more mature ones had a better chance of survival and developed blindness [4]. A randomized, controlled trial disclosed an increased ROP rate in the high oxygen group compared to the low oxygen group [10]. As a result, the recommendation of the use of oxygen became restricted, leading to a fall in ROP blindness. However, there was an unfortunate increase in neonatal mortality [11, 12]. Since then there have been many studies to characterize the best saturation interval that could reduce the incidence of severe ROP without increasing the mortality. The second ROP epidemic occurred in the 1970s, particularly in high-income countries, with the advent of neonatal intensive care units (NICU) [3]. The consequence of better neonatal care was an increase of survival rates of more premature and low BW infants and consequent occurrence of severe ROP in this population [4]. During this period, infants under 1000 g had a survival rate of 50–60% [9]. The third epidemic started in 1990s, and remains until today in middle-income countries due to varying levels of neonatal care. Severe ROP can still be diagnosed in bigger more mature babies where the quality of neonatal care needs improvement [3].

ROP has progressive clinical stages and the incidence of any ROP is about 60–68% for infants less than 1500 g in high-income countries [3]. However, the incidence of severe ROP is a more useful measure to estimate the magnitude of ROP [3]. Severe ROP includes advanced clinical stages requiring treatment to avoid potential blindness. The incidence of severe ROP is used as an indicator of the level of neonatal care [3] and also helps planning efficient screening and treatment programs. The incidence of severe ROP varies between authors and the mean estimate incidence of severe ROP is 7.5% (0–34.8%) in studies from high-income countries and 13.5% (1.3–44.9%) in studies from low- and middle-income countries [3]. Moreover, these discrepancies can occur among NICU from the same city, for example, in Rio de Janeiro, Zin et al. examined babies under 2000 g and rates of ROP needing treatment ranged from 2.1% to 7.8% [13].

Additionally, the incidence of blindness from ROP also varies between countries. Gilbert suggested that the proportion of blindness due to ROP was related to infant mortality rates (IMR) [6]. Countries with high IMR (above 60/1000 live births), such as those in sub-Saharan African, have low incidence of blindness from ROP [6]. The reason is the lack of NICU and/or of basic facilities for pregnant women leading to low neonatal survival rates. Countries with very low IMR (under 9/1000), such as in Western Europe, also have low rates of blindness due to ROP [6]. There are several explanations: low prematurity rates, high neonatal care quality, good supplemental oxygen monitoring, and appropriate ROP management for at-risk infants. Countries with intermediate IMR (9–60/1000) are the ones facing the third ROP epidemic and include those in Latin America, Eastern Europe, India, and China [6]. They have high prematurity rates, improved neonatal survival rates, poor supplemental oxygen monitoring, shortage of ophthalmologists with appropriate skills to diagnose and treat ROP, and insufficient (not universal) timely ROP screening and treatment.

Sixty percent of all preterm births occur in the following countries: India, China, Nigeria, Pakistan, Indonesia, United States, Bangladesh, Philippines, Congo, and Brazil [14]. Overall, 65% of visually impaired survivors and 39% of neurodevelopmental impaired cases were estimated to live in middle-income countries in 2010 [2]. The understanding of ROP epidemiology is crucial to address regional differences and guarantee appropriate ROP management for childhood blindness control.

Patophysiology and Risk Factors

Retinal vascularization begins at 16th week of gestation [15]. Retinal vessels grow centrifugally from the optic disc, reaching nasal periphery by 36 gestational week and temporal periphery by 40th gestational week [15]. Their normal development occurs in a hypoxic environment in utero called physiologic hypoxia-driven angiogenesis [16, 17]. When the infant is born prematurely and/or with low birth weight, the hypoxic environment changes with the higher oxygen offer. As a result, the retinal vascularization is delayed, which increases the risk of abnormal retinal vessels [16, 17].

ROP develops in two phases, the first one with a relatively hyperoxic environment and vaso-obliteration and the second one with a hypoxic environment and vasoproliferation. The first phase involves cessation of vessel growth and some loss of endothelial formed cells driven by higher availability of oxygen compared to the intrauterine period, particularly when supplemental oxygen is used. As a result, the downregulation of hypoxia-inducible factors such as vascular endothelial growth factor (VEGF) and erythropoietin (EPO) occurs. In addition to this, there is loss of factors from maternal fetal interface with poor endogenous production. They are also involved in vessel growth, such as growth hormone, insulin-like growth factor 1 (IGF-I), and insulin-like growth factor binding protein 1 (IGF-BPI) [9, 16–19]. Serum levels of IGF-1 correlate with fetal and postnatal growth, more importantly, early IGF-1 deficit and slow postnatal weight gain were associated with a higher risk of severe ROP [20, 21].

The second phase usually occurs after 32 postmenstrual weeks but can present a wide range of onset [17, 22, 23]. The metabolic needs of the developing retina are not being supplied and the retina becomes relatively hypoxic. As a result, VEGF and EPO expression becomes upregulated and vascular growth resumes. However, these pathological vessels lack astrocytic ensheathment are abnormal leaky, do not reperfuse the avascular retina, and can grow into the vitreous. The neovascular proliferation may lead to a sight-threatening tractional retinal detachment, macular dragging, vitreous and retina hemorrhages [17, 18].

There are several risk factors associated *with* ROP which can be divided in two categories: prenatal factors, including gestational age at birth (GA) and birth weight (BW), and postnatal factors, comprising exposure to supplemental oxygen, loss of maternal nutrition (including essential fatty acids), decreased IGF-I, IGF-BPI, among other factors [17–21].

Prenatal factors are the two major risk factors. The lower the GA and/or BW, the higher are the chances of ROP development and progression. Notably, in middle-income countries, bigger and heavier infants can also progress to ROP advanced clinical stages [4, 13, 24, 25].

Exposure to unmonitored oxygen is a well-known risk factor. Campbell suggested a link with oxygen in 1951 and Patz et al. disclosed that higher oxygen levels were associated with retrolental fibroplasia in a clinical trial in 1952 [26, 27]. Several studies followed confirming this association and a policy of restricted oxygen therapy was adopted [16]. However, Cross reported an increase in *preterm* mortality in 1973: for every case of blindness prevented, 16 infants died [12].

Nowadays, there is still no consensus about the appropriate level of oxygen saturation (Spo2) for extremely preterm to maximize survival and minimize morbidity. Infants exposed to lower levels of oxygen (<90% Spo2) during the first few weeks of life may be at greater risk of death, cerebral palsy, patent ductus arteriosus, pulmonary vascular resistance, and apnea, whereas infants exposed to higher levels of oxygen (>90% Spo2) may be at greater risk of ROP and chronic lung disease [16].

It has been postulated that increased oxygen saturation during phase two of ROP may reduce VEGF levels and arrest progression to severe ROP [16]. This concept was tested in the Supplemental Therapeutic Oxygen for Pre-threshold ROP (STOP-ROP), but there was no significant difference between infants in the group with Spo2 target of 89–95% and of 96–99% [28]. The supplemental oxygen group had more pneumonia and worsening chronic lung disease. Therefore, it is likely that different oxygen saturation may be needed throughout hospitalization.

Long-term results from Neonatal Oxygenation Prospective Meta-analysis (NeoPROM) found no significant difference between a lower Spo2 target (85–89%) compared to a higher Spo2 target (91–95%) on death or major disability at corrected age of 18 to 24 months [29]. The lower Spo2 target was associated with a higher risk of death [relative risk 2.8 (95% confidence interval (CI) 0.6%–5.0%)] and necrotizing enterocolitis [relative risk 2.3% (95% CI, 0.8%–3.8%)], but a lower risk of ROP needing treatment [risk difference – 4.0% (95% CI, −6.1−−2.0%)]. There is also clinical evidence linking oxygen fluctuation with increased risk of ROP [30]. Experts' recommendation is to avoid hypoxemic episodes and to target Spo2 between 90% and 94% in very preterm infants from high-income countries and between 88% and 94% from middle-income countries, where more mature babies are at risk for severe ROP [30].

Omega-3 long-chain polyunsaturated fatty acid and docosahexaenoic acid are fatty acids transferred from the mother to the fetus during the third trimester. Animal studies have shown an important role in retinal vessels and neuronal survival [17]. IGF-I is a polypeptide that promotes fetal growth and is synthetized in the liver of the fetus/preterm infants from maternal nutrient supply. Animal models have also shown a critical role in VEGF signaling [17]. Low fatty acids and low IGF-I driven by maternal–fetus transfer interruption in premature birth could induce retina neovascularization [17]. Supplementation therapy are potential targets although have not yet demonstrated to reduce incidence of ROP [30].

Human recombinant EPO, a cytokine factor that regulates fetal erythropoiesis, has been used in preterm infants to prevent anemia. In vitro EPO is as potent as

VEGF in inducing angiogenesis [17]. Two Cochrane reviews found divergent results relating EPO to ROP. The oldest one found association between the use of EPO and an increased risk of any ROP with a similar trend for severe ROP [31]. Conversely, the recent one found no increased risk of ROP with EPO therapy [32].

Other specific approaches such as antenatal corticosteroids prior to preterm delivery [30, 33–35], prevention of hypothermia in preterm infants [36], caffeine for very preterm infants [37], lactoferrin supplementation [38] have been associated to decreased incidence of severe ROP although more studies are necessary.

Healthcare of preterm newborns requires multidisciplinary neonatal team approach, where skilled neonatal nurses play a central role. Zin et al. disclosed that the rate of ROP requiring treatment could vary according to infant-to-nurse ratio. A neonatal unit with a 2:1 infant-to-nurse ratio had 4% of infants requiring ROP treatment whereas other with 17:1 infant to nurse ratio had 12% treatable ROP [4, 13].

ROP is a multifactorial disease with the most important risk factors being high prematurity, low birth weight, and oxygen exposure. Genetic mutations may also be involved in the disorder as in the Wnt signaling pathway [9, 39] and in Norrin, Frizz-led 4, and Lrp5 genes [40]. Primary prevention includes addressing preterm birth causes, improving antenatal care, adopting basic neonatal best care practice, balancing oxygen control, provisioning sufficient nutrition, and universalizing adequate ROP screening and monitoring.

Classification

The International Classification published in 1984 and revisited in 2005 and 2021 [41–43] described ROP as seen by standard binocular indirect ophthalmoscopy done by an experienced ophthalmologist, in the NICU. The disease was defined based on location, severity, and extension as discussed below.

Location

ROP is a disorder affecting part of the posterior segment of the eye called retina. The most important structures of the retina are the optic disc and the macula. Three concentric zones of retinal involvement have been described to help define the anteroposterior location of the retinopathy [42]. This is a relevant concept because the more posterior is the retinopathy, the nearer it is to the optic disc and to the macula and the worst the visual prognosis.

Zone I consists of a circle with the radius extending from the center of the optic disc to twice the distance from the center of the macula. Zone II extends centrifugally from the edge of zone I to the nasal ora serrata/periphery. Zone III is the residual crescent of retina anterior to zone II (Fig. 63.1) Recently, it has been defined the posterior zone II region, which begins at the margin between zone I and zone II and extends into zone II for 2 disc diameters. Also, the term *notch* was described to represent the incursion by the ROP lesion of 1-2 clock hours into a more posterior zone. For instance, the infant's eye exam could be described as "zone I secondary to *notch*".

Severity

There are five stages used to describe the abnormal vascular response at the junction of the vascularized and avascular retina. When there is no ROP, the ophthalmologist can describe the preterm infants's eye examination as an incomplete or immature retina vascularization (Fig. 63.2), which needs monitoring until complete vascularization. If more than one ROP stage is present, the eye is classified by the most severe stage.

Stage 1: Demarcation Line

There is a thin, flat, and white line separating the vascular retina posteriorly from the avascular retina anteriorly (Fig. 63.3).

Stage 2: Ridge

There is a ridge with height and width that extends above the plane of the retina separating the vascular retina posteriorly from the avascular retina anteriorly. The ridge's color may change from white to pink (Fig. 63.4).

Stage 3: Extraretinal Fibrovascular Proliferation

There is a neovascularization, which can be extrarretinal - from the ridge into the vitreous (the structure that fills the eye's posterior segment) - or flat (Fig. 63.5).

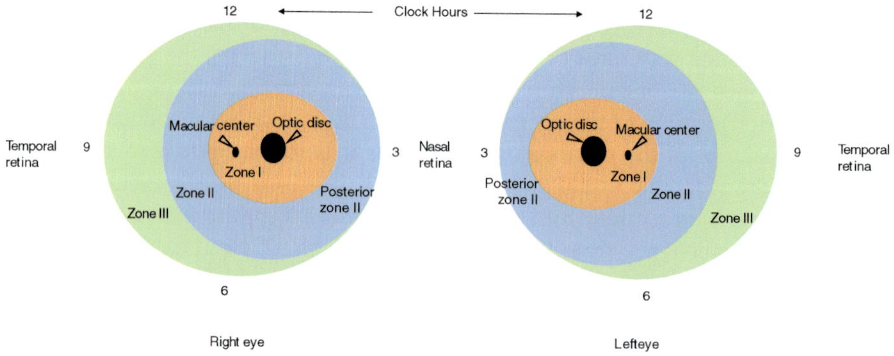

Fig. 63.1 Zone location and clock hours extension for ROP classification, adapted from IC ROP revisited [41, 43]

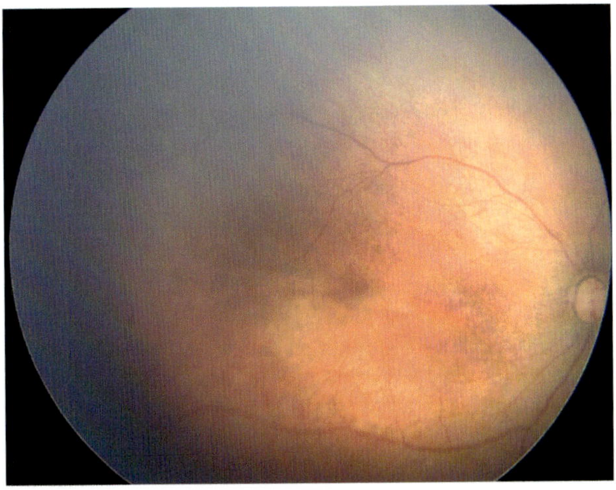

Fig. 63.2 Right eye: peripheral avascular retina

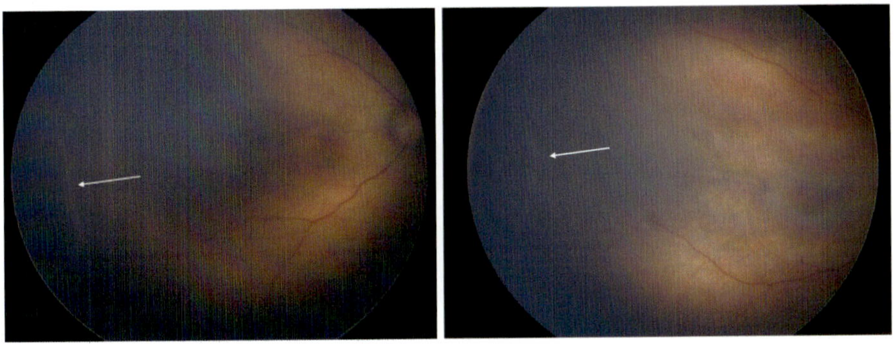

Fig. 63.3 White arrow indicates demarcation line: thin, flat and white line separating the vascular retina posteriorly from the avascular retina anteriorly

Stage 4: Partial Retinal Detachment

There is a partial retinal detachment. It can be divided as 4a when the detachment is extrafoveal and 4b when it is foveal. The fovea is the center of the macula, responsible for the most detailed vision (Fig. 63.6).

Stage 5: Total Retinal Detachment

There is a total retinal detachment. Stage 5A occurs when the optic disc is visible by ophthalmoscopy. Stage 5B occurs when the optic disc is not visible because of retrolental fibrovascular tissue or closed-funnel detachment. Stage 5C occurs when 5B is accompanied by anterior segment changes.

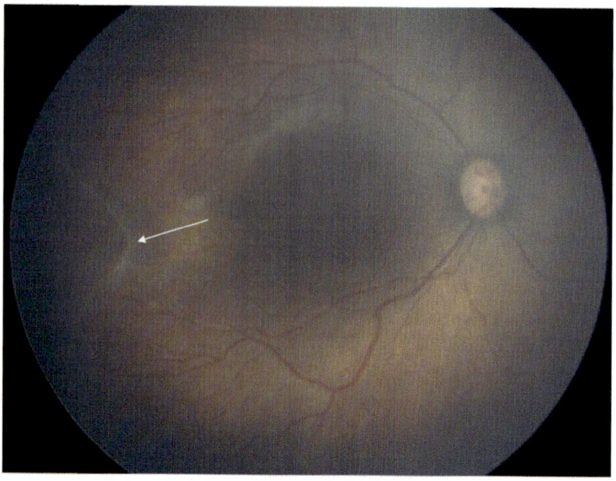

Fig. 63.4 Stage 2: white arrow indicates ridge with height and width that extends above the plane of the retina separating the vascular retina posteriorly from the avascular retina anteriorly

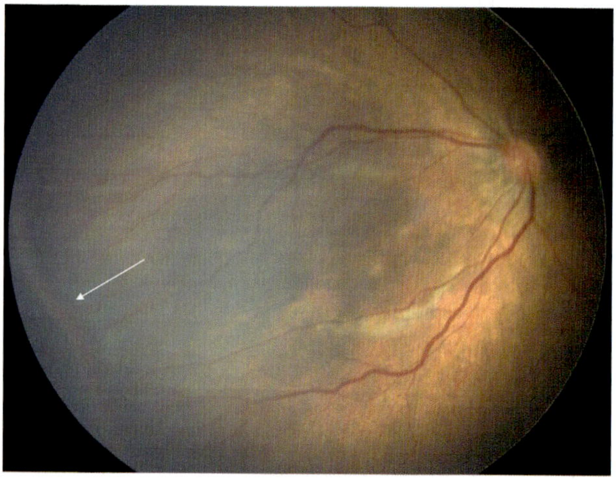

Fig. 63.5 Stage 3: white arrow indicates extraretinal fibrovascular proliferation. There is a neovascularization from the ridge into the vitreous

Extension

The extent of the disease is recorded as 12 sectors using clock-hour designation.

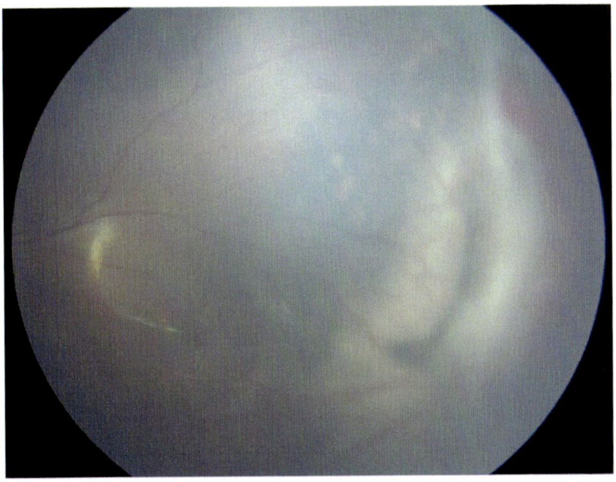

Fig. 63.6 Stage 4a: extrafovealpartial retinal detachment.

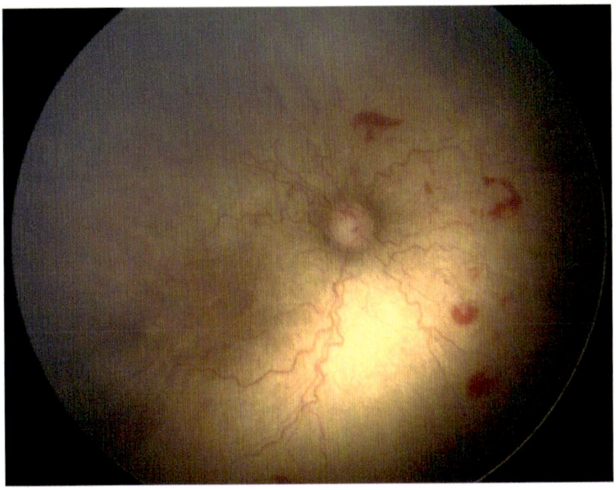

Fig. 63.7 Plus disease - increased venous dilation and arteriolar tortuosity of the posterior retina vessels in at least two quadrants. AROP: posterior location, prominence plus disease and ill-defined nature of retinopathy, hemorrhages

Plus and Preplus Disease

Plus disease is an additional sign indicating ROP severity and include increased venous dilation and arteriolar tortuosity of the posterior retina vessels (zone I) (Fig. 63.7). At the clinical practice, the symbol "+" is frequently used to indicate presence of plus disease. Preplus disease occurs when there are vascular abnormalities, but they are insufficient for the plus disease criteria (Fig. 63.8).

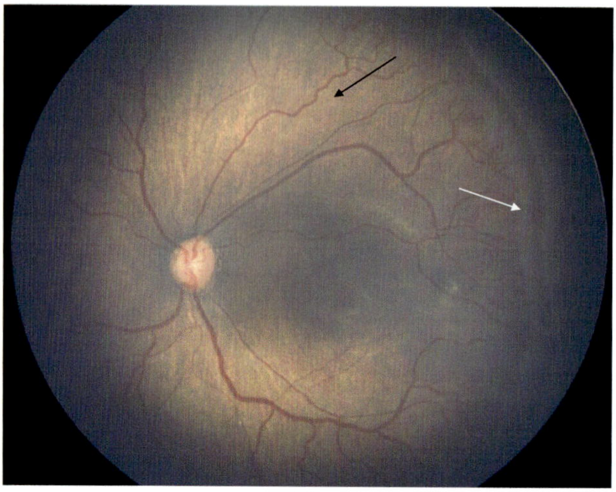

Fig. 63.8 Black arrow: pre plus - venous dilation and arterial tortuosity insufficient for plus disease criteria. White arrow indicates extraretinal fibrovascular proliferation (Stage 3)

Aggressive ROP

There is a rapidly progressing and severe form of ROP that may not develop through the classic stages [41]. The clinical signs are prominence plus disease, ill-defined nature of retinopathy and vascular changes such as shunting, and hemorrhages can occur (Fig. 63.7) Previously, it was named as agressive-posterior ROP, however, because of the increasing recognition that it may develop beyond the posterior retina and in larger preterm infants, the Third International Classification recommends the term aggressive ROP.

ROP Regression, long-term sequelae and reactivation

The regression occurs when there is a failure of the retinopathy to progress to next stage and starts a process of involution of the vasoproliferative phase to a fibrotic phase. It can be spontaneous or after treatment and normally occurs at the junction of vascular and avascular retina with a broad spectrum of involutional sequelae. Location and extent of peripheral avascular retina should be documented. One severe sequelae is the displacement of the macula or the optic disc, known as *dragging* (Fig. 63.9). Long-term sequelae may be seen in patients with a history of premature birth, even without a history of ROP and they include: late retinal detachments, retinoschisis (separation of the retina's layers), persistent avascular retina, fovea alterations (blunting, smaller). Finally, ROP may reactivate after treatment, including new lesions and vascular lesions. It is recommended to use the term "reactivated" and then the new classification, for instance "reactivated stage 2".

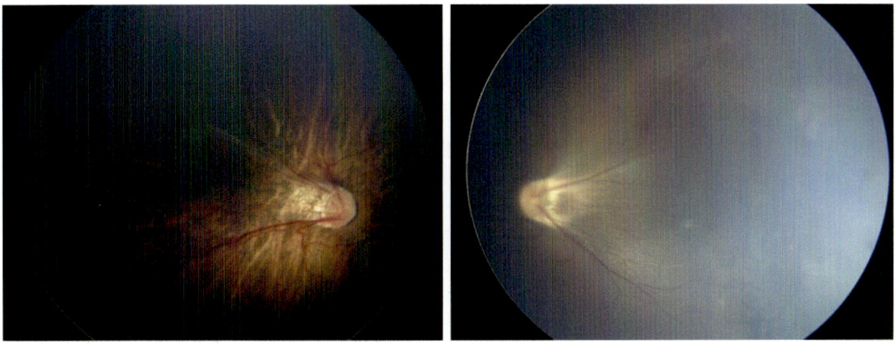

Fig. 63.9 Dragging: displacement of the macula or the optic disc

Table 63.1 ROP screening criteria for high-, middle-, and low-income countries

Country	Criteria	Observation
High-income countries screening criteria for ROP		
United Kingdom [44]	Must be screened: <31 weeks GA or < 1251 g BW	Should be screened: < 32 weeks GA or < 1501 g BW
United States [45]	< 30 weeks GA or < = 1500 g BW	>30 weeks GA or 1500–2000 g BW if illness[a]
Canada [46]	< =30 weeks GA or < = 1250 g BW	>30 weeks GA or 1500–2000 g BW if unstable clinical course at high risk for ROP
Low- and middle-income countries screening criteria for ROP		
India [48]	< 34 weeks GA or < 2000 g BW[a]	34–36 weeks GA With risk factors for ROP
Brazil [49]	< = 32 weeks GA or < = 1500 g BW	More mature infants with risk factors or < =35 weeks in NICU with poor survival rates (< = 80% among infants with BW < 1500 g)
Kenya [47]	< = 34 weeks GA or < 1750 g BW	<36 weeks GA with unstable clinical course

GA gestational age. *BW* birth weight
[a]According to Chan-Ling et al., current Indian guidelines are under revision and will likely suggest modified BW criteria to <1750 g BW [18]

Screening, Monitoring, and Examination

Universal screening for all at-risk infants and appropriate monitoring until vascularization is completed (approximately 40 weeks of gestation age) are two priorities for ROP blindness control.

Screening

Who to Screen?

Screening criteria can vary between countries because of differences in neonatal care quality: High-income countries usually include narrower screening criteria and low- and middle-income countries have wider ones [24] (Table 63.1).

High-Income Countries

The current inclusion criteria in high-income countries are generally satisfactory as they include almost all the infants requiring ROP treatment [24]. The United States and Canada include lower GA and BW criteria than the United Kingdom (UK) but require knowledge of the additional illness risk factors for ROP.

- The Royal College of Paediatrics & Child Health (RCPCH) in collaboration with the Royal College of Ophthalmologists (RCOphth), British Association of Perinatal Medicine (BAPM), and the premature baby charity BLISS [44]:
  - All infants less than 32 weeks GA (up to 31 weeks and 6 days) or less than 1501 g BW should be screened for ROP. One criterion is to be met for inclusion.
  - Infants less than 31 weeks GA or less than 1251 g BW must be screened for ROP. Again, one criterion is to be met for inclusion.
- The American Academy of Pediatrics (AAP), American Academy of Ophthalmologists (AAO), and American Association for Pediatric Ophthalmology and Strabismus (AAPOS) [45]:
  - All infants less than 30 weeks GA or less or equal 1500 g BW should be screened for ROP.
  - Selected infants with GA > 30 weeks or BW 1500–2000 g who are believed by their attending pediatrician or neonatologist to be at risk for ROP (infants with hypotension requiring inotropic support, oxygen supplementation for more than a few days or without monitoring) should also be screened.
- The Canadian Paediatric Society [46]:
  - All infants less or equal 30 weeks GA or less or equal 1250 g BW should be screened for ROP.
  - Selected infants with GA > 30 weeks or BW 1500–2000 g and unstable clinical course and believed to be at high risk for ROP should also be screened.

Low- and Middle-Income Countries

There are different screening criteria not only between low- and middle-income countries but also among NICUs from the same city [13, 24, 47].

- The Rashtriya Bal Swasthya Karyakram, Ministry of Health & Family Welfare, Government of India [48]:
  - All infants less than 34 weeks GA or less than 2000 g BW should be screened for ROP.
  - Selected infants with 34–36 weeks GA and risk factors for ROP should also be screened. The risk factors are cardiorespiratory support, prolonged oxygen therapy, respiratory distress syndrome, chronic lung disease, fetal hemorrhage, blood transfusion, neonatal sepsis, exchange transfusion, intraventricular hemorrhages, apneas, poor postnatal weight gain.
  - According to Chan-Ling et al., current Indian guidelines are under revision and will likely suggest commencing ROP screening for infants <34 weeks GA or < 1750 g BW, as well as 34–36 weeks GA or 1750–2000 g BW in the presence of risk factors for ROP [18].
- Brazilian Society of Pediatrics, Brazilian Council of Ophthalmology, and Brazilian Society of Pediatric Ophthalmology Guidelines Proposal for Screening and Treatment of ROP [49]:
  - All infants less or equal 32 weeks GA or less or equal 1500 g BW should be screened for ROP.
  - Selected infants with respiratory distress syndrome, sepsis, multiples blood transfusions, and intraventricular hemorrhages should also be screened.
  - There is evidence suggesting a wider criteria with GA < =35 weeks in NICU with poor survival rates (< = 80% among infants with BW < 1500 g) [13].

Other low- and middle-income countries have been following criteria according to the BW and GA of babies developing treatable disease [47].

When to Screen?

The onset and progression of ROP is determined predominantly by postmenstrual age (PMA) [24]. Rarely ROP requires treatment before 31 weeks PMA [24]. The ET-ROP trial laser early treatment group showed that mean age for treatment of Type 1 ROP (pre-threshold) and threshold disease was 35.2 weeks PMA and 37 weeks PMA, respectively [50]. Even in more mature infants, the mean PMA for ROP treatment follows this concept as their stage progression tend to be compressed [24].

Several guidelines suggested to start screening between 4 to 6 weeks old [49, 51], 6 to 7 weeks old [52], or even 2 to 3 weeks old [48]. However, recent evidences have suggested the commencement tailored to the infants' GA [24, 45] as can be seen in Table 63.2.

Monitoring

The follow-up and discharge should be recommended by the ophthalmologist according to retinal findings. The following schedule is a suggestion [45] (Table 63.3):

Table 63.2 Age at first ROP screening examination

	Age at first ROP screening examination			
Gestational age (in weeks)	Postnatal age (in weeks)		Postmenstrual age (in weeks)	
22	8a	9b	30a	31b
23	7a	8b	30a	31b
24	6a	7b	30a	31b
25	5a	6b	30a	31b
26	4a	5b	30a	31b
27ab	4		31	
28ab	4		32	
29ab	4		33	
30ab	4		34	
31a	4		35	
32a	3		35	
33a	2		35	
34a	2		36	
35a	2		37	

a Ref. [24]
b Ref. [45]

Table 63.3 ROP follow-up and discharge criteria

Follow-up examination	ROP classification
One week or less	Zone I: avascular retina, no ROP Zone I-II boundary: immature vascularization Zone I: Stage 1 or 2 Zone II: Stage 3 Suspected AP-ROP
One to two weeks	Posterior zone II: avascular retina Zone II: Stage 2 Zone I: regressing ROP
Two weeks	Zone II: avascular retina Zone II: Stage 1 Zone II: regressing ROP
Two to three weeks	Zone III: Stage 1 or 2 Zone III: regressing ROP
Discharge criteria	
1. Full retina vascularization in close proximity to the ora serrata 360°	
2. PMA > 35 weeks and zone III retinal vascularization attained without previous zone I or II ROP	
3. PMA > 45 weeks and no type 1 disease or worse ROP is present	
4. PMA > 65 weeks if intravitreal anti-VEGF injection was used for ROP treatment	
5. ROP regression	

Examination

Preparation of the Eye

Effective mydriasis of the pupil is crucial for the accurate diagnosis and ROP staging. The available mydriatic eye drops are either parasympathetic blockers which affect the pupillary sphincter muscle, such as tropicamide and cyclopentolate, or sympathetic stimulants which affect the pupillary dilator muscle such as phenylephrine [44].

The UK ROP Guideline reported a range of mydriatic regimen in the literature: phenylephrine 1%, phenylephrine 2.5%, cyclopentolate 0.2%, tropicamide 0.5%, tropicamide 2.5%. They recommend the combination of phenylephrine 2.5% and cyclopentolate 0.5% instilled one drop each in two to three doses, each 5 minutes apart, 1 hour prior to examination [44].

The above guideline cited studies reporting renal failure with tropicamide 0.5%/phenylephrine 0.5%, transient ileus with cyclopentolate 0.2%/phenylephrine 1%, bradycardia with tropicamide 1%, and heart failure with phenylephrine 10%/cyclopentolate 1%. Slow gastric emptying emesis, abdominal distension, and feeding related to bradycardia were also mentioned to be greater after screening [44]. The Brazilian recommendation is 1 drop of 0.5% proxymetacaine (anesthetic), followed by a single drop of 2.5 phenylephrine and 2 or 3 drops of 0.5% or 1.0% tropicamide five minutes apart. The exam should be performed at least 30–40 minutes after the first drop (artigo Ian) [53].

Care and Comfort During Examination

ROP examination can be uncomfortable and distressing; therefore, comfort care techniques are indicated: administering sucrose solution, nesting or swaddling, using a pacifier, and, eventually, using a topical anesthetic eye drop (proparacaine hydrochloride) [44].

Treatment

The objective of ROP treatment is to eliminate neovascularization stimulus driven by the avascular peripheric retina. As previously discussed, the avascular retina is a hypoxic environment and upregulates VGEF liberation, leading to neovascularization and eventually to abnormal vascular proliferative tissue formation and retina fold.

When to Treat?

The Early Treatment for ROP Cooperative Group (ET-ROP) revised and changed ROP treatment criteria and timing [54]. In Cryotherapy for ROP Cooperative Group (Cryo-ROP) study, treatment was performed when the ocular findings, known as threshold disease, indicated a risk of approximately 50% for retinal detachment [55] (Table 63.4).

Conversely, ET-ROP study compared early treatment of high-risk pre-threshold with conventional threshold treatment and concluded early treatment of high-risk pre-threshold ROP significantly reduced unfavorable structural and functional outcomes [54] (Table 63.4).

The recommendation became treating any eye meeting the criteria of type I pre-threshold and closely observing (wait and watch) any eye meeting the criteria of type 2 pre-threshold, as defined below (Table 63.4).

How to treat?

There are several techniques to perform ROP treatment and eliminate (or try to) retinal avascular VEGF stimulus. The first ROP treatment explored was cryoablation of avascular retina in Japan in the 1960–1970s. The Cryo-ROP was the first robust evidence of successful results with transscleral cryotherapy, which was concluded prematurely due to the demonstration of an overwhelming benefit of the treatment

Table 63.4 Criteria for ROP needing treatment according to Cryo-ROP, ET-ROP, and BEAT-ROP

Criteria for ROP needing treatment		
Cryo-ROP [55]	ET-ROP [54]	BEAT ROP [56]
Threshold disease 5 or more contiguous or 8 cumulative 30° sectors (clock hours) of stage 3 ROP in zone I or II in the presence of plus disease	*Type 1 ROP* Zone I, any stage ROP, plus disease Zone I, stage 3 ROP, no plus disease Zone II, stage 2 or 3, plus disease	Zone I or posterior zone II, stage 3 ROP, plus disease
	Type 2 ROP: wait and watch Zone I, stage 1 or 2 ROP, no plus disease Zone II, stage 3 ROP, no plus disease	

[55]. The study compared cryotherapy with no treatment and followed up the patients for 15 years [57].

However, diode laser photocoagulation largely supplanted cryotherapy in the 1990s because of better precision and less morbidity. Cryotherapy long-term results revealed unfavorable functional and structure outcomes [18, 57, 58]. The comparison between both treatments showed better visual acuity and refractive error outcomes in laser photocoagulation patients compared to cryotherapy patients [59].

Currently, diode trans-pupillary laser treatment is the preferable technique used for ROP treatment in high-, middle-, and low-income countries [44–46, 48, 49]. The procedure takes about 1 to 2 hours and as it is traumatic and painful, it requires sedation and analgesia [18]. Laser burns produce immediately a whitish spot (Fig. 63.10) and chronically hyperpigmented retina scars in the periphery retina (Fig. 63.11). Stage 4 ROP has shown positive results with lens-sparing vitrectomy (surgery that removes the vitreous component and spares the crystalline lens) [60]. Stage 5 ROP has a poor prognosis.

Intravitreal anti-VEGF injection holds great promise in the treatment of ROP, especially in more posterior (near the optic disc) disease, as salvage treatment when laser fails or when laser is difficult, such as in opaque media, sick and unstable infants [18]. The Bevacizumab Eliminates the Angiogenic Threat of ROP Cooperative Group (BEAT-ROP) investigated the efficacy of anti-VEGF therapy for Zone I or posterior Zone II, stage 3, plus disease ROP with results favoring anti-VEGF injection [56].

Nevertheless, there are many uncertainties about the use of anti-VEGF for ROP regarding systemic toxicity (in organs as brain, kidney and lungs), long half-life in the body, late ROP reactivation, correct dosage, and volume [18]. Recent Cochrane review concluded, although with low quality of evidence, that intravitreal anti-VEGF used as monotherapy reduces the risk of refractive errors during childhood

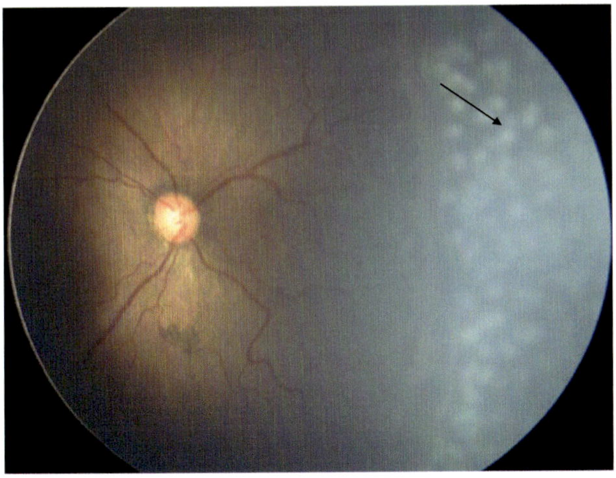

Fig. 63.10 Recent laser burns produce immediately a whitish spot

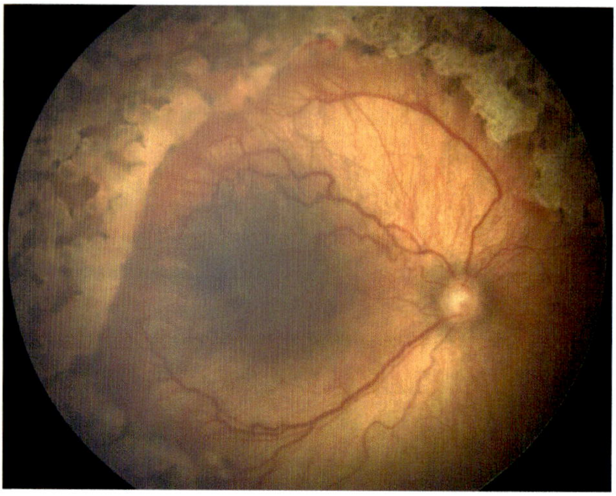

Fig. 63.11 Old hyperpigmented retina scars in the periphery retina

but does not reduce the risk of retinal detachment or recurrence of ROP in infants with type 1 disease [61].

There are four candidate anti-VEGF drugs for ROP treatment: bevacizumab (trade name: Avastin), ranibizumab (trade name: Lucentis), pegaptanib (trade name: Macugen), and aflibercept (trade name: Eylea) [18]. Chan-ling et al. reported the wide range (0.25 mg to 0.625 mg) of drugs dosage in previous data [18]. Recent study suggested that 0.004 mg may be the lowest dose of bevacizumab effective for ROP, but further investigation is warranted [62].

The American Academy of Pediatrics reports that considerations may be given to treatment of infants with zone I, stage 3 and plus disease ROP with intravitreal anti-VEGF and that it is essential to obtain an informed consent because of the unanswered questions involving dosage, timing, safety, visual and systemic outcomes [45]. Moreover, they advocate that infants treated with anti-VEGF should be monitored closely until retinal vascularization is complete or if not complete until the examiner be assured of no reactivation occurrence. There are reports of avascular retina even 4 years after intravitreal anti-VEGF treatment.

Long-Term Outcomes

Improving treatment criteria and options have changed visual and structural outcomes for severe ROP [63]. Visual outcomes are related to visual acuity and structural outcomes are related to retinal anatomy. Structural retinal abnormalities are pigmentary changes, degenerations, macular dragging, retinal folds, and detachment [57, 64].

In the Cryo-ROP study, 15 years of follow-up showed unfavorable visual outcome in 44.7% and unfavorable structural outcomes in 10% of treated eyes. In non-treated eyes, 64.3% and 51.9% had unfavorable visual and structural outcomes, respectively. Visual ($p < 0.001$) and structural outcomes differences were statically significant ($p < 0.001$) [57].

In the ET-ROP study, 6 years of follow-up showed unfavorable visual outcomes in 24.6% and unfavorable structural outcomes 8.9% of early-treated eyes. In conventionally treated eyes 29.0% and 15.2% had had unfavorable visual and structural outcomes, respectively. Visual outcomes differences were not statically significant ($p = 0.15$) but structural outcomes were ($p < 0.001$) [64].

Myopia is a major long-term complication and has been associated with prematurity, laser treatment, and/or severe ROP [63]. Others complications are cataract, constriction of visual field, strabismus, and reduced contrast sensitivity, although it should be emphasized that neurologic deficits in preterm infants may also have a role in the last three complications [63, 65].

Ophthalmologic follow-up for diagnosis of these potential problems after discharge is indicated. Although there is not a consensus about the timing of follow-up examination, the AAP, AAO, and AAPOS indicate examination within 4 to 6 months after discharge [45, 63] .

New ROP Approaches

There are several ongoing discussions about ROP screening, monitoring, and treatment such as algorithms for ROP prediction, telemedicine programs, new diagnostic imaging technologies, and intravitreal anti-VEGF injections. ROP screening programs have usually high sensitivity but low specificity, in other words, catch almost all at-risk infants, but most examined infants do not develop severe disease. In fact, approximately less than 10% of screened infants will need treatment [3]. As a result, there are many unnecessary ROP examinations and a high opportunity cost regarding the ophthalmologist time.

In an effort to improve the specificity, postnatal growth-based ROP risk models were developed [66]. One algorithm is named WINROP (Weight, IGF-1 levels, Neonatal, ROP) and intend to detect slowdowns in postnatal weight gain, predict severe ROP, and reduce the number of examinations [21, 66]. It uses a cumulative-deviations statistical approach in multiple steps with the weekly infant's weight, along with GA and BW [21, 66]. Another less complex model is named ROP Score which uses a logistic regression equation with the infant's GA, BW, and weight gain at 6 weeks' postnatal age, along with information about blood transfusion and oxygen mechanical ventilation [66, 67].

Two others logistic regression-based models are PINT ROP and CHOP ROP. The first model, PINT ROP, is based in infants with BW < 1000 g and included BW, GA, and daily rate of weight gain to predict the risk of severe ROP. Additional predictors such as ethnicity, perinatal and postnatal comorbidities, medical and surgical interventions are also evaluated [68]. The second model, CHOP ROP, is based in infants with BW < 1501 g [69]. The model had 100% sensitivity for type 1 ROP, reducing the number of examinations by 6.8% [70].

GROP is the most recent algorithm and is a hybrid modeling approach combining GA, BW, weight comparison with expected growth [71]. They predicted 100% sensitivity for type 1 ROP and reduced the number of examinations by 30.3% [71]. Noteworthy, WINROP, PINT ROP, CHOP ROP, and GROP were modeled to high-income countries populations. Consequently, their use may not be generalizable to poorer countries with more mature infants at-risk and where IGF-1 may play a less important role [66].

The association of wide-field digital retinography and telemedicine imaging interpretation is another emerging alternative to expand ROP screening. It enables retinal photographic documentation and expert's discussion around different centers; facilitates in training ophthalmologists with tele-education; decreases ophthalmologist's opportunity cost in treating less than 10 infants for every 100 screened; increases access for ROP care in areas with scarce specialized human resources and enables parents to better understand their infant's eye disease [72–74]. Studies have shown that telemedicine screening is more cost-effective in terms of cost per quality-adjusted life year than standard ophthalmoscopy for ROP management in the United Kingdom and the United States [75, 76]. *Our group has studied telemedicine screening for ROP under Brazilian health system perspective and concluded that the combination of telemedicine with standard ophthalmoscopy is more cost-effective than isolated standard ophthalmoscopy, especially due to an increase in ROP care access, which is still not universal in Brazil.*

Challenges to using wide-field imaging and telemedicine for ROP screening include a narrow field of view, quality of some images, and two-dimension image. There are studies addressing artificial intelligence with computer-based imaging analysis that try to read and classify the retinography (photograph of the infant's retina) [73]. Recent review reported high accuracy for the detection of clinically significant ROP, serving as a useful adjunct but not replacement for binocular ophthalmoscopy [72].

There are real-world successful examples of telemedicine for ROP as Karnataka Internet Assisted Diagnosis for ROP (KIDROP) in India [73, 77]. The program comprises 126 NICU and has completed over 150,000 screening sessions [73]. Other example is in Chile, with a national telemedicine network for ROP among 11 NICU [78]. New future screening approach could be risk models determining which infants require fundus photography and digital images determining which infants require eye examination by an ophthalmologist [66].

New diagnostic imaging tools can elucidate ROP pathophysiology and eventually provide information on new therapies or new risk predictions [74, 79]. Optic coherency tomography (OCT) provides cross-sectional images of the retinal layers and when performed in neonates can diagnose subclinical findings not seen by standard binocular ophthalmoscopy, such as preretinal tissue known as popcorn retinopathy, epiretinal membranes, cystoid macular changes, retinal layer schisis, precise localization of retinal detachment, vascular changes of plus disease, and cellular and subcellular changes related to ROP [74, 79]. OCT may clarify when functional outcomes do not correlate to structural outcomes in ROP.

Fluorescein angiography can evaluate retinal vascular flow can also identify subclinical findings not seen by binocular ophthalmoscopy, specially shunting in vascularized retina, or leakage from neovascular tissue [74]. It can have an important role in monitoring efficacy of anti-VEGF treatment in ROP [74].

Finally, as previously mentioned, anti-VEGF therapy for ROP brings many uncertainties and a large clinical trial comparing anti-VEGF treatment with laser is needed, regarding data on short- and long-term visual acuity, refractive error, and neurodevelopment. Others information such as best drug, safest dose, potential systemic side effects also need better understanding.

Conclusions

ROP is one of the leading causes of childhood visual impairment (low vision and blindness). The goal to control visual morbidity due to ROP should be based on primary prevention through improvement in neonatal care quality and on secondary prevention through early detection of at-risk infants and timely treatment and follow-up. Multidisciplinary care with neonatologists, nurses, physiotherapist, ophthalmologists, and parents is crucial for ROP management.

References

1. Muhit M, Gilbert C. A review of the epidemiology and control of childhood blindness. Trop Doct. 2003;33(4):197–201.
2. Blencowe H, Lawn JE, Vazquez T, Fielder A, Gilbert C. Preterm-associated visual impairment and estimates of retinopathy of prematurity at regional and global levels for 2010. Pediatr Res. 2013;74(Suppl 1):35–49.
3. Zin A, Gole GA. Retinopathy of prematurity-incidence today. Clin Perinatol. 2013;40(2):185–200.
4. Quinn GE. Retinopathy of prematurity blindness worldwide: phenotypes in the third epidemic. Eye Brain. 2016;8:31–6.
5. Dale N, Sosken P. Developmental outcome, including setback, in young children with severe visual impairment. Dev Med Child Neurol. 2002;44:613–22.
6. Gilbert C. Retinopathy of prematurity: a global perspective of the epidemics, population of babies at risk and implications for control. Early Hum Dev. 2008;84(2):77–82.
7. Terry T. Fibroblastic overgrowth of persistent tunica vasculosa lentis in infants born prematurely. Trans Am Ophthalmol Soc. 1942;40:262–84.
8. Ryan H. Retrolental Fibroplasia. Am J Ophthalmol. 1952;35(3):329–42.
9. Quinn G, Fielder A. Chapter 44. Retinopathy of prematurity. In: Taylor and Hoyt's Pediatric ophthalmology and strabismus. London: Elsevier Inc; 2017. p. 443–55.
10. Kinsey VE, Hemphill FM. Etiology of retrolental fibroplasia and preliminary report of the Cooperative Study of Retrolental Fibroplasia. Trans Am Acad Ophthalmol Otolaryngol. 1955;59:15–29.

11. Bolton DP, Cross KW. Further observations on cost of preventing retrolental fibroplasia. Lancet. 1974;1(7855):445–8.
12. Cross K. Cost of preventing retrolental fibroplasia. The Lancet. 1973:954–6.
13. Zin AA, Moreira ME, Bunce C, Darlow BA, Gilbert CE. Retinopathy of prematurity in 7 neonatal units in Rio de Janeiro: screening criteria and workload implications. Pediatrics. 2010;126(2):e410–7.
14. Howson CP, Kinney MV, Lawn JE, March of Dimes P, Save the Children W. Born too soon: the global action report on preterm birth. Geneva: World Health Organization; 2012.
15. Ophthalmology AAo. Pediatric ophthalmology and strabismus. Basic and clinical science course of the AAO. 2019–2020:475p.
16. Fleck BW, Stenson BJ. Retinopathy of prematurity and the oxygen conundrum: lessons learned from recent randomized trials. Clin Perinatol. 2013;40(2):229–40.
17. Smith LE, Hard AL, Hellstrom A. The biology of retinopathy of prematurity: how knowledge of pathogenesis guides treatment. Clin Perinatol. 2013;40(2):201–14.
18. Chan-Ling T, Gole GA, Quinn GE, Adamson SJ, Darlow BA. Pathophysiology, screening and treatment of ROP: A multi-disciplinary perspective. Prog Retin Eye Res. 2018;62:77–119.
19. Smith LE. Through the eyes of a child: understanding retinopathy through ROP the Friedenwald lecture. Invest Ophthalmol Vis Sci. 2008;49(12):5177–82.
20. Hellstrom A, Engstrom E, Hard AL, Albertsson-Wikland K, Carlsson B, Niklasson A, et al. Postnatal serum insulin-like growth factor I deficiency is associated with retinopathy of prematurity and other complications of premature birth. Pediatrics. 2003;112(5):1016–20.
21. Lofqvist C, Andersson E, Sigurdsson J, Engstrom E, Hard AL, Niklasson A, et al. Longitudinal postnatal weight and insulin-like growth factor I measurements in the prediction of retinopathy of prematurity. Arch Ophthalmol. 2006;124(12):1711–8.
22. Good WV, Hardy RJ, Dobson V, Palmer EA, Phelps DL, Quintos M, et al. The incidence and course of retinopathy of prematurity: findings from the early treatment for retinopathy of prematurity study. Pediatrics. 2005;116(1):15–23.
23. Austeng D, Kallen KB, Hellstrom A, Tornqvist K, Holmstrom GE. Natural history of retinopathy of prematurity in infants born before 27 weeks' gestation in Sweden. Arch Ophthalmol. 2010;128(10):1289–94.
24. Wilson CM, Ells AL, Fielder AR. The challenge of screening for retinopathy of prematurity. Clin Perinatol. 2013;40(2):241–59.
25. Gilbert C, Fielder A, Gordillo L, Quinn G, Semiglia R, Visintin P, et al. Characteristics of infants with severe retinopathy of prematurity in countries with low, moderate, and high levels of development: implications for screening programs. Pediatrics. 2005;115(5):e518–25.
26. Campbell K. Intensive oxygen therapy as a possible cause of retrolental fibroplasia: a clinical approach. Med J Aust. 1951;2(2):48–50.
27. Patz AHL, De La Cruz E. Studies on the effect of high oxygen administration in retrolental fibroplasia. I Nursery observations. Am J Ophthalmol. 1952;35(9):1248–53.
28. Prematurity. S-R-STOfPRo. Supplemental therapeutic oxygen for prethreshold retinopathy of prematurity (STOP-ROP), a randomized, controlled trial. I: primary outcomes. Pediatrics. 2000;105(2):295–310.
29. Askie LM, Darlow BA, Finer N, Schmidt B, Stenson B, Tarnow-Mordi W, et al. Association between oxygen saturation targeting and death or disability in extremely preterm infants in the neonatal oxygenation prospective meta-analysis collaboration. JAMA. 2018;319(21):2190–201.
30. Darlow BA, Husain S. Primary prevention of ROP and the oxygen saturation targeting trials. Semin Perinatol. 2019;43(6):333–40.
31. Aher SM, Ohlsson A. Early versus late erythropoietin for preventing red blood cell transfusion in preterm and/or low birth weight infants. Cochrane Database Syst Rev. 2012;10:CD004865.
32. Ohlsson A, Aher SM. Early erythropoiesis-stimulating agents in preterm or low birth weight infants. Cochrane Database Syst Rev. 2017;11:CD004863.
33. Higgins RD, Mendelsohn AL, DeFeo MJ, Ucsel R, Hendricks-Munoz KD. Antenatal dexamethasone and decreased severity of retinopathy of prematurity. Arch Ophthalmol. 1998;116(5):601–5.

34. Travers CP, Clark RH, Spitzer AR, Das A, Garite TJ, Carlo WA. Exposure to any antenatal corticosteroids and outcomes in preterm infants by gestational age: prospective cohort study. BMJ. 2017;356:j1039.
35. Wyllie J, Perlman JM, Kattwinkel J, Wyckoff MH, Aziz K, Guinsburg R, et al. Part 7: Neonatal resuscitation: 2015 international consensus on cardiopulmonary resuscitation and emergency cardiovascular care science with treatment recommendations. Resuscitation. 2015;95:e169–201.
36. Lyu Y, Shah PS, Ye XY, Warre R, Piedboeuf B, Deshpandey A, et al. Association between admission temperature and mortality and major morbidity in preterm infants born at fewer than 33 weeks' gestation. JAMA Pediatr. 2015;169(4):e150277.
37. Schmidt B, Roberts RS, Davis P, Doyle LW, Barrington KJ, Ohlsson A, et al. Long-term effects of caffeine therapy for apnea of prematurity. N Engl J Med. 2007;357(19):1893–902.
38. Manzoni P, Rinaldi M, Cattani S, Pugni L, Romeo MG, Messner H, et al. Bovine lactoferrin supplementation for prevention of late-onset sepsis in very low-birth-weight neonates: a randomized trial. JAMA. 2009;302(13):1421–8.
39. Hartnett ME, Morrison MA, Smith S, Yanovitch TL, Young TL, Colaizy T, et al. Genetic variants associated with severe retinopathy of prematurity in extremely low birth weight infants. Invest Ophthalmol Vis Sci. 2014;55(10):6194–203.
40. Ells A, Guernsey DL, Wallace K, Zheng B, Vincer M, Allen A, et al. Severe retinopathy of prematurity associated with FZD4 mutations. Ophthalmic Genet. 2010;31(1):37–43.
41. Prematurity ICfCoRo. The international classification of retinopathy of prematurity revisited. Arch Ophthalmol. 2005;123:991–9.
42. Prematurity. I-CfCoRo. An international classification of retinopathy of prematurity. Arch Ophthalmol. 1984;102:1130–4.
43. Chiang MF, Quinn GE, Fielder AR, Ostmo SR, Paul Chan RV, Berrocal A, et al. International Classification of Retinopathy of Prematurity, Third Edition. Ophthalmology. 2021 Jul 8:S0161-6420(21)00416-4. https://doi.org/10.1016/j.ophtha.2021.05.031. Epub ahead of print. PMID: 34247850.
44. Health RCoOaRCoPaC. United Kingdom retinopathy of prematurity guideline. 2008.
45. Fierson WM, Ophthalmology AAOPSo, American Academy of O, American Association For Pediatric O, Strabismus, American Association Of Certified O. Screening examination of premature infants for retinopathy of prematurity. Pediatrics. 2018;142(6):e20183061.
46. Jefferies AL. Canadian Paediatric Society FaNC. Retinopathy of prematurity: An update on screening and management. Paediatr Child Health. 2016;21(2):101–4.
47. Bowe T, Nyamai L, Ademola-Popoola D, Amphornphruet A, Anzures R, Cernichiaro-Espinosa LA, et al. The current state of retinopathy of prematurity in India, Kenya, Mexico, Nigeria, Philippines, Romania, Thailand, and Venezuela. Digit J Ophthalmol. 2019;25(4):49–58.
48. India RBSKMoHFWGo. Guidelines for universal eyes screening in newborns including retinopathy of prematurity. 2017.
49. Zin A, Florencio T, Fortes Filho BJ, Nakanami CR, Gianini N, Graziano RM, Moraes N. Proposta de diretrizes brasileiras do exame e tratamento de retinopatia da prematuridade (ROP). Arq Bras Oftalmol. 2007;70(5):875–83.
50. Good WV, Group. E-RC. Final Results of the Early Treatment for retinopathy of prematurity (ET ROP) randomized trial. Trans Am Ophthalmol Soc. 2004;102:233–50.
51. Fierson WM, American Academy of Pediatrics Section on O, American Academy of O, American Association for Pediatric O, Strabismus, American Association of Certified O. Screening examination of premature infants for retinopathy of prematurity. Pediatrics. 2013;131(1):189–95.
52. Medicine. JWPoTRCoOatBAoP. Retinopathy of prematurity: guidelines for screening and treatment. The report of a Joint Working Party of The Royal College of Ophthalmologists and the British Association of Perinatal Medicine. Early Hum Dev. 1996;46(3):239–58.
53. Curi I, Nakayama S, Pereira EM, Hopker LM, Ejzenbaum F, Barcellos R, et al. Brazilian guideline for pediatric cycloplegia and mydriasis. Arquivos Brasileiros de Oftalmologia. 2021.

54. Group. E-R-ETfRoPC. Revised indications for the treatment of retinopathy of prematurity: results of the early treatment for retinopathy of prematurity randomized trial. Arch Ophthalmol. 2003;121(12):1684–94.
55. 1988 CRYO-ROP preliminary resultsmulticenter-trial-of-cryotherapy-for-retinopathy-of-prematurity-1988.pdf.
56. Group M-HHKKCAB-RC. Efficacy of Intravitreal Bevacizumab for Stage 3+ ROP N England. J Med. 2011;364(7):603–15.
57. Palmer EA, Hardy RJ, Dibson V, Phelps DL, Quinn GE, Summers CG, et al. 15-year outcomes following threshold retinopathy of prematurity: final results from the multicenter trial of cryotherapy for retinopathy of prematurity. Arch Ophthalmol. 2005;123(3):311–8.
58. O'Keefe M, Burke J, Algawi K, Goggin M. Diode laser photocoagulation to the vascular retina for progressively advancing retinopathy of prematurity. Br J Ophthalmol. 1995;79(11):1012–4.
59. Shalev B, Farr AK, Repka MX. Randomized comparison of diode laser photocoagulation versus cryotherapy for threshold ROP 7 years. Am J Ophthalmol. 2001;132(1):76–80.
60. Prenner JL, Capone A Jr, Trese MT. Visual outcomes after lens-sparing vitrectomy for stage 4A retinopathy of prematurity. Ophthalmology. 2004;111(12):2271–3.
61. Sankar MJ, Sankar J, Chandra P. Anti-vascular endothelial growth factor (VEGF) drugs for treatment of retinopathy of prematurity. Cochrane Database Syst Rev. 2018;1:CD009734.
62. Wallace DK, Kraker RT, Freedman SF, Crouch ER, Bhatt AR, Hartnett ME, et al. Short-term outcomes after very low-dose intravitreous bevacizumab for retinopathy of prematurity. JAMA Ophthalmol. 2020;138(6):698–701.
63. Holmstrom G, Larsson E. Outcome of retinopathy of prematurity. Clin Perinatol. 2013;40(2):311–21.
64. Early Treatment for Retinopathy of Prematurity Cooperative G, Good WV, Hardy RJ, Dobson V, Palmer EA, Phelps DL, et al. Final visual acuity results in the early treatment for retinopathy of prematurity study. Arch Ophthalmol. 2010;128(6):663–71.
65. Davitt BV, Christiansen SP, Hardy RJ, Tung B, Good WV. Early treatment for retinopathy of prematurity cooperative G. Incidence of cataract development by 6 months' corrected age in the Early Treatment for Retinopathy of Prematurity study. J AAPOS. 2013;17(1):49–53.
66. Binenbaum G. Algorithms for the prediction of retinopathy of prematurity based on postnatal weight gain. Clin Perinatol. 2013;40(2):261–70.
67. Eckert GU, Fortes Filho JB, Maia M, Procianoy RS. A predictive score for retinopathy of prematurity in very low birth weight preterm infants. Eye (Lond). 2012;26(3):400–6.
68. Binenbaum G, Ying GS, Quinn GE, Dreiseitl S, Karp K, Roberts RS, et al. A clinical prediction model to stratify retinopathy of prematurity risk using postnatal weight gain. Pediatrics. 2011;127(3):e607–14.
69. Binenbaum G, Ying GS, Quinn GE, Huang J, Dreiseitl S, Antigua J, et al. The CHOP postnatal weight gain, birth weight, and gestational age retinopathy of prematurity risk model. Arch Ophthalmol. 2012;130(12):1560–5.
70. Binenbaum G, Ying GS, Tomlinson LA, Postnatal G. Retinopathy of prematurity study g. validation of the children's hospital of philadelphia retinopathy of prematurity (CHOP ROP) model. JAMA Ophthalmol. 2017;135(8):871–7.
71. Binenbaum G, Bell EF, Donohue P, Quinn G, Shaffer J, Tomlinson LA, et al. Development of modified screening criteria for retinopathy of prematurity: primary results from the postnatal growth and retinopathy of prematurity study. JAMA Ophthalmol. 2018;136(9):1034–40.
72. Fierson WM, Capone A Jr, American Academy of Pediatrics Section on O, American Academy of Ophthalmology AAoCO. Telemedicine for evaluation of retinopathy of prematurity. Pediatrics. 2015;135(1):e238–54.
73. Quinn GE, Vinekar A. The role of retinal photography and telemedicine in ROP screening. Semin Perinatol. 2019;43(6):367–74.
74. Valikodath N, Cole E, Chiang MF, Campbell JP, Chan RVP. Imaging in retinopathy of prematurity. Asia Pac J Ophthalmol (Phila). 2019;8(2):178–86.

75. Castillo-Riquelme MC, Lord J, Moseley MJ, Fielder AR, Haines L. Cost-effectiveness of digital photographic screening for retinopathy of prematurity in the United Kingdom. Int J Technol Assess Health Care. 2004;20(2):201–13.
76. Jackson KM, Scott KE, Zivin JG, Bateman DA, Flynn JT, Keenan JD, et al. Cost-utility analysis of telemedicine and ophthalmoscopy for retinopathy prematurity management Kevin Jackson. Arch Ophthalmol. 2008;126(4):439.
77. Vinekar A, Gilbert C, Dogra M, Kurian M, Shainesh G, Shetty B, et al. The KIDROP model of combining strategies for providing retinopathy of prematurity screening in underserved areas in India using wide-field imaging, tele-medicine, non-physician graders and smart phone reporting. Indian J Ophthalmol. 2014;62(1):41–9.
78. Ossandon D, Zanolli M, Stevenson R, Agurto R, Ortiz P, Dotan G. A national telemedicine network for retinopathy of prematurity screening. J AAPOS. 2018;22(2):124–7.
79. Maldonado RS, Toth CA. Optical coherence tomography in retinopathy of prematurity: looking beyond the vessels. Clin Perinatol. 2013;40(2):271–96.

Chapter 64
Necrotizing Enterocolitis

Renata Bastos Lopes, Maria Elisabeth Lopes Moreira, and Fernanda Hermeto

Introduction

Preterm birth is one of the biggest challenges in perinatal care [1]. In recent years, new therapies, such as the use of surfactant to treat hyaline membrane disease and antenatal corticosteroids to accelerate lung maturation, have had a significant impact in mortality of premature infants [2]. However, despite the reduction in mortality, some morbidities related to prematurity have not significantly changed. Bronchopulmonary dysplasia (BDP), retinopathy of prematurity (ROP), and necrotizing enterocolitis (NEC) remain major issues in current neonatology [3].

Necrotizing enterocolitis is the most frequent and lethal gastrointestinal disorder affecting preterm infants. Complications such as intestinal necrosis, sepsis, and death often cannot be avoided, even when disease is detected early and aggressively treated [4, 5]. The prevalence of NEC varies among different neonatal intensive care units (NICUs), being reported between 3% and 11% in very low birth weight (VLBW) preterm [6, 7]. There is an inversely proportional relationship between the incidence of NEC and gestational age at birth, with VLBW (birth weight less than 1500 g) and extremely low birth weight (ELBW or birth weight less than 1000 g) premature babies being the most at risk for the disease [2, 8–10]. Mortality related to NEC varies from 20% to 50%, and can reach 100% in severe cases [11–13].

The pathophysiology of necrotizing enterocolitis remains incompletely understood. However, it is believed to be a disease with multifactorial

R. B. Lopes (✉) · F. Hermeto
Neonatology Department, Perinatal Maternity Hospital, Rio de Janeiro, RJ, Brazil
e-mail: renata.lopes@perinatal.com.br

M. E. L. Moreira
Instituto Fernandes Figueira - Fiocruz, Clinica Perinatal Laranjeiras, Rio de Janeiro, RJ, Brazil
e-mail: bebeth@iff.fiocruz.br

© Springer Nature Switzerland AG 2022

R. A. Moreira de Sá, E. B. d. Fonseca (eds.), *Perinatology*,
https://doi.org/10.1007/978-3-030-83434-0_64

pathophysiology. Factors such as genetic predisposition, intestinal immaturity, imbalance of vascular tone, abnormal intestinal colonization, and immunological factors of the intestinal wall may contribute to the development of the disease [14]. Molecular studies suggest that the individual inflammatory response plays an important role in the pathogenesis of the disease [15, 16]. Besides prematurity, other risk factors are involved in the pathophysiology of NEC, such as asphyxia, bacterial infection, mesenteric ischemia, and feeding practices in the NICU [4].

Epidemiology

The incidence of enterocolitis is inversely proportional to the gestational age. The incidence is clearly related to prematurity, with a significant drop in newborns with gestational age greater than 35–36 weeks and birth weight greater than 1500 g. A study by the Canadian neonatal research network demonstrated an incidence of 5.1% in newborns under 33 weeks of gestational age, with significant variation among the participating units (1.3% to 12.9%) [6]. In the United States, a population study showed an incidence of 2.6% in patients younger than 33 weeks of gestational age [7]. Full-term infants who develop NEC usually have risk factors related to mesenteric hypoperfusion, such as congenital heart disease, sepsis, hypotension, and polycythemia [17].

NEC-related mortality can reach 50%, varying from center to center and depending on patient's characteristics. Higher mortality is observed in surgical cases [12]. There is also a form of the disease with specific characteristics, called fulminant enterocolitis, with a fast and fatal course, affecting a large part of the bowels, and it is present in approximately 7% of NEC cases. Patients with fulminating NEC usually are more premature and have a lower birth weight compared to patients with non-fulminating NEC [18].

Risk Factors

Antenatal Risk Factors

The main risk factor for NEC is preterm birth, since approximately 90% of cases occur in newborns under 35 weeks of gestational age. Babies born after 35 weeks who present with NEC are more likely to have had perinatal asphyxia, sepsis, or congenital malformations, leading to mesenteric ischemia. Enterocolitis is a multifactorial disease, and intestinal reperfusion injury is one of the factors involved. It results from an ischemic insult triggering a local inflammatory process, leading to damage to the intestinal mucosa and vasculature in areas where the intestine is less irrigated. Any maternal condition that impairs placental and fetal circulation can increase the risk for NEC [19].

Maternal use of drugs may be a significant risk factor for NEC. Cocaine can lead to placental vasoconstriction, uterine contraction, and intrauterine growth restriction, as well as causing sympathomimetic effects directly on the fetal circulation [20]. Downard C et al. (2012) demonstrated that nicotine impairs the initial placental vascular development, which can cause placental insufficiency and intrauterine growth restriction [21]. Furthermore, drugs used for tocolysis, such as indomethacin and sulindac, nonsteroidal anti-inflammatory drugs (NSAIDs), and prostaglandin inhibitors, have also been associated with an increased risk for NEC [22, 23].

Although maternal hypertensive disease can cause placental disease, the relationship with NEC is unclear. Bashiri et al. (2003) consider that pregnancy-induced hypertension (PIH) is an independent risk factor for NEC development in VLBW newborns [24]. Cetinkaya M. et al. (2012) described an association of NEC and pre-eclampsia [25]. In a Brazilian study, Vieira et al. (2013) demonstrated that the presence of pre-eclampsia increased the risk for NEC by 2.84 times in VLBW infants [26].

Chorioamnionitis may damage placental circulation and cause fetal inflammation. García-Muñoz et al. (2014) showed that newborns exposed to clinical chorioamnionitis had a higher risk of NEC (11.2% × 7.7%) after adjustment in a multivariate model [27]. A recent study observed that the presence of histopathological chorioamnionitis with evidence of fetal involvement increased the risk for NEC [28].

Postnatal Risk Factors

Perinatal asphyxia is a known risk factor for NEC [29]. Manogura et al. (2008) showed that a 5-minute Apgar score less than 7 and a higher umbilical cord artery base deficit were related to NEC [30]. Intestinal pathological study from infants with NEC frequently demonstrates coagulation necrosis and other evidence of ischemic injury, which may support the possibility of a strong role for secondary hypoxic-ischemia in the pathogenesis of this disease [31]. In a recent study, Yong et al. (2016) demonstrated that ischemia has a primary role [32].

A patent ductus arteriosus (PDA) is a common pathology in premature babies and may be present in over 80% of ELBW infants [33]. A moderate PDA shunt may cause hemodynamically significant changes such as lower systemic blood pressure and lower mean and diastolic superior mesenteric artery velocities. The inability to increase mesenteric flow, in the presence of a PDA, may increase the risk for intestinal ischemia, feeding intolerance, and NEC [34]. The association between PDA with use of indomethacin and NEC in premature newborns has been reported, although no randomized controlled trial has confirmed that [35–37]. In a recent study, Louis et al. (2016) showed no association between the use of indomethacin for PDA ligation and NEC [38].

Although infant formulas for preterm population have been design to mimic the composition of human milk, some protective properties present in breast milk, such as secretory IgA, lysozyme, and oligosaccharides have not yet been reproduced. The incidence of NEC is lower in newborns who receive breast milk when compared to those receiving formula [39]. Human milk contains antimicrobial and anti-inflammatory properties; however, studying its protective action against the development of NEC is a challenge, due to the difficulty to standardize a human milk–based diet. Variations may be present, such as exclusive breast milk, donor human milk, additives in human milk, and breast milk supplemented by formula for preterm infants [40]. A meta-analysis suggested that the use of human milk reduces the incidence of NEC and that the use of breast milk fortifier does not increase this incidence [41]. A prospective study comparing an exclusive human milk diet with bovine-based formula one showed a 77% lower incidence of NEC in the group that received only human milk [42].

Feeding practices have been linked to the development of NEC. However, the wide variation in nutritional strategies among neonatal ICUs makes it difficult to study this issue [40]. Retrospective studies have shown that a rapid increase in feeds appears to be a risk factor for NEC [43], but a meta-analysis has not confirmed this hypothesis [44].

Blood transfusions are required for many preterm infants throughout the NICU stay, especially for the ELBW babies [45]. It is not clear whether the transfusion of red blood cells is an independent risk factor for NEC or the newborns who received the transfusion are manifesting initial symptoms of the disease [46]. Some theories have been proposed to explain this association: systemic inflammatory reaction, increased blood viscosity, and changes in mesenteric blood flow during transfusion [47]. Bailey et al. (2016), using the Near Infrared Spectroscopy (NIRS), observed that splanchnic tissue oxygenation was significantly lower during the red blood cell transfusion compared to cerebral oxygenation [48]. Marin et al. (2014), using the same method, demonstrated that, during blood transfusion, mesenteric oxygenation was lower during and after diet, and this reduction remained for 15 hours. However, when diet was interrupted during transfusion, there was a positive trend in mesenteric oxygenation [49]. In 2013, a case–control study showed that red blood cell transfusion 48 hours before the appearance of NEC appears to be an independent risk factor for the development of this disease in premature infants [47]. However, in 2014, a prospective observational study enrolling 585 infants born at <33 weeks gestational age did not find a significant relationship between blood transfusion and NEC [50]. Patel et al. (2016) in secondary analysis of a multicenter and prospective study investigating blood transmission of cytomegalovirus in three neonatal intensive care units in the United States demonstrated that severe anemia was an independent risk factor for the occurrence of NEC. However, blood transfusion was not a risk factor for the disease [46].

Pathophysiology

The pathogenesis of NEC is not clearly defined, but is likely multifactorial. Currently, it is believed that there is a combination of factors, such as genetic predisposition, intestinal and immunologic immaturity, imbalance of vascular tone, abnormal intestinal colonization, and local immunological factors of the intestinal wall that lead to the development of the disease [51].

Genetic Predisposition

Familial and genetic susceptibility to necrotizing enterocolitis and other neonatal morbidities have been studied. Twin analyses have shown that familial factors contribute to susceptibility for NEC and intraventricular hemorrhage (IVH), but without conclusive findings to define the genetic contribution [52].

Intestinal Immaturity

Immaturity in intestinal motility, absorption, digestion, and immune defenses probably predispose the premature intestine to injuries. Acidic gastric juice production is deficient in the preterm newborn and this has been shown to be associated with NEC, especially in patients using H2-blocker therapy [53].

Animal studies suggest that premature infants have an overexuberant inflammatory response to some type of insult, which may vary between infants. This initial insult results in disruption of the intestinal epithelium, bacterial translocation, and an exaggerated immune response by immature intestinal epithelium cells. The intestinal epithelium plays a major role in protection against potential pathogens and acts as both a biochemical and physical barrier. In premature infants, the physical barrier is not fully developed, increasing intestinal permeability to bacteria. In preterm infants, the mucin layer, which creates an adherent barrier to bacteria, is less mature and, hence, less effective, allowing for increased bacterial adherence and permeability. Immunologic function of the neonatal intestinal tract is also immature in many ways, including not producing secretory IgA, which functions to bind luminal bacteria, in the first weeks of life [19].

Intestinal Microbiota Versus Bacterial Colonization

Intestinal colonization occurs after birth and can be variable [54]. The early neonatal period represents a crucial moment for gut colonization to occur properly, resulting in better intestinal homeostasis. In the weeks after birth, the gut acquires a nascent microbiome, and starts its transition to bacterial population equilibrium. This early-in-life microbial population quite likely influences later-in-life host biology.

Studies suggest that the microbiota of the premature infant differ significantly from the full-term newborn [55, 56]. The latter, when born by vaginal delivery and fed exclusively with breast milk, is the reference of a normal intestinal flora [57]. Premature newborns may have different colonization patterns according to the environment they are constrained. The NICU environment, with a predominance of pathogenic organisms, can negatively affect intestinal colonization by commensal bacteria [58, 59]. In addition, they are frequently exposed to antibiotics, which has been associated with an increased risk of sepsis and NEC [60, 61]. With the development of new technologies for analyzing the intestinal microbiota, there has been great progress in understanding the intestinal colonization of premature infants [54]. It is possible that the initial colonization of the premature gut with an inappropriate microbiota is a risk factor for NEC.

A prospective study identified a specific bacterial flora in the analysis of meconium in patients with NEC. The presence of *Clostridium perfringens* in meconium in newborns was related to NEC from the first day of life until the onset of the disease [62]. It is noted that NEC rarely occurs in newborns less than a week old, suggesting a relationship of intestinal colonization and NEC onset.

Endothelial Dysfunction

The physiologic characteristics of the newborn intestinal circulation are unique when compared with the adult condition. Intestinal vascular resistance within newborn gut is very low and this reduction is mediated by an increased production of nitric oxide (NO) by the gut vascular endothelium. The low vascular resistance alters the capacity of this vasculature to respond to systemic circulatory changes, such as hypotension and hypoxemia. The essential role of endothelium production of NO in maintaining newborn intestinal hemodynamics might be important in the pathogenesis of NEC. Factors such as bacterial translocation, production of platelet-activating factor, and intestinal stasis can damage the vascular endothelium, leading to a decrease in the production of NO, hence the reduction in intestinal blood flow being directly related to NEC [63].

Inflammatory Mediators

Pathogenesis of NEC involves the final route of inflammatory mediators production, leading to development of intestinal injury. Endotoxins, platelet-activating factor (PAF), tumor necrosis factor (TNF) and other cytokines, along with prostaglandins, leukotrienes, and NO appear to be involved. It is believed that the excessive inflammatory response of the immature intestine, a hallmark of NEC, is secondary to a developmental immaturity in the preterm infant's innate immune system [64, 65].

Probiotics

Probiotics modify the intestinal mucosa, increase intestinal motility, and control the production of inflammatory cytokines [66]. They effectively reduce the incidence and mortality related to NEC [67]. A recent meta-analysis involving 1514 preterm babies showed significantly lower risk of NEC (risk reduction of 36%) for patients using probiotics [68]. A randomized controlled study using probiotics, prebiotics, and placebo revealed a lower incidence of NEC in the group that received probiotics [69].

Some issues related to the use of probiotics have not yet been clarified: dose and type of species for the composition of the solutions, the lack of evidence in large randomized studies regarding long-term follow-up, and safety regarding mortality and infection related to the use of these solutions.

Clinical Presentation

Clinical presentation of NEC varies, from an insidious beginning, with gradual progression in days, to an abrupt and fulminant presentation, with shock and dysfunction of multiple organs in a few hours. The timing of occurrence of NEC is related to gestational age. The more immature the newborn is, the later the disease usually presents [70].

Systemic clinical manifestations are, in most cases, nonspecific, and include apneas, tachycardia, tachypnea, pallor, lethargy, thermal instability, and hyperglycemia.

Gastrointestinal symptoms in early disease, such as food intolerance, increased gastric residual, and bloody stools may be present. As the disease progresses, the abdomen may evolve with a change in color, becoming erythematous and painful. In cases of intestinal perforation, it is usually bluish, more tense, and painful. Extreme premature newborns may present a bluish discoloration of the scrotum in cases of perforation [70].

Laboratory

Laboratory findings are also nonspecific and usually demonstrate a state of increased systemic inflammation. Anemia is often present. Leukogram findings range from leukopenia with neutropenia to leukocytosis with left shift. The presence of thrombocytopenia is frequent and also a factor of worse prognosis. Blood culture is positive in 40–60% of NEC cases, with Gram-negative bacteria being more common [70]. Metabolic acidosis and hyponatremia may be present. C-reactive protein is usually increased and its rule is related not to the diagnosis but to the monitoring of the disease, with an expected fall when the patient improves. The high permanence of CRP can indicate complications, such as abscesses, stenosis, or fistula [19]. Recurrence can occur in 5–6% of cases, being associated with the presence of congenital heart disease, rotavirus infection, and allergy to breast milk [70, 71].

Radiographic Findings

The presence of intestinal pneumatosis, the most common radiological finding in the disease, confirms the diagnosis of NEC. Air in the portal space may also be present and is usually associated with a more advanced disease, indicating a worse prognosis. The occurrence of pneumoperitoneum indicates intestinal perforation. Nonspecific findings, such as gas distension, fixed sentinel loop, and global gas decrease, may also be present [72].

An NEC classification system was initially proposed by Bell in 1978 [77] but has undergone changes since its initial publication. It brings together clinical findings, physical examination of the gastrointestinal system, with radiographic findings for the definition, and classification of disease stages. This classification is widely used to define the diagnosis, categorize NEC, and guide the treatment to be performed.

Treatment

Clinical Management

Most patients with NEC can be managed with clinical support. In the clinical and radiographic suspicion of NEC, the enteral diet should be suspended and the patient should be kept with an orogastric tube, in order to provide an intestinal rest. It is necessary to provide intravenous fluids and parenteral nutrition to insure adequate nutrients support and minimize catabolic state. Broad-spectrum antibiotics are also indicated and coverage for anaerobes should be started in the presence of intestinal perforation. Blood culture and urine culture should be collected to better define the duration and type of antibiotic, which varies from 7 to 14 days. The support of the other systems will depend on the clinical presentation and the individual need of each patient. Hemodynamic support with volume, vasoactive amines, and hydrocortisone may be necessary. Patients may progress with respiratory failure, requiring respiratory support with positive pressure and mechanical ventilation. Anemia, thrombocytopenia, and coagulopathy may be present, requiring transfusion of red blood cells, platelets, plasma, and cryoprecipitate. In the absence of intestinal perforation, serial abdominal radiographs should be performed every 8–12 hours in order to identify pneumoperitoneum for possible surgical indication [51].

Surgical Treatment

The surgical approach basically comprises two types of intervention: exploratory laparotomy or insertion of a peritoneal drain. Surgical treatment aims to remove necrotic intestinal tissue, preserve healthy intestinal tissue, and stabilize the patient's clinical condition. To date, there is no clinical resource that can predict the extent of intestinal necrosis and the exact moment for surgical intervention. The ideal approach would be when the necrosis process could be detected early, with complete removal.

The indications for surgery are pneumoperitoneum, significant clinical deterioration despite maximum clinical treatment, persistent thrombocytopenia, ascites, and persistent radiological image.

Laparotomy with resection of necrotic intestinal tissue and the performance of an enterostomy are widely used as the surgery of choice for NEC. The purpose of performing the enterostomy is to allow the recovery of the remaining intestine, avoiding the anastomosis of inflamed loops and possible complications. However, 23–34% of these ostomies present complications, such as dehiscence, abrasions on the skin, stenosis, prolapse, infection, and fistula [73, 74].

For a long time, laparotomy was the initial intervention of choice for the surgical management of NEC. Over time, peritoneal drainage has become an alternative to laparotomy [70].

There are still controversies in the literature as to whether the peritoneal drainage presents better results compared to laparotomy. In 2006, a prospective multicenter observational study, involving 16 American centers, showed a result of death or greater neurological sequelae in the group submitted to peritoneal drainage. However after multivariate analysis, there was no statistical difference between the groups [75].

Two randomized controlled clinical trials, comparing peritoneal drainage with laparotomy, showed similar results in relation to death, the need for parenteral nutrition, and the length of stay in the hospital [76, 77].

Complications

Mortality from NEC remains high, up to 50%, and is inversely proportional to gestational age [12, 51]. Other complications include post-NEC stenosis, enterocutaneous fistulas, cholestasis, and short bowel syndrome with intestinal and liver failure.

Post-NEC strictures usually appear 3–8 weeks after the acute condition and are diagnosed by a contrast exam. The colon is the main site of stenosis, but they can also appear in the ileum [78, 79].

Infants with surgical necrotizing enterocolitis have a higher risk of neurodevelopmental impairment. A retrospective analysis of the NICHD Neonatal Research Network showed that patients who had NEC requiring surgical treatment had the worst results, with 53% of mortality before discharge and 82% of neurological sequelae, although statistically similar to infants who had spontaneous intestinal perforation [80].

References

1. Howson CP, Kinney MV, Mcougall L, Lawn JE, the Born Too Soon Preterm Birth Action Group. Born Toon Soon: Preterm birth matters. Reprod Health. 2013;10(Suppl 1):S1.
2. Stoll BJ, Hansen NI, Bell EF, Walsh MC, Carlo WA, Shankaran S, et al. Trends in care practices, morbidity, and mortality of extremely preterm neonates, 1993-2012. JAMA. 2015;314(10):1039.
3. Patel RM, Kandefer S, Walsh MC, Bell EF, Carlo WA, Laptook AR, et al. Causes and timing of death in extremely premature infants from 2000 through 2011. N Engl J Med. 2015;372(4):331–40.
4. Srinivasan PS, Brandler MD, D'Souza A. Necrotizing enterocolitis. Clin Perinatol. 2008;35(1):251–72, x.
5. Ahle M, Drott P, Andersson RE. Epidemiology and trends of necrotizing enterocolitis in Sweden: 1987-2009. Pediatrics. 2013;132(2):e443–51.
6. Yee WH, Soraisham AS, Shah VS, Aziz K, Yoon W, Lee SK, et al. Incidence and timing of presentation of necrotizing enterocolitis in preterm infants. Pediatrics. 2012;129(2):e298–304.
7. Guthrie SO, Gordon PV, Thomas V, Thorp JA, Peabody J, Clark RH. Necrotizing enterocolitis among neonates in the United States. J Perinatol. 2003;23(4):278–85.
8. Hsueh W, Caplan MS, Qu X-W, Tan X-D, De Plaen IG, Gonzalez-Crussi F. Neonatal necrotizing enterocolitis: clinical considerations and pathogenetic concepts. Pediatr Dev Pathol. 2003;6(1):6–23.
9. Llanos AR, Moss ME, Pinzòn MC, Dye T, Sinkin RA, Kendig JW. Epidemiology of neonatal necrotising enterocolitis: a population-based study. Paediatr Perinat Epidemiol. 2002;16(4):342–9.
10. Battersby C, Longford N, Costeloe K, Modi N, for the UK Neonatal Collaborative Necrotising Enterocolitis Study Group. Development of a gestational age–specific case definition for neonatal necrotizing enterocolitis. JAMA Pediatr. 2017;171(3):256.
11. Fanaroff AA, Stoll BJ, Wright LL, Carlo WA, Ehrenkranz RA, Stark AR, et al. Trends in neonatal morbidity and mortality for very low birthweight infants. Am J Obstet Gynecol. 2007;196(2):147.e1–8.
12. Fitzgibbons SC, Ching Y, Yu D, Carpenter J, Kenny M, Weldon C, et al. Mortality of necrotizing enterocolitis expressed by birth weight categories. J Pediatr Surg. 2009;44(6):1072–5; discussion 1075-1076.
13. Berrington JE, Hearn RI, Bythell M, Wright C, Embleton ND. Deaths in preterm infants: changing pathology over 2 decades. J Pediatr. 2012;160(1):49–53.e1.
14. Zhou P, Li Y, Ma L-Y, Lin H-C. The role of immunonutrients in the prevention of necrotizing enterocolitis in preterm very low birth weight infants. Nutrients. 2015;7(9):7256–70.
15. Neu J, Mihatsch W. Recent developments in necrotizing enterocolitis. JPEN J Parenter Enteral Nutr. 2012;36(1 Suppl):30S–5S.
16. Sharma R, Tepas JJ. Microecology, intestinal epithelial barrier and necrotizing enterocolitis. Pediatr Surg Int. 2010;26(1):11–21.
17. Lambert DK, Christensen RD, Henry E, Besner GE, Baer VL, Wiedmeier SE, et al. Necrotizing enterocolitis in term neonates: data from a multihospital health-care system. J Perinatol. 2007;27(7):437–43.
18. Lambert DK, Christensen RD, Baer VL, Henry E, Gordon PV, Besner GE, et al. Fulminant necrotizing enterocolitis in a multihospital healthcare system. J Perinatol. 2012;32(3):194–8.

19. Dominguez KM, Moss RL. Necrotizing enterocolitis. Clin Perinatol. 2012;39(2):387–401.
20. Ganapathy V. Drugs of abuse and human placenta. Life Sci. 2011;88(21–22):926–30.
21. Downard CD, Grant SN, Maki AC, Krupski MC, Matheson PJ, Bendon RW, et al. Maternal cigarette smoking and the development of necrotizing enterocolitis. Pediatrics. 2012;130(1):78–82.
22. Sood BG, Lulic-Botica M, Holzhausen KA, Pruder S, Kellogg H, Salari V, et al. The risk of necrotizing enterocolitis after indomethacin tocolysis. Pediatrics. 2011;128(1):e54–62.
23. Kamath-Rayne BD, Habli M, Rodriguez Z, Wu M, Gresh J, DeFranco EA. Antenatal exposure to sulindac and risk of necrotizing enterocolitis. Am J Obstet Gynecol. 2015;212(1):96.e1–7.
24. Bashiri A, Zmora E, Sheiner E, Hershkovitz R, Shoham-Vardi I, Mazor M. Maternal hypertensive disorders are an independent risk factor for the development of necrotizing enterocolitis in very low birth weight infants. Fetal Diagn Ther. 2003;18(6):404–7.
25. Cetinkaya M, Ozkan H, Koksal N. Maternal preeclampsia is associated with increased risk of necrotizing enterocolitis in preterm infants. Early Hum Dev. 2012;88(11):893–8.
26. Vieira AA, David BBL, Lino RRG, Duarte L, de Barros Duarte L, Bueno AC. Evaluation of perinatal factors that influence the incidence of necrotizing enterocolitis in very low birth weight infants. Rev Bras Ginecol Obstet. 2013;35(8):363–7.
27. García-Muñoz Rodrigo F, Galán Henríquez G, Figueras Aloy J, García-Alix PA. Outcomes of very-low-birth-weight infants exposed to maternal clinical chorioamnionitis: a multicentre study. Neonatology. 2014;106(3):229–34.
28. Been JV, IGIJG R, Kornelisse RF, Lima Passos V, Kramer BW, TAJ S, et al. Histologic chorioamnionitis, fetal involvement, and antenatal steroids: effects on neonatal outcome in preterm infants. Am J Obstet Gynecol. 2009;201(6):587.e1–8.
29. Gane B, Bhat BV, Adhisivam B, Joy R, Prasadkumar P, Femitha P, et al. Risk factors and outcome in neonatal Necrotising enterocolitis. Indian J Pediatr. 2014;81(5):425–8.
30. Manogura AC, Turan O, Kush ML, Berg C, Bhide A, Turan S, et al. Predictors of necrotizing enterocolitis in preterm growth-restricted neonates. Am J Obstet Gynecol. 2008;198(6):638.e1–5.
31. Young CM, Kingma SDK, Neu J. Ischemia-reperfusion and neonatal intestinal injury. J Pediatr. 2011;158(2):e25–8.
32. Chen Y, Chang KTE, Lian DWQ, Lu H, Roy S, Laksmi NK, et al. The role of ischemia in necrotizing enterocolitis. J Pediatr Surg [Internet]. 2016. Jan [cited 2016 May 14]; Available from: http://linkinghub.elsevier.com/retrieve/pii/S0022346815008404.
33. Fujii AM, Brown E, Mirochnick M, O'Brien S, Kaufman G. Neonatal necrotizing enterocolitis with intestinal perforation in extremely premature infants receiving early indomethacin treatment for patent ductus arteriosus. J Perinatol. 2002;22(7):535–40.
34. McCurnin D, Clyman RI. Effects of a patent ductus arteriosus on postprandial mesenteric perfusion in premature baboons. Pediatrics. 2008;122(6):e1262–7.
35. Fowlie PW, Davis PG, McGuire W. Prophylactic intravenous indomethacin for preventing mortality and morbidity in preterm infants. In: The Cochrane Collaboration, editor. Cochrane Database of Systematic Reviews [Internet]. Chichester, UK: John Wiley & Sons, Ltd; 2010. [cited 2016 May 14]. Available from: http://doi.wiley.com/10.1002/14651858.CD000174.pub2.
36. Jones LJ, Craven PD, Attia J, Thakkinstian A, Wright I. Network meta-analysis of indomethacin versus ibuprofen versus placebo for PDA in preterm infants. Arch Dis Child - Fetal Neonatal Ed. 2011;96(1):F45–52.
37. Mirea L, Sankaran K, Seshia M, Ohlsson A, Allen AC, Aziz K, et al. Treatment of patent ductus arteriosus and neonatal mortality/morbidities: adjustment for treatment selection bias. J Pediatr. 2012;161(4):689–694.e1.
38. Louis D, Torgalkar R, Shah J, Shah PS, Jain A. Enteral feeding during indomethacin treatment for patent ductus arteriosus: association with gastrointestinal outcomes. J Perinatol [Internet]. 2016 25 [cited 2016 May 14]; Available from: http://www.nature.com/doifinder/10.1038/jp.2016.11.

39. Ramani M, Ambalavanan N. Feeding practices and necrotizing enterocolitis. Clin Perinatol. 2013;40(1):1–10.
40. Good M, Sodhi CP, Hackam DJ. Evidence-based feeding strategies before and after the development of necrotizing enterocolitis. Expert Rev Clin Immunol. 2014;10(7):875–84.
41. Kuschel CA, Harding JE. Multicomponent fortified human milk for promoting growth in preterm infants. Cochrane Database Syst Rev. 2004;1:CD000343.
42. Boyd CA, Quigley MA, Brocklehurst P. Donor breast milk versus infant formula for preterm infants: systematic review and meta-analysis. Arch Dis Child Fetal Neonatal Ed. 2007;92(3):F169–75.
43. Anderson DM, Kliegman RM. The relationship of neonatal alimentation practices to the occurrence of endemic necrotizing enterocolitis. Am J Perinatol. 1991 Jan;8(1):62–7.
44. Morgan J, Young L, McGuire W. Slow advancement of enteral feed volumes to prevent necrotising enterocolitis in very low birth weight infants. Cochrane Database Syst Rev. 2015;10:CD001241.
45. For the Brazilian Network on Neonatal Research, dos Santos AMN, Guinsburg R, de Almeida MFB, Procianoy RS, Marba STM, et al. Factors associated with red blood cell transfusions in very-low-birth-weight preterm infants in Brazilian neonatal units. BMC Pediatr [Internet]. 2015 Dec [cited 2016 May 14];15(1). Available from: http://www.biomedcentral.com/1471-2431/15/113.
46. Patel RM, Knezevic A, Shenvi N, Hinkes M, Keene S, Roback JD, et al. Association of red blood cell transfusion, anemia, and necrotizing enterocolitis in very low-birth-weight infants. JAMA. 2016;315(9):889.
47. Wan-Huen P, Bateman D, Shapiro DM, Parravicini E. Packed red blood cell transfusion is an independent risk factor for necrotizing enterocolitis in premature infants. J Perinatol. 2013 Oct;33(10):786–90.
48. Bailey SM, Hendricks-Muñoz KD, Mally PV. Variability in splanchnic tissue oxygenation during preterm red blood cell transfusion given for symptomatic anaemia may reveal a potential mechanism of transfusion-related acute gut injury. Blood Transfus [Internet]. 2015 [cited 2016 May 14]; Available from: http://www.bloodtransfusion.it/articolo.aspx?idart=002871&idriv=000103.
49. Marin T, Josephson CD, Kosmetatos N, Higgins M, Moore JE. Feeding preterm infants during red blood cell transfusion is associated with a decline in postprandial mesenteric oxygenation. J Pediatr. 2014;165(3):464–471.e1.
50. Sharma R, Kraemer DF, Torrazza RM, Mai V, Neu J, Shuster JJ, et al. Packed red blood cell transfusion is not associated with increased risk of necrotizing enterocolitis in premature infants. J Perinatol. 2014;34(11):858–62.
51. Neu J, Walker WA. Necrotizing enterocolitis. N Engl J Med. 2011;364(3):255–64.
52. Bhandari V, Bizzarro MJ, Shetty A, Zhong X, Page GP, Zhang H, et al. Familial and genetic susceptibility to major neonatal morbidities in preterm twins. Pediatrics. 2006;117(6):1901–6.
53. Guillet R, Stoll BJ, Cotten CM, Gantz M, McDonald S, Poole WK, et al. Association of H2-blocker therapy and higher incidence of necrotizing enterocolitis in very low birth weight infants. Pediatrics. 2006;117(2):e137–42.
54. La Rosa PS, Warner BB, Zhou Y, Weinstock GM, Sodergren E, Hall-Moore CM, et al. Patterned progression of bacterial populations in the premature infant gut. Proc Natl Acad Sci. 2014;111(34):12522–7.
55. Wang Y, Hoenig JD, Malin KJ, Qamar S, Petrof EO, Sun J, et al. 16S rRNA gene-based analysis of fecal microbiota from preterm infants with and without necrotizing enterocolitis. ISME J. 2009;3(8):944–54.
56. Arboleya S, Sánchez B, Solís G, Fernández N, Suárez M, Hernández-Barranco A, et al. Impact of prematurity and perinatal antibiotics on the developing intestinal microbiota: a functional inference study. Int J Mol Sci. 2016;17(5):649.

57. Arboleya S, Sánchez B, Milani C, Duranti S, Solís G, Fernández N, et al. Intestinal microbiota development in preterm neonates and effect of perinatal antibiotics. J Pediatr. 2015;166(3):538–44.
58. Morowitz MJ, Poroyko V, Caplan M, Alverdy J, Liu DC. Redefining the role of intestinal microbes in the pathogenesis of necrotizing enterocolitis. Pediatrics. 2010;125(4):777–85.
59. Baranowski JR, Claud EC. Necrotizing enterocolitis and the preterm infant microbiome. Adv Exp Med Biol. 2019;1125:25–36.
60. Shah P, Nathan E, Doherty D, Patole S. Prolonged exposure to antibiotics and its associations in extremely preterm neonates - the Western Australian experience. J Matern Fetal Neonatal Med. 2013;26(17):1710–4.
61. Alexander VN, Northrup V, Bizzarro MJ. Antibiotic exposure in the newborn intensive care unit and the risk of necrotizing enterocolitis. J Pediatr. 2011;159(3):392–7.
62. Heida FH, van Zoonen AGJF, Hulscher JBF, te Kiefte BJC, Wessels R, Kooi EMW, et al. A necrotizing enterocolitis-associated gut microbiota is present in the meconium: results of a prospective study. Clin Infect Dis. 2016;62(7):863–70.
63. Reber KM, Nankervis CA, Nowicki PT. Newborn intestinal circulation. Physiology and pathophysiology. Clin Perinatol. 2002;29(1):23–39.
64. Nanthakumar N, Meng D, Goldstein AM, Zhu W, Lu L, Uauy R, et al. The mechanism of excessive intestinal inflammation in necrotizing enterocolitis: an immature innate immune response. PLoS One. 2011;6(3):e17776.
65. Nanthakumar NN, Fusunyan RD, Sanderson I, Walker WA. Inflammation in the developing human intestine: a possible pathophysiologic contribution to necrotizing enterocolitis. Proc Natl Acad Sci U S A. 2000;97(11):6043–8.
66. Deshpande G, Rao S, Patole S. Probiotics for prevention of necrotising enterocolitis in preterm neonates with very low birthweight: a systematic review of randomised controlled trials. Lancet Lond Engl. 2007;369(9573):1614–20.
67. Olsen R, Greisen G, Schroeder M, Brok J. Prophylactic probiotics for preterm infants: a systematic review and meta-analysis of observational studies. Neonatology. 2015;109(2):105–12.
68. Balasubramanian H, Ananthan A, Rao S, Patole S. Probiotics for preterm infants in India - systematic review and meta-analysis of randomized controlled trials. Indian J Pediatr. 2020;87:817–25.
69. Dilli D, Aydin B, Fettah ND, Özyazıcı E, Beken S, Zenciroğlu A, et al. The propre-save study: effects of probiotics and prebiotics alone or combined on necrotizing enterocolitis in very low birth weight infants. J Pediatr. 2015;166(3):545–551.e1.
70. Sharma R, Hudak ML. A clinical perspective of necrotizing enterocolitis: past, present, and future. Clin Perinatol. 2013;40(1):27–51.
71. Srinivasan P, Brandler M, D'Souza A, Millman P, Moreau H. Allergic enterocolitis presenting as recurrent necrotizing enterocolitis in preterm neonates. J Perinatol. 2010;30(6):431–3.
72. Bell MJ, Ternberg JL, Feigin RD, Keating JP, Marshall R, Barton L, et al. Neonatal necrotizing enterocolitis. Therapeutic decisions based upon clinical staging. Ann Surg. 1978;187(1):1–7.
73. Musemeche CA, Kosloske AM, Ricketts RR. Enterostomy in necrotizing enterocolitis: an analysis of techniques and timing of closure. J Pediatr Surg. 1987;22(6):479–83.
74. Weber TR, Tracy TF, Silen ML, Powell MA. Enterostomy and its closure in newborns. Arch Surg Chic Ill 1960. 1995;130(5):534–7.
75. Blakely ML, Tyson JE, Lally KP, McDonald S, Stoll BJ, Stevenson DK, et al. Laparotomy versus peritoneal drainage for necrotizing enterocolitis or isolated intestinal perforation in extremely low birth weight infants: outcomes through 18 months adjusted age. Pediatrics. 2006;117(4):e680–7.
76. Moss RL, Dimmitt RA, Barnhart DC, Sylvester KG, Brown RL, Powell DM, et al. Laparotomy versus peritoneal drainage for necrotizing enterocolitis and perforation. N Engl J Med. 2006;354(21):2225–34.
77. Rees CM, Eaton S, Kiely EM, Wade AM, McHugh K, Pierro A. Peritoneal drainage or laparotomy for neonatal bowel perforation? A randomized controlled trial. Ann Surg. 2008;248(1):44–51.

78. Guner YS, Friedlich P, Wee CP, Dorey F, Camerini V, Upperman JS. State-based analysis of necrotizing enterocolitis outcomes. J Surg Res. 2009;157(1):21–9.
79. Abdullah F, Zhang Y, Camp M, Mukherjee D, Gabre-Kidan A, Colombani PM, et al. Necrotizing enterocolitis in 20,822 infants: analysis of medical and surgical treatments. Clin Pediatr (Phila). 2010;49(2):166–71.
80. Wadhawan R, Oh W, Hintz SR, Blakely ML, Das A, Bell EF, et al. Neurodevelopmental outcomes of extremely low birth weight infants with spontaneous intestinal perforation or surgical necrotizing enterocolitis. J Perinatol. 2014;34(1):64–70.

Chapter 65
Persistent Pulmonary Hypertension of the Newborn

Fernando de Freitas Martins

Abbreviation List

AA	Arachidonic Acid
cAMP	Cyclic Adenosine Monophosphate
CDH	Congenital Diaphragmatic Hernia
cGMP	Cyclic Guanosine Monophosphate
COX-1	Cyclooxygenase 1
DA	Ductus Arteriosus
ECMO	Extracorporeal Membrane Oxygenation
ET-1	Endothelin
FiO2	Inspired Oxygen Fraction
FP	Foramen Ovale
HFV	High-frequency Ventilation
HRF	Hypoxic Respiratory Failure
iNO	Inhaled Nitric Oxide
LV	Left Ventricle
MAP	Mean Airway Pressure
MAS	Meconium Aspiration Syndrome
MLCK	Myosin Light Chain Kinase
NO	Nitric Oxide
NOS	Nitric Oxide Synthase
O_2	Oxygen
OI	Oxygenation Index
$PaCO_2$	Partial Arterial Carbon Dioxide Pressure
PaO_2	Partial Arterial Oxygen Pressure

F. de Freitas Martins (✉)
Neonatology Department, Fernandes Figueira Institute, Oswaldo Cruz Foundation, Neonatal Intensive Care Unit, Perinatal Clinic, Rio de Janeiro, RJ, Brazil
e-mail: fernando@perinatal.com.br

© Springer Nature Switzerland AG 2022

R. A. Moreira de Sá, E. B. d. Fonseca (eds.), *Perinatology*,
https://doi.org/10.1007/978-3-030-83434-0_65

PDE3	Phosphodiesterase 3
PDE5	Phosphodiesterase 5
PEEP	Pulmonary End Expiratory Pressure
PGE_1	Prostaglandin E1
PGI_2	Prostacyclin , Prostaglandin I2
PGIS	Prostacyclin Synthase
PHT	Pulmonary Hypertension
PPAR- γ	Peroxisome Proliferator-activated Receptor-γ
PPHN	Persistent Pulmonary Hypertension of the Newborn
PVR	Pulmonary Vascular Resistance
RDS	Respiratory Distress Syndrome
rhSOD	Recombinant Human Superoxide Dismutase
ROCK	RhoA-RhoKinase
ROS	Reactive Oxygen Species
RV	Right Ventricle
sGC	Soluble Guanylate Cyclase
SOD	Superoxide Dismutase
SVR	Systemic Vascular Resistance
TR	Tricuspid Regurgitation
TTN	Transient Tachypnea of Newborn
V/Q	Ventilation /Perfusion
VOCC	Voltage Operated Calcium Channels

Persistent pulmonary hypertension of the newborn (PPHN) is one of the most challenging acute disorders of postnatal transition and is related to substantial morbidity and mortality. PPHN occurs when pulmonary vascular resistance (PVR) fails to decrease after birth, remaining abnormally elevated. This leads to severe hypoxemia due to right-to-left extra pulmonary shunting of blood through fetal circulatory pathways: Foramen Ovale (FO) and Ductus Arteriosus (DA). This condition was first recognized in the late 1960s and because of the fetal pattern of right-to-left shunting was previously called persistent fetal circulation [1, 2].

Prevalence of PPHN has been estimated between 0.4 and 6.8 per 1000 live births [3] in developed countries with mortality rate of ~10% [4, 5]. Perinatal asphyxia, meconium aspiration syndrome (MAS), and sepsis account for the majority of cases. Occasionally, PPHN occurs as the primary diagnosis with no other identifiable underlying pathology. Improved obstetric care has considerably reduced the incidence of these perinatal pathologies but PPHN continues to be an important clinical problem, accounting for up to 4% of all admissions in tertiary neonatal units [6]. Mortality and morbidity rates are related to the severity of hypoxemia, treatment response and associated diseases [7].

The transition from fetal to neonatal cardiopulmonary circulation is a complex process that involves both cellular and hemodynamic mechanisms. A comprehensive knowledge of these physiologic concepts is important to better define diagnostic and therapeutic strategies.

Physiology Concepts

- Pulmonary Vascular Resistance (PVR): Resistance to pulmonary blood flow determined by pulmonary vascular tone.
- Systemic Vascular Resistance (SVR): Resistance to systemic blood flow determined by systemic vascular tone.
- Afterload: Pressure that the heart must work against to eject blood during systole.
- Preload: Preload is the amount of sarcomere stretch experienced by cardiomyocytes, at the end of ventricular filling during diastole. Indirectly represents the blood volume coming to a cardiac chamber.
- Vascular tone: Degree of constriction experienced by a blood vessel.
- Pulmonary hypertension (PHT): Cardiopulmonary disorder characterized by elevated mean pulmonary artery pressure (mPAP) and prolonged exposure of the right ventricle (RV) to high afterload. Physiologically, mPAP is directly related to pulmonary blood flow (PBF), PVR, and pulmonary capillary wedge pressure (PCWP) by the equation:

$$\mathrm{mPAP} = \left(\mathrm{PBF} \times \mathrm{PVR}\right) + \mathrm{PCWP}$$

- Although PHT may result from high PBF (e.g., large left-to-right shunts, severe chronic anemia) or rise in PCWP (e.g., left ventricular dysfunction), the vast majority of cases are secondary to high PVR. In neonates, PHT is almost always secondary to dysregulation of PVR. The usual presentation is in the immediate postnatal period as acute pulmonary hypertensive crises, and is referred to as PPHN.

Classification of PPHN

Based on etiology, PPHN can be classified into seven groups [Fig. 65.1]:

1. *Idiopathic:* No lung disease is present and PVR is increased due to abnormal vascular remodeling leading to pulmonary vasoconstriction. Idiopathic PPHN is caused by impaired pulmonary vascular relaxation in the absence of parenchymal lung disease. Histopathological changes include increased vascular smooth muscle proliferation in the pulmonary blood vessels that extend into intra-acinar arteries. One of the mechanisms of idiopathic PPHN is due to premature closure of the DA in utero, which forces blood through the constricted pulmonary vasculature leading to increased sheer stress and remodeling. Nonsteroidal anti-inflammatory drugs (NSAIDs) [8] and selective serotonin reuptake inhibitors (SSRIs) [9] taken during pregnancy have been associated with PPHN in the offspring. This condition is also called black lung PPHN due to the characteristic appearance on chest X-ray due to lack of lung disease and decreased pulmonary vascularity.

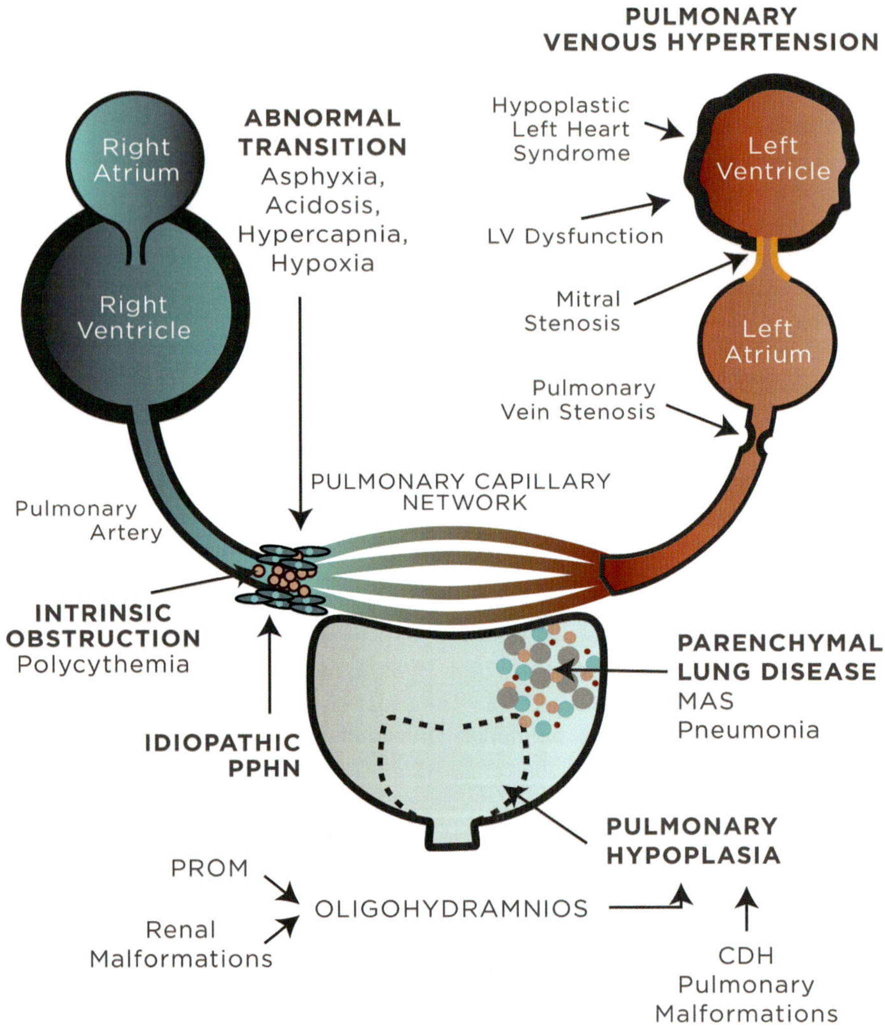

Fig. 65.1 Etiology groups of persistent pulmonary hypertension of newborn (PPHN). PROM Premature rupture of membranes, CDH Congenital diaphragmatic hernia, MAS Meconium aspiration syndrome

2. *Abnormal Transition at Birth:* Perinatal asphyxia, respiratory distress syndrome (RDS), and transient tachypnea of newborn (TTN) may result in impaired pulmonary vasodilation at birth. Abnormal pulmonary transition at birth can lead to hypoxemia, hypercarbia, and metabolic acidosis, all of which cause pulmonary vasoconstriction and increased intra and extra-pulmonary shunting. Decreased lung volume can cause physical constriction of the intrapulmonary blood vessels further impeding pulmonary blood flow. Optimizing lung recruitment to functional residual capacity (FRC) and effective ventila-

tion often lead to reversal of the pathophysiological process associated with these conditions. Preterm infants with severe RDS and infants born by cesarean section without labor experience a slower decrease in PVR compared to term infants born by vaginal delivery.

3. *Parenchymal Disorders:* Sepsis, pneumonia, and MAS cause parenchymal lung disease with variable degrees of chemical pneumonitis, surfactant inactivation, and release of proinflammatory mediators that increase levels of vasoconstrictors such as endothelin and thromboxane. Ventilation–perfusion (V/Q) mismatch associated with these conditions causes hypoxemia, worsening pulmonary vasoconstriction. The decrease in SVR associated with sepsis, combined with exacerbation of PVR due to hypoxemia increase the right to left shunt at the DA and foramen ovale (FO).
4. *Abnormal Lung Development:* Pulmonary hypoplasia due to oligohydramnios secondary to renal anomalies and dysfunction or prolonged rupture of membranes, or congenital diaphragmatic hernia (CDH) and other pulmonary malformations. Pulmonary hypoplasia leads to impaired parenchymal and pulmonary vascular development. In addition, CDH is often associated with abnormalities of cardiac development and function. Left ventricular dysfunction and pulmonary venous hypertension frequently complicate the clinical course in infants with CDH [10].
5. *Intravascular Obstruction:* Polycythemia. The increased blood viscosity secondary to polycythemia is responsible to difficult, decreased pulmonary flow and secondary hypoxia.
6. *Pulmonary Hypertension in the Initial Phase of RDS.* Extremely premature infants are at risk of PHT and hypoxic respiratory failure (HRF) in the first few days of postnatal life. The fetal PVR is high during the canalicular stage of pulmonary development. Due to paucity of pulmonary vascular network the cross-sectional area of the immature pulmonary vascular bed is reduced. Pulmonary vasculature at mid-gestation is less responsive to oxygen mediated pulmonary vasodilation. These infants typically respond poorly to inhaled pulmonary vasodilators such as Inhaled Nitric Oxide (iNO) [11, 12].
7. *Pulmonary Venous Hypertension.* Secondary to conditions present with HRF and that can be clinically indistinguishable from pulmonary arterial hypertension.[13] The chest X-ray appearance shows increased pulmonary vascularity and fluid congestion. The decrease in pulmonary blood flow is due to backpressure from impaired venous drainage into the left atrium. Left-sided obstructive congenital heart disease (mitral atresia, hypoplastic left heart syndrome, critical coarctation of aorta), total anomalous pulmonary venous connection with obstruction, pulmonary vein stenosis can all present with varying degrees of pulmonary venous hypertension. Left ventricular dysfunction due to asphyxia, sepsis or CDH can also present with pulmonary venous hypertension. The diagnosis depends on echocardiographic evaluation. iNO is contraindicated in these conditions as it increases pulmonary edema and causes deterioration of gas exchange.[14].

Fetal Circulation

The fetus is in a state of physiological PHT. In utero, the fetus receives oxygenated blood from the placenta through the umbilical vein. Oxygenated umbilical venous blood enters the right atrium and is diverted to the left atrium through the FO. Owing to high PVR in the fetus, most of the right ventricular output crosses the DA into the descending aorta, so the organ of gas exchange (placenta) receives approximately 30–45% of combined ventricular cardiac output. The lungs receive between 8% and 21% of the combined ventricular output through the pulmonary arteries. The high PVR in the fetus is maintained by a combination of anatomical, physical, biochemical, and humoral factors. Compression of pulmonary blood vessels by the fluid-filled alveoli, lack of rhythmic distension of the lungs, and narrowing of the vascular lumen by the cuboidal configuration of the endothelial cells, all play a role in maintaining the elevated PVR in the fetus. Hypoxic pulmonary vasoconstriction is maintained due to the low resting arteriolar and alveolar oxygen tension. Humoral mediators such as endothelin-1 and arachidonic acid metabolites such as leukotrienes and thromboxane and lack of vasodilators such as nitric oxide (NO) and prostacyclin (PGI2) contribute to high PVR. The low placental/systemic vascular resistance in the fetus is maintained by high levels of estrogen, prostaglandins, and NO produced by the placenta [15].

Transitional Circulation

At birth, following initiation of respiration (mechanical distension of the lung, decrease in carbon dioxide tension, and increase in alveolar oxygen tension), PVR drops dramatically leading to an increase in pulmonary blood flow by 8–10-fold, which facilitates the transition to gas exchange by the lungs. SVR increases due to the removal of the placenta from circulation. These changes lead to a progressive decrease and later reversal of shunts at the FO and DA. Pulmonary endothelial NO, acting via the cyclic guanosine monophosphate (cGMP) pathway, and PGI2, acting through the cyclic adenosine monophosphate (cAMP) pathway, mediate pulmonary vasodilation following birth [15].

The failure of this normal physiological pulmonary transition leads to the syndrome of PPHN often manifesting as HRF.

Cellular Biochemical Physiology

Several cellular pathways involved in regulation of pulmonary vascular tone have been identified over the last two decades [16]. It is important for clinicians to be aware of these pathways, which modulate pathophysiological progression, clinical impact and therapeutic strategies.

- *Nitric Oxide/Cyclic Guanosine Monophosphate (NO/cGMP) Pathway*: NO is synthesized by endothelial nitric oxide synthase (NOS) from the terminal nitrogen of L-arginine, diffuses toward the smooth muscle cell where it stimulates soluble guanylate cyclase (sGC) to increase intracellular cGMP. The mechanism whereby increased cGMP regulates pulmonary vascular tone includes activation of K+ channels, causing smooth muscle cell membrane hyperpolarization and inactivation of voltage-operated calcium channels (VOCC). Closure of VOCC causes a decrease in cytosolic Ca++ concentration and vasorelaxation. Intracellular concentration of cGMP is downregulated by phosphodiesterase 5 (PDE5) activity. Inhibition of this enzyme by drugs like Sildenafil causes vasodilation [Fig. 65.2] [17, 18]..
- *Prostacyclin/Cyclic Adenosine Monophosphate (PGI_2/cAMP) Pathway:* Prostacyclin is synthetized in endothelial cell by cyclooxygenase 1 (COX-1) and Prostacyclin Synthase (PGIS) from Arachidonic Acid (AA). Both COX-1 and COX-2 are found in the lung, but COX-1 in particular is upregulated during late gestation. This upregulation leads to an increase in PGI_2 production in late gestation and early postnatal life. In the smooth muscle cell PGI_2, through PGI_2 receptor (IP), stimulates adenylate cyclase to increase intracellular cAMP levels, which similar to cGMP, leads to vasorelaxation through a decrease in intracellular calcium concentrations [19]. Intracellular concentration of cAMP is downregulated by phosphodiesterase 3 (PDE3) activity. Inhibition of this enzyme with drugs like milrinone causes vasodilation [Fig. 65.2].
- *Endothelin (ET-1) Pathway:* ET-1 acts on ET-A receptors in the smooth muscle cell and increases ionic calcium concentration leading to intense vasoconstriction. A second endothelin receptor (ET-B) on the endothelial cell stimulates NO release and vasodilation. Bosentan is a competitive antagonist of ET-1 at the ET-A and ET-B receptors, but exerts a greater effect on ET-A receptors, causing a total decrease in pulmonary vascular resistance [Fig. 65.3] [20].
- *RhoA-RhoKinase (ROCK) Pathway:* Increased ROCK activity leads to phosphorylation of Myosin Light Chain Kinase (MLCK), which in turns causes increases in intracellular calcium and causes vascular contraction. The ROCK Pathway plays an important role in hypoxic pulmonary vasoconstriction and as a mediator of the impaired angiogenesis and increased contractility associated with chronic fetal pulmonary hypertension [6].
- *Superoxide Dismutase (SOD) Pathway:* NO is a free radical and avidly combines with superoxide anions to form a toxic vasoconstrictor, peroxynitrite. The bioavailability of NO in a tissue is determined by the local concentration of superoxide anions. Hyperoxic ventilation can increase the risk of formation of superoxide anions in the pulmonary arterial smooth muscle cells and limit the bioavailability of NO. [21].

Hemodynamic Physiology

High PVR is the hallmark pathophysiological feature in PPHN, irrespective of the underlying etiology. Hemodynamic and clinical consequences may be similar between patients, however the variability in phenotypic presentation depends on the

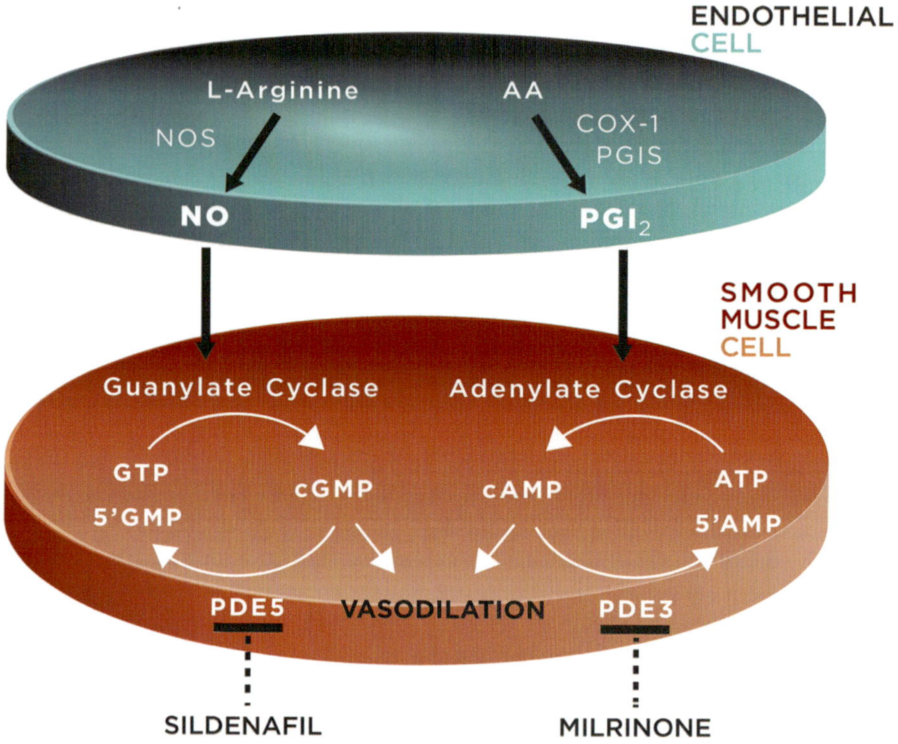

Fig. 65.2 Nitric oxide (NO) and prostacyclin (PGI_2) pathways. In the vascular endothelium, NO is synthesized by NO synthase (NOS) from the terminal nitrogen of L-arginine and cyclooxygenase (COX-1) and prostacyclin synthase (PGIS) synthesize PGI_2 from arachidonic acid (AA). Once in vascular smooth muscle cells NO stimulates soluble guanylate cyclase (sGC) to increase intracellular cGMP and PGI_2 stimulates adenylate cyclase which increases intracellular cAMP. Both cGMP and cAMP indirectly decrease free cytosolic calcium, resulting in smooth muscle relaxation. Phosphodiesterases (PDE) 3 and 5 hydrolyze respectively cAMP and cGMP, regulating the intensity and duration of their vascular effects. Inhibition of these PDE with such agents as Sildenafil and Milrinone may enhance pulmonary vasodilation

presence or absence of fetal shunts and the ability of the myocardium to adapt to alterations in cardiac loading conditions. In many patients, the consequences may include a vicious cycle of reduced pulmonary blood flow (PBF), hypoxemia, acidosis, ventilation–perfusion mismatch, and cardiac dysfunction. The type and severity of secondary hemodynamic disturbances may vary among patients depending upon the severity and duration of the increased PVR as well as underlying etiology.

Significant pulmonary vasoconstriction, even in the absence of other secondary hemodynamic alterations, causes severe ventilation–perfusion mismatch leading to the clinical picture of HRF. This may be aggravated by inability of the immature neonatal right ventricle (RV) to compensate for the increased afterload, leading to further decrements in pulmonary blood flow. RV dysfunction may lead to worsening of hypoxemia and acidosis, which potentiates pulmonary vasoconstriction and

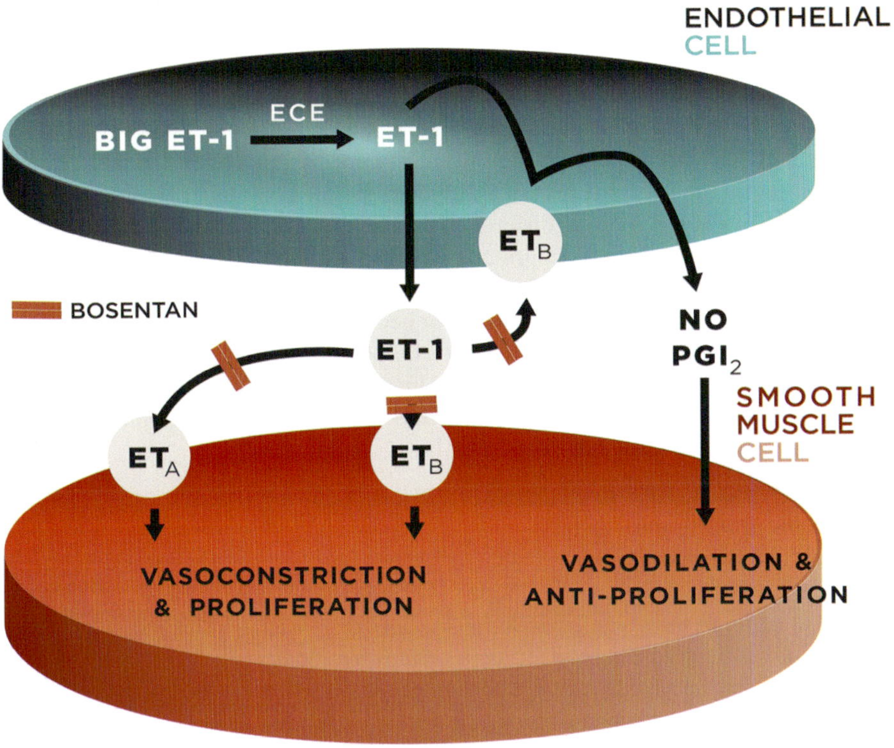

Fig. 65.3 Endothelin (ET-1) pathway. Big ET-1 is cleaved to ET-1 by endothelin-converting enzyme (ECE) in endothelial cells. ET- 1 binds its specific receptors ETA and ETB with differential effects. On smooth muscle cells, binding of ET-1 to ETA or ETB leads to vasoconstrictive and proliferative effects. ETB are transiently expressed on endothelial cells after birth; binding of ET-1 to ETB on endothelial cells leads to downregulation of ECE activity and increased production of Nitric Oxide (NO) and Prostacyclin (PGI2), leading to vasodilation and antiproliferation. Bosentan blocks ET-1 binding to ETA and ETB receptors causing vasodilation and antiproliferative effect

blunts the effect of pulmonary vasodilator therapies. Elevated PVR and the consequent decreased pulmonary blood flow causes low left ventricular preload, forcing the left ventricle (LV) to compensate by increasing its contractility and heart rate in an attempt to maintain LV output. The adequacy of compensation is variable and occurs at an expense of increased myocardial oxygen consumption. RV dilatation may cause leftward deviation of the interventricular septum, thereby reducing the LV filling capacity and compliance. Systolic dysfunction of the RV, by virtue of ventricular–ventricular interaction through shared myocardial fibers between the two ventricles, may adversely affect LV systolic function. Further, non-PVR-related factors might also contribute to the myocardial dysfunction. These factors include the underlying etiology (e.g., sepsis, perinatal asphyxia), systemic hypovolemia, invasive ventilation with high mean airway pressure (MAP), and medications (e.g., pulmonary vasoconstriction from high-dose epinephrine and dopamine, low preload secondary to systemic vasodilatation from milrinone) [6] [Fig. 65.4].

Clinical Presentation

PPHN presents with varying degrees of HRF. Distinguishing between PPHN and cyanotic heart lesions at bedside sometime is challenging, but is essential since management for these disorders are quite different. A complete, detailed clinical investigation for the identification of risk factors [Table 65.1] and a thorough physical examination could help to differentiate both diagnoses [Table 65.2] before a cardiology performed echocardiogram is possible.

Timely echocardiographic evaluation, to rule out a critical cyanotic congenital heart defect [22], is of critical importance for neonates suspected to have PPHN. The possibility of a duct-dependent pulmonary blood flow disorder should be considered in all neonates presenting with HRF during the neonatal period, particularly when symptoms fail to resolve after resuscitation and standard treatment.

Clinical signs suggestive of congenital heart defect:

- Absence of suggestive risk factors for PPHN
- No signs of respiratory distress
- Presence of heart murmur
- Reduced femoral pulse
- Abnormal heart image on chest X-ray
- Blood pressure gradient between upper and lower body
- Lack of response to high oxygen concentrations (Hyperoxia Test)
- No effect or deterioration after exposure to nitric oxide

The characteristic findings of PPHN are labile hypoxemia and pre–post-ductal saturation gradient (manifested clinically as differential cyanosis). Infants with PPHN have wide swings in arterial oxygen saturation levels due to acute changes in pulmonary blood flow and right-to-left shunt associated with episodic changes in PVR in response to minimal stimulation. A pre- to post-ductal gradient of greater than 10% is common in infants with PPHN. Physical examination findings are often minimal with a loud second heart sound and systolic murmur of tricuspid regurgitation (TR). A chest X-ray is often helpful to diagnose the underlying cause and to assess response to changes with ventilator therapy.

Echocardiography

Echocardiogram is the gold standard exam used to confirm the diagnosis of PPHN. It is also useful to monitor disease progression and response to therapies. It is a simple, noninvasive, bedside test, which can be performed even in the most unstable patient. Echocardiographic definition of PPHN in neonates is based on findings consistent with supra-systemic pulmonary pressure. Peak systolic RV pressure calculated from measured peak velocity of tricuspid regurgitant jet, presence of pure

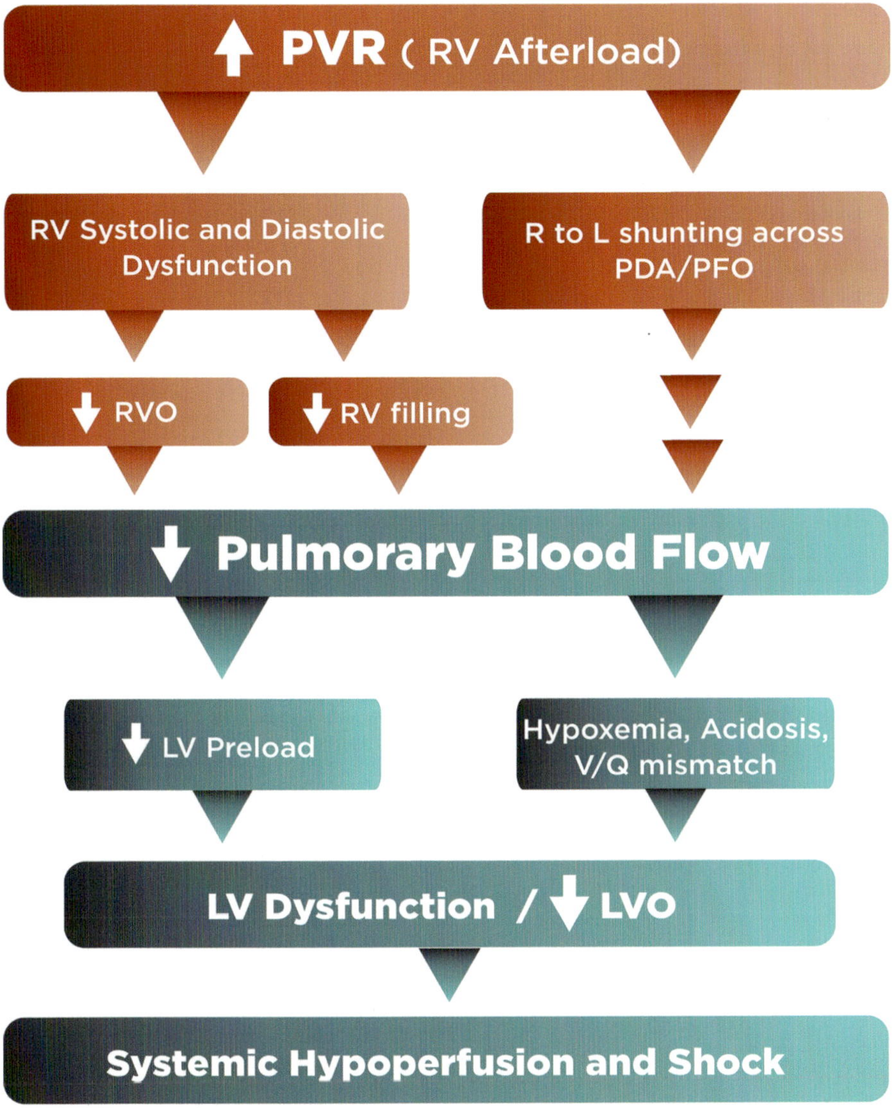

Fig. 65.4 Hemodynamic pathophysiology in neonates with persistent pulmonary hypertension. High PVR may causes a sequence of circulatory alternations of varying degree of severity where decreased pulmonary perfusion results in V/Q mismatch and hypoxemia that leads to cardiac dysfunction, systemic hypoperfusion and shock. Despite the possible benefit that the right-to-left shunt across PDA may cause offloading the pulmonary circulation, preventing RV failure, and maintaining systemic perfusion. It can also augment hypoxemia by reducing pulmonary blood flow. PVR: Pulmonary vascular resistance; RV Right ventricle, R to L Right to left, PDA Patent ductus arteriosus, PFO Patent foramen ovale, RVO Right ventricle output, LV Left ventricle, V/Q Ventilation/perfusion, LVO Left ventricle output

Table 65.1 Risk factors for pulmonary hypertension in term and preterm infants

Term and late preterm infants	Preterm infants
Meconium-stained amniotic fluid Cesarean section Chorioamnionitis Maternal obesity, diabetes, asthma Perinatal infection/asphyxia Hypothermia Hypocalcemia, acidosis Polycythemia Pain, stress Trisomy 21 Antenatal exposure to drugs (serotonin reuptake inhibitors, cyclooxygenase inhibitors) Male gender African or Asian maternal ethnicity	Chorioamnionitis Sepsis Prolonged rupture of membranes Oligo(an)hydramnios Lower gestational age/birth weight Small for gestational age Severe bronchopulmonary dysplasia Prolonged invasive respiratory support

Table 65.2 Differential diagnosis of hypoxemia in newborn infants

	PPHN	Cyanotic CHD	Lung disease without PPHN
History	Negative or presence of risk factors	Antenatal diagnosis	Fetal distress, maternal infection
Respiratory distress	Present	Usually absent	Present
Oxygen saturation	Labile saturations/ pre–post-ductal difference	Fixed low saturations, minimal response to oxygen	Improves with oxygen
Hyperoxia test	$PaO_2 > 100$ mmHg	$PaO_2 < 100$ mmHg	$PaO_2 > 150$ mmHg
$PaCO_2$	Often elevated	Normal/low	Elevated
Hyperventilation/ hyperoxia	PaO_2 improves with hyperventilation	$PaO_2 < 100$ mmHg	$PaO_2 > 150$ mmHg
Chest X-ray	Decreased vascular markings	Abnormal cardiac image and pulmonary vascularity	Abnormal
Echocardiogram	Normal anatomy	Structural cardiac abnormalities	Normal anatomy

CHD Congenital Heart Disease, *PaO2* Partial Pressure of Arterial Oxygen

right-to-left shunt at the ductal or atrial level, and paradoxical interventricular septal motion at end-systole are echocardiographic parameters most frequently associated with PPHN. The RV systolic pressure can be estimated using the modified Bernoulli equation as $4v^2$ + right atrial pressure, where v = maximal velocity of the TR jet in m/s. Changes in pulmonary arterial pressure, myocardial function, and blood flow patterns across the ductus and FO can be monitored over time by echocardiography. Echocardiograms can assess response to therapy in infants with PPHN [23, 24].

Figure 65.5 presents the main echocardiographic findings used to diagnose and monitor PPHN treatment. A detailed description of the application of echocardiography in the assessment and management of PPHN is found in Boode WP et al. [25]

Assessment of Severity of HRF and Monitoring Response to Therapy

Besides the echocardiogram markers of PHT, there are some clinical indexes used to evaluate infants with PPHN/HRF. These indexes express the relationship between disease severity and oxygenation. They are based on the difference between the amount of respiratory support/oxygen offer and the level of blood oxygenation.

1. *Oxygenation index (OI)*: $FiO_2 \times MAP \times 100/PaO_2$

Severity of HRF based on OI:

- Mild: ≤ 15
- Moderate: 15 to ≤ 25
- Severe: 25 to ≤ 40
- Very severe: >40

2. *Alveolar–arterial oxygen gradient (A–a gradient or A–aDO₂)*: This estimates the partial pressure gradient of oxygen from the alveolus to the aorta.

$$\text{A} \quad \text{aDO2} = \left(\text{FiO2 x}\left(\text{Barometric Pressure} \quad \text{Water Vapor Pressure}\right) \quad \text{PaCO2 / R}\right)) \quad \text{PaO2}$$

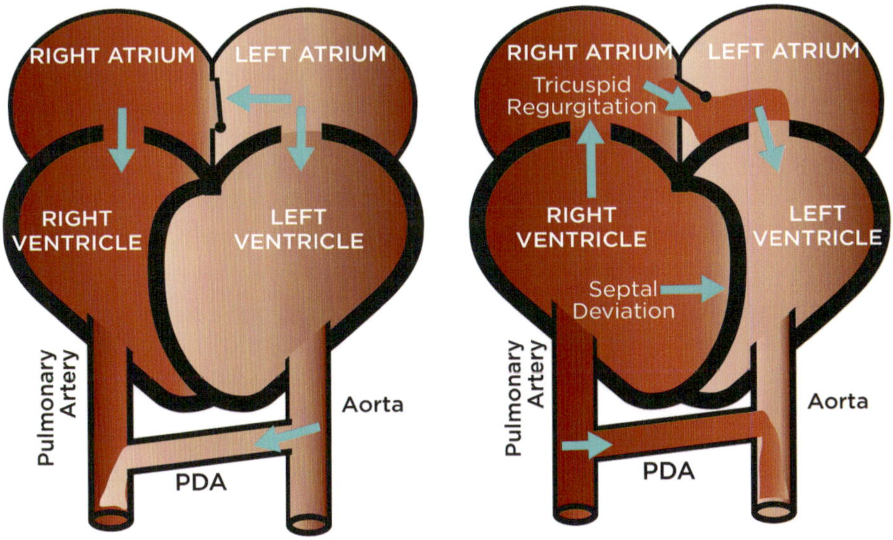

Fig. 65.5 Echocardiographic findings in infants in normal transitional circulation (left) and in PPHN (right). In normal transitional circulation the higher pressures/volume in the left heart chambers determines left to right flow at FO and at PDA. In PPHN patients, due to the increased PVR, pressures in the right atrium and ventricle remain elevated causing right to left shunt at FO and at PDA. Right ventricle increased pressure/volume causes tricuspid regurgitation and interventricular septum bulging to the left decreasing left ventricle volume

Where barometric vapor pressure at sea level is 760 mmHg; water vapor pressure at 37 degrees Celsius is 47 mmHg; R is the respiratory quotient ($R = 1$, in an infant receiving exclusive intravenous dextrose and approximately 0.8 when on mixed diet).

The normal $A\text{–}aDO_2$ is 4–20 mm of Hg.

3. *P/F ratio:* Is the ratio of PaO_2 (mmHg) to FiO_2:

Severity assessment based on P/F ratio:

- Mild: > 200 to ≤300
- Moderate: > 100 to ≤200
- Severe: < 100 mmHg

4. *Oxygen saturation index (OSI):* All of the above indices require arterial blood gas for evaluation and hence the need for arterial access. OSI is a noninvasive index of gas exchange and is calculated as follows:

   $OSI = MAP \times FiO_2 \times 100/\text{Preductal } SpO_2$

   OSI has been shown to correlate well in infants with HRF, $OI \approx 2 \times OS$ [15]

PPHN Treatment

The goals of therapy in PPHN are to improve oxygenation, to provide adequate oxygen delivery to the tissues and to treat any underlying condition. To achieve these therapeutic objectives we have to promote adequate lung recruitment and pulmonary blood flow while avoiding (minimizing) pulmonary mechanical/inflammatory injuries and hemodynamic instability secondary to treatment.

Therapeutic strategies could be gathered in interventions that aim to (1) establish supportive measures, (2) increase oxygen supply, (3) decrease oxygen demand, (4) facilitate adequate pulmonary gas exchange, (5) induce pulmonary vasodilation.

1. Supportive Measures

After initial clinical stabilization in the delivery room and transportation to the Neonatal Intensive Care Unit according to standard algorithms [26], timely supportive measures are vital in successful management of PPHN. Care should be taken to maintain normothermia and correct metabolic abnormalities, such as hypoglycemia, hypocalcemia, acidosis, and polycythemia. Intravenous nutrition with adequate glucose infusion rate and appropriate calcium and amino acid supplementation should be administered preferably through a central line.

Metabolic or respiratory alkalosis are related to vasodilation but therapeutic strategies like hyperventilation and infusion of alkali that were used in the past should be avoided because of adverse effects on cerebral perfusion and increased risk of sensorineural deafness [3]. On the other hand, acidosis (pH < 7.25) promotes exaggerated hypoxic pulmonary vasoconstriction. Acidosis and elevated lactate are markers of tissue hypoxia and suggestive of inadequate systemic blood flow, as are prolonged capillary filling time, low pulse volume, and systolic hypotension. In the presence of metabolic acidosis therapeutic strategies should focus on improvement on oxygenation and perfusion on the target organs.

2. Increase Oxygen Supply

2.1 Oxygen Therapy

Providing adequate oxygenation forms the mainstay of PPHN therapy. However, the target oxygen concentration ideal for optimizing outcomes for neonates with PPHN is not established. Although oxygen is the best pulmonary vasodilator for treatment in PPHN, conversely hyperoxemia can also occur if too much oxygen is given, leading to increased oxidative stress and reactive oxygen species (ROS) formation, enhancing vasoconstrictive effects in the pathogenesis of PPHN [27, 28]. Given the current state of evidence, avoidance of both hypoxia and hyperoxia, and maintenance of oxygen levels within physiologically normal range (PaO_2 between 60 and 100 mmHg, oxygen saturation 90–97%) appear to be the safest and most appropriate clinical approaches in neonates with PPHN [6, 29].

2.2 Surfactant Therapy

Surfactant deficiency or inactivation is commonly observed in diseases associated to PPHN. Administration of exogenous surfactant may be useful to improve oxygenation in diseases with significant parenchymal lung disease like MAS, pneumonia, and sepsis. A study of surfactant lung lavage in MAS patients showed an improvement in oxygenation, a decrease in MAP, and oxygen gradient between alveoli and arteries; however, it did not improve the duration of mechanical ventilation, use of iNO, length of hospitalization, or overall complications [30].

2.3 Optimize Hemodynamics

Adequate pulmonary and systemic blood circulation is a necessary condition for adequate supply of oxygen to all tissues. Systemic blood pressure is a surrogate marker of adequacy of tissue perfusion. Systemic hemodynamics should be optimized with volume expansion and cardiotonic therapy to support both left and right ventricular function and to enhance systemic O_2 transport.

PPHN is frequently associated with hypotension and low cardiac output, in part because increased RV afterload with interventricular septum deviation toward LV may restrict left ventricular filling and subsequently cause myocardial dysfunction. In infants with PPHN associated with left ventricular dysfunction, the hypoxemic respiratory failure may result from increased left atrial and pulmonary venous pressure, which gives rise to increased pulmonary arterial pressure and causes right-to-left shunting at ductal level but left-to-right shunting at atrial level with little pulmonary vasoconstriction. In such circumstances, pulmonary vasodilators should be used with caution and the treatment must be targeted to improve left ventricular performance and also decrease LV afterload [31].

2.3.1 Volume Expansion

Systemic blood pressure should be maintained at normal values for gestational age. If there is diastolic hypotension and/or poor perfusion indicating hypovolemia, volume replacement with 1–2 fluid boluses of 10–15 ml/kg in 15–30 min of normal saline should be administered. If hypotension persists despite volume replacement, inotropic agents probably are indicated.

2.3.2 Ionotropic Drugs

If hypotension persists despite volume replacement, inotropic agents such as dobutamine or vasopressors such as dopamine or epinephrine are indicated. Dobutamine can cause systemic vasodilation, decreasing SVR, and diastolic arterial pressure which could worse right-to-left shunt. Vasopressors agents are not selective to systemic circulation and may be associated with pulmonary vasoconstriction and elevation of PVR at high doses. Other vasopressors that have the effect of increasing SVR and the potential of decreasing PVR are norepinephrine and vasopressin. Ideally, the choice of drug or combination of drugs to be used in PPHN patients should be guided by the findings of a comprehensive echocardiographic evaluation investigating heart chambers volume, myocadiac function, and interatrial and ductal shunt direction [23, 24].

2.3.3 Systemic Steroids

Hydrocortisone treatment postnatally has been shown to improve oxygenation, increase cGMP levels, and reduce ROS levels in animal studies of PPHN [32]. These data suggest a potential role for hydrocortisone in PPHN. The recommended dosage of hydrocortisone is 1 mg/kg every 8 to 12 hours [33].

3. Decrease Oxygen Demand

3.1 Sedation and Neuromuscular Paralysis

Minimal stimulation, covering eyes and ears and maintaining a low-noise environment are non-pharmacological strategies used to avoid any stimulus that could result in a precipitous drop in oxygen saturations, characteristic of this disease. Agitation may further increase right-to-left shunting, as well as catecholamine release, resulting in increased PVR. If ventilation asynchrony is present despite respiratory support optimization, judicious use of sedation and analgesia with narcotic analgesics, like morphine and fentanyl, is recommended. Fentanyl can have adverse effects such as chest wall rigidity during rapid infusion and rapid onset tachyphylaxis and should be used with caution. The use of benzodiazepines like midazolam should be considered with caution due to the possible hemodynamic (hypotension) and long-term neurologic effects [34]. Some neonatologists induce neuromuscular paralysis in PPHN infants to reduce spontaneous breathing efforts and body movements and facilitate ventilation. Despite the information obtained from a recent survey that muscle relaxation is preferred by around one-fifth of individual neonatologists [35] guidelines have recommended avoiding paralysis in ventilated neonates for reasons such as decreased functional residual capacity and oxygenation, associated tachycardia, increased risk of intraventricular hemorrhage, and of muscle atrophy [36].

4. Facilitate Adequate Pulmonary Gas Exchange/Respiratory Support

Neonates with significant PPHN are expected to require invasive respiratory support. The ventilation strategy should be focused to establish optimal alveolar recruitment and adequate carbon dioxide clearance, while avoiding lung hyperexpansion and the secondary hemodynamic consequences of decreased venous return (RV preload) and increased PVR. Gentle ventilation strategies with optimal PEEP, relatively low peak inflation pressure or tidal volume, and a degree of permissive hypercapnia are recommended to ensure adequate lung expansion while limiting barotrauma and volutrauma. Both lung underinflation and overinflation will lead to elevation of PVR [37]. In newborns with severe lung disease, high-frequency ventilation (HFV) is frequently used to optimize lung inflation and minimize lung injury. Optimal lung expansion is essential for adequate oxygenation as well as the effective delivery of iNO [38].

5. Induce Pulmonary Vasodilation

5.1 Inhaled Nitric Oxide

Since 1999, when it was approved by the FDA for use in near-term and term infants with PPHN, iNO has been the mainstay of PPHN treatment. It causes potent and selective pulmonary vasodilation without decreasing systemic vascular tone. In the intravascular space, it combines with hemoglobin to form methemoglobin, which prevents systemic vasodilation. iNO reduces V/Q mismatch by entering only in ventilated alveoli and redirecting pulmonary blood by dilating adjacent pulmonary arterioles.

Hypoxic near-term and term infants responded to iNO within 30–60 min [39]. iNO also reduces the need for extracorporeal membrane oxygenation (ECMO) in PPHN patients [40]. iNO treatment for PPHN reduces the incidence of death or need for ECMO with a Relative Risk of 0.66 (Confidence Interval 0.57–0.77) [41].

iNO treatment should be initiated at a dose of 20 parts per million (ppm), as it identifies the majority of "responsive" cases and is rarely associated with side effects. Doses higher than 20 ppm have been associated with more adverse effects like methemoglobinemia with no clinical benefits [40]. The indication for treatment with iNO would be an OI 15–25 with echocardiographic evidence of PPHN or a higher OI with or without evidence of right-to-left shunt. Due to rebound vasoconstriction and resultant PHT due to abrupt withdrawal, iNO needs to be weaned gradually [29].

5.2 Phosphodiesterase Inhibitors

5.2.1 Sildenafil

Sildenafil, a highly specific PDE5 inhibitor, has the potential to independently decrease PVR through cGMP-mediated vasodilation pathway and improve oxygenation in infants with PPHN. Systematic reviews of 49 studies concerning the safety of Sildenafil administration revealed no evidence of serious adverse events in infants. Studies have shown that oral Sildenafil (dose range: 1–3 mg/kg every 6 h) improves oxygenation and reduces mortality in centers where iNO is not available. Sildenafil may reduce the rebound PHT noted during iNO weaning [29, 42].

5.2.2) Milrinone

Milrinone is a PDE3 inhibitor and has been shown to decrease pulmonary artery pressure and resistance in infants with PPHN. Also exerts inotropic and vasodilatory properties and improves diastolic performance. The properties of dual "inodilator" effects make it particularly effective in treatment of PPHN with associated LV dysfunction. As with any systemic vasodilator, hypotension is a clinical concern and blood pressure needs to be closely monitored [43, 44].

5.3 Prostaglandins

Prostaglandins activate adenylate cyclase (AC) to increase cAMP concentrations in vascular smooth muscle cells which produces vasodilation through a decrease in intracellular calcium concentration. Two classes of prostaglandin have therapeutic applications for treatment of PPHN: prostacyclin (prostaglandin I_2, PGI_2) and prostaglandin E_1 (PGE_1).

5.3.1 Prostaglandin I_2 (Prostacyclin)

Studies have shown that intravenous or inhaled PGI_2 (iloprost) may be used as a rescue therapy for infants with severe PPHN. However, systemic hypotension may raise some concern in intravenous use. All PGI_2 analogs have the limitation of an extremely short half-life. Inhaled iloprost may be a therapeutic option in newborns with PPHN when iNO and ECMO are not available [31].

5.3.2 Prostaglandin E_1 (Alprostadil)

The prostaglandin PGE_1 (Prostin) is widely used as a continuous intravenous infusion to maintain ductal arteriosus patency in newborns. The possible therapeutic effects in PPHN patients include the pulmonary vasodilator effects of PGE_1 and the beneficial effect that ductal patency offers in providing a pop-off that permits alleviation of increased afterload in the otherwise volume and pressure loaded RV [24, 45]. PGE_1 is also available in inhalation form. A small pilot phase I–II study in PPHN patients demonstrated that inhaled PGE_1 was a safe, selective pulmonary vasodilator in HRF [46].

5.4 Endothelin Receptor Antagonist (Bosentan)

Endothelin-1 (ET-1), which is synthesized by vascular endothelial cell, acts on two kinds of endothelin receptor to cause vasoconstriction. An increased ET-A-mediated vasoconstriction with loss of ET-B-mediated vasodilation may be associated with the pathogenesis of PPHN. Bosentan is a nonselective ET-1 antagonist acting on both ET-A and ET-B receptors with possible benefits of vasodilation and antiproliferation. Studies have found conflicting results in the use of Bosentan in PPNH, especially for those who received iNO. Bosentan should be used as an adjunctive therapy, not first line, in the treatment of PPHN, because the clinical response time for this drug is more than 6 hours after administration. The recommended dosage of Bosentan is 1 to 2 mg/kg twice daily, following pediatric dosing guidelines [47, 48].

6. Emerging Strategies

Novel therapies, targeting intrinsic signaling pathways responsible for vascular regulation behind the pathophysiology of pulmonary vascular disease in infants, are under investigation to treat PPHN. Several approaches have been proposed such as antioxidants, L-citrulline, soluble guanylate cyclase (sGC) activators, Rho-kinase inhibitors, and peroxisome proliferator-activated receptor-γ (PPAR- γ) agonists.

6.1 Antioxidants

An increase ROS such as superoxide and hydrogen peroxide in the smooth muscle and adventitia of pulmonary arteries has been demonstrated in the PPHN lamb model and it may promote vasoconstriction. The administration of recombinant human superoxide dismutase (rhSOD) diminished ROS production and improved endothelial NOS function in fetal lambs and might be useful in the treatment of PPHN [31].

6.2 L-citrulline

To date, evidence reveals that an impaired L-citrulline–L-arginine–Nitric Oxide Pathway is involved in the pathogenesis of chronic hypoxia-induced PHT. Hypoxia may reduce NO production through uncoupling NOS in pulmonary arterial endothelial cells, which results in decreasing NO formation from L-arginine. Application of L-arginine can improve NO signaling and assist vascular regulation. However, oral L-citrulline supplementation is even more effective in increasing serum L-arginine concentrations. Therefore, oral L-citrulline supplementation may be a novel strategy for treatment of PHT associated with chronic hypoxia [31].

6.3 Soluble Guanylate Cyclase Activators

Soluble guanylate cyclase (sGC) involved in NO-cGMP signaling pathway can enhance cGMP-mediated vasodilation effect. Decreased activity of sGC may reduce the cGMP production and contribute to PPHN. When facing with hyperoxic exposure, the sGC becomes oxidized and it may reduce sGC function and impair its ability to produce cGMP-mediated vasodilation. Cinaciguat, a sGC activator, has been shown to improve cGMP production after oxidative stress and ameliorate pulmonary vasodilation in fetal lambs with PPHN. Additionally, a better Cinaciguat improvement of cGMP production is observed under hyperoxic condition, which makes it a promising treatment option for severe PPHN with hyperoxic exposure [31].

6.4 Rho-kinase (ROCK) Inhibitors

Vascular smooth muscle contraction is regulated by cytosolic Ca levels. Elevation of Ca increases formation of the calcium–calmodulin (CaM) complex, and myosin light-chain kinase (MLCK) is activated. MLCK phosphorylates the myosin light chain (MLC), enhancing cross-bridge cycling and inducing vascular smooth muscle contraction. A small GTP-binding protein RhoA increases Rho-kinase (ROCK) activity leading to phosphorylation of MLC and vascular contraction. The RhoA-Rho-kinase pathway plays an important role in hypoxic pulmonary vasoconstriction. RhoA-Rho-kinase is an important mediator of elevated myogenic tone contributing to high PVR in fetal lambs. ROCK inhibition increased left pulmonary artery blood flow and decreased PVR. ROCK inhibitors such as Fasudil may have therapeutic potential in infants with PPHN [45].

6.5 Peroxisome Proliferator-Activated Receptor-γ (PPAR-γ) Agonists

Both ROCK and PPAR-γ regulate smooth muscle cell proliferation and contribute to vascular remodeling in pulmonary hypertension. PPAR-γ is an essential regulator of pulmonary arterial smooth muscle cell proliferation and vascular tone. PPAR-γ agonists produce vasodilation through inhibition of ROCK and there may be a potential role for PPAR-γ agonists in the management of PPHN [45].

Extracorporeal Membrane Oxygenation (ECMO)

ECMO is a supportive measure that essentially gives time for the neonatal heart and lung to recover from the underlying pathology. It is a modified cardiopulmonary bypass used as a rescue therapy in patients with persistent hypoxemia (OI > 40) and hemodynamic instability despite the use of other therapeutic strategies. The association of adequate respiratory and hemodynamic support based on physiologic principles and the use of therapies like HFOV, surfactant, iNO, and other vasodilators, leads to a progressive decline in the use of ECMO for neonatal respiratory disorders.

Follow-Up

The long-term outcomes of infants with PPHN are mainly determined by their underlying diseases and the therapeutic interventions they receive at birth. The management for PPHN, including hyperoxic exposure, prolonged mechanical ventilation, and ECMO, may also adversely affect outcomes. Feeding problems and short-term respiratory morbidities can be seen in 24% of PPHN survivors [49]. Furthermore, in long-term follow up, high risk of neurodevelopmental disabilities ranging from 14% to 46% has been reported, which includes sensorineural hearing loss, cerebral palsy, and delays in either cognitive or motor performance [31].

A recent population-based study have assessed post-discharge mortality and morbidity burden for PPHN patients measured by hospital readmissions during the first year of life in late preterm and term infants with different etiologies and severities of PPHN [50]. After adjusting for gestational age and other demographic variables, investigators have found a more than threefold higher rate of post discharge mortality or hospital readmission in infants with PPHN during the first year of life compared with infants without PPHN. Infants with severe PPHN, CDH, or pulmonary anomalies had the highest readmission rates. However, even infants with only mild PPHN or etiologies that are assumed to be short term, such as MAS, sepsis, or RDS, had a significantly increased hospital readmission rates compared with infants without PPHN.

The morbidity burden found in infants with PPHN diagnosis points indicate that is important to ensure long-term multidisciplinary follow up care for these infants.

Conclusion

PPHN is a serious event affecting both term and preterm infants. In the past 20 years, we have been gathering knowledge about the mechanisms of vascular regulation of the developing pulmonary circulation. This has a positive impact for the therapeutic approaches to neonates with PPHN. In particular, iNO has been proved to be a selective, effective, and safe pulmonary vasodilator. Successful clinical management requires detailed clinical evaluation and judicious care of all aspects of the associated lung and cardiac diseases.

Despite all these important improvements in treatment, PPHN continues to be related to significant short- and long-term morbidities and mortality. Researchers now are focusing on building knowledge about cellular responses in the remodeled pulmonary vasculature. This will likely elucidate additional signaling pathways and lead to new therapeutic strategies.

References

1. Drummond WH. Persistent pulmonary hypertension of the neonate (persistent fetal circulation syndrome). Adv Pediatr Infect Dis. 1983;30:61–91.
2. Gersony WM. Commentary: patent ductus arteriosus and the respiratory distress syndrome--a perspective. J Pediatr. 1977;91(4):624–5. https://doi.org/10.1016/s0022-3476(77)80520-9.
3. Walsh-Sukys MC, Tyson JE, Wright LL, Bauer CR, Korones SB, Stevenson DK, et al. Persistent pulmonary hypertension of the newborn in the era before nitric oxide: practice variation and outcomes. Pediatrics. 2000;105(1 Pt 1):14–20. https://doi.org/10.1542/peds.105.1.14.
4. Lipkin PH, Davidson D, Spivak L, Straube R, Rhines J, Chang CT. Neurodevelopmental and medical outcomes of persistent pulmonary hypertension in term newborns treated with nitric oxide. J Pediatr. 2002;140(3):306–10. https://doi.org/10.1067/mpd.2002.122730.
5. Hosono S, Ohno T, Kimoto H, Shimizu M, Takahashi S, Harada K. Developmental outcomes in persistent pulmonary hypertension treated with nitric oxide therapy. Pediatr Int. 2009;51(1):79–83. https://doi.org/10.1111/j.1442-200X.2008.02664.x.
6. Jain A, McNamara PJ. Persistent pulmonary hypertension of the newborn: advances in diagnosis and treatment. Semin Fetal Neonatal Med. 2015. https://doi.org/10.1016/j.siny.2015.03.001.
7. Bendapudi P, Rao GG, Greenough A. Diagnosis and management of persistent pulmonary hypertension of the newborn. Paediatr Respir Rev. 2015;16(3):157–61. https://doi.org/10.1016/j.prrv.2015.02.001.
8. Alano MA, Ngougmna E, Ostrea EM Jr, Konduri GG. Analysis of nonsteroidal antiinflammatory drugs in meconium and its relation to persistent pulmonary hypertension of the newborn. Pediatrics. 2001;107(3):519–23. https://doi.org/10.1542/peds.107.3.519.
9. Chambers CD, Hernandez-Diaz S, Van Marter LJ, Werler MM, Louik C, Jones KL, et al. Selective serotonin-reuptake inhibitors and risk of persistent pulmonary hypertension of the newborn. N Engl J Med. 2006;354(6):579–87. https://doi.org/10.1056/NEJMoa052744.
10. Chandrasekharan PK, Rawat M, Madappa R, Rothstein DH, Lakshminrusimha S. Congenital diaphragmatic hernia - a review. Matern Health Neonatol Perinatol. 2017;3:6. https://doi.org/10.1186/s40748-017-0045-1.
11. Kumar VH, Hutchison AA, Lakshminrusimha S, Morin FC 3rd, Wynn RJ, Ryan RM. Characteristics of pulmonary hypertension in preterm neonates. J Perinatol. 2007;27(4):214–9. https://doi.org/10.1038/sj.jp.7211673.
12. Chock VY, Van Meurs KP, Hintz SR, Ehrenkranz RA, Lemons JA, Kendrick DE, et al. Inhaled nitric oxide for preterm premature rupture of membranes, oligohydramnios, and pulmonary hypoplasia. Am J Perinatol. 2009;26(4):317–22. https://doi.org/10.1055/s-0028-1104743.
13. Holcomb RG, Tyson RW, Ivy DD, Abman SH, Kinsella JP. Congenital pulmonary venous stenosis presenting as persistent pulmonary hypertension of the newborn. Pediatr Pulmonol. 1999;28(4):301–6. https://doi.org/10.1002/(sici)1099-0496(199910)28:4<301::aid-ppul10>3.0.co;2-m.

14. Baird JS, Havalad V, Aponte-Patel L, Ravindranath TM, October TW, Starc TJ, et al. Nitric oxide-associated pulmonary edema in children with pulmonary venous hypertension. Pediatr Cardiol. 2013;34(4):817–25. https://doi.org/10.1007/s00246-012-0538-7.
15. Mathew B, Lakshminrusimha S. Persistent pulmonary hypertension in the newborn. Children (Basel). 2017;4(8). https://doi.org/10.3390/children4080063.
16. Gao Y, Raj JU. Regulation of the pulmonary circulation in the fetus and newborn. Physiol Rev. 2010;90(4):1291–335. https://doi.org/10.1152/physrev.00032.2009.
17. Storme L, Aubry E, Rakza T, Houeijeh A, Debarge V, Tourneux P, et al. Pathophysiology of persistent pulmonary hypertension of the newborn: impact of the perinatal environment. Arch Cardiovasc Dis. 2013;106(3):169–77. https://doi.org/10.1016/j.acvd.2012.12.005.
18. Steinhorn RH. Neonatal pulmonary hypertension. Pediatr Crit Care Med. 2010;11(2 Suppl):S79–84. https://doi.org/10.1097/PCC.0b013e3181c76cdc.
19. Wedgwood S, Gerard K, Halloran K, Hanhauser A, Monacelli S, Warford C, et al. Intestinal dysbiosis and the developing lung: the role of toll-like receptor 4 in the gut-lung axis. Front Immunol. 2020;11:357. https://doi.org/10.3389/fimmu.2020.00357.
20. Maneenil G, Thatrimontrichai A, Janjindamai W, Dissaneevate S. Effect of bosentan therapy in persistent pulmonary hypertension of the newborn. Pediatr Neonatol. 2018;59(1):58–64. https://doi.org/10.1016/j.pedneo.2017.02.003.
21. Lakshminrusimha S, Saugstad OD. The fetal circulation, pathophysiology of hypoxemic respiratory failure and pulmonary hypertension in neonates, and the role of oxygen therapy. J Perinatol. 2016;36(Suppl 2):S3–S11. https://doi.org/10.1038/jp.2016.43.
22. Weiss DM, Kaiser JR, Swearingen C, Malik S, Sachdeva R. Association of antegrade pulmonary artery diastolic velocity with spontaneous closure of the patent ductus arteriosus in extremely low-birth-weight infants. Am J Perinatol. 2015;32(13):1217–24. https://doi.org/10.1055/s-0035-1554795.
23. Giesinger RE, More K, Odame J, Jain A, Jankov RP, McNamara PJ. Controversies in the identification and management of acute pulmonary hypertension in preterm neonates. Pediatr Res. 2017;82(6):901–14. https://doi.org/10.1038/pr.2017.200.
24. Giesinger RE, McNamara PJ. Hemodynamic instability in the critically ill neonate: an approach to cardiovascular support based on disease pathophysiology. Semin Perinatol. 2016;40(3):174–88. https://doi.org/10.1053/j.semperi.2015.12.005.
25. de Boode WP, Singh Y, Molnar Z, Schubert U, Savoia M, Sehgal A, et al. Application of neonatologist performed echocardiography in the assessment and management of persistent pulmonary hypertension of the newborn. Pediatr Res. 2018;84(Suppl 1):68–77. https://doi.org/10.1038/s41390-018-0082-0.
26. Escobedo MB, Aziz K, Kapadia VS, Lee HC, Niermeyer S, Schmolzer GM, et al. American Heart Association focused update on neonatal resuscitation: an update to the American Heart Association guidelines for cardiopulmonary resuscitation and emergency cardiovascular care. Pediatrics. 2019;2020:145(1). https://doi.org/10.1542/peds.2019-1362.
27. Farrow KN, Groh BS, Schumacker PT, Lakshminrusimha S, Czech L, Gugino SF, et al. Hyperoxia increases phosphodiesterase 5 expression and activity in ovine fetal pulmonary artery smooth muscle cells. Circ Res. 2008;102(2):226–33. https://doi.org/10.1161/CIRCRESAHA.107.161463.
28. Farrow KN, Steinhorn RH. Pulmonary hypertension in premature infants. Sharpening the tools of detection. Am J Respir Crit Care Med. 2015;191(1):12–4. https://doi.org/10.1164/rccm.201411-2112ED.
29. Nair J, Lakshminrusimha S. Update on PPHN: mechanisms and treatment. Semin Perinatol. 2014;38(2):78–91. https://doi.org/10.1053/j.semperi.2013.11.004.
30. Gadzinowski J, Kowalska K, Vidyasagar D. Treatment of MAS with PPHN using combined therapy: SLL, bolus surfactant and iNO. J Perinatol. 2008;28(Suppl 3):S56–66. https://doi.org/10.1038/jp.2008.163.
31. Lai MY, Chu SM, Lakshminrusimha S, Lin HC. Beyond the inhaled nitric oxide in persistent pulmonary hypertension of the newborn. Pediatr Neonatol. 2018;59(1):15–23. https://doi.org/10.1016/j.pedneo.2016.09.011.
32. Perez M, Lakshminrusimha S, Wedgwood S, Czech L, Gugino SF, Russell JA, et al. Hydrocortisone normalizes oxygenation and cGMP regulation in lambs with persistent pulmo-

nary hypertension of the newborn. Am J Physiol Lung Cell Mol Physiol. 2012;302(6):L595–603. https://doi.org/10.1152/ajplung.00145.2011.
33. Peeples ES. An evaluation of hydrocortisone dosing for neonatal refractory hypotension. J Perinatol. 2017;37(8):943–6. https://doi.org/10.1038/jp.2017.68.
34. Ng E, Taddio A, Ohlsson A. Intravenous midazolam infusion for sedation of infants in the neonatal intensive care unit. Cochrane Database Syst Rev. 2003;1:CD002052. https://doi.org/10.1002/14651858.CD002052.
35. Nakwan N, Chaiwiriyawong P. An international survey on persistent pulmonary hypertension of the newborn: a need for an evidence-based management. J Neonatal Perinatal Med. 2016;9(3):243–50. https://doi.org/10.3233/NPM-16915133.
36. Johnson PN, Miller J, Gormley AK. Continuous-infusion neuromuscular blocking agents in critically ill neonates and children. Pharmacotherapy. 2011;31(6):609–20. https://doi.org/10.1592/phco.31.6.609.
37. Wung JT, James LS, Kilchevsky E, James E. Management of infants with severe respiratory failure and persistence of the fetal circulation, without hyperventilation. Pediatrics. 1985;76(4):488–94.
38. Kinsella JP, Abman SH. Clinical approaches to the use of high-frequency oscillatory ventilation in neonatal respiratory failure. J Perinatol. 1996;16(2 Pt 2 Su):S52–5.
39. Finer NN, Barrington KJ. Nitric oxide for respiratory failure in infants born at or near term. Cochrane Database Syst Rev. 2000;2:CD000399. https://doi.org/10.1002/14651858.CD000399.
40. The Neonatal Inhaled Nitric Oxide Study Group (NINOS). Inhaled nitric oxide and hypoxic respiratory failure in infants with congenital diaphragmatic hernia. Pediatrics. 1997;99(6):838–45. https://doi.org/10.1542/peds.99.6.838.
41. Barrington KJ, Finer N, Pennaforte T, Altit G. Nitric oxide for respiratory failure in infants born at or near term. Cochrane Database Syst Rev. 2017;1:CD000399. https://doi.org/10.1002/14651858.CD000399.pub3.
42. Steinhorn RH, Kinsella JP, Pierce C, Butrous G, Dilleen M, Oakes M, et al. Intravenous sildenafil in the treatment of neonates with persistent pulmonary hypertension. J Pediatr. 2009;155(6):841–7. e1. https://doi.org/10.1016/j.jpeds.2009.06.012.
43. James AT, Corcoran JD, McNamara PJ, Franklin O, El-Khuffash AF. The effect of milrinone on right and left ventricular function when used as a rescue therapy for term infants with pulmonary hypertension. Cardiol Young. 2016;26(1):90–9. https://doi.org/10.1017/S1047951114002698.
44. James AT, Bee C, Corcoran JD, McNamara PJ, Franklin O, El-Khuffash AF. Treatment of premature infants with pulmonary hypertension and right ventricular dysfunction with milrinone: a case series. J Perinatol. 2015;35(4):268–73. https://doi.org/10.1038/jp.2014.208.
45. Lakshminrusimha S, Mathew B, Leach CL. Pharmacologic strategies in neonatal pulmonary hypertension other than nitric oxide. Semin Perinatol. 2016;40(3):160–73. https://doi.org/10.1053/j.semperi.2015.12.004.
46. Sood BG, Keszler M, Garg M, Klein JM, Ohls R, Ambalavanan N, et al. Inhaled PGE1 in neonates with hypoxemic respiratory failure: two pilot feasibility randomized clinical trials. Trials. 2014;15:486. https://doi.org/10.1186/1745-6215-15-486.
47. Steinhorn RH, Fineman J, Kusic-Pajic A, Cornelisse P, Gehin M, Nowbakht P, et al. Bosentan as adjunctive therapy for persistent pulmonary hypertension of the newborn: results of the randomized multicenter placebo-controlled exploratory trial. J Pediatr. 2016;177:90–6. e3. https://doi.org/10.1016/j.jpeds.2016.06.078.
48. Nakwan N. The practical challenges of diagnosis and treatment options in persistent pulmonary hypertension of the newborn: a developing country's perspective. Am J Perinatol. 2018;35(14):1366–75. https://doi.org/10.1055/s-0038-1660462.
49. Rosenberg AA, Lee NR, Vaver KN, Werner D, Fashaw L, Hale K, et al. School-age outcomes of newborns treated for persistent pulmonary hypertension. J Perinatol. 2010;30(2):127–34. https://doi.org/10.1038/jp.2009.139.
50. Steurer MA, Baer RJ, Oltman S, Ryckman KK, Feuer SK, Rogers E, et al. Morbidity of persistent pulmonary hypertension of the newborn in the first year of life. J Pediatr. 2019;213:58–65. e4. https://doi.org/10.1016/j.jpeds.2019.06.053.

Chapter 66
Intracranial Hemorrhage

Danielle Negri de Souza Lopes, João Henrique Carvalho Leme de Almeida, and Márcia Cristina de Azevedo Gomes

Background

In the last decades, there was an increase in the survival rates of infants in the edge of viability due to improvement of perinatal and neonatal care. Despite a large number of extremely preterm (less than 28 weeks) that now survive, the overall frequency of the GMH-IVH has declined [1].

Approximately 26% of infants born weighting 501–750 g, and 12% weighting 751–1000 g develop severe forms of hemorrhage [2]. Although most long-term neurocognitive deficits will occur after severe hemorrhage (Grade III and IV), milder bleedings can also lead to some long-term compromise [3, 4].

Perinatal brain injury may lead to significant long-term neurodevelopmental impairment, including cognitive, neurologic, motor, and sensory disability. Perinatal brain injury affects infants born at all gestational ages, but its incidence and morbidity increases with decreasing gestational age [5].

The improvement in neonatal imaging area, cerebral monitoring, and newborn hemodynamics, in association with better knowledge of inflammatory and genetic mechanisms allow us to advance the understanding of premature infants intracranial hemorrhage (ICH). The challenge now is early detection and prevention strategies [6].

D. N. de Souza Lopes (✉)
Neonatology Department, Perinatal Maternity Hospital, Rio de Janeiro, RJ, Brazil
e-mail: daninegri@perinatal.com.br

J. H. C. L. de Almeida
Neonatology Department, Instituto Nacional da Saúde da Mulher, da Criança e do Adolescente Fernandes Figueira, Fundação Oswaldo Cruz, Rio de Janeiro, RJ, Brazil

M. C. de Azevedo Gomes
Clínica Perinatal, Neonatal Intensive Care, Rio de Janeiro, RJ, Brazil

© Springer Nature Switzerland AG 2022

R. A. Moreira de Sá, E. B. d. Fonseca (eds.), *Perinatology*,
https://doi.org/10.1007/978-3-030-83434-0_66

Definition and Classification

Intracranial hemorrhage in the premature infant is an acquired lesion with potential impact on morbidity, mortality, and long-term neurodevelopmental outcome [6]. The GM-IVH hemorrhage is directly related to the immature cerebral structures specially on cellular and vascular proliferation zones of the brain, like germinal matrix.

The hemorrhage can be defined according to the region of the brain:

1. Epidural, subdural, or subarachnoid
2. White matter or cerebellar zone
3. In cerebral ventricles, vessels of subependymal germinal matrix or choroid plexus

The germinal matrix hemorrhage is the most common, and can progress to ventricular bleeding or into periventricular white matter. With maturation, germinal matrix region becomes less prominent, and by term is essentially absent.

The GMH–Intraventricular hemorrhage can be classified in four grades:

Grade I: The hemorrhage is confined to the germinal matrix region
Grade II: The hemorrhage may extend and rupture into the adjacent ventricular system
Grade III: The hemorrhage into the ventricle associated with dilatation
Grade IV: The hemorrhage extends into the white matter

Germinal Matrix–Intraventricular Hemorrhage

Of all types of cerebral hemorrhages, germinal matrix–intraventricular hemorrhage (GM-IVH) is the most common and distinctive pathology diagnosed by cranial ultrasound (CUS) in premature infants [7] (Figs. 66.1, 66.2, and 66.3). The rate and severity are inversely proportional to the gestational age and birth weight [2, 8]. The IVH complications (periventricular hemorrhagic infarct [PVHI], posthemorrhagic

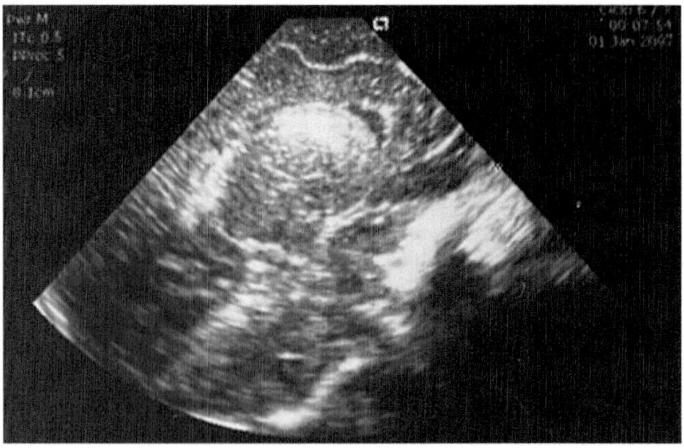

Fig. 66.1 Germinal matrix hemorrhage

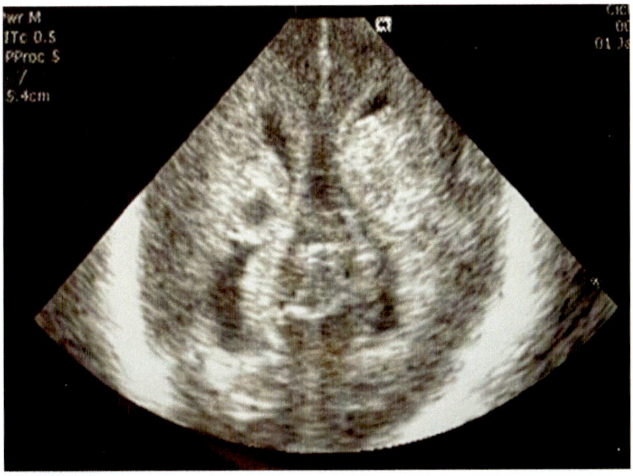

Fig. 66.2 Intraventricular hemorrhage

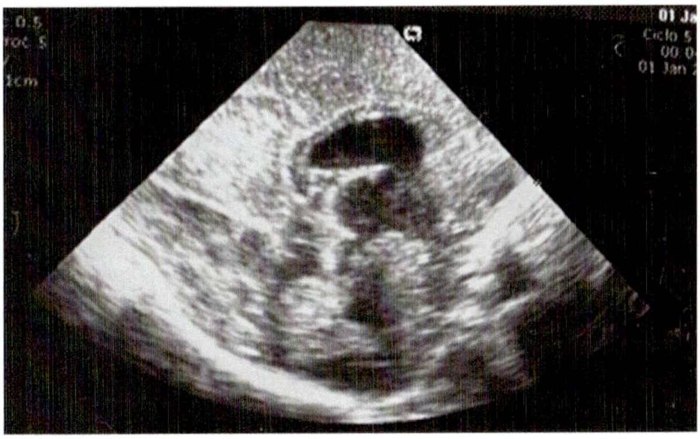

Fig. 66.3 White matter hemorrhage

hydrocephalus [PHH]), the associated cerebellar hemorrhagic injury (CHI), and periventricular leukomalacia (PVL) are critical determinants of neonatal morbidity, mortality, and also long-term neurodevelopmental sequelae [7, 9].

Although advances in perinatal medicine have led to a significant reduction in the overall incidence of GM-IVH in premature infants (i.e., from 50% in the late 1970s to the current 15–25%) [1, 10]. GM-IVH continues to be a significant problem in the neonatal intensive care unit.

GM-IVH in premature infants is typically diagnosed during the first days of life, 50% on the first day, and 90% within the first 4 days. Between 20% and 40% of these infants undergo progression of hemorrhage during NICU stay [7]. GM-IVH is usually clinically asymptomatic and diagnosed by routine screening CUS in 25% to 50% of cases, whereas symptoms in the rest of the cases are manifested by either a subtle and intermittent signs or acute catastrophic presentation [6] (Fig. 66.2).

Mechanisms of the germinal matrix–intraventricular hemorrhage:

1. Vascular anatomic vulnerability of the premature infant
2. Hemodynamic factors- Autoregulation of cerebral blood flow
3. Cytokines and vasoactive angiogenic and growth factors

4. Coagulation and platelet abnormalities
5. Genetic factors

IVH in premature infants arises from fragile capillaries in the subependymal germinal matrix, which are rich in immature vessels and poorly supported by connective tissue. Until its involution between 28 and 36 weeks' gestation, the germinal matrix remains vulnerable to hemorrhage [6]. On top of that, a poor homeostasis and impaired autoregulation has also been described in the preterm infant who is not able to compensate for changes in blood pressure and cerebral blood flow. This situation of a passive-pressure system coupled with varying intrathoracic pressures during respiratory distress syndrome and mechanical ventilation in very sick infants may predispose to IVH [11, 12].

Clinical Manifestations of GMH-IVH

As discussed, many infants are asymptomatic and only diagnosed at routine CUS. In some cases, the diagnosis is difficult as clinical manifestations are not clear or nonspecific, attributable to other prematurity-related conditions. Furthermore, these manifestations can differ in term and preterm newborns.

Postnatal GMH-IVH clinical manifestations in preterm infants can be divided into three groups with three different postnatal presentations [13]:

1. In 25–50% of cases, babies remain asymptomatic. In such cases, this clinically silent GMH-IVH is detected by routine ultrasound screening.
2. The most common presentation can evolve in a few hours to several days. It is characterized by nonspecific findings including an altered level of consciousness, apneas, hypotonia, decreased spontaneous and elicited movements, and subtle changes in eye position and movement.
3. The most severe clinical presentation is also the least common and can evolve over minutes to hours with a catastrophic deteriorated course. In such cases, signs include (a) stupor or coma; (b) irregular breathing pattern, hypoventilation, or even apnea; (c) decerebrate posturing; (d) generalized seizures, especially tonic; (e) flaccid weakness; and (f) cranial nerve abnormalities, including pupils unreactive to light.

Other features include a bulging anterior fontanelle, hypotension, bradycardia, a falling hematocrit, metabolic acidosis, and inappropriate antidiuretic hormone secretion [14].

In recent years, NICUs have incorporated noninvasive bedside methods to monitor brain function, as near infrared spectroscopy (NIRS) and amplitude-integrated EEG (aEEG). NIRS measure cerebral oxygenation and provides a good method to estimate cerebral blood flow, a key component on the physiology of GMH-IVH. Amplitude-integrated EEG can diagnose subclinical seizure activity and help to direct CUS examination.

Manifestations in Term

The origin and location of IVH in term differs from that of preterm infants [15, 16]. They occur in the choroid plexus (35%); thalamus (24%); GM (17%); periventricular cerebral parenchyma (14%) and 10% not determined.

In term infants, the incidence of symptomatic intracranial hemorrhages (epidural, subdural, subarachnoid, intraventricular, and intraparenchymal) is 0.27 to 0.49 per 1000 live births [17, 18] and severe IVH is very uncommon [19].

The term newborn with IVH typically presents focal neurological signs such as epileptic seizures, asymmetry of tone and abnormal movements. In addition, irritability or depressed level of consciousness, apnea, vomiting with dehydration, or a full fontanelle can be a possible clinical presentation.

Best Evidences for Prevention

Antenatal Steroids

The use of antenatal steroids in perinatal medicine is one of the most cost-effective therapies utilized in the last 20 years. It decreases the rate and severity of respiratory distress syndrome, improve survival and decrease the incidence of IVH. Several studies have already demonstrated reductions from 30% to 50% in the incidence and severity of IVH after antenatal steroid administration, even when optimal timing (1–7 days before delivery) is not achieved [20].

Perinatal Centers and Delivery Room Management

There is good evidence to show that birth at perinatal centers prepared for both high-risk mothers and infants is an advantage in terms of survival and may reduce the incidence of IVH [21]. Resuscitation with a well-prepared team is very critical at this moment, where the transition from intrauterine to extrauterine life will require many cardiovascular adaptations, particularly for an extreme low birth infant. Infants will be admitted to NICU, without the need from transport, providing the best of care.

Delayed Cord Clamping

Studies comparing early versus late cord clamping (>30, 45, or 60 seconds) show a reduction in the incidence of intracranial hemorrhage, necrotizing enterocolitis, number of transfusions and neonatal mortality [22–26]. However, the evidence for the effect of late clamping on the population of very low birth weight newborns is not yet fully established. Inder et al. published a study with 148 preterm <32 weeks comparing two periods, before and after late cord clamping, and observed a reduction in the incidence of intracranial hemorrhage [27]. Tarnow-Mordi et al. in a systematic review of the literature and meta-analysis comparing early and late clamping of the umbilical cord in 2834 premature infants <37 weeks demonstrated 30% reduction in the mortality rate. Nevertheless, they found no significant differences in the main major neonatal morbidities and there was no reduction in the incidence of intracranial hemorrhage [27].

Long-Term Development

Outcome of GMH-IVH is directly proportional to the degree and severity of the hemorrhage. Most studies shown that Grade I and II IVH have a good prognosis, not very different from infants without IVH. Grade III and IV are characterized either by ventricular dilatation or bleeding extending to the white matter. Grade III IVH may progress to obstruction, hydrocephaly, and the need for a shunt. This is related to a greater incidence of neurodevelopment impairment. The prevalence of cerebral palsy increases with IVH severity and is seen in 8%, 11%, 19%, and 50% for grades I to IV, respectively [28–30].

Periventricular Leukomalacia

Periventricular leukomalacia is the most common cause of cerebral palsy in premature newborns and cause severe and permanent consequences, with significant social and economic impact. Since its original description by Virchow in 1867, much progress has been made in studies of its causes, now assigned to the specific anatomical features of prematurity compromised by injuries caused by hypotension, hypocarbia, and infection [31].

History

The term periventricular leukomalacia was first described in 1962 by Banker and Larroche referring to a sequence of histological changes in the white matter of premature infants [32]. These changes began with a process of necrosis by coagulation and liquefaction followed by intensive activity of macrophages and resulting in cavitation with formation of cysts 2 weeks after the beginning of the lesion. The possibility of further research arose in 1982 with the discovery that these cysts could be detected by ultrasound [31, 33].

With the technological advancement of imaging diagnostic, it has been shown that the ultrasound findings of leukomalacia have little correlation with the pathological findings and the images detected by MRI [31]. In recent years, greater use of brain MRI findings has shown that, in extremely premature infants, white matter injury is more common, and more diffuse than previously thought. Volpe proposed that this lesion with a diffuse aspect should be called "**Cerebral Leukoencephalopathy**" [34].

Incidence

Like intraventricular hemorrhage, periventricular leukomalacia mainly affects premature infants born less than 32 weeks of gestational age, with a higher incidence the lower the gestational age. White matter changes may not be seen on the initial ultrasound examination and may not be detected until a latter brain ultrasound or MRI scan is performed on the newborn [35]. The periventricular leukomalacia is detected in brain ultrasound at 6 weeks of life in approximately 10% of with very low birth weight newborns [35].

In newborns with less than 28 weeks of gestation that reach term, early imaging exams obtained in the first 2 weeks of life showed the occurrence of grade 3 or 4 intraventricular hemorrhage and periventricular leukomalacia in 9.7% of cases. When brain MRI is used as a follow-up exam between 35 weeks and 42 weeks of corrected postmenstrual age, moderate or severe white matter lesions are detected in 19.3% of cases [36].

According to Younge et al. (2017), the incidence of periventricular leukomalacia in newborns at the limit of viability (between 22 and 24 weeks of gestational age) remained stable at 6–7% between the years 2000 to 2011 [37].

The overall incidence of periventricular leukomalacia in newborns weighing 500 to 1500 grams can vary from 3% to 15%, with most studies using ultrasound to evidence cystic formation [31]. In studies that use brain magnetic resonance as a diagnostic method and that is more sensitive to demonstrate white matter damage, the incidence can reach 20% [38]. About 10% of infants with very low weight develop cerebral palsy and the cause of severe handicap in 90% of cases is periventricular leukomalacia. In addition, 50% of these newborns will evolve with neurocognitive abnormalities that will be recognized at school age and will persist into adulthood, such as mental retardation, specific learning disorders, motor disabilities, and hearing and/or visual impairment.

There are also reports of periventricular leukomalacia occurring not only in late preterm newborns (over 32 weeks of gestational age) but also in full-term newborns. In the latter, periventricular leukomalacia is associated with perinatal asphyxia, complex congenital heart disease, chromosomal abnormalities, and use of oxygenation by an extracorporeal membrane and is manifested with delayed development and a wide spectrum of neurological sequelae, especially the classic spastic diplegia [31].

Physiopathology

The anatomical characteristics of immature brain tissue is an important risk factor for preterm newborns to develop periventricular leukomalacia. Cerebral vessels of white matter are few and still immature before 32 weeks of gestation, with reduced perfusion and therefore predisposed to the occurrence of tissue ischemia [38, 39].

In response to systemic hypotension, premature infants are unable to increase cerebral perfusion in the border areas of the brain where the cerebral vascular network is immature. Therefore, a series of cascading events due to hypoxia and ischemia might result in brain damage On the other hand, infection, presents on about one-third of preterm birth, might worsen the brain injury [35].

The reduced blood flow in the premature white brain substance increase the risk for brain injury as well. Unlike older children and adults in which blood flow remains constant independent of blood pressure, in premature infants the self-regulation does not occur adequately and cerebral circulation becomes susceptible to variations in systemic pressure. Any drop in blood pressure, will be able to cause cell necrosis in the white matter areas.

A similar effect will occur when there is a vasoconstriction caused by hypocarbia [31]. As many premature infants depend on mechanical ventilation in the first weeks of life, hypocarbia associated with the use of this technology has been identified as one of the causes of cystic periventricular leukomalacia [40].

Before 32 weeks of gestational age, most of the oligodendrocytes are in the initial phase of development (90% are preoligodendrocytes) and extremely sensitive to lesions caused by free radicals released by the ischemic process, due to the presence of excessive amount of iron and fragile antioxidant defenses. The excessive concentration of iron that is an oxidizing agent may explain the increased incidence of periventricular leukomalacia after episodes of intraventricular hemorrhage [31]. A late effect of ischemia is the necrosis of axons and neurons, which releases glutamate into the extracellular compartment and causes destruction of preoligodendrocytes and also enhances the action of free radicals [41] (Fig. 66.4).

Chorioamnionitis is associated with preterm deliveries and has been identified as one of the contributing factors to the pathophysiology of periventricular leukomalacia in extremely preterm infants. Its incidence can vary from 66% at 24 weeks of gestation to 16% at 34 weeks and causes a fetal inflammatory response with the production of cytokines. Such substance increases the permeability of the blood–brain barrier and facilitate the inlet of new cytokines and bacterial antigens, activating the microglia and causing destruction of the preoligodendrocytes by free radicals and by the cytokines themselves [31, 42] (Fig. 66.5).

Other maternal and neonatal risk factors have been identified in association with periventricular leukomalacia, such as pre-labor premature rupture of membrane, preeclampsia, hyaline membrane disease, and hyperbilirubinemia. However, the clinical relevance of these factors in the context of this neurological sequela needs to be better understood and, therefore, research are needed [43].

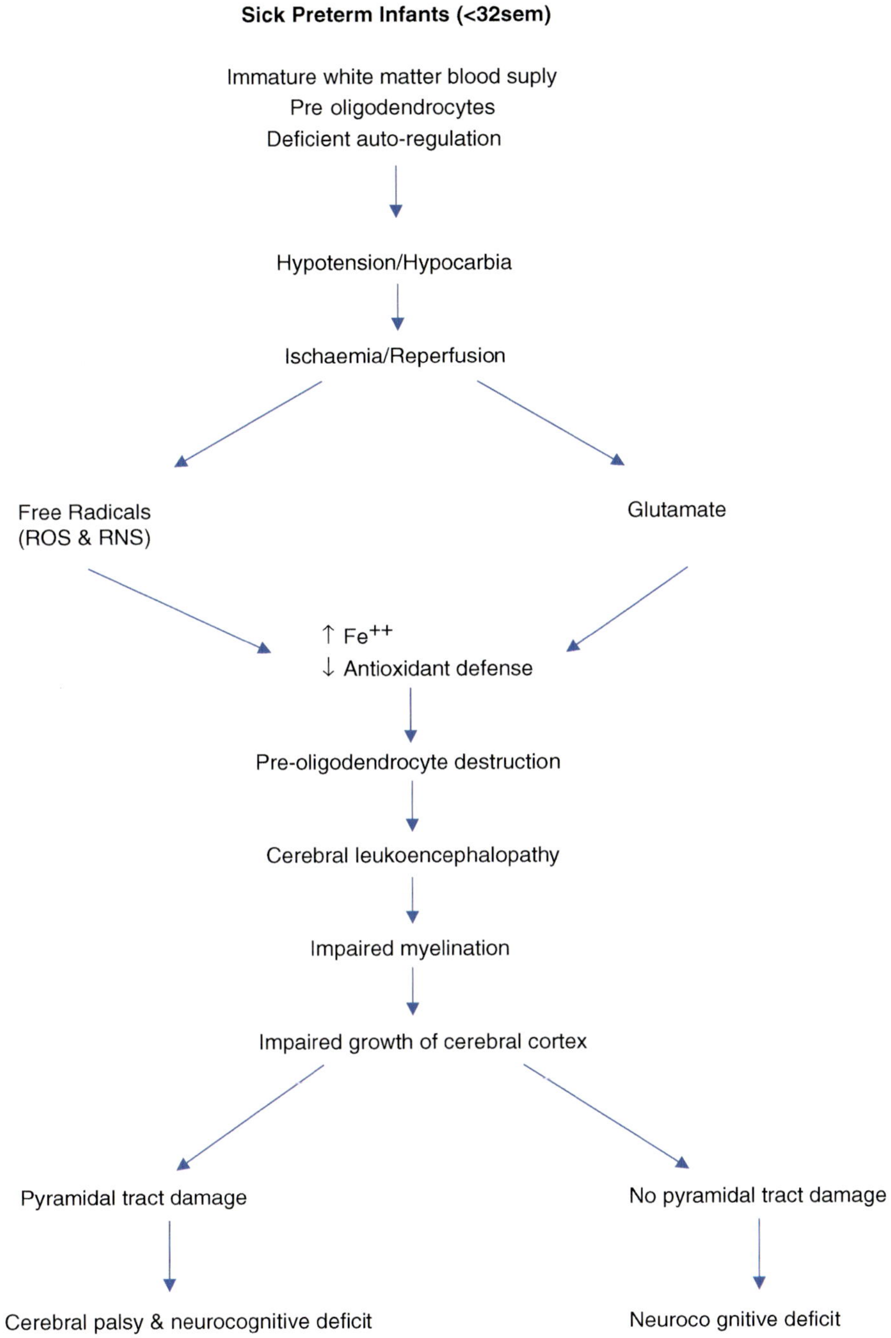

Fig. 66.4 Pathogenesis of cerebral palsy and neurocognitive deficits in the preterm infant

Diagnostic Imaging

After the ischemic insult, changes in the eco-density of the brain tissue may be visible initially between 24 and 48 hours by cerebral ultrasound. In some patients they may be transient and disappear, but in others premature these lesions may persist after 7 days and evolve into periventricular cysts after 18 days (between 10 and 39 days) (Figs. 66.6 and 66.7). The cysts are usually absorbed and disappear 2–3 months after the initial injury. White matter necrosis, atrophy, tissue resorption, and gliosis are often followed by ventriculomegaly, which may be the only

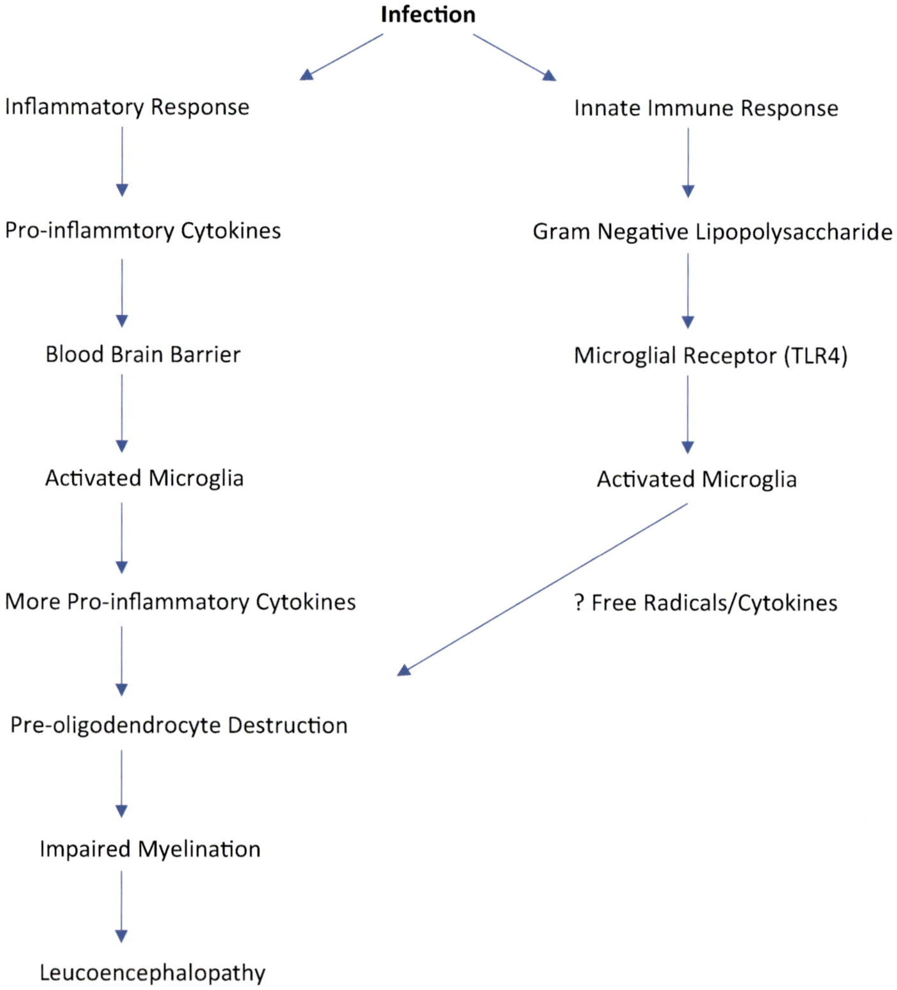

Fig. 66.5 Pathogenesis of infection-induced white matter damage. It is probable that in most infants, infection works in concert with the ischemia/reperfusion pathway

manifestation. The presence of cysts at birth indicates the onset of the ischemic process in the intrauterine environment [31, 44].

The risk of cerebral palsy is influenced by the extent and location of the cystic formation. Large cysts in the occipital–parietal region have the worst prognosis while isolated cysts in the frontal region usually evolve with milder consequences (Fig. 66.8) [45].

The study of the clinical outcomes in premature infants with cysts detected on ultrasound examination shows that 60% develop cerebral palsy mainly involving the medial part of the corticospinal neural cord that innervate the legs, causing the typical cerebral palsy of prematurity called diplegia spastic. The latter is characterized by spasticity of the lower limbs with minimal or absent involvement of the upper limbs [46, 47].

Ultrasound is the established method for the diagnosis of periventricular leukomalacia both in the initial assessment as well as in the follow-up of these lesions in premature newborns. Sequential examinations are recommended for specific diagnosis and normal findings in ultrasound examinations performed at 1 week of life and 1 month after birth exclude the presence of periventricular leukomalacia [43]. The greatest difficulty with ultrasound examination is the inability to detect diffuse changes in white matter, which can occur in many extremely premature infants.

The MRI has shown a good correlation between anatomical abnormalities and functional disabilities, being more effective in demonstrating the extent of the white matter lesion. However, it is a high-cost exam and not as practical as brain ultrasound that can be performed at the bedside [38, 46, 47].

Clinical Outcomes

The extent of the white matter lesion correlates with long-term neurodevelopment-related outcomes. Moderate and severe abnormalities of white matter detected by brain MRI in preterm infants born earlier than 30 weeks are predictive of severe

Fig. 66.6 Cystic leukomalacia

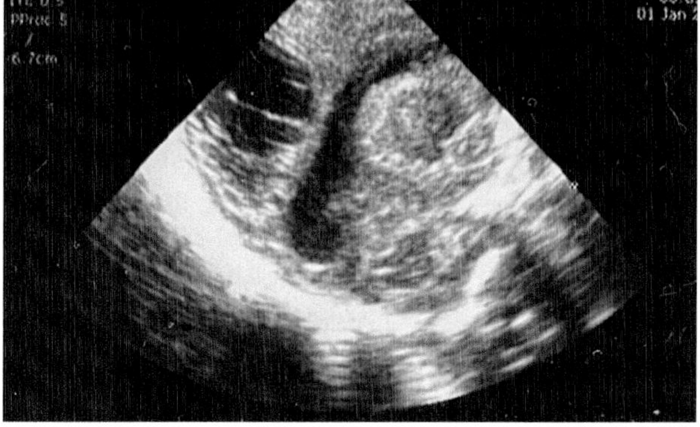

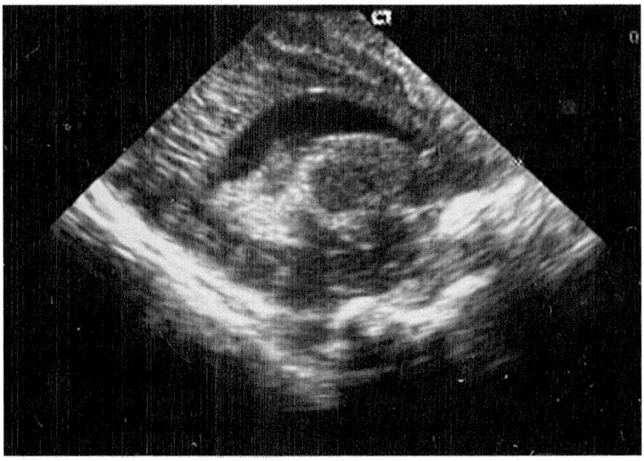

Fig. 66.7 Periventricular leukomalacia

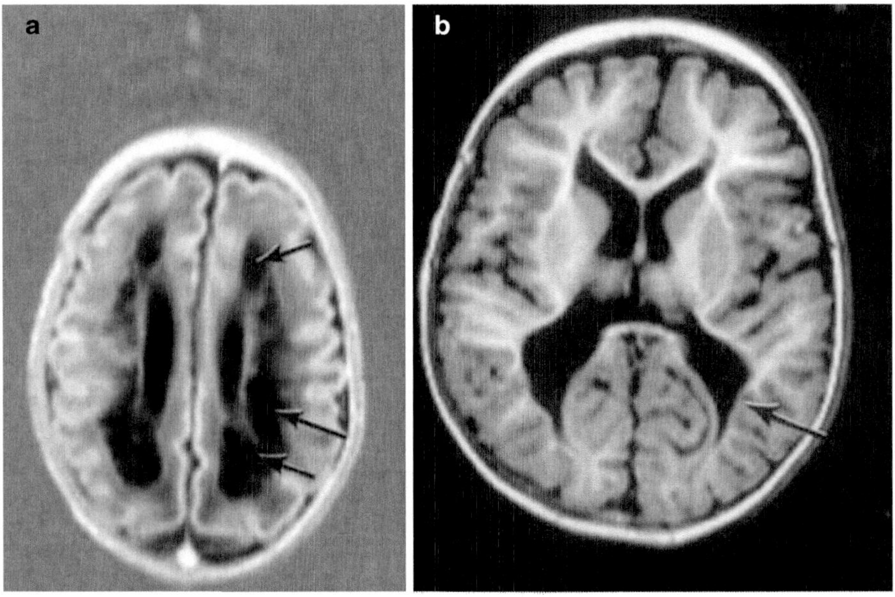

Fig. 66.8 (**a**) MRI inversion recovery sequence of a 32-week infant shortly after birth. Arrows show extensive periventricular cyst formation. (**b**) MRI inversion recovery sequence at 15 months showing irregular ventricular dilatation, most marked posteriorly (arrow) with little myelination [48]

adverse outcomes to neurodevelopment at 2 years of age, including cognitive and motor delay, sensorial neurodeficiencies, and cerebral palsy.

In addition, severe changes in white matter are strongly associated with low intelligence coefficients and severe motor delay at 7 years of age. Preterm infants diagnosed with periventricular leukomalacia are at increased risk for the development of spastic diplegia or quadriplegia [49].

References

1. Philip AG, Allan WC, Tito AM, et al. Intraventricular hemorrhage in preterm infants: declining incidence in the 1980's. Pediatrics. 1989;84:797–801.
2. Lemons JA, Bauer CR, Oh W, et al. Very low birth weight outcomes of the national institute of child health and human development, neonatal research network, January 1995 through December 1996. Pediatrics. 2001;107:el.
3. Laptook AR, O'Shea TM, Shankaran S, Bhaskar B. Adverse neurodevelopment outcomes among extremely low birth weight infants with a normal head ultrasound:prevalence and antecedents. Pediatrics. 2005;115:673–80.
4. Patra K, Wilson-Costello D, Taylor HG. Grades I-II intraventricular hemorrhage in extremely low birth weight infants:effects on neurodevelopment. J Pediatr. 2006;149:169–73.
5. Larroque B, Ancel PY, Marret S, et al. Neurodevelopmental disabilities and special care of 5-year-old children born before 33 weeks of gestation (the EPIPAGE study): a longitudinal cohort study. Lancet. 2008;371:813–20.
6. Bassan H. Intracranial hemorrhage in the preterm infant: understanding it. Preventing It Clin Perinatol. 2009;36:737–62.
7. Volpe JJ. Intracranial hemorrhage: neurology of the newborn. 5th ed. Philadelphia: W.B. Saunders Co.; 2008. p. 481–588.
8. Levene MI, Fawer CL, Lamont RF. Risk factors in the development of intraventricular haemorrhage in the preterm neonate. Arch Dis Child. 1982;57:410e7.
9. du Plessis AJ, Volpe JJ. Intracranial hemorrhage in the newborn infant. In: Burg FD, Ingelfinger JR, Wald ER, et al., editors. Gellis & Kagan's current pediatric therapy, , vol 16. Philadelphia: W.B. Saunders Company; 1999. p. 304–8.
10. Hamrick SE, Miller SP, Leonard C, et al. Trends in severe brain injury and neurodevelopmental outcome in premature newborn infants : the role of cystic periventricular leukomalacia. J Pedriatr. 2004;145(5):593–9.
11. Perlman JM, McMenamin JB, Volpe JJ. Fluctuating cerebral blood-flow velocity in respiratory-distress syndrome. Relation to the development of intraventricular hemorrhage. N Engl J Med. 1983;309:204e9.
12. Perlman JM. The relationship between systemic hemodynamic perturbations and periventricular- intraventricular hemorrhage historical perspective. Semin Pediatr Neurol. 2009;16:191e 9.
13. Inder TE, Perlman JM, Volpe JJ. Preterm Intraventricular Hemorrhage/Posthemorrhagic hydrocephalus. In: Volpe JJ, editor. Volpe's Neurology of the Newborn. 6th ed. Philadelphia: Elsevier; 2018. p. 637.
14. Vries LS, Leijser LM, Germinal matrix hemorrhage and intraventricular hemorrhage (GMH-IVH) in the newborn: Pathogenesis, clinical presentation, and diagnosis (up to date Mar 2020).
15. Wu YW, Hamrick SE, Miller SP, et al. Intraventricular hemorrhage in term neonates caused by sinovenous thrombosis. Ann Neurol. 2003;54:123.
16. Inder TE, Perlman JM, Volpe JJ. Intracranial hemorrhage: Subdural, Subarachnoid, Intraventricular (Term Infant), Miscellaneous. In: Volpe JJ, editor. Volpe's Neurology of the Newborn, 6. Philadelphia: Elsevier; 2018. p. 593.
17. Hanigan WC, Powell FC, Miller TC, Wright RM. Symptomatic intracranial hemorrhage in full-term infants. Childs Nerv Syst. 1995;11:698.
18. Hayden CK Jr, Shattuck KE, Richardson CJ, et al. Subependymal germinal matrix hemorrhage in full-term neonates. Pediatrics. 1985;75:714.
19. Szpecht D, Frydryszak D, Miszczyk N, et al. The incidence of severe intraventricular hemorrhage based on retrospective analysis of 35939 full-term newborns-report of two cases and review of literature. Childs Nerv Syst. 2016;32:2447.
20. Roberts D, Brown J, Medley N, Dalziel SR. Antenatal corticosteroids for accelerating fetal lung maturation for women at risk of preterm birth. Cochrane Database Syst Rev. 2017 Mar 21;3(3):CD004454.

21. Mohamed MA, Aly H. Transport of premature infants is associated with increased risk for intraventricular hemorrhage. Arch Dis Child Fetal Neonatal Ed. 2010;95:F403–7. 49.
22. McDonald SJ, Middleton P, Dowswell T, Morris PS. Cochrane in context: Effect of timing of umbilical cord clamping in term infants on maternal and neonatal outcomes. Evid Based Child Health. 2014;9(2):398–400.
23. Fogarty M, Osborn DA, Askie L, Seidler AL, Hunter K, Lui K, Simes J, Tarnow-Mordi W, Delayed versus early umbilical cord clamping for preterm infants: a systematic review and meta-analysis. Am J Obstet Gynecol. 2017.
24. Fogarty M, Osborn DA, Askie L, Seidler AL, Hunter K, Lui K, Simes J, Tarnow-Mordi W. Delayed vs early umbilical cord clamping for preterm infants: a systematic review and meta-analysis. Am J Obstet Gynecol. 2018 Jan;218(1):1–18.
25. Tarnow-Mordi W, Morris J, Kirby A, Robledo K, Askie L, Brown R, Evans N, Finlayson S, Fogarty M, Gebski V, Ghadge A, Hague W, Isaacs D, Jeffery M, Keech A, Kluckow M, Popat H, Sebastian L, Aagaard K, Belfort M, Pammi M, Abdel-Latif M, Reynolds G, Ariff S, Sheikh L, Chen Y, Colditz P, Liley H, Pritchard M, de Luca D, de Waal K, Forder P, Duley L, El-Naggar W, Gill A, Newnham J, Simmer K, Groom K, Weston P, Gullam J, Patel H, Koh G, Lui K, Marlow N, Morris S, Sehgal A, Wallace E, Soll R, Young L, Sweet D, Walker S, Watkins A, Wright I, Osborn D, Simes J, Australian Placental Transfusion Study Collaborative Group. Delayed versus immediate cord clamping in preterm infants. N Engl J Med. 2017;377(25):2445–55.
26. Chapman J, Marfurt S, Reid J. Effectiveness of delayed cord clamping in reducing post-delivery complications in preterm infants: a systematic review. J Perinat Neonatal Nurs. 2016;30(4):372–8.
27. Chiruvolu A, Tolia VN, Qin H, Stone GL, Rich D, Conant RJ, Inzer RW. Effect of delayed cord clamping on very preterm infants. Am J Obstet Gynecol. 2015;213(5):676 e1–7.
28. Mukerji A, Shah V, Shah PS. Periventricular/intraventricular hemorrhage and neurodevelopmental outcomes: a meta-analysis. Pediatrics. 2015;136:1132–43.
29. Payne AH, Hintz SR, Hibbs AM, et al. Neurodevelopmental outcomes of extremely low-gestational-age neonates with low-grade periventricular-intraventricular hemorrhage. JAMA Pediatr. 2013;167:451–9.
30. Beaino G, Khoshnood B, Kaminski M, et al. Predictors of cerebral palsy in very preterm infants: the EPIPAGE prospective population-based cohort study. Dev Med Child Neurol. 2010;52:e119–25.
31. Blumenthal I. Periventricular lucomalacia: a review. Eur J Pediatr. 2004;163:435–42.
32. Deng W, Pleasure J, Pleasure D. Progress in periventricular leucomalakia. Arch Neurol. 2008;65:1291–5.
33. Banker BQ, Larroche JC. Periventricular leukomalacia of infancy. Arch Neurol. 1962;7:368–410.
34. Volpe JJ. Cerebral White matter injury of the premature infant – more common than you think. Pediatrics. 2003;112:176–80.
35. Novak CM, Ozen M, Burd I. Perinatal brain injury mechanisms, prevention e outcomes. Clin Perinatol. 2018;45:357–75.
36. Hintz SR, Barnes PD, Bulas D, et al. Neuroimaging and neurodevelopmental outcome in extremely preterm infants. Pediatrics. 2005;135:e32–42.
37. Younge N, Goldstein RF, Bann CM, et al. Survival and neurodevelopmental outcomes among periviable infants. N Engl J Med. 2017;376:617–28.
38. Inder TE, Wells SJ, Mogridge NB, Spencer C, Volpe JJ. Defining the nature of the cerebral abnormalities in the premature infant: a qualitative magnetic resonance imaging study. J Pediatr. 2003;143:171–9.
39. Khwaja O, Volpe JJ. Pathogenesis of cerebral white matter injury of prematurity. Arch Dis Child Fetal Neonatal. 2008;93:F153–61.

40. Stensel M, Stüwe-Kunz L, Bührer C, Roll C. Spontaneous hypocarbia without mechanical ventilation in preterm infants with cystic periventricular leukomalacia. Acta Peddiatrica. 2020;00:1–7.
41. Volpe JJ. Neurobiology of periventricular leukomalacia in the premature infant. Pediatr Res. 2001;50:553–62.
42. Yoo BH, Park CW. Chaiworapongsa intrauterine infection and the development palsy. Br J Obstet Gynaecol. 2003;110:124–7.
43. Resch B, Resch E, Maurer-Fellbaum U, Pichler-Stachl E, Riccabona M, Hofer N, Urlesberger B. The whole spectrum of cystic periventricular leukomalacia of the preterm infant: results from a large consecutive case series. Childs Nerv Suyt. 2015;31:1527–32.
44. Novak CM, Ozen M, Burd I. Perinatal brain injury mechanisms, prevention and outcomes. Clin Perinatol. 2018;45:357–75.
45. Pierrat V, Duquennoy C, van Haastert IC, Ernst M, Guilley N, De Vries LS. Ultrasound diagnosis and neurodevelopmental outcome of localised and extensive cystic periventricular leucomalacia. Arch Dis Child Fetal Neonatal Ed. 2001;84:F151–6.
46. Krägeloh-Mann I, Toft P, Lunding J, Andresen J, Pryds O, Lou HC. Brain lesions in preterms: origin, consequences and compensation. Acta Paediatr. 1999;88:897–908.
47. Staudt M, Pavlova M, Böhm S, Grodd W, Krägeloh-Mann I. Pyramidal tract damage correlates with motor dysfunction in bilateral periventricular leukomalacia. Neuropediatrics. 2003;31:257–64.
48. Counsell AS, Rutherford MA. Magnetic resonance imaging of the newborn brain. Curr Paediatr. 2002;12:401–13.
49. Imamura T, Ariga H, Kaneko M, et al. Neurodevelopmental outcomes of children with periventricular leukomalacia. Pediatr Neonatol. 2013;54:367–72.

Chapter 67
Resuscitation of the Newborn Development of Algorithms, Present Status and Future Perspectives

Shamik Trivedi, Siw Helen Westby Eger, and Ola Didrik Saugstad

Need for Resuscitation

Every year an estimated 130–140 million neonates are born worldwide. A small percentage require resuscitation with positive pressure ventilation (PPV) support to start breathing. It is important to distinguish between stabilization and resuscitation. All neonates need to be stabilized after birth. They should be dried, kept warm, and positioned correctly with immediate skin-to-skin contact with their mother if possible. Around 85% of those who are born at term initiate spontaneous respiration within 10–30 seconds (s) and 10% respond during drying and stimulation.

Basic resuscitation could be defined as use of PPV either with bag and mask or continuous positive airway pressure (CPAP) with or without oxygen supplementation. Advanced resuscitation includes one or more of the following: PPV following endotracheal intubation, chest compressions, need of medication, or volume therapy.

Overall, 3% or more need PPV to initiate spontaneous ventilation, 2% will be intubated to support respiratory function, 0.1% or even less will require chest

S. Trivedi
Ann & Robert H. Lurie Children's Hospital of Chicago and Prentice Women's Hospital, Division of Neonatology, Feinberg School of Medicine, Northwestern University, Chicago, IL, USA

S. H. W. Eger
Department of Pediatrics and Adolescence Medicine, Oslo University Hospital, Oslo, Norway

O. D. Saugstad (✉)
Ann & Robert H. Lurie Children's Hospital of Chicago and Prentice Women's Hospital, Division of Neonatology, Feinberg School of Medicine, Northwestern University, Chicago, IL, USA

Department of Pediatric Research, Oslo University Hospital and University of Oslo, Oslo, Norway
e-mail: odsaugstad@rr-research.no

© Springer Nature Switzerland AG 2022

R. A. Moreira de Sá, E. B. d. Fonseca (eds.), *Perinatology*,
https://doi.org/10.1007/978-3-030-83434-0_67

compressions and/or medications. Only 1/12,000 term or near-term deliveries would need volume therapy immediately after birth [1].

Approximately 15 million neonates are born preterm and often require special handling and interventions. The European registry e-newborn has demonstrated that neonates born between gestational age (GA) 24–28 weeks required resuscitation in approximately 95% of the cases, decreasing to 57% at 32 weeks. Neonates born at 23 weeks needed resuscitation in approximately 90% of deliveries, indicating not all of these infants were resuscitated [2].

Development of the Resuscitation Algorithm

Experts representing accreditation bodies across the world meet twice a year to discuss resuscitation guidelines for neonates, children, and adults. Together they comprise a group known as the International Liaison Committee on Resuscitation (ILCOR) whose goal is to provide a forum for discussion of all aspects of cardiopulmonary and cerebral resuscitation worldwide [1, 3–5]. Founded in 1992, members from eight major resuscitation organizations (American Heart Association, European Resuscitation Council, Heart and Stroke Foundation of Canada, Australia and New Zealand Committee on Resuscitation (ANZCOR), Resuscitation Council of Asia, Resuscitation Council of Southern Africa, and InterAmerican Heart Foundation) meet at ILCOR to discuss mechanism for collecting, reviewing, and sharing international scientific data on resuscitation [1, 3–5].

Evidence-based review of resuscitation science occurs every 5 years with the end results being the development of the Consensus on Science and Treatment Recommendations (CoSTR) [1, 3–5]. Individual councils take the information from the CoSTR and construct specific resuscitation guidelines for their country. In the US, American Heart Association (AHA) and American Association of Pediatrics (AAP) experts work jointly to develop the Guidelines for Cardiovascular Care and Emergency Cardiac Care of the neonate, which are based on the CoSTR [1, 3, 4]. For neonates, they ask the Neonatal Resuscitation Program (NRP) steering committee to review the guidelines and translate into everyday practice through the Textbook of Neonatal Resuscitation with associated training material [5–7]. Currently, neonatal providers in the USA are using the algorithm developed in the NRP, seventh edition textbook, which went into practice nationwide on January 1, 2017 [5]. A number of national and local algorithms based mostly on ILCOR have been published all over the world.

Anticipation, Preparation, and Initial Stabilization

Delivery room handling, identification of maternal and infant risk factors, antenatal care decisions such as steroid administration and mode of delivery, and provision of effective interventions are vital information to gather prior to resuscitation that can affect outcome. Ideally, both obstetrics and neonatal teams should provide antenatal counselling together, especially if the fetus is at high risk for extremely preterm birth or there is concern for an antenatal diagnosis consistent with a genetic disease or congenital malformation. The parents should be counselled about the possible outcome, with the focus of presenting a consistent approach for the neonate as this leads to better rapport between neonatologist, obstetrician, nurses, and parents.

Ideally, a neonatologist would attend all the deliveries that are likely to require resuscitation. This is the reality in some cases since the presence of antenatal and intrapartum risk factors increase the likelihood for resuscitation. This anticipation enables health-care professionals skilled in neonatal resuscitation to be present, which may decrease time to resuscitation and improve the prognosis. However, the need for neonatal resuscitation cannot always be predicted and history has to be obtained while resuscitation is under way. Therefore, all health-care professionals in maternity or neonatal units should be skilled in airway management, mask ventilation, and cardiac compressions. There should also be staff skilled in intubation and drug administration available at all times.

Equipment and Preparation

All delivery suites should be equipped to deal with advanced resuscitation (Table 67.1).

If there is time before delivery, review obstetric records and speak to the family. In the delivery room, turn on the resuscitation unit heater, check the room temperature, and that equipment is present and working. For neonates, especially those in the need of intervention at birth, actions taken during time after birth, the so-called "Golden hour" may have important implications for long-term outcomes [8]. The concept of "golden hour" uses evidence-based interventions and treatment in term and preterm neonates for improved outcome [8, 9]. Recently published studies support the concept of golden hour in preterm neonates with decreased neonatal mortality and morbidity [10]. The standard approach is derived from the best available evidence with aim of practicing gentle but timely and effective interventions (Fig. 67.1) [11].

Initial Stabilization

The initial steps of resuscitation are to provide warmth by placing the neonate under a radiant heat source and position the neonate correctly with the head in a "sniffing" position to open the airway. It is important to start the timer on the resuscitation bed the moment the neonate is delivered and not when the cord is clamped. As soon as the neonate is placed on the resuscitation bed, assess the HR, respiration, color, and tone within the first 30 seconds. In term neonates, remove the wet towel and cover with a dry, preheated towel. In preterm neonates, specifically less than 28 weeks

Table 67.1 Recommended equipment

Resuscitation Bag	Masks (different sized masks available for preterm neonates)
Laryngoscopes	Blades (Sizes-00, 0, 1)
Endotracheal tubes (size: 2.0, 2.5, 3, 3.5, 4 mm)	Endotracheal tube stylets (introducers)
Oropharyngeal tubes	Magill forceps for nasal endotracheal tubes
Nasogastric tubes	Masks and Gloves
Occlusive wrap/plastic bag for preterm neonates	Portable thermal mattress
Tape, scissors	Syringes, needles, specimen bottles
Intraosseous needles	Umbilical venous line and tray
Equipment for needle decompression, chest tube placement	EKG monitor and pulse oximeter
Stethoscope	Medications (epinephrine, surfactant, normal saline, dextrose)

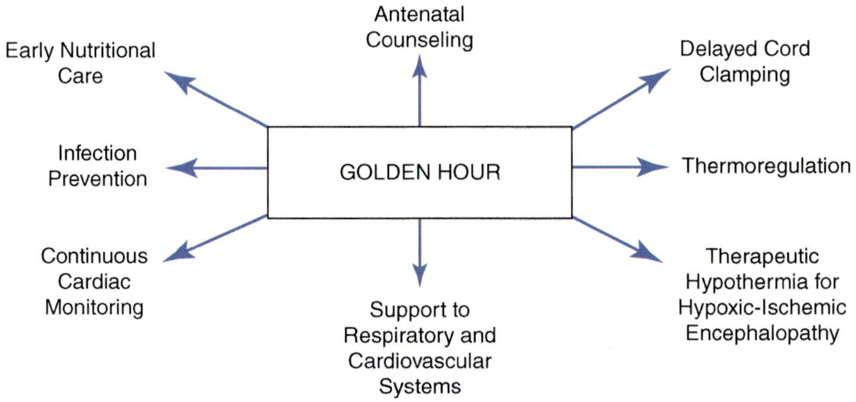

Fig. 67.1 Components of "golden hour"

gestation, it is recommended that the neonate is placed directly into a clear plastic bag under a radiant warmer without drying to reduce the risk of hypothermia.

The neonate should be stimulated to breathe by rubbing the chest or the spine, preferably in a caudocranial direction, which may lead to extension of the spine contributing to opening the lungs. In the next 30 seconds, respiratory support should be established if needed, and if available, a pulse oximetry probe is placed. The first Apgar score should be awarded at 1 minute of age. The Apgar score is used to describe a neonate's condition during the first few minutes of life assessing the neonate's heart rate (HR), respiration, muscle tone, reflex, and color at 1 and 5 minutes of life [12].

These recommendations are important to optimize the short- and long-term neonatal outcome. However, in many cases it is unrealistic to reach all of these goals in such a short period of time. In a neonate who does not breathe adequately, it is imperative to assess the cause of the poor transition to postnatal life.

Monitoring: Heart Rate Assessment

The NRP algorithm is heavily focused on accurate assessment of a neonate's HR [3, 4, 6]. Initiation or withholding an intervention may be solely based on a neonate's HR [1, 4]. Indications for starting PPV are HR less than 100 beat per minute and or insufficient ventilation to sustain such an adequate HR. There is a highly significant odds ratio for death in the first week of life or for development of moderate or severe hypoxic-ischemic encephalopathy (HIE) if the 5 min HR ≤ =60 bpm with OR 16.5 (95% CI 3.1–86.5) and 11.6 (95% CI 6.9–19.5) respectively [13].

There is a concern for providing unnecessary intervention due to a false result. In addition, an increase in the newborn's HR is considered the most sensitive indicator of a successful response to each intervention [1, 3, 13]. Therefore, it is apparent that a rapid, reliable, and accurate method should be used in the delivery room [5, 7]. Historically, assessment of a neonate's HR was obtained by palpation of the umbilical cord and/or auscultation with a stethoscope. Due to evidence showing that auscultation is more accurate and reliable, palpation is no longer recommended [4, 7, 14]. However, auscultation also has its disadvantages and can be inaccurate. In a randomized controlled trial conducted by Kamlin et al., results showed that auscultation underestimated the actual HR in comparison to electrocardiograph (ECG) monitoring [14]. The study was conducted on vigorous term neonates not requiring resuscitation and thus did not assess for accuracy of detection in preterm or non-vigorous neonates. However, when comparing the two detection techniques in simulated manikins, auscultation inaccurately detected HR compared to ECG when the HR was less than 100 [14].

Pulse oximetry is often used in the delivery room to assess oxygenation if there is clinical concern for persistent cyanosis and hypoxia based on the time of life [6]. In order to detect the oxygen saturation, the HR must be detected first and there is a known variable response time. When compared to ECG, pulse oximetry takes longer to detect a HR in both term and preterm neonates as well as underestimates the actual HR in the first 2 minutes of life [15, 16]. ILCOR in 2015 suggested that ECG should be the primary tool to detect HR at birth. NRP recommends ECG monitoring for all preterm neonates less than 32 weeks and any infant receiving positive pressure ventilation. In conjunction, pulse oximetry should be used for detection of oxygen saturation [1]. However, a recent study conducted by Shah et al. showed ECG monitoring in neonates receiving PPV led to less intubations, a higher rate of chest compression, with no difference in mortality [15]. A problem with the ILCOR recommendations is that most delivery rooms in the world per 2020 do not have access to ECG. At this time we therefore consider auscultation to be the gold standard of HR detection immediately after birth for all neonates, regardless of GA [16]. The

NeoTap device, a mobile device application, calculates the pulse rate by counting 3 beats [17].

Suctioning

According to ILCOR, routine intrapartum oropharyngeal and nasopharyngeal suctioning for neonates born with clear or meconium-stained amniotic fluid is no longer recommended [1, 3]. In fact, it has been demonstrated that routine oropharyngeal suctioning of term neonates born vaginally significantly reduces oxygen saturation for the first minutes of life after birth [18]. Suctioning may damage the pharyngeal mucosa and is a powerful vagal stimulus that may trigger a reflex bradycardia. Enthusiastic suctioning is based on the frequently held misconception that what is coming out of the neonates' mouth is inhaled amniotic fluid. It is not; it is fetal pulmonary fluid that has been in the lungs prior to birth, and it will do no harm if it stays there a few moments longer or is swallowed. Routine suctioning is therefore not recommended for neonates born at any GA. Wiping the face, nose, and mouth with a towel is sufficient in most cases, provided there is no airway obstruction [19].

Upper airway suctioning is indicated if there is blood or other extraneous material. If suctioning is required based on clinical assessment, you must suction the mouth before the nose (M before N) to reduce the risk of aspiration. It is recommended by NRP to clear the airway with a bulb syringe or a suction catheter if airway obstruction is evident or the newborn is in need of positive ventilation [6]. If suctioning is done mechanically, the negative pressure should be limited to 100 mm Hg [6]. In addition, suctioning the stomach is not needed routinely after C-section despite previous widespread practice. This practice may open the esophagus leading to more air leaks into the stomach when PPV with bag and mask is needed [20].

Oxygenation in the Delivery Room

Supplementation with pure oxygen (100% oxygen) was a part of the delivery room support of neonates for 200 years. However, human and animal data in the 1990s showed that air (21% oxygen) is as efficient as pure oxygen for neonatal resuscitation. Based on these results, the WHO recommended in 1998 that air could be used instead of pure oxygen for basic neonatal resuscitation [21]. From the turn of the century, evidence showed a brief exposure of pure oxygen in the delivery room could trigger inflammation and oxidative stress lasting for weeks. Several meta-analyses demonstrated a significantly lower mortality for term and near-term neonates resuscitated with air compared to pure oxygen. In addition, the time to first breath increased when resuscitation was carried out with pure oxygen [22]. In 2010, ILCOR therefore gave a similar recommendation as WHO: "In term neonates receiving resuscitation at birth with positive pressure ventilation, it is best to begin with air rather than 100% oxygen" [23].

In preterm resuscitation, starting with low FiO_2 and working up is in our opinion better than starting high and working down in terms of reducing oxidative stress [24–26]. It is recommended to start with 30% oxygen, and increase/decrease the oxygen based on published recommendations of target values for preductal SpO_2 [3]. See Table 67.2 for suggested SpO_2 targets the first 10 min of life [3].

The case for preterm neonates less than 32 weeks GA is more ambiguous. Meta-analyses showed no difference in death or major outcomes, including bronchopulmonary dysplasia (BPD), intraventricular hemorrhage (IVH), retinopathy of prematurity (ROP), or necrotizing enterocolitis (NEC) regardless of if initial oxygen was high (60–100%) or low (21–30%) even though it was noted that none of these studies examined the most commonly used initial oxygen: 40–50% [27].

Oei et al. showed that regardless of initial FiO_2, neonates who did not reach oxygen saturation (SpO_2) of 80% by 5 minutes of age were at significantly increased risk of IVH and death [27]. Whether these infants were unable to reach target SpO_2 due to inherent clinical instability or whether they were given less oxygen than required is uncertain.

Based on present knowledge the following recommendations can be given for newborns in need of PPV in DR (Table 67.3) [26].

Delayed Cord Clamping

At the time of delivery, the universal custom was to immediately clamp the umbilical cord. This allowed for immediate resuscitation of a preterm neonate and reduced risks such as hypothermia [28]. In recent years, there is an increase in practice of delaying clamping the cord (DCC) in vigorous neonates for a length of time after delivery due to the benefits seen in preterm and term neonates. The actual delay in time varies widely across the world from 30 seconds to 3 minutes [28]. The WHO and Royal College of Obstetricians and Gynaecologists (RCOG) recommend DCC for at least 60 and 120 seconds respectively [29, 30]. The American College of Obstetricians and Gynecologists (ACOG) recommends a delay in umbilical cord

Table 67.2 Target SpO_2 per minute of life (from Ref. [3])

Minute of Life	Target SpO_2
1 minute	60–65%
2 minutes	65–70%
3 minutes	70–75%
4 minutes	75–80%
5 minutes	80–85%
10 minutes	85–95%

Table 67.3 Starting percentage of FiO_2 by gestational age (GA)

GA weeks	Recommendations
Greater than 31 weeks	Start with air
28–31 weeks	Start with air or 30% FiO_2
Less than 28 weeks	Start with 30% FiO_2

clamping in vigorous term and preterm infants for at least 30–60 seconds after birth [31], and NRP as well defines DCC as 30–60 seconds after birth assuming there is no concern for the mother–fetus dyad [4, 5]. The benefit primarily stems from the increase in blood volume, as 70–80% of blood volume from the placenta is transferred to the healthy-term neonate in the first minute of life [20].

Benefits for preterm neonates include higher blood volume leading to a decreased need for blood transfusions [28]. They have consistently higher blood pressures improving hemodynamic stability, in some studies decreased IVH, and a lower risk of NEC [28]. Regarding mortality, data from studies are equivocal, demonstrating no effect to a small effect with a recent metanalysis showing a significant reduction in mortality [32]. Risks associated with DCC are polycythemia and hyperbilirubinemia, both stemming from the increase in blood volume. There is an increase in the need for phototherapy, however the incidence of needing a partial/full exchange transfusion is the same in both immediate and DCC groups [28, 33]. Although the data stems from studies of preterm neonates who did not undergo resuscitation, NRP nevertheless recommends DCC for most vigorous preterm infants.

In term neonates, DCC may decrease the risk of iron deficiency, improve iron storage with possible effect on neurodevelopmental outcome [31, 34]. Similarly, to preterm neonates, there is the associated risk of hyperbilirubinemia and clinical jaundice, however, it is not associated with an increase in morbidity. Vain et al. found that position of the newborn baby before cord clamping does not seem to affect volume of placental transfusion. According to these authors, mothers could safely be allowed to hold their baby on their abdomen or chest [35]. Delayed compared to early cord clamping improved scores in the fine-motor and social domains at 4 years of age, especially in boys, in a low-risk population of term born children [36].

From the maternal perspective, concern for postpartum hemorrhage led to the medical management of immediate cord clamping. In multiple studies, DCC did not increase postpartum hemorrhage in mothers without any concern for placenta abnormality prenatally [31]. DCC is contraindicated in the setting of multiple gestation, intrauterine growth restriction, concern for abnormal umbilical cord perfusion, or any placenta abnormality [4].

Cord clamping after the onset of ventilation is physiologic and in animal models seem to restore hemodynamics changes more smoothly with less post-hypoxia rebound hypertension possibly protecting the brain from cerebrovascular injury [37].

Temperature Regulation

Thermoregulation in the delivery room is a vital step in the resuscitation of a neonate in both low and high income countries. The WHO defines the goal temperature between 36.5 °C and 37.5 °C with mild hypothermia 36 °C–36.4 °C, moderate hypothermia 32 °C–35.9 °C and severe hypothermia less than 32 °C [38]. Through the main avenues of heat loss (evaporation, convective, conductive, radiation), the neonate is at significant risk for developing hypothermia in the delivery room. The risk is inversely related to the neonate's GA; the most preterm neonates due to their low fat stores, underdeveloped epidermal thickness, and higher surface area-to-weight ratio require the closest attention [39]. There is clear data showing an increased morbidity and mortality if a neonate, regardless of GA, is admitted to the NICU with moderate hypothermia (temperature less than 36 °C) [3].

In preterm neonates, with hypothermia there is an increased risk for respiratory distress syndrome (RDS), late-onset sepsis, IVH, and metabolic derangements (hypoglycemia, hyperkalemia, metabolic acidosis) [40]. The Canadian Research Network demonstrated that the lowest rate of morbidity in preterm neonates less than 33 weeks' gestation occurred when the admission temperature ranged between 36.5 °C and 37.2 °C [41]. Strict monitoring and thermoregulation are imperative in preterm neonates. Over the years, measures employed individually to avoid hypothermia such as total body occlusive wrapping, exothermic warming mattress, warmed humidified resuscitation gas, polyethylene caps, and increasing delivery room temperature produced variable results [3]. Combining the measures is most successful in reducing the rate of hypothermia, with multiple studies demonstrating an increase in admission temperature to the NICU when compared to single or a few of the interventions [3]. For all deliveries, NRP recommends increasing environmental temperature to 23 to 25 °C [6].

As with many therapeutic measures in medicine, finding the right balance is the key to success. Implementing these strategies in the delivery room decreases the incidence of neonates admitted to the NICU with hypothermia, however, there is an associated increased risk of developing hyperthermia. Studies show hyperthermia on admission (defined as greater than 37.5 °C) increases morbidity and mortality [40]. There are concerns for maternal morbidity, for example increase in infection risk due to elevated temperatures in the operating delivery. A single-center, randomized, control trial did not find an increase in endometritis or wound infection with a higher operating room temperature [42].

Meconium Delivery

The approach to managing the neonate post-delivery through meconium stained fluid (MSAF) has fluctuated over the years. In the 1970s, neonates delivered via MSAF underwent intrapartum suctioning at the perineum and then intubation and suctioning on the resuscitation bed to decrease the risk of developing meconium aspiration syndrome (MAS) [3, 43, 44]. In the first edition of NRP, published in 1986, the recommendation was to suction the trachea via intubation for all infants who delivered through thick meconium. This was the standard of care for much of the following two decades.

Providers started to question whether the benefit outweighed the risk of intubation and suctioning in vigorous neonates. In the 2000s, Wiswell et al. demonstrated no difference in MAS or other respiratory outcomes such as the need for mechanical ventilation, duration of therapy, or mortality in vigorous neonates who were randomized to the non-intubation cohort [45]. Similarly, Vain et al. investigated the widely practiced suctioning at the perineum and concluded routine suctioning did not decrease MAS, need for mechanical ventilation, or duration of oxygen therapy [46]. NRP (fifth edition) and AAP/ACOG updated their consensus statements and recommended against routine intrapartum suctioning and to only attempt tracheal suctioning in non-vigorous neonates.

In non-vigorous neonates, routine tracheal suctioning may delay appropriate resuscitation. Intubation can be harmful, especially if performed by an inexperienced provider. Determined to evaluate ongoing clinical practice, Chettri et al. performed a randomized controlled trial in term neonates and revealed routine tracheal suctioning in non-vigorous neonates did not affect development of MAS and its associated complications [47]. The goal is to provide the appropriate NRP steps if a neonate is non-vigorous. Based on all the data available, ILCOR decided the information available is insufficient to recommend routine tracheal suctioning in all neonates delivered through MSAF [3]. Even though tracheal suctioning is not a "knee-jerk reflex," a meconium aspirator can be useful during resuscitation and should be used if the appropriate clinical situation arises.

10. Noninvasive Ventilation

In term and preterm neonates who require respiratory support, the goal is to provide appropriate noninvasive ventilation with the hope of preventing intubation. Options include a flow-inflating bag (FIB), self-inflating bag (SIB), or T-Piece resuscitator, all of which have their own benefits and shortcomings. The main advantages of using a FIB or a T-Piece resuscitator are the ability to provide CPAP and free-flowing oxygen [6]. In spontaneously breathing neonates with respiratory distress, CPAP can help establish and maintain functional residual capacity (FRC), allowing for better gas exchange at the alveoli [3, 48, 49]. The use of early CPAP in the delivery room has shown to decrease the need for mechanical ventilation, need for surfactant, and reduce death or bronchopulmonary dysplasia (BPD), however, did not statistically affect the risk of developing BPD alone [3, 48, 49]. If it is required clinically, NRP recommends starting CPAP at 5–6 cm H_2O [3]. In contrast, the SIB does not require a continuous compressed gas source to provide respiratory support, therefore useful in low resource settings or if the gas source is not readily available, such as in a mother's postpartum room.

As mentioned above, if a neonate has a HR less than 100 bpm, inadequate respiratory effort or apneic, the recommendation is to begin PPV [6]. Even though all three interfaces provide PPV, NRP recommends using positive end-expiratory pressure (PEEP) while providing PPV in preterm neonates [6]. The SIB is the most ubiquitous interface used worldwide, albeit it does not reliably deliver PEEP [3]. When comparing PPV using a T-piece resuscitator (providing PEEP) to SIB (no PEEP), there is no difference in HR at 2 minutes of life and the time it takes to attain a HR greater than 100 bpm, oxygen saturation at 5 minutes of life, need for intubation/surfactant. In addition, there is no difference in the APGAR score, air leaks, or development of BPD in the very low birth weight (VLBW) subset [50, 51]. Even though the evidence available shows no statistically significant difference in many short- and long-term outcomes, the benefit of PEEP on establishing and maintaining FRC is valuable and therefore recommended. In low-resource settings, using the SIB can be effective and lifesaving.

Sustained inflation (SI) followed by CPAP in the delivery room did not decrease the need for respiratory support, however increased pneumothorax with no change in survival without BPD in preterm infants between 25 and 29 weeks GA [52], and potential increase in mortality [53]. The quality of the evidence and conflicting conclusions from a Cochrane review provided ILCOR pause in recommending the practice [3].

Advanced Airway

Effective PPV during neonatal resuscitation is critical to improving a neonate's outcome [3, 54]. After initiating maneuvers to improve delivery of positive pressure via bag and mask ventilation using the MRSOPA pneumonic: **M**ask adjustment, **R**eposition head, **S**uction, **O**pen mouth, increase **P**ressure; an advanced airway is the recommended intervention to stabilize the neonate. Historically, an advanced airway referred to intubation using an endotracheal tube (ETT), however, the practice of using a laryngeal mask airway (LMA) in neonatal resuscitation has increased. NRP seventh edition defines an advanced airway as either an ETT or a LMA [6]. The smallest-size LMA is recommended for neonates greater than 34 weeks' gestation and/or 2 kilograms. If intubation, a difficult skill to achieve, is unattainable due to the airway anatomy or provider's skill, LMA is an extremely useful device. In comparison to intubation using an ETT, LMA insertion was effective in achieving appropriate vital signs and successful resuscitation [54, 55]. In low-resource settings where the primary provider in a neonatal resuscitation may not have the skill to intubate or difficulty maintaining the skill, LMA insertion can be lifesaving [1, 54, 56].

In the situation where a LMA is not an option due to size of the neonate/GA, placing the appropriate sized ETT quickly and accurately is important to improving the clinical status of a deteriorating neonate. NRP seventh edition recommends a 2.5-, 3.0-, and 3.5-sized ETT to be used in neonatal resuscitation [1, 6], thereby any infant larger than 2.0 kg to receive a 3.5-sized ETT. Proper depth insertion is imperative to prevent unplanned extubation if tube placement is too high or unilateral lung ventilation with associated risks (unilateral surfactant administration) if the tube placement is too low. In previous iterations, NRP recommended depth insertion using Tochen's rule (weight in kilograms plus 6 cm measured from the lip), based on an autopsy study conducted in the 1970s on 40 neonates ranging from 24 to 40 weeks' gestation. Ongoing investigation in preterm neonates, assessing this tip-to-lip distance calculation, demonstrated inadequate tube placement in up to quarter of the neonates using clinical and radiographic confirmation [57]. To prevent the associated morbidities with improper tube position, it is crucial to utilize a better estimate for adequate placement defined as mid-tracheal location.

The nasal–tragus length (NTL), measured from the base of the nasal septum to the tragus of the ear, plus 1 cm has shown to improve proper placement of the ETT compared to Tochen's rule in both preterm and term neonates [58, 59]. Therefore, depth insertion should be determined using NTL + 1 cm when orally intubating both preterm and term neonates [1, 6, 7].

Chest Compressions /Drugs/ Volume

Progressing through the NRP algorithm, if there is continued bradycardia with HR less than 60 bpm after 30 seconds of effective ventilation via an advanced airway, the neonatal resuscitation team should initiate chest compressions [6]. The emphasis on having an advanced airway prior to initiation of chest compressions is an update for NRP seventh edition as many bradycardia events in neonates are due to asphyxia [7]. Historically, chest compressions were completed using the two-finger technique or the two-thumb encircling technique. In 2010, NRP recommended using the two-thumb encircling technique due to evidence at the time. Reviewing the literature for NRP seventh edition, in comparison to the two-finger technique, randomized and nonrandomized clinical trials demonstrated that the two-thumb encircling technique generated higher blood pressure and coronary perfusion pressure and less compressor fatigue [1]. The goal is to provide effective chest compressions for 60 seconds before pausing to delineate the innate HR, rhythm, and pulse check. Chest compressions are routinely done at the side of the resuscitation warmer. However, ergonomics may play a key role in rescuer fatigue and quality of delivered chest compressions. Manikin studies demonstrate chest compressions delivered from the head of the neonate are sustained for a longer period of time compared to the side of the neonate [60]. In addition, it allows for greater real estate on the neonate, especially an extremely low-birth-weight premature neonate, requiring emergent vascular access.

PPV is carried out with a frequency of 40–60 breaths per minute. However, once chest compressions are initiated, the goal ratio of ventilations to compressions is 3:1 resulting in 90 compressions and 30 ventilations. Other resuscitation guidelines such as pediatric advanced life support (PALS) utilize a ratio of 30:1 or 15:2 depending on the number of providers. The reasoning for utilizing a 3:1 ratio in newly born infants stems from the underlying physiology of asphyxia due to intrapartum-related events leading to bradycardia in many neonates. If the resuscitation team is able to improve ventilation and oxygenation, the HR should increase. Animal studies, primarily in pig models, show no advantage in higher compression to ventilation ratios in regard to gas exchange during cardiopulmonary resuscitation (CPR), time to return of spontaneous circulation (ROSC), short-term survival [61]. Employing simulated manikins to assess which ratio is superior, physicians and nurses performing chest compressions achieve more consistent compression depth, less fatigue, and highest ventilation rates using a 3:1 ratio compared to a 15:2 [62]. Incorporating technology to measure respiratory dynamics such as tidal volume and ventilation rates in simulated manikins, higher compression ratios (9:3 and 3:1) resulted in lower tidal volumes delivered [63]. Even though the data is considered low-grade evidence, ILCOR and subsequently NRP recommend using a 3:1 ratio if chest compressions are initiated during a delivery room resuscitation.

Even though data is lacking, it is still recommended to do chest compressions with 100% oxygen. However, piglet studies have demonstrated similar outcomes using air [64]. Although it seems reasonable to believe that the latter produces less oxidative stress, a change in the guidelines from 100% to for instance 21% O_2 should wait till clinical data are available demonstrating a benefit with lower FiO_2.

Once chest compressions are initiated, a member of the resuscitation team should be prepared for emergent intravenous access using an umbilical venous catheter or intraosseous needle. Once access is achieved Epinephrine (1:10,000) at 0.1–0.3 ml/kg to improve cardiac contractility and rate can be given every 3 to 5 minutes. If concern for hypovolemia, normal saline (0.9% NaCl) can be given at 10 ml/kg. If there is concern for bleeding/hemorrhagic shock, quickly ordering packed red blood cells (PRBC) and administering a 10 ml/kg bolus is imperative.

Respiratory Management for the Preterm Infant

Methods for optimal delivery room management for preterm neonates have become more evidence based with the main focus on optimizing heart and lung function, administration of surfactant, and avoid hypothermia due to an increased risk for neonatal mortality and morbidity. RDS is still one of the most common complications of preterm birth and the incidence increases with decreasing GA [65]. Gradually over the years, its management has evolved, resulting in improved survival for the smallest neonates but with possible increasing rates of BPD [66]. Stabilization of preterm neonates with RDS may require inflation of the lung with blended air/oxygen. Protocols for lung protection, including initiation of noninvasive ventilation with CPAP, and titration of oxygen, should be implemented soon after birth.

Neonates with RDS have difficulty maintaining alveolar aeration after birth, although most try to breathe for themselves, and therefore any support of transition is "stabilization" rather than "resuscitation." Updated European Resuscitation Guidelines highlighted recent evidence-based approaches to supporting babies during the immediate postnatal period, including newborn life support [67]. When dealing with preterm neonates with RDS, we must allow the neonate to pass gradually through the transition if possible whilst exposing them to a minimum number of interventions that may cause harm [68].

Newer protocols for surfactant administration including optimal timing, mode of delivery, and the best preparation are aimed for avoiding exposure to mechanical ventilation. A strategy of initiation of noninvasive ventilation with CPAP from birth with early selective surfactant administration for babies showing signs of RDS is recommended. The European consensus guidelines on the management of RDS advice rescue surfactant as the standard approach, especially for neonates less than 26 weeks of gestation [69]. These guidelines were recently updated stating that natural surfactants are broadly equivalent and should be used [70]. However, promising data using synthetic surfactant with surfactant protein B and C analogs have recently been published [71, 72]. Hopefully, such compounds can be used, resulting in reduced cost and need for animal derived products.

Low-Income Countries

Approximately 7-800,000 neonatal deaths mostly occurring in low-income countries are due to intrapartum-related events (asphyxia). Neonatal resuscitation training was estimated to reduce term intrapartum-related deaths by 30% [73].

The ILCOR algorithm presupposes some experience in delivery room resuscitation and certain technical standards. This algorithm therefore is difficult to apply worldwide, particularly in low-income areas. For that reason, the Helping Babies Breathe (HBB) algorithm, a simpler algorithm focusing on basic resuscitation in low-income areas, was launched in 2010 by The Global Implementation Task Force of AAP in collaboration with private nonprofit and for-profit industry organizations. It is based on International ILCOR guidelines for neonatal resuscitation and WHO guidelines for basic neonatal resuscitation renewed in 2012 [74]. They are adapted to meet the needs of low-resource settings with a focus on basic steps of resuscitation (stimulation, temperature control, mask and bag ventilation) that can be done without access to intensive care or high-tech equipment. It uses modern educational methods including picture-based learning material for those unable to read as well as simulation and practical training in peers. It includes an implementation guide with a plan for scaling up using a low-cost, train-the-trainer principle.

The HBB program focuses on practical training of basic steps using low-tech simulation-based training. The premise is based on receiving support within the first 60 seconds of life – the so-called "golden minute." HBB is implemented in more than 80 countries and is expanding worldwide. The primary results are promising.

We, as others, found a significant early reduction in mortality [75]. However, long-term follow-up is lacking and the sustainability of the results is unknown. In addition, HBB does not include advanced resuscitation. Recently, promising results using an uncuffed LMA compared to bag and mask ventilation were demonstrated in Uganda. The time needed to achieve a HR > 100 bpm was shorter for LMA [56].

Teaching and Debriefing

Teaching a neonatal resuscitation course should convey an evidence-based approach to care of the neonate at birth and facilitate effective team-based care for healthcare professionals. It should be a blended learning approach, including classroom and/or online teaching and testing, case-based simulations, and hands-on case-based simulation/debriefing that focus on critical leadership, communication, and team-work skills. All participants must demonstrate clinical skills regarding neonatal resuscitation in simulation training demonstrating familiarity with all the equipment.

NRP has teamed up with HealthStream in the United States to provide its online educational content while improving the services available [7]. The electronic simulation (eSim) cases allow providers to practice simulation style cases prior to attending an initial certification or renewal course. The cases focus on gathering the appropriate supplies, resuscitate the neonate utilizing the NRP diagram and post-resuscitation care. More importantly, the program provides feedback to the provider after the case [7].

Difficult cases impact the whole medical team and it is imperative to discuss what went well and areas for improvement. With regard to ongoing training, one of the most important aspects is a careful debriefing. This allows any problems, whether clinical, procedural or mechanical, to be dealt with. Actions that follow debriefing might include more training for an individual or modification to a piece of equipment [76].

Future Aspects

Improved women and maternal health is a key to reducing the need for newborn resuscitation. Providing education at an early age to girls improves their health and postpones the age of first delivery. Combining potent measures such as adequate antenatal care and a safe environment for deliveries can reduce intrapartum-related events in the future. Introduction of simple and inexpensive measures may reduce neonatal mortality substantially [77, 78]. For example, utilizing air instead of 100% oxygen for resuscitation allowed for a simplified ubiquitous algorithm such as HBB, which, as mentioned above, rapidly spreads in low-income areas. There are still unsolved questions regarding the optimal oxygenation requirement in DR especially in extremely low-birth-weight neonates.

The potential future direction for HR assessment at birth is exciting. Philippos et al. summarized possible methods for assessing HR including Doppler ultrasound with forehead reflectance photo plethysmography and wearable low-power context-aware ECG monitoring systems with Bluetooth capabilities for data transmission to a smartphone [79]. A wireless ECG sensor can be worn around a finger and transmit HR data via Wi-Fi. Even techniques that measure HR without touching the skin could be a future option. Perhaps most convenient for clinicians will be a digital stethoscope that can transmit HRs to a smartphone [79].

In 2020, ILCOR revised recommendations for newborn resuscitation is published. We need a constant focus on this issue and improvement based on solid evidence.

References

1. Perlman JM, Wyllie J, Kattwinkel J, Wyckoff MH, Aziz K, Guinsburg R, et al. Part 7: neonatal resuscitation: 2015 international consensus on cardiopulmonary resuscitation and emergency cardiovascular care science with treatment recommendations. Circulation. 2015;132:S204–41.
2. Haumont D, Modi N, Saugstad OD, Antetere R, NguyenBa C, Turner M, et al. Evaluating preterm care across Europe using the eNewborn European Network database. Pediatr Res. 2020;88(3):484–95.
3. Wyllie J, Perlman JM, Kattwinkel J, Wyckoff MH, Aziz K, Guinsburg R, et al. Part 7: neonatal resuscitation: 2015 international consensus on cardiopulmonary resuscitation and emergency cardiovascular care science with treatment recommendations. Resuscitation. 2015;95:e169–201.
4. Wyckoff MH, Aziz K, Escobedo MB, Kapadia VS, Kattwinkel J, Perlman JM, et al. Part 13: neonatal resuscitation: 2015 American Heart Association Guidelines update for cardiopulmonary resuscitation and emergency cardiovascular care (reprint). Pediatrics. 2015;136(Suppl 2):S196–218.
5. Sawyer T, Umoren RA, Gray MM. Neonatal resuscitation: advances in training and practice. Adv Med Educ Pract. 2017;8:11–9.
6. Weiner G, Zaichkin J, Kattwinkel J. Textbook of neonatal resuscitation. 7th ed. Itasca: American Academy of Pediatrics and American Heart Association; 2016.
7. Zaichkin J, McCarney L, Weiner G. NRP 7th edition: are you prepared? Adv Neonatal Care. 2016;16(4):255–63.
8. Reynolds RD, Pilcher J, Ring A, Johnson R, McKinley P. The Golden hour: care of the LBW infant during the first hour of life one unit's experience. Neonatal Netw. 2009;28(4):211–9; quiz 55-8.
9. Sharma D. Golden hour of neonatal life: need of the hour. Matern Health Neonatol Perinatol. 2017;3:1–27.
10. Ashmeade TL, Haubner L, Collins S, Miladinovic B, Fugate K. Outcomes of a neonatal golden hour implementation project. Am J Med Qual. 2016;31(1):73–80.
11. Vento M, Cheung PY, Aguar M. The first golden minutes of the extremely-low-gestational-age neonate: a gentle approach. Neonatology. 2009;95(4):286–98.
12. Apgar V. A proposal for a new method of evaluation of the newborn infant. Curr Res Anesth Analg. 1953;32(4):260–7.
13. Saugstad OD, Ramji S, Rootwelt T, Vento M. Response to resuscitation of the newborn: early prognostic variables. Acta Paediatr. 2005;94(7):890–5.
14. Kamlin CO, O'Donnell CP, Everest NJ, Davis PG, Morley CJ. Accuracy of clinical assessment of infant heart rate in the delivery room. Resuscitation. 2006;71(3):319–21.

15. Shah BA, Wlodaver AG, Escobedo MB, Ahmed ST, Blunt MH, Anderson MP, et al. Impact of electronic cardiac (ECG) monitoring on delivery room resuscitation and neonatal outcomes. Resuscitation. 2019;143:10–6.
16. Saugstad OD, Soll RF. Assessing heart rate at birth: auscultation is still the gold standard. Neonatology. 2016;110(3):238–40.
17. Binotti M, Cavallin F, Ingrassia PL, Pejovic NJ, Monzani A, Genoni G, et al. Heart rate assessment using NeoTapAdvancedSupport: a simulation study. Arch Dis Child Fetal Neonatal Ed. 2019;104(4):F440–F2.
18. Carrasco M, Martell M, Estol PC. Oronasopharyngeal suction at birth: effects on arterial oxygen saturation. J Pediatr. 1997;130(5):832–4.
19. Kelleher J, Bhat R, Salas AA, Addis D, Mills EC, Mallick H, et al. Oronasopharyngeal suction versus wiping of the mouth and nose at birth: a randomised equivalency trial. Lancet. 2013;382(9889):326–30.
20. Marshall S, Lang AM, Perez M, Saugstad OD. Delivery room handling of the newborn. J Perinat Med. 2019;48(1):1–10.
21. WHO. Basic newborn resuscitation: a practical guide. Geneva: WHO; 1998. Report No.: WQ 450 98BA.
22. Saugstad OD, Ramji S, Vento M. Resuscitation of depressed newborn infants with ambient air or pure oxygen: a meta-analysis. Biol Neonate. 2005;87(1):27–34.
23. Kattwinkel J, Perlman JM, Aziz K, Colby C, Fairchild K, Gallagher J, et al. Part 15: neonatal resuscitation: 2010 American Heart Association guidelines for cardiopulmonary resuscitation and emergency cardiovascular care. Circulation. 2010;122(18 Suppl 3):S909–19.
24. Oei JL, Finer NN, Saugstad OD, Wright IM, Rabi Y, Tarnow-Mordi W, et al. Outcomes of oxygen saturation targeting during delivery room stabilisation of preterm infants. Arch Dis Child Fetal Neonatal Ed. 2018;103(5):F446–F54.
25. Dekker J, Martherus T, Lopriore E, Giera M, McGillick EV, Hutten J, et al. The effect of initial high vs. low fio2 on breathing effort in preterm infants at birth: a randomized controlled trial. Front Pediatr. 2019;7:504.
26. Saugstad OD, Lakshminrusimha S, Vento M. Oxygenation of the extremely premature infant the first few minutes of life: start low or high? J Pediatr. In Press.
27. Oei JL, Vento M, Rabi Y, Wright I, Finer N, Rich W, et al. Higher or lower oxygen for delivery room resuscitation of preterm infants below 28 completed weeks gestation: a meta-analysis. Arch Dis Child Fetal Neonatal Ed. 2017;102(1):F24–30.
28. Fogarty M, Osborn DA, Askie L, Seidler AL, Hunter K, Lui K, et al. Delayed vs early umbilical cord clamping for preterm infants: a systematic review and meta-analysis. Am J Obstet Gynecol. 2018;218(1):1–18.
29. World Health Organization. Guideline: Delayed umbilical cord clamping for improved maternal and infant health and nutrition outcomes. Geneva: WHO; 2014.
30. Royal College of Obstetricians and Gynaecologists SAC. Clamping of the umbilical cord and placental transfusion, Scientific Impact Paper No. 14. 2015.
31. Committee on Obstetric P. Committee Opinion No. 684: delayed umbilical cord clamping after birth. Obstet Gynecol. 2017;129(1):e5–e10.
32. Backes CH, Rivera BK, Haque U, Bridge JA, Smith CV, Hutchon DJ, et al. Placental transfusion strategies in very preterm neonates: a systematic review and meta-analysis. Obstet Gynecol. 2014;124(1):47–56.
33. Strauss RG, Mock DM, Johnson KJ, Cress GA, Burmeister LF, Zimmerman MB, et al. A randomized clinical trial comparing immediate versus delayed clamping of the umbilical cord in preterm infants: short-term clinical and laboratory endpoints. Transfusion. 2008;48(4):658–65.
34. McDonald SJ, Middleton P, Dowswell T, Morris PS. Effect of timing of umbilical cord clamping of term infants on maternal and neonatal outcomes. Evid Based Child Health. 2014;9(2):303–97.
35. Vain NE, Satragno DS, Gorenstein AN, Gordillo JE, Berazategui JP, Alda MG, et al. Effect of gravity on volume of placental transfusion: a multicentre, randomised, non-inferiority trial. Lancet. 2014;384(9939):235–40.

36. Andersson O, Lindquist B, Lindgren M, Stjernqvist K, Domellof M, Hellstrom-Westas L. Effect of delayed cord clamping on neurodevelopment at 4 years of age: a randomized clinical trial. JAMA Pediatr. 2015;169(7):631–8.
37. Polglase GR, Blank DA, Barton SK, Miller SL, Stojanovska V, Kluckow M, et al. Physiologically based cord clamping stabilises cardiac output and reduces cerebrovascular injury in asphyxiated near-term lambs. Arch Dis Child Fetal Neonatal Ed. 2018;103(6):F530–F8.
38. World Health Organization. Maternal and Newborn Health/Safe Motherhood. Thermal protection of the newborn: a practical guide. Geneva: WHO; 1997.
39. Laptook AR, Salhab W, Bhaskar B. Admission temperature of low birth weight infants: predictors and associated morbidities. Pediatrics. 2007;119(3):e643–9.
40. Trevisanuto D, Testoni D, de Almeida MFB. Maintaining normothermia: why and how? Semin Fetal Neonatal Med. 2018;23(5):333–9.
41. Lyu Y, Shah PS, Ye XY, Warre R, Piedboeuf B, Deshpandey A, et al. Association between admission temperature and mortality and major morbidity in preterm infants born at fewer than 33 weeks' gestation. JAMA Pediatr. 2015;169(4):e150277.
42. Duryea EL, Nelson DB, Wyckoff MH, Grant EN, Tao W, Sadana N, et al. The impact of ambient operating room temperature on neonatal and maternal hypothermia and associated morbidities: a randomized controlled trial. Am J Obstet Gynecol. 2016;214(4):505.e1–7.
43. Carson BS, Losey RW, Bowes WA Jr, Simmons MA. Combined obstetric and pediatric approach to prevent meconium aspiration syndrome. Am J Obstet Gynecol. 1976;126(6):712–5.
44. Gregory GA, Gooding CA, Phibbs RH, Tooley WH. Meconium aspiration in infants--a prospective study. J Pediatr. 1974;85(6):848–52.
45. Wiswell TE, Gannon CM, Jacob J, Goldsmith L, Szyld E, Weiss K, et al. Delivery room management of the apparently vigorous meconium-stained neonate: results of the multicenter, international collaborative trial. Pediatrics. 2000;105(1 Pt 1):1–7.
46. Vain NE, Szyld EG, Prudent LM, Wiswell TE, Aguilar AM, Vivas NI. Oropharyngeal and nasopharyngeal suctioning of meconium-stained neonates before delivery of their shoulders: multicentre, randomised controlled trial. Lancet. 2004;364(9434):597–602.
47. Chettri S, Adhisivam B, Bhat BV. Endotracheal suction for nonvigorous neonates born through meconium stained amniotic fluid: a randomized controlled trial. J Pediatr. 2015;166(5):1208–13.e1.
48. Network SSGotEKSNNR, Finer NN, Carlo WA, Walsh MC, Rich W, Gantz MG, et al. Early CPAP versus surfactant in extremely preterm infants. N Engl J Med. 2010;362(21):1970–9.
49. Subramaniam P, Ho JJ, Davis PG. Prophylactic nasal continuous positive airway pressure for preventing morbidity and mortality in very preterm infants. Cochrane Database Syst Rev. 2016;6:CD001243.
50. Szyld E, Aguilar A, Musante GA, Vain N, Prudent L, Fabres J, et al. Comparison of devices for newborn ventilation in the delivery room. J Pediatr. 2014;165(2):234–9. e3.
51. Dawson JA, Schmolzer GM, Kamlin CO, Te Pas AB, O'Donnell CP, Donath SM, et al. Oxygenation with T-piece versus self-inflating bag for ventilation of extremely preterm infants at birth: a randomized controlled trial. J Pediatr. 2011;158(6):912-8 e1–2.
52. Lista G, Boni L, Scopesi F, Mosca F, Trevisanuto D, Messner H, et al. Sustained lung inflation at birth for preterm infants: a randomized clinical trial. Pediatrics. 2015;135(2):e457–64.
53. Kirpalani H, Ratcliffe SJ, Keszler M, Davis PG, Foglia EE, Te Pas A, et al. Effect of sustained inflations vs intermittent positive pressure ventilation on bronchopulmonary dysplasia or death among extremely preterm infants: the SAIL randomized clinical trial. JAMA. 2019;321(12):1165–75.
54. Grein AJ, Weiner GM. Laryngeal mask airway versus bag-mask ventilation or endotracheal intubation for neonatal resuscitation. Cochrane Database Syst Rev. 2005;2:CD003314.
55. Yang C, Zhu X, Lin W, Zhang Q, Su J, Lin B, et al. Randomized, controlled trial comparing laryngeal mask versus endotracheal intubation during neonatal resuscitation---a secondary publication. BMC Pediatr. 2016;16:1–6.
56. Pejovic NJ, Trevisanuto D, Lubulwa C, Myrnerts Hook S, Cavallin F, Byamugisha J, et al. Neonatal resuscitation using a laryngeal mask airway: a randomised trial in Uganda. Arch Dis Child. 2018;103(3):255–60.

57. Amarilyo G, Mimouni FB, Oren A, Tsyrkin S, Mandel D. Orotracheal tube insertion in extremely low birth weight infants. J Pediatr. 2009;154(5):764–5.
58. Shukla HK, Hendricks-Munoz KD, Atakent Y, Rapaport S. Rapid estimation of insertional length of endotracheal intubation in newborn infants. J Pediatr. 1997;131(4):561–4.
59. Whyte KL, Levin R, Powls A. Clinical audit: optimal positioning of endotracheal tubes in neonates. Scott Med J. 2007;52(2):25–7.
60. Mildenhall LF, Huynh TK. Factors modulating effective chest compressions in the neonatal period. Semin Fetal Neonatal Med. 2013;18(6):352–6.
61. Solevag AL, Dannevig I, Wyckoff M, Saugstad OD, Nakstad B. Return of spontaneous circulation with a compression:ventilation ratio of 15:2 versus 3:1 in newborn pigs with cardiac arrest due to asphyxia. Arch Dis Child Fetal Neonatal Ed. 2011;96(6):F417–21.
62. Hemway RJ, Christman C, Perlman J. The 3:1 is superior to a 15:2 ratio in a newborn manikin model in terms of quality of chest compressions and number of ventilations. Arch Dis Child Fetal Neonatal Ed. 2013;98(1):F42–5.
63. Solevag AL, Madland JM, Gjaerum E, Nakstad B. Minute ventilation at different compression to ventilation ratios, different ventilation rates, and continuous chest compressions with asynchronous ventilation in a newborn manikin. Scand J Trauma Resusc Emerg Med. 2012;20:1–7.
64. Solevag AL, Dannevig I, Nakstad B, Saugstad OD. Resuscitation of severely asphyctic newborn pigs with cardiac arrest by using 21% or 100% oxygen. Neonatology. 2010;98(1):64–72.
65. Reuter S, Moser C, Baack M. Respiratory distress in the newborn. Pediatr Rev. 2014;35(10):417–28; quiz 29.
66. Stoll BJ, Hansen NI, Bell EF, Walsh MC, Carlo WA, Shankaran S, et al. Trends in care practices, morbidity, and mortality of extremely preterm neonates, 1993-2012. JAMA. 2015;314(10):1039–51.
67. Wyllie J, Bruinenberg J, Roehr CC, Rudiger M, Trevisanuto D, Urlesberger B. European resuscitation council guidelines for resuscitation 2015: section 7. Resuscitation and support of transition of babies at birth. Resuscitation. 2015;95:249–63.
68. Saugstad OD. Delivery room management of term and preterm newly born infants. Neonatology. 2015;107(4):365–71.
69. Sweet DG, Carnielli V, Greisen G, Hallman M, Ozek E, Plavka R, et al. European consensus guidelines on the management of neonatal respiratory distress syndrome in preterm infants - 2010 update. Neonatology. 2010;97(4):402–17.
70. Sweet DG, Carnielli V, Greisen G, Hallman M, Ozek E, Te Pas A, et al. European consensus guidelines on the management of respiratory distress syndrome - 2019 update. Neonatology. 2019;115(4):432–50.
71. Johansson J, Curstedt T. Synthetic surfactants with SP-B and SP-C analogues to enable worldwide treatment of neonatal respiratory distress syndrome and other lung diseases. J Intern Med. 2019;285(2):165–86.
72. Sweet DG, Turner MA, Stranak Z, Plavka R, Clarke P, Stenson BJ, et al. A first-in-human clinical study of a new SP-B and SP-C enriched synthetic surfactant (CHF5633) in preterm babies with respiratory distress syndrome. Arch Dis Child Fetal Neonatal Ed. 2017;102(6):F497–503.
73. Lee AC, Cousens S, Wall SN, Niermeyer S, Darmstadt GL, Carlo WA, et al. Neonatal resuscitation and immediate newborn assessment and stimulation for the prevention of neonatal deaths: a systematic review, meta-analysis and Delphi estimation of mortality effect. BMC Public Health. 2011;11(Suppl 3):1–19.
74. Little GA, Keenan WJ, Singhal N, Niermeyer S. International perspectives: helping babies breathe: evolution of a global neonatal resuscitation program for resource-limited areas. NeoReviews. 2014;15(9):e369–e80.
75. Innerdal M, Simaga I, Diall H, Eielsen M, Niermeyer S, Eielsen O, et al. Reduction in perinatal mortality after implementation of HBB training at a District Hospital in Mali. J Trop Pediatr. 2019:1–7.
76. O'Currain E, Davis PG, Thio M. Educational perspectives: toward more effective neonatal resuscitation: assessing and improving clinical skills. NeoReviews. 2019;20(5):e248–e57.
77. Saugstad OD. Reducing global neonatal mortality is possible. Neonatology. 2011;99(4):250–7.

78. Gonzalez R, Merialdi M, Lincetto O, Lauer J, Becerra C, Castro R, et al. Reduction in neonatal mortality in Chile between 1990 and 2000. Pediatrics. 2006;117(5):e949–54.
79. Phillipos E, Solevag AL, Pichler G, Aziz K, van Os S, O'Reilly M, et al. Heart rate assessment immediately after birth. Neonatology. 2016;109(2):130–8.

Index

© Springer Nature Switzerland AG 2022
R. A. Moreira de Sá, E. B. d. Fonseca (eds.), *Perinatology*,
https://doi.org/10.1007/978-3-030-83434-0

C

G

H

I

P

U